# TEXTBOOK
# OF
# MEDICINE

## *CAUTION TO READERS :*

*Medical science is an ever changing science due to world wide research work specially in the field of drugs. Large number of new drugs and many indigenous drugs are also being used. The Editor and publisher of this work have presented all information contained in this work after careful scrutiny, so that the drug information may be accurate.*

*However it is essential that doctors while prescribing any drug specially the newer ones, should check the product information carefully to avoid therapeutic hazards.*

# TEXTBOOK OF MEDICINE

*Edited by*

Prof. (Dr.) G.C. Mookerjee

A.V.S.M., Surg. Commodore, I.N. (Retd.)
M.Sc., M.B. (Cal.), F.R.C.P. (Edin.), F.R.C.P. (Lond.)
F.A.I.I.D. (Bom.), F.C.C.P. (U.S.A.)

Professor & Hony. Consultant in Medicine, Vivekananda Institute of Medical Sciences & Chief, Diabetes Unit, Ramkrishna Seva Pratisthan, Kolkata
Head of the Dept. of Medicine and Chief, Jahangir Kabir Diabetes Research Centre, Islamia Hospital, Kolkata
Hony. Consultant, Assembly of God Hospital & Research Centre, Kolkata
Consultant in Medicine, Armed Forces of India
Formerly, Professor & Head of the Dept. of Medicine, Armed Forces Medical College, Pune, and
Later Principal & Professor of Medicine, N.R.S. Medical College, Kolkata

New Central Book Agency (P) Ltd

LONDON

HYDERABAD ERNAKULAM BHUBANESWAR

NEW DELHI KOLKATA PUNE GUWAHATI

**NCBA**

REGD OFFICE
8/1 Chintamoni Das Lane, Kolkata 700 009, India
email: ncbapvtltd@eth.net

OVERSEAS
NCBA (UK) Ltd, 149 Park Avenue North, Northampton, NN3 2HY, UK
email: ncbauk@yahoo.com

EXPORT
NCBA Exports Pvt. Ltd, 212 Shahpur Jat, New Delhi 110 049
email: ncbaexports@ncbapvtltd.com

BRANCHES

212 Shahpur Jat
**New Delhi** 110 049
email: ncbadel@ncbapvtltd.com

Shop Nos. 3 & 4, Vinayak Towers
681/B Budhwar Peth, Appa Balwant Chowk
**Pune** 411 002
email: ncbapune@ncbapvtltd.com

Shop No. 15, Bharati Towers, Ground Floor
Forest Park, **Bhubaneswar** 751 001
email: ncbabub@ncbapvtltd.com

House No. 3-1-315, 1st Floor
Nimboliadda, Kachiguda, **Hyderabad** 500 027
email: ncbahydb@ncbapvtltd.com

GSS Shopping Complex, 1st Floor
Opposite College Post Office, Convent Road
**Ernakulam** 682 035
email: ncbaernk@ncbapvtltd.com

Radhamayee Complex (Second Floor)
Opp. SBI, Panbazar, Jaswanta Road
**Guwahati** 781 001
email: ncbaguwahati@ncbapvtltd.com

TEXTBOOK OF MEDICINE • G. C. Mookerjee



First Published: 1988
Reprinted: 2001, 2010, 2014

PUBLISHER AND TYPESETTER
New Central Book Agency (P) Ltd
8/1 Chintamoni Das Lane, Kolkata 700 009

PRINTER
New Central Book Agency (P) Ltd
Web-Offset Division, Dhulagarh, Sankrail, Howrah

TECHNICAL EDITOR
Mita Sen, MBBS

PROJECT SUPERVISOR
N. Radhakrishnan

ISBN: 978 81 7381 411 2

Price: ₹ 850.00

**THIS BOOK IS DEDICATED TO
MY WIFE SANTA
AND
MY DAUGHTER INDRANI**

# FOREWORD

Recent advances in medicine have made spectacular strides in medical and surgical treatment of patients especially in the diagnostic field. Laboratory tests have multiplied. Ultrasonic, C.T. Scanning and nuclear magnetic resonance testings are making diagnosis more and more accurate. Newer drugs are alleviating more and more human suffering e.g. $\beta$- blockers, thrombolytic agents, steroids etc. Surgical techniques have improved. Coronary bypass surgery, transplant of tissues, organs and even of brain (fetal brain transplant in parkinson's disease) are now being used successfully. Laser technique has made some surgical operations redundant. Lithotripsy is used to pulverise renal calculi and even gall bladder stones. But these latest techniques are costly and can be used in selective cases only.

Our present day doctors tend to depend a good deal on laboratory tests, and prescribe new and costly drugs too often. In India and in the many third world countries these laboratory tests may not be available in many places, and patients also can ill-afford to pay for them. Clinical examination and clinical acumen, as well as a good background-history of the patient and his illness, will continue to play a major role in medical practice in the years to come. However the doctors should know about new developments in different medical fields so as to enable them to give their patients the best deal. Here is a new text book edited by Prof. G.C.Mookerjee attempting to present these features.

Surgeon Commodore G.C. Mookerjee is a well-read person, veteran clinician, and a long-time teacher. He had been Professor of Medicine in the Armed Forces Medical College, Pune and then Principal & Professor of Medicine in N.R.S. Medical College & Hospital in Calcutta. He has combined his clinical experience and medical knowledge in compilation of the present Text Book of Medicine.

Earlier he has published a book on Liver disease (Mookerjee & Sapra 1973) possibly the first concise Indian book on liver diseases. He has also edited two volumes of "Diagnosis and Management of Common Diseases" published in 1982 and 1983, which had a wide acceptance.

Professor Mookerjee has been fortunate in enlisting support from a wide range of stalwarts collaborators each highly specialised in his own line. Each has contributed up-date knowledge in his respective subject. The result has been a rich and concise hand-book of up-date knowledge of modern medicine. I feel that this book will be a valuable handbook for our advanced medical students and practitioners alike. I also hope that it will find a place in every medical library.

I congratulate Professor Mookerjee for compiling such a scholastic task.

Dr. P.K. Ghosh M.B, DTM (Cal.), TDD (Wales),
MRCP (Lond.), FRCP (Edin.),
FCCP (USA), FIPHA (Ind.).
Formerly, Professor of Medicine
R.G.Kar Medical College, Calcutta
and Ex-Governor EIC American
College of Chest Physicians of the
International Academy of Chest
Physician and Surgeons.

16th June, 1988.

# ACKNOWLEDGEMENT

In addition to the contributors, I also express my grateful thanks to those who assisted me in many ways in preparation of this book :

| | |
|---|---|
| Dr. N.Banerjee | Associate Professor, Vivekananda Institute of Medical Sciences and Visiting Physician Ramkrishna Mission Seva Pratisthan, Calcutta — 26. |
| Dr. D.S.Chopra | Consultant Cardiologist, Marwari Relief Hospital, Calcutta. |
| Dr. Asoke Gupta | Medical Director, Calcutta Medical Centre, 12, Loudon Street, Calcutta — 17. |
| Dr. (Miss) Madhu Chanda Kar | P.G. Research Assistant, Department of Medicine, Medical College, Calcutta. |
| Dr. D.K.Majumdar | Associate Professor, Vivekananda Institute of Medical Sciences and Visiting Physician, Ramkrishna Mission Seva Pratisthan, Calcutta. |
| Dr. Saukat Ali | Hony. Registrar, Jahangir Kabir Memorial Diabetes Clinic, Islamia Hospital, Calcutta. |
| Dr. (Mrs) Mita Sen | Cardiology Department, Islamia Hospital, Calcutta. 54B, Patuatola Lane, Calcutta — 9. |
| Dr. K.K.Sengupta | Allergy Clinic, Calcutta. Calcutta Medical Centre, 12, Loudon Street, Calcutta — 17. |
| Dr. N.A.Shah | Consultant Cardiologist, Gujarati Relief Hospital and Vishudhananda Hospital, Calcutta. |
| Dr. K.K.H.Siddique | Consultant Cardiologist, Islamia Hospital, Calcutta. |
| Dr. M.A.Wali | Prof. of Dermatology, Calcutta and National Medical College & Hospital. |

# PREFACE

It is customary to write a preface when a new book is published, hence my submission. There are many excellent text books and classics on Medicine. Why then another publication of a short text book ?

Since the publication of the book "Diagnosis and Management of Common Diseases", Vol.I & II published in 1982 and 1983 by Allied Book Agency, Calcutta and edited by me, many of my students, friends and colleagues encouraged me to undertake the task of preparing a Short Book on Medical Practice especially tailored for our practitioners. The problems of our practitioners with limited facilities in vast rural areas are really tremendous due to lack of proper transport, sophisticated instruments and adequate laboratory facilities. The standard of medicine in the Western hemisphere today as well as in some Far Eastern countries have gone far ahead, in comparison to facilities available to our doctors, practising in rural areas. Although in large cities and towns there are sophisticated medical centres doing high standard of professional work, yet these facilities are only available to a very few people in developing countries. Even cerebral strokes and heart attacks are being treated in general wards of not-so-well-equipped hospitals. Sometimes even such cases cannot be admitted in a hospital due to shortage of beds or transport problems from villages.

Therefore, our basic doctors must not only be experts in clinical medicine but also should stress the value of preventive aspects to their patients during their practice. Many of our countrymen are not aware that jaundice, typhoid fever, diarrhoea, diphtheria and many infectious diseases including sexually transmitted diseases, can be prevented by taking simple measures. Many newborns may die due to gastro-enteritis. Death of many infants and new-borns can be prevented by simple hygienic measures adopted by mothers.

Our country has many problems. Our doctors have to work against many odds. Our students need to be more clinically efficient, at the same time recent works should be known. With the encouragement and support of many of my friends and colleagues,I finally ventured to undertake the ardous task of editing this text book suitable for **our** students and general practitioners.

The senior contributors of this volume are all eminent teachers and well known experts in their specialities. Among the eminent contributors many of my old colleagues of the Armed Forces, now authorities in their respective subjects, have also contributed several chapters in this volume. The joint-contributors are also practising physicians and scientists, attached to well-known institutions. As the Editor, I feel they have done excellent jobs in their respective areas for the sake of continuing medical education in our country. In my own articles I have expressed my views based on my own experiences wherever necessary. In this kind of book there may be some differences in opinion in certain situations but as the Editor I have tried to iron out controversies as far as possible so as not to confuse the readers. Even then some repetitions as also differences in opinion may have remained.

Though in the Third World latest therapy and new techniques are not available to most people, specially in rural areas, we must keep in touch and learn about the latest, while it must be remembered that latest may not always be final and the last word. In a few years the latest may be found wrong or superseded by newer discoveries. Therefore, an important dictum is to be particularly careful in using a new drug or a latest drug without adequate consideration. Doctors should critically evaluate all information given by visiting medical representatives. Critical reading of literature regarding their products is essential before a new drug is accepted. Students of medicine must not forget the thalidomide disaster. Juniors should treat their patients with established drugs. Tailored drugs should also be avoided as far as possible.

Cost factor is also extremely important in poverty-stricken developing countries. To prescribe antibiotics for acute nasopharyngitis or mild diarrhoeas, is not necessary. Cost of course of broad spectrum of antibiotic along with some cough syrup, for a week, may be equal to the patient's weekly earnings. A latest cephalosporin, cephotaxime (Claforan) costs about three hundred rupees per day. No doubt it is a powerful and most valuable cephalosporin, now also available in India. It has its unique life-saving value in proper situations.

Doctors must consider the patient's economic problem. It is the duty of Government of any country to introduce proper drug policy and ensure treatment of poor people in Government Hospitals. Life saving drugs must be provided free for the poor people.

*Our rural Doctors are often in serious trouble due to lack of proper facilities in rural areas. Hence they are reluctant to go to the villages.*

Today's doctor has to know a lot more, work more hard and take more responsibilities than several decades ago. Doctors practising in 'Developing Countries' also must be good bedside clinicians, as most sophisticated instruments will not always be available to them. They have to treat cerebral strokes and heart problems without I.C.U. in most cases. Hence our medical students require more clinical training.

Up-to-date knowledge of drugs is most important as many such drugs can be prescribed even in villages. Many lives can be saved by prescribing modern drugs while adverse effects must be well known.

Again incompatible combination of drugs may not only be dangerous but may also cause fatalities. The medico-legal aspects must not be forgotten. Fatal toxicity of antidepressant drugs due to overdosage (often self-induced or wrong combination) must not be forgotten. Patient and relatives should be cautioned in advance. Combination of amitryptiline (prescribed by doctor) and Nardil (taken by the patient from existing old stock), had caused death leading to legal complication. We should not prescribe chloramphenicol unless there is absolute indication. Barbiturates must not be taken after alcoholic drinks. While prescribing a common drug like metronidazole, it is necessary to advise not to take alcohol.

Analgesic nephropathy is well known. Pharmaco-epidemiology or analgesic-risks show that adverse effects of analgesics are quite low, as far as the gastrointestinal or agranulocytic effects are concerned but nephropathy occurs insidiously over many years. So it is safer not to indiscriminately use these drugs specially in elderly and old patients.

Sympathetic approach, close observation and critical evaluation of patients are very important steps, to be a successful practitioner.

*To understand the patient's problem, his psychological background and economic limitations are extremely important.* Listen to the patient carefully. If you are too busy, you will make mistakes.

Finally it must be stressed that even today the clinical approach is the most important instrument of medical practice and students must learn this art from their teachers directly in hospital wards and at bedside. This art cannot be learnt from books. Weaker the clinical skill, larger the number of investigations.

This book has been prepared keeping in view the requirements of our students and practitioners of this part of the world and to guide our basic doctors and rural practitioners. We have tried to up-date the newer advances, at the same time stressed the importance of clinical approach.

*Advanced techniques are expensive and these should not be ordered routinely, most clinical problems can be solved with routine laboratory tests and by consulting more experienced and experts in the speciality.*

I hope this book will be of great value to our students and medical practitioners.

Before I conclude,I wish to thank Sri Nayan Majumdar and Sri Bob Ghosh of Calcutta Medical Centre who have rendered valuable typewriting assistance for this book. To Sri S.B.Chakraborty, M.A. and Smt. Chakraborty I am specially thankful for efficient proof reading.

I am grateful to my good friend Mr. Biren Sarkar, Managing Director of Parker Robinson (Pvt.) Ltd., Calcutta and publisher of my previous work on "Diagnosis and Management of Common Diseases" for his permission to use a few selected material from the second volume with adequate updating. I thank Sri Sarkar for his kind permission.

I also express my sincere appreciation to Kum. Ratna Bhattacharjee, B.A. now a student of D.H.M.S. for her efficient secretarial assistance throughout the preparation of this volume.

I would not have undertaken this heavy task of editing this volume unless, I was really persuaded by Mr.J.N. Sen, his able and dynamic son Mr.Amitabha Sen and his wife Dr.Mita Sen as well as their family friend Sri Aloke Dasgupta, Secretary of Central Calcutta District Social Welfare Organisation who did an excellent job to expedite its publication.

*29th August, 1988*

G.C. MOOKERJEE
(EDITOR)

# CONTRIBUTORS

1. Lt. Gen. I.M.Ahuja PVSM
MBBS (Madras), MD (Pune), FRCP (Lond.), Ph.D. Cardiology (Pune)
Formerly, Professor and Head of the dept. of Medicine, Armed Forces Medical College, Pune.
Commandant, AMC Centre & School, Lucknow
(4, Sahani Sujan Park, Kandhwa Road, Pune — 40).

2. Dr. S.H. Advani M.D., Physician & Haematologist
Tata Memorial Hospital, Dr. Ernes Borgeo Marg, Parel, Bombay — 400 012.

3. Dr. Anil Adhya D.L.O. (Lond.), FRCS (Eng.)., Calcutta Medical Centre, 12, Loudon Street, Calcutta — 700 017
Visiting ENT Surgeon, Ramakrishna Mission Seva Pratisthan
(124, Hemchandra Naskar Road, Calcutta — 700 014).

4. Major A.C.Anand, M.D., Research Pool Officer, Office of D.G. AFMS, Ministry of Defence, New Delhi — 110 001.

5. Dr. Debabrata Banerjee M.B. (Cal.) MRCP (Lond.), FRCP (Edin.), FCCP, FIIA (USA), Consultant Physician, Formerly Chief Medical Officer & Medical Adviser, Burnpur Hospital and Indian Iron & Steel Co's mining and Industrial group, Asansol, West Bengal.
(3, Ramani Chatterjee Road, Calcutta — 700 029).

6. Dr. M.Bhattacharya, M.D. (Pune), FCCP (USA), Medical Specialist,
Naval Hospital "ASVINI", Indian Navy, Bombay.

7. Dr. C.M.Banerjee MBBS, D.C.H., RCPS (Ireland), Hony. Lecturer, Chittaranjan Seva Sadan, College of Obstetrics, Gynaecology and Child Health and Visiting Paediatrician, Chittaranjan Sisu Sadan and Behala Balanando Brahmachari Hospital, Calcutta — 700 023.
(4/1, Puddopukur square, Kidderpore, Calcutta—700 023).

8. Col. Jagjit Singh Bhalla B.A., MBBS., MD (Medicine), D.C.D., F.C.C.P. (USA)
Senior Adviser in Medicine & Respiratory Diseases, Military Hospital, Namkum, Ranchi, Bihar.

9. Dr. P.N.Biswas, MD., Medical specialist, Central Govt. Health Scheme, Calcutta, Formerly Associate Professor in Medicine, Patliputra Medical College and Physician, Central Hospital, Dhanbad.
(Flat No.17, 16, Dover Lane, Calcutta — 700 029).

10. Prof. (Dr.) A.K. Chatterjee MBBS (Cal.), FRCP (Edin.), FACC (USA), FCCP (USA), Professor & Head Dept. of Medicine, Patliputra Medical College, Dhanbad. (12, Govind Nagar, Bakerbandh, Dhanbad — 826 001).

11. Dr. Ambar Chakraborty MD, MRCP, FICA, Hony. Neuro Physician & Lecturer, Vivekananda Institute of Medical Sciences, Calcutta. (59, Beadon Street, Calcutta — 700 006).

12. Prof. K.S. Chugh MD, FAMS, FICA (USA), FACP (USA), FISN (Neph.), Hony. Consultant to Armed Forces & Head of the Dept. of Nephrology, Post Graduate Institute, Chandigarh — 12.

13. Dr. Subhankar Chaudhury M.D. (Cal.), Nephrology Clinic, Bellevue Clinic, Loudon Street, Calcutta — 700 017.

14. Dr. Niren Das MB. (Cal.), DARCPS (Lond.), FICS, FCCP (USA.), Consultant in Anaesthesia & Pulmonology, Assembly of God Church Hospital & Research Centre, Calcutta — 700 017. (48/7, Purnadas Road, Calcutta — 700 029)

15. Dr. Ramanuj Dasgupta MBBS (Cal.), FRCP (Lond.), FACC, FCCP (USA)., Visiting Cardiologist, Ramakrishna Mission Seva Pratisthan Vivekananda Institute of Medical Sciences. Visiting Cardiologist, Calcutta Medical Research Institute, Visiting Cardiologist, Niramoy Polyclinic, Calcutta (21, Rup Chand Mukherjee Lane, Calcutta — 700 025).

16. Prof. P.S.Das, M.A., Ph.D; Yoga Adviser, Ghosh's Institute of Yoga & Physical Culture & "Castle Corner", 3A, Albert Road, Calcutta — 700 017.

17. Brig. (Dr.) R.N.Dutta, AVSM, FRCP (Edin.), FRC path (Eng.)., Consultant in Haematology to the Assembly of God Hospital & Research Centre, 125/1, Park Street, Calcutta — 700 017. (128, Salt Lake City, Calcutta — 700 064)

18. Dr. B.K.Das AVSM, Brig (Retd.), M.D. (Med.) D.M. (Card.), M.D. (Paed.), DTM & H Ex-Consultant Physician & Cardiologist, Armed Forces. (2, Gariahata Road (South), Flat No.92, Calcutta — 700 068).

19. Dr. Bimal De, MBBS (Cal.), DPM (Lond.), MRCP (Sych.) (Eng.), Consultant Psychiatrist & Chief, The Mental Hospital Calcutta and Mankundu, Consultant Psychiatrist to the Department of Applied Psychology, University of Calcutta. (4, Shakespeare Sarani, Flat : 10F, Calcutta — 700 071).

20. Dr. Subir Kumar Dutta, MBBS, DCP, MD (Path.),
Lecturer, Dept. of Pathology, University College of Medicine, Calcutta.
(2, Ram Chandra Das Row, Calcutta — 700 013)

21. Prof. (Dr.) D.N. Guha Majumdar M.D. (Cal.),
Professor of Medicine & Incharge — Gastroenterology Unit, Dept. of Medicine Institute of Post Graduate Medical Education and Research, Calcutta — 700 020.
(37/C, Block 'B', New Alipore, Calcutta — 700 053).

22. Dr. D.C.Ghosh, FRCP, FCCP,
Prof. of Cardiology, Medical College, Calcutta.
(P/325, C.I.T. Road, Calcutta — 700 054).

23. Dr. S.K. Hajra,
Dept. of Leprology School of Tropical Medicine,
Chittaranjan Avenue, Calcutta — 700 012.

24. Dr. A.A. Hingorani, M.D.
Windsor House Opp. Oval, Churchgate, Bombay — 400 020.

25. Dr. S.Kumar, MBBS, FRCP (Edin.), Physician,
Endocrine Unit, Medical College, Calcutta.
(20/B, Garcha 1st Lane, Calcutta — 700 019).

26. Lt. Gen. N.R.Krishnan, MBBS (Andhra), M.D. (Pune), F.C.C.P., FISE, FICA, FIM, SACERT, FDP, Commandant, Armed Forces Medical College,
Commandant AFMC Pune — 411 040.

27. Dr. (Mrs.) K.A. Kabir, MBBS (Cal.), M.D. (Nag.), FCCP (USA),
Dy. Hony. Visiting Physician, Islamia Hospital,
(Flat 1E "Panchsheel", 41/1B, Jhowtala Road, Calcutta — 700 019).

28. Dr. Barkat Ullah Khan, MBBS, M.D. (Cal.), FCCP (USA),
Hony. Deputy Visiting Physician, Islamia Hospital,
(5, Dedar Bux Lane, Calcutta — 700 016).

29. Mrs. Gouri Krishna, M.Sc. (Home Sci.),
Hony. Dietecian, Ramakrishna Mission Seva Pratisthan.
99, Sarat Bose Road, Calcutta — 700 026.
(9, Hensman Road, T.Nagar, Madas—17).

30. Dr. Narendra Kumar, M.D., Windsor House, Opp : Oval Churchgate, Bombay — 400 020.

31. Prof. (Dr.) G.C. Mookerjee AVSM
M.Sc, M.B. (Cal.)., FRCP (Edin.), FRCP (Lond.), FAIID (Bom.), FCCP (USA),
Professor and Hony. Consultant in Medicine, Vivekananda Institute of Medical Sciences
& Chief Diabetes Unit, Ramakrishna Mission Seva Pratisthan,
Head of the Dept. of Medicine, Islamia Hospital, Calcutta — 700 012.

32. Dr. Sanjib Mukherjee MBBS (Cal.), MRCP (Glasy.), MRCP (Edin.), FRCP (C), FCCP (USA) FIMSA
Consultant Cardiologist, The Calcutta Medical Research Institute, 7/2, Diamond Harbour Road, Calcutta — 700 027.
(42, Gariahat Road, Calcutta — 700 029.)

33. Dr. Sukumar Mukherjee, M.D. (Cal.), FRCP (Lond.), FRCP (Edin.), FCCP (USA),
FIAMS (IND.),
Prof. of Medicine, Medical College, Calcutta.
(1/1A, Tara Road, Calcutta — 700 026).

34. Brig. Monojmohan Roy B.Sc., MBBS, FRCP (Path.), DCP (D path),
Prof. of Pathology, Vivekananda Institute of Medical Sciences,
99, Sarat Bose Road, Calcutta — 26.
Consultant Pathologist, Assembly of God Hospital & Research Centre, 125/1, Park Street, Calcutta — 700 017.
(P/489, Keyatola Road, Calcutta — 700 029).

35. Dr. (Mrs.) Arati Moitra, MBBS, D.A.(Cal.), M.D. (Madras),
Prof. of Anaesthesiology, Medical College, Calcutta.
(DL 131/13, Narayan Co-operative, Sector II, Salt Lake, Calcutta — 700 091).

36. Dr. M.K. Mukherjee, MBBS, I.D.D., D.C.H. (Cal.), M.I.M.S. (Delhi),
Chief Medical Officer, M/s.Bata India Ltd., Batanagar — 743313.

37. Dr. T.P. Mukherjee, MBBS (Cal.), M.D. (Cal.) Dip. Card (Cal.), FCCP (USA), FIAGP (India)
Prof. of Medicine, R.G. Kar Medical College & Hospital, Calcutta — 700 004
(Sector III, Bulidina Special Flat No : 7, Salt Lake City, Calcutta — 700 091).

38. Dr. N.K. Majumdar,
Prof. of Medicine, R.G. Kar Medical College, Calcutta.
(P-285, Darga Road, Calcutta — 700 017).

39. Dr. A.R. Nandi, MBBS (Cal.), MRCP (UK),
Nephrologist, Bellevue Clinic, Calcutta — 17
(19, Hindusthan Road, Calcutta — 700 029).

40. Dr. Jagadish Roy Chaudhury, MBBS, T.D.D.,
Chest Specialist, Kamarhati E.S.I. Hospital.
(BE — 177, Salt Lake City, Calcutta — 700 064).

41. Dr. D.Roychaudhury, M.S. (Cal.),
Prof. of Neurosurgery, Calcutta National Medical College, Calcutta.
(Salt Lake City FE 71 Sector III, Calcutta — 700 091).

42. Mr. Ram Udayan Roy, M.Sc.
Research Asst, Diabetes Clinic, Ramakrishna Mission Seva Pratisthan,
99, Sarat Bose Road, Calcutta — 700 026.

43. Dr. (Col.) P.K.Sethi, MBBS, M.D., FICA (USA), FCCP.
Senior Consultant Neurology, Sir Ganga Ram Hospital, New Delhi — 110 071.
(104, Navjivan Vihar, New Delhi — 110 017).

44. Dr. Sanat Kr. Sarkar, MBBS, D.T.M., D.D.H. (Cal.), D.Phys, Med. (Eng.),
Ex-Prof. and Head of the Dept. of Physical Medicine, Rheumatology, N.R.S.Medical College,
Calcutta — 700 014. & Inst. of Post Graduate Medical Education and Research Centre,
Calcutta — 700 020.
(93A, Beltala Road, Calcutta — 700 026).

45. Prof. N.N. Sarangi, M.D., Ph.D.
Prof. and Head of the Dept. of Neurology, Bangur Institute of Neurology & Institute of Post
Graduate Medical Education and Research, Calcutta.
(Q/2, Belgachia Villa, Calcutta — 700 037).

46. Col. M.L. Sapra, MBBS (Pb.), M.D. (Pune),
Head of Medicine, Dept. and Senior Adviser Medicine, Army Hospital, Delhi Cantt.

47. Dr. Shaymal Sen, M.D. (Cal.), FRCP (Lond.),
Dean, Vivekananda Institute of Medical Sciences,
Prof. of Medicine, Ramakrishna Mission Seva Pratisthan, 99, Sarat Bose Road, Calcutta—26.

48. Brig. A.K. Sensharma, AVSM (Retd.), M.Sc, FRCS (Eng.), FRCS (Edin),
Ultra Medical Cure & Research Centre, 18/7, Ballygunge Place (East), Calcutta — 700 019.

49. Dr. B.K. Sharma, M.D., FAMS, FISN, FICA.
Prof. & Head, Dept. of International Medicine,
Post Graduate Institute of Medical Education & Research, Chandigarh — 160 012.

50. Dr. S.K. Sharma, M.D.
Hony. Radiologist, Calcutta Medical Research Institute,
Chief Radiologist, EKO X-Ray Clinic,
54, Chowringhee Road, Calcutta — 700 071.

51. Dr. K.P. Sengupta, MB, D.Phil, FAMS, FSMF,
Director of Laboratories, Calcutta Medical Centre, 12, Loudon Street, Calcutta—700 017.
(Flat No : 3B, 48/1E, Gariahat Road, Calcutta — 700 019).

52. Lt. Gen. A.R. Subramaniam, Formerly D.S.A.F.M.S., New Delhi.

53. Dr. P.Sen, M.D., FRCP, FICA,
Prof. Director of Medicine, Institute of Post Graduate Medical Education & Research, Calcutta.
(245, Acharya Jagadish Chandra Bose Road, Calcutta — 700 020).

54. Dr. P.K. Talukdar, MBBS, MRCP,
Visiting Physician (Paediatrics), N.R.S. Medical College, Calcutta — 700 014.
(21, Jatin Bagchi Road, Calcutta — 700 029).

55. Dr. (Mrs.) Geeta Talukdar, M.D., Ph.D., FAMSC, FASC.
Incharge — Human Genetics Unit, Centre for Advanced Study in Cell and Chromosome Research Dept. of Botany, University of Calcutta,
35, Ballygunge Circular Road, Calcutta — 700 019.
(6, Mullen Street, Calcutta — 700 019).

56. Lt. Col. Yashpal, MBBS, MD. (Med.)., DM (Neph.), MNAMS (Nephrology), FCCP (USA), F.I.S.N. (Neph), Consultant Nephrologist, Command Hospital, Central Command, Lucknow — 2.

57. Late Hon. Brigadier Dr.K.K. Datey, SEM.
B.A., M.D., F.R.C.P.(Lond.), F.P.C.C.(Hon.), F.A.C.C. (U.S.A.), F.A.M.S. (Ind.), F.A.C.P. (Hon.) (U.S.A.), F.R.C.P. (Edin.), F.M.A.S. (Mah.), F.R.S.A. (Lond.), F.N.A. (Ind.), F.I.C.P.M. (Hol.), D.C.H. (Eng.), F.A.A.B.S. (U.S.A.), D.T.M. & H. (Lond.), F.C.C.P. (U.S.A.), F.I.C.A. (U.S.A.),
Windsor House, Opp. Oval, Churchgate, Bombay — 400 020.

58. Dr. J.R. Barua, MBBS, DCH.
Ex-Professor, Paediatrics, Rangon Medical College, Burma and Ex-Visiting Physician, Chittaranjan Seva Sadan, Calcutta.

59. Dr. S.N.Sengupta, M.D. (Cal.) F.R.C.P. (Edin.), F.C.C.P, F.I.C.A. (U.S.A.),
Ex-Professor and Head of the Dept. of Medicine, B.S. Medicial College, Bankura.
(Res : Taragoti Samanta Road, Kenduadihi, Bankura — 722 101.

60. Dr. Jayanta Chakraborty, M.D.
Hony. Registrar,
Dept. of Medicine, Vivekananda Institute of Medical Sciences, Calcutta.

Please read *Subhankar Chaudhury* in two places of *Subhankar Chakravorty* (page no.xx).

# CONTENTS

CHAPTER I

# ENVIRONMENT, HEALTH & DISEASES

*G C Mookerjee*

## INTRODUCTION:

The meaning of the word 'Health' is soundness and vigour of mind and body and, therefore, any deviation from health, is considered as a state of sickness. The doctor must be able to appreciate whether this departure from normal state of health, is due to psychological or physical factors or due to both reasons. It is quite possible that lack of emotional stability may be attributed to many symptoms which may sometimes be mistaken for organic disease. On the other hand, a patient suffering from organic disease may sometimes ignore it and may not come to the doctor till the disease is fairly advanced. This becomes specially important not only for disease of heart, lungs or gastro-intestinal problems but it is specially significant when the underlying lesion is a carcinomatous condition.

It must also be realised that some normal people in good health are also at a high risk due to genetic or familial causes. This will be evident in a middle-aged person who comes from a family with history of heart attacks and strokes due to atherosclerotic disease. When such an individual indulges in excess of tobacco, alcohol and indiscriminate food habits, his risk to suffer from cardiovascular disorders and diabetes will certainly increase.

Many people with pre-clinical disease may not come to the doctor at all and will never be diagnosed till the disease manifests frank symptoms such as fever, pain, dyspepsia, bleeding, diarrhoea, weakness, fatigue, palpitation, sweating, nausea, vomiting, frequency of urine, constipation or oliguria, etc.

In certain countries as well as in the armed forces, medical inspection and periodic medical check-up is a *must*. Therefore, in these situations diseased state may be discovered in pre-clinical stage. However, the ideal is not always possible and is therefore, the family doctor must be able to decide what kind of physical check-up and investigation is required when a patient comes for consultation. The practice of writing a tonic or disposing him with a few capsules of antibiotics is certainly a bad practice. A little time given during the first visit is the most important action, which the doctor must not fail to offer. Choice of correct investigation is not always very easy and, therefore, an inexperienced doctor usually may indulge in indiscriminate investigation leading to unnecessary waste of patient's time and money.

The health of an individual will also be affected by the environment, where he resides or is exposed to. Thus a westerner from a temperate climate exposed to a hot and humid climate in the tropics may develop a lot of health problems. Exposure to infections is always a great risk. Residence in or exposure to, high altitude poses newer medical problems. Man to-day goes into the depths of the sea and also to great heights in the space. He also indulges in various kinds of sports and games, and obviously additional environmental hazards will be encountered. Therefore, a modern doctor must be well-versed in all these external environmental problems as well as the genetic susceptibility to these disorders must be taken into account. If there is any single factor in disturbing the health of a normal individual it is undoubtedly his environment, Environment can give him physical as well as mental stress and also contribute to infection by virus, bacteria, fungus as well as parasites.

A baby born in prosperous areas of society in a nursing home will have much more advantage to gain ideal health than a baby born in a village of an undeveloped country, where possibly a quack doctor in the only physician available and the domestic environment of the family may be far from ideal. The mother may be malnourished and anaemic, who may not be able to provide enough breast milk to the new-born.

new-born. The father may be financially inadequate to provide sufficient domestic allowance for adequate artificial milk to the baby. The result is a malnourished rickety child, who is more susceptible to infection. Such mothers may develop tuberculosis during their repeated pregnancies. How many of these children will receive adequate immunological protection is also uncertain. It is, therefore, obvious why infections become a great health problem, particularly in developing countries. Though the defence mechanisms of the hosts play a dominant role in fighting environmental infections, the role of modern methods of immunisation cannot be overemphasised.

## RESISTANCE TO INFECTION :

The human body has got several mechanisms to combat infections due to pathogenic organisms. It should be realised that many harmless organisms live in symbiosis in our body in the upper respiratory tract, in the lower bowels and in the skin. These may occasionally infect the tissues when the resistance is extremely low or viral infections have devitalised mucosal membrane. The chief factors which are utilised to fight external infections are as follows :—

(a) **Immunity—**

Immunity is associated with the formation of antibodies, which acquire specific power to inactivate or kill the invading pathogens. Immunity can be defined as active immunity or passive immunity. Active immunity is developed in the tissues due to an infection, e.g., after an attack of smallpox or enteric fever or poliomyelitis. Polio virus sometimes may affect without any clinical manifestation and thus human immunity may be acquired. Similarly, active immunity may be bacterial proteins or inactivated or killed organisms. This is the basis of protective innoculation and vaccination and it is by this method that infections like smallpox, diphtheria, tetanus, polio, whooping cough, etc., are prevented in modern times.

(b) **Susceptibility to infection—**

There are some individuals who are inherently susceptible to infection as they have got certain genetic and acquired weaknesses in their ability to form antibodies. There may be deficiency of gamma globulin which usually is connected to antibody formation.

(c) **Cellular defence—**

During the process of infection in the tissues, there is always a local inflammatory response to fight microbic infection. There is vasodilatation with increased permeability of capillary beds and polymorph white cells accumulate in large numbers, to engulf the attacking organisms and destroy them by their own enzymes. Subsequently, lymphocytes, plasma cells, monocytes and macrophages also take part in clearing local inflammation, but if the invasion is too severe, pus formation may take place. These tissue changes may ultimately clear up or, in case of suppuration, abscess may have to be drained. Sometimes good healing takes place with or without local fibrosis.

(d) **Humoral Defence—**

Humoral defence is really the basis of chemical immunity based on specific globulin fraction of the plasma proteins. During the course of viral or bacterial infection, antibodies form which fight the infection. Details of these processes have been discussed in a separate chapter on 'Immunology'.

In modern times great advances have been made in the field of active immunisation against various preventable diseases. Vaccination against smallpox is well known. Active immunisation against measles has also been prepared. This can be given to susceptibles by S.C. or I.M. injection in single dose in the second year of life. Cholera vaccine is not routinely given but should be injected during an epidemic.

In endemic areas vaccines for typhoids, and paratyphoid organism should be given from childhood and in adults these injections are to be repeated annually.

(e) **Mechanical Defence—**

Mechanical barriers also help to prevent infection as follows :—

(i) Secretion of mucus entangles organisms.
(ii) Ciliary movements brush out invaders.
(iii) Cough reflex itself is a mechanical defence.
(iv) Fibrinous exudate is another example, which limits infection.
(v) Local fibrosis and calcification actively localises infection.
(vi) Skin and mucous membranes are great mechanical barriers.

## INFECTION & DISEASE

Numerous organisms abound in our environment. These are viruses, cocci, bacilli, rickettsial organisms, fungi and parasites of various kinds. Curiously enough, large number of these organisms are harmless to us. Some bacterial organisms known as commensal organisms reside in the human body in symbiosis, while others are capable of producing mild to severe damage to the tissues. The latter group of organisms are called pathogens.

Whenever any pathogenic organisms attack human body, the tissues put up a battle by its humoral as well as its cellular mechanisms. Sometimes organisms may be so virulent that all defence mechanisms may fail to combat the attack. The result is overwhelming infection mainfested by severe symptoms, e.g., high fever, profound weakness, fall of BP, severe shock, cardio-respiratory failure and death.

Various other factors which may influence development of infection are : age, sex, general health of the individual at the time of exposure, racial factor, genetic influence as well as environmental factors. For instance an attack of bacillary dysentery in a patient of high economic status who is in good health may not be a very serious problem, while a similar problem in a poor slum-dweller in a tropical country may be fatal. An idea of the living conditions of poor tropical labourers in some underdeveloped parts of the world may be obtained from a photograph illustrating very adverse living conditions. (Fig. 1.1)

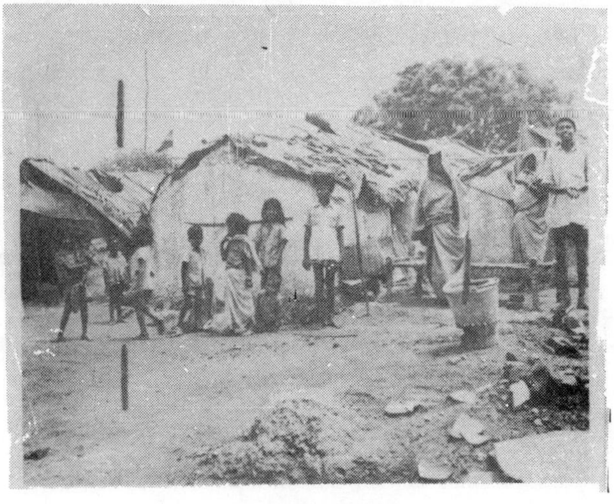

FIG.1.1 Living in slums

Influence of climate is a very important factor. Hot humid climate itself has very adverse effects on the tissues. Loss of water and sodium chloride due to sweating produces dehydration. In hot dry climate evaporation of sweat causes heat loss, but in hot humid weather evaporation of sweat is not satisfactory and may cause paralysis of heat-regulating mechanism.

## MODES OF INFECTION :

1 Airborne—

(a) **Droplets**—Usually due to coughing and sneezing within two metres.

(b) **Dust**—Contaminated hospital beds and linen and floor dust are a rich source. Droplets also can settle down in floor dust, furniture or curtains, and during dusting and cleaning process they may cause shower effect.

2. **Vehicle**—

Contaminated articles of food, milk and water may directly cause infection or via flies and fingers. Flies may bring infection from faecal matter voided in open fields, quite common in villages of this part of the world. Serum, plasma and blood may carry virus via transfusion route.

3. **Vectors**—

Arthropods quite commonly contaminate food, skin and mucous membranes. They may also introduce infection via bites through skin as in malaria, kala-azar and plague.

4. **Contact**—

Contact by touching infected persons or animals and, by kissing or sexual relation may cause infection. Using common towels, hanky, clothes, sharing beds and blankets may also be responsible.

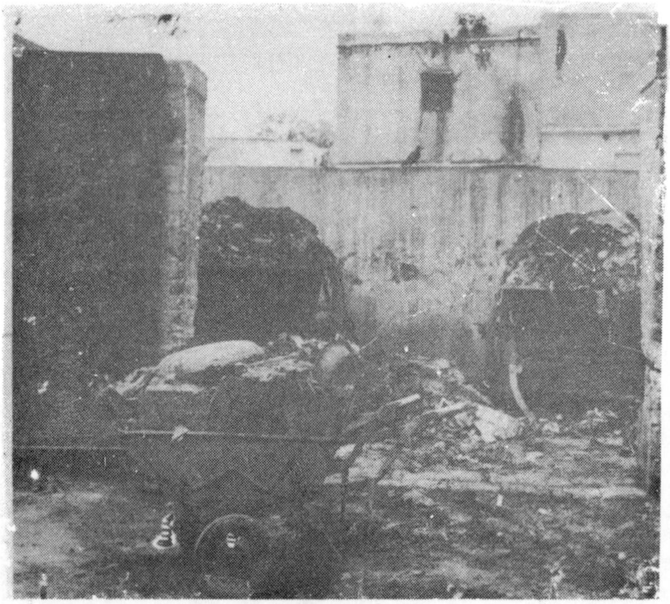

Fig.1.2 : Common modes of infection

### RESERVOIRS OF INFECTION

Humans are a good source of many infections, e.g., enteric fever, amoebic dysentery, giardiasis, bacillary dysentery, meningococcal, streptococcal, staphylococcal infections as well as gonorrhoea and syphilis. Many infections come from birds and animal sources, e.g., trichniosis and tenea soleum from pork, tenea saginata from beef, psittacosis from parrots and ducks and other birds. Tetanus and gas gangrene come from contaminated soil during street accidents.

Mosquitoes transmit malaria from human to human, sandflies transmit kala-azar, trypanosomiasis via tsetse flies. Viral infections are also transmited by humans.

## INCUBATION PERIODS (I.P.) OF COMMON INFECTIOUS DISEASES :

## COURSE OF INFECTIOUS DISEASES:

There are two important stages—

(a) Asymptomatic or Incubation stops.

(b) Symptomatic Phase.

*Incubation Period*—It is the time-interval between the actual exposure to infection and development of symptoms of diseases due to the infection, the period being different in different infections. It is the phase during which germs of diseases mature and multiply in tissues, before any symptoms develop. Table 1.1 gives the details of incubation of diseases due to infection.

TABLE 1.1 Incubation periods (I.P) of common infectious diseases :

| 1. *Diseases with I.P.of less than one week—* | 2. *Diseases with I.P. of one to two weeks—* | 3. *Diseases of I.P. of more than two weeks—* |
|---|---|---|
| Bacillary Dysentery (Shigellosis)<br>Infantile gastroenteritis<br>Diphtheria<br>Meningococcal infection, infections due to Str. pyogenes : e.g., epidemic tonsillitis, scarlet fever, erysipelas and streptococcal puerperal fever.<br>Salmonellosis (usually about 24 hours). | Enteric fever : Variable 7 to 14 days.<br>Paratyphoid fever: 1 to 10 days.<br>Infectious mononucleosis (glandular fever) : 1 to 21 days.<br>Measles : To the development of exanthem, 10 to 12 days.<br>Pertussis (whooping cough) : To the catarrhal stage, 7 to 14 days.<br>Smallpox : 5 to 14 days.<br>Poliomyelitis | Chicken-pox : 14 to 21 days.<br>Mumps : 17 to 24 days.<br>Rubella (German measles) : 14 to 21 days.<br>Virus hepatitis :15 to 40 days (Virus 'A').<br>Serum hepatitis : 40 to 180 days or longer (Virus 'B'). |

## PREVENTION OF INFECTIOUS DISEASES :

This can be achieved in many cases by control of spread of germs, by public health measures, e.g.,

(a) *Isolation of infectious patients*—e.g., smallpox, tuberculosis, diphtheria, meningitis, etc.

(b) *Quarantine of travellers*—This is an isolation period imposed on travellers, voyagers or sick persons to prevent import of diseases. There are international regulations of control for different diseases in various countries.

(c) *By good public health measures*—i.e., by providing disposal of sewage, by supplying clean waters, by controlling fly-menace, stray dogs and animals. Provision of good food and avoiding overcrowding as well avoiding public nuisance etc.

(d) *Ensuring notification of infectious diseases*—This is another important measure; the list varies in different countries.

(e) *Immunisation* may be active or passive.

(i) **Active Immunisation—**

For protection against some infectious diseases active immunisation is effective but it is to be noted that immunisation for most viral infection are not yet available. Hepatitis-B Vaccine is available, but very expensive. Modern immunisation schedule as practised nowadays is included in the Appendix.

(ii) **Passive Immunisation—**

Passive immunisation by the use of specific human immunoglobulin can be used when there is no time to wait for active immunity to develop. Passive immunisers are used in cases of diphtheria, rabies, tetanus and sometimes for viral hepatitis. The immunity is immediate but does not last beyond three to six months (Refer to Appendix)

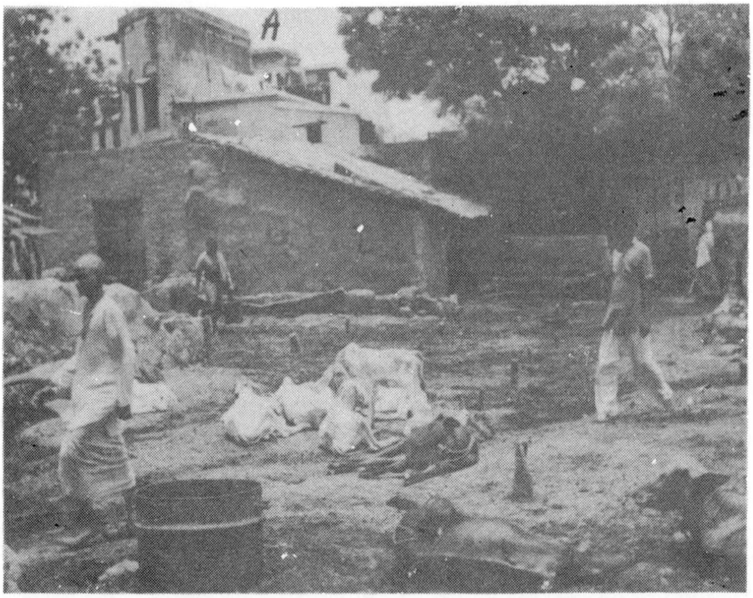

FIG.1.3 Source of health-hazards : (Photograph from a middle class living area in a big city)

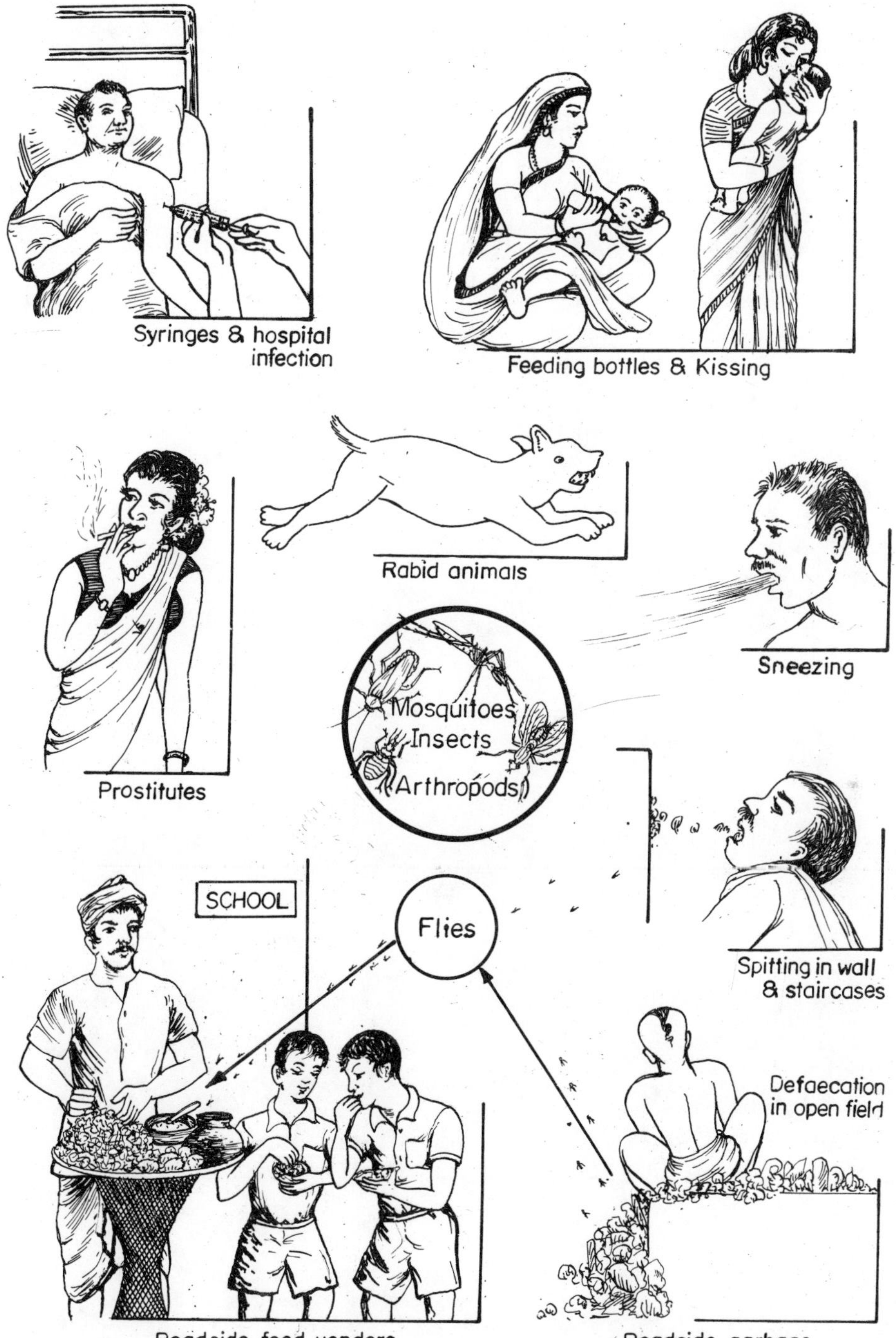


Fig. 1.2 : Modes of infection specially in the Tropics.

CHAPTER 2

# GENETIC FACTORS IN DISEASE

*GEETA TALUKDER*

## INTRODUCTION

The physician is gradually facing a change in the pattern of cases seen in general practice. Congenital anomalies and hereditary diseases are becoming increasingly important with the control of infections. This is especially true for paediatric practice where up to 1 in 20 children admitted to hospitals appears to have a genetic disease. In India, inherited factors had been considered to play a part in the causation of a disease and it is commonly believed that congenital anomalies, mental retardation, epilepsy and various other diseases have a heritable bias. With popularisation of family welfare planning as well, genetic counselling is increasing in popularity and the physician is often faced with the question of recurrence of a hereditary disease and also problems regarding delayed mental and skeletal growth, delayed or abnormal sexual development and the possible effects of consanguineous union. All these fall within the purview of genetic counselling where the basic knowledge of genetics is applied to answer some of these questions.

## BASIC CONCEPTS

All characters in the living organism are inherited through submicroscopic particles, the *genes,* which are carried from parent cell to daughter cell through rod-like bodies—the *chromosomes.* The gene substance is primarily DNA and the conversion of information carried in the DNA molecule of the parent cell to the protein and enzymes of the daughter cells is one of the fascinating discoveries of recent times. The DNA molecule carries the genetic information in a compact form dependent on the arrangement of nucleotides—*the genetic code.* This coded language is translated into protein molecules through the different molecules of RNA—a process of translation.

The DNA molecule is also divided into identical strands by a process of *replication.* The chromosomes are but vehicles by which the genes are carried from cell to cell.

*Mitosis* is the process of cell division in which replication and equal division of chromosomes (karyokinesis) accompanied by division of the cell into two daughter cells occurs (cytokinesis). Usually, thus equal number of chromosomes pass to either side except in gametogenesis where half the number (haploid number) of chromosomes pass to either cell. The normal or diploid number is regained on fertilisation and zygote formation.

The chromosomes of man are 46 in number or 23 pairs of which twenty-two are identical *autosomes* and two are heteromorphic *sex chromosomes* referred to as XX in a female and XY in a male. The chromosomes are studied during metaphase where their structure is visible in stained preparations and can be photographed and drawn. It is customary to arrange them in pairs according to size, i.e., length, shape and presence of the *centromere* (Fig. 2.1). Recent advances in culture techniques have helped in the analysis of chromosomes. The original studies were carried out on bone marrow cells by the so-called squash technique. The initiation of cell division by PHA of the mononuclear leucocytes has given an easier technique. Other tissues used for chromosome analysis are the skin, lymph nodes, amniotic fluid cells and gonadal tissue.

## CLASSIFICATION AND IDENTIFICATION OF CHROMOSOMES

The chromosomes in man are mostly metacentric with the centromere situated near the centre of the arms but there are two groups of acrocentric chromosomes with the centromere placed subterminally. The Y chromosome belongs to this group. The original classification, termed the Denver system, divided the chromosomes into groups A to G according to size. Groups D and E were acrocentric. Individual chromosomes were clearly identified after the development of banding techniques over the last ten years. The following banding techniques are in use :

(1) Q banding observed in cells subjected to UV light after fluorescence dye staining.

(2) G, R and C banding observed by Giemsa staining after treatment with various substances.

(3) N and NOR banding on nucleolar regions.

(4) Orcein banding used mostly in plant cells.

Banding techniques and also autoradiography have helped to identify individual chromosomes and thus minor variations in structure can be detected.

The norms regarding the identification of individual chromosomes have been laid down in successive conferences regarding their nomenclature.

## STUDY OF GENE EFFECT

The gene, however, is not visible and its detection is dependent on its function. It must be emphasised that no gene functions alone and its action is controlled and helped by other genes—termed *suppressor* and *regulator* genes, it being itself termed the *operator* gene. The total effect of the *genotype* on the *phenotype* or external characters depends on the activity of genes of the two chromosomes—paternal and maternal, at the same position or *locus*. If both alleles are similar they are termed *homozygous*, if dissimilar *heterozygous*. If the gene is capable of expressing itself in the heterozygous state it is termed *dominant* and if in the homozygous state alone it is termed *recessive*.

The detection of dominant gene effect is thus visible if the inheritance pattern or pedigree is studied as the phenotype will be seen to be affected vertically, i.e., through parents to siblings. For recessive inheritance it would be necessary to study affected individuals alone and siblings are more likely to be affected with parents remaining normal. The field of biochemical genetics has developed especially for the detection of recessive gene-linked conditions. Here the end product of a gene action may be found deficient or the precursor substance in excess showing that a particular gene is lacking. If the gene were one of dominant (A) type, the activity of the daughter cell would be carried on by the normal allele but in case of a homozygous recessive (a/a) this would not be possible. Garrod's concept of inborn errors of metabolism is based on this (Fig. 2.2). The heterozygote or carrier detection is achieving great importance in recent years as a prerequisite for genetic counselling. Unfortunately, it is yet not possible to detect the carriers in most of the diseases except in the case of haemoglobinopathies, bleeding disorders and some cases of mucopolysaccharidoses.

*Antenatal diagnosis* of a genetic disease is necessary to detect abnormality in the fetus. While fetal sex, bilirubin levels, lecithin/sphingomyelin ratio and alfafetoprotein have been successfully carried out, other conditions cannot be easily determined. Recently analysis of the DNA of the fetal cells by means of the enzymes DNA polymerase and reverse transcriptase has been utilised to diagnose the presence of the $\alpha$-thalassaemia gene in the fetus.

*Gene mapping* : The location of genes to specific position in chromosomes is important not only for basic research but also for early detection of a disease. The study of inheritance pattern of certain characters, absence and presence of characters related to chromosome lesions has helped to identify the position of

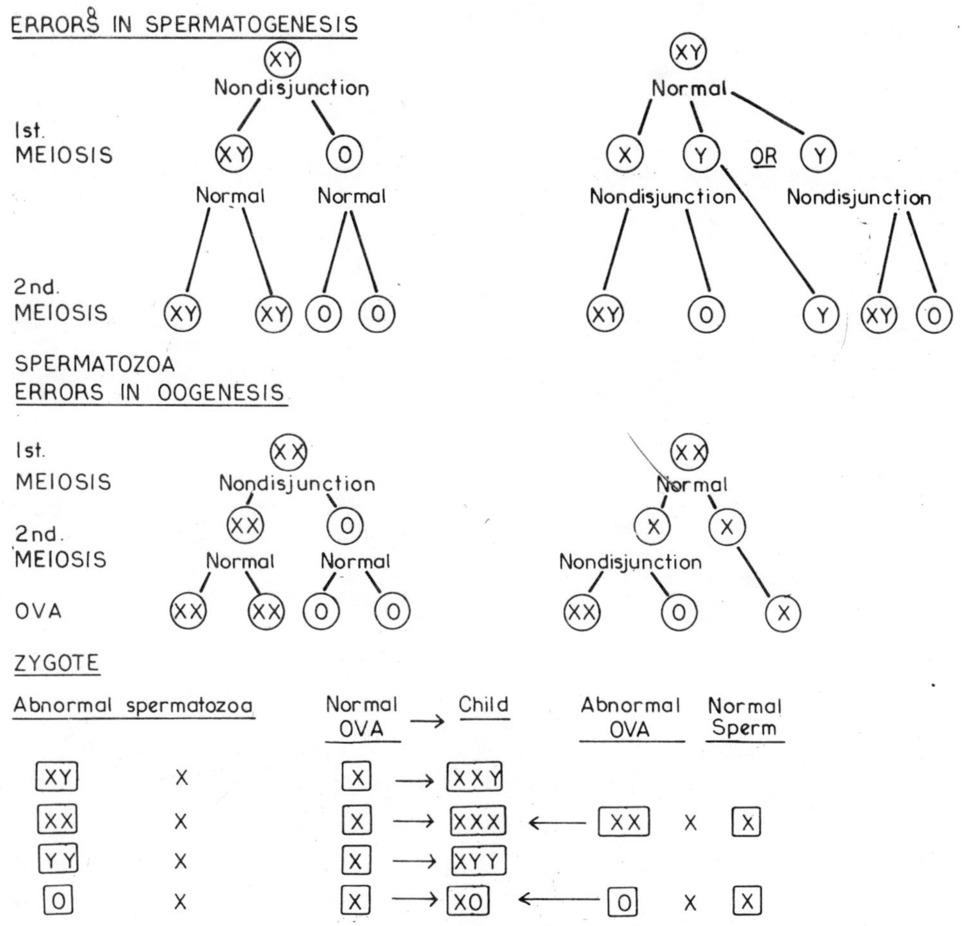


Fig. 2.1 Sex Chromosomal Aberrations

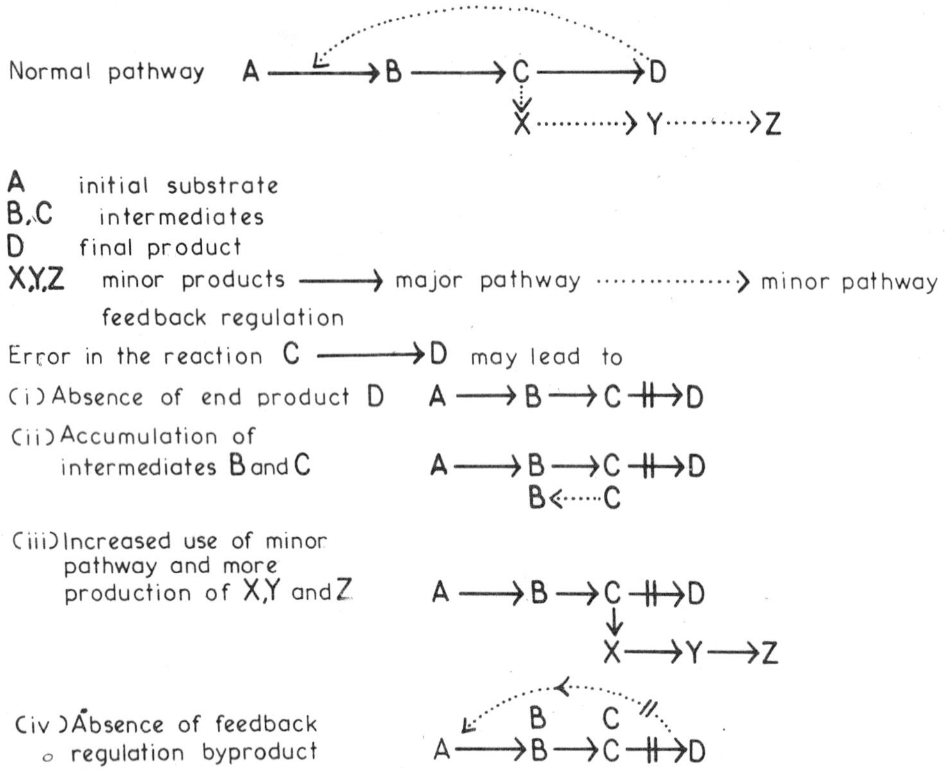


Fig.2.2 Effect of Inborn Errors of Metabolism

loci of a large number of genes, e.g., the Haemophilia gene on the X chromosome and the HY locus on the Y chromosome. In recent years the development of cell hybridization techniques has further helped to localise a very large number of genes on the specific loci of the human chromosome.

*Genetic diseases* can be classified into the following broad categories :

(I) *Diseases due to chromosomal aberrations can be*
Autosomal due to numerical or structural anomalies,
Sex chromosomal due to numerical or structural anomalies.

(II) *Diseases due to single genes of large effect*
Autosomal dominant (AD)
Autosomal recessive (AR)
X-linked dominant (XD)
X-linked recessive (XR)

(III) *Diseases due to polygenic or multifactorial inheritance.*

(I) *Diseases due to chromosomal aberrations* are found in a large number of early abortions (reported up to 60%) and many are probably lost soon after conception. Aberrations in chromosomes may be numerical or structural.

*Numerical aberrations* occur as a result of non-disjunction or anaphase lagging usually during gametogenesis or after zygote formation, producing a zygote with one or more extra chromosomes or less chromosomes—trisomy and monosomy respectively (Fig. 2.1).

*Causation :* The various etiological factors involved in the causation of chromosomal abnormalities are :—

Increased maternal age
Virus infections
Drugs
Radiation
Alcohol
Smoking

*Structural aberrations* involve breakage and rejoining of chromosome segments with or without loss of DNA material. Thus the various types of lesions could be *deletion* where a part of the chromosome is lost, *translocation* where the bit is rejoined on to another chromosome. This includes exchange of segments—*reciprocal translocation, insertion* of a broken segment into another arm of the same chromosome *shift* or to another chromosome *insertion. Robertsonian translocation* involves a break across the centromeric regions of two non-homologous acrocentric chromosomes with subsequent exchange leading to the formation of one large and one small metacentric chromosomes.

## SYNDROMES DUE TO NUMERICAL ANOMALIES OF AUTOSOMES :

*Down's syndrome*—Incidence at birth 1-2/1000 increases if a population of mental retardates is observed.

The syndrome is characterised by growth retardation, hypotonia, mental retardation, broad flat face with slanting eyes and epicanthus, short nose, high arched palate, furrowed tongue, flat occiput, dysplastic ears and pelvis, short broad hands with incurved 5th finger. Congenital heart lesions, umbilical hernia and congenital pyloric stenosis, megacolon and intestinal atresia are additional defects. The association of the disease with increased maternal age is observed in a large number of cases.

In 90% cases the defect is due to the presence of an extra chromosome (21 trisomy). In 10% a translocation of the distal part of chromosome 21 occurs onto another chromosome usually 21, 22, 13, 14 or 15.

*Other autosomal trisomies*

*Trisomy 13 (Pataus syndrome)* is less common and shows mental and physical growth failure with coloboma, microphthalmia, low set deformed ears, microcephaly, hypertelorism, arhinencephaly, cleft lip and palate, polydactyly and defects of the urinary system, heart and gonads.

*Trisomy 18 (Edward's syndrome)* is associated with growth and mental retardation, open skull sutures, dolicocephaly, retroflexion of head, hypertelorism with high arched eyebrow, short sternum, micrognathia, defects of heart, Meckel's diverticula, horseshoe kidney, pes equinus and external genital defects.

*Trisomy 8* : Mental retardation, prominent forehead, short broad nose, short upper lip, hypotonia, renal and pelvic defects, slender hands and feet, long first fingers and toes.

*Trisomy 9* : Microcephaly, malformation of cerebellum, small palpebral fissures, micrognathia, developmental defects of tibia and fibulas, small pelvis and scrotum, reduction in number and size of toes.

Table 2.1 gives the summarised findings of major chromosomal aberrations.

## SYNDROMES DUE TO ERRORS OF SEX CHROMOSOMES

The Y chromosome has been found to carry only two genes—that for hairy pinnae and the H-Y antigen. However, the presence is necessary for the formation of the testis initially. In the absence of it the child develops phenotypically female. Sexual development is caused by interaction probably of a large number of autosomal genes which regulate gonadal development, as well as the development of secondary sex characters and steroid hormones. Thus a wide variety of sexual aberrations occurs due to causes which may or may not display chromosomal errors.

The syndromes showing sex chromosomal errors are mainly as follows:—

(1) *Turner's syndrome* is characterised by short stature, retarded growth, lack of secondary sex characters, wide apart eyes, shield chest, short neck, short 4th metacarpal, cubitus valgus and heart lesions. The uterus is usually rudimentary with streak gonads showing fibrous tissue with no follicles.

The chromosomal pattern is usually 45 XO with absence of one chromosome. Other aberrations of the X chromosome like deletion or isochromosome X may also be seen.

(2) *Klinefelter's syndrome* is characterised by hypogonadism, tall stature, testicular atrophy with additional features often present like gynaecomastia, feminine habitus, mental impairment and lack of secondary sex characters. Chromosome pattern shows 47XXY with an extra X chromosome. Rarer cases show mosaicism or increased number of X chromosomes (48XXXY, 49XXXXY).

(3) XYY usually associated with mental subnormality, hypogonadism and gynaecomastia and skeletal defects.

(4) *Intersexuality and intersex states:*

True hermaphrodites are extremely rare and may show mosaicism or chimaerism of two separate cell lines—male and female. The internal genitalia would then also display lateral hermaphroditism or ovotestis. However, the majority of intersexes show only one cell line either 46XX or 46XX with no mosaicism. Other causes of intersexuality are:—

(i) Adrenogenital syndrome which may be iatrogenic or autosomal recessive.

(ii) Testicular feminisation syndrome which is autosomal dominant and probably due to an end organ resistance so that a normal 46XY develops as a female with usually well developed breasts.

TABLE 2.1 : Major syndromes associated with chromosome defect mainly autosomes

| Syndrome | Chromosome abnormality | Main features |
|---|---|---|
| Down's syndrome | trisomy 21 translocation 21/21, 21/14, 21/15, 21/22 | characteristic facies, mental retardation, hypotonia, congenital heart and pyloric stenosis. |
| Patau's syndrome | trisomy 13 | mental and physical retardation, microcephaly, microphthalmia, clefts of face, feet defect, polydactyly, congenital heart disease. |
| Edward's syndrome | trisomy 18 | motor and mental retardation, flexion defects of fingers, micrognathia, micropthalmia, congenital heart. |
| | trisomy 8 | moderate mental defect, strabismus, clinodactyly, spinal defect, delayed puberty. |
| | trisomy 9 | microcephaly with high forehead, deep-set eyes, short receding chin, cardiac and cerebral defects, hypogonadism, osteoarticular defects. |
| | trisomy 22 | microcephaly, short beaked nose, micrognathia, large malformed ears, severe mental and skeletal retardation, cardiac defects, imperforate anus. |
| Lejeune's syndrome 'criduchat' syndrome | 5p deletion | mental retardation, microcephaly hypertelorism, cat's cry, ocular, cardiac and renal defects. |
| de Grouchy's syndrome | 18p deletion | mental retardation abnormal facies,—ocular ear, and central nervous system defects. |

TABLE 2.2 : Some conditions known to be inherited as autosomal dominant (AD)

| | |
|---|---|
| Achondroplasia | Ankylosing spondylitis |
| Aperts syndrome | Deafness, dominant forms |
| Brachydactyly | Elliptocytosis |
| Cleidocranial dysostosis | Epidermolysis bullosa |
| Craniofacial dysostosis | Huntington's Chorea |
| Crouzons disease | Ehlers—Danlos syndrome |
| Holt-Oram syndrome | Marfan's syndrome |
| Oculodigital syndrome | Methaemoglobinaemia |
| Osteogenesis imperfecta | Mytonic dystrophy |
| Treacher Collins syndrome | Neurofibromatosis |
| Hereditary exostosis | Polyposis coli |
| Hepatic porphyria | Nail Patella syndrome |
| Von Willebrand's Disease | Waardenberg syndrome |

(II)**Diseases due to single** genes of large effect

(i) *Diseases due to dominant inheritance* may be diagnosed by the occurrence of vertically inherited syndromes, i.e., transmission from affected parent to child. Occurrence of unaffected parent is very rare and indicative of fresh mutation. Occasionally minor anomalies may be undetected like in polydactyly due to incomplete penetrance of a gene. Alternately a gene may be polymorphic and show differential expressivity as in osteogenesis imperfecta. Table 2.3 gives a list of a few of the conditions inherited as autosomal dominant.

(ii) *Diseases due to recessive inheritance* are seen to occur in children of unaffected carrier parents. More than one sib is often affected showing a horizontal transmission pattern. A few of the conditions inherited by this mode are given in Table 2.3.

While the affected individual would display the phenotypic and biochemical aberrations associated with the syndrome, the carrier parents are difficult to identify. Some of these conditions are fairly well investigated in India, e.g., thalassaemias (Table 2.4).

(iii) *Diseases due to X-linked inheritance.* The Y-chromosome carries only two genes so far identified—one for hairy pinnae and the other for H-Y antigen. The X-chromosome carries a large number of genes including those for colour blindness, AHG, G6PD, PGK, to mention a few. Thus carrier mothers having one defective gene will not be affected due to the presence of a normal gene on the X-chromosome. The male, on the other hand, has a 50% chance of inheriting an abnormal X-chromosome from the mother and will display the disease. Thus the majority of XL diseases are XR but show up in males. Very few diseases are XD and would show up even in the female (Table 2.5).

(III) *Diseases due to polygenic inheritance:*—The incidence of diseases transmitted by simple Mendelian ratios does not comprise more than 2-4/100 population. The majority of common diseases appears to occur as a result of the interaction of genetic predisposition to external factors. For example, peptic ulcer occurs twice as commonly among sibs as compared to control but is nevertheless precipitated by stress conditions. The same cause may apply to coronary heart disease, essential hypertension and diabetes. Unless and until a single gene-enzyme basis of the various patterns of these conditions is established, it would be necessary to depend upon family studies of affected persons and also to compare incidence rates among twins, racial groups and other factors like enzymes, blood groups or proteins. The present knowledge regarding certain congenital anomalies is also dependent on family studies.

*Coronary heart disease:*—The existence of serum hyperlipidaemia inherited as AD or AR has shown that possibility exists regarding prediction of the possibility of development(Table 2.6).

*Essential hypertension* is believed to be caused by multifactorial inheritance as blood pressure levels are distributed continuously in the population with no evidence of bimodality. Other people are, however, of the view that a single dominant gene is responsible.

*Peptic ulceration* as well as duodenal ulcer is found to be twice as common in close relatives but the precipitating factors appear to be different. An association with different blood groups and HLA antigens also complicate the picture. However, the heritability of both appears to be 40%, being higher for duodenal than for gastric ulcer.

*Diabetes mellitus* : The juvenile and adult onset types appear to be distinct clinically and AR and AD varieties have been reported. However, the present state of knowledge points to a multifactorial mode of inheritance with a heritability of 75% for the early onset and 35% for the late onset type. The detection of prediabetic state by various methods including plasma insulin antagonists is likely to be of use in the early detection of cases.

*Mental retardation:*—About 20% of all cases of mental retardation are due to genetic defects. The commonest chromosomal aberration detected is Down's syndrome. However, familial mental retardation with or without microcephaly has also been found to occur. Apart from specific syndromes like Laurence-

TABLE 2.3 : Some conditions known to be inherited as autosomal recessive (AR)

| | |
|---|---|
| Adrenogenital syndrome | Albinism |
| Alkaptonuria | Alpha antitrypsin deficiency |
| Aminoaciduria | Ataxia telangiectasia |
| Phenylketonuria | Chediak Higashi syndrome |
| Tyrosinosis | Fanconi syndrome |
| Maple syrup urine disease | Lysosomal enzyme deficiency |
| Cystinuria | Mucopolysaccharidosis |
| Histidinaemia | Lipidosis |
| Cystic fibrosis | Ganglioside storage disease |
| Laurence Moon Biedl syndrome | Glycogen storage disease |
| Immunodeficiency syndromes | Thalassaemias |
| Haemoglobinopathies | Wilson's disease |

TABLE 2.5 : Some conditions known to be X linked

| | |
|---|---|
| X linked dominant (XD) | X linked recessive (XR) |
| Vitamin D resistant rickets | Colour blindness |
| Incontinentia pigmenti | Testicular feminisation |
| Oral facial digital syndrome | Muscular dystrophy |
| Brown teeth | Haemophilia A and B |
| | Lesch Nyhan syndrome |
| | Glucose 6 phosphate dehydrogenase deficiency |

TABLE 2.4 : Clinically important haemoglobinopathies

| Disease | | Genetics | Clinical severity |
|---|---|---|---|
| Sickle cell syndromes | Sickle cell anaemia | Homozygote S | Severe |
| | Sickle $\beta$ Thalassaemia | S × $\beta$Thalcompound heterozygote | Severe to moderate |
| | Sickle C disease | S × C compound heterozygote | Mild to moderate |
| | Sickle cell trait | A × S heterozygote | No symptoms |
| $\alpha$-thalassaemia | Hydrops fetalis 4Hb | $\alpha$-deletions | Lethal |
| | $\alpha$-thal-1 heterozygote | 2Hb deletions | Mild |
| | or 2 heterozygote | 1Hb deletions | None |
| $\beta$-thalassaemia | $\beta$ thalassaemia major Cooley's anaemia | Homozygote thal | Severe |
| | $\beta$ thalassaemia major or Cooley's anaemia | Homozygote | Severe |
| | Hb Lepore heterozygote | $\delta\beta$ fusion gene | Mild to severe |
| | $\beta°$, $\beta+$ and $\delta\beta°$ thal trait | Heterozygous compound | Mild |
| | HbE or D thal | heterozygotes | Severe |
| Unstable haemoglobin diseases | Congenital nonspherocytic haemolytic Heinz body | Heterozygous dominant | Mild to severe |
| M-haemoglobin | Familial methaemoglobinaemia | Heterozygous dominant—5 variants | Moderate |

TABLE 2.6 : Genetic causation of coronary heart disease

| Type of hyperlipidaemia | Cholesterol level | Triglyceride level | Lipoprotein types | Inheritance pattern | Population frequency | Age of onset in males | Remarks |
|---|---|---|---|---|---|---|---|
| Familial hyper-cholesterolaemia | raised | Usually normal | IIa or IIb | AD 85-92% below 25 years | 0.2-0.5% | 46 | LDL recept or defect |
| Polygenic hyper-cholesterolaemia | raised | normal | IIa or IIb | Polygenic | 5% | 58 | ? heterogenous |
| Familial hyper-triglyceridaemia | normal | raised | IV or V | AD 26% | Below 1% | 57 | |
| Familial combined hyperlipidaemia | raised in 2/3 | raised in 2/3 | IIa, IIb, IV, rarely V | AD 18% | Below 1.5% | 52 | 33% have increased cholesterol 33% increased TG 33% increased TG and cholesterol |

TABLE 2.7 : Summarised findings of mucopolysaccharoidosis (modified McKusick 1972)

| Type Name | Mental & & motor retardation | Growth retardation | Coarse facies | Bone changes | Joint | Liver | Corneal opacity | Inheritance |
|---|---|---|---|---|---|---|---|---|
| IH Hurler | +++ | ++ | +++ | +++ | ++ | ++ | + | AR |
| IS Scheie | – | – | ± | + | + | ± | + | AR |
| IH/S Hunter-Scheie | ± | + | ++ | ++ | ++ | + | + | AR |
| IIA Hunter | + | + | + | ++ | + | + | ± | XR |
| IIB Vacant | | | | | | | | |
| IIIA Sanfilippo A | +++ | – | + | + | + | ++ | – | AR |
| IIIB Sanfilippo B | +++ | – | + | + | + | ++ | – | AR |
| IIIC Sanfilippo C | +++ | – | + | + | ± | ++ | – | AR |
| IV Morquio | – | +++ | + | +++ | + | + | + | AR |
| VIA Maroteaux Lamy | – | ++ | ++ | ++ | + | + | + | AR |
| VIB Maroteaux Lamy | – | + | + | + | + | + | + | AR |
| VII $\beta$-glucuronidase deficiency | + | ± | ± | + | – | ++ | ± | AR |

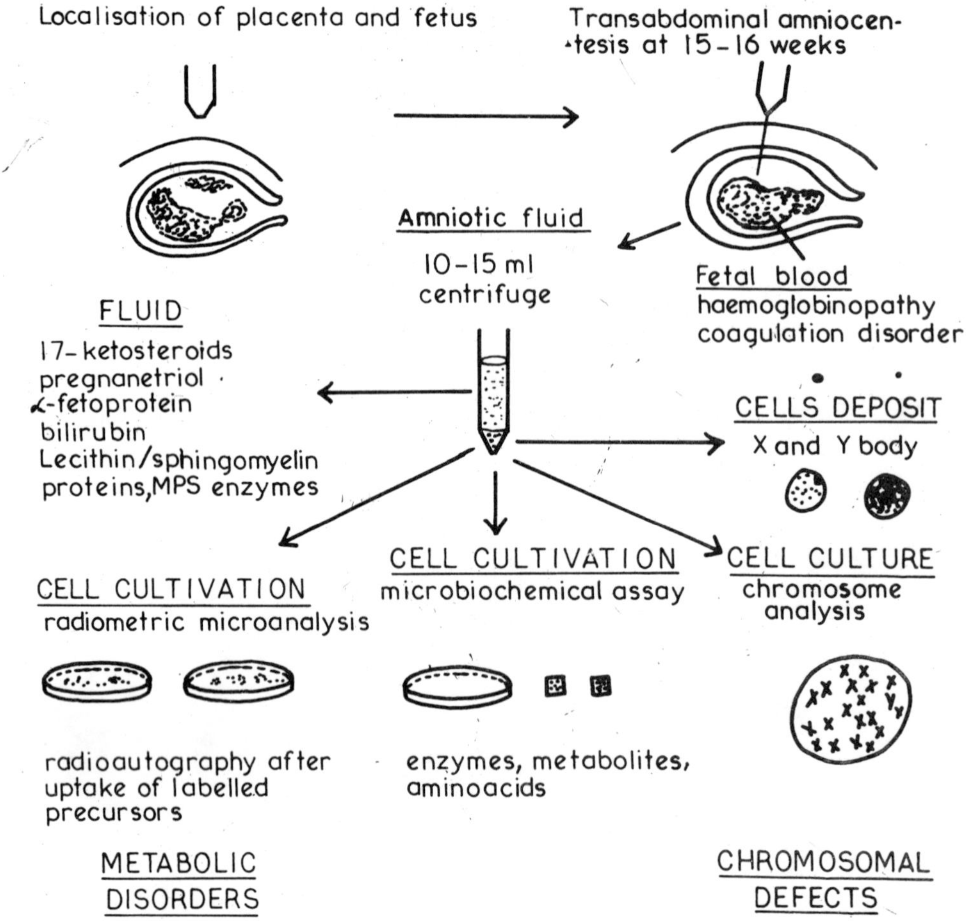


Fig.2.3 Methodology of Prenatal Analysis of fetal Genetic Disease

Moon-Biedl, Sickle's, etc., due to AR, other factors like birth trauma, perinatal infection, drugs, radiation are common causes to be taken into account.

*Investigations of the genetic basis of inherited disease* depend primarily on the diagnosis as, although only a few of the genetic diseases are known, it is not possible to analyse each and every case fully. Thus, it is deemed advisable even in the most advanced countries to have specialised centres for detection of groups of genetic diseases. This is especially applicable for metabolic disorders and for antenatal diagnosis (Fig 2.3). Diagnosis is assisted by:—

1. *Complete physical examination* of affected person (propositus, proband), parents, brothers and sisters (siblings) and children. A complete pedigree chart is usually necessary to determine the inheritance pattern—AD, AR, XR, XD. Occasionally, minor malformations may be overlooked.
2. Radiological examination.
3. Buccal smear examination for X and Y bodies.
4. Chromosome analysis by leucocyte, bone marrow or skin culture and identification of chromosome by banding patterns.
5. Biochemical investigations:
   Urine examination for amino acidurias, mucopolysaccharidosis, alkaptonuria (See Table 2.7).
   Blood—Aminoacidurias
   Coagulation studies
   Enzyme analysis
   Haemoglobinopathies

## GENETIC COUNSELLING

The physician is often faced with the prospect of advising parents who have had a defective child or sibs of affected persons want to know of the risks of having affected children or developing the disease.

(i) For counselling for chromosomal disorders the chromosome analysis of the parents and affected child is necessary.

For trisomy 21, in 95% cases the error is a trisomy and the risk of recurrence increases with mother's age. After 30 years of age, risk in mother increases from 1 : 1350 to 1 : 800. For translocation Down's the parents may also have a translocation defect. Here if the lesion is D/G in the baby and mother, recurrence risk is 10%.

If D/G occurs in baby and father, recurrence risk is 5%;
If 21/22 in baby + mother risk is 7%;
If 21/22 in baby + father risk is 3%;
If 21/21 in baby and either parent risk is 100%.

Other autosomal anomalies are very rare and risk of recurrence in parents with normal karyotype is 1%.

(ii) Counselling for dominant or recessive conditions (Table 2.8) is dependent on pedigree analysis and follows Mendel's laws. In dominant conditions the parents are usually unaffected and the child a heterozygous fresh mutant. Alternatively, an affected person has an affected parent although the degree of expression may not be the same. Usually, if affected persons marry a normal person, 50% of the children are affected. Certain AD diseases have an advanced age of onset, e.g., Huntington's chorea making advice difficult.

Autosomal recessive and X-linked disorders usually need biochemical tests as well as pedigree analysis for counselling. The heterozygote carrier may or may not show less than normal level of enzymes or metabolites in the blood or tissues. Thus, there is also possibility of a diseased individual marrying a carrier. Usually 25% children from the marriage of two heterozygotes are affected, 25% are normal and 50% are

TABLE 2.8 : Proportion of normal and affected progeny of affected parents with different modes of inheritance

| Mode of Inheritance | Progeny of affected male | | Progeny of heterozygous female | |
|---|---|---|---|---|
| | Normal | Affected | Normal | Affected |
| **Male Progeny :** | | | | |
| Autosomal recessive | 1 | 0 | 1 | 0 |
| Autosomal dominant | 1/2 | 1/2 | 1/2 | 1/2 |
| Autosomal dominant (male limited) | 1/2 | 1/2 | 1/2 | 1/2 |
| X-linked recessive | 1 | 0 | 1/2 | 1/2 |
| X-linked dominant | 1 | 0 | 1/2 | 1/2 |
| **Female Progeny :** | | | | |
| Autosomal recessive | 1 | 0 | 1 | 0 |
| Autosomal dominant | 1/2 | 1/2 | 1/2 | 1/2 |
| Autosomal dominant | 1/2 | 1/2 | 1/2 | 1/2 |
| Autosomal dominant (male limited) | 1/2 | 1/2(c) | 1/2 | 1/2(c) |
| X-linked recessive | 0 | 1(c) | 1/2 | 1/2(c) |
| X-linked dominant | 0 | 1 | 1/2 | 1/2 |

(c) indicates a carrier, usually unaffected.

TABLE 2.9 : Empiric risks for some common congenital defects (in per cent)

| Disorder | Incidence | Sex ratio M:F | Normal parents having a second affected child | Affected parent having an affected child | Affected parent having an affected child |
|---|---|---|---|---|---|
| Anencephaly | 0.20 | 1:2 | 2 | - | - |
| Cleft palate only | 0.04 | 2:3 | 2 | 7 | 15 |
| Cleft lip ± Cleft palate | 0.10 | 3:2 | 4 | 4 | 10 |
| Club foot | 0.10 | 2:1 | 3 | 3 | 10 |
| Congenital heart disease (all types) | 0.50 | - | 1-4 | 1-4 | - |
| Diabetes mellitus (early onset) | 0.20 | 1:1 | 8 | 8 | 10 |
| Dislocation of hip | 0.07 | 1:6 | 4 | 4 | 10 |
| Epilepsy (idiopathic) | 0.50 | 1:1 | 5 | 5 | 10 |
| Hirschsprung's disease | 0.02 | 4:1 | | | |
| male index | | | 2 | - | - |
| female index | | | 8 | - | - |
| Manic-depressive psychoses | 0.40 | 2:3 | - | 10-15 | - |
| Mental retardation (idiopathic) | 0.30-0.50 | 1:1 | 3-5 | - | - |
| Profound childhood deafness | 0.10 | 1:1 | 10 | 6 | - |
| Pyloric stenosis | 0.30 | 5:1 | | | |
| male index | | | 2 | 4 | 13 |
| female index | | | 10 | 17 | 38 |
| Schizophrenia | 1-2 | 1:1 | - | 16 | - |
| Scoliosis (idiopathic, adolescent) | 0.22 | 1:6 | 7 | 5 | - |
| Spina bifida | 0.30 | 2:3 | 4<br>After two children 10% | 3 | - |

again carriers. In actual life, however, the figure indicates averages and actual statistical probability depends on the size of the family.

(iii) Multifactorial inherited disorders are the most difficult to predict as in certain families they may follow Mendelian ratios while in others no such pattern is visible. Spinal cord defects, for example, are fairly common in India and may show autosomal dominant mode of inheritance or X-linked inheritance. Thus, the possibility of 1 in 20 risk in general population increasing to a recurrence risk of 3%-6% after one child and 1 in 8 after two children (see Table 2.9) may not apply to all cases. Here it is necessary to undertake detailed pedigree analysis followed by alfa fetoprotein assays during subsequent pregnancy.

Affected parent Aa

| Normal parent aa | | A | a |
|---|---|---|---|
| | a | Aa affected | aa normal |
| | a | Aa affected | aa normal |

Autosomal dominant conditions (AD)

Normal carrier parent

| Normal carrier parent | | A | a |
|---|---|---|---|
| | A | AA normal | Aa unaffected carrier |
| | a | Aa unaffected carrier | aa affected |

Autosomal recessive conditions (AD)

Affected male ($X^HY$)

| Normal female | | $X^H$ | Y |
|---|---|---|---|
| | X | XX carrier daughter | XY normal son |
| | X | $XX^H$ carrier daughter | XY normal son |

Carrier female ($X^hX$)

| Normal Male | | $X^h$ | X |
|---|---|---|---|
| | X | $X^hX$ carrier daughter | XX normal daughter |
| | Y | $X^hY$ affected son | XY normal son |

X-linked recessive conditions (XR)

Fig. 2.3 : Showing Chi-square method of predicting Mendelian ratios of inheritance.

**Neoplasms :** Table 2.10 gives a few of the conditions where neoplasia is seen to be inherited. Apart from these it is important to know that all malignant neoplasms are associated with aneuploidy and chromosome aberrations in the tumour itself. However, the cells of other tissues like the blood do not show the same abberrations. The aneuploidy is non-specific and marker chromosome characteristic of any particular neoplasm does occur but is again non-specific.

Specific chromosome aberration is only seen in CML where a minute chromosome 22 with a deleted short arm is termed the $Ph^1$ or Philadelphia chromosome. The deleted arm is often translocated on the chromosome 9 or 6.

Retinoblastomas are also associated with aberration of chromosome 13 and characterised by differential inheritance patterns for the unilateral and bilateral variants.

TABLE 2.10 : Some inherited disorders associated with neoplastic change

| Disorder | Neoplasm |
|---|---|
| **Autosomal Dominant :** | |
| Basal cell naevus syndrome | Basal cell carcinoma |
| Diaphysial achalasia | Sarcoma |
| Epiloia | Tumours of retina, kidney and heart |
| Neurofibromatosis | Neurofibromata, CNS tumours |
| Phaeochromocytoma and thyroid carcinoma syndrome | Thyroid carcinoma |
| Polyposis coli | Colonic carcinoma |
| Retinoblastoma | |
| Tylosis | Oesophageal carcinoma |
| **Autosomal recessive :** | |
| Albinism | Carcinoma skin |
| Ataxia telangiectasia | Lymphoreticulosis |
| Blooms syndrome | Leukaemia |
| Chediak Higashi syndrome | Lymphoma |
| Fanconis anaemia | Leukaemia |
| Xeroderma pigmentosum | Skin carcinoma |
| **X-linked recessive** | |
| Brutons agammaglobulinaemia | Lymphoreticulosis |
| Wiskott-aldrich syndrome | Lymphoreticulosis |

## CHAPTER 3

# IMMUNOLOGY IN MEDICINE

*K. P. SEN GUPTA*

## INTRODUCTION :

Phylogenetically immunological mechanism has developed in the body as a means of specific recognition and evasion of the harmful foreign substances by a process of natural selection. Since self-recognition mechanisms appear early in evolution, primitive defence mechanism is manifested by phagocytosis of foreign particles by cells. These cells do not respond by proliferation to ensure more effective protection on subsequent contact. The protective mechanism involves an evolution of the host making its own tissues antigenically different from their parasitic relatives around, so that these could be recognised as foreign.

The characteristic cells of the immune system are macrophages and lymphocytes. The former are distributed throughout the body both circulating in the blood and fixed in tissues as cells of the reticuloendothelial system in the spleen, the lymph nodes, the lungs, the bone marrow and in the connective tissue. These cells are phagocytic, contain digestive enzymes in lysosomes to degrade ingested material and serve an important part in the immune mechanism by way of processing and catabolism of antigen or presenting them to the lymphoid cells or retaining them. They also play an important part in natural immunity as phagocytosis or pinocytosis, and, thereby, digest or store them without any harmful effect on the host. The macrophages also play an important role in the initiation of immune response by the lymphoid cells by concentrating antigen in the follicles and medulla of lymph nodes, white pulp of the spleen and in the gut-associated lymphoid tissue and bringing it into contact with the lymphocytes. They can also release soluble factors to influence the activity of lymphocytes. Some antigen may be retained at the surface of macrophages where it is seen as a depot antigen for the maintenence of immune response.

The lymphocytes are the basic cellular unit of the immune system because of their ability to recognise and respond to antigens. They are the antigen sensitive cells. These cells are present in circulation as well as in various lymphoid tissues-thymus, lymph nodes, spleen, gut-associated lymphoid tissue, adenoids and tonsils and bone marrow.

All lymphocytes originate from the bone marrow (or liver in the foetus) as blast cells. These cells differentiate to precursor cells—some of them migrate to the thymus where they proliferate and differentiate and finally come out as T-lymphocyte (T-cell). These are long lived lymphocytes with a life span for months or years. The emergent populations are heterogenous and are composed of subsets of cells with potential for different 'effector' functions. Other precursor cells migrate to the gut-associated lymphoid tissue (Peyer's patches and appendix) from which B-lymphocytes (B-Cell) are produced. These are precursor of the antibody producing cells, plasma cells via plasmoblasts on contact with antigen. B-cells are short lived lymphocytes. These are relatively less mobile but more fixed in the lymphoid organs whereas T-cells are more mobile and are found in circulation to the extent of 70% to 80%. The major lymphoid tissue and organs associated with immune response are lymph nodes, spleen and gut-associated lymphoid tissue. Fig. 3.1 shows the structure of lymph node and also white pulp of spleen. The cortical area of the lymph node and the area around central arteriole of the white pulp of the spleen are under the influence of thymus and are called thymus dependent area. During the induction of cell-mediated immune response the cells that undergo proliferation in response to antigenic stimulation are T-cells. On the other hand, B-cells are found in cortical lymphoid follicles, germinal centres, medullary junctions and medullary cords of lymph nodes and the red pulp of the spleen. In humoral response, immunoglobulins *(vide infra)* are secreted by plasma cells. Each plasma cell produces only one type of immunoglobulin.

This subdivision of lymphocytes into T-cell and B-cell is due to the existence of two parallel types of immune responses in defence against infectious diseases and other antigens. These lead to the initiation of an adaptive immune response specific for the inducing antigens.

The genes controlling the ability to produce an immune response are called immune response genes. In a human being these have been associated with chromosome 6. This is called HLA region and has close link with the major histocompatibility system (MHS) *(vide infra)*.

## ANTIGENS :

Antigens are substances of various chemical types, but differ significantly from the normal body components (foreign or not self-depending on chemical groupings). These are capable of acting as a specific stimulus to the immune system to produce a response specifically directed at the inducing substance, but not other allied substances. The antigenic determinants are areas of the antigenic molecules of specific chemical character, which has the specific binding site on antibody molecule. Antigenic molecule may, thus, consist of many such relatively smaller areas, or antigenic determinants against each of which specific antibody is directed. The surface of an antigenic molecule could, therefore, have a large number of antigenic determinants which could be different from one another or cover one another in a mosaic form. Immune response to a single type of antigen can produce a large number of antibody responses and of various types.

Haptens are usually simple chemicals, but unable to induce immune response, except when attached to a carrier molecule. These are usually small molecules. Each has a single antigenic determinant.

Certain bacterial antigens and cell surface antigens produce antibodies which reveal serological cross-reactions indicating sharing of antigens. Such examples are Forssman antigen present between red cells and bacteria—Pneumococci and Salmonella, between E. coli and human blood group B, and between Treponema pallidum and cardiolipin extract from mammalian heart.

Immunogenecity of an antigen depends on molecular size. A protein substance less than molecular wt. of 5000 is less likely to be antigenic. Lipids alone are not antigenic, but combined with protein or polysaccharides as lipoprotein or lipopoly-saccharides, they are antigenic. Proteins and poly-saccharides of high molecular weight are antigenic. Tyrosine is a helpful constituent for polypeptide to be a good immunogen, but it is not essential. Some chemicals of low molecular weight combine with tissue protein to form complexes and act as a hapten with carrier proteins and behave as a complete antigen. The physical state and particle size are also important in affecting the antigenicity.

Certain antigens can stimulate immunoglobulin producing cell (B-cell) *(vide infra)* while other require co-operation of T-cell (Thymus dependent cell) *(vide infra)* for activation of B-cell. Hence, immunologically the former antigen can be identified as T-independent antigens and the latter as T-dependent antigens. In the latter importance of T-cell factors has been stressed *(vide infra)*.

## IMMUNOGLOBULINS : ANTIBODIES :

Antibody is a soluble protein molecule with ability to bind specifically and combine with essentially only one type of antigenic determinant. Antibodies form a group of structurally related protein molecules known as gamma globulin. Because of their immunological functions they are known as immunoglobulins. Their distribution is seen in serum electrophoresis (Fig. 3.2).

## CHEMICAL STRUCTURE :

Immunoelectrophoresis subdivides them into five classes on the basis of marked antigenic difference in their heavy chains. These are referred to as IgG, IgM, IgA, IgD and IgE. Their different characteristic properties and functions are summarised in Table (3.1). The basic immunoglobulin structure is given in Fig. (3.3).

Each molecule has 12 units, each unit consisting of a polypeptide chain with 160 aminoacids of molecular weight of 12000. Each light chain has two basic units and each heavy chain has four basic units. Light chains are thus about half the length of heavy chains. They are joined together by interchain disulphide bridges. There are two types of light chain, kappa (k) and lambda (l). Each antibody has either two kappa or two lambda chains while the heavy chains are constant for each class. The heavy chains are designated as $\gamma$ (gamma) in IgG, $\mu$ (miu) in IgM, $\alpha$ (alpha) in IgA, $\delta$ (delta) in IgD and $\epsilon$ (epsilon) in IgE. The two light and five heavy chain types—all differ from each other in aminoacid sequence. The mid-region of each immunoglobulin is particularly susceptible to the action of the enzyme papain, which splits the molecule just at a site left to the disulphide bridge on the heavy chain into three almost equal fragments. Two of the fragments on the left side are similar in structure and carry two antigen binding sites termed as Fab fragments (ab=antigen binding). Most of the sites concerned with biological activity are carried on Fc fragment, and the latter is unique to each antibody class (Fig. 3.3). Some of the biological activities of antibody, such as complement activity and chemotaxis to neutrophils at the Fc region are antigen dependent and result from changes in the Fc region which occur after the antigens have bound to the Fab sites. Other properties, such as placental transfer, gut transfer, and binding of IgE to mast cells are independent of antigen and are determined by the nature of Fc region.

Immunoglobulins differ from all other proteins in that the terminal half of the light chain and terminal quarter of heavy chain present within Fab fragment vary from one portion to another in their aminoacid sequence. This variable sequence of aminoacids varies except the position of glycine component which acts as a pivot on the variable regions of molecule. The variable (V) regions of heavy ($V_H$) and light ($V_L$) chain together make up the antigen combining site and are responsible for specificity of antibody. In the constant (C) region there is a constant sequence of aminoacids at the C terminal of the chain and is responsible for biological properties of antibodies. This is class specific. The light chains of the constant region ($C_L$) are different from each other, but all the heavy chain classes share the same variable region ($V_H$).

Antigen sensitive B-cells present heavy chain immunoglobulins as receptors on them. The receptor appears to be an IgM subunit as monomeric form in 20% of cells but not as pentameric form as in serum. In addition to monomeric IgM receptor about 70% of cells also have IgD receptor on their surfaces. IgD is widely distributed over the cells while it is present in very minute quantities in serum. About 5% of cellsalso carry receptor of IgG, IgA or IgE in addition to monomeric IgM receptor. B-cell membrane also possesses receptor for Fc fragment of IgG molecule and a receptor for activated complement component C3b. These receptors may be involved in the genetic control of immune responsiveness by B-cells *(vide infra)*. Antigen tends to bind preferentially to certain areas of lymphocyte membrane rather uniformly all over the cell surface.

Distribution of Ig in the serum is quite different from those present as the receptors on B cell. In the serum IgG, IgA, IgM, IgD and IgE are present in order of concentration while on the surface receptors IgM in combination with IgG or IgA is most frequent while IgE combination on receptors is the least. IgM and

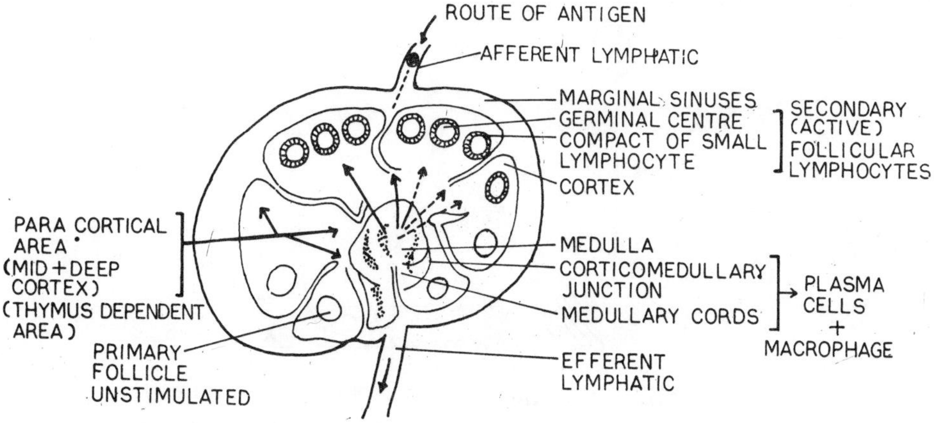


Fig. 1a

Fig 3 1 (a) shows the structure of lymph l nodes

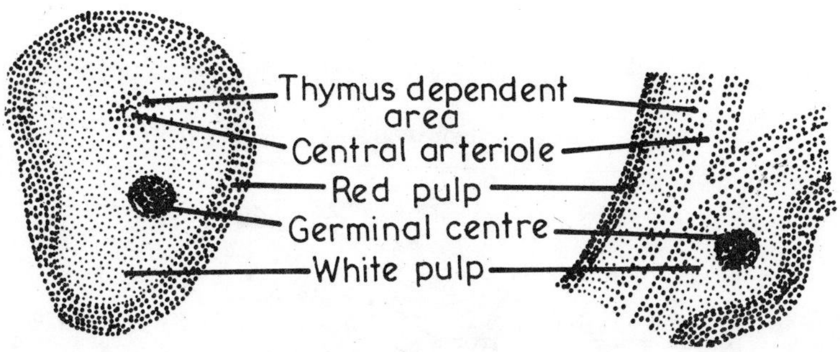


Fig. 1b

Fig.3.1 (b) shows splenic architecture

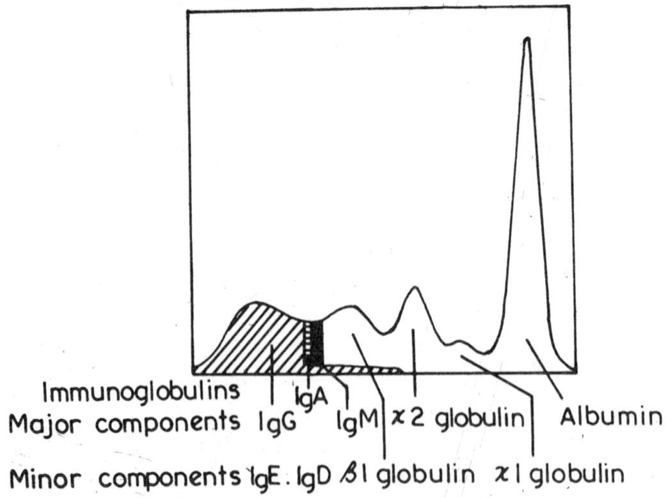


Fig.3.2 Showing immunoglobulin components in serum electrophoresis.

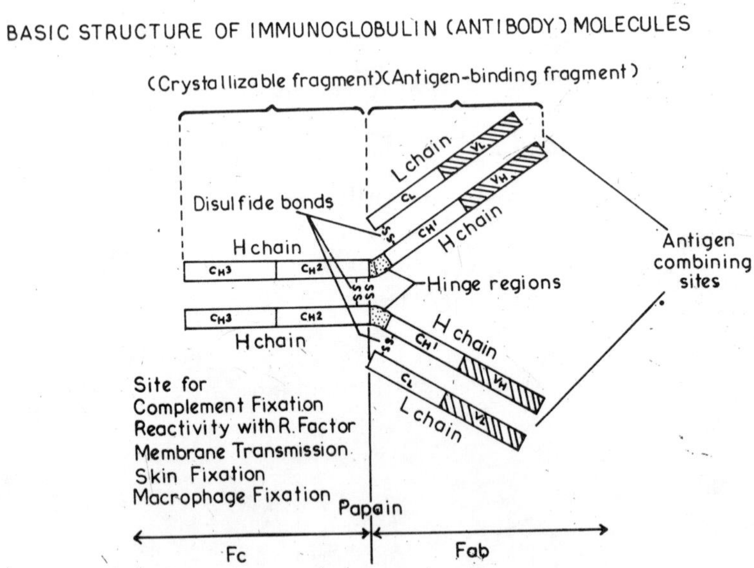


Fig. 3.3 Basic Structure of Immunoglobulin (Anti Body) Molecules

IgD are present predominantly. The nature of the Ig receptor marks out the future course of the cell, in that B-cells which carry IgM and IgD, give rise to plasma cells producing IgM class, while those carrying IgM and IgG or IgA or IgE will give rise to plasma cells producing IgG or IgA or IgE. The amount of Ig classes in serum only indicates the numbers of plasma cells of each class.

TABLE-3.1
PROPERTIES OF IMMUNOGLOBULINS IN MAN

| | IgG | IgM | IgA | IgD | IgE |
|---|---|---|---|---|---|
| Mol. weight. | 145,000 Monomer | 850,000 Pentamer | 385,000 Dimer (170,000) Monomer | 160,000 Monomer | 200,000 Monomer |
| Half life in days in plasma. | 19-24 | 5 | 6 | 2.8 | 1.5 |
| Light chain. | K + L | K + L | K + L | K + L | K + L |
| Heavy chain | $\gamma$ | $\mu$ | $\alpha$ | $\delta$ | $\epsilon$ |
| Normal adult levels (mg/dl) in plasma. | 600-1600 | 50-150 | 60-330 | 0.5-40 | 10-140 ng |
| % Total Immunoglobulin in plasma. | 70-80 | 3-10 | 10-20 | 0.4 | ? |
| Proportion : i) in blood (%) | 40 | 90 | 40 | ? | very low |
| ii) in extracellular fluids (%) | 60 | 10 | 0 | — | — |
| Presence in secretion. | NIL | NIL | 100% | — | — |
| Transfer to offspring. | via placenta | No transfer | via milk | No transfer | No transfer |
| Functional significance. | Major system immunoglobulins. | Appear early in immune response. Appear early in development. | Present on mucosal surface as dimer in circulation as monomer. | ? | Allergenic response, e.g., epithelial surfaces. |
| Characteristic properties. | Precipitation Antitoxin Complement fixation, Late antibody. | Agglutinins Opsonins Lysin, Complement fixation Early antibody. | Surface protection. | Not known | Reagenic antibody. |

| | IgG | IgM | IgA | IgD | IgE |
|---|---|---|---|---|---|
| No. of antigen binding sites. | 2 | 5-10 | 2 | 2 | 2 |
| Complement activation | | | | | |
| i) by classical pathway. | ++ | ++ | — | — | — |
| ii) by alternate pathway | — | — | + | + | + |
| Receptor site on : | | | | | |
| 1. Macrophage | + | — | — | — | — |
| 2. Neutrophil | + | — | — | — | — |
| 3. Lymphocyte | + | — | — | — | — |
| 4. Mast cell | — | — | — | — | + |
| 5. Basophils | — | — | — | — | + |
| 6. Platelet | + | — | — | — | — |

+ Positive, -Negative

## ADAPTIVE IMMUNE RESPONSE :

Adaptive immune response specific for an introduced antigen generally takes two forms—
A. Humoral Immune Response—Humoral antibody production, i.e. immunoglobulin production.
B. Cellular Immune Response—Production of lymphokines and other types of T-lymphocytes.

### A. HUMORAL IMMUNE RESPONSE :

It is during the fifth month of intrauterine life that immunoglobulin producing cells appear in the spleen and lymph nodes. Subsequently, both IgM and IgG are synthesised by the foetus with IgM predominant. Thus, B-cells begin their life as IgM producer. Hence, during the primary immune response B-cells secrete IgM antibody. They later switch over to the synthesis of IgG antibody. It is during the development of some clones and even perhaps within the individual cells that this 'switch' event occurs from production of IgM to that of other immunoglobulins. This IgM-IgG 'switch' seems very likely to depend upon the influence of T-cell on the B-cell population.

When an antigen in either soluble or particulate form is introduced for the first time into a host, there is a rapid increase in synthesis of protein, in the cells of the lymphoid organs indicated by adherence of the antigen to B-cell receptors. This immune response takes 7-14 days and antibodies eventually can be detected in the blood at low levels and for a short duration. This is called *primary immune response*. When the same antigen is introduced for the second time, there is slight fall of circulating antibody at that time due to rapid mopping up of antibody with the antigen. This can be detected by a fall in the level of antibody in the blood. After 1-2 days a marked rise in the level of antibody begins reaching a peak within 3-5 days. This high level is maintained for a long period, even months. This is recognised as *secondary immune response*. The interval between primary and secondary antigenic stimulation should not be less than 10 days. The shorter interval will not only reduce the rise in antibody level, but may lead to tolerance. The longer interval allows the immune system to increase the number of antibody forming cells following second introduction of the same antigen (Fig. 3.4).

Soluble antibodies (immunoglobulins) as components of serum proteins originate from B-cells via plasmoblasts through plasma cells. The latter synthesize and secrete immunoglobulins. During primary immune response IgM is the first formed antibody in the serum. In the secondary immune response IgG is the usual predominant type of immunoglobulin and IgM is usually much less.

### B. CELLULAR IMMUNE RESPONSE :

In this response antigen is either fixed in the cells of the tissues or is a modified part of the body's own tissues cells. T-lymphocytes are sensitised by the antigens in the peripheral circulation since large number of circulating lymphyocytes are T-cells. The T-cells that produce cell-mediated immune response, recirculate through the body (Fig. 3.5). About 90% of the cells go through the artery via the post-capillary venules and the efferent lymphatics of the lymph node to the thoracic duct or via the periarteriolar sheath to the marginal sinus of the white pulp of the spleen to the venous system back to the circulation. Only 10% of cells leave the capillaries of various parts of the body, moving through various tissue spaces into the lymphatics. This is particularly important for the gut-associated lymphoid tissue. 70%-80% of T-cells participate in recirculation and this occurs about once in 24 hours. This continuous movement of T-cells ensures that antigens or microbes entering the body come in contact with specific reactive cells since all T-cells carry on their surface antibody-like receptors specific for the particular antigen. These sensitised lymphocytes first differentiate into large cells within 4 days of sensitisation. Then they begin to divide into new subpopulations which go to other lymph nodes as immunologically active cells. Subsequently, the immunologically active cells are found in the peripheral blood.

The cellular immune response in human depends on intact thymus during foetal and neonatal life since it is in the thymus where primitive immunocytes differentiate and proliferate with the ability to induce immunological competence in the lymphocytes. The changes associated with this can be detected in murine animals as membrane antigens as Thy (theta), Th and Ly. Functional activity of the Ly marker can be defined as helper cell activity, cytoxic T-cell and suppressor T-cell *(vide infra)*.

On second contact with the same antigen the sensitised T-cells are differentiated into several subpopulations. Some are able to secrete lymphokines. These consist of a variety of soluble mediators of cell-mediated immunity. These have effect on macrophages, lymphocytes and blood vessels. The important ones are macrophage migration inhibition factor (MIF), macrophage activating factor (MAF), chemotactic factor (CF), mitogen factor (MF), skin reactive factor (SRF). Other T-cells are cytotoxic T-cells which take part in eradication of virus infected cells or bringing about the elimination of spontaneously rising neoplastic cells. Some other cells work as 'memory' T-cells and 'helper' cells or 'suppressor' cells for B lymphocytes in connection with humoral immune response (Fig. 3.6). The T-cell- B-cell co-operation is thought to be mediated through a soluble substance, T-cell factor, which mediates the interaction without direct contact with B-cell surface receptors. Some of the factors have no specificity for antigen and will promote all thymus dependent antibody responses. Other antigen specific factors strictly carry a binding site for antigen in one hand, and another binding site for the 'acceptor' site of B-cell to initiate them for immunoglobulin production. In addition, the role of macrophages in the co-operation between T-cell and B-cell is required in connection with particular antigens like virus or bacteria or fungus, to process and present it correctly to T-cell and B-cell. These sensitised cells then proceed to interact in the follicles of the lymph node or white pulp of the spleen. 'Suppressor' T-cells, on the other hand, balance the immunological response from becoming excessive by interacting with 'helper' T-cells, T-cells releasing lymphokines and possibly with B-cells. Since the 'suppressor' T-cells specifically block immune response, they can only do so acting in direct competition with the 'effector' immunocytes for antigens or by producing soluble mediators as in case of 'helper' T-cells. Thus, immunological unresponsiveness or tolerance can develop as a result of elimination of active clones of immunocytes or from an increase in the activity of these suppressor' T-cells. Decline in the activity of 'suppressor' T-cells is accompanied by an increase in the production of various auto-antibodies and thus indicates the loss of self-tolerance.

## C. THE COMPLEMENT SYSTEM :

Complement was known as heat labile serum component. Complement is now known as a complex group of serum proteins. Its components interact with certain antigen antibody complex or microbial protein. This activates complement to initiate the primitive process of inflammation and phagocytosis. The latter helps in termination of infection. Complement components are not all synthesised by a single type of cell, but the main sources of the components are the intestinal epithelia, macrophages, liver and spleen. Complement has nine factors or components (C1-C9), C3 being most abundant (1200 $\mu$g/ml).

### INITIATION STAGE :

The activation of complement fragments occurs by immune complexes formed by antigen, antibody (IgG or IgM) and participation of Fc fragment. During activation the cleavage of larger fragments occurs along with combination with other components while small fragments go to the body fluid. Moreover, the activation of complement occurs at cell surface in the vicinity of antibody molecule. The first three components C1, C4 and C2 circulate in an inactive form as proenzymes. Component C1 reacts with Fc fragment of Ig and after its interaction with antigen, the complement binding site is exposed. Subsequently, C1 comprised of three distinct proteins ($C1_q$, $C1_r$ and $C1_s$) held together by calcium ion ($Ca^{++}$) interacts. This may be regarded an initiation stage of the classical pathway. (Fig. 3.7)

### ACTIVATION STAGE :

C1 acts on C4 and C2 resulting in C42 complex (C3 convertase) and release of C2-kinin, a chemical mediator of inflammation. C42 (C3-convertase) activates C3 with release of C3a, anaphylotoxin, which releases histamine from mast cells and basophils. C3b attached to the cell surface, as in the case of microbes, helps in phagocytosis by macrophages and chemotaxis for neutrophils. It also releases platelet activating factor from platelets and helps inflammation while C3 inactivator regulates the release of C3b. Another pathway of activation of complement occurs with C1, C4 and C2, and also without Fc fragment of antibody. This can be initiated by immunoglobulin (IgD, IgA or possibly IgE) and also by various polysaccharides including endotoxin, zymosan, and factor from cobra venom. Normally, zymosan reacts non-specifically with a protein called properidin (P) and a glycine rich glycoprotein called Factor B or C3 proactivator (C3PA) as well as C3 itself and the resulting complex inactivates C3. Inactivation of C3 is associated with production of C3a and C3b in the serum. Those substances in the presence of magnesium ion convert C3 proactivator to C3 activator, which splits C3 into large C3b and small C3a. The factor B then binds with C3b to form a complex C3b, B. This acted on by factor D produces the active convertase complex C3bB which catalyses the conversion of C3 to C3b by the feedback circuit. C3b inactivator cleaves the C3b into two fragments (3c and 3d).

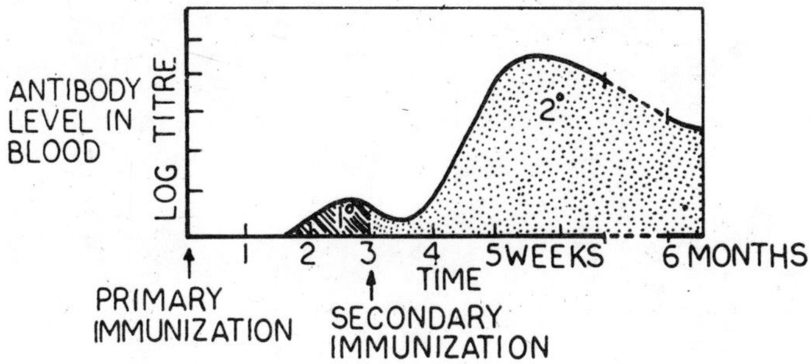


Fig.3.4 Antibody Level in Blood

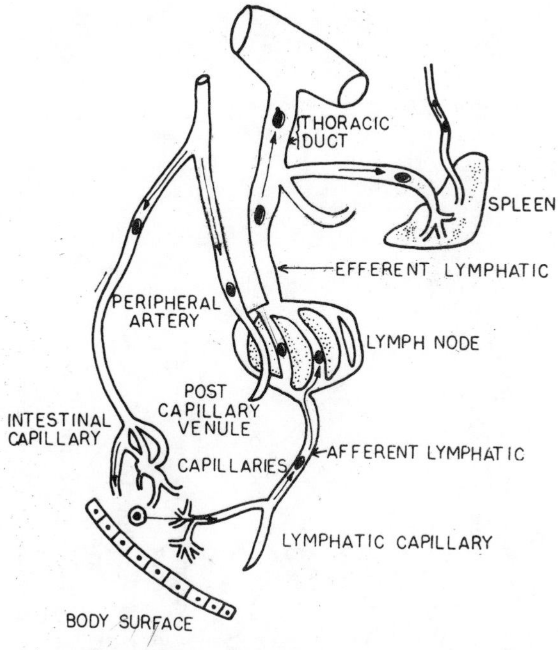


Fig. 3.5 Circulation of sensitised T-lymphocytes.

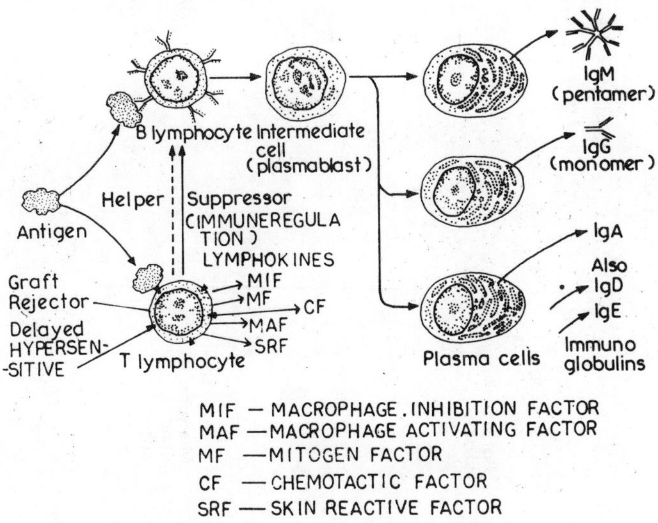


Fig.3.6 Showing Immune-regulatory Mechanism.

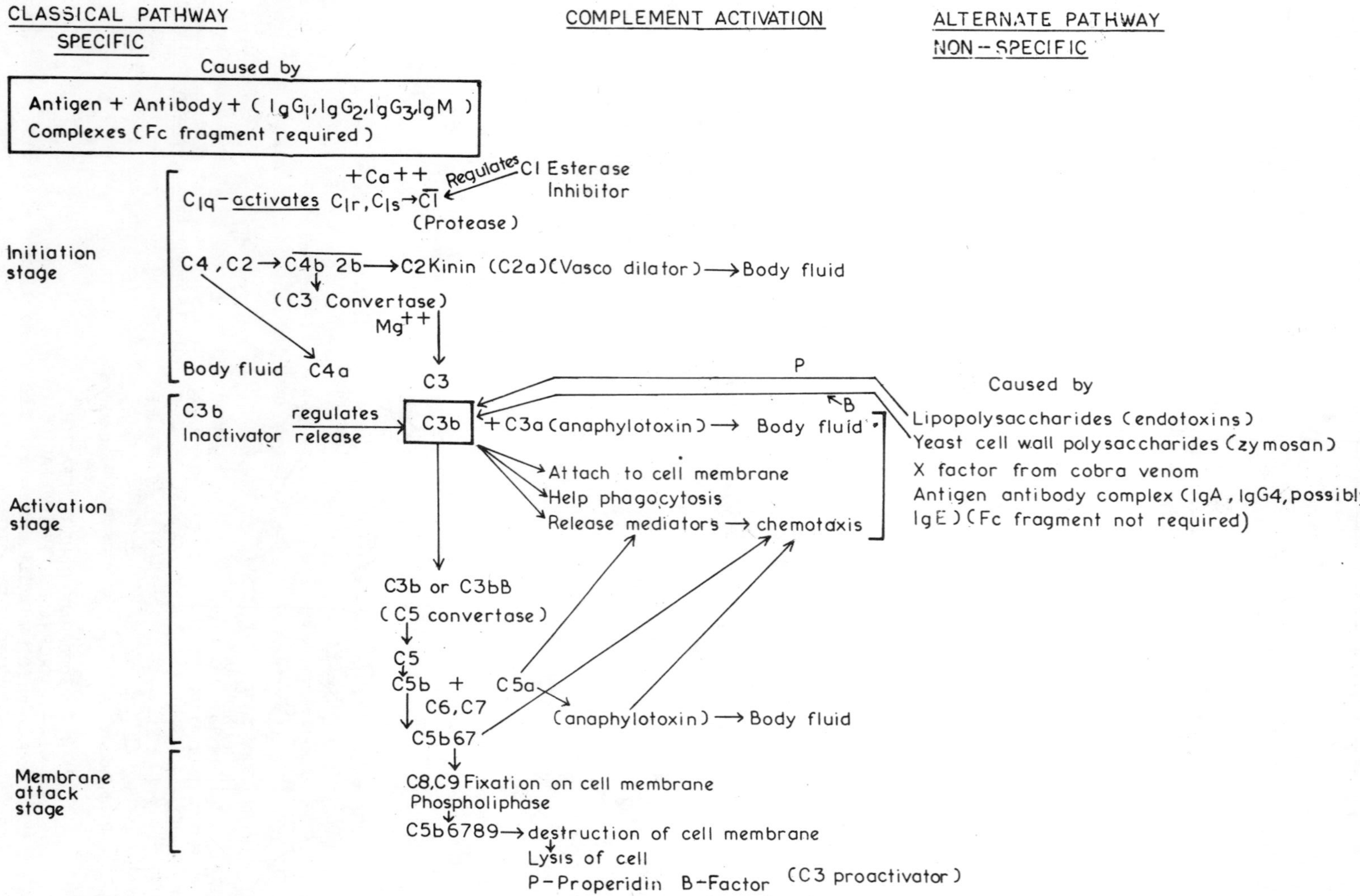


Fig.3.7 Activation of Complement Fragments : Stages of Classical pathway

MEMBRANE ATTACK STAGE:

Following fixation C3b in association with its activating enzyme C3 convertase forms another enzyme, C5 convertase. The latter acts on C5; a small subunit C5a, another anaphylotoxin, is split off. This is also a potent polymorphonuclear neutrophil chemotactic agent and is released into the body fluid. The larger C5b remains bound to C6 and C7 as the activating complex C5b67. This has the property of chemotaxis for neutrophils. Finally, there is fixation of C8 and C9 with liberation of phospholipase leading to damage to the cell wall and its lysis. This is the basis of red cell lysis in complement fixation test. Some thin walled pathogens, e.g., trypanosomes and malaria parasites are killed by complement. This is also observed with gram negative bacteria in association with lysozyme. Activation of complement system is controlled by the lability of the activated components, by esterase inhibitor and C3b inactivator. Functions of complement are (i) ability to kill various types of gram negative bacteria or virus after its interaction with antibody with their cell wall and making them susceptible to lysozymal action, (ii) helping destruction of tumour cells in the presence of antibody, (iii) chemotaxis for neutrophils at the site of antigen antibody interaction with the help of C567 complex, (iv) release of substance C3a or C5a known as anaphylotoxin, release of histamine and contraction of smooth muscle, (v) helping phagocytosis with the components of C1 and C3, (vi) formation of plasma kinin from C2 component and increase of permeability, (vii) action on platelets releasing platelet activating factor (PAF) and release of 5HT helping vascular changes and exudation in inflammation, and (viii) helping the destruction of cells by interaction with antigen-antibody complex on the surface membrane of the cell.

## THE CLONAL SELECTION THEORY (BURNET) :

The cells of antibody forming systems have arisen by random mutation resulting in the emergence of small number of cells or clones of differentiated cell, so as to be capable of producing one or very small number of specific antibodies. The antigen sensitive cells are lymphocytes. They have the ability to recognise and to respond to antigen through their surface receptors which are specific for the particular antigen. It is *via* its surface specific receptors that lymphocyte recognises the presence of antigen. Following such selection and combination the lymphocytes produce a clone of cells which share the same specificity and make up. Some differentiate into antibody-producing cells (B-cells) or into T-cell clones carrying out cell-mediated immunity. Some of the cells of the clone become 'memory' (T or B) cells and are capable of reacting with the same antigen on future occasions, i.e., during secondary response.

Under certain circumstances contact with antigen *via* specific receptors can lead to the death of lymphocytes rather than their proliferation. This happens when contact by such differentiated lymphocytes with self or foreign material occurs before the cells have attained maturity. This would lead to suppression rather than stimulation of antibody formation against the particular antigen. This is regarded as immunological tolerance. In the early stage of development of immune system in the embryo there is particular susceptibility to tolerance induction. It is probably then that lymphocytes act with self determinants and are eliminated.

Initial contact with self antigens leading to elimination of self reactive clones or 'forbidden clones' in thymus. This organ then acts as censor of the T-lymphocytes.

The unblocking of a cell inherently capable of producing antibody against self antigen would explain auto-antibody formation. Thus, autoimmune disease is a failure of destruction of self reacting population of antibody forming cells.

Table 3.2 is a summary of characteristics of macrophages, T-cells and B-cells.

TABLE-3.2

CHARACTERISTICS OF CELLS CONCERNED IN IMMUNE RESPONSE.

| MACROPHAGES | THYMUS DERIVED LYMPHOCYTES (T-cells) | LYMPHOCYTES FROM GUT ASSOCIATED LYMPHOID TISSUE (B-cells) |
|---|---|---|
| Phagocytosis and catabolism of excess antigen. Processing of the antigens in the follicles and medulla of lymph nodes correctly for T or B cells. Release soluble factors (lymphocyte activating factor, LAF) stimulating lymphocytes. Act as depot antigen. Phagocytosis of antigen-antibody complexes with the help of receptors for Fc component and for C3b. | Secrete soluble factors (lymphokines) to regulate the various activities of macrophages and facilitation of B-cells response to T-dependent antigen. As 'helper' cell assist B-cells in their proliferation and differentiation towards antibody formation through a soluble substance termed T-cell factor. As 'suppressor' cell exert a balancing inhibitory influence on immune response. Responsible for some forms of immunological tolerance. Long-lived, 5-10 years in man. Major contributor to immunological memory. Molecule from the HLA acts as surface receptor for T-cell. | Synthesis and production of Immunoglobulins. Binding of antigen through various Ig receptors on the surface. Carry receptors for Fc portion of IgG (Fc receptors) and for fixed complement (C3b receptor), thus regulating B-cell activity. Short-lived, mostly sessile in the lymphoid organs. Contributory to immunological memory of B-cells. Antibody receptors on B-cells are of one or two Ig classes—one of which is always IgM or other is IgD or IgA or IgG alone. |

## DEFECTS IN IMMUNOGLOBULIN SYNTHESIS :

### A. IMMUNOGLOBULIN DEFICIENCY :

Immunological deficiency could manifest as a disease from primary defect in the genesis of immunological competent cells from the bone marrow, thymus or gut-associated lymphoid tissue. Moreover, this deficiency could also be acquired in some other disease processes affecting normal functioning of some part of the lymphoid tissues.

In 1953 Bruton first discovered a case of hypogamma-globulinaemia in a boy of 8 years. At the age of 4 years he developed septic arthritis, and, subsequently, a series of bacterial infection. Low gamma globulin was revealed by serum electrophoresis. This boy failed to elicit immune response to triple or double antigens. This brought into prominence the primary immune deficiency. Specific immune deficiency may be due to effect in the stem cell, precursor T or B cells, defect in thymus or gut associated lymphoid tissues

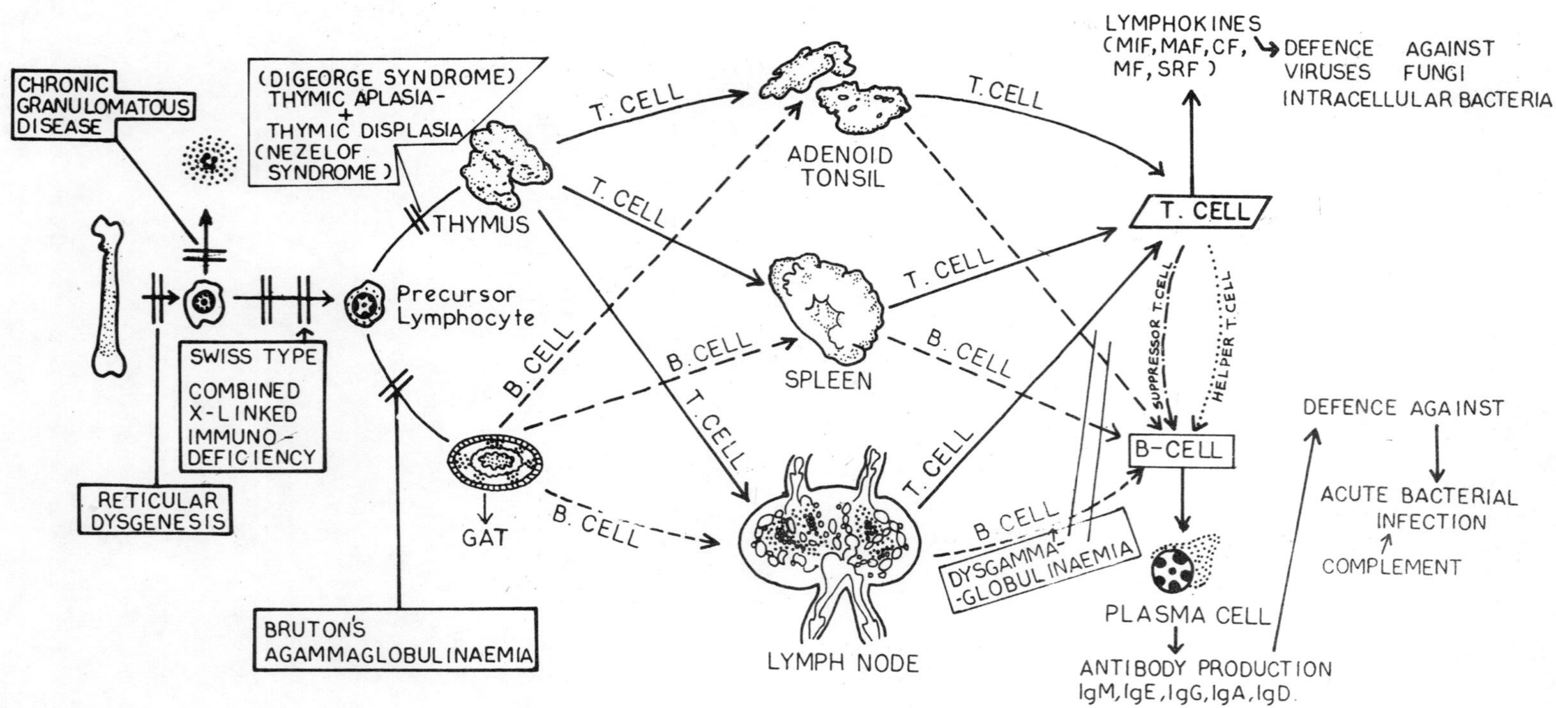


GAT — GUT ASSOCIATED LYMPHOID TISSUE
T-CELL–THYMUS DEPENDENT LYMPHOCYTE
B-CELL– GUT ASSOCIATED LYMPHOCYTE
MIF — MIGRATION INHIBITION FACTOR (MACROPHAGE)
MAF—MACROPHAGE ACTIVATING FACTOR
MF —MITOGENIC FACTOR
SRF — SKIN REACTIVE FACTOR

Fig.3.8 Defects in Immunoglobulin Synthesis

(Fig. 3.8). Stem cell immune deficiency may or may not be associated with generalised hypoplasia of the bone marrow. These could be genetically inherited and may be sex linked or autosomal recessive character. Pure B cell deficiency is frequently inherited and sex linked. Pure immunoglobulin deficiency may affect all the immunoglobulins or IgG and IgA with an increase of IgM or IgA alone. Pure T-cell deficiency may be associated with some defect in humoral antibody production through the defect in helper T-cell. This defect is due to lack of development of 3rd and 4th branchial arches in the embryonic life and is associated with the absence of parathyroid gland and resultant hypocalcaemia. This may also occur as a familial isolated developmental defect. Diseases due to primary immuno-deficiency, their pathogenesis, clinical and pathological features, and treatment are given in Table 3.3. Table 3.4 indicates the line of investigations in suspected cases of immuno-deficiency. Secondary immunological deficiency can occur in a large number of diseases affecting the lymphoid tissue or due to excessive loss of protein through kidney or intestine. These are given in Table 3.5.

**B. RAISED IMMUNOGLOBULINS :**

*Multiple myeloma* is a malignant proliferation of a specific group or clone of plasma cells invading the bone marrow and eroding it. Such a clone will produce a particular type of immunoglobulin whether IgG or more rarely IgA, IgD or even IgE. This raised monoclonal immunoglobulin produced by the clone of malignant plasma cell will have single electrophoretic mobility and appears as a compact band (M-type protein). This is also known as myeloma protein. Hence, clinical conditions showing such a single 'M' band protein in serum electrophoresis are called monoclonal gammopathy. This is, however, generally associated with decrease synthesis of normal immunoglobulin.

In multiple myeloma such monoclonal rise is typical of IgG, IgA or IgD or IgE while in Waldenström's macroglobulinaemia the monoclonal gammopathy is of IgM immunoglobulin.

In addition to homogenous myeloma protein in the serum, another characteristic protein appears in urine. This is known as Bence-Jones protein. These proteins are light chains of myeloma protein which pass out from the circulation into urine before the whole immunoglobulin molecule could be synthesised. Presence of M-type of protein in electrophoresis could also be present in cases with disseminated cancers or as mainfestation of cold agglutinins. Moreover, presence of 'M' type of protein is not always indicative of multiple myeloma but should be correlated with other clinical and radiological observations. These are i) presence of symptoms related to 'M'-type of protein, ii) presence of enlargement of lymph nodes, spleen or liver, iii) presence of radiological disease in flat bones, iv) presence of myeloma cells and plasma cells in marrow smear. On the other hand, absence of any change in clinical, radiological features and normal marrow smear for three years of follow-up, indicate that this particular case is not a multiple myeloma even in the presence of 'M' band protein.

*Heavy chain disease* is a variant of malignant lymphoma where there is overproduction of heavy chain of IgG. These are secreted unconjugated into circulation and also in urine. There is a large amount of an abnormal protein both in serum and in urine. In this disease, bone marrow shows typical plasma cells and an aggregate of reticulum cells. In the skin atypical granuloma consisting of reticulum cells surrounded by lymphocytes and plasma cells is formed but these patients are unable to produce immunoglobulins normally, and, therefore, liable to suffer from repeated bacterial infection.

## TABLE-3.3

## PRIMARY SPECIFIC IMMUNE DEFICIENCY DISEASES.

| TYPE | PATHOGENESIS | PATHOLOGICAL CHANGES. | CLINICAL FEATURES. | TREATMENT |
|---|---|---|---|---|
| COMBINED IMMUNO-DEFICIENCY SYNDROMES.<br>a) Swiss type. | Bone marrow defect of blast cells. | Absence of all immunoglobulin in sera. Total lymphocyte count less than 500/cmm. Thymus is small and consists of stromal cells and epithelial cells, absence of Hassal's corpuscles. Almost complete absence of follicular tissue in lymph nodes and Peyer's patches, and also plasma cells. Lack of adenosine diaminase in 25% cases. | Autosomal recessive. Both sexes involved. Fatal within 2 years. Tests for CMI negative. They usually suffer from bacterial, fungal and viral infection. Die from progressive vaccinia when vaccinated. | Bone marrow graft. |
| b) X-linked. | Same | Same | Same. Only in boys | |
| DEFECT IN CELL-MEDIATED IMMUNITY ONLY.<br>a) Di Georges' syndrome. | Complete lack of T-cells.<br>Thymic Aplasia (Due to defect in development in embryonal 3rd and 4th branchial arch). | Normal immunoglobulin level. Isoagglutinins present. Cell-mediated responses lacking. Hypocalcaemia (due to lack of parathyroid).<br>Lymphopenia (marked).<br>Depletion of cells in the thymic zone of lymph nodes but plasma cells present.<br>Thymus small and without Hassal's corpuscles. | Children can be stimulated by polio virus but cannot reject homograft. Although develop humoral antibodies, they are unable to cope with viral, fungal and bacterial infection. | Fetal thymic graft. |

| | | | | |
|---|---|---|---|---|
| b) X-linked. | Same | Same | Same. Only in boys | |
| b) Neselof syndrome. | Thymic dysplasia. | Parathyroid normal. No hypocalcaemia. Thymus small without Hassal's corpuscles. Immunoglobulins present. Peyer's patches and germinal centre of lymph nodes absent. Tonsils minute but plasma cells present in them. | Autosomal recessive. Other pattern same. | |
| ANTIBODY DEFICIENCY SYNDROME<br>a) Congenital X-linked hypogamma globulinaemia (Bruton). | Complete lack of B-cells. | Very low immunoglobulins-IgG less than 1mg/ml (normal 10mg/ml). IgA + IgM present 1% of normal value. Isoagglutinins lacking. Lymph nodes-absence of germinal centre in the cortex with no plasma cells. Normal proliferation of lymphoid tissue in the thymus dependent area.<br>Peyer's patches and appendix-relatively depleted of lymphoid tissue.<br>Thymus absolutely normal histologically. Circulating lymphocytes normal. | Only male children affected. Symptoms start between 4 and 12 months of life. Unable to develop antibodies against conventional antigens.<br>Children subjected to repeated bacterial infection like pneumococci, staphylococci and Haemophilus influenzæ. | Passive immunoglobulins. |
| b) Ataxia telangiectasia. | | Usually low or absence of IgA with low or absence of IgG. Thymus small with absence of Hassal's corpuscles.<br>Lymph nodes scanty, lack of follicles with lymphocyte depletion. Marked depletion of IgA producing plasma cells in the intestinal mucous membrane. | Autosomal. Manifestation usually by 2 years. Oculocutaneous lesions. Cerebellar ataxia. Recurrent severe infections particularly of respiratory tract. | |

| TYPES | PATHOGENESIS | PATHOLOGICAL CHANGES | CLINICAL FEATURES | TREATMENT |
|---|---|---|---|---|
| c) Wiskott-Aldrich syndrome | Defect in recognition or processing of antigens. | High IgA + IgE with normal IgG. Isoagglutinins absent. Diminished response to diphtheria and virus antigens. Thymus normal in structure but smaller in size. Lymph nodes-depletion of lymphocytes in thymic area with normal germinal centre and plasma cells. | Only male children. Eczema, recurrent infection, multiple skin sensitivities and a high frequency of precipitating antibodies in serum against milk. | |
| COMPLEMENT DEFICIENCY a) Hereditary angioneurotic oedema. | Lack of alpha—2 globulin which acts as an inhibitor (esterase) to C1. | Lack of alpha-2 globulins. During attack-low level of C2 because this being the natural substrate of esterase. After the attack C2 returns to normal. Intradermal injection of C1 precipitates severe attack of angioneurotic oedema. | Autosomal dominant. Oedematous swelling of the skin without itch. Nausea, vomiting, G. I. haemorrhage, asphyxia, laryngeal oedema. Duration of attack—48-72 hours. | Transfer Factor or Drug-Levamisole or Periodic transfusion with whole plasma—15/ml/kg body. |
| b) Deficiency of C2 of complement. | Inadequate clearing of Immune complexes. | Sera of the patient show defect some bactricidal property. | Autosomal recessive. Associated with other diseases, like SLE, glomerulonephritis, Henoch—Schonlein purpura. | |

TABLE-3.4

INVESTIGATION OF IMMUNE DEFICIENT DISEASE:

1. Clinical history and examination.
2. General clinicopathological and biochemical tests.
3. Sweat electrolytes.
4. Electrophoresis of serum proteins.
5. Quantitation of immunoglobulins.
6. Assay of complement.
7. Assay of phagocytosis.
8. Study of cell-mediated immunity response to P.P.D., candidal extracts, mumps skin test and DNCB test.

TABLE-3.5

SECONDARY IMMUNE DEFICIENCY SYNDROMES:

1. Immunoglobulin synthesis.
   a) Primary hypogammaglobulinaemia—lymph nodes show absence of plasma cells.
   b) Secondary— i) Nephrotic syndrome.
   ii) Protein-losing enteropathy. Affect IgG, not IgA or IgM.
   iii) Malnutrition.
2. Cell-mediated Immunity—Malnutrition including Kwashiorkor.
   Hodgkin's disease.
   Sarcoidosis.
   Crohn's disease.
   Rheumatoid arthritis.
   Primary biliary cirrhosis.
   Acute and chronic viral infection, e.g., Rubella.
   Measles.
   Chronic bacterial infection, e.g., lepromatous leprosy.
   Various malignant disorders.
   Primary endocrine deficiency, e.g., hypoadrenalism, hypoparathyroidism, hypothyroidism, diabetes mellitus.

## IMMUNOLOGICAL MECHANISM IN INFECTIOUS DISEASES:

Immunity against parasitic organisms and their metabolic products follows after actual contact with the above antigens. In this connection macrophages play an important part in protection against invading micro-organisms. Macrophages possess Fc and C1 receptors on the cell surface. These help phagocytosis of microbes coated with antibody. After phagocytosis of these microbes or their products they are processed by lysosome, which are the site of synthesis of a wide range of hydrolytic enzymes, capable of digesting proteins and other macromolecules. Immunogenic substances are directly delivered to the lymphoid cells in the neighbourhood. Macrophages thus control the rate of and the type of antigen delivered, and, therefore, have a monitoring influence on induction of immunity. In the later stage of infection the macrophages operate in close association with humoral and cell-mediated immunity. Neutrophils also play some part in association with antibody and complement.

Micro-organisms can evade the innate immune mechanism of the host in various ways; thus, the distinction between pathogenic and non-pathogenic organisms breaks down. This can occur under different circumstances, e.g., congenital or acquired defects in humoral or cell-mediated immunity, depressed number of functioning macrophages and neutrophils, after immunosuppressive drugs, after deep ray, after extensive burns and after splenectomy. The various immune mechanisms involved in different types of bacterial, viral, fungal and helminthic infection are given below:

A. **Bacterial Infections—**

a) **Humoral Immune Mechanism.**

i) Neutralisation of toxins by antitoxins—This is seen in infection by exotoxin producing bacteira, e.g., Coryn. diphtheriae, Vibrio cholerae, Clostridium tetani, Cl. welchii and Cl. botulinum. In these cases immunity is acquired by immunisation or by previous infection. In their absence this can be produced passively by antisera which has the ability to neutralise the toxins and tide over the first stage of infection.

ii) In cases of micro-organisms which do not secrete exotoxins, antibody and complement help in phagocytosis. It has been pointed out earlier that macrophages and neutrophils have receptors for Fc fragment of IgG and also for C3b of complement. These make the bacteria susceptible to phagocytosis. Other effects of antibody reacting with the surface of microbes cause cell lysis by activation of complement system and help agglutination or clumping. Clumped bacteria have limited metabolic activity from lack of sufficient nutrient material, e.g., lack of iron in some bacteria. Role of IgA or IgE prevents the adherence of microbes to the gut wall. Some organisms, such as streptococci, carry a substance known as M-protein, mucopeptide polysaccharide complex. The latter resists digestion by the hydrolytic enzyme. Other bacteria resist killing by macrophages. They are the important sites of bacterial growth of Myco. tuberculosis, Myco. leprae, brucella and listeria.

IgA immunoglobulin is selectively produced by the mucous membrane of the intestine, the respiratory tract and the urogenital tract where the IgA producing plasma cells are frequently found in the lamina propria. It acts as anti-toxin together with IgG. Infection of mucosal surfaces by bacteria or viruses is caused by adhesion of these micro-organisms to the epithelial surface. IgA antibody (as dimer) prevents their adhesion to the mucous membrane. This may also bring cell lysis by activation of complement system. In the submucous tissue, where this antibody as a monomer lacks secretory piece, and by agglutination helps localisation of bacteria.

b) **Cell-mediated Immune Response.**

In certain bacterial infection like mycobacteria, brucella and listeria in addition to humoral immunity, non-specific cellular reactions involving macrophages and polymorphonuclear neutrophils are observed during re-infection by their increased resistance. This could be enhanced by the liberation of some

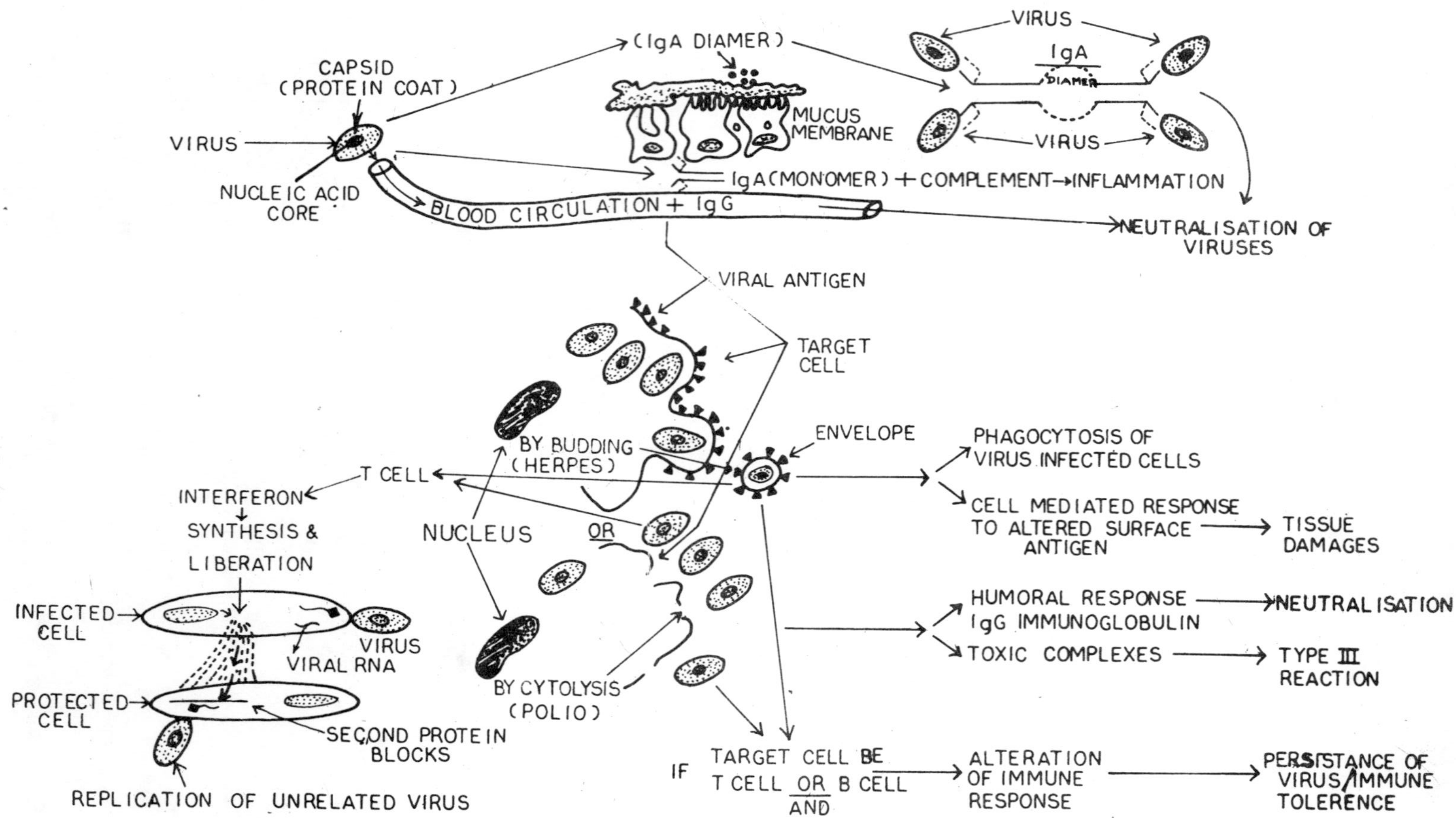


Fig.3.9 Cell-mediated Immune Response

of the lymphokines directed to the macrophages by the T-cells. This has been proved experimentally by transfer of lymphoid cells from the stimulated recipient to the unstimulated one. The macrophages of the recipients then acquire enhanced bactericidal action. Thus, cellular immunity through T-cells exerts its influence on the recipient on its macrophages in a non-specific manner by increasing their resistance.

**B. Viral Infections—**

a) **Humoral Immune Response.**

Humoral antibody (IgG) plays only a minor role to prevent viral infection since it can only neutralise the viruses from their entry into host cells like poliomyelitis and influenza. Most of the viruses during primary infection are absorbed on the cell surface, the viruses envelop, then fuse with the plasma membrane so that viral contents are set free in the cytoplasm. Some viruses (herpes, measles, vaccinia) spread from one cell to the adjacent one without being extracellular. Secretory IgA (dimer) antibodies could react with viral antigens on the cell surface, but complement system cannot be activated because of the presence of secretory piece and hence cytolysis could not occur there. IgA (as monomer) in the tissue can react with complement and in contact with virus can produce inflammation. When the virus gets into the circulation IgG antibody neutralises the viruses to some extent before they reach the target cells. Antiviral humoral immunity is usually of long duration and in some cases life-long, perhaps, due to persistence of a small amount of virus in the body. Mutation of viral body in repeated epidemics renders the immunity developed by earlier epidemic ineffective due to antigenic variant. This is commonly seen in influenza epidemic. The emergence of this antigenic variant is probably due to suppressive effect of selective antibody and emergence of mutant.

b) **Cell-mediated Immune Response.**

Importance of cell-mediated immune response came from the observations that children with primary immune T-cell deficiency states are susceptible to viral infection. Since viruses multiply intracellularly, the recovery from these virus infections, like herpes, pox and measles viruses, requires destruction of cells. This may be brought about in various ways depending on the maturation of virus in the cell. Many viruses, e.g., polio or papilloma virus, replicate and produce fully infecting intracytoplasmic particles. These are nucleocapsids consisting of basic nucleic acid covered with its protein coat (capsid). These are liberated from the cell by cytolysis, come in contact with specific antibody and are neutralised or disintegrated. In cases of other viruses, like influenza, herpes, nucleo-capsids are liberated by budding through altered cell membrane incorporated with viral antigen on it as an envelope (Fig.3.9) leaving the cell alive and intact. In addition, the foreign viral antigen appears on the surface of the infected cell. These generate in host cell-mediated immune response. Sensitized T-cells make intimate contact on the virus infected cells with antigen on the cell surface. The target cell membrane is damaged when the T-cell moves away leading to a leakage of cell component with an influx of water. The target cell swells up and dies. Moreover, activation of macrophages and their accumulation at the site of infection are mediated by release of lymphokines. There they either phagocytose or kill virus-infected cells. In whatever way the cell destruction is brought about, virus material and cell debris are phagocytosed and disposed of by the activated macrophages. These events also occur in lymph nodes to which virus or viral antigens were brought in by the lymphatics. Another type of mononuclear cells (M-cell) which are not macrophages or T-lymphocytes, have the ability to destroy the target cells with the assistance of specific antibody. They recognize antibody coated cells *via* Fc receptor.

*Interferon*— Viruses are classical interferon producer. Interferon has been found to be produced by T lymphocytes as a result of viral antigenic stimulation *in vitro*. The infected cells liberate interferon for a few hours, even for a day. Interferon acts on uninfected cells, causing them to synthesise a second protein that remains within the cell, but protects it against all viruses. Interferon has no direct action on the virus itself and does not interfere with viral entry into the susceptible cells. Interferon is non-virus in effect, but species-specific. Interferon liberated by the infected cells can reach other neighbouring cells by diffusion and protects them from virus infection, whether on epithelial surface or in solid tissue.

C. Protozoal Infections—

*Malaria*—During exoerythrocytic stage of malarial infection in the liver initiated by sporozoites, i.e., during the latent period, the parasite avoids stimulating antibody response. This is also true for trophozoites growing inside the red blood cells and causing the disease. Their sojourn in the red blood cells gives them protection against circulating antibodies and sensitised lymphocytes. The merozoites liberated from infected cells are only exposed briefly to the circulating antibodies before entering the fresh red blood cells. Immunity is incomplete, and, as a result, the host fails to eradicate the parasite completely. The major antibody class involved in the acquired resistance to malaria is IgG. In people living in endemic areas this immunoglobulin shows high levels and rapid increase in synthesis on stimulation. Acquired immunity of this type is effective only against parasites at the stage when it is within the red blood cells and only in later stage of this life cycle of the parasite when the red cell membrane becomes more permeable to immunoglobulin. Only 5% of IgG, however, is found to react with malarial antigens because the major part of IgG constitutes the antibody of soluble malarial antigens but plays no role against toxic malarial products.

During recovery the antibodies are directed against the relevant stage of parasite, particularly, the merozoites and also against relevant antigen on it. Protective antibodies, therefore, coat the merozoites and prevent their absorption into red blood cells and help phagocytosis by the macrophage. The latter is due to binding of IgG to Fc receptor on the macrophage. This form of phagocytosis could be an important mechanism in acquired immunity in malaria.

Malarial infection is associated with depressed T-lymphocyte response to blastoid transformation and also B-lymphocyte response to certain bacterial antigen. Malarial parasite can change their character and evade the host-immune response developed earlier.

**D. Helminthic Infections—**

Protective immune mechanism can act only in the early part of the helminthic life cycle. The main immunological stimulus is derived from the antigen derived from the adult worm and the continuous presence of adult worm is essential for the immune state of the host. This immune state prevents infection from parasite entering the body through the skin and their subsequent dissemination through the blood stream. This is true for filarial infection where microfilaria are poorly antigenic. Children infested with Ascaris lumbricoides are associated with urticarial rashes, asthma and high level of IgE antibody in their blood. Tropical eosinophilia is referred to be associated with larva migrans of particular helminth. In this there is an increased IgE with pulmonary eosinophilia and peripheral eosinophilia. This could be due to immediate type of hypersensitivity type 1 *(vide infra)* in the pathogenesis.

## HYPERSENSITIVITY REACTION :

Immune reactions indicate a means of protection against infection due to development of specific resistance. Certain immunological reactions produce tissue damage during antigen and antibody reaction, instead of protection, by direct action or due to release of pharmacologically active substances. These are known as hypersensitivity reactions.

Broadly, there are two forms of hypersensitivity reactions—

A) Reactions mediated by humoral antibodies (immediate type)

1. Type I Reaction   2. Type II Reaction
3. Type III Reaction.

B) Reaction mediated by cell-mediated immune response: Type IV Reaction (Delayed type of hypersensitivity).

## A) REACTIONS MEDIATED BY HUMORAL ANTIBODIES :

### 1. TYPE I REACTION : ANAPHYLACTIC REACTION.

In man there are two types of anaphylactic reactions. These depend upon the portal of entry of the antigen. (a) The *systemic reactions* occur when the antigen is infected parenterally as in the case of foreign sera, drugs—like penicillin or even bites of insects or during desensitisation with pollen extracts. This is manifested by bronchospasm, laryngeal oedema, dyspnoea, cyanosis and fall of blood pressure. Cutaneous wheal or urticaria occurs during absorption through intestinal mucosa. There may be diarrhoea and nausea. (b) The *local reactions* are due to pollen, dander, house dust, animal food, etc. These act on the respiratory mucosa causing asthma or hay fever, on the conjunctiva causing conjunctivitis, and on the nasal mucosa causing rhinorrhoea.

The IgE class antibody involved in this reaction has strong affinity for tissue of the same species (homocytotrophic). After sensitisation when an individual again comes into contact with antigen, anaphylactic reaction sets off. In this reaction there is not sufficient IgE antibody in circulation to mop up the antigen. Initial binding of IgE to the Fc fragment of mast cell and its subsequent interaction with antigen on the cell membrane of the mast cell with entry of calcium releases pharmacological mediators, e.g., histamine, slow reacting substance of anaphylaxis (SRS-A), serotonin, plasma kinin, prostaglandins and eosinophil chemotactic factor of anaphylaxis (ECF-A) and platelet activating factor (PAF). Recent works indicate that two adjacent IgE molecules must be bridged by an antigen before degranulation of mast cell can occur. Monovalent antigen will only block the antibody IgE and will not set off the reaction.

Histamine from its precursor histidine in the granules of mast cells causes vasodilation. It also liberates 5-HT or serotonin which causes contraction of smooth muscles and increases capillary permeability. SRS-A has contracting effect on smooth muscles of blood vessels. Plasma kinin liberates bradykinin, acts like histamine and also like an enzyme aryl sulphatase, which inactivates SRS-A. ECF-A is related to repair of tissue damage in this reaction.

### 2. TYPE II REACTION : CYTOTOXIC FOR CYTOLYTIC REACTION :

This is initiated by an antigenic component which is a part of or a small molecule attached to the cell surface. The antibodies either IgG or IgM class are directed against their antigens bringing about cytotoxic or cytolytic effect involving complement. These are observed in haemolytic disease of the new-born, sedormid purpura and certain bacterial infections.

Haemolytic disease of the new-born is caused by Rhesus incompatibility between mother and foetus, when a Rh (-ve) mother carries Rh (+ve) foetus in the first pregnancy, the latter having inherited Rh antigen from its Rh (+ve) father. If the foetal red cells enter maternal circulation in sufficient quantity at the time of delivery, anti-Rh (+ve) (IgM and IgG) antibodies are found 6-8 weeks after delivery, but not during the course of the first pregnancy although the foetal red cells are introduced into the mother's circulation throughout pregnancy but not in sufficient amount to elicit immunological response.

In the subsequent pregnancy the only circulating anti-Rh IgG antibodies from the maternal circulation pass across the placental circulation and react with Rh antigen of foetal red cells. These antibody coated cells are then phagocytosed and destroyed by the macrophages in the foetal liver and spleen. This results in haemolytic anaemia. In such cases if there be ABO incompatibility between the mother and foetus along with Rh incompatibility, the small number of foetal cells that cross the placenta are rapidly haemolysed by maternal antibodies against the foetal red cells. So Rh sensitisation will not occur. Thus, ABO incompatibility in the first and subsequent pregnancies will protect mother from Rh immunisation until she carries ABO compatible foetus.

### 3. TYPE III REACTION : TISSUE DAMAGE BY IMMUNE COMPLEXES :

This reaction falls into two categories—1) Local reaction—Arthus phenomenon. 2)Systemic reaction—Serum sickness.

1. LOCAL REACTION—*Arthus phenomenon* is a local reaction at the site of entry of antigen. This occurs in the wall of small blood vessels in the presence of large amount of IgG antibody forming microprecipitate both intravascular and extravascular tissue with activation of complement. This results in inflammation with liberation of vaso-active amines causing vasodilatation and chemotaxis for neutrophils. This is seen at the site of injection of insulin in diabetes or in asthmatic reaction in allergic alveolitis following inhalation of mouldy hay, after frequent immunisation with toxoids and following intradermal injection of fungal antigen in cases of Farmer's lungs.

2. SYSTEMIC REACTION—*Serum sickness* was initially described in individuals treated with anti-diphtheritic horse serum foreign to the host. The individual may develop anaphylactoid reaction within a few minutes, if there be previous contact with antigen and residual antibody be present in circulation. The anaphylactoid reactions are due to IgE antibodies attached to the mast cells and subsequent setting off a chain of events, but the tissue damage is caused by combination of excess of antibody with soluble antigen forming complexes deposited on the blood vessels, where they activate the complement leading to inflammation and chemotaxis or neutrophils. The intensity of reaction depends upon the concentration of complexes and on the type of the antibody on activating the complement since IgM, IgG, IgG2 and IgG3 can activate complement but not other antibodies (IgG4 and IgA dimer). Apart from typical serum sickness, in a number of infectious diseases the development of tissue damage occurs in this mechanism and could be featured as a failure in cell-mediated immunity, but not in humoral immunity. Certain organisms like mycobacteria or viruses need cell-mediated immunity for their eradication. The infecting organism proliferates as a result of specific failure of T-cell function and soluble bacterial or viral antigen is released into the circulation. The latter will stimulate B-cell to produce large amount of humoral antibodies because of lack of 'suppressor' to T-cell. The latter will react with antigen and form immune-complexes in the wall of blood vessels.

Antigens derived from infective micro-organism have been demonstrated in the immune-complexes in the glomeruli in malarial infection in children, in the skin as cutaneous vasculitis in lepromatous leprosy (erythema nodosum leprosum), in kidney deposits of certain surface antigen of hepatitis B virus. Immune-complex glomerulonephritis occurs as a part of infection by virus, bacteria and parasite, autoimmune disorder and immune-reaction to drugs like penicillin, streptomycin and sulphonamide. Arthritis as manifestation of an immune-complex disease is associated with drug for hypertension, SLE, following recovery from meningococcal infection and viral disease such as rubella.

B) TYPE IV REACTION. REACTION CAUSED BY CELL-MEDIATED IMMUNE RESPONSES :

Initial antigenic stimulus produces virgin T-cells to sensitised T-lymphocytes. These cells are always passing through the tissue since 70%-80% of circulating lymphocytes are T-cells. These sensitised T-cells may have some receptor-like from their cell wall or may be a substance secreted by the cell on its surface in a soluble form. On subsequent challenge a single sensitised lymphocyte at the site of antigen deposition sets up reactions bringing in a small number of sensitized lymphocytes which also act with antigen. They release pharmacologically soluble mediator, lymphokines. The latter first act directly as being chemotactic for macrophages and then act directly by causing a decreased electrostatic charge on the surface of these cells as a result of which they tend to aggregate in the lesion. The non-sensitized lymphoid cells from the bone marrow are also drawn into the site of reaction directly. These cells are related enzymatically to the macrophages. The latter activate complement through their Fc receptor and receptor for C1, and initiate inflammation. This is the mechanism of delayed hypersensitivity in man. This can be demonstrated against bacteria, e.g., myco.tuberculosis, myco.leprae, brucella; viruses, e.g., vaccinia, paramyxovirus, herpes; fungi, e.g., candidiasis, histoplasmosis, coccidiomycosis; and protozoa, e.g., leishmania. Similar phenomenon is also observed in allograft (homograft) reaction. This reaction is also observed with chemicals, like dinitrochlorobenzene, picryl chloride, and phenylhydrazine, following contact with skin and following contact of metals, e.g., mercury, nickel, chromium with skin.

Certain insect bites like mosquitoes produce red induration which is due to delayed hypersensitivity and is directed to an antigen present in the saliva of mosquitoes. Reactions to stings from bees, wasps and hornets are usually anaphylactic.

Table (3.6) is a summary of the mechanism of pathogenesis of the diseases caused by hypersensitivity reactions.

## IMMUNOLOGICAL UNRESPONSIVENESS OR TOLERANCE :

In every immune response the resultant expression of immunological phenomenon depends on the balance between the conventional reactive immunocytes or 'effector' cells and the 'suppressor' cells which specifically block the immune response. These cells would appear to act either by direct competition for antigen or by producing a soluble mediator that can inhibit other immunological mechanisms. Therefore, elimination of active clones of "effector' cells or increase in activity of those 'suppressor' cells leads to immunological tolerance. This is specific for the inducing antigen.

It was observed by Medwar and his group that tolerance can readily be induced to a large variety of antigens when the latter are injected neonatally in very small amount. In the adult large amount of antigen is required to paralyse the large quantity of mature lymphoid tissues of the body. In cases of soluble protein, another form of tolerance known as 'low zone' tolerance can be produced. In 'low zone' tolerance unresponsiveness involves T-cell only while in 'high zone' tolerance, unresponsiveness of both T-cell and B-cell can be produced. Immunogenic dose is, however, in between these two doses.

This would only indicate in that 'low zone' tolerance there is still present reactive B-cell in the host. The stimulation to the B-cell by some self antigen will induce antibody formation to the self antigen, hence, produces autoimmunity. This 'low zone' tolerance can be broken by introducing a few determinants to the tolerated antigen.

Clonal selection theory envisages that the clonal elimination of the 'effector' cells is the cause of tolerance. Self-tolerance is thus the result from elimination of all self-reactive lymphocytes of the system at an early stage by contact with self-molecule.

## TABLE-3.6
## HYPERSENSITIVITY REACTIONS

| | ANTIGEN (Ag) | ANTIBODY (Ab) | MECHANISM | EFFECT ON TISSUES. | DISEASES. |
|---|---|---|---|---|---|
| Type I. ANAPHYLATIC PHENOMENON. | A) *Local*—pollen, house dust, animal dander, insect bites.<br>B) *Systemic*—serum protein, drugs, e.g., penicillin. | IgE Reagenic antibody. | Complement required at the initial stage. Ag + Ab attached to membrane of mast cells (basophils).Release—<br>Bradykinin<br>Histamine<br>SRS-A<br>Enzyme<br>Plasmaglobulin (Kinin)<br>ECFA<br>PAF | 1. Capillary permeability.<br>2. Vasoconstriction and vasodilatation.<br>3. Contraction of plain muscles.<br>4. Accumulation of eosinophils. | Asthma, hay fever, conjunctivitis, rhinitis, diarrhoea, oedema, urticaria, (helminthic infection) P.K. reaction. |
| Type II. CYTOTOXIC OR CYTOLYTIC REACTION. | Drug or substances derived from viruses attached to cell surface. | IgG<br>IgM | Ab + Ag fixed on cell surface, activation of complement acting directly or through 'killer'cell (K-cell). | Cytolysis or phagocytosis (red cells, platelets). | Haemolytic disease of new-born. Autoimmune or drug induced haemolytic anaemia. Hashimoto's thyroiditis, thyrotoxicosis. Myasthenia gravis. Transfusion reaction. Liver necrosis in serum hepatitis (?). |

| | ANTIGEN (Ag) | ANTIBODY (Ab) | MECHANISM | EFFECT ON TISSUES. | DISEASES. |
|---|---|---|---|---|---|
| Type III. IMMUNE COMPLEX REACTION. | A) *Systemic* : serum virus, bactrin parasites, drugs.<br>B) *Local* : fungus insulin. | IgM<br>IgG1<br>IgG2<br>IgG3 | 1. *Intravascular Phase.* Soluble complexes (excess of Ab, soluble Ag) activating circulating complement.<br>2. *Extravascular Phase.* Soluble Ag activating *fixed* complement. | A) Systemic diseases—inflammation of vessels of the tissue involved.<br>B) Local inflammation of vessels. | Glomerulonephritis (malaria, LCM, treponema), arthritis, vasculitis.<br>Erythema Nodosum Leprosum, SLE, Inject. of antibacterial and antitoxic serum.<br>Pulmonary aspergillosis. Farmer's lung. |
| Type IV. CELL MEDIATED (DELAYED HYPERSENSITIVITY TYPE) REACTION. | *Bacteria* (M. tuberculosis M. leprae, *viruses:* smallpox, chicken pox, herpes simplex, yellow fever, measles).<br>*Fungi:* Aspergillus, Candida, mucor. | *No Ab* but sensitised T-cell. | Second contact with sensitised T-cell Lymphokines (MIF, MF, MAF, CF, SRF).<br>Accumulation and activation of macrophages.<br>Increase in lysosomal enzyme activity.<br>Enhanced antimicrobial activity. In case of virus infection—killing virus infected cells by direct contact or by production of *Interferon.* | Granuloma formation. | Bacterial (Tuberculin or Fungal skin test).<br>Rejection of allografts or xenografts.<br>Resistance to viral infection. |

In some cases, tolerance is caused by an active suppression of the immune response by suppressor T-cells, rather than by elimination of specific antigen sensitive clones. This may explain the increase in autoantibody in man which occurs with age. This is attributed to the gradual lack of regulation of antibody response by T-cells.

Self antigens, which are inaccessible to either reactive or suppressor lymphocytes due to certain anatomical situation, can also behave immunogenically. Such a situation exists because of tissue/blood barrier in the nervous system, or of lack of vascularisation in case of cornea and lens of the eyes, or of intracellular localisation as in the case of thyroid colloid, islet cell cytoplasm, adrenal cytoplasm, biliary tract, smooth muscles, and skeletal muscles. Tissue damage by external agents in these situations leads to inflammation, and may bring about contact with antigen with immune-system for the first time. This also leads to autoimmunity. The lists of antigen and the diseases produced by autoimmune state are given in Table (3.7).

## AUTOIMMUNE DISEASES :

Burnet accounts for development of autoimmune disease as a failure of destruction of the self reactive population of antibody forming cells, since a breakdown of natural tolerance occurs in autoimmunity. There are at least two main ways by which this tolerance mechanism can be overcome. The most important one is the evasion of nomal tolerance to self antigen *(vide supra)* due to anatomical peculiarity or intracellular localisation. The autoimmune phenomenon is also associated with infection with micro-organisms some of which contain antigens which crossreact with human tissue, for example, nephritogenic strain of type 12 Group A streptococci with glomeruli, or Group A streptococci with human heart tissue, or polysaccharide antigen of E. coli 014 with human colonic mucosa. Some drugs may act as hapten with body's tissue protein resulting in antigenic complex. This immune reaction results in damage to the cells coated with drug, for example, haemolytic anaemia in cases of hypertension treated with methyl-Dopa or SLE-like disease in cases treated with hydralazine, procainamide, isoniazide, phenylbutazolidin etc. Second category is the breakdown of tolerance mechanism by drugs, or infection against affecting antibody-forming cells, or due to deficiency or genetically controlled tolerance mechanisms by 'suppressor' T-cells.

### Pathogenesis :

Presence of circulating autoantibodies demonstrated by serological or tissue staining techniques, indicates their occurrence in diseases. The latter, however, do not provide adequate data as to their role in the disease process. In a number of diseases autoantibodies have been detected against a number of body antigens (Table 3.7). Some of these autoantibodies are directly involved in the tissue damage in these diseases by type II, type IV and type III hypersensitive reactions. The type II and type IV reactions are mainly directed against the organs and may be grouped under organ specific reactions while type III reactions occur in diseases where it is more generalised and is not particular to any specific organ. Hence this may be regarded as non-organ-specific reaction. Table 3.8 is a summary of these types of reactions and the mechanisms involved in these diseases.

TABLE-3.7

SELF ANTIGENS IN AUTOIMMUNITY (Taussig, 1979).

| ANTIGEN | DISEASE |
|---|---|
| a) *Soluble, circulating Immunoglobulin* (IgG) | Rheumatoid arthritis, SLE, Sjogren's disease, Scleroderma, Hashimoto's |
| Thyroglobulin | thyroiditis, thyrotoxoicosis |
| Clotting factors | SLE |
| Complement (C3b) | Rheumatoid arthritis. |
| b) *Soluble, non-circulating:* Intrinsic factor. | Pernicious Anaemia. |
| c) *Cell surfaces (excl. receptors)* | |
| Erythrocytes | Autoimmune haemolytic anaemia |
| Platelets | Idiopathic thrombocytopenia |
| Leucocytes | Idiopathic neutropenia, SLE |
| Thyroid cells | Thyroiditis, primary myxoedema |
| Cardiac muscle | Rheumatic fever |
| Spermatozoa | Infertility |
| Zona pellucida of ovum | Infertility |
| d) *Cell surface receptors* | |
| TSH receptor | Thyrotoxicosis |
| Acetylcholine receptor | Myasthenia gravis |
| Insulin receptor | Insulin-resistant diabetes |
| e) *Extracellular* | |
| Salivary gland ducts | Sjogren's disease |
| Glomerular and alveolar basement membrane | Goodpasture's syndrome |
| Epidermal basement membrane | Bullous pemphigoid |
| Desmosomes | Pemphigus vulgaris |
| Reticulin | Coeliac disease |
| f) *Intracellular* | |
| Nucleic acid, nucleoprotein | SLE, rheumatoid arthritis |
| Mitochondria | Primary biliary cirrhosis, Sjogren's disease. |
| Microsomes | Thyroiditis, pernicious anaemia |
| Thyroid colloid | Thyroiditis |
| Adrenal cytoplasm | Addison's disease |
| Islet cell cytoplasm | Juvenile diabetes, polyendocrine syndrome of females |
| Skeletal muscle A-band (actin, myosin) | Myasthenia gravis. |
| Smooth muscle (actin) | Active chronic hepatitis |
| Cardiolipin | Syphilis, Leprosy, Malaria |

## TABLE-3.8

### MECHANISM OF TISSUE DAMAGE IN AUTOIMMUNITY

A) ORGAN SPECIFIC TYPE:

a) Type II reaction : Tissue damage by autoantibody with cell surface.

a) Cytotoxic effect, e.g., Autoimmune haemolytic anaemia, Paroxysmal cold haemoglobinuria, Idiopathic thrombocytopenic purpura, Hashimoto's thyroiditis.

b) Cell surface receptors, e.g., Thyrotoxicosis, Myasthenia gravis.

c) Stimulation of cellular secretions, i.e., active secreted molecule, e.g., Atrophic gastritis in Pernicious anaemia.

d) Non-circulating extracellular antigen, e.g., glomerulonephritis in 5% cases.

b) Type IV reaction : Tissue damage mediated by T-cells sensitized against autoantigens.

Thyroiditis
Atrophic gastritis
Juvenile diabetes
Multiple sclerosis
Rheumatoid arthritis (RA).

B) NON-ORGAN SPECIFIC TYPE :

Type III reaction : Tissue damage by antigen and antibody complexes initiated by complement fixation in and around blood vessels, e.g., SLE, RA.

## HLA SYSTEM AND IMMUNE RESPONSES

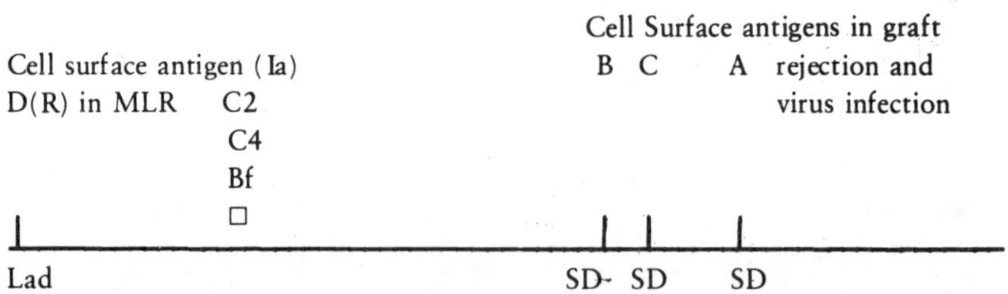


Ia Immune associated antigen

C2
C4 are factors for classical complement pathway.

Bf—factor B for alternate pathway.

MLR—Mixed lymphocyte reaction.

Lad—Lymphocyte defined antigen.

SD—Serologically defined antigens.

The WHO committee coined the name HLA meaning H for human (or histocompatibility), with L for leucocyte, the cell type first studied, and A for the first system (*not* for antigen).

Extensive research during last fifteen years indicates that certain genes controlling the ability of *immune-competent* cells to respond to antigen are genetically closely related to those genes controlling certain important cell surface antigens. HLA-A, -B, -C or —D(R) antigens are coded for by four of the genes in HLA region in chromosome 6 (Fig 3.10). Since each individual inherits a maternal and paternal MHS chromosome, eight distinct HLA antigens can be present on human tissue cells (two each of the A, B, C and D antigens). Since all four loci are highly polymorphic, with many alleles at each locus, it is very unlikely that two unrelated persons will have HLA-identical. The major histocompatibility region of human controls the expression of three groups of gene products, e.g., complement components, and two sets of polymorphic cell surface glycoproteins. The cell surface antigens are known as histocompatibility antigens and the group of genes that determine the expression of these antigens as major histocompatibility system (MHS).

Thus, HLA region induces the structural gene for the C2 and C4 components of complement and also of factor B for alternate pathway. The two groups of cell surface antigens (HLA-A, -B, -C). These are coded by genes located at closely linked HLA-A, -B, -C loci. Immune associated antigens (Ia) are coded by HLA-D(R) locus. These antigens have been implicated in regulating the interaction between immune-competent cells. Both groups of antigens have been connected with an individual susceptibility to diseases. HLA-A, -B and -C are expressed on the surfaces of almost all the cells except red cells, sperm, and placental trophoblast. HLA-DRw antigens are present only on B lymphocyte and monocytes, not on T-cells and are firmly attached to the cell surface. From the study of the allogenic graft rejection, importance of MHS-gene products on the T-cell reaction to antigen was realized. T-cells do not respond to antigen unless the antigen is presented on the surface of an appropriate cell macrophage. The interaction of T-cells with antigen must involve the receptor. This recognition of T-cells to specific antigen is governed by MHS gene products expressed on the cells presenting the antigen. This is also known as MHS restriction. The macrophages carrying HLA-D coded molecule are able to present the antigen to T-cells for response but the product of HLA-D region is needed for specific recognition of antigen by T-cells and their subsequent proliferation. Thymus grafting experiments indicate that MHS-antigens on the thymus epithelial cells are critical in determining the pattern of subsequent MHS restrictions. Individual T-cells coming out of thymus have been pre-selected to interact preferentially with antigens with only one product of the MHS. This is true for primary interaction and also for secondary clonal proliferation either to 'memory' T-cells or to 'effector' T-cells with specificity preserved towards the original priming antigen. Other T-cell reactions that are subjected to MHS restriction include helper T-cells interacting with B-cells in antibody response and T-cells interaction with macrophages in delayed type of hypersensitivity reactions. MHS products are also involved in antigen recognition by the suppressor T-cells. Thus, each T-cell is restricted by the products of one locus of the MHS. In the heterozygous state different T-cells are restricted by the different allelic products of a particular locus. This can only occur provided these are on T-cell specific receptors for recognition of specific products of MHS.

The antigens detected by serological methods are referred to as serologically defined antigens or SD antigens. HLA-A, -B and -C are three types of antigens. Mixed lymphocyte reaction (MLR) is performed by mixing the blood lymphocytes of the individuals in culture. If the two have identical genes at HLA-D locus then there will not be any blastoid transformation. The lymphocytes responding to MLR are T-cells while those which carry the HLA-D antigens and therefore stimulate the reaction, are B cells. Since the HLA-D antigen can be detected by lymphocyte stimulation, they are known as lymphocyte defined or LD antigen ('Lads : lymphocyte activated determinants). The diseases associated with HLA have been studied to a great extent and can be broadly divided to two, i) those diseases that are primarily associated with the HLA-D locus and ii) those that show mainly HLA-A, -B, or -C associations. The first major class involved autoimmune or immunologically associated diseases, e.g., thyrotoxicosis, coeliac disease, chronic hepatitis and myasthenia gravis etc. Juvenile-onset diabetes is associated both with i) DRw3 and ii) DRw3 and B8 sets of antigens and DRw4 or Dw4. Rheumatoid arthritis is associated only with DRw4 or Dw4. Myasthenia gravis is also found with DRw4 antigen. There are at least two diseases which are not associated with any immune development, e.g., haemochromatosis and psoriasis. The latter is associated with Cw6, B13, B27 and Bw37 antigen while haemochromatosis with A3 antigen (Table 3.9)

None of the HLA associations with disease found so far is absolute. There are four main reasons for this: i) environmental factors determine whether a susceptible individual actually will contract the disease; ii) genetic factors may contribute to disease susceptibility but this may not be connected with HLA system; iii) if the association be really due to a so-far-undetectable-at-a-closely-linked locus, this allele occurs at much lower frequency than the one detected at HLA-A, -B, -C or -D locus; iv) it is often likely that diseases studied are heterogenous and the HLA association is only with a particular subset of individuals having the disease. In such cases the HLA association itself contributes to the better definition of the diseases.

Thus, the HLA system contains remarkable clusters of genes controlling cell surface determinants and immune functions. The functions so far defined as controlled by genes in the HLA region concern cell surface determinants involved in the interaction between cells in the immune system, immune-response differences and certain complement components.

## TABLE 3.9

### ASSOCIATIONS BETWEEN HLA AND DISEASE.

| Disease | HLA antigen* |
|---|---|
| Ankylosing spondylitis | B27 |
| Reiter's disease | B27 |
| Juvenile rheumatoid arthritis | B27 |
| Yersinia arthritis | B27 |
| Multiple sclerosis | B7, A3 |
| | DW2 |
| Myasthenia gravis | B8 |
| Psoriasis vulgaris | BW37, B27 |
| Juvenile diabetes | B8 |
| | BW15 |
| Graves' disease | B8 |
| Addison's disease | B8 |
| Coeliac disease | B8 |
| De Quervain's thyroiditis | BW35 |
| Hodgkin's disease | B5, A1, B8 |
| Acute lymphocytic leukaemia | A2, B12 |
| Acute anterior uveitis | B27 |
| Dermatitis herpetiformis | B8 |
| Thyrotoxicosis | B8 |
| Chronic active hepatitis | B8 |
| Systemic lupus erythematosus | BW15 |
| Paralytic Poliomyelitis | A3, B7 |
| Ragweed allergy | HLA linked Ir gene. |

*The letters A,B and D refer to HLA loci, and the numbers following are serologically detected antigens coded by those loci; W. for Workshop, indicates an antigen which is not fully characterised.

# APPENDIX

## I. INVESTIGATIONS FOR IMMUNOLOGICAL STATUS OF A PATIENT:

### 1. INVESTIGATION FOR HUMORAL IMMUNE RESPONSE.

a) Quantitative estimation of immunoglobulin by radial diffusion technique. Non-specific antisera against IgG, IgA, IgM, or $\beta$ or $\alpha$ globulin are incorporated into agar gel, holes are cut and sera are placed in them. A ring forms because antigen diffuses into the gel where it precipitates at optimal proportions with immobilised antibody. The size of the ring is at any time proportional to the antigen concentration in the gel.

b) Immunoelectrophoresis enables the identification of proteins in complex mixtures as in serum, by electrophoresis followed by analysis by immune precipitation.

c) Estimation of highest antibody titre following injections of tetanus toxoid.

### 2. INVESTIGATION FOR CELL-MEDIATED IMMUNE RESPONSE (CMI) :

A) *In vivo* test for CMI.

a) Active sensitisation by a hapten.

This is done with 2:4 dinitrochlorobenzene (DNCB). Skin is at first sensitized with 0.05 ml of 10% DNCB in acetone. Subsequently, after two weeks 0.1% and 0.05% DNCB in acetone applied on the same site and covered with dressing. After 48 hours the reading of the test is done as follows : + (erythema only), ++ (erythema and induration), +++ or more is regarded as evidence of active sensitisation.

b) Delayed type of hypersensitivity to ubiquitious antigens. In this strength and doses of antigen used are given in parenthesis. Positive response is determined by erythema and induration of any diameter above 10mm at the end of 48 hours. Any reaction within few minutes to few hours may be regarded as Arthus reaction.

i) Tuberculin (P.P.D.) or OT (1 in 10,000 or 1 in 1000 in 0.1ml)
ii) Candida (1 in 1000 in 0.1ml).
iii) Trichophyton (1 in 1000 in 0.1ml).
iv) Varidase (streptokinsase) (5 units in 0.1 ml) (Lederle).
v) Mumps skin antigen (100 $\mu$g) (E.Lilly).

B) *In vitro* tests for CMI.

| Type of tests | Methods | Action on type of lymphocytes | | Method used for assessment |
|---|---|---|---|---|
| | | T-Cell | B-Cell | |
| 1. Lymphocyte | i) Phyto-agglutinin (PHA). | + | ? | Usually measured by |

| Type of tests | Methods | Action on type of lymphocytes | | Method used for assessment |
|---|---|---|---|---|
| | | | | uptake of H3 Thymidine. |
| Transformation. | ii) Pokeweed Mitogen (PWM). | +(?)* | + | |
| 2. Lymphokine Production. | i) Mitogen factors (MF) | + | + | |
| | ii) Macrophage inhibition | + | + | Inhibition of macrophage migration. |

*requires T helper cell function.

3. ESTIMATION OF PROPORTION OF T-CELL AND B-CELL IN THE PERIPHERAL BLOOD:

| | Tests used | | | | |
|---|---|---|---|---|---|
| | E-rosette | EAC-rosette | Fl. anti-Ig sera. | EA-rosette | Fl. T-cell antisera. |
| T-Cell | + | - | - | - | + |
| B-Cells | - | + | + | + | - |

E-rosette—sheep erythrocytes form rosette with T-cell.

EAC-rosette—erythrocytes coated with specific antibody (IgG or IgM) and complement component (C3) form rosette.

Fl. anti-Ig sera—Fluorescene conjugated antihuman globulin.

EA-rosette—erythrocyte sensitised with antibody.

Fl. T-cell antisera—Fluorescene conjugated antisera against T-Cells (sera from rabbits immunised with human foetal thymocytes and subsequent absorbtion into B-Lymphocyte leukaemic cells).

## II. INVESTIGATION OF IMMUNOLOGICAL DISEASES:

### 1. DIAGNOSIS OF AUTOIMMUNE DISEASES.

i) Detection of cellular antigen by using fluorescene conjugated antibodies against the antigen (direct immunofluorescence techniques) as in Hashimoto's thyroiditis.

ii) Detection of serum autoantibodies can be done by in direct immunofluorescence in appropriate tissue slices with highest dilution of test serum. This can be measured against thyroid, stomach, adrenal, salivary gland and other tissue antigens.

iii) Individual complement components may be measured by radial immunodiffusion. Levels of C3, C4 or both are depressed.

## 2.DIAGNOSIS OF IMMUNE COMPLEX DISEASES:

i) Decrease in the level of total complement level, or C3 or C4 indicates involvement of classical pathway whereas drop in C3PA would indicate activation of the alternate pathway. These can be estimated quantitatively by single radial immunodiffusion.

ii) Estimation of C1q binding: Radioactively labelled C1q component of complement added to test serum, binds to antigen antibody complexes. Addition of polyethylene glycol precipitates the labelled C1q which reacts with the immune complexes. The radioactivity of the precipitate gives the measurement.

iii) Rajii cell binding : Rajii cells are lymphoblastoid cells which have receptors for complement and Fc receptors for IgG. When test serum is added to Rajii cells, immune complexes bind mainly to complement receptors. Radioactively labelled rabbit anti-IgG sera added, binds to antibody moiety of the complex and radioactivity is then counted.

iv) Cryoprecipitation—cryoglobulin forms a gel when incubated at 4°C. This is centrifuged, then washed, redissolved at 37°C and reprecipitated at 4°C. Then it is characterised. Monoclonal cryoglobulins are IgG, IgA and IgM and may be associated with lymphoma. Mixture of IgM and IgG—anti IgG complexes are found in rheumatoid arthritis.

CHAPTER 4

# DISORDERS OF BLOOD

*R. N. DUTTA*

## EMBRYOLOGY OF BLOOD FORMATION

### Site of formation

In the foetus, blood is formed in mesenchymal tissue, subsequently mainly in the liver and partly in the spleen. From the fifth month onward bone marrow progressively takes over this function of blood formation. In a full-term neonate, bone marrow is the only site for blood formation especially the red cells, polymorph-neutrophils and platelets. It is possible that all blood cells derive from stem cell in the marrow. From this stem cell in the marrow arise the red cell series, granular cells and platelets. If the stem cell matures and differentiates in the thymus, it becomes small lymphocytes responsible for cellular immunity and are called 'T' lymphocytes. If the stem cell passes through and differentiates in the gut associated lymphoid tissue, then by division and maturation it becomes plasma cells. Large lymphocytes arising from gut-associated lymphoid tissues can produce immunoglobulins and are called B-lymphocytes.

## BONE MARROW

The marrow is found in the medullary cavities of all bones and could be red or yellow. Red is active marrow while yellow is inactive composed mostly of fatty adipose tissue. Red marrow is active and produces the red cell series of cells, myeloid series and platelet series. During the first few years of life, all the bones of the body have red marrow. By the third year, fat cells start appearing, and as one ages, the fatty tissue replaces the red marrow from all the bones in the distal parts of the body. By the age of 18 years, red marrow is found only in the vertebrae, ribs, sternum, skull bones and innominate bones of the pelvis and, to some extent, in the proximal epiphyses of femur and humerus. Bone marrow comprises essentially of blood vessels, developing haemopoietic cells, fat cells and a matrix of cancellous bone.

## CELLS OF BONE MARROW AND BONE MARROW BIOPSY

### 1. Stem Cell

It is a large cell (25 to 35 $\mu$m). The nucleus is large and cytoplasm is rather small. Chromatin is very fine and regular with 3 to 4 nucleoli. Cytoplasm is blue and is very thin around nucleus. This is the parent cell for red cell, myeloid, lymphoid, monocyte and platelet series.

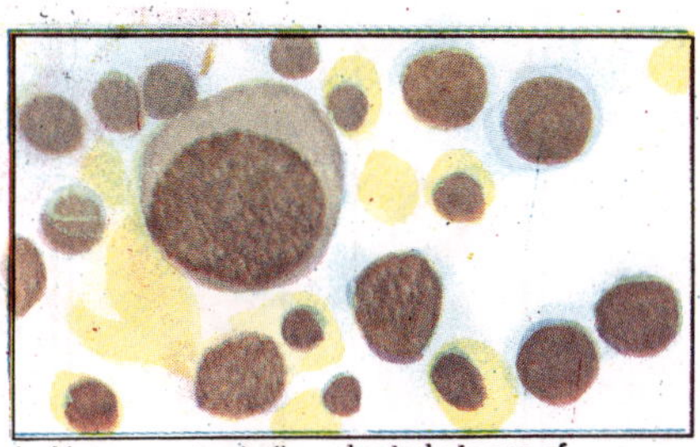

1. Normocytes: all nucleated stages of development.

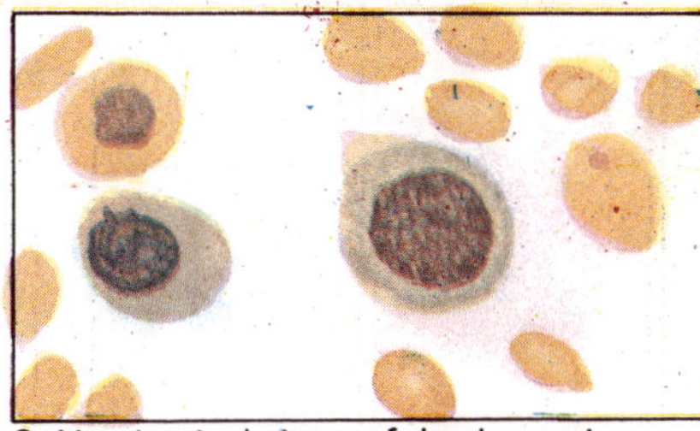

2. Megalocytes: stages of development.

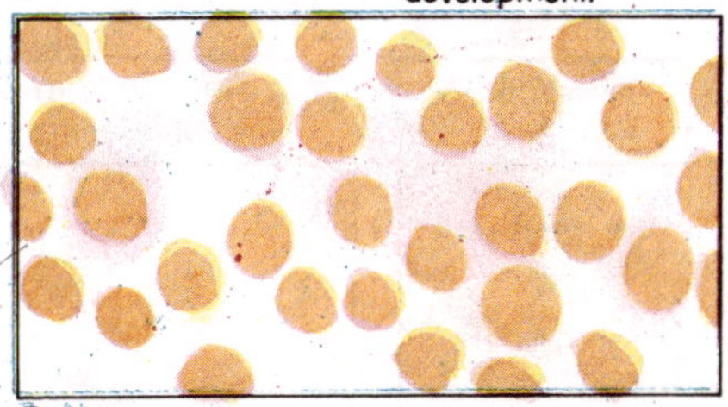

3. Normocytes.

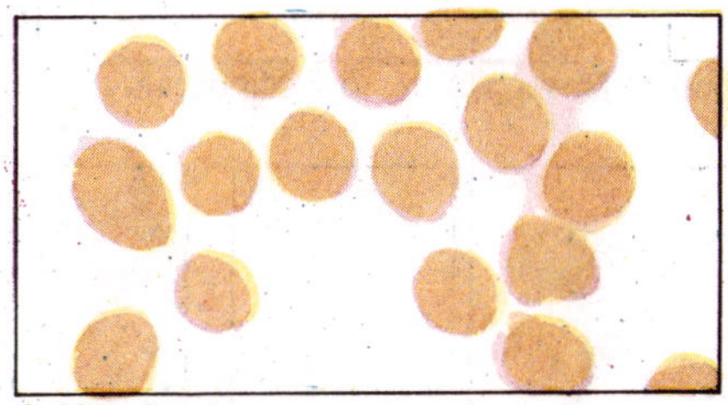

4. Megalocytes.

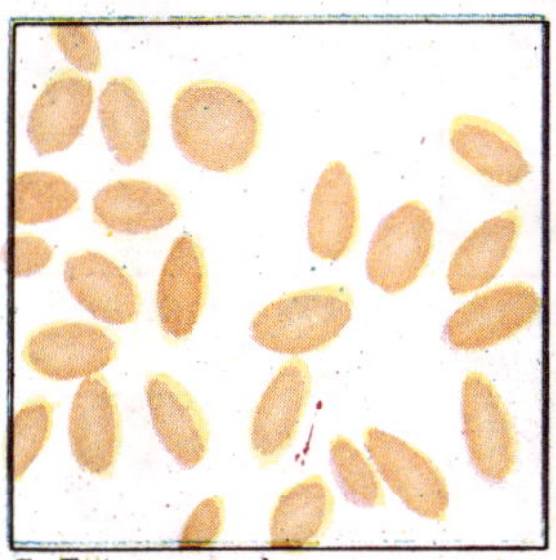

5. Elliptocytosis.

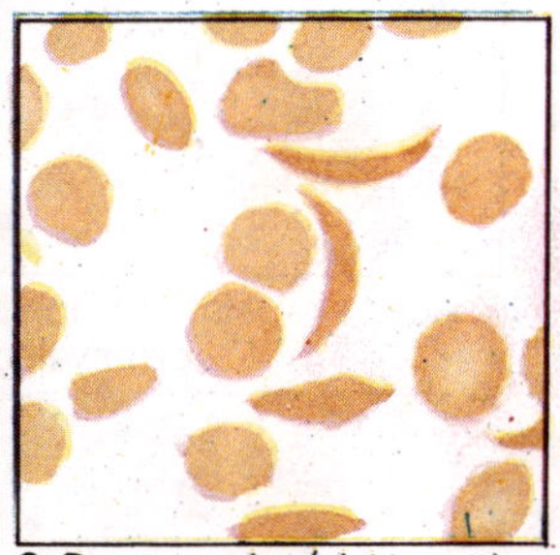

6. Drepanocytes. (sickle-cell)

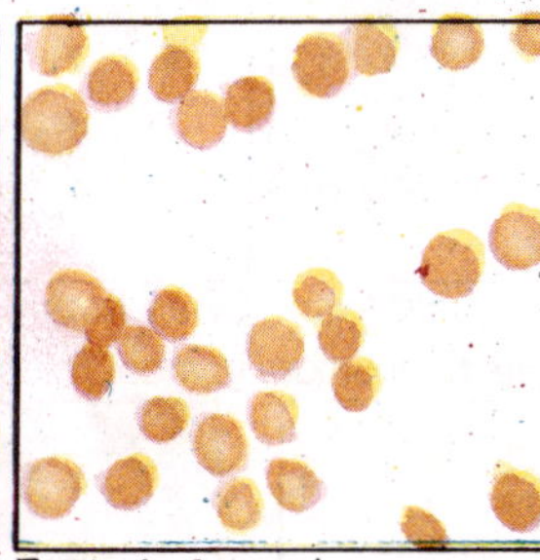

7. Microspherocytes

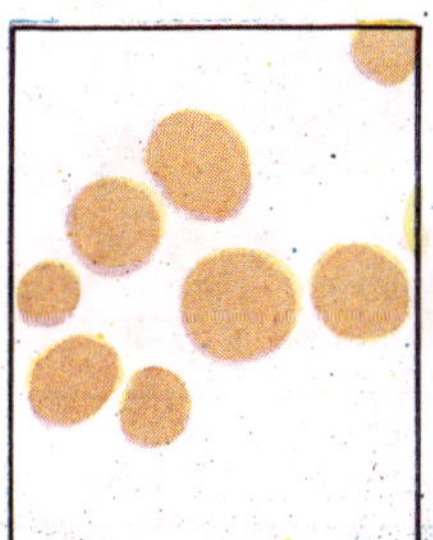

8. Anisocytosis.

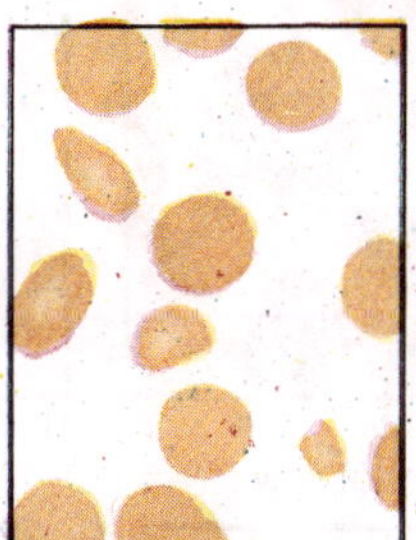

9. Poikilocytosis.

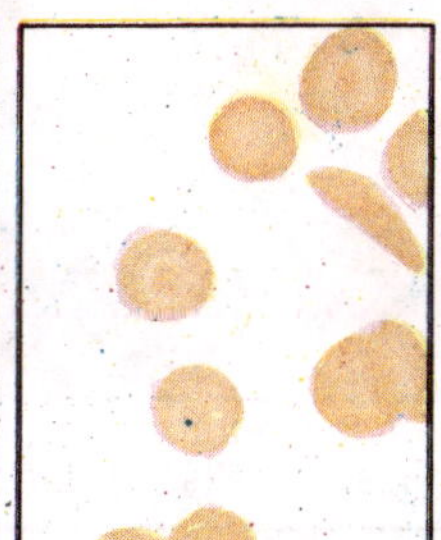

10A. Target cells.

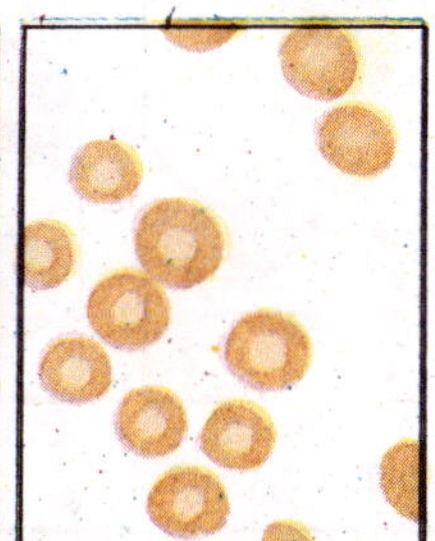

10B. Anulocytes.

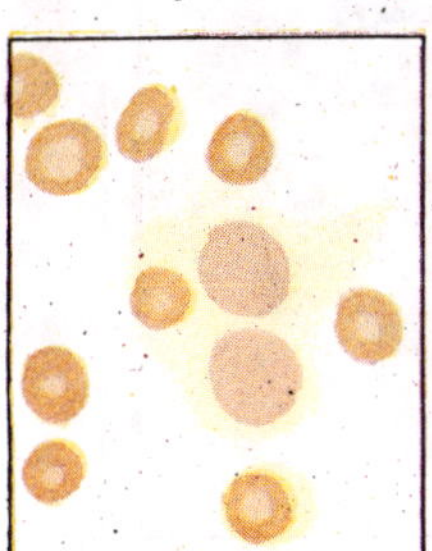

11A. Polychromasia.

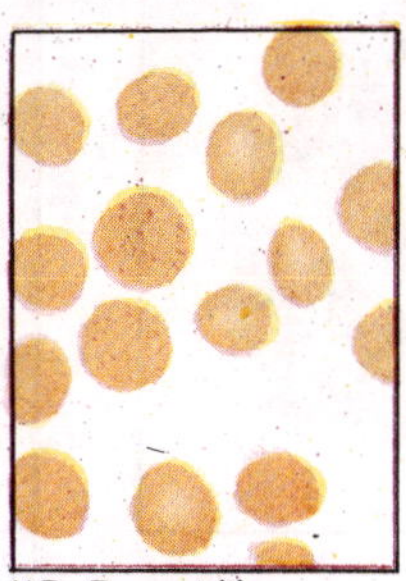

11B. Basophilic stippling.

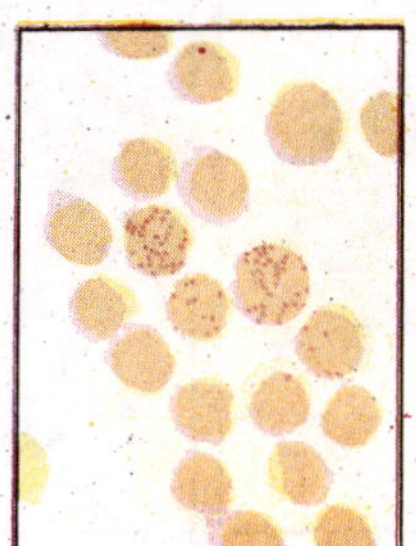

12. Proerythrocytes: Wolfer's vital staining.

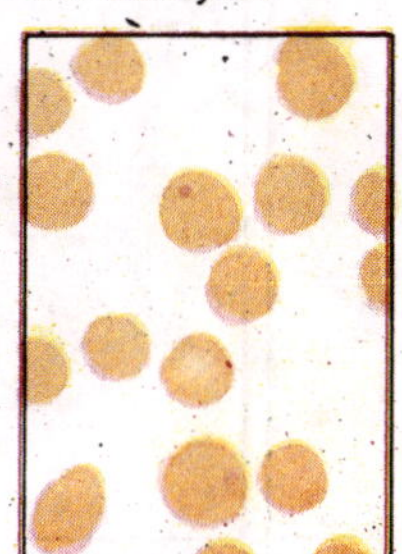

13. Normocytes: Giemsa staining.

Plate-I Red Cells :

Precursors, Normal and abnormal cells.

PLATE II

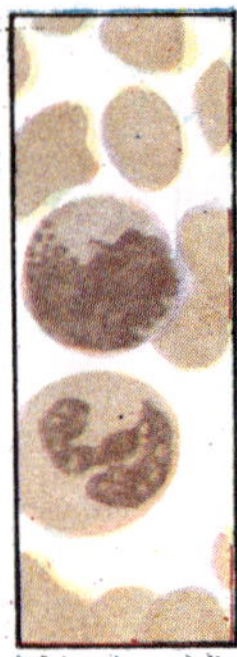

1. Neutrophils

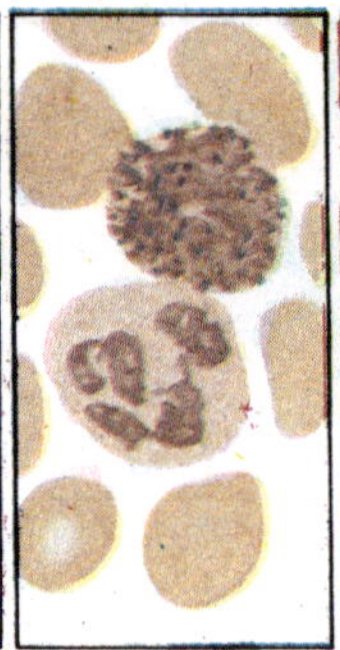

2. Basophils

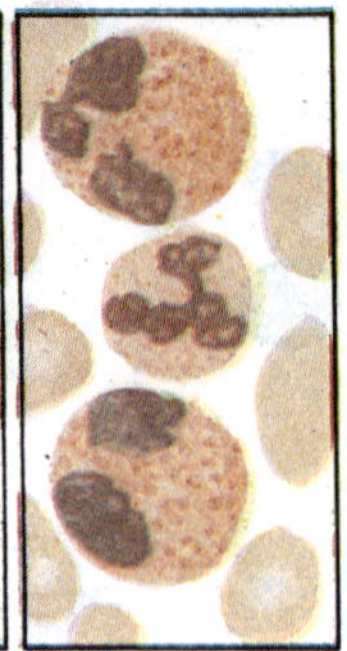

3. Eosinophils

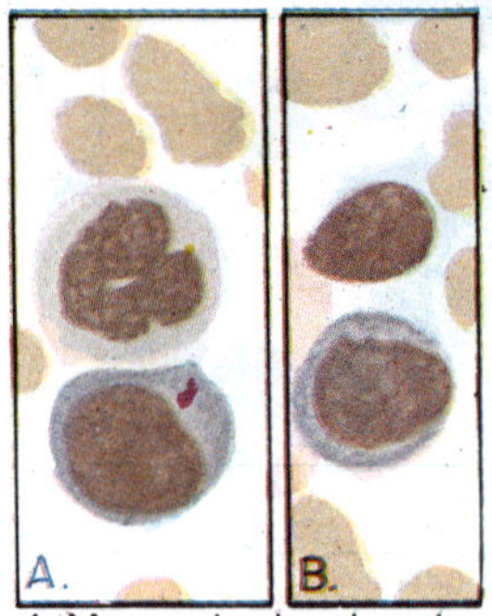


4. Monocytes, lymphocytes, plasma cells.

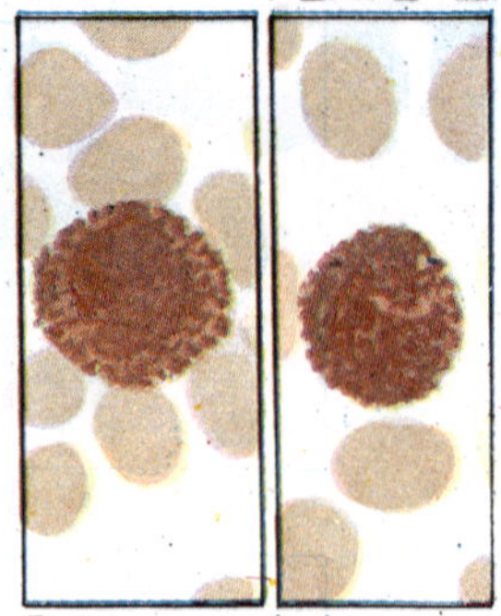

5. Basophils in blood. Pappenheim staining.

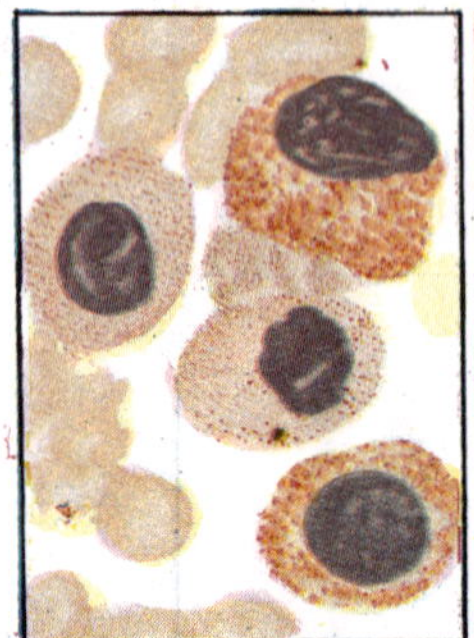

6A. Homozygotic form

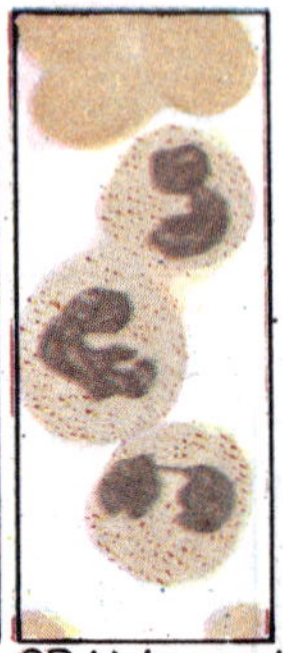

6B. Hetrozygotic form

Pelger-Huet's anomally in man.

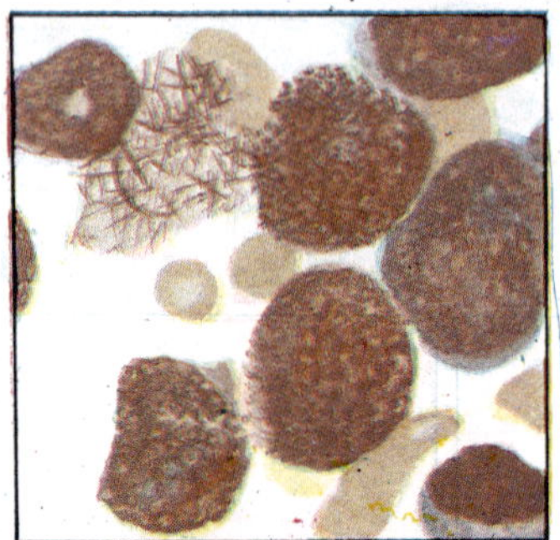

7. Auer's rods in neutrophillic promyelocytes.

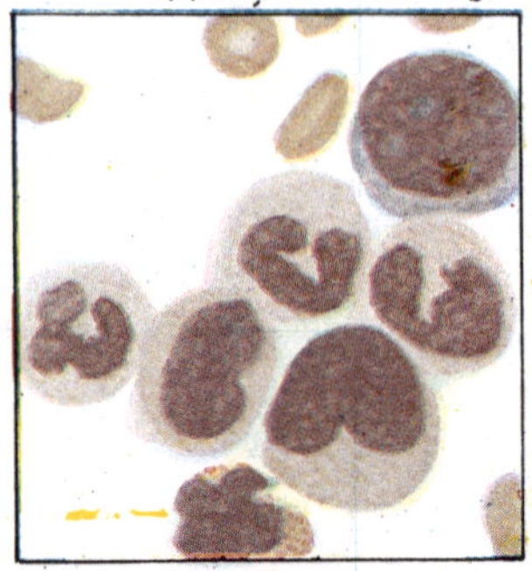

8. Chronic myelogenous Leukaemia.

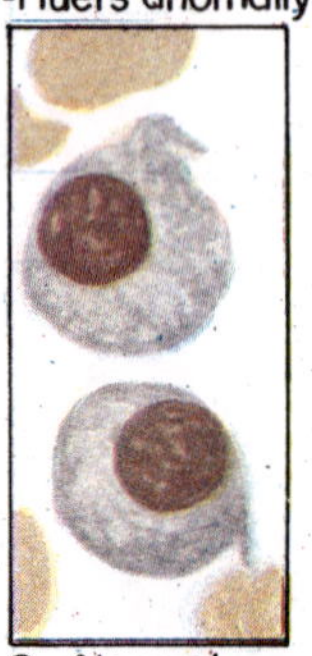

9. Normal plasma cells.

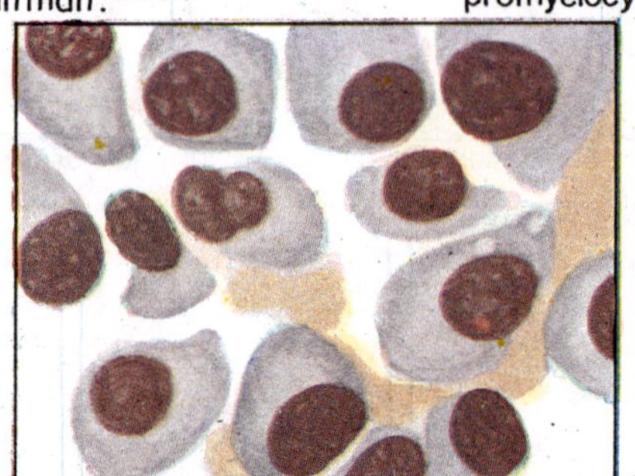

10. Plasmocytoma. Plasma cells in bone marrow.

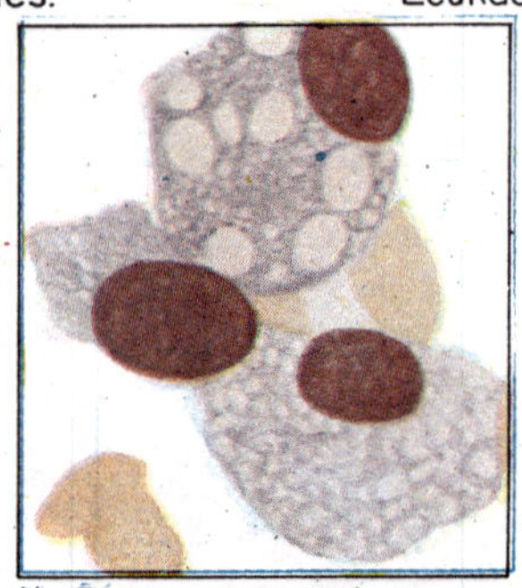

11. Plasmocytoma. Vacuolated plasma cells.

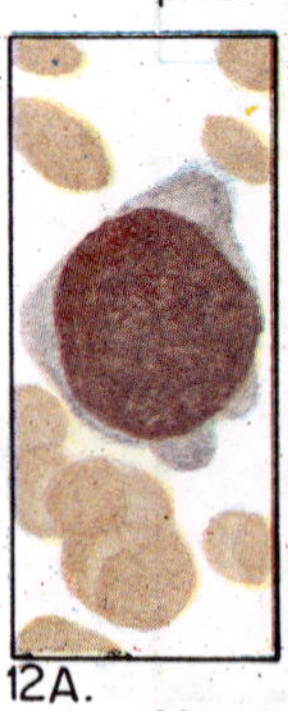

12A.

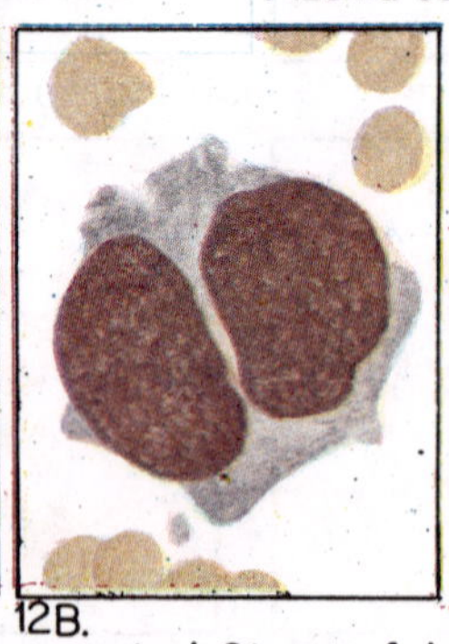

12B.

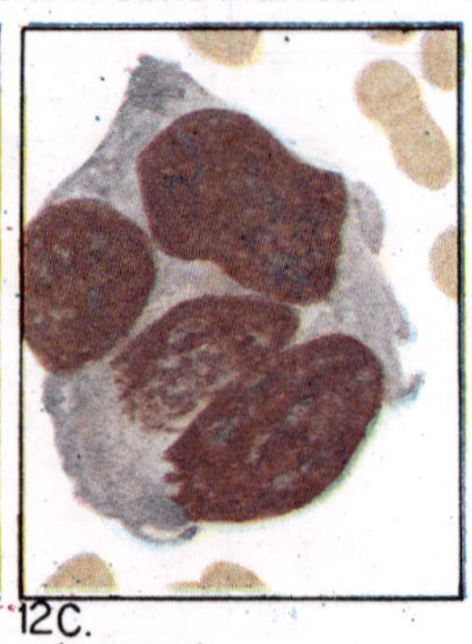

12C.

Megakaryocytes: Stages of development.

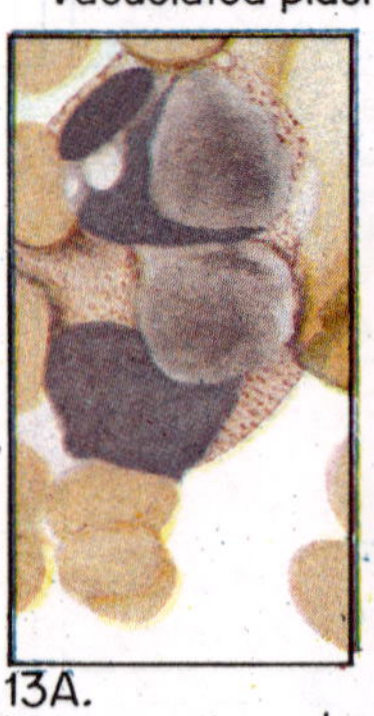

13A.

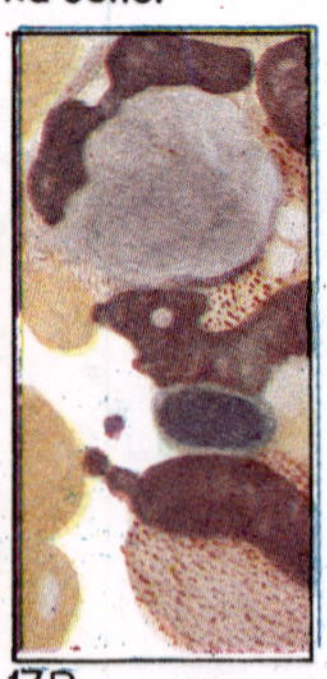

13B.

Lupus erythematosus. L.E. cells.

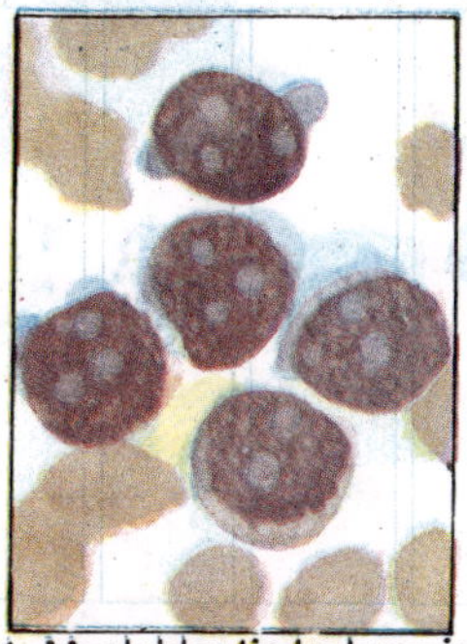

1. Myeloblastic leukaemia.

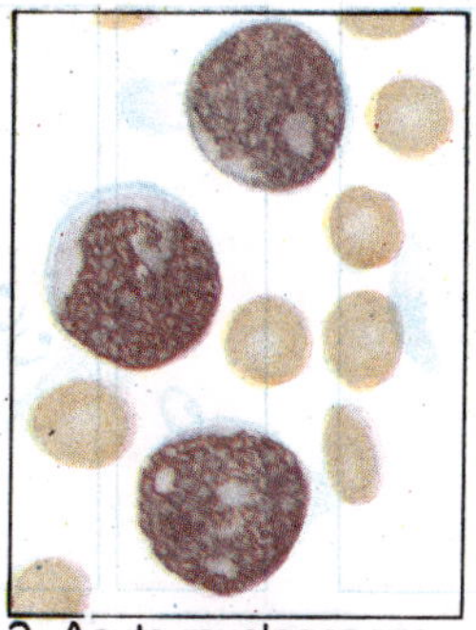

2. Acute myelogenous leukaemia.

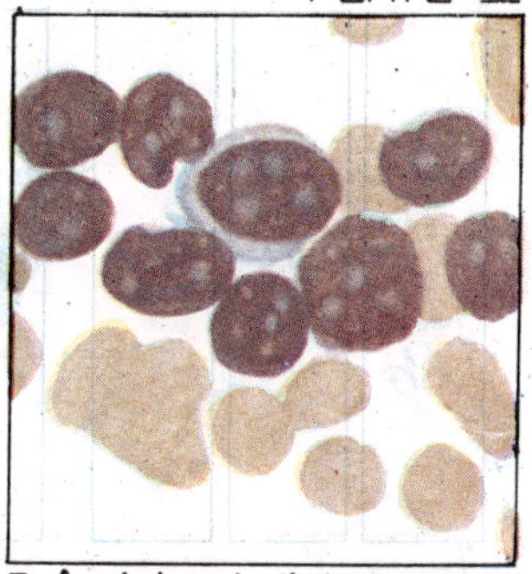

3. Acute lymphatic leukaemia. Peripheral smear.

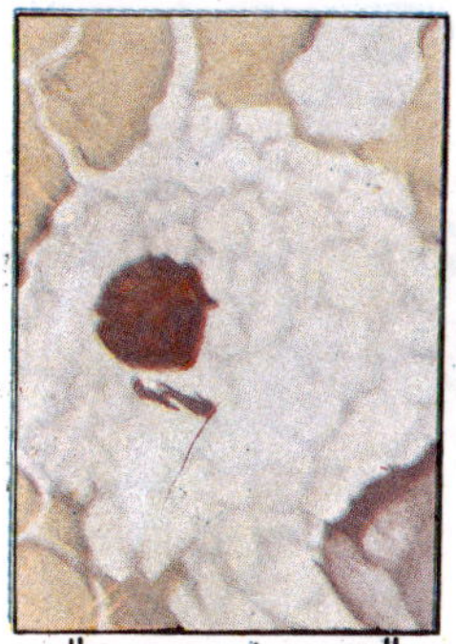

4. "Gaucher's cells".

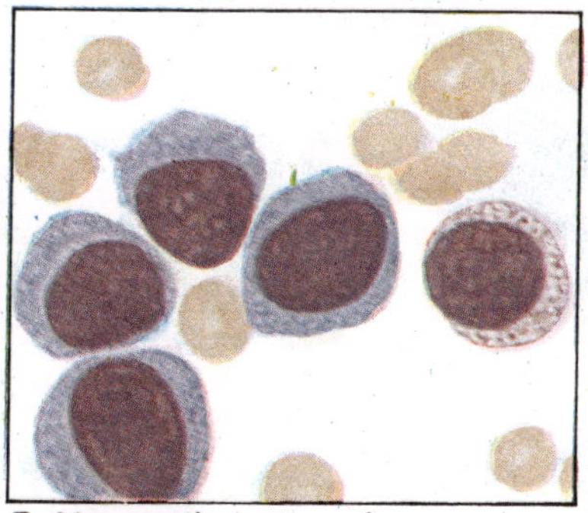

5. Monocytic leukaemia.

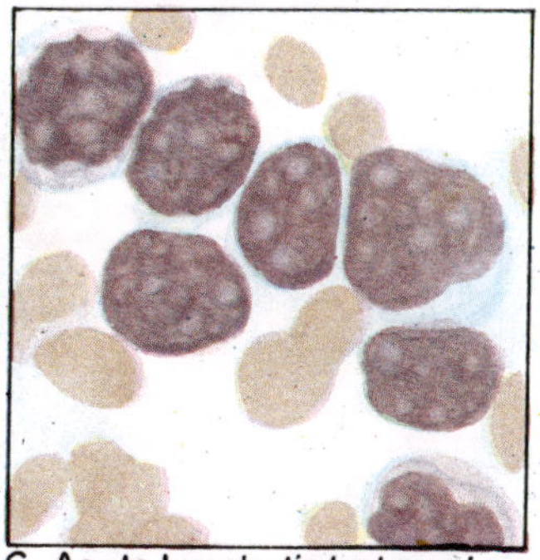

6. Acute lymphatic leukaemia. Bone marrow.

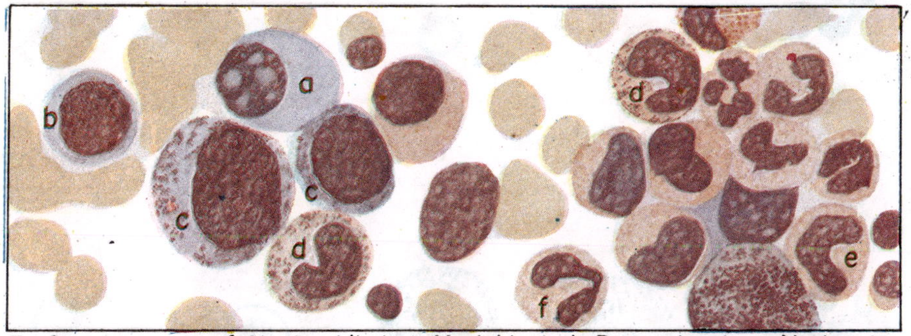


7. Development of Neutrophils: a. Myeloblast b. Promyelocyte c. Myelocyte d. Metamyelocyte e. Juvenile f. Neutrophil

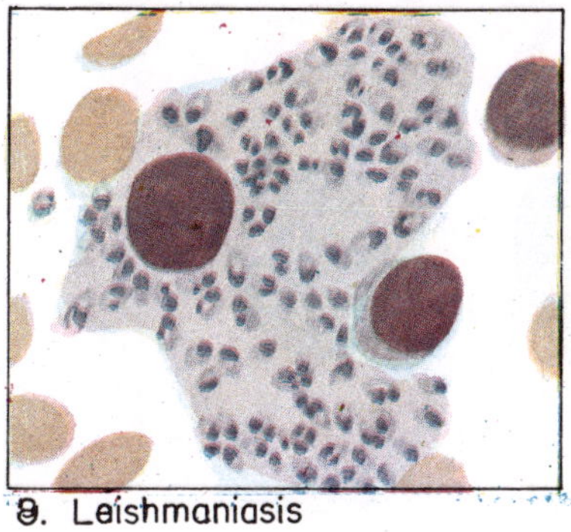

8. Leishmaniasis

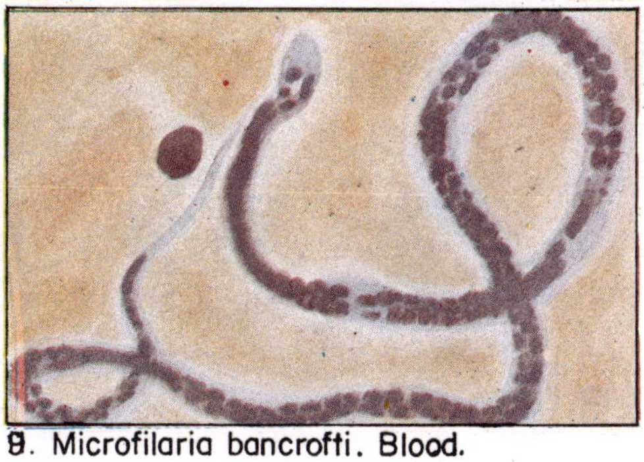

9. Microfilaria bancrofti. Blood.

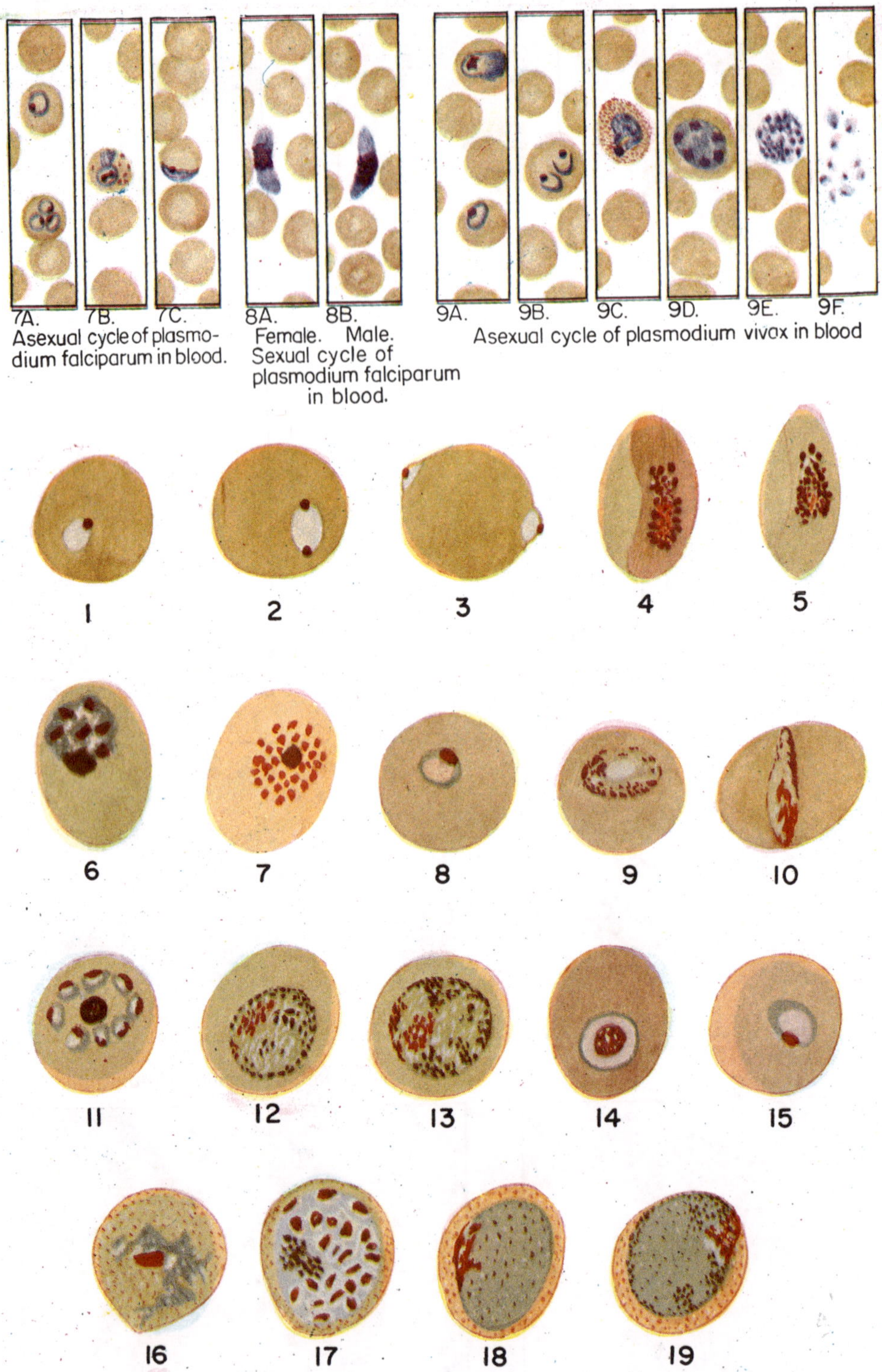


Plate-IV

Presence of trophozoites and similar growing forms of a sexual parasites in red cells.

(For reference see Pgs. 216, 219).

## DEVELOPMENT OF BLOOD CELLS

Table 4.1 shows the development of blood cells from stem cells in the marow and Table 4.2 shows origin and development of lymphocytes.

### TABLE 4.1 : DEVELOPMENT OF BLOOD CELLS

- Stem Cell
  - Normoblastic series
    - Early
    - Intermediate
    - Late
  - Myeloid series
    - Myeloblast
    - Promyelocyte
    - Myelocyte
    - Metamyelocyte
  - Platelet series
    - Mega karyoblast
    - Mega karyocyte
    - Platelet
  - Monocyte series
    - Monoblast
    - Monocyte
  - Lymphoid series
    - Lymphoblast
    - Lymphocyte

### TABLE 4.2 : DEVELOPMENT OF LYMPHOID SERIES OF CELLS

- Stem cell
  - Thymus
    - 'T' Lymphocyte (Cellular immunity)
  - Gut associated lymphoid tissue
    - Large Lymphocyte
      - 'B' Lymphocyte (Humoral immunity and immunoglobulin production)
      - Plasma Cell (Antibody formation)

**2. Red Cell Series**

There are many names given to the progenitor of this series like erythroblast, rubriblast, normoblast. These are interchangeable names, whilst megaloblast is an abnormally developed normoblast.

The mature red cells in the circulation arise from stem cells through series of division of early cells, progressive ripening of the nucleus and diminution of cell size and progressive haemoglobinisation (Pl. I, Figs. 1 & 3)

**Early normoblast** has a fine chromatin network in a large open nucleus and a blue cytoplasm. Its size is about 16 to 18 μm in diameter (Pl. I, Fig. 1)

**Intermediate normoblast** is about 12 to 15 μm in diameter. The nuclear chromatin is now coarse and condensed. In the cytoplasm, traces of haemoglobin have now appeared. This now divides into late normoblast.

**Late normoblast :** is 10 μm in diameter (Pl. I, Fig. 1). It has a dark dense nucleus and a cytoplasm which is now haemoglobinised. The nucleus in this cell breaks up through pyknotic degeneration and is extruded. The cell then becomes a non-nucleated reticulocyte which is a young red cell. The nucleus could also be lost by dissolution. Reticulocytes contain a fine reticular material which can be demonstrated by supra-vital staining with brilliant cresyl blue. They are about 0.5% to 1.5% in the peripheral blood. They are slightly larger than red cells and they increase in number whenever there is increased marrow activity. It is increased in haemolytic and haemorrhagic anaemias, and in dyshaemopoietic and iron deficiency anaemias under proper treatment. The cells mature in 2 to 4 days' time to become red cells. (Pl. I, Figs. 11A, 12)

**Red Cell** in the peripheral blood is disc-shaped, biconcave disc, size being 7.2μm in diameter. It is highly flexible and stains eosinophilic with Romanowsky stain. The cell membrane is not inert but dynamic and takes active part in gas transfer. The red cells contain inside haemoglobin which is responsible for oxygen transport. Life of red cells is about 120 days. (Pl. I Fig. 3)

**Haemoglobin :** The basic structure of haemoglobin consists of two different pairs of identical chains and each chain has one haem molecule. In adults haemoglobin there are two alpha chains combined with two beta chains ($\alpha_2\beta_2$). Alpha chain has 141 amino acids and $\beta$ chain has 146 amino acids (or residues). Haem molecule (or red pigment) is a combination of porphyrin with ferrous iron. Haemoglobin F (or foetal haemoglobin) is found in intrauterine life up to few months after delivery. By six months' time it falls to a low level of 5 per cent. In adults, only 1%-2% is present. It has two alpha chains and two gamma chains ($\alpha_2\gamma_2$). Each gamma chain has 146 amino acids. Hb F is found elevated in some haemoglobin disorders like thalassaemias, F haemoglobinopathy. It may be raised in other conditions also like paroxysmal nocturnal haemoglobinuria, aplastic anaemia, sideroblastic anaemia. There are many varieties of haemoglobin disorders due to haemoglobin molecular variation known as haemoglobinopathies.

**Control of erythropoeisis**

A decrease in oxygen content of arterial blood stimulates erythropoeisis through a substance called erythropoietin in the plasma. Erythropoeitin, a glycoprotein, with a molecular weight of 40,000 to 65,000 is perhaps formed in kidney in response to lowered oxygen tension in the blood. It acts on bone marrow stimulating the primitive cells to early normoblasts and perhaps helps in haemoglobin synthesis. Some endocrinal glands like thyroid, pituitary and gonads play some role in the erythropoeisis.

**3. Myeloid series**

**Myeloblast**— It has a large nucleus with open fine chromatin network with 2 to 5 blue, sharply defined nucleoli. The cytoplasm is blue and has no granules; size 15 to 20 μm. It is peroxidase negative (Pl. III, Fig. 7A)

**Promyelocyte**— It has no well-defined nucleoli, nucleus is still open and large in relation to cytoplasm. The cytoplasm has hardly any granules, which may be peroxidase positive; size 10-12 μm. Colour of the cytoplasm is blue and is less intense than myeloblast (Pl. II, Fig. 7b).

**Myelocyte**— It has no nucleoli and the cytoplasm has granules which are peroxidase positive. Cells may be large, even up to 20 μm. Chromatin of nucleus is thick and coarse (Pl. III, Fig. 7c)

**Metamyelocyte**—It has an indented nucleus with coarse chromatin. Cytoplasm is pink and has granules which are peroxidase positive. Size of the cell is less than myelocyte and nuclear chromatin are more clumped. The granules in the cytoplasm are more numerous and evenly placed (Pl. III, Fig. 7)

**Juvenile Cell**— Its nucleus could be in band shape or U-shape. It is slightly smaller than metamyelocyte and has coarse granules in the cytoplasm (Pl. III, Fig. 7e).

**Mature Polymorph neutrophil**—It is about 10 to 12 μm in size. Its nucleus has 2 to 5 lobes connected by thin strands of chromatin. The cytoplasm is pink and has azurophil granules. Neutrophils of females have a drum stick attached to a lobe of the nucleus. Males do not have them. The drum stick is present in some neutrophils and not in all (Pl. II, Fig. 1; Pl. III, Fig. 7f).

**Eosinophils**— It has coarse brick coloured granules with a two lobed nucleus often shaped like a spectacle. Size is about 15-16 μm. The granules appear from myelocytic stage (Pl. II, Fig. 3).

**Basophils**— It has coarse, deeply stained basophilic granules overlapping and overlying the single nucleus and hiding its detailed structure (Pl. II, Figs. 2, 5).

### 4. Platelet series

Platelets are budded out of megakaryocytes which is the largest cell in the marrow. First cell, that is, megakaryoblast is smaller than megakaryocyte. Its size is about 30 μm and has scanty cytoplasm. Repeated nuclear division takes place without cell division so that the cell becomes polypoid. Megakaryocyte is about 40 to 100 μm and is of irregular shape having a cluster of large nuclei. No nucleoli are present. The cytoplasm is abundant and is pale grey in colour with many azurophil granules. Active platelet, which is a cytoplasmic fragment, could be seen at the periphery of the cytoplasm. Megakaryocytes push out psuedopodia between sinusoidal cells and get the cytoplasm pinched out which becomes platelets in the blood (Pl. II, Figs. 12A, B & C).

### 5.Monocyte Series

Monoblast :— It has a size of 15 to 20 μm. Its size is irregular because of amoeboid movement. The cytoplasm is greyish blue, may contain fine azure granules and may be vacuolated. The nucleus is rarely regular and shows some indentation or convolution. (Pl. III, Fig. 5)

Monocyte :— Monoblast gives rise to promonocyte and then to monocyte which is found on the peripheral blood. The nucleus is large, eccentric and indented or irregular. Cytoplasm is fairly large and is pale, grey blue ground glass appearance and usually contains dust-like lilac coloured granules. Its size is 15 to 20 μm and is the largest cell in the peripheral blood. When its confronts a suitable inflammatory stimulus, it changes into a histiocyte. They have a pronounced amoeboid movement and phagocytic activity (Pl. II, Fig. 4a).

### 6. Lymphoid Series of Cells

Small lymphocytes are closely connected with thymus. By the ninth week of intrauterine life, the lymphocytes start developing in the region of thymus and are seen in the blood by 12th week and in spleen and lymph nodes by 20th week.

Lymphocytes enter the circulation mainly through the thoracic duct. About 20% are large and the rest are small lymphocytes. There are two types of lymphocytes, B lymphocytes, with a life span of 100 to 200 days and are associated with gut lymphoid tissue and second group with a life span of 2 to 3 days, T lymphocytes, which are the large lymphocytes. Small ones are the B lymphocytes which are capable of producing immunoglobulins and are responsible for humoral immunity, while the thymus or T lymphocytes are responsible for cellular immunity.

**Lymphoblast :** This is a large cell, 15 to 20 μm size having a large nucleus with one or two blue coloured nucleoli with sharp margin. Cytoplasm is homogenous and blue (Pl. III, Fig. 3).

**Prolymphocyte :** Here the nucleoli are indistinct, otherwise look like lymphoblast. They differ from it in that the chromatin strands are thicker. Nuclei may or may not be demonstrable.

**Mature lymphocyte :** There are two types in the peripheral blood, small and less numerous large ones. The difference is only in the size and bulk of cytoplasm. Small lymphocyte is 10 μm in size, has a dense round nucleus and a thin rim of blue scanty cytoplasm. Few purplish red granules may be seen. Large lymphocyte is about 15 to 20 μm in diameter. It has a large cytoplasm which is pale blue with few purple red granules. Nucleus is round or may be slightly indented (Pl. II, Fig. 4b).

**7. Plasma Cell Series**

About 2%-3% of bone marrow cells are plasma cells, though they are not usually seen in the peripheral blood. Plasma cell is about 15 +m in diameter having an eccentric nucleus whose chromatin is dense and arranged in cart-wheel manner. A pale area is seen in the cytoplasm near the nucleus on the side of greater cytoplasm. Vacuoles may be seen in the cytoplasm (Pl. II, Fig. 9) . In chronically inflammed tissues, plasma cells in large number are seen which may contain eosinophilic (acidophilic) smooth hyaline spherical bodies called Russell bodies in their cytoplasm. These bodies are composed mainly of gamma globulin and it is thought that plasma cells are the chief manufacturers of antibodies. Plasma cell are formed from the stem cell in the bone marrow (some authors think that they are formed from lymphocytes) and then migrate to tissues depending upon its immunoglobulin secretion. Plasma cells synthesizing IgA migrate to gastrointestinal tissues while cells producing IgG and IgD go to tonsillar tissue.

## BONE MARROW BIOPSY

It is an important and integral part of haematological examination. In some cases like iron deficiency anaemia or chronic myeloid leukaemia it may not be necessary, but in all other haematological cases bone marrow biopsy is essential. Aspiration biopsy is the method that is used commonly nowadays and trephine biopsy, i.e. removal of portion of marrow is hardly ever used these days except in cases of myelosclerosis when the latter is indicated.

**Site for aspiration bone marrow biopsy** is either sternum or iliac crest. In adults, sternum is the site of choice, while in children iliac crest is preferable. Vertebral puncture can also be carried out in children.

**Sternal Puncture :** Under proper aseptic condition the manubrium, a little to the right, is injected with local anaesthesia. The sternal puncture needle with the stillete on (there are many varieties of sternal puncture needle) is pushed on vertically with a rotatory movement till the marrow cavity is reached. The guard is often fixed prior to introduction of the needle. When the marrow cavity is reached, then the stillette is withdrawn and a well fitting 2ml or 5ml all-glass sterile syringe is attached and the marrow fluid is aspirated by gentle suction. The needle is immediately withdrawn and puncture site is pressed hard by the assistant for few minutes and then sealed either with collodion or tribenzene.

The author's procedure is to place the marrow fluid thus withdrawn at the end of 6 to 8 slides and then drain away the fluid blood by tapping the end of the slide against the table. What is left on the slide is mostly marrow material. Another slide is held at an angle of 30° over the marrow material and smears are drawn very quickly.

**Iliac crest puncture** site is the thickened area of the crest just posterior to the anterior superior iliac spine. The needle, after local anaesthesia, is pushed through the crest on a plane at right angles to the upper surface. Correct depth is indicated by lessening of resistance. The marrow fluid in this technique will be much less; material in the needle should be utilised for making smears.

**Vertebral spine puncture :** Rarely it is resorted to and that also only in children, whose spines can be seen and felt. The vertebral column is made prominent by the patient sitting up and bending forward or using the same position as in the withdrawal of C.S.F. fluid. The needle is inserted at right angle to the surface. Only few drops of material can be obtained.

**Contraindications of aspiration biopsy :** Haemophilia and other coagulation disorders are absolute contraindications.

**Complications :** In few cases especially in children, while carrying out sternal marrow biopsy, heart or great vessels have been punctured where death occurs suddenly due to cardiac tamponade.

### Examination of the marrow material

The smears are stained either by Leishman or Giemsa-Leishman stain and examined by the oil immersion lens. Following points are studied : (1) Cellularity, (2) predominant cell type in red cell and white cell series, (3) plasma cells, (4) platelet series, (5) any abnormal cells, (6) parasites. This is qualitative assessement and is good enough to come to any conclusion. Rarely one may have to resort to differential cell count.

### Clinical value of bone marrow examination

This examination confirms or gives positive result in cases of pernicious anaemias, megaloblastic anaemias, aleukaemic-leukaemias, differentiation of acute types of leukaemias, lipoidosis like Nieman-Pick's disease, Gaucher's disease, myelomatosis, myeloid reticulosis, myelosclerosis, erythroleukaemia, kala-azar (L.D.bodies). It also helps in confirming the diagnosis of idiopathic thrombocytopenic purpura.

**Assessment of Prognosis :** In a case of lymphatic leukaemia, types of cell often help in the assessment of prognosis. The more premature the cells are, the poorer is the prognosis though the peripheral blood may contain mature lymphocytes. In agranulocytosis, marrow having adequate number of myeloid series of cells indicates certain recovery.

**Peripheral Blood :** The values of peripheral blood vary according to age and sex. In a new-born, the red cell count is approximately 5-6$\times 10^{12/l}$. whilst in a child of one year it is $4.5 \pm 0.8 \times 10^{12/l}$. In an adult man it is 4-6.6 $\times 10^{12/l}$ whilst in women it is about 3.5-4.5 $\times 10^{12/l}$. Haemoglobin in infants is about 16-18g/dl whilst in man, it is 13-16g/dl and in women 12-14.5g/dl. The total white cell count in the peripheral blood in infants is about 15.0-16.0 $\times 10^{9/l}$ whilst in adults, it varies from 5-10 $\times 10^{9/l}$. The polymorph neutrophils consititute 40-70 per cent, lymphocytes 20-45 per cent, monocytes 2-9 per cent, eosinophils 1-5 per cent and basophils 0-1 per cent.

**Absolute Values of Red Cells :** These are calculated from packed cell volume (PCV), haemoglobin (Hb) and red cell count.

(1) M.C.H.C.—Mean corpuscular haemoglobin concentration and represents concentration of haemoglobin in each red cell. It is calcutated as follows :

$$\frac{Hb}{PCV} \times 100$$ and varies from 32-36g/dl in a normal individual.

(2) M.C.H. — Mean corpuscular haemoglobin. It represents average weight of haemoglobin in the cell and is calculated as follows :

$$\frac{\text{Hb} \times 10}{\text{R.B.C COUNT IN MILLION}}$$

It varies from 27 to 32 pg (picogramme).

(3) M.C.V.—Mean corpuscular volume. It tells us the average volume of red cells and is calculated as follows :

$$\frac{\text{P.C.V.} \times 10}{\text{Red Cell in million}}$$

Value range in normal varies from 76-94 fl.

(4) P.C.V.—Packed cell volume which is obtained by centrifuging a Wintrobe tube for 30 mins. at a speed of 3500 revolutions per min. One can use a micro-haematocrit tube in the microhaematocrit method which allows the determination of P.C.V. with small quantity of blood and is highly accurate. It is one of the simplest, most accurate and most valuable of all haematological investigations.

Its value in man is 40%-54% and in woman range is 35%-47%.

Table for normal values is given in the chapter on Anaemia.

(5) Peripheral Smear : One of the most important haematological examinations to assess the disorders of blood in a patient is the peripheral smear examination. The smear must be thin and should have a good tail. It should be properly stained. One examines the smear first by low power and then under oil immersion. All the cellular series in the smear are examined one after another and evaluated.

**Red Cell Series :**

(a) Its size and shape are examined. Small sized cells are called microcytes. Larger than normal size are called macrocytes (Pl. I, Fig. 4). Normocytes are normal sized cells (Pl. I, Fig. 3). Variation of size is called anisocytosis (Pl. I, Fig. 8). It may be due to increase in small sized cells or macrocytes or both. It could also be a round cell instead of a biconcave disc. It is then called spherocyte. It is round, small and densely stained in cases of hereditary spherocytosis (Pl. I, Fig. 7).

b) Its Shape—If the cell is pear or tear drop shaped, it is called poikilocyte (Pl. I, Fig. 9). It could be oval or elliptical in shape as in *Ovalocytosis* (Pl. I, Fig. 5). or *Elliptocytosis*. In sickle-cell anaemia, it is *sickle-shaped* (Pl. I, Fig. 6). It could be *'Burr'* cell with spinous projections on the surface which is seen in renal failure. *Schistocytes* are fragmented red cells whilst *acanthocytes* are spur cells — both are seen in haemolytic anaemia.

(c) Staining properties— Normal red cells are stained reddish, brick-coloured with a light staining area in the centre. Perpihery is densely stained. Hypochromasia means less staining which is seen in various types of anaemia. If it is a thin rim of stained material at the periphery and rest of the red cell is absolutely pale, it is called leptocytes. It is mostly seen in iron deficiency anaemia of severe degree. If there is a stained rim of Hb in the periphery and a central pale area in which a rounded central drop of stained material is seen like a "target"in shooting range, it is called "Target cell" as seen in thalassaemia and other haemoglobinopathies. Hyperchromasia is seen in young red cells like reticulocytes. It indicates an active marrow. It is also called Polychromasia (Pl. I, Fig. 11A) and has the same significance as reticulocytosis.

(d) Inclusion bodies— **Punctate Basophilia:** It is seen in chronic lead poisoning and indicates damage to red cells. These are blue staining dots in the red cells. Occasionally, they are seen in severe anaemia and following splenectomy. (Pl. I, Fig. 11B)

**Siderocytes** are red cells containing iron granules. They give Prussian blue reaction with ferrocyanide. It is seen in sideroblastic anaemia, lead poisoning and in some haemolytic anaemias. When stained by Romanowsky stain, it is called *Pappenheimar bodies* seen following splenectomy and in cases of haemolytic anaemias.

**Howell-Jolly bodies** are nuclear remnants. They are seen as small, round, dark staining particles usually one, occasionally more. Seen after splenectomy and sometime in cases of leukaemia.

**Cabot rings** are ring-shaped or twised or convoluted threads blue in colour and are seen in cases of megaloblastic anaemia.

**Malarial parasites** are also seen in the red cells either in ring forms, shizonts, merozoites or gametes.

**White cell series** increase or decrease in number could be assessed. Increase in polymorphonuclear leucocytes with a shift to the left indicates infection. Toxic granules are basophilic coarse granules seen in the cytoplasm of neutrophils. Polymorph neutrophils also increase in moderate to severe haemorrhage, in burns, in extensive tissue injuries, damage, coronary thrombosis, and generally after an initial phase of shock.

The polymorph neutrophils may show Pelger-Huet abnormality where the nuclei are dumb-bell-shaped and have coarse chromatin (Pl. II, Figs. 6A, 6B). They do not segment further. It is a non-sex linked, rare, dominant hereditary abnormality. Hyper segmented neutrophils or macropolycytes are abnormally large (15 to 25 $\mu$m) with more than 4 nuclear lobes. They are associated with Vit $B_{12}$ or folic acid deficiency.

**Atypical mononuclear cells**

**Turk cells** are about 15 $\mu$m in diameter and have deeply stained narrow rim of cytoplasm and a large round nucleus seen in patients with infection. Now it is thought that this hyperbasophilic medium sized mononuclear cell (probably lymphoid series) appears in the blood after immunization, infection, hypersensitivity reaction and onset of autoimmune disorder. It is now considered to be derived from lymphoid tissue responding to an antigenic stimulation. *Sezary cell* has PAS positive coarse granules and is seen in Sezary syndrome.

**Glandular fever cell** is an atypical mononuclear cell with pseudopodia flowing around nearby red cells. It has a round nucleus and large pale blue cytoplasm.

**Eosinophilia** indicates an absolute increase in the number of eosinophils as seen in pulmonary or tropical eosinophilia. It is seen in allergic condition, parasitic infection and in certain skin diseases. It is occasionally seen in Hodgkin's disease.

**Abnormal increase** in number and presence of premature white cells help in the diagnosis of leukaemias.

**Platelet series :—** Shape, size, granularity as well as number can be estimated from a peripheral blood film.

### TABLE 4.3 : NORMAL HAEMATOLOGICAL VALUES

| | |
|---|---|
| 1. **Haemoglobin :** | — |
| Infants | — 16-18 gm/dl. |
| Men | — 13-16 gm/dl. |
| Women | — 11-14.5 gm/dl. |

2. **Red Cells :**
    - Infants — $5\text{-}6 \times 10^{12/l}$
    - Men — $4\text{-}6.6 \times 10^{12/l}$
    - Women — $3.5\text{-}4.5 \times 10^{12/l}$
3. **PCV :**
    - Men — 40-54%
    - Women — 35-47%
4. **M.C.V. :** — 76-94 fl.
5. **M.C.H.** —27-32 picogramme (pg)
6. **M.C.H.C** 32-36 g/dl
7. **Reticulocytes** — 0.2-2.5%.
8. **E.S.R. :**
    - Males — 0-10 mm 1st hour (Westergreen)
    - Females — 0-20 mm 1st hour (Westergreen)
9. **White Cells :**
    - Infants — $15\text{-}16 \times 10^{9/l}$
    - Adults — $5\text{-}10 \times 10^{9/l}$
10. **Differential Leucocyte count :**
    - Adults : Neutrophils — 40-75%
        - Lymphocytes — 20-45%
        - Monocytes — 2-9%
        - Eosinophils — 1-5%
        - Basophils — 0.0-1%
11. **Platelets** — 150,000-400,000 per $mm^3$ (1.5-4 $\times 10^{9/l}$
12. **Bleeding time** (Ivy's method) up to 10 mins.
13. **Coagulation time** (Lee & White method at 37°C) 5-11 mins.
14. **Prothrombin time** — 12-14 secs.
15. **Plasma fibrinogen** — 150-400 mgm/100 ml.
16. **Serum iron** — 60-160 μg/100 ml.
17. **Total Iron binding capacity** (TIBC) — 280-400 μg/100 ml.

# ANAEMIA

## DEFINITION

The term 'anaemia' referes to a state in which there is a reduction in the quality or quantity of red cells below normal level. Anaemia, therefore, must occur

(i) when the production of red cells is poor in quality or quantity,

(ii) when blood loss or destruction outstrips the available supply of new red cells.

To know that a person is anaemic, one must know the normal haematological values (Table 4.3).

## CLINICAL FEATURES

Due to diminished oxygen carrying power of the blood, anaemic patients show a group of clinical symptoms and signs whose occurrence and severity depend on the degree of anaemia, rapidity of development but are independent of the type of anaemia. The clinical features are (i) general feeling of fatigue, breathlessness on exertion, tiredness, lassitude, easy fatigability, (ii) headache, **insomnia**, (iii) pallor of skin and mucous membrane, (iv) palpitation, tachycardia and functional systolic murmurs, (v) anorexia and dyspepsia, (vi) general muscular weakness, tingling and numbness, pins and needles in the fingers and toes and in severe cases, (vii) there may be oedema ankles. It may also be remembered that general symptoms can occur at a high Hb level with rapidly developing anaemia. Children as well as young adults can tolerate a much greater degree of chronic anaemia than older patients.

## CLASSIFICATION OF ANAEMIA

I. Anaemias due to deficiency of haemopoietic principles.

A. Iron deficiency anaemia
- (i) Chronic nutritional hypochromic anaemia
- (ii) Post-haemorrhagic anaemia
- (iii) Hypochromic anaemia due to malabsorption of iron
- (iv) Sideroblastic anaemia

B. Vit $B_{12}$ and folic acid deficiency anaemia.
- (i) Nutritional megaloblastic anaemia
- (ii) Megaloblastic anaemia of pregnancy
- (iii) Megaloblastic anaemia complicating pathological conditions of G.I. tract like extensive gastric resection, intestinal anastomosis, tropical sprue
- (iv) Addisonian pernicious anaemia
- (v) Megaloblastic anaemia of liver disease
- (vi) Megaloblastic anaemia of infancy
- (vii) Megaloblastic anaemia due to anti-convulsant drugs
- (viii) Megaloblastic anaemia complicating leukaemia

C. Vit C deficiency—Anaemia of scurvy

D. Thyroxin deficiency anaemia of myxoedema.

II. Anaemias due to excessive haemolysis :

A. Intracorpuscular causes due to congenital abnormalities of erythrocytes. They are:

(i) Haemoglobinopathies like thalassaemia, sickle-cell disease

(ii) Enzyme deficiencies like Glucose-6-Phosphate dehydrogenase deficiency

(iii) Hereditary spherocytosis

(iv) Paroxysmal nocturnal haemoglobinuria

B. Extracorpuscular defects due to infective, toxic or allergic factors. Also associated with other diseases.

C. Due to erythrocyte antibodies (immune mechanism) like isoantibodies, cold and warm antibodies.

III. Anaemias due to aplasia or hypoplasia of the bone marrow.

(i) Idiopathic

(ii) Secondary

IV. Symptomatic or secondary anaemias : Cause for anaemia in this group is often multiple or uncertain. With a number of well-defined disorders, severity of anaemia depends entirely on the underlying disorder and hence it is also called symptomatic. In most cases, like chronic infection, chronic renal disorders, rheumatoid arthritis, other collagen disorders, liver diseases, tuberculosis, causes for anaemia are many or often uncertain in origin. Anaemia associated with these disorders is often normocytic and normochromic in type, although in some cases it could be macrocytic or microcytic in type as well.

## 2. ANAEMIAS DUE TO DEFICIENCY OF HAEMOPOIETIC PRINCIPLES

### 3. Anaemia due to deficiency of iron

This is the commonest type of anaemia encountered in our country. It is widely prevalent in all ages and sexes as well as in all parts of India. General incidence of iron deficiency anaemia varies according to the economic and social status of the individual. Its incidence is higher in the poorer section of the society though it is also met with in the higher income group.

In India incidence varies from place to place. In the South, 25-50 per cent of pregnant women during the last trimester of pregnancy and approximately 50 per cent of infants and young children suffer from iron deficiency anaemia. In Gujarat, in a village community of 1441 people, 29.55 per cent were found to be suffering from iron deficiency anaemia whilst in a survey of low income group at Poona, 51.43 per cent showed a similar type of anaemia, whereas a similar study from Kerala showed that 14.2% of the females were suffering from iron deficiency anaemia. A study from New Delhi showed that out of 71 children, 51 were suffering from manifestations of hypochromic anaemia. In view of its widespread incidence a detailed discussion on the iron metabolism and its disorders is considered necessary.

### Iron Metabolism and its Disorders

#### (a) Body Iron Content

There are about 4 to 5 gms of iron in the adult human body. About two-thirds of it are found in the red cells. One ml of red cell contains approximately 1 mgm of iron, so that an adult has about 2 gms of iron in the red cell mass. About 0.15 gm is present as myoglobin and respiratory enzymes. Stores of iron are found in the reticulum cells of liver, spleen and bone marrow and the amount varies from 0 to 1g or more. Stored iron is in two forms in the body, ferritin and haemosiderrin. Plasma iron forms only a small proportion of the total (3-4 mgm). Plasma iron functionally is of great importance since all iron exchange takes place through this pool. Iron is always bound to transferrin, a $\beta_1$-globulin to prevent the toxic reaction of unbound iron and its precipitation at the PH of body fluids. Transferrin acts as a transfer protein carrying iron to and from various tissues without itself being utilised or assimilated. Iron is continuously circulating through plasma bound to transferrin and major part of this iron is derived from the daily destruction of about 20 ml of red cells which liberates 20 mgm of iron. There is also a further 10-15 mgm of iron derived from stores and tissues carried through plasma daily. Plasma iron is rapidly removed by the active haemopoietic tissues in the bone marrow but part goes to stores and new tissue formation. There is an increase in iron absorption when erythropoiesis is stimulated by bleeding, haemolysis or by high altitude.

(b) **Body Iron Balance**

Iron metabolism occurs within a closed system in the body. Iron is conserved by the body, the small amount lost daily is made good by absorption from the gut.

(i) **Iron Loss**

**Faecal loss**—is about 0.4 to 0.5 mgm daily. Urinary loss—is normally less than 0.1 mgm daily. These urinary losses are uninfluenced by body iron content. Urinary iron losses may be greatly increased by the use of iron chelators.

**Skin loss**—losses from growth of hair, nails and from desquamation of epithelial cells have been estimated at 1-5 mg daily. It has also been suggested that in hot humid climate of tropical countries, thermal sweating may account for several milligrams of iron loss daily but this has not been supported by isotope studies.

**Menstrual iron loss**—an additional daily loss of about 0.8 mgm of iron is incurred by a menstruating woman.

Thus basal losses of body iron in man amount to less than 1.0 mgm daily. In females, it is about 1.5 mgm daily.

**Pregnancy**—Total iron requirement during pregnancy is as follows—Foetal need is about 280 mgm of iron. Expanding maternal red cell mass requires about 200 mgm of iron and a further 125 mgm of iron for blood loss and placenta during delivery. Although, basal iron losses are offset by amenorrhoea, to this must be added an average daily loss of 162-370 mgm of iron throughout pregnancy.

Thus total iron requirement is about 800 mgm; since after delivery mother's red cell mass comes down to normal level again, which permits 140 mgm of iron becoming available to her, the total iron outlay during pregnancy is around 650 mgm.

(ii) **Iron Absorption**

This is the principal means of body iron regulation. Mechanism of absorption is complex and still is not well understood. Many factors are known to influence iron absorption and they are (a) luminal factors, (b) systemic factors and (c) mucosal cell factors.

(a) **Luminal factors :—**

Dose—depends on the amount of iron presented.

Valency—ferrous iron is much more readily absorbed than ferric.

6

Substances increasing absorption—are reducing agents like Vit C orally, Succinic acid orally as well as intravenously increases iron absorption. Iron chelates with fructose and combines with aminoacids such as histidine and cysteine and gets readily absorbed.

Substances decreasing absorption—are those which form insoluble compound with ferric iron like dietary phytates, phosphates, iron chelators such as desferrioxamina. Food iron absorption—an average diet contains approximately 10-20 mgm of iron per day mostly in organic form but there is some in inorganic form also. Iron is widely distributed in vegetables and meat, concentration being higher in the latter. 11 to 14 per cent of dietary iron is absorbed. Liver iron is well absorbed, iron in egg yolk, spinach and rice is less well absorbed and still less in wheat and soyabeans. It is difficult to define the precise role of dietary iron deficiency in the etiology of a condition so multifactorial as iron deficiency anaemia. There is apparently no co-relation between dietary iron and iron deficiency anaemia. The availability of food iron for absorption depends not only on its form in the natural state but also in the case with which digestion releases iron containing compounds from the foods and the presence of iron-binding substance in food which may increase or decrease iron absorption.

Stomach and iron absorption—Importance of stomach in iron absorption could be seen from the fact that the incidence of gastric atrophy and achlorhydria is higher in patients with this type of anaemia than in normal people. It is well established that hydrochloric acid is an important factor in its absorption. The ingested iron is liberated from food by peptic digestion and becomes bound to chelators which with the help of HCL keep it in soluble form. Iron is absorbed in the duodenum and jejunum. Regulation of iron absorption takes place in this portion of the intestine. There is a significant impairment of non-haem iron absorption in patients with histamin fast achlorhydria. Gastric acid also may influence iron absorption through lowering of pH.

(b) **Systemic factors modifying iron absorption :**

Body iron stores—a decrease of body iron induces increased iron absorption from the alimentary tract. This may occur in iron deficiency state without anaemia. Conversely, iron absorption is diminished in states of iron overload.

Erythropoietic activity—Iron absorption increases with increased erythropoietic activity which occurs during bleeding, haemolysis or staying in high altitudes. Similarly, iron absorption is reduced when erythropoiesis is depressed.

Plasma transferrin level—There is a correlation between unsaturated transferrin levels and iron absorption.

Humoral factors—Recent investigations suggest that there is a heat stable humoral factor which regulates iron absorption.

(c) **Mucosal cell factors**—After iron has been taken up by the mucosal cells, it is either bound to an intracellular protein resembling transferrin which carries across the mucosal cell to plasma or it is incorporated into ferritin in the epithelial cells. Iron requirement of the body regulates the iron absorption. Precise mechanism is still speculative. It could be a messenger iron from plasma that is incorporated in the epithelial cell, which in turn will synthesize ferritin and prevent the absorption of unnecessary iron which is eventually shed in the the G.I. tract. The cells in iron deficiency have no ferritin and in iron repletion body has abundant ferritin. The function of the ferritin is to trap absorbed iron into mucosal cells. In iron deficiency states with no intestinal ferritin, iron would pass unhindered into the body; conversely in iron overload, iron would be held back in the cell and be shed with it into the intestinal lumen at the end of its three-day life span. Recent experiments show that the synthesis of muscosal ferritin is controlled by the amount of iron in body iron stores. In man, there are two stages of iron absorption from the gut, *viz.*, a rapid stage starting 10 minutes after administration of an oral dose and lasting 3 to 4 hours and subsequent slow plasma phase lasting several hours. Absorbed iron is transported in the plasma bound to transferrin. The latter circulates in interstitial spaces and exchanges iron with all cells of the body. Normally transferrin iron is delivered to developing red cells. Iron liberated from transferrin and not taken up by young red cells, is incorporated into an intracellular exchangeable pool of low molecular weight complexes. This pool plays a vital role in the regulation of iron absorption and is in equilibrium with body iron pools. After having considered the salient points in the iron metabolism, it would now be proper to discuss various types of iron deficiency anaemia and their management.

## CHRONIC NUTRITIONAL HYPOCHROMIC ANAEMIA

It is the commonest type of anaemia in this country. Its widespread incidence is well recognised in all strata of the society but it is seen mostly in women, children and infants and in men belonging to the low socio-economic group.

### Causes of iron deficiency

Iron absorption may be inadequate which in turn may be due to low iron content in the diet or to an impairment of intestinal absorptive mechanism. On the other hand, loss of iron through haemorrhage may occur at a greater rate than replacement from a normal diet by a normal absorption mechanism. In women of the child-bearing age, this anaemia is seen more frequently because of enhanced demand for iron resulting from menstrual blood loss, foetal requirment and lactation. There may be insufficiency of iron in the diet also. Other causes in the country in both sexes are helminthiasis, especially ankylostomiasis, malabsorption syndrome, tropical sprue, parasprue, steatorrhoea and gastrointestinal bleeding. Gastrectomy is also responsible for iron deficiency anaemia.

### Clinical features

The symptoms are gradual and progressive unless treated. The general clinical features of anaemia already described (*vide supra*) will be seen along with other evidences of nutritional deficiencies like glossitis, angular stomatitis, koilonychia and dysphagia. The glossitis is usually referred to as chronic atrophic glossitis because of atrophy of the papillae and mucous membrane, makes the tongue smooth and glazed. The atrophy begins at the edges and later affects the whole tongue. Koilonychia or nail changes are seen as brittleness, dryness, flattening and thinning followed later on by concavity (spoon-shaped nail). Dysphagia occurs in severe cases. Post-cricoid dysphagia is the least common consequence of iron deficiency. This is occasionally associated with the presence of an oesophageal web. In a long-standing case, sometime spleen can become palpable. Hypochlorhydria or achlorhydria is commonly present. Paraesthesias may be complained of but no definite C.N.S. findings are detected. A combination of glossitis, dysphagia and anaemia is called Plummer-Vinson syndrome (Kelly-Paterson syndrome).

Blood examination shows a hypochromic, microcytic anaemia with an M.C.H.C. value less than 31%. Anisocytosis and poikilocytosis are present but not marked. Bone marrow shows normoblastic reaction. Serum iron level is low. Iron binding capacity (T.I.B.C.) is invariably raised. A raised T.I.B.C. is a useful diagnostic criterion since the only other disease in which it may be raised is viral hepatitis. T.I.B.C. is frequently reduced below normal in infection, neoplasm and rheumatoid arthritis and this helps to distinguish anaemia in these diseases from those due to iron deficiency. Percentage of transferrin that is bound to iron (i.e. serum iron concentration to T.I.B.C. expressed as a percentage) is a very useful index for the diagnosis of iron depletion.

**Diagnosis**

The differential diagnosis from other types of anaemia can be arrived at from the blood examination. Peripheral smears immediately suggest the diagnosis which is confirmed by an M.C.H.C. value less than 31%, low serum iron level, high T.I.B.C. and a reduced transferrin saturation. A value of 16 per cent or lower for the transferrin indicates lack of iron stores.

## HYPOCHROMIC ANAEMIA IN INFANCY AND CHILDHOOD

Iron deficiency is frequently found between the ages of 6 months and 5 years, the highest incidence being at the age of 12 months. There are two factors which predispose to iron deficiency in infancy, namely, inadequate iron stores at birth and inadequate amount of iron in the diet. Prolonged milk feeding especially breast-fed and artificially fed infants become anaemic due to iron deficiency. Low birth weight, nutritional anaemia in mother, infections in infants and intestinal malabsorptions are some other etiological factors which lead to iron deficiency. Clinical features are similar to those of adults, but are not easy to recognise. Anaemia leads to impairment of general health and vitality and an increased incidence of infection.

## IRON DEPLETION WITHOUT ANAEMIA

In recent years, this state has been well documented. The diagnosis of this stage can be made when the Hb concentration is within the normal range but the serum iron concentration is below normal and transferrin saturation is below 16 per cent. In pregnant women, the depletion of iron stores is the rule rather than the exception. It is generally agreed, however, that iron depletion without anaemia does not cause symptoms and there are no good reasons to treat these people with iron.

## TREATMENT OF IRON DEFICIENCY ANAEMIAS

In iron deficiency anaemia, there is a depletion of the body's usually considerable iron reserves. As a consequence, the iron through intestinal tract is rapidly absorbed. Ferrous salts are more effective than ferric salts. Treatment should start with oral administration of ferrous sulphate (600 mgm) which contains 120 mgm of elemental iron daily in 3 daily doses after meals. This is the cheapest and safest method. To replenish the depleted body stores, administration of iron should continue for 4-6 months after the haemoglobin has become normal. Patient should be warned that the stool will be black. If the response to this dose is not adequate, then the following should be considered.

(a) The patient has not taken the tablets. One of the common reasons advanced by patients that the tablets cause gastro-intestinal symptoms such as pain, diarrhoea or constipation. These patients who cannot tolerate the ferrous sulphate, other types of preparations like ferrous carbonate, chloride, fumarate, gluconate or succinate can be tried. All these preparations are equally effective.

(b) That patient has malabsorption syndrome. In such patient iron may be injected I.M. or I.V. in dose of 100-250 mgm daily. Ferrivenin is suitable for the I.V. route whilst Imferon and Jactofer (iron sorbital-citric acid) are efficient and well tolerated by I.M. route. Another preparation, Iron Polymaltose (Ferrum Hausmann) has also been used for parenteral therapy. In order to cut down the hospital stay and to avoid repeated injection to pregnant women especially within a limited time that is available before labour or operation, many workers have tried giving infusion of total dose of iron in one sitting (T.D.I.). But because of many side effects which have been reported, treatment by T.D.I. should not be taken lightly. Total amount of iron required can be calculated as :

(Normal Hb — patients Hb) × 0.255
= gm. Iron required.

(c) That initial dose was incorrect or that $B_{12}$ or folate deficiency is also present. It should be remembered that there is a high incidence of overt or latent folic acid deficiency in pregnancy and this usually manifests when haemoglobin level reaches 7-8 gms per cent. Some Indian firms have brought out intramuscular iron preparations combined with folic acid.

(d) If the iron deficiency was due to haemorrhage, the bleeding may still continue from the gut.

A rise of 1% Hb level per day is expected and in an average case blood level is restored in 4 to 8 week's time. The purpose of the treatment with iron is not only to restore the red cell volume to normal but also to replenish iron stores. The former is easy but the latter is difficult. If the patient absorbs 10 per cent of 120 mgm iron ingested each day as ferrous sulphate then it will take approximately three months to raise the iron stores to about 1g. In practice it has been found that the percentage of iron absorbed is often less than this and the patient should therefore be persuaded to continue taking iron for 6 months. Failure rate with oral iron therapy is high because of not taking the tablets regularly. Iron medication should be supplemented by a well-balanced diet. There are a large number of iron and folic acid preparations in the market. These are costly and should not be used in pure iron deficiency anaemias. The addition of trace elements like copper, manganese and cobalt is of no clinical value. When the Hb is below 5 g per 100 ml. it is normally advisable to keep the patient in bed. Whether to transfuse blood or not will be decided on the clinical condition of the case.

**In infants** the treatment of iron deficiency anaemia requires the administration of a liquid iron preparation as well as introduction of iron containing food in the diet. The dose should be about 6 mgm iron per mg body wt. daily.

## POST HAEMORRHAGIC IRON DEFICIENCY ANAEMIA

It may be acute or chronic.

**Acute**—Sudden loss of a large volume of blood more than 1 litre due to trauma or bleeding can lead to haemodilution during the recovery phase which is reflected by a fall in Hb level and red cell count. When the circulating blood volume is partially restored, the acute symptoms of shock subside. During convalescence, general symptoms and signs of anaemia may be present. During recovery, the red cells are formed more rapidly than Hb and the M.C.H.C. falls unless adequate iron is available. Treatment consists of bed rest, blood transfusion of adequate amount to restore the blood volume and combat the oligaemic shock. The cause of the blood loss should be sought and treated. Iron, afterwards, should be given.

**Chronic**—Anaemia results from repeated loss of small amounts of blood. Common causes are bleeding peptic ulcer, piles, carcinoma, ankylostomiasis or menorrhagia. Frequent medication with aspirin can also cause alimentary bleeding. Frequent and persistent blood loss can cause a progressive fall in Hb. The clinical and haematological features are similar to those found in chronic nutritional hypochromic anaemia. In addition, the clincial features of the causative disorder will be present. Treatment is to arrest the source of blood loss by appropriate measures where possible and the administration of iron and a good diet.

## SIDEROBLASTIC ANAEMIA

Abnormal utilisation of iron with failure of haem synthesis by the marrow may cause a refractory anaemia. In this condition, there is a peripheral blood picture of chronic iron deficiency anaemia with excessive accumulation of iron containing granules in the erythroblasts and reticulocytes of the bone marrow and haemosiderosis of the liver and other tissues. The condition may be congenital or acquired. The congenital form is sex-linked and found in boys. Iron therapy does not help. The secondary type may be caused by drugs such as isoniazid or be associated with chronic general diseases. Some cases respond to treatment with pyridoxine, Vit C and folic acid. Those who do not respond to above therapy, blood transfusion is the only treatment which should be given very cautiously to avoid transfusion siderosis.

## MEGALOBLASTIC ANAEMIA

Occurs due to deficiency of Vit $B_{12}$ or folic acid or both. Deficiencies of both vitamin $B_{12}$ and folate produce identical changes in cells of bone marrow and peripheral blood. Normal erythropoiesis is changed to a megaloblastic character. In the peripheral blood, red cells are macrocytic (Pl. I, Fig. 4.4). The megaloblasts in the marrow are larger and have a fine reticular structure of the nucleus than normal red cell precursors (Pl. I, Fig. 4.2). Causes of megaloblastic anaemia are—

(i) Due to lack or defective production of intrinsic factor as in Addisonian pernicious anaemia. Total or partial gastrectomy also leads to a deficiency of Vit $B_{12}$.

(ii) Poor nutrition or diet leading to nutritional megaloblastic anaemia where chief deficiency being folic acid.

(iii) Resection, short circuit or disease of small intestine.

(iv) Blind loop syndrome or jejunal diverticulosis where there is an abnormal growth of bacteria which utilises Vit $B_{12}$ leading to its deficiency.

(v) Pregnancy where there is a higher requirement of folic acid and at the same time patient suffers from anorexia and vomiting *pari passu* with a low food intake.

(vi) Due to drugs like methotrexate and cytosine arabinoside which interferes with dihydrofolate reductase system or DNA synthesis or anticonvulsant drugs like phenytoin sodium or pirimidone.

Vit $B_{12}$ acts as a co-enzyme and helps in the synthesis of methionine. Although Vit $B_{12}$ is required for the proper functioning of every cell, signs and symptoms of deficiency are usually seen in haematological, gastrointestinal and neurological systems. Vit $B_{12}$ is produced entirely by intestinal bacteria and none is present in plants. Man gets this Vit $B_{12}$ also by eating animal food. Vit $B_{12}$ is absorbed through distal half of small intestine after combining with the intrinsic factor. Intrinsic factor is produced in the stomach by the parietal cells which produce HCL. Daily requirement of Vit $B_{12}$ is about 3-5 $\mu$g and the normal diet contains an excess of Vit $B_{12}$. This vitamin is mainly stored in the liver and an average healthy adult has a total body content of about 3 mgm. Loss of Vit $B_{12}$ takes place through desquamation of epithelium and through excretion in bile. Rate of loss of Vit $B_{12}$ is approximately 0.1 per cent of the total body content each day. The factors which cause deficiency of Vit $B_{12}$ are failure to secrete the intrinsic factor and a failure to absorb Vit $B_{12}$ as a result of abnormalities of ileum. Folic acid or pteroylglutamic acid is absorbed mainly in the proximal half of the small intestine and is converted into an active form (tetrahydrofolate) in the body by reduction. The active form acts as a co-enzyme in the purine and pyrimidine synthesis for the formation of DNA and RNA. The chief cause of folate deficiency in pregnancy is greatly increased DNA and RNA synthesis associated with growth of fetus, placenta and uterus and increased red cell volume of mother. Folate requirements increase three times during pregnancy. Several other factors also play a part in the production of folate deficiency in pregnancy like anorexia and vomiting along with a reduced food intake. Folate deficiency also occurs in malabsorption syndrome where it is associated with iron and Vit $B_{12}$ deficiencies. Failure to absorb folate may occur in regional ileitis or resection of jejunum where it is absorbed chiefly.

## NUTRITIONAL MEGALOBLASTIC ANAEMIA & MEGALOBLASTIC ANAEMIA OF PREGNANCY

This is seen commonly in tropical countries including India due to dietary deficiency mainly of folic acid. The anaemia is made worse during pregnancy. The disease is most common in second and third decades. Though folic acid deficiency is the main causative factor, in some of the cases Vit $B_{12}$ also may be required thereby causing a dual deficiency anaemia. Symptoms are mostly due to anaemia. Diarrhoea and vomiting may occur but are usually due to an intercurrent infection to which subjects are particularly liable. Sore tongue is relatively uncommon and C.N.S. symptoms have not been described. Oedema of the feet and ankle, a low blood pressure, cardiac haemic murmurs and fever are common. Blood changes—The anaemia is megalocytic (Pl. I, Fig. 4). The R.B.C. count is reduced more than haemoglobin, so the colour index, M.C.H., M.C.V., all are high whilst the M.C.H.C. is normal. There may be some thrombocytopenia, sometime there is leucopenia. In uncomplicated cases, serum iron is normal or high and T.I.B.C. is depressed and the bone marow haemosiderin is increased. The bone marow is megaloblastic (Pl. I, Fig. 2) There may be giant metamyelocytes, hypersegmented granulocytes and twin nucleated granulocytes. Megakaryocytes are usually reduced and show depression of platelet formation.

Treatment—Folic acid in doses of 15 mgm to 20 mgm or more a day is the treatment of choice and causes a rapid and satisfactory response. Some cases need both Vit $B_{12}$ and folic acid for complete recovery. Relapses should be prevented by providing adequate diet containing 100 g of protein preferably derived from meat, fish or eggs.

## MEGALOBLASTIC ANAEMIA DUE TO PATHOLOGICAL CONDITIONS OF G.I. TRACT

It is seen in tropical sprue and para sprue, and idiopathic steatorrhoea. The anaemia in these conditions is due to failure of absorption of folate or Vit $B_{12}$ or both.

Anaemia can also occur subsequent to resection or short circuiting of a large segment of the small intestine. Vit $B_{12}$ is only absorbed from the lower portion of the ileum whereas folate is mainly absorbed through proximal half of small intestine.

Clinical picture is mainly that of the underlying condition along with general symptoms of anaemia. Achlorhydria is uncommon. Folate level in the blood and urine is measured by means of microbiological assay after giving a large dose of folic acid orally.

Vit $B_{12}$ absorption is measured by giving the fasting patient a small dose of Vit $B_{12}$ labelled with radioactive cobalt. A large dose of non-radioactive Vit $B_{12}$ is injected two hours after and urine is collected for 24 hours. Radioactivity of urine is then measured. In normal subjects more than 16 per cent of the oral dose should be excreted in urine. In P.A., when the radioactive $B_{12}$ is given with an intrinsic factor, excretion is more than 16 per cent whereas in a malabsorption case, the result is low due to the diseased ileum. In tropical sprue and para sprue, folic acid therapy produces excellent response. It should be given I.M. for first two or three days and orally in a dosage of 20 mgm a day thereafter. Vit $B_{12}$ should also be given. Iron may also become necessary. If anaemia is due to resection or short circuiting of a large segment of small intestine, then the primary deficiency is Vit $B_{12}$ which should be administered in large doses.

## ADDISONIAN PERNICIOUS ANAEMIA

It is uncommon in our country but is the commonest type of megaloblastic anaemia in Western countries. It is due to failure of secretion of the intrinsic factor. This disease affects the females more than males between the ages of 40 and 65 years.

**Clinical manifestations**—It is commonly observed that degree of anaemia is quite considerable before the patient consults the doctor. In addition to the symptoms due to anaemia, patient complains of soreness of tongue and occasional diarrhoea. Four most common presenting symptoms are weakness, dyspnoea, paraesthesia and sore tongue. Apart from pallor, the most common sign is atrophic glossitis. Fever is seen in some percentage (22%) of cases and spleen is seldom enlarged.

In about 7% of cases, neurological features are also seen. The usual syndrome described is sub-acute combined degeneration of the cord as posterior and lateral columns are both affected. Dementia may also occur. Gastric analysis invariably shows achlorhydria which is histamine or pentagastrin fast.

Peripheral blood shows a macrocytic anaemia. M.C.V. is increased and M.C.H.C. is normal. There is marked anisocytosis and poikilocytosis (Pl. I, Figs. 8 & 9). Serum bilirubin is raised. There is leucopenia, reduction involving the granulocytes which are mature, some having more lobes than five in their nuclei (hypersegmented). There is also thrombocytopenia.

**Treatment**—Hydroxycobalamine should be given in a dose of 1000 microgram two to three times a week in the first week and then once a week until blood count becomes normal. Then 100-1000 $\mu$g IM daily once a month for the patient's lifetime

If sub-acute combined degeneration of cord is present, then patient should be given 1000 microgram of Vit $B_{12}$ twice weekly for about six months and then switching over to monthly injections.

It is important that a patient of pernicious anaemia is given a maintenance therapy of Vit $B_{12}$, 1000 microgram every four to eight weeks for the rest of his life. Oral $B_{12}$—intrinsic preparation is not recommended for the treatment of P.A.

### Megaloblastic anaemia due to drugs

Drugs as earlier stated (Page 68, vi) interfere with the dihydrofolate reductase mechanism. Therefore, folic acid should be given for treatment. When anticonvulsant drugs are given, simultaneous folic acid therapy should also be given to the patient.

## MEGALOBLASTIC ANAEMIA IN INFANCY

Infants whose diet is deficient in proteins, folate and ascorbic acid and who are suffering from infection and diarrhoea may become anaemic which is megaloblastic or dimorphic in character. In India, this type of anaemia in infants is due to protein calorie malnutrition. This anaemia responds to folic acid along with a good high protein diet.

## THE HAEMOLYTIC ANAEMIAS

Whenever there is an increased destruction of red cells, haemolytic anaemia results. This anaemia may be due to an intracorpuscular defect or due to an extracorpuscular abnormality. Anaemia will occur if destruction exceeds the regeneration of red cells. In this condition there will be an increased reticulocytosis and an increase in serum bilirubin level. Peripheral smear will show schistocytes and nucleated red cells. There may be microspherocytes (Pl. I, Fig. 7). Target cells (Pl. I, Fig. 10A). may be seen in cases of haemoglobinopathies. Osmotic fragility may be increased in some cases. Antiglobulin test will be positive in acquired haemolytic anaemias.

**Classification of Haemolytic Anaemia :**

1. **Intracorpuscular defects :**
   Hereditary spherocytosis
   Hereditary ovalocytosis or elliptocytosis
   Haemoglobinopathies like sickle cell anaemia, thalassaemia,
   E-thalassaemia and other disorders like HbC, HbD, HbH
   G-6-PD deficiency or other enzyme deficiency
   Paroxysmal nocturnal haemoglobinuria
2. **Extracorpuscular abnormality** (infective, toxic, allergic or associated with other diseases)
   Immune acquired haemolytic anaemia (warm or cold) types
   Haemolytic disease of the new-born
   Drug induced haemolytic anaemia
   Incompatible blood transfusion
   Due to burns, lead or infection

## HEREDITARY SPHEROCYTOSIS
### (Acholuric Jaundice)

It is an inherited disorder of red cells where the red cells are abnormal in shape being spherocytic and rigid. The defect is in the red cell membrane which permits the sodium to move easily inside the cell along with chloride and water. The sodium pump mechanism is at fault in this disease. Such cells are more fragile and get destroyed in the splenic sinuses. When the rate of destruction exceeds that of regeneration from the bone marrow, anaemia occurs.

Usually, the symptoms start in childhood. But in some cases, the symptoms are mild in childhood but become evident when the patient becomes adult in the form of anaemia or mild persistent jaundice. Occasionally, patient may come with symptoms of gall stones. On examination, an enlarged spleen directs the suspicion towards the disease.

Sometime patient comes with crises when the anaemia becomes severe and is accompained by fever and other constitutional symptoms. Crises often occurs following infection but may occur without any cause. Ulceration of leg occurs occasionally in a long-standing case.

Blood picture shows anaemia with an increased reticulocyte count. Peripheral smear shows large number of microspherocytes which is fairly diagnostic. Increased osmotic fragility confirms the diagnosis. Family history is also very important for diagnosis. Red cells labelled with 51 Cr show themselves to have short life and an increased uptake in the spleen.

Treatment is by splenectomy. Improvement is seen immediately and anaemia disappears. It is indicated in all those cases who have symptoms. Though the spherocytes still persist in the blood, splenectomy removes the danger of early destruction of spherocytes. Splenectomy in children may be deferred till the child is 6 yeats old. Operation should be carried out during a period of remission and not in crises.

## HEREDITARY ELLIPTOCYTOSIS OR OVALOCYTOSIS

It is an inherited autosomal disorder where the red cells are elliptical or oval. It is not a common disorder and produces mild symptoms of haemolytic anaemia. Spleen is often palpable. Splenectomy often results in a clinical cure.

## HAEMOGLOBINOPATHIES OR ABNORMAL HAEMOGLOBIN DISORDERS

Adult haemoglobin—A ($\alpha_2\beta_2$) comprising 98 per cent of total Hb consists of four polypeptide chains, two alpha and two beta chains. There is also 1 to 3 per cent $A_2$ in adult blood consisting of two alpha and 2 delta chains ($\alpha_2\ \delta_2$). Hb A is written as $\alpha_2^A\ \beta_2^A$. In foetus, the Hb F has two alpha chains and two gamma chains ($\alpha_2\ \gamma_2$). There are 141 amino acids in alpha chain and 146 amino acids in beta chain.

There are 3 types of Hb disorders that one meets with: (1) there is an alteration in the amino acid sequence or structure of the polypeptide chain as in sickle cell anaemia, (ii) the amino acid sequence is normal, but the rate of production is impaired or absent as in thalassaemias, (iii) there is persistence of Hb F in the adult life. More than 100 varieties of haemoglobinopathies have been described but most of them are rare. In India commonest haemoglobinopathy is thalassaemia and in West Bengal, E-thalassaemia. Sickle cell anaemia has been described amongst tribals and aborigines of India. Other haemoglobin disorders like D, J, L. Q and M have also been described. We will only consider thalassaemia as it is the commonest and sickle cell anaemia because of its importance amongst tribal population.

**Thalassaemia :** It is commonest haemoglobinopathy in India. In eastern part, it is E-thalassaemia and in western India it is $\beta$-thalassaemia or sickle cell-thalassaemia or a combination with other Hb disorders. In all of them, there is a decreased rate of synthesis of beta chains. Heterozygotes are called thalassaemia minor and the homozygotes, thalassaemia major. There is a wide spectrum of severity in thalassaemia ranging from normal haemoglobin concentration on one hand to still birth on the other. In thalassaemia minor, disability is much less whereas in major, manifestation of disease could be very great, though there is a wide variability in manifestations. In $\beta$-thalassaemia, there is little or no Hb A, there is an increase in $A_2$ which helps in the diagnosis and also that of Hb F.

Patients of thalassaemia major are very anaemic and depend entirely on packed red cell transfusion for survival. Because of persistent bone marrow hyperplasia, there is osteoporosis, may be even pathological fracture, head bossing, prominent malar eminences giving rise to Mongoloid facies.

Patients are often stunted, puberty is greatly delayed but they are normally intelligent. Mild jaundice may be present. Splenomegaly is an important sign and it could be large enough to cause abdominal distension and discomfort. They are susceptible to infection. Leg ulcer and gallstones can occur. X-ray of skull shows hair-on-end appearance. Extramedullary haemopoiesis can occur which causes spinal cord compression. Liver is enlarged much later but more quickly if splenectomy is carried out early.

Blood picture often is similar to severe iron deficiency anaemia. Target cells are seen in fair number. Normoblasts (esp. late variety) are present. Osmotic fragility shows increased resistance. Bone marrow aspiration shows normoblastic hyperplasia.

Diagnosis is confirmed by Hb electrophoresis.

**Treatment :—** Repeated packed red cell or washed red cell transfusion is the mainstay of the treatment. Iron deposition which was seen in earlier years producing ultimately haemosiderosis, could be avoided by using iron chelating agent like desferrioxamine. Present trend is to keep the haemoglobin at a higher level of 10-12 gm/dl to allow proper development. Splenectomy may be considered when it is huge and causing mechanical difficulties or hypersplenism. Splenectomy should only be considered after the age of 6 years. As there is folic acid deficiency it is advisable to give folic acid in higher dosage along with other members of Vitamin B Complex group.

## SICKLE CELL HAEMOGLOBINOPATHIES

The importance of Hb-S is for its clinical severity. In homozygous Hb-S, the sickle cell anaemia, most patients die in infancy or within first 10 years of life. It is seen amongst the aboriginal tribes of India, especially those of Nilgiri Hills of south India like Irules, Kothas, Kurumba and Toda aboriginals. It is also seen in aboriginals of Orissa, central India, Gond, Goshti of western India. Tribal groups from Gujarat, U.P., Bastar district of Madhya Pradesh also show sickle cell trait.

Clinical manifestation is uncommon during first six months of life. When the foetal haemoglobin gets replaced, clinical symptoms develop which is evident as anaemia and jaundice in early childhood. Repeated debilitating crises lasting 5 to 7 days are usually associated with shock and prostration and may simulte a perforation of abdominal organ or other surgical emergencies localising either in abdomen or bones or joints. Spleen is often enlarged in early stages but may shrink later on due to repeated infarction. Bacterial infection is the commonest cause of early childhood morbidity and mortality. The hand-foot syndrome is due to micro-infection of medulla of the carpal and tarsal bones. Overlying skin is tender and swollen with a rise in temperature. The lesion is symmetrical and healed without therapy but may recur. When pooling of blood suddenly occurs in the spleen, splenic sequestration syndrome in the form of oligaemic shock occurs. Blood transfusion can only save the life. There may occur cerebral, pulmonary or vascular accidents due to occlusion of vessels by sickled cells. Aplastic crises can occur due to sudden cessation of marrow activity due to an infection. Gallstone and leg ulcer are common. Liver is often enlarged, spleen in adult is not palpable. Cardiac complications are common; skeletal X-rays show often rarefaction and osteoporosis. Aseptic necrosis of femoral or humoral head may occur due to repeated bone infection and may cause severe arthritis

**Blood Picture**—Anaemia is often severe due to reduction of red cell life span. The anaemia is normocytic normochromic. There may be elongated cells in the smear or sickle cells. Cover slip preparation confirms sickling. Hb electrophoresis confirms the diagnosis.

**Treatment** of sickle cell anaemia consists of proper management, especially, of painful crises by complete rest, use of analgesics, early treatment by appropriate antibiotics and partial exchange transfusion. No specific treatment has yet been evolved for sickling disorder, though urea in high doses and cyanates have been tried to prevent sickling. Cyanate therapy shows some success in this field but has the drawback of several toxic symptoms and is still in the trial stage.

## G-6-P D DEFICIENCY

(Glucose-6-Phosphate dehydrogenase deficiency)

It is an inherited disorder which is transmitted by a sex-linked gene of intermediate dominance. Males are always full reactors and intermediate expression is seen in a female when she is heterozygous.

Amongst Indians, 5 to 9 per cent are G-6-PD deficient. Whenever any oxidising drug like aspirin, quinine, chloromycetin, sulphonamide group, primaquin or any such drug is taken, oxidised Hb cannot be reduced back due to the absence of the enzyme G-6-PD. Such oxidised red cells are unstable and break down producing an acute haemolytic episode. The severity of the haemolytic episode, in general, is related to the dose of the drug. Patient may become jaundiced. The haemolytic episode is self-limiting. When the incriminating drug is withdrawn, the haemolysis stops. New-borns, who are G-6-PD deficient, may have severe degrees of jaundice necessitating even exchange transfusion. Such cases may be mistaken for Rh incompatibility. Predisposing factor in them is mostly some infection, bacterial or viral.

**Laboratory test for diagnosis** :—Common screening tests for G-6-PD deficiency are brilliant cresyl blue dye test or methaemoglobin reduction test.

Other enzyme deficiencies like pyruvate kinase producing haemolytic anaemia have also been reported, but they are very rare.

## PAROXYSMAL NOCTURNAL HAEMOGLOBINURIA (PNH)

In this condition, there is an acquired defect of the red cell membrane which renders them unusually sensitive to the complement of normal serum. Because of it, there is haemolytic anaemia with haemoglobinuria and also haemosiderinuria along with leucopenia and thrombocytopenia. Haemolytic crises are common with crises of haemoglobinuria, especially during sleep. Increased haemolysis in the night may be due to changes in the pH of blood because of retention of $CO_2$ during sleep. PNH has definite relationship with aplastic anaemia. Occasionally acute leukaemia following PNH has also been described. Diagnosis of the disorder is by seeing haemoglobinuria in the urine and confirmation by acid serum test (Ham's test) and sucrose lysis test. Treatment is to give blood transfusion during the episodes of haemoglobinuria. Because of occasional haemolytic reaction following transfusion, due to the activation of complement by a factor in the donor plasma, it ia advisable to give packed red cells or washed packed red cells.

## PAROXYSMAL COLD HAEMOGLOBINURIA

This occurs due to a cold auto-haemolysin and is related to syphilis, often of congenital type. It is usually cured by antisyphilitic treatment.

## ACQUIRED HAEMOLYTIC ANAEMIA

(Immune Haemolytic Anaemia)

There are two types either due to warm or cold agglutinins.

### Warm Immune Haemolytic Anaemia

This is due to warm antibody of Ig G type reacting with red cells at 37°C. It could be either idiopathic or following lymphoma, chronic lymphatic leukaemia, multiple myeloma, acute leukaemia or collagen disorder like S.L.E., Polyarteritis nodosa or Rheumatoid arthritis. It could also be due to drugs. Patients report with anaemia, hepatosplenomegaly and often mild icterus. Peripheral smear examination shows evidences of haemolytic anaemia, spherocytosis and reticulocytosis. Diagnosis is confirmed by direct antiglobin test (Coomb's). Treatment is usually with corticosteroids. In severe cases, most compatible red cell transfusion is given taking into consideration patient's ABO and Rh group, as crossmatching is difficult. Majority patients achieve remission with a high dose of prednisolone 60 to 100 mgm daily. 30% resistant cases may need splenectomy. Some 10 per cent cases who are resistant to cortico-steroids and splenectomy, may need cytotoxic drug like cyclophosphamide or imuran to achieve remission.

### Cold Immune Haemolytic Anaemia

This disorder is due to an IgM complement fixing antibody. It acts best at 4°C and leaves the red cell surface at warmer temperature. Normally, it is present in low titres (1:32) but in patients suffering from this anaemia, titre goes up as high as 1:150,000 at 4°C. Because of high titre, it starts acting at body temperature producing haemolytic anaemia. It was seen classically in Indian soldiers moving from plains to high altitude and very cold climate as Leh. The first symptoms to appear are Raynaud's phenomenon, acrocyanosis, especially during the winter. They complain of weakness and dizziness. In some cases, there may be hepatosplenomegaly and in severe cases, icterus. Direct antiglobin test will be positive for complement components but negative for immunoglobulin. Therefore, the human antiglobulin serum should be a broad-based one with complement antibodies. The test has to be carried out keeping all equipment including syringes at 37°C, otherwise antibodies will be absorbed into red cells at room temperature.

Treatment is unsatisfactory. Patient should be protected from cold and given blood transfusion. If necessary, corticosteroid therapy may be tried but is usually ineffective. Few cases with very high titre may respond.

## HAEMOLYTIC DISEASE OF NEW-BORN

(Erythroblastosis foetalis)

This is due to blood group incompatibility, mostly due to ABO group but is also seen due to Rh incompatibility between parents.

In ABO, the mother usually belongs to O group and father belongs to any other group excepting O.

In Rh incompatibility, mother is rhesus negative (Rh or D negative) and father is rhesus positive (Rh or D positive). Due to earlier sensitisation either through transfusion or previous child birth, mother forms Rh antibodies which are of IgG type and can cross the placental barrier. These antibodies combine with Rh positive cells of foetus in utero and cause haemolysis. Usually the first born child escapes any morbidity but subsequent ones may suffer. Very severe haemolysis produces hydrops foetalis or still birth. Less severe one is the cause of erythroblastosis foetalis where the peripheral blood of the neonate shows large number of erythroblasts. Present nomenclature is Haemolytic Diseases of the New-born (HDN). ABO incompatibility in marriage can produce HDN but the morbidity and mortality are less severe than Rh incompatibility. The baby is born with jaundice, peripheral smear shows erythroblasts and reticulocytosis, Hb is less than normal, serum bilirubin is high and direct antiglobin test is positive. Treatment is by exchange transfusion in all severe cases. In recent years, Rh negative mothers (not sensitised) and primipara are given high titre anti-D immunoglobin intramuscularly within 72 hours of delivery. By adopting this procedure, it has been possible to prevent sensitization of Rh negative mother following child birth.

## ACUTE HAEMOLYTIC ANAEMIA FOLLOWING INCOMPATIBLE BLOOD TRANSFUSION :

A mismatched or incompatible blood may be transfused due to (i) clerical error, (ii) technical fault, (iii) wrong labelling and (iv) nursing error. Whenever such wrongly matched blood is transfused, patient complains of warm sensation along the vein, severe constriction in the chest, pain in the back and loin. If sufficient quantity has been transfused, then it may lead to haemoglobinuria, oliguria leading to anuria. Immediately on detecting the error or onset of the symptoms, compatible blood should be transfused. Quantity should be twice the amount of incompatible blood transfused. Idea is to prevent renal ischaemia and acute cortical necrosis. Most, if not all, patients, make a miraculous recovery following compatible blood transfusion.

Procedure for investigation of a case of haemolytic anaemia has been discussed in detail in the chapter dealing with investigation of anaemia which may be referred to (Pages 79, 81, 82, 83, IV).

## ANAEMIAS DUE TO APLASIA OR HYPOPLASIA OF THE BONE MARROW

Here the anaemia is due to a failure of bone marrow to regenerate cells. Marrow shows varying degrees of hypocellularity to complete aplasia. The condition is refractory to treatment. In few cases, bone marrow may show normal cellularity or hypercellularity. There may be failure of one or two types of the cell especially affecting the granular series of cells or thrombocytes. When all the cells are affected, pancytopenia results.

About half or more cases of bone marrow failure develop without cause. Rarely there are congenital or familial pancytopaenia in children (Fanconi syndrome), bone marrow failure with thymoma or with paroxysmal nocturnal haemoglobinuria. Agents responsible for bone marrow depression fall into two categories.

(a) Those which regularly produce bone marrow damage if a sufficient dose is given. They are ionising radiations, radioactive elements, benzene and its derivatives, cytotoxic agents, antimetabolites and other toxic agents like inorganic arsenicals.

(b) Agents occasionally associated with bone marrow damage :

| | |
|---|---|
| Antibiotics | Chloramphenicol, streptomycin, sulphonamides |
| Anticonvulsants | Mesantoin, tridione, phenylacetylurea, dilantin |
| Antirheumatic drugs | Phenylbutazone, gold salts. |
| Other drugs | Mepacrine, acetazolamide, organic arsenicals, bismuth, mercury, carbon tetrachloride, chlorpropamide, carbimazole, insecticides, hairdyes, chlorpromazine. |

**Clinical features**—The symptoms may appear suddenly when marrow aplasia is secondary to radiation or antimitotic treatment. In idiopathic cases the onset is usually insidious, with severe anaemia, weakness, fatigue, dyspnoea, palpitation, pounding headache and fever. Infections become a serious problem associated with severe granulocytopenia. A low platelet count is frequently attended by bleeding. Lymph nodes and spleen are usually not enlarged but splenomegaly may develop after many transfusions due to transfusion siderosis. Blood picture shows a normochromic normocytic anaemia with low leucocyte and platelet counts but without any nucleated cells or reticulocytosis. Bone marrow may be hypocellular, normocellular or hypercellular, the latter can be explained on the basis of ineffective haematopoiesis. Serum iron is elevated, iron binding capacity is moderately reduced. Differentiation from subleukaemic leukaemia or myelophthisic anaemia is made by bone marrow examination. This differentiation may be difficult but LAP (leukocyte alkaline phosphatase) stain of peripheral film and chromosomal study for Philadelphia chromosome may be helpful.

**Treatment**—Prevention of exposure to a possible toxic agent should be the first aim of treatment. In most instances, however, the evidence on which a drug is incriminated is purely circumstantial. The patient should be advised against the use of hair dyes, insecticides, plant sprays and all drugs except those specifically prescribed. The medication should be kept simple and potential marrow toxic drugs should be avoided.

Supportive care consists of careful mouth hygiene, caution against picking the nose, use of a soft tooth-brush, avoidance of intramuscular or subcutaneous injections, care of arm veins and avoidance of constipation. Antimicrobial therapy should be given for the treatment of specific infections. Blood transfusion should be type specific and given only when Hb level has fallen below 8 gms/dl. Two or three units of blood can be given on successive days after two to three weeks. The development of transfusion haemosiderosis and of sensitisation to minor blood groups, leucocytes or platelets is thus postponed as long as possible. Platelet transfusions and corticosteroids help in the haemorrhagic manifestations and in thrombocytopaenia.

Corticosteroids, i.e. prednisolone 20 to 40 mg per day and testosterone preparation like oxymetholone (4-5 mg/kg body weight daily orally) are known to induce remissions in the children and adults.

Oxymetholone should be continued for several months, but the dosage should be halved when there is evidence of remission. Treatment with blood transfusion, oral antibiotics and haematinics should be continued for at least six months before being abandoned.

Splenectomy should be of value if the spleen is enlarged and is destroying cells at an accelerated rate or if it is depressing the bone marrow function.

In pure red cell aplasia, the use of immunosuppressive drugs like cyclophosphamide, or 6-mercaptopurine may induce a remission. If thymoma is present, thymectomy may help. Bone marrow transplantation should be tried in aplastic anaemia when all other measures have failed. In some centres, bone marrow transplantation is being carried out earlier because of successful results. Recent results suggest that bone marrow transplantation has become the treatment of choice in cases of aplastic anaemia. Best result is obtained from a twin, otherwise from an HLA matched family member. As the marrow transplantation is best with immunological problems; only centres having the expertise and facilities to manage Graft versus Host reaction should carry out the marrow transplantation. Recent reports suggest successful use of antithymocyte globulin injections in some cases.

## SYMPTOMATIC OR SECONDARY ANAEMIA

Most infectious and chronic systemic diseases such as renal or hepatic disease, rheumatoid arthritis, the connective tissue disorders, malnutrition, malignancy, lymphomas, and endocrine deficiencies, are accompanied by anaemia during the course of illness. Usually it is mild, but can be severe in leukaemia and renal failure. In most cases the anaemia is normocytic and normochromic, occasionally it may be microcytic and also hypochromic. In general, the pathogenesis of anaemia can be explained by a combination of mild haemolytic component with decreased erythropoiesis or relative bone marrow failure. In renal disease, anaemia increases with rise in blood urea above 70 mg/dl though there is no precise correlation with urea retention. There is reduced span of red cells; sometimes frank haemolytic process occurs when microangiopathy is present. Haemorrhage often makes a contribution terminally but the prime mechanism is marrow failure. The anaemia of hepatic disease is frequently complicated by chronic blood loss and in patients with alcoholic cirrhosis by folate deficiency. After elimination of iron and folate deficiencies, normocytic anaemias remain. Increased plasma volume exaggerates the depression of erythrocyte value by haemodilution. The anaemia in endocrinopathies is attributed to general hypometabolism. The causes of anaemia in a widespread malignant disease are many and varied. Loss of appetite, malabsorption or blood loss from the G.I. tract or increased haemolysis are some of the factors. Further metastasis in the bone marrow may cause myelophthisic anaemia. The term "myelophthisic anaemia" is applied to those anaemias associated with space occupying lesions of the bone marrow. The anaemia may be moderate to severe, the white blood cell count may be elevated or depressed; thrombocytopenia may or may not be present. Normoblasts are found in the peripheral blood often in large numbers; young granulocytes may also be seen but are less prominent. Red blood cell survival is shortened, and the anaemia is caused because the bone marrow, although stimulated, does not increase erythrocyte production enough to compensate for the haemolysis. The old idea that normal marrow is crowded out by the invading cells is no longer tenable. The diagnosis should be suspected whenever there occurs leucoerythroblastic anaemia, i.e. immature red cells and white cells appear in the peripheral blood. The number of nucleated red blood cells present is out of proportion to the degree of anaemia. Treatment and prognosis depend on the causative disorder.

## INVESTIGATION IN A CASE OF ANAEMIA

While investigating a case of anaemia, fundamental questions that need to be answered are :—

1. Is the patient anaemic ?
2. What is the type of anaemia ?
3. What is the exact cause for this anaemia ?

In order to answer the above-mentioned three questions correct investigations of any anaemic patient consist of two types of examination.

1. Clinical examination.
2. Haematological examination.

These will be discussed in detail keeping in view the above-mentioned three questions which need to be answered before a case could properly be diagnosed and treated.

### CLINICAL EXAMINATION

**It consists of :—**

(a) Present history,
(b) Personal and social history,
(c) Past history,
(d) Family history, and
(e) Physical examination.

(a) **Present history**

In most cases, a patient is suspected to be anaemic from his or her present complaints like tiredness, lassitude, easy fatigability, weakness, lack of concentration, dyspnoea on slight or moderate exertion, tingling or numbness in the extremities and, rarely, pallor. If any of the above symptoms is present, than the patient is suffering from anaemia.

It must also be remembered that chronic anaemia, especially of iron deficiency, slowly mainfests itself. Therefore, the patient's body has enough time to adapt its vital organs to a lower level of oxygen and may not be complaining of any general ill-health till the haemoglobin level has really fallen below 8 gms per dl. This is classically seen in our country amongst multipara women during their pregnancy and also in large number of people belonging to the weakest economic stratum of our society. It may not often be possible to diagnose anaemia from the clinical history alone and laboratory examination has to be resorted to confirm the same. Clinical history is also very important in cases where anaemia has already been established. It frequently gives an indication as to the cause for the anaemia.

Patient may give history of blood loss like haematemesis, melena, bleeding piles, haematuria, haemoptysis or epistaxis. In women there may be history of metrorrhagia or menorrhagia.

Patient may complain of gastric discomforts, dyspepsia-like symptoms or pain of peptic ulcer. He may complain of loss of appetite, weight loss and dysphagia. There may be history of diarrhoea, constipation, passing of mucus, soreness of tongue or history of previous abdominal operation. Gastrointestinal symptoms are common in anaemia and when present are usually due to the etiological condition rather than to anaemia itself, although severe anaemia may cause some degree of anorexia, nausea and flatulence. Such conditions as peptic ulcer, hiatus hernia or neoplasm cause bleeding. Chronic amoebiasis, intestinal parasitic worms, especially hookworm infestations can cause anaemia. But the diarrhoea itself could be due to anaemia as it is known to occur in megaloblastic anaemia. In women, during the child-bearing age, common cause of anaemia is due to iron deficiency. If the anaemia is of rapid onset, then one should always try to find out whether the patient is loosing blood either extravascularly or intravascularly, or is suffering from acute leukaemia.

Any history of prolonged bleeding after trivial injuries, haemarthrosis or subcutaneous haemorrhages, purpuric spots, etc., should also be enquired into. While enquiring about purpuric spots, one must not forget to ask the patient about any recent history of drug ingestion, joint or abdominal pain.

While enquring about the symptoms of an urogenital system, patient should be asked about the colour of the urine (haemoglobinuria), its quality and frequency (polyuria, especially nocturnal). If haemoglobinuria is present, then one should try to find out whether it occurred after an exposure to infection or cold or after heavy exertion like a long distance run or march or after taking a drug.

Symptoms of C.N.S. in anaemia are mostly numbness, tingling and paresthesia. They are usually bilateral and symmetrical occurring first in hand and feet in megaloblastic anaemia with Vit $B_{12}$ deficiency.

(b) **Personal and social history**

Patient's personal history like addiction to drugs, alcohol or his occupation, especially as a painter or exposure to toxic chemicals, irradiation is important for finding out the etiology of anaemia. His habit and diet especially, if he is a vegetarian or habituated to alcohol is important. Alcoholic liver is increasingly recognised as being associated with folic acid deficiency and megaloblastic anaemia. A detailed history is necessary if patient shows clincial features suggestive of dietary deficiency.

(c) **Past history**

Past history of recurrent episodes of anaemia points towards a haemolytic anaemia especially, if associated with mild icterus. Similarly, past history of anaemia associated with the history of taking drugs or with an infection of malaria suggests the possibility of G-6-PD deficiency. Therefore, particular attention to past history is important.

(d) **Family history**

Family history is also helpful in diagnosing all the hereditary blood disorders like hereditary spherocytosis, or haemoglobinopathies. Even in cases of G-6-PD or other enzyme deficiencies, family history is a good pointer. In this connection it is good to remember that racial history is also important in the investigation of blood disorders e.g. a Bengali suffering from haemoglobinopathy is likely to be suffering from HbE disease whereas one from Gujarat or from Maharashtra probably will be suffering from beta thalassaemia. Similarly, aboriginals like Todas or from Maharashtra will be suffering from sickle cell anaemia or sickle cell thalassaemia disease. A Sikh, on the other hand, may suffer from D Punjab or from C haemoglobin disease.

(e) **Physical examination**

To confirm that the patient is suffering from anaemia, one must look for pallor. Here one must remember that in our country we are dealing mostly with dark-complexioned people. Therefore, in India, when a patient looks definitely pale, then he usually has anaemia of moderate severity. In milder cases of anaemia, one should examine the conjunctiva, nail beds, palm creases and mucous membrane of the mouth. It is difficult to assess the degree of anaemia from conjunctival pallor especially in milder cases of anaemia.

After having established that the patient is suffering from anaemia, one proceeds to find out the cause of anaemia. Physical examination on many occasion gives the necessary clue to the cause of anaemia.

A thorough general examination is necessary with special emphasis on the following features :

a. Skin

(1) Colour : If muddy—ankylostomiasis, K. A.
Dark pigmented–Malaria
Lemon Yellow—hereditary spherocytosis, haemolytic anaemias and, uncommonly, pernicious anaemia.

| | |
|---|---|
| Extreme pallor | —in leukaemia and aplastic anaemia |
| Plethoric redness | —Polycythaemia |
| Bronzing or darkening of skin | —Haemochromatosis or haemosiderosis |
| Greyish yellow colour | —Hodgkin's disease (May produce jaundice due to biliary obstruction). |

(ii) Ulceration : Especially of legs seen in sickle cell anaemia, thalassaemia. Ulceration also is known to occur in mycosis fungoides, leucosarcoma, Hodgkin's disease.

(iii) Telangiectasis : As in Osler-Rendu disease or in urticaria pigmentosa.

(iv) Purpura : Primary as in E.T.P.H. or secondary to infection, drugs, scurvy, allergy, etc.

(v) Herpes Zoster : Sometime occurs in lymphatic leukaemia.

(vi) Exfoliative erythrodermia, leukaemia especially of chronic lymphatic variety.

**b.Nails**

(i) Koilonychia—Iron deficiency anaemia (May be only brittleness, striation and longitudinal ridging)

(ii) "Watch-glass" clubbed fingers in polycythaemia

(iii) Flattening of nail in chronic leukaemia.

**c. Lymph glands**

One must especially search for enlarged lymph glands in a case of anaemia. Various infections like tuberculosis, infectious mononucleosis and proliferative disorders, both benign and malignant, should be kept in mind.

**d. Conjunctiva**

As already stated earlier pallor is detected better in conjunctiva than in skin. Icterus is also better appreciated in the sclera than in the skin. If icterus is present along with anaemia, one must consider various types of haemolytic anaemia.

**e. Lesion of mucous membranes :**

(i) m.m. of oral cavity : pallor, petechae, dark pigmentations can be detected here easily.

(ii) Gum—Bleeding may be the first presenting symptom of monocytic leukaemia. It is also common in severe thrombocytopenia.
Hypertrophy is seen in monocytic leukaemia, multiple myeloma, oedema of palate and bleeding of gums are usual in aplastic anaemia and terminal stages of all leukaemias. Buccal mucosa is red and swollen in polycythaemia. Swollen and bleeding gums are also seen in scurvy.

(iii) Ulceration of fauces : Occurs in aplastic anaemia, agranulocytic angina, lymphoblastic and monocytic leukaemia.

(iv) Glossitis : A smooth red tongue, occasionally painful, occurs in iron deficiency anaemia. A raw red tongue or an atrophic tongue occurs in nutritional anaemia.

**f. Abdomen**

(a) Spleen—It is enlarged in many conditions associated with anaemia. Sometime, it helps in the diagnosis. Mild to moderate enlargement of spleen is found in most cases of haemolytic anaemia with the exception of sickle cell anaemia. Rather on many occasions, hereditary spherocytosis has often been suspected on finding a spleen in a case who has a lemon yellow discolouration and is asymptomatic and afebrile. In our country, though malaria and kala-azar are no longer that common as in yester years yet these two conditions should always be excluded in a case of splenomegaly with anaemia. In certain parts of India like Gujarat, parts of Maharashtra and in Bengal, beta-thalassaemia and E-thalassaemia are not uncommon conditions and should be thought of, especially in a child or young individual with a moderate enlargement of spleen. There are many conditions which are not common and may have to be considered on some occasions like polycythaemia vera and I.T.P. where other symptoms are very suggestive. Moderate to huge enlargement of spleen is seen in various types of leukaemia, malignant lymphomas, Hodgkin's disease, myelosclerosis, Gaucher's disease, malaria, kala-azar, portal hypertension. With marked enlargement of spleen especially when it has enlarged beyond the umbilicus, there may be pressure on adjacent organs along with a feeling of nausea, vomiting, flatulence, dyspepsia and epigastric pain. Signs and symptoms of hypersplenism may also develop.

(b) Liver—Liver may be enlarged either be due to anaemia or due to other causes. To investigate a case of hepatosplenomegaly along with anaemia, one should consider the possibility of leukaemias and reticulosis group along with malaria.

(g) **Cardiovascular System**

Signs of this system are mostly due to anaemia or coincidental heart disease. A systolic ejection murmur is invariably present in anaemia of moderate to severe degree.

(h) **Bony tenderness**

It is present in leukaemias, metastatic bone carcinoma, multiple myeloma and myelosclerosis. Bony tenderness is usually demonstrated in the sternum, but may occur in any bones containing red marrow especially skull, clavicles and pelvic bones.

(j) C.N.S.

Tingling, paresthesia of toes and sensory loss of stocking and glove distribution suggests Vit $B_{12}$ neuropathy.

(k) **Fundus oculi**

Fundus shows changes like haemorrhages in severe anaemia, thrombocytopenia and leukaemia; in the last condition, infiltration of retina sometime can also be seen.

(l) **Rectal examination**

Wherever it is considered necessary, it should be carried out, especially in the elderly.

(m) **Vaginal examination**

Where indicated.

## HAEMATOLOGICAL EXAMINATION

First step in the haematological examination is to carry out:

(i) Hb estimation
(ii) Peripheral smear examination
(iii) Total Leucocyte count (TLC) and differential count (DLC)
(iv) PCV, MCV, MCHC and ESR.

Hb examination confirms the presence of anaemia. TLC and DLC help in many conditions like infectious mononucleosis, leukaemia especially chronic myeloid and lymphoid leukaemias, and erythraemic myelosis.

Differential leucocyte count should be carried out in a nicely drawn thin smear with a good tail. Of all the preliminary investigations in a case of anaemia, examination of a good peripheral blood smear is the single most important investigation which in a competent hand helps in the diagnosis of 90% of anaemia cases.

While examining the peripheral smear one must examine thoroughly all the cellular elements one after another.

It is not possible to give in detail all the conditions that one can diagnose from the examination of the peripheral smear because they are too many, but some examples are cited below :

**Red cells—**

(i) Iron deficiency anaemia—microcytes and ring staining red cells. One can assess the degree of iron deficiency also (Pl. I, Fig. 10B).
(ii) Megaloblastic anaemia—Macrocytes and megalocytes, marked anisocytosis, poikilocytosis (Pl. I, Figs. 4, 8, 9). Leucocytes may show more than 5 lobes in the nuclei.
(iii) Acute haemolytic anaemia—Fragmented red cells, reticulocytes, basophilic stippling, Cabbot's ring, Howell-Jolly bodies, large number of nucleated red cells, occasionally erythrophagocytosis.
(iv) Thalassaemia—Large number of target cells (Pl. I, Fig. 10A)
(v) Sickle cell anaemia—Sickle-shaped cells (Pl. I, Fig. 6).
(vi) Hereditary spherocytosis—Microspherocytes (Pl. I, Fig. 7).
(vii) Elliptocytosis and ovalocytosis—Elliptical and oval red cells (Pl. I, Fig. 5).
(viii) Malaria infection—Malarial parasites in the blood.

**White cell series**

(i) Number—Normal, increased or decreased.
(ii) Immature forms—Myeloblasts or lymphoblasts or monoblasts.
(iii) Abnormal character—Pelger-Huet abnormality, G.F. cells.
(iv) Abnormal increase in any of the series of white cells—Polymorphs, eosinophils, basophils.

**Platelet series**

(i) Number—Normal, increased or decreased.
(ii) Shape—Any abnormality in shape and size.

**Absolute values**

After the preliminary examination of a slide of peripheral smear, one knows how to proceed further. MCV shows the size of the cells whilst M.C.H.C. confirms presence of iron deficiency. The diagnosis is confirmed by further special tests:

PCV is important in certain situations, especially in condition of polycythaemia where it is a better indicator than Hb or RBC for diagnosis and to assess the condition of the patient, during treatment and for post-treatment assessment.

**Reticulocyte count**

It is also a preliminary step in confirming the observed acute haemolytic process in the peripheral smear. It is also carried out as a routine procedure in anaemia cases who are under treatment to see the response to therapy.

**Special tests in**

I. Iron deficiency anaemia

(a) Bone marrow always
(b) Serum iron and iron binding capacity of blood.
(c) Stool—for the cause of iron deficiency.
(d) In certain situation—X-ray of the G.I. tract

II. Megaloblastic anaemia (usually nutritional)

(a) Bone marrow always
(b) F.T.M. especially after injection of histamine
(c) Radiological investigation of small intestine (if necessary)
(d) Estimation of Folate level and of the absorption of folic acid from alimentary tract
(e) Vit $B_{12}$ assay and Schilling test
(f) Jejunal biopsy through oral route in cases of malabsorption syndrome where diagnosis is in doubt
(g) Stool examination

N.B.—All these investigations as outlined above may not be necessary in many megaloblastic anaemias where history and clinical examination will be of great help, viz. pregnancy, parasprue, tropical sprue, blind or stagnant loop syndrome, partial gastrectomy etc.

III. Anaemia associated with purpura

(a) Hess or Torniquet test for capillary fragility
(b) Platelet count

(c) Bleeding time and clotting time
(d) Clot retraction
(e) Platelet factor 3 release
(f) Platelet adhesion and aggregation

IV. Haemolytic Anaemia

A. To find out evidence of increased haemolysis
(i) Serum bilirubin
(ii) Reticulocyte count
(iii) Bone marrow
(iv) Increased urobilinogen in the urine
(v) Osmotic fragility test

B. Haemolysis—is it intra or extra vascular ?
(i) Direct and indirect antiglobin test
(ii) Plasma haemoglobin
(iii) Schum's test
(iv) Haemosiderin in urine
(v) Life span of red cells (51 Cr method)

Cause for haemolysis

C. If intravascular, then
(i) Peripheral smear and osmotic fragility would help in hereditary spherocytosis, ovalocytosis and elliptocytosis.
(ii) The above-mentioned tests in (i) and also tests for sickling help in the diagnosis of sickle cell anaemia.
(iii) Tests in (i) and supravital staining—Hb H
(iv) Screening test for G-6-PD deficiency
(v) Alkalie denaturation test for Hb F (confirmed by HB electrophoresis)
(vi) Hb electrophoresis for other abnormal haemoglobins

D. If extravasular, then
(i) Tests for autoantibodies
(ii) Tests for iso antibodies
(iii) Titration of cold agglutinins
(iv) Acidified serum test
(v) Sucrose lysis test
(vi) Donath-Landsteiner test
(vii) Tests for methaemoglobin and sulphaemoglobin
(viii) Drug antibody

## BLEEDING DIATHESIS DUE TO DEFECTS IN THE COAGULATION FACTORS

**Introduction :**

Whenever normal haemostatic mechanism becomes faulty, prolonged bleeding episode occurs. Causes for such haemorrhagic episodes are many and varied but could be divided into three broad categories. They are (i) vascular response (ii) platelet plug formation and (iii) fibrin deposition. Normal haemostasis depends on these three factors. Commonest cause for bleeding disorders seen in clinical practice is from vascular causes followed by coagulation factor defects. Blood coagulation is an enormously complex sequence of physico-chemical reaction which transforms fluid blood into a firm fibrin clot and thereby stops bleeding from an injured vessel. This process requires the initiation of a platelet plug, followed by reinforcement with the fibrin derived from the activation of the intrinsic coagulation system. Simultaneously, natural inhibitors and accelerators are brought into action.

A clotting defect is commonly present in one of the three ways:

(i) A patient may have bled abnormally
(ii) or may be referred because he is known to suffer from a bleeding diathesis
(iii) or defective clotting is noted when he is being investigated for other causes.

**Haemostatic mechanism :**

In order to understand the management one should have some conception of the normal haemostatic mechanism. Normal sequence of haemostatic machanism could be summarised briefly as follows :—

Bleeding occurs when blood vessels and tissues are injured. Immediately, there occurs vasoconstriction of the injured vessel. Thromboplastic materials are released from the damaged tissues. Plasma, as it flows over the damaged tissues, contains factor XII (contact factor), which is activated and this triggers the activation of the intrinsic system.

Factor VII of the plasma activates the tissue thromboplastic substances or the extrinsic system. The activated extrinsic thromboplastin, in the presence of calcium then interacts with factors V, X and converts plasma prothrombin into thrombin. In the meantime, plateletes have started adhering to damaged endothelium of the vessel. The thrombin produced by the extrinsic thromboplastic system and ADP now coming into contact with plateletes adhering to the sub-endothelial collagen causing them to aggregate into a plug. Plateletes, in their turn, release a number of substances which encourage further aggregation of plateletes and laying down of fibrin to reinforce the platelet plug. The plug grows continuously till it seals the defect completely.

In the meantime, the intrinsic thromboplastic mechanism has been activated leading to the production of relatively larger amounts of thrombin. Thrombin thus produced converts fibrinogen to fibrin. The fibrin absorbs much of the excess thrombin and the remainder is neutralised by anti-thrombin. Platelet plug which contracts and the fibrin lattice work which effectively anchors the platelet plug seals the defect in the vessel.

Thus we see that after activation of the contact factor, three main mechanisms are involved in this phenomenon, viz. (i) Extrinsic and intrinsic procoagulant action. (ii) Platelet interaction through the haemostatic plug and (iii) the fibrinolytic system.

Sequence of events in normal coagulation is based on cascade or waterfall theory which could be diagrammaticaly depicted as follows :

a) **Intrinsic system : Test P.T.T.K.**

Factor XII —Surface Contact— XIIa
Factor XI ———— XIa
Factor IX ———— IXa
Factor VIII ———— VIIIa
Factor X ———— Xa + Platelet Lipid
+ Factor V
+ $ca^{++}$
Prothrombin ———— Thrombin

b) **Extrinsic System : Test Prothrombin time**

Extrinsic Thromboplastin

Factor X $\underline{+ \text{ VII}}$ Xa + factor V + $Ca^{++}$ + platelet

Prothrombin ——— Thrombin

c) **Fibrin formation and fibrinolysis**

Fibrinogen $\underline{\text{Thrombin}}$ fibrin monomer + a & b peptides

Fibrin monomer $\underline{\text{factor XIII A}}$ Fibrin clot

Fibrin ——————— X Y

D E fragments

**Investigation of Bleeding Disorders :**

First principle in the diagonsis is to establish that an abnormal bleeding diathesis exists. Second step after that is to establish the basic compartment to which the case exactly belongs. In order to avoid unnecessary investigations, it is of great importance to take an accurate personal and family history. Special notes will be taken of the amount, course and previous history of bleeding, family history of bleeding disorders and response to haemostatic stress like dental extraction, injury and surgery. Clinical examination helps greatly. Haemarthrosis means a coagulation defect while petechae means a platelet or a vascular abnormality.

Patient should be questioned in detail for the evidence of clinically spontaneous bleeding. While taking history evidence should be sought whether the defects are lifelong or acquired. The haemostatic response to the injury should be assessed like the duration of post-traumatic bleeding.

Generally, cutaneous purpura or superficial bruises, especially over commonly injured surfaces, suggest an abnormality of the vascular component of haemostasis. Deeper, larger bruises, haematomas, bleeding into joint, prolonged or continuous bleeding from mucous membranes, cuts and wounds suggest a defect in the blood coagulation mechanism. Purpura or petechae associated with urticaria, eczema, swollen painful joints or abdominal cramps suggest a Henoch-Schönlein type of purpura, Bruising on the back of hands or feet of an older person is likely to represent senile purpura. A male patient with bleeding into joints or deeper tissues and with positive family history is suggestive of Haemophilia or Christmas disease. A pale, pudgy infant who resents being moved or handled suggests scurvy, as does swollen bleeding gums in an elderly patient who has been living on a "frying-pan" diet. If the patient is pale with hepatosplenomegaly and bleeding swollen gums with purplish infiltration in the skin, he may be suffering from leukaemia. Bleeding in a jaundiced patient or in an alcoholic is due to the deficiency of Vitamin K dependent factors like II, VII, IX and X. Excessive bleeding or oozing following delivery or associated with surgery or trauma is due to hypofibrinogenopenia.

In large number of cases one could make a tentative diagnosis regarding the etiology of the bleeding and then confidently proceed to carry out only limited number of tests to confirm the diagnosis.

Whenever a patient has presented a bleeding complaint following screening, examination should immediately be carried out to help in arriving at a proper diagnosis which will, in turn, help in treating the patient correctly.

**Screening tests are as follows :**

1) Peripheral blood smear examination
2) Capillary resistance test (Tourniquet or Hess test)
3) Bleeding time (B. T.)

4) Clotting time (C. T.)
5) One stage prothrombin time (P. T.)
6) Kaolin activated partial thromboplastin test (P.T.T.K.)
7) Thrombin clotting time test
8) Platelet count
9) Clot retraction

1. **Peripheral Smear :** Importance of peripheral smear need not be stressed. It will rule out haemolytic anaemia and indicate or point towards an incriminating cause for the occurrence of bleeding like D.I.C.; peripheral smear has already been discussed in detail earlier in the chapter on investigation of anaemia (Pages 81, 82).

2. **Positive capillary resistance test:**—Indicates either vascular defect or thrombocytopenia. When the Hess test is negative these two components out of three major ones responsible for haemostasis can be taken as normal though it must be remembered that this test is rather crude and often carried out in an unstandardised manner. This test may be positive even though B.T. is normal. It means that the capillary wall in such cases cannot withstand increased pressure though the mechanism to arrest bleeding is normal.

3. **Bleeding time (B.T.):**—Is increased in cases of thrombocytopenia and also in cases of Von Willebrand's disease. In the latter, the B.T. is prolonged and the factor VIII level is also low.

This test should be carried out under standard conditions like Ivy's method.

4. **Whole blood clotting time (C.T.):**—This test should always be carried out at 37°C according to Lee and White method. Even then it is of limited value as it is very insensitive and a normal result does not exclude a severe coagulation abnormality. For example, in a patient with anticoagulant therapy with grossly abnormal coagulation mechanism the clotting time may be within normal range. Similarly in cases of hypofibrinogenopenia, the fibrinogen must be grossly deficient to produce an increased clotting time. In many cases of haemophilia, C.T. may be normal.

A prolonged C.T. may be due to a deficiency (Haemophilia or Christmas disease) or an inhibitor, like circulating anticoagulants as heparin. The distinction is obviously important in the beginning of the investigation of a case, if clinical examination does not reveal it. The simplest way to find out is to compare the C.T. of a patient's sample, control sample and an equal mixture of the two. If the C.T. of the mixture approximates to that of the normal control, it suggests that the defect is due to a deficiency of a clotting factor and if the mixture behaves more like the patient plasma alone, then the inference is that there is an inhibitor in the plasma.

5. **Prothrombin time (one stage):**—Is a non-specific indicator of the extrinsic blood coagulation mechanism. An increase in prothrombin time indicates a deficiency either of prothrombin, factor V, factor VII or X or a combination of them. Common causes of prolonged one stage prothrombin time are, (i) anticoagulant therapy, (ii) obstructive jaundice, (iii) haemorrhagic disease of new-born, (iv) liver disease, (v) congenital deficiency of one or more factors II, V, VII or X, (vi) Fibrinogen deficiency, and (vii) malabsorption states.

6. **Kaolin activated partial thromboplastin test** (P.T.T.K.):—It is a sensitive technique to detect deficiencies of intrinsic factors viz. V, VIII, IX, X and XII and also anti-coagulants. The test is most useful in detection of haemophilia and Christmas disease but does not differentiate between the two. It is a very simple and easy test which can be carried out in any laboratory.

7. **If the prothrombin time is found to be abnormal, then it is advisable to carry out the following tests:—**

a) Thrombin clotting time of plasma:— If the thrombin clotting time is prolonged then it could be D.I.C. (Disseminated Intravascular Coagulation) or increased fibrinolysis, decrease in fibrinogen or presence of an anti-coagulant. It is important to differentiate between D.I.C. and increased fibrinolysis, as the treatment for these two conditions is different. In both these conditions P.T., P.T.T.K. and thrombin time will be prolonged. But in D.I.C., platelet count will be low whereas in case of fibrinolysis it will be normal. Peripheral smear shows evidence of haemolytic anaemia in D.I,C. Presence of F.D.P. (Fibrinogen Degradation Product) indicates increased fibrinolysis. This can easily be verified in any laboratory by means of protamine sulphate test and ethanol gelation test.

b) If the P.T. is prolonged but the thrombin clotting time is normal and clot is firm, then there is a deficiency of any of the factors II, V, VII and X.

For finding out defects of individual coagulation factors., detailed tests are necessary for which a specialised laboratory is considered essential.

8. **Platelet count:**—It is an essential screening test to confirm or exclude cases of thrombocytopenia. It is preferable to use a plastic or a siliconised syringe and a plastic vial for a proper platelet count. It is also desirable to carry out count promptly and an average of two countings should be taken. Phase contrast microscope is always preferable for proper platelet countings. Best, of course, is an electronic counter.

9. **Clot retraction:**—It is a useful screening test for platelet function. Contraction of clot depends on the adequate number of normal functioning platelets. A definite quantity of blood is allowed to clot at 37°C in a water bath and is observed at 1 and 2 hours after clotting. Some degree of quantitation can be achieved by measuring the amount of serum expressed from the clot after 2 hours of incubation.

## CAUSES FOR ABNORMAL BLEEDING TENDENCY

1. **Vascular defects:**—
   (a) Infection like typhoid fever, smallpox, measles
   (b) Drugs like aspirin, quinine
   (c) Anaphylactoid purpura and allergic purpura
   (d) Vitamin deficiency like scurvy
   (e) Inherited disorder like Osler-Rendu-Weber disease (hereditary haemorrhagic telangiectasie)

2. **Platelet defects:**—
   (a) Idiopathic or secondary thrombocytopenic purpura
   (b) Thrombocytosis as in myeloproliferative disorders
   (c) Functional like thromboasthenia, thrombocytopathy, uraemia and gamma globulinaemia

3. **Coagulation factor defects:**—
   (a) Factor VIII deficiency—haemophilia
   (b) Factor IX deficiency—Christmas disease
   (c) Factor V deficiency—para haemophilia
   (d) Von-Willebrand's disease
   (e) Factor II deficiency—hypoprothrombinaemia
   (f) Factor I deficiency—acquired or congenital fibrinogenopenia

**Vascular defects:**

Purpura simplex—Seen especially in fair, child-bearing healthy females. Seen mostly in arms, legs and trunks, especially following minor trauma. There is no obvious coagulation abnormality. Patient should be reassured and given large doses of Vits C and P. She should be advised to avoid aspirin.

In senile purpura because of loss of supportive connective tissue, any mild to moderate injury ruptures the small vessels and produces ecchymotic patches, especially at the back of hand, forearm and thigh. Requires no treatment.

### Anaphylactoid Purpura
(Henoch-Schönlein purpura)

This condition is due to an unknown allergen. Some cases result from bacterial infection. It can occur in all ages but is seen mostly in children and young adults. Most cases start with purpura followed by abdominal pain due to serosanguinous effusion into the gut wall and joint pain. Abdominal pain may be severe enough to simulate abdominal emergency. Affected joint or joints may be swollen due to periarticular swelling. There may be haematuria, albuminurea and casts. Renal signs may persist for longer period leading to chronic nephritis. Occasionally, angio-neurotic oedema around eyes (usually one) may also be found. Treatment is mainly symptomatic. Offending drug or food should be identified and discontinued. Corticosteroid therapy may help, especially the joint manifestations.

### Hereditary Haemorrhagic Telangiectasia
(Osler-Rendu-Weber disease)

In this inherited condition, both sexes are equally affected which is transmitted as an autosomal dominant trait. Multiple dilated non-contractile capillaries and arterioles are present in the skin and mucous membrane. It is an uncommon disorder in this country. It is commonly seen in the mucous membrane of nose and mouth but may be present in G.I. tract, bronchi and kidneys. Telangiectatic spots could be pin-size or larger. They bleed easily and lead to epistaxis, haematemesis, haemoptysis or bleeding at any site where they are present. Retinal and cerebral haemorrhages have been reported. Platelet count and tests for coagulation disorders are normal. Treatment of local sites includes pressure. packing and topic haemostatic agents and may be cauterisation.

### Platelet Defects (Quantitative)
Idiopathic Thrombocytopenic Purpura (I.T.P.)

Cause for the decrease in quantity of platelets is not known. Whenever the count drops to $40 \times 10^{9/l}$ and below, bleeding occurs spontaneously. With values above $40 \times 10^{9/l}$ spontaneous bleeding is uncommon. The disorder can occur at any age but is commonly seen in children and young adults.

It is considered that I.T.P. is an autoimmune disorder where an autoantibody reacts with platelet antigen. Bleeding can occur from any site. It could be acute or chronic. *Acute cases* occur mostly in young children between 2 and 6 years. In most cases, there is an acute febrile episode following 2 to 3 weeks after bleeding episode from skin and mucous membranes with low platelet count. It is a self-limiting disease and corticosteroids do not help in this condition. *Chronic I.T.P.* occurs in all ages but commonly in adults. It occurs most commonly in women with no previous history of infection. Onset is insidious. Platelet count is moderately low. There is no significant anaemia or splenomegaly. Purpura occasionally may be absent for some time and reappear again. It does not remit spontaneously. Bleeding time is increased, there is positive tourniquet test and platelet count is low. Antiplatelet antibodies may be demonstrated. Bone marrow shows increased number of megakaryocytes. Principle of treatment is corticosteroid therapy and splenectomy. Prednisolone in the doses of one mgm per kg body weight per day for six weeks should be tried. In most cases, remission can be induced. Splenectomy is the most effective treatment in 60 to 80 per cent cases where a sustained remission occurs. About 10 to 20 per cent cases will obtain a partial remission.

Remaining 10 per cent cases will show no improvment and these are the cases where immunosuppressive agents may be employed. Drugs used are vincristine, cyclophosphamide or imuran (azathioprine). Recently, intravenous immunoglobulin therapy was found to induce remission in this condition.

### Secondary Thrombocytopenic Purpura

Majority of cases of thrombocytopenia met in the clinical practice occur following leukaemias, aplastic anaemias, multiple myeloma, secondary carcinomas, myelosclerosis, disseminated lupus erythematosis, drugs like quinine, quinidine, chlorothiazide, aspirin, sulphonamides, meprobamate, phenobarbitone, and phenylbutazone. Less common causes are following respiratory infection, infectious mononucleosis, measles,diphtheria and sub-acute bacterial endocarditis. Massive blood transfusion may cause thrombocytopenia. Cytotoxic drug therapy can also cause thrombocytopenia. Treatment consists of identification of the causative factor and specific measures against it. Platelet transfusion in cases of leukaemia and cytotoxic drug therapy may be necesssary. Drugs may cause thrombocytopenia either by direct toxic action or by hypersensitivity reaction or by a combination of both. In such cases, corticosteroid therapy may be beneficial.

### Thrombotic thrombocytopenic purpura

It is a disorder due to hypersensitivity and manifests itself as purpura, thrombocytopenia, haemolytic anaemia, leucocytosis. Manifestations are due to multiple unabsorbed intravascular thrombosis. Treatment consists of steroids, splenectomy and sometime anticoagulant, if disseminated intravascular coagulation is also present.

**Thromboasthenia** (Glanzmann's disease)

This disorder is transmitted as an autosomal recessive gene. Here, the bleeding time is prolonged in spite of normal platelet count. Patient complains of bruising even after minor trauma and prolonged bleeding after cuts or bruises. It is a rare condition in this country. In some cases, fibrinogen may also be low.

### Bleeding disorders due to coagulation factor deficiency

### Factor VIII deficiency or Haemophilia

This is hereditary bleeding diathesis linked with X-sex chromosome, recessive in character transmitted by females and manifested in male progeny due to deficiency of factor VIII (or anti-haemophilic globulin). Daughters of female carriers carry the trait. Male haemophilics pass on the trait to their daughters but not to their sons. When the concentration of factor VIII is 30 per cent of normal or above, a haemophilic will not bleed. But when it drops below 30 per cent, he will bleed following trauma or surgery. Below 5 per cent of normal, he will bleed spontaneously.

The bleeding tendency is noticed when the child is a toddler or little older. Bleeding can occur from any site but is commonly present as epistaxis or from G.I. tract or as haematuria. Sometime, there are subcutaneous ecchymotic patches or bleeding in the joints, commonly knee or elbow joints which are swollen and painful. Mild unnoticed trauma initiates the bleeding which continues unless treated. Bleeding can occur in central nervous system particularly in severe haemophilics. Repeated haemorrhages into joints may lead to organisation of blood and crippling ankylosis. One suspects the disease from history, hereditary features and from prolonged coagulation time. Bleeding time is normal, so also platelet count; prothrombin time is normal but kaolin activated partial thromboplastin test is prolonged. Assay of factor VIII shows it to be markedly deficient in such cases.

**Treatment :** When bleeding occurs, patient must be rested, his pain must be relieved by appropriate analgesics but not aspirin which is to be avoided. Locally, measures to stop the bleeding should be undertaken by means of adrenaline, thrombophobe or fibrin foam. Bleeding from gums or tooth socket or nose should be plugged with adrenaline. If there is a bleeding in the joint, it should splinted in an optimum position. Aspiration of joint should be avoided till bleeding stops after therapy. Cold packs or ice bags can be applied over the joint to relieve the pain. To prevent fibrous ankylosis early movement should be encouraged.

Mainstay of the treatment is by transfusion of one of the preparations of factor VIII concentrate or by fresh frozen plasma and fresh blood.

Cryoprecipitate, which is prepared easily from fresh frozen plasma, contains factor VIII and fibrinogen. Amount transfused varies according to the location and severity of haemorrhage. Haemarthrosis should be treated by cryoprecipitate till factor VIII level rises up to 50% of normal and to be repeated every 12 hours for about two days. For major surgery, factor VIII level should be raised to 100% and also for life threatening haemorrhage and to be repeated every 8 hours. Second subsequent amount could be half of the first dose and is to be continued till bleeding stops. Prior to transfusion of cryoprecipitate, Phenergan 50 mgm I.V. should be given to prevent urticarial reaction.

In the case of non-availability of cryoprecipitate fresh frozen plasma is the next best preparation to stop the bleeding. Fresh blood should be used to replace the lost blood. It is now possible to treat haemophiliacs at home with the cryoprecipitate. Recently, D.D.A.V.P., structural analogue of the natural anti-dieuretic hormone vasopressin with two changes has been used in the treatment of mild haemophilia as it can produce an increase of factor VIII level in the blood.

Every haemophilia patient must carry a card indicating that he is haemophilic and showing his blood group. Children can attend ordinary school provided they are exempted from games and physical training. They should avoid all traumas.

### Christmas disease

This disorder also is X-linked recessive gene transmitted by females and manifested in males. It is diagnosed by thromboplastin generation test. They are deficient of factor IX. Treatment is by plasma containing factor IX or by fresh frozen plasma. It is a milder disease than haemophilia with much less disability.

### Von-Willebrand's disease

Initally, it was thought to be a vascular defect as there was abnormal bleeding time with a normal platelet count. Subsequently, it was thought to be primarily a qualitative platelet defect because of impaired glass adhesiveness. Recently, with the association of low factor VIII level found in this condition, it is now classified as a coagulation defect. This disorder is a hereditary autosomal dominant bleeding diathesis characterised by a prolonged bleeding time and low factor VIII activity and defective platelet adhesion. In this condition, transfusion of plasma, cryoprecipitate or even old plasma shows a prolonged and progressive rise of factor VIII. It is thought that the defective factor in Von-Willebrand's disease is a factor VIII related protein or antigen. Bleeding episodes in this condition are less severe than those of haemophilia. Treatment of haemorrhage may be initiated with 10 ml/kg/day of plasma. Aspirin should not be given to these cases. D.D.A.V.P. has also been used in these cases successfully.

### Acquired deficiencies

There are many acquired conditions like liver disease, Vit K deficiency as in obstructive jaundice or malabsorption syndrome, circulating anticoagulant and disseminated intravascular coagulation (D.I.C.) or consumption coagulopathy. Of all the acquired conditions most important in clinical practice is the D.I.C.

### Disseminated Intravascular Coagulation (D.I.C.)

(Consumption coagulopathy or defibrination syndrome.) In this condition, there is an activation of haemostatic mechanism due to many and varied clinical conditions which cause intravascular clotting. This in turn leads to deficiency of clotting factors and lowering of platelet count which is utilised for clotting process. The process could be acute or chronic. Acute condition usually arises following abortion, abruptio placentae or following surgery on heart or lungs.

It has also been noted following septicaemias, incompatible blood transfusion, pulmonary embolism or after viper bite. Chronic cases arise mostly following leukaemia, especially promyelocytic leukaemia, adenocarcinomas, retained dead foetus, congenital heart disease and vascular malformations like giant haemangiomas.

Clinically, bleeding which starts after trauma, surgery or childbirth does not stop and this in turn leads to organ damage, especially that of kidneys and brain. Peripheral smear examination will show increased erythrocytic fragmentation with evidences of haemolytic anaemia. Thrombin clotting time, prothrombin time and activated partial thromboplastin tests—all will be prolonged. Platelet count will be low. Fibrinogen degradation product (FDP) will be found in the blood with a low fibrinogen content. Treatment is to remove the offending agent and transfusion of cryoprecipitate factor VIII-fibrinogen complex. It may be necessary to give platelet transfusion. If there is accompanying fibrinolysis, epsilon aminocaproic acid (EACA) or amicar is to be given. If there is continuing hypofibrinogenopenia and thrombocytopenia, one may have to resort to heparin therapy but a careful laboratory control would be imperative to avoid over-treatment. Heparin should only be used when the bleeding cannot be controlled with cryoprecipitate or fresh frozen plasma therapy along with platelets.

### Vitamin K deficiency

This vitamin is essential for the production of prothrombin, factor VII, factor IX and factor X. Following deficiency of Vit K, hypoprothrombinaemia results very rapidly within two weeks' time as the body stores are small. Prothrombin time (one stage) test becomes prolonged. It occurs in (i) obstructive jaundice, (ii) malabsorption syndrome, (iii) haemorrhagic diseases of new-born (iv) as a result of therapy with anticoagulants like warfarin or phenindione. Treatment is by administration of Vit K preparation either water soluble compound or synthetic analogues. If the bleeding is severe, fresh frozen plasma may have to be transfused.

### Liver Disease

In chronic liver disease, there will be defective synthesis of coagulation factors like fibrinogen (factor I), prothrombin (factor II) factors V, VII, IX and X. The vitamin K dependent factors are first depressed and is evident by prolonged prothrombin time (one stage). In several liver diseases, factor V and fibrinogen are also affected. In portal hypertension with splenomegaly, platelets may also be depressed. Therefore, patient may have severe bleeding episode when such a patient is subjected to surgery, especially for porta-caval shunt. Aspiration liver biopsy may produce troublesome bleeding episodes. These patients do not respond to Vit. K therapy. Fresh frozen plasma transfusion helps in such cases.

**Thrombosis**

Vascular wall, platelets and plasma factors are involved in increased thrombotic episodes in clinical practice.

Vascular factor as in arteriosclerosis is associated with increased thrombosis. There occurs an increase in the platelet count in such platelet disorders like thrombocythaemia following splenectomy and in myeloproliferative disorders like chronic myeloid leukaemia. This may lead to thrombosis. Theoretically, over-transfusion with cryoprecipitate can produce thrombosis due to increase in the coagulation factors.

Antithrombin III deficiency can induce increased thrombosis. It controls the counter-balancing force to coagulation and has a capacity to inactivate large amounts of thrombin as well as factors Xa, XIIa and IXa but not factor VIIa. It can be inherited or acquired following cirrhosis, hepatitis, stroke and in diabetes mellitus. Birth control pills which are known to induce thrombosis do so by reducing anti-thrombin III.

## DISORDERS OF WHITE CELLS

**Agranulocytosis** is a condition where the leucocytes go down below $1 \times 10^{9/l}$ with absence or near absence of neutrophil polymorphs. Causes are mostly drugs like amidopyrine (as in analgin, novalgin, cibalgin), neomercazole, sulphonamides, chloromycetin, streptomycin, largactil, equanil, stemetil, siquil, anti-bacterials like ristocetin, salazopyrin, PAS, INH, primaquin, chlorothiazid, metronidazole, pronestyl, following cytotoxic drug therapy or irradiation, or there could be no obvious cause as in idiopathic agranulocytosis.

Drugs could cause neutropenia by their direct toxic action on the bone marrow or by hypersensitivity reaction. In case of hypersensitivity reaction, the drug combines with a protein to form an antigen which in turn produces drug antibody in the blood. The antibody acts as a leucoagglutinin and causes agglutination of leucocytes. Bone marrow shows depletion of myeloid series of cells and disappearance of neutrophils. Peripheral blood shows neutropenia with or without anaemia or thrombocytopenia. There is usually relative increases in lymphocytes. History of drug intake would help in the diagnosis. Onset could be sudden or gradual. Patient may present himself with fever, sore throat, buccal and throat ulceration. This may lead to toxaemia and septicaemia. Death is usually due to infection. Treatment consists in withdrawal of the incriminating drug and a broad spectrum antibiotic cover like ampicillin and cloxacillin. If ulceration in the mouth and throat prevents oral therapy, intramuscular injection will have to be resorted to. White cell, especially granulocyte transfusion is specifically indicated in such a condition. Granulocytes can be collected through a cell separator machine. In the absence of such a machine, fresh blood transfusion should be given. Administration of corticosteroids, especially in the hypersensitivity neutropenia cases would be helpful. Recently, lithium carbonate which is now known to be granulocyte producing stem cell stimulator can be given a trial with a dosage of 250 mgm three times daily orally to a 60-70 kg adult individual. Careful nursing, preferably barrier nursing is advocated in such cases.

## LEUKAEMIAS

In this group of disorders which share a common feature of an uncontrolled proliferation of haemopoietic cells in the bone marrow and other tissues of the body accompanied by, but not always, an increase of similar cells in the peripheral blood. Abnormal proliferation could involve white cells, red cell precursors or those of megakaryocytes. Though the term 'leukaemia' originally meant uncontrolled proliferation of white cells, later two conditions are now also included under this group of disorder as they are related. This is a progressive and fatal disease in the vast majority of cases though in recent years some been achieved in inducing complete remission and especially cure, particularly in cases of acute lymphoblastic leukaemia.

**AETILOGY** of leukaemia is still not definitely known, but certain theories have been postulated which are as follows.

(i) **Viral** — Evidences point out that RNA virus can cause animal leukaemia. Similar virus may be responsible for human leukaemia. Now evidence is coming that RNA viruses have link with leukemogenicity in human cells.

(ii) **Ionising radiation** — Acute myelogenous leukaemia and chronic myelogenous leukaemia may develop following irradiation. Japanese populations exposed to radiation from atomic bomb generally developed leukaemia. Relationship of diagnostic X-rays to the aetiology of leukaemia remains uncertain.

(iii) **Chemicals and drugs** — Benzene exposure, phenylbutazone, arsenic and chloramphenicol have been related to the future development of leukaemia. Initially, drug exposure produces aplasia and then subsequently leukaemia.

(iv) **Genetic factors** — There is an increased frequency of leukaemia in identical twins of a leukaemia patient, in Mongolism, in Fanconi's anaemia and in Klinefelter's syndrome.

(v) **Immunological** — Immunodeficiency may favour development of neoplasia.

## CLASSIFICATION:

Leukaemia could be acute or chronic.

**Acute :**

**1. Acute lymphatic leukaemia.**

**2. Acute non-lymphocytic leukaemia** —Acute myeloblastic
(Acute Myelogenous leukaemia)
- Acute myelomonocytic
- Acute progranulocytic
- Acute granulocytic
- Erythro-leukaemia
- Acute monocytic or histiocytic

**3.Unclassified & Miscellaneous.**

**Chronic**

1. Myelocytic
2. Lymphocytic
3. Hairy cell leukaemia.

Generally, acute forms are fatal within six months if untreated. The blood shows large number of blast cells. In chronic form, patient may not die for many years and the blood picture is characterised by more differentiated and mature cells. The acute leukaemias are seen more frequently in children whilst chronic forms are more frequent in the adults and old.

Incidence of leukaemia seems to have increased in our country in recent years. This may partly be due to better diagnostic facilities and partly due to longer life expectancy than in earlier years.

## ACUTE LEUKAEMIAS

### Acute lymphoblastic leukaemia (A.L.L.)

This leukaemia is commonly seen in children, especially in the first 5 years of life. Fever, malaise, gingivial, nasal, cutaneous bleeding are present in 50 per cent cases. There is lymphadenopathy in majority of cases with or without hepatosplenomegaly. Leukaemic cellular accumulation can lead to various types of manifestations including C.N.S. signs and symptoms. White cell count can be high varying from 30,000 to 1,30,000/mm$^3$ or low as in cases of aleukaemic leukaemia. Usually, more than 40-50 per cent of the cells are blast cells (Pl. III, Figs. 3 & 6). It is confirmed by bone marrow examination. Recently, on the basis of morphology, A.L.L. has been differentiated into three broad types. $L_1$—acute leukaemia of childhood where mainly microlymphoblasts are seen and $L_2$—acute undifferentiated leukaemia where there is pleomorphic population of lymphoblasts and prolymphocytes. Occurs in adolescents and adults. $L_3$ is Burkitt type composed of Burkitt's lymphocytes. Most of $L_1$ and $L_2$ fit with the null cell category. Sometime, one may have to resort to P.A.S. (periodic acid schiff's) staining and peroxidase staining to differentiate it from an acute non-lymphatic leukaemia case.

**Treatment** is by chemotherapeutic agents.

**Remission Induction :—** Vincristine is given once a week in the dosage of .033-.025 mgm/kg body weight for 3 to 4 weeks. It is advisable to test the ankle and knee jerks after injection to check up on motor weakness as well as paresthesia. This is combined with prednisolone 2-3 mgm/kg body weight P.O. and also cytosin arabinoside (cytosar) continuously for 5 days by I.M./I.V. in the dosage of 3 mgm/kg body weight. 90% children will achieve a complete haematological remission with this therapy. As there will still be blast cells in the body, it is always advisable to continue the maintenance therapy.

**Maintenance therapy** with 6-mercaptopurine 2-5 mgm/kg body weight per orally (P.O.) daily and twice a week methotrexate in the dosage of 0.5 mgm/kg body weight intramuscularly is to be continued to prolong the remission. Some people give periodic induction therapy to reduce the body load of leukaemic cells.

**C.N.S. Infiltration :—** It is necessary to irradiate C.N.S. sanctuaries of leukaemic cell to produce a complete cure in A.L.L. From 6 weeks onward, intrathecal methotrexate is given weekly up to a maximum of 10 mgm for at least 8 such injections or more till C.S.F. becomes free of cells. Some people like to give cranio-spinal irradiation as well. Recommended dose is 2400 rads although lower dose has been used also.

**Immunotherapy:—** In order to reduce or retard the accumulation of small clones of cells, administration of vaccines of irradiated leukaemia cells or Bacillus Calmette Guerin (BCG) has been advocated and have been found to be useful.

**Supportive therapy:—**In the form of fresh blood transfusion, platelet rich plasma or granulocyte transfusion may become necessary. To control infection it may be necessary to use broad spectrum antibiotics. Acute lymphoblastic leukaemia with its chronic counterpart seems to be a part of a general spectrum of lymphoproliferative disorders which include the lymphomas and infectious mononucleosis. Recent observation of linking Epstein-Barr virus specific IgM antibodies in the first degree relatives of children with A.L.L. suggests that the condition may be an uncontrolled response to an infection by a low grade virus.

**Acute Myeloblastic Leukaemia** (AML)

This is slightly less common than A.L.L. and can occur in any age group, though frequency is increased in those over 40 years of age. Males are more affected than females. The myelogenous leukaemias are defined by the direction of differentiation and by the degree of maturation of the leukaemic cells. French-American and British (FAB) group has suggested to subdivide AML into six types ($M_1$ to $M_6$). $M_1$, $M_2$, $M_3$ granulocytic in type reflect an evolution from myeloblast to progranulocyte. $M_1$ is myeloblast (Pl. III, Fig. 4.1) without maturation. $M_2$ is myeloblast with maturation (Pl. III, Fig. 2). $M_3$ is acute progranulocytic leukaemia, with hypergranular cells frequently containing Auer bodies (Pl. II, Fig. 7). $M_4$ is acute myelomonocytic leukaemia where both myeloid series and monocytic cells are seen. $M_5$ is monocytic leukaemia with monocytic differentiation (Pl. III, Fig. 5). $M_6$ is erythroleukaemia, red cell precursors being the predominant cellular element. Erythroblast may also be present in the peripheral blood. Special stains like P.A.S., peroxidase, NASDA will help in the differentiation. Erythroleukaemia is also called Erythraemic Myelosis or Di Guglielmo's syndrome. Clinically, patients are anaemic, febrile with easy fatigability. Patient may bleed from gums or from other sites. Sometime there may be no symptom and diagnosis is made while finding out the cause for pallor or hepatosplenomegaly or bleeding from gums. Enlargement of liver and spleen is seen in 50% cases. Lymphadenopathy is uncommon in AML. Leukaemic infiltration of organs will produce symptoms referable to it. Localised tumour masses may have a greenish appearance which occurs in skin, orbit or other tissues. These are called chloromas. Greenish colour is due to myeloperoxidase. Bleeding may occur from any site. And intracranial haemorrhage may lead to headache, dimness of vision, blindness or death. Peripheral blood will show an elevated leucocyte count. Myeloblasts are present in the peripheral blood. There is accompanying anaemia and thrombocytopenia. When marrow is examined, it is seen to be infiltrated with a large number of blast cells *pari passu* with a reduction of normal precursors. The megakaryocytes may be increased and marrow is often hypercellular.

**Treatment** of AML is not as successful as A.L.L. Various types of protocol have been suggested of which a combination of Daunorubicin, cytosine arabinoside, 6-thioguanine is the best available one to induce a remission. Some combine vincristine and prednisolone along with the previous three. Dosage also varies with various protocols. Whatever drug combinations are used, they produce pancytopenia. Therefore, supportive therapy should be prompt and available which is only possible in those centres which specialise in leukaemia treatment. The protocol and usual dosage that are used:—Daunorubicin 1-1.5 mgm/kg body weight I.V. on day 1. Days 2-6, cytosine arabinoside 3 mgm/kg body weight I.V. along with 6-thioguanine 2 mgm/kg body weight per orally twice daily from 2 to 6 days. We usually combine prednisolone along with these three drugs in the dosage of 2 mgm/kg for these 5 days. Next 2 to 3 weeks no drugs are given to permit the marrow to recover its function. The same protocol is repeated 5 to 6 times till remission occurs. This is followed by maintenance therapy, of which combination of cytosine arabinoside with 6-thioguanine is the best and simplest. They could be given monthly or weekly.

**Bone Marrow Transplantation** :—In acute leukaemia, bone marrow transplantation has been used as a curative procedure. In some highly specialised centres, 60% of patients with acute myeloid leukaemia in remission transplanted with marrow from HLA-identical sibs or twin are still surviving without any evidence of recurrent leukaemia at the end of two years and it is now considered that many of these patients are cured of their disease. Graft failure due to Graft-versus-Host reaction is the main reason for graft failure. Many techniques are now being progressed to prevent GVH reaction.

### Supportive care

Main dangers to life are bleeding and infection. Anaemia is combated by fresh blood transfusion. Bleeding is due to thrombocytopenia where PRP (platelet rich plasma) or PC (platelet concentrate) will be of great help. Infection is due to granulocytopenia. A combination of two broad-spectrum antibiotics along with white cell transfusion will be of considerable value. Granulocyte transfusion is considered when granulocyte count is less than 500 per $mm^3$ and antibiotics do not help in combating the fever for 2 to 3 days.

For meningeal leukaemia, one has to introduce intrathecally cytosine arabinoside or methotrexate.

### Chemotherapy in cases of relapse

Various combinations have been tried including POMP, Adriamycin, Oncovin and Prednisolone. But the rescue has been ineffective in most cases and prognosis is poor.

## CHRONIC LEUKAEMIAS

### Chronic Granulocytic Leukaemia

Majority of cases occur between the ages of 30 and 50 years though they may occur at any age. It is associated with a chromosomal abnormality in over 90 per cent of cases, the Philadelphia (Ph′) chromosome. This chromosomal abnormality persists throughout the course of the disease irrespective of remission and relapse.

**Clinical features:**— The onset is insidious. There may be anaemia, weakness, malaise, fatigue, night sweats and loss of weight. Spleen is enlarged, occasionally below the umbilicus. Bleeding can occur from any site due to occurrence of thrombocytopenia. Fever may be present when the disease has progressed for some time. Most important signs are pallor, huge enlargement of spleen (sometime massive) and may be associated with hepatomegaly. Deposits of tumour cells commonly under skin, breast, orbit called 'chloromas' can occur. Lymphadenopathy, though uncommon, can occur.

Blood examination reveals a total leucocyte count more than 100 × $10^{9/1}$. Normal looking granulocytes form the predominant cells. Earlier cells like metamyelocytes, myelocytes and promyelocytes are also seen (Pl. II, Fig. 4.8). In chronic phase, myeloblasts usually do not exceed 5 per cent. Presence of increased eosinophils and basophils, which may occur, indicates poor prognosis. Platelets will also be increased. Bone marrow presents a hypercellular marrow. M:E ratio may be 45-50:1 compared to normal 4-5:1. There is granulocytic cellular preponderance. Leucocyte alkaline phosphatase activity is markedly reduced or absent.

**Treatment:**—Busulphan (Myleran), an alkylating agent, remains the drug of choice in this condition till now. It is given orally commencing with a dosage of 4 mgm daily but may have to be increased in certain cases (those who are Ph′ negative) to 6 mgm daily till a haematological remission occurs or the total count drops below 10 × $10^{9/1}$. Some advocate continuing maintenance therapy with 2 mgm myleran daily and others deprecate it as it will induce marrow depression because of its cumulative effect. Radiation therapy is no longer popular now. Patients usually survive 4 to 5 years. Transformation of chronic granulocytic leukaemia to 'blastic' or acute phase usually occurs after 3 to 4 years of treatment. Recurrent infection, lymphadenopathy, bleeding and infection are the usual complications one may see during transformation. Peripheral blood shows a large number of 'blast' cells and the marrow may show 40 to 50 per cent of blast cells. In the acute accelerated phase, therapy will be like acute leukaemias, though the response to treatment has been very poor. Patients usually die of infection or bleeding.

### Chronic Lymphatic Leukaemia (C.L.L.)

It is a disease of older people who may remain asymptomatic for a long period. Various lymphoid tissues of the body like lymph glands, tonsils, bone marrow become infiltrated with mature lymphocytes. These mature lymphocytes are long lived ones. Majority of the C.L.L. are B type, some are T type and the rest are neither B nor T type i.e. "null" types.

**Clinical features:**—About 25 per cent of patients are asymptomatic and are detected on a routine check-up for other conditions. There may be symptoms of anaemia along with generalised lymphadenopathy. Hepatosplenomegaly is often present. There may be bleeding from any site due to thrombocytopenia and erythrodermia or skin infiltration of leukaemic cells. There may be fever due to infection. Enlarged retroperitoneal or mesenteric glands can present gastrointestinal symptoms.

Peripheral blood shows a high total leucocyte count varying from 50-100 × $10^{9/1}$, though normal count in few cases could also be present. Most of the cells are mature small lymphocytes. Anaemia is usually present which is normocytic normochromic. Bone marrow shows infiltration with lymphocytes which is variable and may have some relationship to prognosis.

A clinical staging system has been introduced by Rai et al as follows:—

| | Clinical Stage | | Medium survival months |
|---|---|---|---|
| Stage 0 | Absolute lymphocytosis $15 \times 10^{9/l}$ | ... | 150 |
| Stage 1 | Absolute lymphocytosis + lymphadenopathy | ... | 105 |
| Stage 2 | Absolute lymphocytosis + lymphadenopathy + enlarged spleen and/or liver | ... | 71 |
| Stage 3 | Absolute lymphocytosis + lymphadenopathy + anaemia (Hb < 11 gm/dl) | ... | 19 |
| Stage 4 | Absolute lymphocytosis + lymphadenopathy + thrombocytopenia | ... | 19 |

**Treatment**—Asymptomatic patients need not be treated. When patient develops symptoms like pallor, fever, weight loss, enlarged lymph nodes, splenomegaly, thrombocytopenia, then they must be treated. No drug is shown to alter the prognosis in C.L.L. but they do help in arresting the signs of disease activities for some time. Chlorambucil (Leukeran) 0.1 to 0.2 mgm/kg per day or Cyclophosphamide 2 mgm/kg body weight per day along with prednisolone 2 mgm/kg per body per day are effective in arresting the progress of the disease. Patients will improve in general health, lymph glands and spleen will decrease in size, anaemia will disappear and there will be marked drop in the total leukocyte count. The drugs are given on intermittent schedule. Maintenance therapy is not advisable, especially in older groups because of the danger of marrow depression. Irradiation has been also tried in C.L.L. Steroids are particularly useful in cases with autoimmune haemolytic anaemia.

### Hairy Cell Leukaemia

It is an uncommon variety of chronic leukaemia which is important to diagnose because it shows very little response to cytotoxic drugs. Clinically, over and above the usual symptoms of fatigue, loss of weight, the most characteristic sign is splenomegaly which may even be massive. There may be haemorrhage from any site. Liver may or may not be enlarged. Peripheral smear shows characteristic mononuclear cell with hair-like projections. There is usually pancytopenia in peripheral blood. Bone marrow is infiltrated with similar type of hairy cell. Hairy cells are from monocytes or from B lymphocytes. Treatment is splenectomy following which there is complete or partial response. Patients with partial response have not been very encouraging. Treatment by leukapheresis has been considered in this variety also because of long life of hairy cells and slow turnover.

### Leukaemoid Reaction

Here the peripheral blood picture resembles that of leukaemia but the underlying condition is non-leukaemic. Increase of white cell count seldom goes beyond $80 \times 10^{9/l}$ and immature cells are moderately increased. Occasionally 'blast' cells 1% to 2% are also seen. Myeloid leukaemoid reaction occurs mostly in children following an acute infection. Underlying clinical condition differentiates it from leukaemia. A lymphatic leukaemoid reaction is seen in infectious mononucleosis, occasional cases of tuberculosis and rare cases of carcinoma.

**Leucoerythroblastic anaemia:**—This occurs due to infiltration of bone marrow by secondary carcinoma, multiple myeloma, myelosclerosis, Gaucher's disease and marble bone disease.

### Infectious Mononucleosis

It is an infection by an Epstein Barr virus. It is characterised by fever, headache, superficial lymph node enlargement. Occasionally there may be jaundice, skin rash (maculo-papular) and rarely atypical pneumonia, conjunctivitis or purpura haemorrhagica. Spleen may be enlarged and hepatitis is fairly common. Peripheral blood shows an increase in total count varying from 10 to $20 \times 10^{9/1}$ but occasionally may exceed $20 \times 10^{9/1}$. Majority of the cells are lymphocytes. Atypical lymphocytes with blue, foamy cytoplasm and floating pseudopodia flowing around adjoining red cells is very suggestive of the diagnosis which is confirmed by the detection of heterophil antibodies by Paul-Bunnel test or by the sensitized horse red cells as in "Mono" test kit. Treatment is symptomatic and recovery is usual. When there is evidence of autoimmune phenomenon like thrombocytopenia or haemolytic anaemia, steroids will be useful. Antibiotics have no effect on the course of the disease.

## HODGKIN'S DISEASE, MALIGNANT LYMPHOMAS, MULTIPLE MYELOMA, MACROGLOBULINEMIA AND MONOCLONAL GAMMOPATHIES.

### Hodgkin's Disease

It is characterised by painless lymph gland enlargement with or without fever, anaemia and weight loss. Cervical lymph nodes are commonly enlarged but mediastinal, retroperitoneal glands, axillary and inguinal glands can also be enlarged in many cases. There is progressive weight loss.

Cause of the condition is unknown though viral agent like Epstein-Barr virus has been implicated but not confirmed. Sub-types of Hodgkin's disease have been classified as (i) lymphocyte predominance (paragranuloma) (ii) nodular sclerosis (iii) mixed cellularity (granuloma) (iv) lymphocyte depletion (Hodgkin's Sarcoma). Peripheral blood shows a neutrophil leucocytosis sometime with eosinophilia. There may be haemolytic anaemia.

Diagnosis is made by lymph node biopsy where the glandular architecture is replaced by the proliferation of reticular endothelial cells. Presence of Sternberg-Reed mirror image giant cell with prominent nucleoli is diagnostic of the condition. Classification is based on the histological picture that is presented by lymph gland. Nodular sclerosis constitutes 50% of most series and occurs in young adults. Nodules contain plasma cells, neutrophils and eosinophils and SR cells having abundant cytoplasm with lacunar spaces (Lacunar cells). Nodules are surrounded by bands of collagen tissue. Lymphocyte predominance has abundant normal lymphocytes and small number of SR cells. Mixed cellularity has moderate number of SR cells along with plasma cells, neutrophils and eosinophils. Lymphocyte depletion has few lymphocytes but many SR cells.

**Assessment of the disease and planning for therapy**

(Staging)

The 1971 Ann Arbor symposium suggested the following:

Stage I — Involvement of a single lymph node region.

| | | |
|---|---|---|
| Stage II | — | Involvement of 2 or more lymph nodes on same side of diaphragm. |
| Stage III | — | Lymph node involvement on both sides of diaphragm. |
| Stage IV | — | Diffuse or disseminated involvement of one or more extra lymphatic organs or tissues with or without associated lymph node enlargement. |

Each stage is subdivided into A or B category. A—no symptom ; B—with symptoms of fever, weight loss and night sweats.

### Principles of Treatment

Treatment programmes involve both chemotherapy and radiotherapy. When initial diagnosis is made, joint discussion amongst surgeon, haematologist, radiation oncologist, medical oncologist and pathologist is advisable.

**Surgery:**—Primary role is to have the diagnostic biopsy. Abdominal laparotomy with lymph node biopsy, splenectomy, liver biopsies have been performed in staging certain patients prior to extensive lymph node irradiation. Splenectomy is carried out in patients with hypersplenism.

**Radiation therapy:**—Irradiation is still the primary form of treatment for all localised Hodgkin's diseases with few exceptions. Recent analysis shows that stage I and stage II patients treated with irradiation, 71.18 per cent have remained disease-free.

**Chemotherapy:**—May be advocated in addition to irradiation when systemic symptoms are present with localised disease (stage II B) or more advanced disease (stage III, stage IV). With chemotherapy, some patients are in remission for more than 10 years or more and may be cured. Radiotherapy is the treatment of choice for stages I and II, chemotherapy for other stages. Treatment with chemotherapy should be a combination of drugs and not one single drug.

**Remission induction:**—MOPP or MVPP therapy. It consists of mustine hydrochloride 6 mg/m$^2$ I.V. on days 1 and 8, vincristine (now replaced by vinblastine) 1.4 mgm/m$^2$ I.V. on 1 and 8. Procarbazine 100 mgm/m$^2$ per orally daily on days 1 to 14 inclusive. Prednisolone 40 mgm orally daily on days 1 to 14 inclusive. Cycles are to be repeated every 4 weeks.

Other combinations are :

BCNU 100 mgm/m$^2$ I.V. day 1

Vinblastin 5 mgm/m$^2$ I.V. day 1

Cyclophosphamide 600 mgm/m$^2$ I. V. on day 1

Procarbazine 100 mgm/m$^2$ P.O. days 1 to 4

Prednisolone 60 mgm/m$^2$ P.O. days 1 to 4

Cycle repeated every 4 weeks.

There are other regimen like adding bleomycin to MOPP regimen (BLEO-MOPP).

In this condition it is not considered essential to give any maintenance therapy.

### Combined Radiotherapy and Chemotherapy

As 70% of patients with Hodgkin's disease treated with irradiation are likely to be cured, it is not considered essential to further treat them with chemotherapy, as chemotherapy may produce in its wake various complications including depression of immunity.

Perhaps it would be all right to treat stages I and II with radiotherapy, but stage II B (with fever, night-sweats), it would would be preferable to give 2 to 3 cycles of chemotherapy as well. Stages III A—Irradiation with chemotherapy. Stages III B, IV A and B are given usually six courses of combinat chemotherapy followed by irradiation to initially involved sites. It is always advisable to give courses of chemotherapy first to mediastinal tumours as irradiation might damage the lungs.

## NON-HODGKIN'S LYMPHOMAS

**(Lymphocytic, Histiocytic and Undifferentiated)**

This is one of very common malignancy that is met with in our country. This may occur at any age but shows a peak in childhood and after 50 years of age.

**Aetiology**—A viral aetiology has been suggested in some lymphomas like Burkitt's lymphoma where virus is thought to be the cause.

**Clinical features** are similar to Hodgkin's disease except for (a) an early involvement of oropharyngeal lymphoid tissue, skin, G.I. tract and bone (b) leukaemic transformations with high peripheral lymphocyte count (c) increased susceptibility to bacterial, viral and fungal infections associated with hypogammaglobulinemia, and poor humoral antibody responses (d) autoimmune haemolytic anaemia with positive antiglobin test (e) intra-abdominal manifestations occur commonly in children. Diagnosis is made by lymph gland biopsy. Recommended classification is that of Rappaport (1966) but with the recent discovery of T cells and B cells, some authors have proposed revised classification.

Rappaport's classification :—

| | |
|---|---|
| Lymphocytic well differentiated : | (a) Nodular or<br>(b) diffuse. |
| Lymphocytic poorly differentiated : | (a) Nodular or<br>(b) diffuse. |
| Mixed lymphocytic histiocytic : | (a) Nodular<br>(b) diffuse. |
| Histiocytic : | (a) Nodular<br>(b) diffuse |
| Stem cell or undifferentiated diffuse. | |

Most of the nodular lymphomas are of B cell origin. Burkitt's lymphoma has surface markers for B lymphocytes. Only a minority of lymphomas are of T cell type. Mycoisis fungoides, Sezary's syndrome are of T cell type. Probably also Sternberg's sarcoma. Staging is similar to Hodgkin's disease. Diagnosis is from lymph node biopsy, but bone marrow should be examined in all cases as they are commonly involved unlike Hodgkin's.

### TREATMENT

**Radiation therapy**—Irradiation is the primary form of treatment in localized stages. Extended field arrangement on one side of diaphragm is most frequently used.

Surgical treatment is resorted to in gastrointestinal lymphoma by excision followed by chemotherapy, though some authors advocate irradiation. The childhood bowel lymphoma should be treated with chemotherapy from the very beginning as the risk of dissemination is very high. Chemotherapy is the treatment of choice in generalised cases. Combination chemotherapy in the form of cyclophosphamide, vincristine and prednisolone (COP) may be given at 3 weekly intervals. It is given in the following doses :

| | |
|---|---|
| Cyclophosphamide | 1000 mgm/$m^2$ I.V. day 1 |
| | or |
| | 400 mgm/$m^2$/d.p.o. from days 1 to 5 |
| Vincristine | 1.2 mgm.$m^2$/I.V. on day 1 |
| Prednisolone | 100 mgm/$m^2$/d.p.o. from days 1 to 5 |
| | Repeat cycle every 4 weeks. |

Drug Adriamycin has been found to be very useful in this condition. The most commonly used combination nowadays is:

| | |
|---|---|
| Adriamycin | 40 mgm/$m^2$/ I.V. on day 1 |
| Vincristine | 1.4 mgm/$m^2$/I.V. on day 1 |
| Cyclophosphamide | 600 mgm/$m^2$ I.V. on day 1 |
| Prednisolone | 100 mgm/$m^2$/d.p.o. on days 1 to 5 |

Courses are given every 3 to 4 weeks. Bleomycin has now been added. The role of maintenance therapy in this condition remains undecided.

## MULTIPLE MYELOMA

(Pl. II, Figs. 4.10, 4.11)

In this condition, there is a neoplastic proliferation of plasma cells characterised by osteolytic bone lesions and elevation of serum globulin. It is associated with B lymphocytes. Homogenous globulin produced by the neoplastic plasma cells indicates single clone disorder from B-lymphocytes. Benign monoclonal gammopathy is also of B-lymphocyte disorder and should be differentiated from multiple myeloma.

**Clinical features**—Most common presenting symptom is back pain. Pathological fractures are also common. An unexplained anaemia may bring the patient to the doctor. There may be abnormal bleeding tendencies especially from the gums. Infection is the most common complication of M.M. There may be renal insufficiency and it is one of the causes of death in this condition. Bence-Jones proteinuria appears to be the cause of renal failure. Blood shows high E.S.R. and rouleux formation of red cells.

**Diagnosis**—Major criteria are (i) plasmacytomas on tissue biopsy, (ii) bone marrow showing more than 30 per cent plasma cells, (iii) lytic bone lesions, (iv) monoclonal globulin spike with Ig G$>$3.5 g/d1 or Ig A $>$ 2.0 gm/dl; light chain excretions $>$ 1 g per day.

Minor criteria are (i) bone marrow plasma cells 10%-30% (ii) monoclonal globulin spikes with Ig G$<$ 3.5 g/d1 or Ig A$<$ 2.0 g/d1, (iii) lytic bone lesions, (iv) reduction of normal immunoglobulins Ig M$<$50 mgm% Ig A $<$ 100 mgm% or Ig G $<$ 600 mgm%.

Diagnosis is supported by (i)b, (i)c, (i)d or (ii)b, (ii)c, (ii)d or (iii) or a+b+c, a+b+d.

**Treatment**—Chemotherapy should be started when the disease is progressive.

(i) Melphalan (or alkeran) is the drug of choice and is given in an intermittent schedule with high dosage for 4 days, viz. 10 mgm/$m^2$/d or 0.25 mgm/mg/d × 4 days. It is given every 4 weeks. Melphalan increase the survival time. It is often combined with prednisolone which further increases the longevity.

(ii) Prednisolone or prednisone is given in the dosage of 1-2 mgm/kg body wt/d for 4 days, concurrently with melphalan or endoxan.

(iii) Cyclophosphamide or Endoxan orally or i.v. in intermittent dosage of 1 gm/$m^2$ i.v. or orally 60-100 mgm/$m^2$/d or 1.5 to 2.5 mgm/kg/d for 4 days.

(iv) BCNU,CCNU, procarbazin or adriamycin have also been tried in M. M. with limited success.

(v) Radiation therapy is especially effective in the relief of local painful bony lesion and following pathological fractures. Solitary plasmacytomas with absent bone marrow infiltration deserves local irradiation in preferance to chemotherapy. Maintenance therapy in multiple myeloma is not advocated.

**Waldenstrom's Macroglobulinaemia**

This is an uncommon condition seen in men over the age of 50 years. Clinical features of this condition are like those of lymphoma which progress slowly. In this condition, clone of B lymphocytes proliferates and infiltrates bone marrow, lymph nodes, liver and spleen. These lymphocytic cells have plasma-like morphological appearance and produces an abnormal macroglobulin which has antibody specificity as rheumatoid factor, cold antibody or antistreptolysin O.

**Clinical features**—Patient complains of fatigue and bleeding tendency. There may be thrombocytopenia. Lymph glands are moderately enlarged, so also liver and spleen. Raynaud's phenomenon may occur due to hyperviscosity in small peripheral vessels. Visual disturbances due to impaired retinal circulation may occur.

**Diagnosis** is by bone marrow aspiration which shows plasmacytoid lymphocytes and an increase in mast cells. Peripheral blood shows lymphocytosis. Serum electrophoresis shows IgM spike. The 'Sia water test' where a drop of serum in a tube of distilled water produces flocculation is often positive.

**Treatment**—Plasmapharesis or penicillamine therapy may help. Chlorambucil with or without prednisolone may be given at a dose of 0.4—0.8 mgm/kg every 2 to 3 weeks. Supportive therapy with blood transfusion and antibiotics may be necessary.

**Monoclonal Gammopathy**

Due to proliferation of B lymphocytes, monoclonal protein is produced consisting of heavy chains which are incomplete and is called heavy chain disease.

Alpha heavy chain disease occurs in those areas where there is conisderable intestinal infestation which is common in our country. Therefore, it is expected that there may be many undetected alpha heavy chain diseases in our country.

## MYELOPROLIFERATIVE DISORDERS

Under this term, a group of disorders showing hyperplasia or neoplasia of one or more haemopoietic stem cell derivative have taken place. Myeloproliferative disorders occur without any apparent physiological or reactive cause. Controversy still exists about this nomenclature and placing polycythaemia, erythroleukaemia, thrombocythemia, myelofibrosis and chronic granulocytic leukaemia under one head. Chronic granulocytic leukaemia, thrombocythaemia and erythroleukaemia have already been described. We shall now discuss polycythaemia and myelofibrosis.

**Polycythaemia Rubra Vera**

This is a disease of middle age characterized by erythrocytosis with Hb up to 20 gm/dl. It is not due to any known physiological causes which can cause polycythaemia. This disease arises due to abnormal proliferation of stem cell. There is an increased blood volume and blood viscosity. Most of the symptoms are due to the consequence of these two conditions leading to increased red cell mass. Complaints relating to the disturbed cerebral circulation include headache, dizziness, vertigo, a sense of fullness of the head, blurred vision, tinnitus and syncope. Repeated thrombotic episodes and haemorrhages occur during the course of the disease. Spleen may be enlarged. Pruritus does occur and is often very disabling. There is also hyperuricaemia and attack of gout.

Blood examination shows elevated haemoglobin value, increase in red cells, white cells and platelet series of cells; packed cell volume is raised. Nucleated red cells and polychromasia are also present. White cell count may be raised as high as 50,000/mm$^3$ with an increase in basophils and alkaline phosphatase. Platelets are also increased. Bone marrow is hypercellular and normoblastic. There is also an increase in megakaryocytes. In a suspected case with an increase in Hb and P.C.V, the diagnosis is confirmed. If isotope technique is available, red cell mass can be determined to differentiate polycythaemia rubra vera from secondary polycythaemia.

**Treatment :** Repeated phlebotomy is the first choice as it is safe. By plebotomy, one can bring down the Hb and PCV to normal range. Chemotherapy in the form of myleran has also been used for depressing marrow activity. This is the most satisfactory drug. Other drugs also have been used like melphalan and chlorambucil.

Radioactive phosphorus has also been used to depress the marrow activity. Radioactive phosphorus might produce leukaemia on a later date.

**Secondary Polycythaemia**

Occurs in (i) high altitude, (ii) chronic pulmonary disease, (iii) congenital heart disease, (iv) familial polycythaemia and (v) is associated with haemoglobinopathies.

**Myelosclerosis**

This disease is characterised by progressive splenic enlargement and gradual fibrosis of the bone marrow. It could be (i) primary idiopathic or (ii) secondary following tuberculosis, secondary carcinoma, Hodgkin's disease, leukaemia or exposure to benzene or irradiation.

The disease, primary idiopathic myelosclerosis, is a progressive disease affecting people in late middle age. Males and females are equally affected. Along with myelosclerosis, there is extramedullary erythropoiesis (myeloid metaplasia). Onset is gradual and insidious. Patients present with unexplained anaemia, not responding to usual antianaemic drugs. He also complains of abdominal fullness which is due to large enlargement of spleen. Liver enlargement also occurs in more than 50% of cases. Bleeding from any site can occur usually due to thrombocytopenia. Sternal tenderness may be present. X-ray shows patchy sclerosis of medullary cavity, coarsening of trabeculae giving mottled appearance.

Peripheral blood shows leucoerythroblastic anaemia. Anaemia is invariable, may be slight in the beginning. In later stages of the disease Hb may fall to as low as 6 gm/dl due to less production and haemolysis. Anisocytosis is usual and often conspicuous. Hypersplenism also contributes to anaemia. Leucocyte count is raised. Few immature myeloid series of cells will be seen in the peripheral blood. The alkaline phosphatase content is increased. One of the essential diagnostic points is the failure of bone marrow aspiration to draw marrow material resulting in dry tap. Bone marrow biopsy is essential in this condition.

**Treatment**—There is no specific therapy, but anaemia is treated with blood transfusion. Steroids along with androgen are given with a hope to reduce the number of transfusions. Myleran is also given to help in the reduction of the size of spleen. Splenectomy is not considered helpful in this condition unless it is really massive and is producing hypersplenism which in turn raises the demands of too frequent blood transfusion.

**Hypersplenism**

It is a condition where there is enlargement of spleen, anaemia, leucopenia with neutropenia or thrombocytopenia singly or in combination. Splenectomy corrects this disorder. Hypersplenism could be primary or secondary following thalassaemia, malaria, kala-azar and a host of other conditions in which there are enlargement of spleen along with symptoms of hypersplenism.

## BLOOD TRANSFUSION

### ABO Blood Groups

Landsteiner in 1901 discovered ABO blood group system which paved the way for safe blood transfusion and contributed to the present-day knowledge of all blood group systems.

ABO blood group is divided into 4 main blood groups based on the fact that A and B antigens can be present singly or together or may be absent. Identification of these antigens is carried out by means of anti-A and anti-B agglutinins which occur naturally in the sera of persons not having the corresponding antigens. Serum antibodies cannot coexist with the corresponding antigens.

| Blood Group | Agglutinogens in cells | Antibodies in the serum |
|---|---|---|
| A | A | anti-B |
| B | B | anti-A |
| AB | AB | none |
| O | none | Both anti-A and anti-B |

O blood group used to be called universal blood donor as it was thought to be safe to transfuse to any group. Now it is known that those O group who have high titre anti-A or anit-B are dangerous to be transfused to any other group but O blood group. AB group is universal recipient as they do not have any antibodies in their sera.

The blood group antibodies are natural antibodies and react best with the corresponding antigen in cold or at room temperature. They are complete antibodies and require no other additives to bring about agglutination with the corresponding antigen. There is another type of antibody called immune type or incomplete type which appears in the blood as a response to the introduction of a red cell antigen in the body parenterally. These antibodies can react best with antigen at 37° C. These are IgG immunoglobulins which can pass through placental barrier. Immune anti-A or anti-B produced in a pregnant mother can cross the placental barrier and produce haemolytic disease in the new-born due to incompatibility in ABO blood group system with her husband.

ABO blood group is identified by direct and indirect grouping tests. In direct grouping, individual's red cell antigen is identified by using known anti-A or anti-B antisera.

**Table below showing the agglutination reaction :**

| Anti-A | Anti-B | Anti A,B (Group O) | Blood Group |
|---|---|---|---|
| + | – | + | A |
| – | + | + | B |
| + | + | + | AB |
| – | – | – | O |

Anti-A,-B (group O) sera are always used in direct grouping to detect weak sub-groups of A like $A_2$, $A_3$, $A_x$, as these are not detected by anti-A serum. It is important to remember that in A blood group there are two main sub-groups $A_1$ and $A_2$. If $A_1$ blood is given to $A_2$, the recipient will be sensitized to $A_1$ antigen and subsequent transfusion will produce reaction. Sub-group $A_1$ is detected by the extracts of seed doliches bifloras.

Indirect grouping is done by putting up patient's sera against known A, B and O cells.

| Recipient's Sera | A Cells | B Cells | O Cells | Blood Group |
|---|---|---|---|---|
| R. S. against | – | + | – | A |
| R. S. against | + | – | – | B |
| R. S. against | – | – | – | AB |
| R. S. against | + | + | – | O |
| R. S. against | + | + | + | $O_h$ (Bombay group) |

The Bombay blood group was first discovered in Bombay and is a very rare group. Bombay blood group people can be transfused with only Bombay group blood. Distribution of ABO group amongst 10,000 persons belonging to different parts of India was analysed by the author. Phenotype percentage was A group 26.0 per cent, B group 34.3 per cent, AB group 9.6 per cent and O group 30.1 per cent.

**Rh blood group system**

In 1940 Landsteiner and Weiner discovered another important blood group antigen called Rh antigen (Rh stands for Rhesus monkey whose red cells were used to produce anti-Rh sera in rabbits and guinea-pigs). It is an important blood group as many cases of haemolytic disease of the new-born are due to Rh immunisation of the pregnant mother. Those who have Rh antigen are called Rh positive. 95% of the people of India are Rh positive and those who do not possess Rh antigen are called Rh negative. 5 per cent of the Indian population are Rh negative. Rh antigen is not a single one but either closely linked genes on the same chromosome (called C,D,E, c, d,e) or according to Weiner by a series of allelic genes like $R^0$, $R^1$, $R^2$, $R^z$ r, r′, r″ and $r^y$. Convenient notation for Rh phenotype is to use one nomenclature using 5 sera for detection of antigen, namely, anti-C, anti-c, anti-D, anti-E and anti-e. However, for all practical purposes in clinical practice, one only determines whether a person is Rh positive or negative by using anti-D sera. (D positive or D negative). This Rh group is always determined routinely in any transfusion procedure to prevent sensitization.

As Rh (or D) antigen is a strong antigen, if it is introduced parenterally into an Rh negative individual, it will produce anti-Rh antibodies. These antibodies are immune type, IgG antibodies which react best with the corresponding antigen at 37°C. As these are IgG antibodies, they can cross the placental barrier.

Importance of Rh system is in the production of haemolytic diseases of new-born (HDN). HDN is produced whenever IgG antibodies from mother's circulation cross the placental barrier and react with the red cells of foetus. Both ABO as well as Rh incompatibility between husband and wife can lead to HDN. In ABO group usually mother belongs to O blood group and father to A, B or AB blood group. In Rh incompatibility, mother is Rh (D) negative and father is Rh (D) positive and the foetus is Rh (D) positive. If the mother is already immunised due to previous transfusion, miscarriage or still birth, IgG Rh antibodies of sensitized mother will cross the placental barrier and produce HDN. If mother is not immunised, then her first baby will not be affected, but during or just prior to child birth, certain quantity of foetal cells will leak into maternal circulation and sensitise her, and, therefore, in subsequent pregnancies foetal cells will be acted upon by Rh antibodies and produce HDN. Cases of Rh incompatibility produce severe degrees of HDN,whilst cases of ABO incompatibility, which are more common, are milder. HDN due to Rh incompatibility could be very severe like hydrops foetalis, still-birth or erythroblastosis foetalis depending on the maternal antibody titre. In erythroblastosis foetalis, the neonate is jaundiced right from the birth and would require exchange transfusion to be saved. Some cases may be milder with anaemia and jaundice, when exchange transfusion and phenobarbitone to reduce the icterus might save the child. Nowadays with the introduction of high titre anti-D immunoglobulin which is injected to an unsensitized mother within 72 hours of the birth of the child, sensitisation is prevented in subsequent pregnancy and HDN does not occur.

### Techniques of Blood Transfusion

Transfusion of whole blood, its components and its products have become an important established therapeutic procedure throughout the world. Because of its easy operative procedure and therapeutic value, there is a tendency now to misuse this valuable therapeutic measure without considering the risks involved in the transfusion. Further, whole blood should be used rarely as in case of oligaemic shock following haemorrhage. Components like packed red cells, platelet rich plasma (PRP), platelet concentrate (PC), white cells, plasma coagulation factors like factor VIII, factor IX, prothrombin, fibrinogen or products like immunoglobulin, albumin should be used instead.

In the laboratory, blood O is collected from a healthy donor aged between 18 and 60 years who is free from all diseases. There should be no past history of jaundice or recent attack of malaria. Donor blood is tested for Hb which should be 13 gms/dl or above and also for Australia antigen ($Hb_s$ Ag) which is the cause for serum hepatitis. It should be free from $HB_s$ Ag.

The blood is collected in a B.T. bottle or plastic bag containing ACD (Acid Citrate Dextrose) or CPD (Citrate Phosphate Dextrose).

Before the blood is issued, the recipient's blood is cross-matched with donor's blood by (i) saline, (ii) albumin, (iii) indirect antiglobin (Coomb's) techniques and sometime by enzyme method. Donor's cells are put up against recipient's serum (major match) and donor's serum is put up against recipient's cells (minor match) by the above-mentioned three methods. If there is no agglutination in any of the tubes, then the blood is issued for transfusion, It is preferable to issue blood after 72 hours of storage at 4° C as Treponema pallidum cannot survive at that temperature and not to issue after 14 days of storage, though up to 21 days blood can be stored in the bank and issued. If there is a demand for fresh blood, V.D.R.L. test must be carried out first on that blood and issued only after it is found to be negative. Australia antigen should also be tested prior to the issue of the blood.

### Complications of Blood Transfusion

There are many hazards in transfusing blood to a patient. Therefore, it is a good maxim to remember to give transfusion only when the values accrued to a patient from such measures outweigh the inherent risks involved.

Common complications that one meets with following blood transfusions are as follows :

(1) Pyrogen reaction
(2) Allergic reaction
(3) Transmission of diseases like malaria, serum hepatitis
(4) Circulatory overload
(5) Citrate and potassium toxicity

Uncommon complications are :

(6) Incompatible blood transfusion
(7) Transfusion of infected blood
(8) Transfusion haemosiderosis
(9) Air embolism
(10) Thrombocytopenia

(1) **Pyrogen reaction** :—Febrile reaction due to pyrogens which are dead bacterial products contributes the greatest number of reactions. Pyrogen reaction occurs more commonly with bottles and rarely with plastic bags. Febrile reaction due to leucocyte antibodies, platelet antibodies also contributes a fair number of cases. When a patient develops febrile reaction, drip must be slowed, patient to be covered with blankets and given either aspirin or paracetamol to reduce the temperature. To prevent pyrogen reaction, one must use scrupulous aseptic technique in manfacturing ACD bottles and stricter asepsis during the collection of blood.

Leucocyte and platelet antibodies can be removed by packing the red cells and washing them with sterile normal saline. This is necessary especially in thalassaemia cases who get repeated transfusions.

(2) **Allergic reaction** :—It is not often possible to prevent allergic reaction which varies from 1 to 3 per cent. The allergic manifestations could be (a) urticarial rash, (b) giant urticaria, (c) an attack of bronchial asthma, (d) anaphylactoid reaction, or (e) laryngeal oedema or oedema glottis. Often it is due to anti-IgA antibodies in the recipient which reacts with the IgA of donor's plasma.

Treatment is to slow down the drip and give antihistamine drugs like Phenergan I.M. If the reaction is severe like an attack of bronchial asthma, laryngeal oedema or anaplylactoid reaction, then over and above adrenaline, one may have to give hydrocortisone intravenously. In severe cases, transfusion should be stopped.

(3) **Transmission of disease**

(a) **Malaria** :—If malaria occurs following transfusion, patient should be treated fully with camoquin or chloroquine.

(b) **Serum hepatitis** :—It is due to Australia antigen present in the donor's blood. About 2.5 per cent of our donor population carry this virus. Therefore, all donor's blood must be tested for Australia antigen prior to transfusion to prevent such an occurrence. Serum hepatitis is more severe than infectious hepatitis (short incubation virus) and should be prevented. In case it occurs, treatment is similar to that of infectious hepatitis. Recently, high titre immunoglobulin containing antibody to Australia antigen has been given by injection to such patients and has been found to be useful.

(4) **Circulatory overload** : Leads to acute left ventricular failure. It occurs especially in elderly, anaemic individuals and those with cardiac and pulmonary disease. Here the transfusion rate should be very slow to prevent such occurrence. Treatment is to stop the transfusion and give morphine, Lasix and digoxin intravenously. It is better in such cases to give 40 mgm Lasix I.M. prior to transfusion. Venesection may be necessary in desperate cases.

(5) **Citrate and potassium toxicity** :—These are seen mostly in massive transfusion or during exchange transfusion in neonates. To prevent such an occurrence, it is always better to give 10% calcium gluconate intravenously, usually 10 ml after every litre of blood has been transfused and in neonates after every 100 ml of blood exchanged.

(6) **Incompatible blood transfusion** :— It may occur due to wrong labelling of blood, wrong identification of patient with similar name or due to technical error.

When an incompatible blood is given, patient complains of warm sensation along the vein, constrictive feeling or oppression in the chest, severe pain in the loin, chill and rigor, high temperature, tachycardia and fall of blood pressure. Patient then develops haemoglobinuria and jaundice due to destruction of blood, followed by oliguria which then goes on to anuria and uraemia.

**Treatment**—Immediately the condition is recognised, blood transfusion must be stopped and bottle preserved for grouping and cross-matching with a sample from patient's blood collected after the reaction and also with the one collected before the reaction. In order to prevent the occurrence of renal failure one must give to the patient immediately enough of compatible blood. If nearly one bottle of incompatible blood has been transfused, then about two bottles of compatible blood should be transfused immediately. If the urine flow falls below 100 ml/hr, Mannitol 25 gm is to be given I.V. and if necessary to be repeated, but not more than 100 gm to be given within 24 hours. If oliguria or anuria develops, restricted fluid regimen is to be adopted. (Modified Bull's regimen).

7. **Transfusion of infected blood** :—Contamination of blood is to be prevented by strict aseptic measure during blood collection. Blood, after collection, should be refrigerated immediately. Prior to issue of the bottle, one must check for signs of haemolysis in the bottle. Treatment is to combat shock and use of broad spectrum antibiotics. The suspected bottle should be cultured at 4° C room temperature and at 37° C. Immediate slide preparation with a gram stain may help in quick identification.

8. **Transfusion haemosiderosis** :—Occurs where blood is being transfused periodically as in cases of aplastic anaemia and thalassaemia. It is always advisable to give chelating agent like desferrioxamine (Desferal) frequently by I.M. to reduce the iron load.

9. **Air embolism** :—It occurs when the blood bottle becomes empty and air rushes into the vein. It may also occur through a leak in the tube. Higginson's syringe is rarely used these days to introduce positive pressure in the blood bottle. When there is air embolism, patient becomes cyanosed and dyspnoeic. There is a fall of B.P. and ventricular fibrillation may set in. Treatment is to place the patient head down on his left lateral position and hope for the best. In most instances, the blood bottle becomes empty as there is lack of supervision by the nursing staff and the patient is found dead. It is therefore the duty of the nursing staff to see that the bottle is disconnected before it is completely empty. Normal adults can tolerate about 200 ml of air I.V., but a seriously ill patient may not tolerate even 10 ml which may become fatal.

10. **Thrombophlebitis** :—It occurs when transfusion is going on for a longer period, especially following infusion of dextrose saline or dextrose. It is preferable not to continue blood in the same vein after 5% dextrose drip, as not only there may occur thrombophlebitis, but also certain amount of haemolysis of the donor red cells may result following such procedure.

CHAPTER 5

# COLLAGEN DISORDERS

(Syn : Connective tissue diseases; diffuse collagen diseases or collagenoses)

*M. Roy*
*G. C. Mookerjee*

## INTRODUCTION

Connective tissues or collagen tissues may be affected due to autoimmune or allergic disorders, producing varieties of clinical syndromes depending on the tissues involved, e.g., muscles, skin, blood vessels, heart, lungs, joints, kidneys and CNS.

They are acquired diseases that have the following features in common :

(a) There may be widespread degeneration of collagen with or without fibrinoid necrosis. The process may be acute or chronic.

(b) There may be marked constitutional effects with raised ESR, hypergammaglobulinaemia, while some have sub-acute symptoms.

(c) There is considerable interrelationship between the disorders.

(d) Most of these disorders usually respond to adrenal steroids and ACTH, though often temporarily. Their action is presumably anti-inflammatory and inhibitory to auto-antibody formation.

This group of acquired diseases must be distinguished from rare hereditary disorders of connective tissue. In addition to the "big five" collagen disorders, rheumatic fever, rheumatoid arthritis, systemic lupus erythematosus, polyarteritis nodosa and scleroderma, these acquired group of diseases include dermatomyositis, Sjogren's syndrome, glomerulonephritis, etc. The aetiology of these disorders is not clearly understood, though immunological aberrations may be playing a part in most. While the diseases mentioned above have been characterised as distinct entities, these have some common features, e.g., synovitis, pleuritis, myocarditis, myositis, vasculitis, nephritis etc., and because of these overlapping features, their differentiation is often difficult. Further, in some cases the disorder may include characteristics of more than two or three of these diseases providing what is called *overlap syndromes.*

Rheumatic fever and rheumatoid arthritis have been discussed in separate chapters. In the subsequent paragraphs we have presented SLE, polyarteritis nodosa, scleroderma, Sjogren's syndrome, dermatomyositis and overlap syndromes.

## SYSTEMIC LUPUS ERYTHEMATOSIS (S.L.E.)

### GENERAL CONSIDERATIONS

S.L.E. is an inflammatory autoimmune disorder usually with multiple system involvement. The clinical manifestations are considered to be due to antigen-antibody complexes being trapped in capillaries of visceral structures.

The course of the disease may vary from a mild episode to a rapidly fulminating fatal illness. It shows a striking predilection for women. It may occur at any age; most patients are between 10 and 50 years, with greatest clustering between 20 and 40.

There have been some reports of familial occurrence of SLE. Asymptomatic family members often show positive anti-nuclear antibody tests, anti-DNA antibody and increased gammaglobulin in serum; some of them also show features of other collagen diseases. All these suggest that there is an underlying genetically determined abnormality in immunological regulation. It is postulated that there is a defective T-cell function resulting in B-cell overactivity; this leads to production of various types of antibodies, which causes tissue damage due to deposition of immune complexes. Viruses are thought to play a role in the triggering of this disorder in a genetically disposed individual. Patients with SLE have increased antibody to many viral antigens, like measles, rubella, para-influenza etc.

## CLINICAL FINDINGS

**Systemic features** : Fever, anorexia, malaise, arthralgia and weight loss.

**Skin** : Acute erythematous lesions and photosensitivity occurring in several exposed areas (face and scalp) are of diagnostic importance and may lead to vitiligo, alopecia, hyperpigmentation and subsequent scarring. The characteristic butterfly rash affects fewer than 50% of patients. Other cutaneous manifestations include discoid lupus, periungual erythema, nail-fold infarcts and splinter haemorrhages.

*Kidneys* : Four forms of renal disease are observed :

(a) Diffuse proliferative glomerulonephritis (DPG)—usually begins within the first year of the onset of SLE, with 40-50 per cent of patients dying within the first two years due to renal failure.

(b) Membranous glomerulonephritis—usually associated with a nephrotic syndrome and tends to be slowly progressive. This occurs in about 10-15% patients with kidney disease. The lesion is more responsive to treatment than DPG and 5 years survival rate approaches 70%.

(c) Mesangial type glomerulonephritis has a benign course, renal function is unaffected and little or no proteinuria occurs.

(d) Focal proliferative glomerulonephritis—about 75% of patients with renal disease have this lesion, which is responsive to therapy.

*Neurological symptoms*—develop in about 20% of cases and after renal disease. The symptoms include mental changes, severe depression, psychosis and sometimes convulsions. The assessment of CNS involvement is complicated by steroid therapy, which may induce psychoses that may be difficult to differentiate from SLE induced mental syndromes.

*Joint symptoms*—with or without active synovitis occur in about 90% cases and are often the earliest symptoms. The arthritis usually does not lead to any deformity and erosive changes are not seen in X-ray studies.

*Pleurisy and/or pericarditis*—are seen in 60% cases. Bronchopneumonia and pneumonitis are frequent. Myocarditis may lead to cardiac arrhythmia and cardiac failure. A typical varrucous endocarditis (Libman-Sach's type) may be seen at autopsy. But such a lesion has little effect on the dynamics of circulation.

*Other organ involvement*—Less frequent clinical features of SLE include corneal ulceration, retinal exudate, gastrointestinal ulcerations.

## LABORATORY FINDINGS

A number of serological tests provide a firm basis for diagnosis of SLE and for assessment of the clinical course. Examples of important ones are given below :

A) Antibodies of diagnostic importance

| | |
|---|---|
| Anti-native DNA | —Most widely used for diagnosis and for assessing disease activity. |
| Anti-DN protien | —Responsible for production of L.E. cells *in vitro.* |
| Anti-crude nuclear extracts (ribonuclease resistant) | —Highly specific for SLE. Poor correlation with disease activity. |
| Anti-nuclear RN protein | —Found in other collagen diseases and in overlap syndromes. |
| Anti-cardiolipin | —Biological false positive test for syphilis often used as a screening test for detecting asymptomatic SLE patients. |

B) Antibodies which may have direct cytotoxic effects :

| | |
|---|---|
| Anti-red cell surface antigen | —associated with haemolytic anaemia. |
| Anti-lymphocyte | —associated with lymphopaenia. |
| Anti-platelet | —associated with thrombocytopaenia. |
| Anti-coagulants | —associated with haemostatic disorders. |

The LE cell, present in about 60% cases, are also seen in rheumatoid arthritis, drug induced LE and other collagen disorders. Antinuclear antibody which is less specific is seen in most cases. Hypergammaglobulinaemia, a positive Coomb's test and presence of rheumatoid factor are important findings. Biologically false positive serological test for syphilis occurs in about 20% cases.

There is often mild normochromic anaemia and sometimes autoimmune haemolytic anaemia. Leucopenia, lymphopenia and thrombocytopenia often occur. ESR is almost always raised. Cases with renal lesions usually show proteinuria and cellular casts in urine. Severe proteinuria usually indicates serious renal disease.

## COURSE AND PROGNOSIS

In recent times, the disease has a better prognosis than before. In most patients the disease runs a mild chronic course with exacerbations. In some cases the disease runs a virulent course where there is impairment of many vital functions (e.g. kidney, heart, lungs, etc.), often leading to death. The most frequent observed serious complication is progressive renal disease.

## DIAGNOSIS

The diagnosis of SLE can be made with reasonable probability if at least four of the 14 following criteria are present—butterfly rash, discoid lupus, alopecia, photosensitivity, oral ulcers, Raynaud's phenomenon, non-deforming arthritis, LE cells, false positive serological tests for syphilis, psychoses or convulsions, proteinuria, cellular casts, serositis and some haematological findings (haemolytic anaemia or leucopenia or thrombocytopenia)

## ESSENTIALS FOR DIAGNOSIS :

(a) Occurs mainly in women
(b) Rash over areas exposed to sunlight
(c) Joint symptoms
(d) Multiple symptom involvement
(e) Anaemia, lymphopenia, thrombocytopenia

(f) Serological findings—positive anti-nuclear antibody test, LE cell, false positive serological tests for syphilis.

Before making a diagnosis of spontaneous SLE, it is imperative to exclude that the condition has not been induced by a drug. These drugs include procainamide, hydralazine etc. However, such reactions are not frequent. While anti-nuclear antibody tents may become positive in some persons receiving these drugs, clinical manifestations occur in only a few. For differentiating these reactions from spontaneous SLE, four features may help :—

(i) In drug induced disease, the male and female ratio is nearly equal.
(ii) Renal and neurological symptoms are not usually present.
(iii) Absent antibodies to native DNA and depressed serum complement.
(iv) On withdrawal of the offending drug, the clinical features and most laboratory abnormalities disappear though serological abnormalities may persist for months or years.

## TREATMENT

Corticosteroids are chiefly used for amelioration of symptoms and to check the progress of antigen-antibody damage. Other immunosuppressive agents, which are used when steroids fail, are azathiopurine, cyclophosphamide or chlorambucil. The last two agents are also used along with steroids when there is progressive renal damage.

Steroids are used as prednisolone in dosage of 60 mg. per day in adults in four divided doses with usual precautions. Betamethasone or dexamethasone can be used in equivalent dosage. Gradually dosage is tapered to a daily maintenance level for six to 12 months. Local steroid ointments may be used for skin lesions.

Discoid skin lesions may also respond to chloroquin 250 mg. daily, to be used with caution (risk of retinal damage).

Azathiopurine is used in dosage of 2.5 mg/kg. of body weight per day if steroids fail or when steroids may have to be discontinued due to side effects.

The patient requires additional care for control of joint pains, and cardiac failure from time to time.

Salicylates, ibuprofen and indomethacin group of drugs may be added to relief of joint pains.

Physiotherapy and graduated exercises are also useful.

Rest, high protein diet, sedatives, analgesics, haematinics, blood transfusion, diuretics and digitalis may be prescribed as required.

# POLYARTERITIS NODOSA

## INTRODUCTION

The disease is characterised by segmental lesions in the arteries of small to medium size, resulting in a variety of clinical presentations, depending upon the blood vessel involved. The characteristic hallmark of the disease is acute necrotizing inflammation of the arterial media with fibrinoid necrosis and extensive inflammatory cell infiltration of all coats of the vessel and surrounding tissue. Such a lesion may lead to aneurysmal dilatation, rupture or thrombosis; the lesion may heal by fibrosis with or without occlusion of the lumen. Thus the disease may be encountered in the acute, healing and healed phase. Depending upon the blood vessels affected, all the organs of the body may be affected, but especially kidney, heart, liver, gastrointestinal tract, muscle and testes.

Unlike other collagen diseases, polyarteritis nodosa appears predominantly in men (75% of patients) except those with pulmonary involvement. Its onset is usually acute. It is a multisystem disease with a peak incidence between the ages of 30 and 60 years.

The aetiology of polyarteritis nodosa is unknown. The disease occurs in drug abusers and may be induced by sulphonamides, allopurinol etc. History of allergy is often obtained. Hepatitis B surface antigen is demonstrable in the serum in 30% of cases. Immune complex deposition in the walls of the involved vessels has been observed, suggesting that an immunological factor may be important in the aetiopathogenesis. Anti-nuclear antibodies and rheumatoid factor are found infrequently and in low titre.

## CLINICAL FEATURES

About 80% of patients have renal involvement with painless haematuria, proteinuria and hypertension. The vessels involved are the arcuate and the interlobar arteries; in addition glomeruli may show a focal lesion with fibrinoid necrosis. Azotaemia is usually a late finding and renal failure accounts for about 75% of deaths in cases of polyarteritis nodosa.

Cardiac symptoms occur in 60% of cases and are manifested by pericarditis, myocarditis, arrhythmias and myocardial infarction secondary to coronary artery involvement. Hypertension contributes to congestive heart failure.

Acute abdominal pain (in about 50% of cases) may be related to involvement of vessels supplying major abdominal viscera and concurrent peritonitis.

Lung involvement with severe asthma and eosinophilia occurs in about 20% of cases. The symptoms include chest pain, cough, dyspnoea and haemoptysis. Certain patients fall in the category of Wagener's granulomatosis with granuloma formation, occurring in conjunction with renal disease, but without widespread vascular lesions characteristic of polyarteritis nodosa.

Fifty per cent of patients of this disease show CNS involvement manifested by seizures, focal haemorrhagic signs, organic mental symptoms, hemiparesis, cranial nerve involvement and peripheral neuropathy.

The relatively low incidence of clinical orchitis does not reflect the higher incidence of small testicular vessel involvement seen at autopsy thereby suggesting the testis as a site for diagnostic biopsy.

Myositis is manifested by pain and tenderness in about 20% of cases. It is caused by vasculitis which may be confirmed by muscle biopsy.

Haematological findings include mild anaemia, leucocytosis and eosinophilia. The last is seen in about 30% of cases, more frequently in those with pulmonary involvement. ESR is almost always raised.

The course is variable and unpredictable. Spontaneous remissions may occur. In a large percentage of cases the disease runs a fulminant course resulting in death in months or years.

Diagnosis depends on recognizing multisystem involvement (Fig. 5.1). Biopsy of a tender muscle is positive only in about 20% cases; testicular biopsy is positive in a lesser percentage of cases with tender testes. Visceral angiography may help but is often not useful.

## TREATMENT

There is no satisfactory or specific treatment, although corticosteroids are used to relieve acute symptoms and may have to be continued as in cases of SLE. Careful watch is necessary as it may aggravate hypertension, addition to its well-known adverse effects. Control of hypertension and cardiac failure should be carried out in the usual fashion. Analgesic and anti-

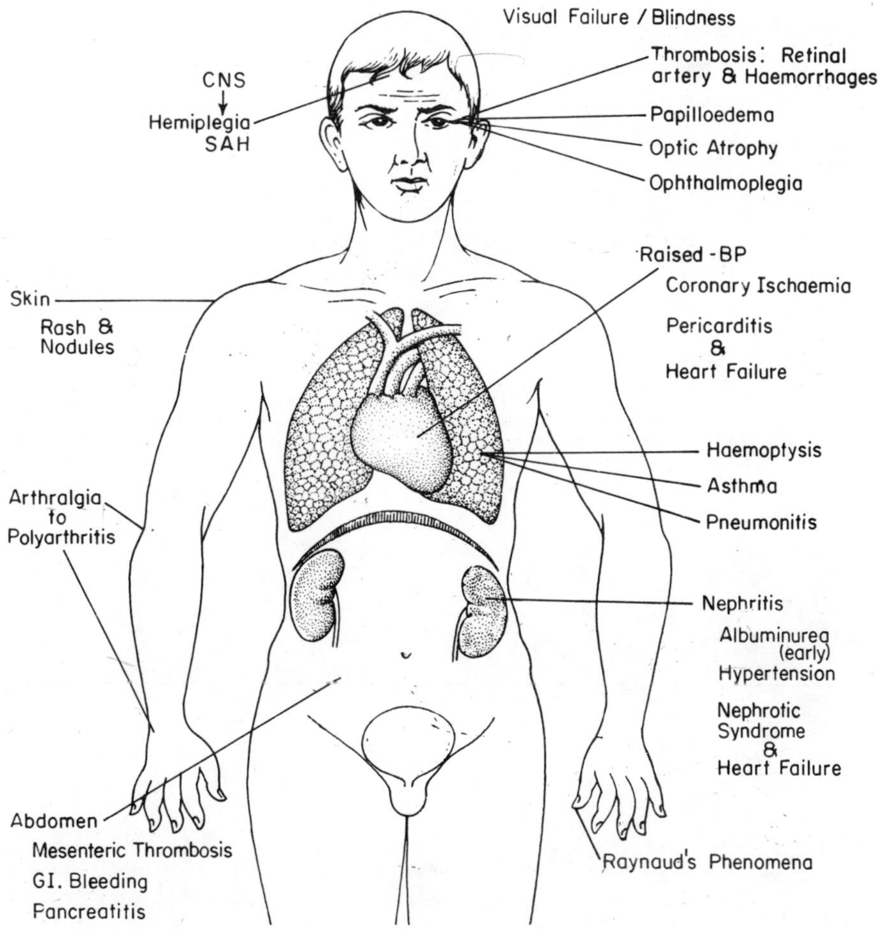


Fig. 5.1 Manifestations of P.A.N.

rheumatic drugs, well-balanced diet are recommended. Acute progressive cases rapidly deteriorate in spite of all treatment and may end in fatality within a year. Some cases may show chronic and recurrent course.

## POLYMYOSITIS - DERMATOMYOSITIS

### INTRODUCTION

This group of diseases is a less distinct clinical entity than other connective tissue diseases. It may occur at any age, predominantly in women. The incidence is not known, as mild cases are often missed. This group of diseases can be conveniently classified as

(a) Polymyositis without organ involvement

(b) Dermatomyositis with typical skin rashes

(c) Polymyositis or dermatomyositis associated with malignancy.

Symmetrical proximal muscle weakness of the arms or legs is characteristic. The axial group of muscles are also affected, especially in the cervical region which may result in difficulty in raising the head. In severe cases, pharyngeal muscles and the diaphragm may be affected, leading to aspiration pneumonia. The muscles are not tender and muscle pain is usually absent. Muscle biopsy shows varying stages of degeneration and regeneration. Focal lymphocytic infiltration and scattered plasma cells are seen in the interstitium. In later stages, atrophy and fibrosis supervene and the histological differentiation between primary and secondary muscle diseases is often difficult.

In dermatomyositis besides muscle involvement, there is a characteristic skin rash in 50% of adult cases and in almost all cases in children. The rash is reddish purple in colour with minimal scaling. The rash, which may be confluent or patchy, is distributed chiefly in areas exposed to sunlight. Periorbital oedema and a purplish suffusion over the eyelids are classical signs. In the acute stage, the dermis shows infiltration by lymphocytes, plasma cells and histiocytes, followed later by fibrosis. In advanced cases the dermis is hyalinised and epidermis is atrophic thus resembling scleroderma. Calcium may be deposited in the subcutaneous and periarticular areas. Other features such as oesophageal dysfunction, myocardial involvement and synovitis may occur thus indicating an overlap syndrome.

In about 20% cases of this group, a concomitant tumour in the lung, uterus, ovary, prostate, breast or colon is found. Removal of the tumour may result in improvement of the muscular and skin symptoms. This association is frequent, particularly in older patients, and, therefore, in all cases of polymyositis/dermatomyositis, periodic check should be done to detect an underlying tumour.

### DIAGNOSIS AND LABORATORY FINDINGS

Muscle biopsy is important in confirming a diagnosis of myositis. Elevation of muscle enzymes, e.g., SGOT, LDH, CPK and Aldolase, are most useful in diagnosis and in estimation of disease activity. Increased urinary levels of myoglobin and creatine are early and sensitive indicators of muscle injury. Electromyogrophy shows non-specific changes and polyphasic potentials of short duration and high frequency active potentials compatible with inflammatory muscle disease.

The serum may show non-specific hypergammaglobulinaemia, antinuclear antibodies and rheumatoid factor. ESR is usually elevated.

## TREATMENT

Chiefly symptomatic. Steroids may be used but do not alter the course of the disease but it may relieve acute symptoms. Sometimes dermatomyositis may be an external manifestation of internal malignancy. Hence a search should be made to exclude it.

# SCLERODERMA

(Syn : Progressive Systemic Sclerosis)

## INTRODUCTION

This is a chronic disorder characterised by diffuse fibrosis of the skin and internal organs ; that is why the progressive systemic sclerosis is a better term than scleroderma. The disease occurs predominantly in young women with an insidious onset between 20 and 40 years of age. The disease may appear in several forms:

(a) a localised type, not associated with visceral disease, usually benign,

(b) a relatively benign slowly progressive disease characterised by calcinosis, Raynaud's phenomenon (episodes of periodic vasoconstriction, causing a gray cyanotic appearance of fingers and toes with numbness, followed by vasodilatation, limpness and painful swelling of the digits), oesophageal involvement, sclerodactyly and telangiectasia—often referred to as CREST syndrome,

(c) in some cases, other systems are also involved,

(d) some have an overlapping syndrome called mixed connective tissue disease (MCTD) where serological and clinical features of both of two or more of collagen diseases and

(e) rapidly progressive type in which functions of major viscera are adversely affected, leading to death within a few years.

The cause of this disease is not known but these are certain evidences indicating an autoimmune mechanism. About 60% of patients have a positive antinuclear antibody test, most characteristically antibodies against nuclear antigen. Immunological and histopathological findings have not contributed significantly to the understanding of the mechanism of tissue injury in this disease. A generalised increase in collagen deposition and vascular changes in organs are common denominators of the disease. The vascular change consists of intimal proliferation in small arteries and arterioles.

## CLINICAL FEATURES

*Skin*—in the early phase (oedematous phase), there is increased deposition of collagen and glycoprotein in the dermis to give the skin a pale, eosinophilic homogenous appearance on microscopical examination. In the later phase (sclerotic phase), the skin appears taut and waxy. The epidermis and the cutaneous appendages and sub-cutaneous fatty tissue undergo atrophy. In the advanced phase, the skin is dry and atrophic; the epidermis is thinned and the sub-epithelial connective tissue is densely hyalinised with complete loss of appendages. Immunoglobulins and complement have not been found in these lesions. The skin lesions are most prominent on the hands and face, but as the disease progresses, they may extend to the arms, chest, neck, back and abdomen.

*Gastrointestinal tract*—Oesophageal hypomotility and gastric reflux are present in 90% cases. Large mouthed diverticuli occur in jejunum, ileum and colon. The lower two-thirds of oesophagus and other parts of the G.I. tract show smooth muscle atrophy and increased collagen deposition. Mucosal ulceration is common in the lower two-thirds of oesophagus. Inflammatory infiltrates of plasma cells and leucocytes are mainly in lamina propria. Small blood vessels often have intimal proliferation and a non-necrotizing vasculitis. Majority of patients with small bowel involvement have malabsorption.

*Lung*—Dyspnoea and chronic bronchitis are frequent and reflect interstitial lung disease. Interstitial fibrosis of the lung, mainly in the lower lobes, leads to thickening of alveolar septa with proliferation of the alveolar lining cells; these cause alveolar-capillary block and disturbance of the alveolar diffusing capacity. Thickening of pulmonary arterioles is associated with pulmonary hypertension, and in some cases, cor pulmonare, which is an important cause of death. With prolonged pulmonary involvement, radiological changes include diffuse fibrosis, sparing the apices and hilar regions. An increased incidence of alveolar cell carcinoma, usually peripheral in location, has been reported in lungs affected by the disease.

*Cardiovascular system*—Involvement includes pericarditis, myocardial fibrosis and right-sided cardiac failure secondary to pulmonary hypertension.

*Kidney*—The major renal lesion consists of fibrinoid necrosis of interlobular arteries and smaller arterioles, associated with intimal proliferation and narrowing of the lumen and perivascular fibrosis. The glomeruli are not significantly affected. Renal angiography shows characteristic narrowing and tortuosity of the interlobular arteries.

Renal failure, usually a late complication, is responsible for death in 50% of cases. Hypertension may precede renal disease though vascular and glomerular disease itself may lead to acute onset of malignant hypertension.

*Musculoskeletal system*—Due to skin involvement, stiffness and arthralgias are frequent. In some cases joint symptoms may suggest rheumatoid arthritis. Like rheumatoid arthritis the synovium in scleroderma shows oedema, infiltration by plasma cells and by lymphocytes leading to fibrosis, but distribution of cartilage characteristic of rheumatoid arthritis is absent. Muscles may be affected by interstitial fibrosis, focal inflammatory infiltration and atrophy; the serum CPK level may be moderately increased.

### TREATMENT

Unfortunately response to treatment is poor though steroids are given in the same way as for SLE. Symptomatic therapy is continued to relieve dysphagia with drugs like bethanicol 5-10 mg. before meals.

Physiotherapy and balanced diet are both essential. Symptomatic treatment for joint pains should be continued.

## SJOGREN'S SYNDROME

### INTRODUCTION

This is a chronic autoimmune disease characterised by the triad of xerostomia (dry mouth), keratoconjunctivitis sicca and a rheumatoid disease. Xerostomia and keratoconjunctivitis sicca constitute the Sicca syndrome. About 50% patients have rheumatoid arthritis and the rest have SLE or scleroderma. The greatest incidence is between 40 and 60 years and 90% of the patients are women.

The oral and conjuctival mucous membranes become dry and tend to get inflamed. The parotid glands are often bilaterally enlarged. Dry mouth often leads to increased fluid intake resulting in polyuria. Dryness of the upper respiratory tract may result in tracheobronchitis and other respiratory complications. Dryness in vaginal mucosa may result in dysparunia. In about 25% of cases there is renal tubular acidosis and urinary concentrating defect is common. Gastric, pancreatic and small intestinal secretions may also be reduced.

## DIAGNOSIS AND LABORATORY FINDINGS

The diagnosis depends on:

(a) tests for exocrine gland functions,

(b) serological tests and

(c) histopathological studies.

Function of the lacrimal gland is often assessed by Schirmer test. In this test strips of filter paper are inserted behind the lower eyelids. Wetting of the strip 15 mm or more outside the lid is considered normal and less than 5 mm as definitely abnormal. An early sign is the low level of lysozome in tear fluid. The salivary gland function can be assessed by radionuclide scanning, salivary flow measurements or sialography. An easy method of assessing salivary gland function is to ask the patient to eat dry crisp biscuit; the patient finds it difficult due to dryness of the mouth.

*The important immunological findings are :—*

1. High titre of rheumatoid factor in 90% cases, even in the absence of rheumatoid arthritis.
2. Antinuclear antibodies in 70% cases.
3. Antibodies to salivary duct epithelium demonstrated by immunofluorescence studies in about 50% cases.
4. Precipitating antibodies which react with extract of nuclei of certain lymphoid cell lines. Detected by agar-gel techniques, these antibodies are present in 50%-60% cases.
5. A variety of autoantibodies are often encountered, e.g., antibodies reactive with thyroglobulin, gastric parietal cells, smooth muscles etc.
6. Polyclonal hyperglobulinaemia.
7. Depressed cellular hypersensitivity as indicated by PPD reactivity and DNCB (dinitro-chlorobenzene) test—in about 30% cases.

A variety of lymphoproliferation, benign or malignant, may be found in Sjogren's syndrome. Malignant lymphoma and Waldenstrom's macroglobulinaemia occur as complications in some cases. Amyloidosis rarely occurs.

*Microscopic examination* of the salivary glands usually shows a characteristic infiltrate composed of lymphocytes and plasma cells with atrophy of the parenchyma. Biopsy of parotid glands should be reserved for patients with a typical presentation. Labial biopsy, a simple procedure is a valuable diagnostic aid; presence of lymphoid foci is confirmative and is often positive in about 75% cases.

Laboratory finds include mild anaemia, leucopenia and eosinophilia. The disease is usually benign and may be consistent with normal span of life.

## TREATMENT

It is chiefly supportive and symptomatic. Hazardous occupation which may injure skin and joints should be avoided. Bleeding, if severe, requires blood transfusion.

Initially it should be established that the syndrome is not a manifestation of internal malignancy. Hence all efforts should be made to exclude it.

Prednisolone as for SLE may be given, which may result in remission in a few cases. Maintenance dose is continued depending on its effect especially on muscular function.

Immunosuppressive agents like azathiopurine and methotrexate, if steroids have to be discontinued.

Physiotherapy must be seriously carried out. Artificial tear drops (carbonymethyl cellulose 0.5% Soal.) may be used for dry eyes. Goggles are also protective. Glycerine mouth washes keep the oral mucosa moist.

## OVERLAP SYNDROMES AND MIXED CONNECTIVE TISSUE DISEASE (MCTD)

Overlap syndromes have clinical or serological features or both of two or more of the following diseases :

Rheumatoid arthritis,
Systemic lupus erythematosis,
Sclerodema and
Polymyositis.

With detailed immunological and clinical scrutiny, the incidence of such overlap syndromes has common pathogenic mechanism. One particular type of overlap syndrome which has clinical features of SLE, scleroderma and polymyositis has been identified as MCTD. However there are no unique findings to justify this combination as an independent disease entity.

CHAPTER 6

# VIRUS-DISEASES

*G. C. Mookerjee*
*M. Roy*

## INTRODUCTION TO VIRAL INFECTIONS

Viruses, the smallest micro organisms in nature (measured in mm) are not visible by light microscopy, but can be studied by electron microscopy (EM). The virus particle (Virion: elementary body) consists of a central core of genetic material either RNA or DNA, surrounded by a protein capsule (capsid).

The virus particle in itself does not contain the mechanism for survival and replication and is completely dependent on the host cell where it controls metabolic processes and utilises the metabolites, i.e., it is an obligatory intracellular parasite.

The virus particle adheres to and penetrates the wall of all susceptible cell and the genetic material is incorporated in the DNA/RNA system of the cell. In the affected cell, virus proteins are synthesised and virus-DNA/RNA replication is "switched on" and normal host cell-protein synthesis may be "switched off". Thus within the cell, an amorphous pool of virus protein and genetic material is found; at this stage the virus is not properly formed, so it is not infective. Later the protein and genetic materials come together to form virus particles. If the normal host cell protein synthesis had been "switched off", the cell degenerates and dies with liberation virus particles, capable of infecting new cells.

The reactions occurring in the host are important in understanding the evolution of virus diseases.

1. Changes in the infected cells may be as follows:
   a) No apparent change in the cell but the virus remains latent for reinfection later on or may cause slow damage.
   b) Cell degeneration with loss of function leading to death of cells.
   c) Fusion of adjacent infected cells to form cells, e.g., in measles.
   d) Cells proliferation followed by death of cells, e.g., common warts.
   e) Formation of inclusion bodies within the cytoplasm (e.g. rabies, cytomegalic virus infection) or in the nucleus.
   f) No apparent change, but malignant proliferation may occur.
2. Production of interferon by the infected cells. Interferon is a protein (not an antibody) produced by the infected cell. It acts against any virus by interfering with synthesis of viral protein. This is the first and very important line of defence.
3. Immune response in the host giving rise to:
   a) Antibodies to virus,
   b) Cell mediated immunity, and
   c) Occasional virus antibody responsible for arteritis or glomerulonephritis.
4. Inflammatory response—Vascular and exudative response follow the usual patterns. Polymorphs are not a feature unless there is considerable tissue necrosis or secondary bacterial infection.

The evolution of a typical acute virus infection can be understood in terms of virus replication, release and spread within the body and the host reactions.

The typical evolution of a virus infection is produced by a successive wave of viruses. However, great majority of virus infections are clinically latent or mild, because replication and spread are prevented by body's defence mechanisms. Severe disease occurs where there is a specially virulent virus where the body's resistance is inadequate.

Virus infections can be classified as (i) Acute, (ii) Latent, (iii) Slow, and (iv) Oncogenic.

Examples of latent virus infections are herpes simplex and herpes zoster. In these diseases, the virus lies latent in cells (e.g. H. simplex) or in specialised cells (in dorsal root-ganglia after an attack of chicken-pox). In this stage the host is not infectious to others. But at any time non-specific "triggering" may occur to produce the disease.

In slow virus infection, affection of the nervous system occurs after an incubation period of several years, e.g., Kuru in New Guinea. It is possible that other chronic diseases of the nervous system may be of slow virus origin.

In human beings there is strong presumptive evidence that some tumours may be caused by viruses (oncogenic virus infection), as for example:

1) Common warts (verruca vulgaris)—infection due to papo-virus;
2) Infectious mononucleosis—Epstein-Barr virus of herpes groups;
3) Burkitt's lymphoma—possibly due to Epstein-Barr virus.

Biochemically viruses can be broadly divided into two types as follows:

| (a) RNA VIRUSES : | | (b) DNA VIRUSES : |
|---|---|---|
| Arboviruses | Hepatitis | Adenoviruses |
| Myxoviruses | Measles | Herpes viruses |
| Picoviruses | Rubella | Papo-viruses |
| Reoviruses | Rabies viruses | Pox-viruses. |

But this classification has little clinical utility.

Viruses are so numerous and they affect human tissues in such a manner that it is difficult to classify them even on clinical basis. Table 6.1 presents a list of viruses and that with clinical syndromes produced by them.

Identification of viruses is also very difficult. Some viruses produce unmistakable clinical picture, e.g., smallpox, chicken-pox, herpes zoster, measles, etc. Others may produce acute respiratory tract infection, gastroenteritis, jaundice, acute haemorrhagic fever or encephalitis of varying severity.

As mentioned already viruses may remain dormant in tissues for many years and may cause a disease after years. Some viruses may induce malignant changes in tissues.

**TABLE 6.1: LIST OF VIRUSES CAUSING VARIOUS DISEASES ENUMERATED AS FOLLOWS:**

| | | |
|---|---|---|
| 1. ARBOVIRUSES | : | These are arthropod-borne viruses which may cause encephalitis, encephal meningitis and yellow fever. |
| 2. ADENOVIRUSES | : | These viruses discovered from adenoids and fauces may cause acute upper respiratory tract infection, including common cold, conjunctivitis, even pneumonitis. |

| | |
|---|---|
| 3. HERPES VIRUSES : | Chicken-pox, herpes zoster, herpes simplex and cytomegalovirus. |
| 4. MYXOVIRUSES : | These are well-known influenza viruses A.B. and C.<br>Type A & B : Known to cause epidemics periodically.<br>Type C : Common flu-infection and can cause epidemics also.<br>These viruses can be cultured from throat-swab in amniotic sac of chick embryo. |
| 5. POX-VIRUSES : | Smallpox, vaccinia and molluscum contagiosum. |
| 6. PICORNA VIRUSES : | Coxsachie, ECHO, Rhino and poliomyelitis viruses. |
| 7. PAPO-VIRUS : | Human wart producing virus:<br>papilloma, polyoma and vacuolating viruses. |
| 8. REO-VIRUSES : | The name comes from respiratory (R), enteric (E), orphan (O).<br>It may cause acute upper respiratory tract (URT) as well as diarrhoeal disorders. |
| 9. RHINO VIRUSES : | Virus of common cold and numerous strains are known. Isolation by tissue culture. |
| 10 ECHO VIRUS : | The name comes from enteric (E), cytopathogenic (C), human (H), orphan (O). ECHO virus may cause acute U.R.T., gastroenteritis and meningitis. Isolation by culture in monkey kidney. |
| 11. COXSACKIE VIRUS : | The name is due to the town of Coxsackie in U.S.A. where the disease was first detected. |

It produces various syndromes which are divided into two groups:

| Group A: | Group B: |
|---|---|
| Acute U.R.T. infections (Herpangina) | Aseptic meningitis |
| Aseptic meningitis | Myocarditis |
| Poliomyelitis like neurological complication | Epidemic myalgia (Bornhom disease) |

**The main techniques of diagnosis are:**

**Virus culture in living animal tissues:** Various viruses can be grown in different tissues, e.g., yolk sac and chorio-allantoic membrane of eggs, monkey kidneys, Hela cell lines (derived from malignant tissue cell culture) etc. Once the viruses are grown they can be seen by electron microscopy.

By light microscope only inclusion bodies can be seen in the cells.

**Laboratory demonstration of rising antibody level:** By examining two successive serum specimens, the first one is collected within the first few days, and the other after about two weeks. Usually the fourfold rise in antibody titre is strongly supportive evidence of very recent viral infection. However, there are some newer research techniques for the rapid diagnosis of the virus infections. Viruses like herpes-simplex virus, vaccinia and varicella can be diagnosed by electron-microscope. Hepatitis-B virus can be identified by radioimmunoassay and rabies can be diagnosed by immunofluorescence.

Serological methods, e.g., virus neutralisation test, haemaglutinin test and complement fixation test are also employed.

**Antibody production:** Viral infections usually stimulate production of globulin antibodies in the blood. These antibodies ultimately protect against future viral infections by the same virus and normally cause termination of the infection. In case of viruses like measles, smallpox, rubella and mumps, one attack usually confers a permanent immunity while the viruses affecting respiratory tract usually exist in many strains, and, therefore, repeated attacks may occur by a number of different antigenic strains.

**Therapeutic problems:** From therapeutic angle antibiotic or antibacterial drugs do not have any effect on these viruses. In certain cases, human immunoglobulins are available which act as specific antibodies to a number of viruses such as measles and virus A hepatitis. Some antiviral drugs are now available, e.g., di-iododeoxy-urirdine for the treatment of herpetic infection of the eyes and methisazone for prevention of smallpox. Convalescent sera obtained from human donors have been sometimes used in the treatment of chicken-pox in immuno suppressed patients. In most cases treatment is symptomatic and supportive.

The most important point about viral diseases is that though most are self-limited, yet some of them can be fatal and in the initial stages it is difficult to recognise them. Hence spread of infection may occur rapidly among contacts including hospital staff. Air travel also has added further hazards to its intercontinental spread.

Some of the common viral diseases are discussed in the present chapter while others like poliomyelitis, encephalitis, respiratory viral infections, viral hepatitis, yellow fever, lymphogranuloma inguinale etc. are included elsewhere in different chapters.

# MEASLES

*G. C. Mookerjee*
*P. K. Talukdar*

## INTRODUCTION

It is a highly infectious acute viral disease manifested by fever, conjunctivitis, respiratory catarrh and typical skin rash preceded by appearance of Koplik's spot in mouth. It occurs all over the world, and, though mild in well-to-do classes, may be a serious disease in poorer classes with undernutrition and may cause mortality of five to ten per cent. It occurs more commonly in school group age. Measles virus belongs to paramyxovirus group and can be isolated by tissue culture. Incubation period is 7 to 21 days.

**Pathology:** The virus produces mononuclear reactions with giant cell formation in the affected skin and mucous membrane of respiratory tract.

**Clinical manifestations:** Measles is remarkably punctual in its appearance of symptoms and signs. The invasion takes place via droplets. The patient is usually capable of spreading infection up to fifth day of appearance of the rash. An attack usually renders permanent immunity. Measles vaccination in developed countries has reduced its incidence in these areas.

On the tenth day of contact, the susceptible child will develop fever with upper respiratory catarrh. The next day both will be more marked and conjunctivitis will appear; with high fever there may be convulsion. Often the child has diarrhoea at this stage. The catarrh and the cough could be very troublesome and the latter is often barking in nature.

On the twelfth day of contact Koplik's spot will appear on the buccal mucous membrane, opposite molar teeth. At the beginning the few sparce spots may be hidden opposite the upper molar teeth. Within the next 24 hours or so, clusters of white spots surrounded by erythema will appear. Patches of erythematous spots may be seen on the soft palate on the 14th day of contact; on the 4th day of onset of disease the rash will appear first on the face.

The fever and cough continues. The rash is erythematous maculopapules which gradually becomes confluent and blotchy. The rash gradually spreads downwards along the trunk and limbs and in another 3 to 5 days it will reach up to the feet (plate). The temperature then subsides, the catarrh and cough abates. The erythema and the elevation of the rash disappear and there appears a typical blackish brown discolouration at the site of the rash, mainly on the chest and abdomen and at times on the limbs. This is called post-measles staining. The cough in a subdued form may persist for another 2 to 3 days. But the child takes another 7 to 10 days to come to his usual normal form. This period of convalescence may be longer depending on the severity of the disease and the nutritional status of the child.

The whole manifestation may vary from mild to severe form and sometimes haemorrhagic rash may appear. Measles in undernourished children may take severe form and so it may be in children suffering from leukaemia or having immunosuppressive therapy.

## COMPLICATIONS

Most complications occur in malnourished and debilitated children and in cases where haphazard treatment has been given in the pre-eruptive stage. Activation of primary complex to progressive primary tuberculosis. In these cases, the rash subsides but the cough and fever continues. Fever may be mostly in the evening; history of contact is of diagnostic help. Mantoux test may be fallacious and falsely negative. BCG test may show accelerated reaction. The chest X-ray will confirm the disease. Secondary infections like otitis media, bronchopneumonia and skin infection are not uncommon.

## ENCEPHALITIS

Sign of encephalitis, e.g., cerebral irritation, meningism, high fever, cranial nerve palsies etc. may appear in the initial stage with convulsion. The change in sensorium and associated neurological findings will differentiate it from febrile convulsion which is quite common at the early stage and has quite different and better prognosis than encephalitis.

**Sub-acute sclerosing pan-encephalitis:**

Appears at the latter part of the disease, is slowly progressive and has a very bad prognosis.

## CLINICAL DIAGNOSIS

The typical and punctual appearance of the symptoms and signs make the diagnosis easy on clinical grounds. In pre-eruptive stage history of measles in one of the sites or in the locality should make one think of the diagnosis. In endemic cases suspicion is the only help, and observation for a couple of days will confirm the diagnosis. Koplik's spot must be looked for. Rash is typical with poor health and nutrition.

In should be noted that diagnosis before appearance of rash is missed because of failure to look for Koplik's spots. Differential diagnosis of rash should be made from drug reactions, rubella and glandular fever.

## LABORATORY DIAGNOSIS

Swabs from throat can be inoculated into Hela cells and human amnion. Inclusion bodies, syncitia and giant cell formation can be found. Haemagglutinin and C.F. tests are also possible.

## PROGNOSIS

Mortality is low unless complications supervene, especially in undernourished children.

## TREATMENT

For a healthy child measles should be no problem. Where there is history of previous febrile convulsion or history of fits, temperature should be regulated by cold head-wash and oral phenobarbitone should be given prophylactically.

Isolation of cases has limited value as by the time diagnosis is made most contacts are already infected, still it is practised to avoid further spread.

Child with high temperature requires plenty of fluids, adequate nutrition and sometimes drugs like paracetamol to reduce high temperature. Routine administration of antibiotics is not essential unless child is undernourished or in poor health or has developed complications, e.g., laryngotracheobronchitis, broncho-pneumonia or otitis media. These cases should be treated with antibiotics, e.g., erythromycin, ampicillin, penicillin, or amoxycillin etc. Avoid tetracyclines in small children as repeated or prolonged use may cause dental discolouration.

Acute obstructive laryngitis may occur in severe cases and these children may require hospitalisation, moist oxygen inhalation but its judicious use is life saving.

## IMMUNISATION

Measles vaccine is now available which consists of a single dose of attenuated live-virus vaccine, given in single dose. I.M. protection lasts about ten to twelve years in 90% cases. Rarely vaccine infection may be accompanied by mild reactions similiar to a mild attack of measles without, or sometimes with, minimal skin rash.

Occasionally convulsion or encephalitis has been repeated. Active immunisation with measles vaccine should not be given in children suffering from fever, respiratory infection tuberculosis, leukaemia. Hodgkin's disease or a patient on corticosteroid or immunosuppressive therapy. Passive immunisation is rarely used but may be done with gamma globulin. In early stage of incubation 250 mg to 750 mg of gamma globulin is given I.M. depending on the age of the child

This method is usually adopted for contacts who are at risk due to poor health, especially of the age group of one to three years.

# RUBELLA

(Syn: German Measles)

*G. C. Mookerjee*

## INTRODUCTION

A mild viral infection is associated with transient outbreak of rash, fever and lymphadenopathy, particularly affecting posterior cervical glands.

The virus belongs to RNA class and can be grown by tissue cultures from throat.

Incubation period 14-21 days.

The virus can be recovered from throat for about one to two weeks after the rash as well as it is excreted in urine. Viraemia precedes fever and a rash patient is capable of infecting contacts a few days before and possibly one or two weeks after rash.

## CLINICAL FEATURES

The chief presenting features are fever-congested throat, reddish macular pin-point rash and lymphadenopathy. In small children the disease is very mild but in adults it may be a little more exaggerated in form. Pin-point reddish macules may be noted in palatine mucosa, which may vesiculate soon.

The rashes usually last 24 to 48 hours and even may pass unnoticed. A careful mother may bring the child to the doctor and the clinician makes the diagnosis by noting enlarged slightly tender suboccipital and posterior auricular lymphadenopathy.

Presence of scarlatiniform or morbilliform rash makes the diagnosis certain.

Rash and fever are more pronounced in older children and adults; fever may rise up to 38°C or 40°C. The disease is self-limited and settles down in 3 to 5 days.

*Complications:* Rare in small children. However the rare complications of Rubella are:

a) Encephalitis
b) Polyneuropathy
c) Polyarthropathy
d) Purpura

In pregnant women there is definite possibility of foetal complications leading to embryonic damage, known as Rubella-embryopathy. The foetal complication may include:

a) Congenital heart disease,
b) Cerebral defects and retarded growth,
c) Ocular defects, e.g., cataract and retinal damage
d) Deafness or deaf-mutism, and
e) Hepatosplenomegaly and purpura.

The possibility of these defects is difficult to predict but chances of foetal damage are maximum in earlier weeks of pregnancy.

In the first four weeks the incidence of foetal complications may be up to 50%, while after 16 weeks it may be around 5%.

Abortion may also occur, and in such case rubella virus can be cultured from tissues of the aborted foetus.

## DIAGNOSIS

The diagnosis is clinical, although viral culture is confirmatory. Rubella virus culture is not simple. It is detected by adding ECHO-virus in tissue culture which competes with its cytopathic effect. If haemoglutination inhibition and complement inhibition tests are negative, Rubella can be excluded.

Rubella IgM may persist in blood for 10 to 12 months and hence does not confirm recent infection. As these tests are not available everywhere, careful clinical observation is most important to decide medical termination of pregnancy (MTP).

The decision of M.T.P. should be taken depending on the weeks of pregnancy, parental attitude, age of mother, number of living children, religious and legal aspects.

During the first four weeks possibility of defective embryonic development is very high, and hence M.T.P. should possibly be a safe choice unless risk is taken due to other factors. After 16 weeks the possibility of foetal defect is much less.

## TREATMENT

a) **Preventive:** Measles vaccine is now available but not to be used during pregnancy. Duration of immunity is not impressive. During pregnancy, where it is decided to allow the pregnancy to continue, give an injection of gamma globulin. Dose 1500mg I.M.

Smaller children and teenagers should be allowed to be exposed, though development of rubella may not produce life long immunity.

b) **Therapy:** Entirely symptomatic. Antibiotics may rarely be needed. Steroids are not helpful. Clinical diagnosis, however, should be made with precision by taking into consideration the presence of rash with posterior cervical tender lymphadenopathy. It should be differentiated from:

a) Mild attack of measles—Koplik's spot, acute coryza and longer-lasting dusky red rashes;

b) Scarlet fever—Rare in eastern hemisphere; sore throat is usually marked and circumoral pallor is present. $\beta$-haemolytic streptococci isolated from throat;

c) Drug rash—History of drugs and absence of cervical lymphadenopathy (Refer to section on dermatology).

# CHICKEN-POX

*P. K. Talukdar*

A highly infectious virus disease mainly occurring in children but adults may also be affected. The disease is manifested by typical rash on the mucous membrane of the palate and skin also has benign and self-limiting course.

The same virus in the patient may remain dormant in the posterior root ganglion for years and in a congenial situation may flourish and multiply production. (Clinical manifestations of herpes zoster) Infection takes place by droplets through nasopharynx either by direct contact or by fomites. Incubation period is 2 to 3 weeks.

Initial symptoms are mild fever with malaise for a couple of days followed by appearance of rash usually first on the trunk. Several crops may appear in the next 2 to 5 days. The crops of rash first appear as macules then papule and quickly transform into vesicles. The first rash noticed is often a vesicle on the chest or back, is very superficial unilocular and has a tear drop appearance, becomes turbial and ultimately scabs. Distribution of the rash is central, on the trunk, face, buccal mucous membrane and proximal part of all limbs. Patient is infectious in the initial pre-eruptive stage for a day or two, and in the early stage of appearance of rash scabs are not infectious.

Haemorrhagic chicken-pox is a severe and rare form of the disease, characterised by bleeding from the gum and mucous membrane, in the rash and in surrounding. Haemorrhagic form of chicken-pox occurs usually in patients with leukaemia and in patients on steroid therapy. This is a serious condition and has bad prognosis.

## COMPLICATIONS

Secondary bacterial infection is predisposed by scratching. The rashes of chicken-pox are very superficial and on healing leaves no scar. But if secondary infection occurs there will be deeper involvement of skin and consequent scarring.

### Chicken-pox pneumonia

Uncommon in children pneumonitis may occur in elder patients with severe attack. It coincides with the appearance of the rash. Symptoms and signs of pneumonitis like cough, dyspnoea, cyanosis with crepitations will be there.

X-ray shows nodular opacities throughout the lung fields. Clinical recovery occurs in 7 to 10 days but the radiological signs may take months to clear.

### Chicken-pox encephalomyelopathy

It usually occurs on the 2nd to 7th day of appearance of rash, characterised by headache, vomiting and loss of consciousness.

Evidence of neuritis and myelitis may be there. CSF may be normal or may show increased cell count and raised protein. Prognosis is good.

## TREATMENT

Most cases of chicken-pox need no treatment. Application of soothing lotion will help the skin irritation and prevent scratching. If the irritation is marked, oral antihistaminics in addition will add to the comfort. Scratching should be avoided to prevent scarring. For chicken-pox pneumonia there is no specific treatment, but broad spectrum antibiotics should be used if secondary organisms are suspected. For neurological complications steroid may be of help but should not be used till 6 to 7 days have gone by from the onset of chicken-pox, as earlier use of steroid may cause discrimination of virus producing *severe with haemorrhagic chicken-pox other systemic involvement like heart, liver, etc.*

# SMALLPOX

*G. C. Mookerjee*

## INTRODUCTION

**Smallpox** is a very serious and highly contagious viral infection, due to poxvirus group which exists in two different forms of virulence. The virulent type is called variola major or classical smallpox while the less virulent form is called variola minor or alastrim. There are four viruses known to affect man. The virulent infection is due to variola major while the other three which cause milder disease are variola minor, cow-pox and vaccinia. Variola major is the classical epidemic smallpox.

During the last decade the disease is gradually being wiped out due to excellent eradication programme by the W.H.O. Smallpox is now non-existent in the world. The last case reported from India was on 21st May, 1975, and the last endemic smallpox in the globe was in Somalia in 1977. Since no case has been reported in the world after 1977. The expert group constituted by the Director-General of Health Services, Government of India, recommended that "it will be prudent to discontinue compulsory smallpox vaccination and there need not be any national vaccination programme" but I wonder, whether it requires withdrawal of the 1981 Act regarding primary vaccination.

The profession is watching with anxious interest about this bold decision of W.H.O. Even if the disease is controlled, its accidental contamination through laboratory accidents should be remembered.

## INCUBATION PERIOD

Incubation period of pox is usually 12 days, varying between 8 and 16 days, for alastrim it is 10 to 15 days.

## CLINICAL PICTURE

The most salient features are severe constitutional symptoms, characterised by high temperature, prostration, typical rash and its mode of appearance and spread. The stages are: Prodromal and eruptive phases.

### Prodromal Phase

High temperature, headache, vomiting, severe backache and musculo-arthritic pain. Prodromal rashes may appear in groin, axilla and trunk. These look like drug rash.

### Eruptive Phase

The classical rashes appear on the third day, initially in the oral mucosa and then in forehead and face. The crops of rash spread, centripetally. These are more in extensor surface of limbs, more profuse distally than proximally. They are more in upper limbs in back of hands and forearms than in legs and feet. In chest and abdomen they are not so profuse. Extensor surfaces are more involved. Back of trunk is more involved than the front.

## CLINICAL TYPES

The follwing clinical types are known—

1. **Confluent type—**

Severe form with high temperature, profuse rash and profound toxaemia; mortality may be 50%.

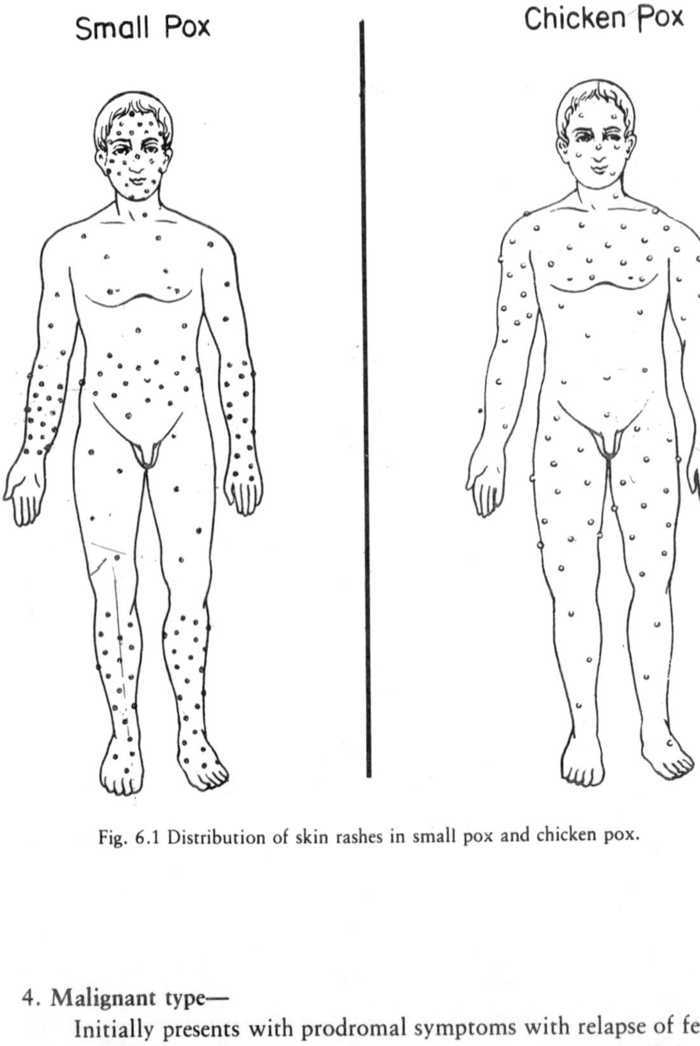


Fig. 6.1 Distribution of skin rashes in small pox and chicken pox.

2. **Discrete type—**

Distribution of rash is illustrated in Fig. 6.1. Toxaemia is moderate to severe. Mortality rare, if good supportive treatment is given. On recovery permanent pockmarked appearance proclaims past smallpox.

3. **Haemorrhagic type—**

Rashes may be purpuric or internal haemorrhage may occur before rash appears in some cases. When rashes occur early, there may be purpura in the skin on second or third day, which is often extensive. Associated with or following purpura, haematemesis, malaena, haemoptysis, haematurea or uterine bleeding may occur. Cases are mostly fatal. Danger to contacts must be noted, if diagnosis is missed. High temperature and severe toxaemia are pointers, especially during epidemic.

4. **Malignant type—**

Initially presents with prodromal symptoms with relapse of fever and petechial rash and erythema. Severe erythema resembling sun-burnt appearance may mislead the diagnosis. The classical evolution of rash is absent. Pustules do not appear but vesicles may coalesce to form bullous formation. Mortality is high usually during second week.

5. **Modified smallpox—**

It occurs usually after many years of vaccination in people who do not revaccinate. Disease is mild and all cases usually recover. Sometimes rashes are so few and far between that it is missed. This type may be called 'variola sine eruption'.

## VARIOLA MINOR

This is also known as Alatrim or Kaffirpox. It is due to a less virulent strain of the virus (attenuated virus). It used to be endemic in South America and Africa as well as in Europe.

The disease runs a mild course and prognosis is good.

## MATURATION OF RASH

Inititally these are maculo-papular, which change to deep-seated multilocular vesicles in 48 to 72 hours. In further period of 48 to 72 hours these become pustules.

The pustules gradually dry up in 7 to 14 days and form crusts due to healing. The crusts ultimately separate out and fall off, leaving behind permanent pockmarks.

The initial febrile phase settles down after appearance of rash but again there is reappearance of fever when pustulation occurs. In some cases there is confluence of profuse rashes, leading to ulceration and sloughing of skin.

## DIAGNOSIS

Immediate isolation is necessary if there is any suspicion about possibility of diagnosis. Once rashes develop it is not difficult to diagnose by experienced eyes. Future students however will not have this experience, hence should be very cautious, before it is ruled out. Hence there will be some need of laboratory aid at times. There is a type of pox-disease whch affects monkeys but fortunately not humans.

## LABORATORY DIAGNOSIS

Smallpox viruses are large viruses which can be seen in light microscope as Guarneiri bodies or elementary bodies of Paschen. These are intracytoplasmic inclusions of real pox viruses.

The following methods should be adopted if required for diagnosis:

(a) Fluid from vesicles or pustules should be collected by fine needles into a tuberculin or insulin syringe for testing. Microscopic examination for inclusion bodies may help but not always.

(b) Scrappings from base of papules, vesicles or pustules are also useful for viral culture. Crusts can be separated by fine forceps and collected carefully, to be sealed in a closed glass container for test in special centres.

(c) Blood samples may be collected for virus culture during first few days or measurement of antibody in serum after 2 weeks. In the latter case it will be too late to diagnose.

(d) The most dependable test is to culture the virus from blood, scrappings, aspirated fluid or pus. The culture of smallpox virus can be done in fertile hen's egg and suitably incubated. The virus grown is recognised by electron microscope. This, however, will take a few days, up to one week for diagnosis.

There is another method of detection of antigen, by gel diffusion technique but it does not discriminate smallpox and vaccinia. However, it can be done within 12 hours and may be positive in 90% cases.

## MANAGEMENT

The most important duty of the attending doctor is proper isolation of the case, where infectious diseases (I.D.) hospital is not available. If an I.D. hospital is available patient must be sent there without delay and health authorities should be notified and contacts should be vaccinated forthwith.

In the recent past a drug known as Marboran (methesazone) was found to be effective in trials carried out in India. The dose is 3g. twice daily for one day only. However, it may be vomited and not tolerated by all especially when given for three days as recommended by Alstead and Girdwood (1979). Hence it cannot replace vaccination and close contacts are carefully watched for three weeks.

Once the disease has started, the patient should be treated symptomatically to relieve headache and pain by analgesics. Care of skin is essential.

Hyperpyrexia needs attention. Paracetamol, aspirin and chlorpromazine group of drugs may be used. Lotio calamine with local anti-histaminic drugs may be applied as soothing agents for skin. Sandalwood pastes are also useful. Oral penicillin, sulpha-drugs, and broad spectrum antibiotics may help in crusting off the pustules, if given as soon as pustules are appearing.

In the past, travellers moving to foreign countries from Asia and Africa and those coming to the places required vaccination certificate as per international regulations. But with the eradication of smallpox from the globe, no country in the world now insists on vaccination certificate from the travellers, except two countries, namely, Chad and Kampuchea.

Similarly no vaccination certificate is necessary at the moment for admission to school or other purpose.

The profession is now watching the disappearance of one dreaded disease from the world with great interest.

## MUMPS

An acute infective disease of virus origin of the salivary glands commonly the parotids but the other salivary glands may also be affected.

## CLINICAL FEATURES

Infection comes through nose or mouth from the patient in the first few days of illness. Incubation period is about 3 weeks.

Onset of the disease is with fever, usually mild but at times may be very high. Often the patient complains of earache which is really the pain over the parotid region. In a day or two swelling of the parotid appears on one side. Subsequently in another day or two the fever may shoot up with appearance of swelling of the other parotid. The condition may be very painful with increase in pain from the movement of the jaw, or the sight or thought of food. The swelling lasts for 7 to 10 days and then gradually subsides. Often the submandibular salivary glands are swollen with or without the parotids being involved. In severe cases there may be marked oedema of the soft tissue of the neck particularly with the submandibular gland involvement, the cause of which is not exactly known.

## COMPLICATIONS

*Aseptic meningitis:* May appear at any stage of the disease at times without any involvement of the salivary glands. Headache, vomiting, fever, neck and back stiffness with increased CSF pressure, increased cell count, mostly lymphocytes and increased protein. Uneventful recovery is usual.

## PANCREATITIS

Appears at the later part of first week with fever, vomiting, pain, abdomen and rigidity gradually subsides in 3 to 4 days.

## ORCHITIS

Appears in the second week in pubertal or postpubertal males.

Fever with pain in abdomen with testicular swelling on the affected side, which is hot and very tender, is the usual clinical manifestations. The condition subsides in a week. There may be permanent testicular damage and subsequent sterility. In female patients oophoritis may occur with abdominal pain, fever and rigidity.

## LABORATORY DIAGNOSIS

It is usually clinical. However, salivary secretions taken from parotid duct openings can be inoculated into the amniotic sac of fertile hen's egg and amniotic fluid is tested for haemagglutination. Hela cell culture may reveal as to pathic effect.

## TREATMENT

Rest for 10 to 15 days with symptomatic treatment for pain and fever is all that is needed. Early ambulation may precipitate complications.

# VIRAL HAEMORRHAGIC FEVER (VHF)

*G. C. Mookerjee*

This is another group of viral fever which has been termed as exotic. These have been found to occur in Africa, South America as well as in the Far East and some parts of tropical Asia including India.

These viral fevers can be classified as follows:

I. **ASIAN VHF**
Kyasanur forest disease
Korean haemorrhagic fevers
Crimea-Congo haemorrhagic fever

II. **AFRICAN VHF**
Lassa fever
Marburg disease
Etoba viral disease
Crimea-Congo haemorrhagic fever

III. SOUTH AMERICA
Argentine haemorrhagic fever
Bolivian haemorrhagic fever

IV. EUROPE
Crimea-Congo fever

Almost all these viral infections have flu-like onset and are never suspected to be dangerous in their initial phases, but soon it is manifested by high fever, toxaemia, as well as haemorrhagic manifestations with high rate of mortality.

The contacts are in great danger, especially nurses and doctors. Many deaths of medical attendants as well as laboratory workers have been recorded.

In 1969 in the mission hospital of Lassa, a small town of Nigeria, a nurse developed flu-like fever and ultimately was evacuated to a larger hospital where she died due to VHF. Another nurse, who was attending on her, also died due to similar disease. When a third nurse became ill with similar clinical picture, she was evacuated to USA at Yale University for viral investigation. Dr. Gordi Casals, who isolated the virus, named Lassa virus (should have been named 'Casals' virus), also fell ill but recovered. Further research was undertaken in USA and later it was found to be due to a virus similar to lymphocytic choriomeningitis (RNA virus).

These viral fevers were previously limited to their own native places but due to modern fast travel facilities and frequent intercontinental travels, possibility of world-wide spread of these VHFs has increased tremendously.

Laboratory diagnosis of these fevers is not possible except where facilities for viral investigation exist and inadvertent infection of laboratory staff is also a great danger.

The danger is considered so great that in U.S.A. plastic negative pressure isolation chambers have been designed (Texler etal).

Laboratory diagnosis can be made by fourfold rise of antibody titres in two paired samples, taken in early first week and second week of infection or by viral culture in egg-embryo and electron microscopic appearance. Some salient features of these fevers are presented in Table 6.1

## GLANDULAR FEVER

*G. C. Mookerjee*

### INTRODUCTION

Glandular fever is clinically characterised by fever and sore throat, associated with peripheral lymph-gland enlargement. Causative organism is Epstein-Barr virus. Incubation period is 5 to 14 days.

The disease is insidious in onset but occasionally may have high fever to start with. In 15% to 20% of the cases, skin rash appears after fourth day form of maculo-papular erythema, looking like drug-rash. Occasionally there is jaundice. Spleen becomes palpable in 50% of cases.

The following clinical types are recognised :

#### 1. GLANDULAR TYPE

Oneset of the disease is proclaimed by fever 38° to 40°C (101° to 103° F) for four or five days, then rash appears. stage of eruption lasts from fourth to tenth day, chiefly involving trunks; subsequently glandular enlargement progresses.

Glands become enlarged and tender. Besides neck glands, peripheral and mediastinal glands may also complicate the picture.

2. FEBRILE TYPE

Most cases have fever, sore throat, constitutional symptoms and progressive glandular enlargement Maculo-papular rash, more marked in trunks, may appear from fourth to tenth day.

3. ANGINOSE TYPE

Sore throat may be severe, with occasional membrane formation (D.D.-Diphtheria) and oedema of oral mucosa and gums causes great distress, along with constitutional symptom. Oral ulcers may bleed.

4. ICTERIC FORM

Onset is mild febrile type, then develops jaundice and hepatosplenomegaly.

5. MENINGOENCEPHALITIC TYPE

There are classical features of meningitis or meningoencephalitis.

Papilloedema, iridocyclitis and peripheral neuritis may complicate the clinical picture.

In mild cases fever is present for three to seven days but in severe cases it may continue up to three weeks. In the beginning, the illness may be confused with septic sore throat or diphtheria. There may be extensive inflammation and oedema of the peritonsillar areas covered with creamy exudative membrane. In rare cases, there may be severe complications such as epistaxis, G.I. tract haemorrhage, purpuric rash, haemolytic anaemia, myocarditis, pericarditis, lymphocytic meningitis and encephalitis.

## DIFFERENTIAL DIAGNOSIS

Infectious mononucleosis comes in D.D. of many unrelated situations and needs careful investigation.

1. PUO, especially in children with poor health, mistaken for tuberculosis
2. Sore throat, diphtheria and agranulocytosis
3. Exanthematous fevers and drug rash
4. Lymphatic leukaemia
5. Meningoencephalitis
6. Secondary syphilis
7. Toxoplasmosis and cytomegalic inclusion disease
8. Viral hepatitis

## LABORATORY DIAGNOSIS

Blood picture shows leucocytosis with predominance of lymphocytes though initially polymorphs may be raised. Later there is flooding of non-granular series of white cells up to 60 to 80 per cent. These include lymphocytes, typical lymphocytes and monocytes.

Diagnosis can be confirmed by a positive Paul-Bunnell reaction, which detects presence of heterophil antibodies, capable of agglutinating sensitised red cells of sheep's blood. In glandular fever, antibody titre rises up to 1/200 or more in 80% cases. The test, however, is usually positive by the end of first week or even later but it may remain positive for several weeks or months.

## PROGNOSIS

Most cases recover with supportive treatment but rarely haemorrhage or severe complications may occur.

## TREATMENT

Mild cases will improve with symptomatic treatment and antibodies need not be used unless there is frank secondary infection or the patient is in poor health being susceptible to secondary infection. In anginose cases, it is wise to start broad-spectrum antibiotics, e.g., tetracyclines.

"On no account ampicillin be given because of the high risk of the sensitization rashes" (Alstead and Girdwood); short course of steroids may be prescribed in anginose cases. Prednisolone (30 to 40mg daily) or dexamethasone (3 to 4mg daily) should be prescribed in severe cases for 48-72 hours, then gradually reduced under close supervision. Lumbar-puncture should be done when meningitis is suspected. Respiratory complications may require antibiotics, oxygen inhalation but rarely tracheotomy.

Oral hygiene is important. Antiseptic gargles with hydrogen-peroxide mouth-wash after feeds may be soothing but should not be overdone. Paracetamol and diazepam may be given to relieve pain and promote sleep.

# BORNHOLM DISEASE

(Syn: Epidemic Myalgia, Epidemic Pleurodynia)

*G. C. Mookerjee*

## INTRODUCTION

The disease is characterised by severe muscular pain especially in chest wall associated with high fever. The causative organism is coxsachie viruses specially $B_3$ and $B_5$. The name is of an island where the disease was discovered.

Incubation period is two to five days.

## CLINICAL FEATURES

Onset usually with sight fever, bradycardia and nasopharyngitis and stitch-like muscular pain which becomes severe causing chest movements specially painful. Severe muscular pain causes difficulty of breathing and symptoms mimick pleurisy; temperature may be high (102° to 104°F) but being a self-limited disease symptoms settles down within a week. Leucopenia is usual. Prognosis is usually good but sometimes arthritis, meningitis, orchitis, pleurisy, pericarditis and jaundice may complicate the issue. However, recovery occurs in due course.

## TREATMENT

Absolute bed rest is necessary. Symptomatic and supportive therapy as in cases of influenza or upper respiratory tract infection should be given.

Antibiotics are not necessary in mild cases unless there are secondary respiratory invaders.

Analgesics and sedatives like aspirin, paracetamol diazepam or barbiturates should be prescribed. In severe cases mafenamic acid may be prescribed along with aspirin and paracetamol.

# DENGUE

(Syn: Break-bone fever, Dandy fever)

*G. C. Mookerjee*

## INTRODUCTION

This is another viral infection which is due to arborvirus group and this is transmitted through mosquitoes of genus Aedes and causes severe muscle and joint pains with fever.

## CLINICAL FEATURES

Onset is usually abrupt with fever bradycardia and joint pain. Headache and retro-orbital pain may be severe. The special feature is development of measly rash and saddle-back temperature (Fig. 6.1). Initially there is some degree of erythema for first two or three days of fever. Then temperature settles down to normal but relapses again (saddle-back temperature chart) with the appearance of measly rash spreading from periphery to centre. Acute symptoms usually settle down by the time rash is well-developed. Orchitis is a troublesome and serious complication. Leucopenia is common. Haemorrhagic type of dengue fever is rarely encountered.

## TREATMENT

As in case of Bornholm's disease.

# PHLEBOTOMOUS FEVER

(Syn: Sandfly fever)

*G. C. Mookerjee*

## INTRODUCTION

It is another arborvirus infection transmitted by female sandfly, phlebotomous papatsii causing short-term fever. Incubation period is two to four days. Infection is spread by the female sandfly, who acquires the infection from the reservoir, infected human. The patient is infective for 24 hours before and after infection, but infected sandfly remains infective for the rest of her short life of about three weeks.

## CLINICAL FEATURES

Onset is sudden with fever, headache, conjunctivitis, photophobia, lacrymation. Musculoskeletal pain is often severe like dengue. Upper respiratory tract complication may occur but leucopenia is typical.

The symptoms settle down within a week.

### TREATMENT

Same as dengue fever.

## FOOT & MOUTH DISEASE

*G. C. Mookerjee*

### INTRODUCTION

Though it is a disease of domestic animals, e.g., cattle, goat and sheep yet the keepers may rarely be affected. The causative organism is a virus. Incubation period is two to five days.

### CLINICAL FEATURES

In humans the disease starts with fever, headache and dry oral mucosa. This is followed soon by excessive salivation and appearance of vesicles in oral mucosa, palms and soles. Keratoconjunctivitis may rarely complicate. The disease is self-limiting but may prolong for two to three weeks.

### TREATMENT

Usually symptomatic, as there are no specific drugs for it. Local application of 1% gentian violet or potassium permanganate may be given. Vitamin C may be useful along with bland non-spicy diet.

## HERPES VIRUS GROUP

*G. C. Mookerjee*

### INTRODUCTION

This is a group of virus which can cause human infection but usually the clinical manifestations are not so severe. The important members of herpes virus group are:

| | |
|---|---|
| Herpes virus simplex | Epstein-Barr virus |
| Herpes zoster virus | Cytomegalovirus |

### HERPES SIMPLEX

Herpes simplex infections are not uncommon. They produce ulcerative stomatitis, which is sometimes very chronic in its behaviour; sometimes it affects small babies producing conjunctivitis, skin and genital tract lesions. Sometimes herpetiform rash occurs around the lips and these are highly infectious. Spread of infection may occur by contact and also via utensils, books and furniture contaminations. The rash consists of vesicles around the lips, face and even neck. Rash elsewhere may rarely occur in trunk and limbs. Widespread palate and buccal mucosa. The lesions are small ulcers covered with white exudate causing difficulty in eating and drinking. They may produce discharge of saliva dribbling out of mouth and this can cause real problem, especially in children.

## COMPLICATIONS

In rare instances there may be keratoconjunctivitis, vomiting, high fever and convulsions in children. Some of these cases develop extension of oral and skin lesion and may end in fatality, especially in small children. Extensive skin lesions are known as Kaposi's varicelliform rash, looking like generalised vaccinia virus infection.

Herpes encephalitis is another serious complication which may present with convulsion, meningism and coma.

## DIAGNOSIS

Virus grows in fertile egg in the chorioallantoic membrane.

## TREATMENT

The treatment is supportive and symptomatic. Glucose and vitamin C appear to produce relief, especially in cases of extensive oral ulcers. Some drugs like Idoxuridine (IND), cytosine arebinoside (cytarabine) and adomine arobinoside (vidarabine) are active antiviral agents *in vitro* but their role in human infections is still uncertain; local applications of trifluoro-thymidine are reported to be of value in conjunctivitis. These drugs are also toxic and may produce gastric irritation and bone marrow damage. Local applications of 1% gentian violet or potassium permanganate may be given after meals. Efcorlin pellets may sometime help.

Usually the patient has uneventful recovery in most cases with local and symptomatic treatment. Avoid trauma to the vesicles. Non-adherent dressing with zinc oxide ointment may be useful. Secondary infection should be treated by antibiotics.

Disseminated zoster with severe complication may be treated by i.v. cytosine arabinose (Conn—*Current Therapy*, 1978, p. 670: method of Dr. R.L. Pitts).

Post-herpetic neuralgia is most difficult to treat. Steroids may help. Ophthalmic complication needs careful management by ophthalmic surgeon.

## HERPES ZOSTER (Syn: Herpes varicellae)

This is a virus which can cause both chicken-pox and herpes zoster. It is believed that after an attack of chicken-pox the virus may remain dormant for many years and may cause herpes zoster.

The virus attacks posterior roots of spinal nerves or sensory ganglia of cranial nerves (usually V nerve). This results in appearance of rash in the areas of nerve supply, associated with symptoms of pain.

## DIAGNOSIS

The virus grows on human tissue culture but not on eggs and it can be recognised by electron microscopy. However, clinical recognition is important.

## TREATMENT

During the eruption stage local soothing agents, e.g., lotio calamine may be helpful. Local use of 5% idoxuridine to vesicles is also recommended but it should not be used for ocular lesions. In case local sepsis occurs due to rupture of vesicles, doxycycline 100 mg twice daily with local antiseptic case is necessary. Systemic use of high doses of corticosteroids has been advocated but risk of dissemination of virus and its spread in the central nervous system limit its use.

Cytosino arabinoside is being used for zoster encephalitis, an experimental therapy.

Treatment of post-herpetic neuralgia is really a serious problem. Systemic steroid if there is no contraindication may be useful. Intra-lesional triamcinolone acetonide has been recommended (Conn 1978, p. 670). Surgical treatment, e.g., rhizotomy or cordotomy is too drastic but has to be considered in severe cases.

## CYTOMEGALO VIRUS

This is a very important condition as it may cause mental retardation of newborn due to involvement of cerebral tissues of foetus if the infection occurs during pregnancy. Intrauterine foetal infection ultimately damages its brain. The neonate may be affected due to jaundice, fever, hepatosplenomegaly and also may develop cerebral damage leading to mental deficiency.

## DIAGNOSIS

The virus can be isolated from throat swab, urine and cervical secretions, and inclusion bodies can be detected.

## TREATMENT

It is unfortunate that no vaccine is available for this kind of viral affection. Experimental works are being carried out to produce the protective vaccine against this kind of viral affections.

# RABIES

*T. P. Mukherjee*

## INTRODUCTION

It is an acute infective disease caused by filtrable neurotropic virus known as Rhabdovirus being transmitted to man from warm blooded mammals due to bites and licks over abrâded skin.

## AETIOLOGY

Two varieties of source of infection are evident.

a) In wild life, wolves, jackals, foxes, mongooses and vampire bats harbour the infection and spreading occurs due to bites.
In Texas some people were affected due to vampire bats, possibly via aerosol showering effect and not bites.

b) In urban areas, dogs are chiefly responsible but cats and cattle may also do it if they are bitten by infected animals.
At the site of injury the virus remains active for 36 hours. From there it goes to C.N.S. through perineural nerve sheath. In C.N.S. the virus forms a specific lesion known as 'negri bodies' which is red eosinophilic mass, surrounded by chronic inflammatory cells. From there it has centripetal distribution to autonomic nervous system to lacrimal and salivary glands. In the salivary gland the virus multiplies being excreted through saliva.

## CLINICAL FEATURES

*Incubation period*—Ten days to one year or more severity of bite and its site.

It is shorter in children, may be within ten to twenty days. Face wounds—about four weeks; hands—five to six weeks; and legs—about two months.

In animals maximum incubation period is four months. The clinical features are divided into three groups.

1) *Prodromal stage,*
2) *Stage of irritability, and*
3) *Stage of stuporose condition.*

*Prodromal stage:* It is characterised by paresthesia or swelling, both at the site of injury. Headache, anorexia, prostration, fever and raised pulse rate and respiratory rate usually proclaim the illness. Later, patient is irritable and tries to catch imaginary objects and soon passes to the stage of irritation (viral encephalitic phase). Rabies clinically has all the features of viral encephalitis, characterised by extreme prostration, fits, hallucination, and cannot even tolerate gentle breeze when a hand-fan is waved in front of his face. He suffers from dyspnoea and convulsion and accordingly this type is graded as grade I to grade III.

*Stage of excitement:* It is termed as acrophobia, the special sign was discovered and practised in I.D. Hospital, Calcutta.

Deep tendon reflexes may either be absent or exaggerated (bizzare pattern); when the patient wants to swallow a glass of water, he experiences pain in the throat due to spasm of larynx and a sense of choking, contraction of platysma and neck muscles sometimes, with convulsion. This painful experience is remembered in lucid interval, and when a glass of water is offered at that time, he refuses to drink and hence this is known as hydrophobia.

*Stage of paralysis:* Very soon this patient passes to the stage of stuporose condition or comatose state. Patient may remain alive even up to a week in this comatose condition when death ends the scene.

One American technician contracted rabies but he survived with the help of cardio-respiratory resuscitation giving rise to a ray of hope in the mind of the clinician dealing with this dreadful disease.

## PROGNOSIS

Almost all cases of rabies end in fatality. In the whole world three probable cases of rabies have survived. But in the animal kingdom, not all the animals die. Abortive cases do escape.

## DIFFERENTIAL DIAGNOSIS

In early stage it may mimic Datura poisoning. A definite history of dog-bite excludes it. Pseudorabies is rarely seen among people dealing with domestic animals who had seen cases of rabies. They mimic almost all the features of rabies and hence this is termed as pseudorabies.

Gullaine-barrie syndrome may sometimes be mistaken for rabies. Early involvement of brainstem is an important differentiating point.

*Management:* (1) Segregation is very essential because the patient spits living virus. Attendants are afraid that they may be bitten but human to human transmission is yet unknown.

(2) Supportive measures are the only treatment.

*Prevention:* Prevention is better than cure. In India so far we have not been able to save a single patient, hence more emphasis on prevention is to be given. It is observed that virus remains alive at the site of injury for 96 hours.

Hence local treatment of the wound is very essential. Possibly, antiviral agent like cetavlon, cauterising the wound with strong solution of potassium permanganate or phenol is necessary.

Wound may invite tetanus. Hence prevention with tetanus toxoid is also to be given.

Recognition of rabid dogs is not difficult. They become restless, irritable, give up food and even do not obey their masters. They bite at slightest provocation and later almost run amuck to assault anyone in the way. However there is a variety of rabies affecting domestic dogs which is called 'paralytic type'. In this type a dog is quiet, lies exhausted and likes to remain near the master. It is dangerous and may bite when provoked and it may be difficult to suspect rabies in such cases.

Rabid dog or/animal cannot live more than 10 days from the day of incubation. Hence offended animals should be observed for 10 days, if available, and then the treatment should be initiated. In case of wild animals, street dogs, treatment should be started immediately. Besides, in those cases where chance of rabies is possible, e.g., unprovoked bites, maximum tissue laceration, head and neck involvement, preventive treatment should be started early and may be discontinued later on if the animal remains alive.

Two types of vaccines are available:

One is derived from the nerve tissue known as nerve tissue virus (N.T.V.) and the other is derived from duck embryo known as (D.E.V.). D.E.V. is used in U.S.P.H.S. This is least toxic but immunity is not of high standard, dose of injection is minimum. It may require twenty-one injections. This is not advocated by W.H.O.

N.T.V. is advocated by W.H.O. and used in our country which contains live attenuated virus. It sometimes produces allergic encephalomyelitis or reactivation of the virus causing real rabies.

Dose of N.T.V. varies accordingly.

Grade I—Head-neck involvement
Multiple bite marks
Maximum tissue lacerations
Bite by wolves and jackals.
Dose—10 c.c. Sub. cut. Inj. × 14 such.

Grade II—Involvement of lower extremity
Bite over the garments
More than two teeth marks
Dose—5 c.c. Sub. cut. inj. round about umbilicus × 14 such.

Grade III—In children one or two teeth marks
Dose—2c.c. Sub. cut × 14 such.

It is also observed that epijoitic and enjoitic cases of Rabies occur, hence for full prevention we have to take help of veterinary surgeons also.

Antirabic antisera are now available from both human or animal sources. Half of the dose is infiltrated round about the site of injury and other half is given I.M. after proper skin test. This method will protect the patient initially till the vaccine induces adequate immunity.

*T. P. Mookherjee*

CHAPTER 7

# BACTERIAL INFECTIONS

*G. C. Mookerjee*

## INTRODUCTION

Bacteria are microscopic unicellular organisms, which may invade living tissues producing disease. All bacteria are not pathogenic to us while some are constantly living in symbiosis in the skin, mucous membranes and large intestines. However, these are usually harmless to the host but may become pathogenic and cause disease at times.

The infecting organisms are conveyed by water, droplets, or through contacts of infected materials but a healthy body can resist the invasion by its complex defence mechanism. When the defence mechanism breaks down the invading organism can enter the body with or without producing local inflammatory reactions at the site of entry.

Credit of our knowledge of bacteriology goes to the great scientist Von Leeuwenhock, who discovered light microscope. That bacteria can cause disease was established by Robert Koch, which is valid even today as Koch's postulates; these are as follows:

1) Bacteria causing disease must be found in the blood, tissues or discharges (e.g. pus, urine, stool or CSF etc.).
2) Organisms isolated from the above sources should grow in pure culture in appropriate culture media.
3) The organisms grown as such should be able to produce the same disease when inoculated in animals or humans.

The type of damage varies, depending on the bacteria and the response it produces, by its pathogenicity and the nature of toxins produced.

Besides damage to tissues due to exotoxins or endotoxins, bacterial infections may produce tissue damage by other means as follows:

1) **Immunologic response:**

These may be cell-mediated hypersensitivity as in mycobacterial infection (tuberculosis and leprosy). In some others it may cause damage by deposition of immune-complex materials in blood vessels and joints, e.g., glomerulonephritis and rheumatic fever.

2) **Extensive tissue damage and blood invasion:**

Organisms may multiply freely in the blood stream (septicaemia) and may cause dissemination of pus all over the tissues (pyaemia). The organisms may cause disturbance in blood clotting mechanism by causing fibrin deposition in walls of blood vessels and then encouraging consumption of clotting factors. Disseminated intravascular coagulation (DIC) is a well-known and dangerous complication.

3) The other complications may be cardiovascular decompensation due to myocarditis, haemorrhage in suprarenal cortex, cerebral damage, toxic capillary damage and hyperpyrexia. The degree of toxaemia varies in different infections related to its pathogenicity and host resistance.
4) Previously existing viral infection, steroid therapy, malnutrition etc. cause overwhelming infection, severe toxaemia and even fatality.

## CLINICAL FEATURES

All bacterial infections have some common clinical features. However, depending on the severity of the infection and the invasive nature of the organisms, there are bound to be considerable variations depending on the toxic effects affecting various organs. Organisms have also predilections for certain organs as well as produce distant effects by their exotoxins or endotoxins. Sometimes the invasion is so rapid that the disease starts with a stormy onset while in other instances the development is insidious and the full clinical picture of the disease develops in five to seven days. The clinical characteristics of common infectious diseases have been discussed in respective chapters laying more stress on common diseases but not omitting relatively rare ones.

Therefore, while examining a patient who is suspected to have viral or bacterial infections the following clinical features require careful assessment:

**Fever:** The normal temperature of the human body in resting state taken by a clinical thermometer in the mouth varies between 36.0°C and 37.0°C (96.8°F and 99°F). It is interesting that as soon as the temperature touches 99°F usually most people feel a peculiar malaise and a feeling of warmth. Axillary temperature may have to be taken sometimes when the patient is non-cooperative or in childhood but is likely to be unreliable unless kept in the axilla for a period of two minutes. Axillary temperature is usually about 0.15°C lower than oral temperature, though there is much variation depending on the environmental temperature. Rectal temperature may have to be taken especially when the patient is in a coma or in the operation theatre. Skin temperature in different areas varies widely depending on the environmental warmth. Normal body temperature is minimum when the person is at rest in the earlier hours of the morning, while it rises by about 0.5 °C to 1°C by the evening or following muscular exercise. In women the body temperature rises on the day of ovulation and usually remains slightly at a higher level during the second half of the menstrual cycle. Newborns and infants have poor thermal control, and, therefore, must be protected from the environmental influence. Mechanism of maintenance of body temperature has been discussed fully in the chapter on effects of heat but it must be remembered that it is a complex mechanism depending on metabolism and neuro-endocrine factors to balance the environmental heat gain and heat loss through conduction, convection, evaporation and radiation.

The rise of temperature during various infections occurs due to the effects of pyrogenic protein substance liberated from polymorphonuclear leucocytes during their lysis in the process of combating viral and bacterial toxins. Pyrogens are also produced as a result of liberation of bacterial proteins due to phagocytosis and liberation of pyrogenic materials from RE cells. In mild infections temperature may or may not be very high but in severe infections the temperature may rise above 40°C to 41°C. It must be remembered by all medical students that temperature above 40°C should be considered medical emergency and temperature above 41°C may sometimes produce permanent brain damage. In these cases it is essential to record rectal temperature which may be even higher than recorded by oral or axillary route.

Although in clinical practice mercury made clinical thermometers are used there are special instruments which can accurately measure internal and external body temperature simultaneously and continuously for purposes of research and investigation. These are special instruments by which temperature is recorded by using thermocouples or thermisters.

Clinicians may be able to understand the nature of bacterial or parasitic infection by observing the nature of fever, its variations, periodicity as well as associated symptoms like shivering (rigor) as well as alternations in pulse and respiration. A relatively slow pulse associated with slowly rising temperature over a week and gradually increasing toxaemia is almost diagnostic of enteric group of fevers. On the other hand, if the temperature is hectic (swinging) along with slow pulse, one should suspect possibility of intracranial abscess or meningitis. In such circumstances careful examination of neck rigidity may be rewarding. Fever starting with rigor and possibly clattering of teeth and feeling of severe cold is suggestive of malaria, urinary tract infection or possibly onset of acute pneumonia. In malaria there may be alternate day rise of fever or every third day depending on the parasite concerned. On a hot humid day a patient is brought with temperature of 40°C or 41°C possibly with dry skin, it is almost certainly a case of heat-stroke. However, if the spleen is also enlarged, one should not forget the possibility of malaria in tropical countries. A patient of kala-azar will show a double rise of temperature and usually will have no toxaemia or much toxic symptoms although temperature may be as high as 39°C to 40°C. Prolonged fevers are often difficult to diagnose when there are no obvious physical signs. A special chapter has been devoted to the subject of P.U.O. (pyrexia of undetermined origin). Common causes of such fevers are chronic malaria, tuberculosis, amoebic liver-abscess,brucellosis, relapsing fever, kala-azar, Hodgkin's disease and hidden pus in some parts of the body. Students must not forget that a deep-seated stitch abscess after a major surgery or even a gluteal abscess as a result of badly given injection may produce swinging and high temperature. Sub-acute bacterial endocarditis is also a very important cause of long continued fever. Renal infections are often accompanied by loin pain and cystitis along with swinging temperature and rigor. However, chronic pyelonephritis may not have much associated symptoms other than continued pyrexia.

## PULSE & RESPIRATION

Most infections are associated with raised pulse and respiration. While relative bradycardia usually occurs in viral infection, enteric fevers are due to raised intracranial pressure. With rise of temperature of about 1°C pulse may rise by 15 beats per minute while it may be 20 to 30 in small children. Unusually rapid pulse rate denotes severe septic condition, rheumatic fever or toxic carditis. Unusually high respiration rate with breathing difficulty and fever is a pointer to pulmonary pathology.

It is most important for the medical students to make provisional diagnosis in every case by obtaining information from the history of the case, as well as from the clinical findings and then to order appropriate investigations to confirm the diagnosis. Ordering irrelevant investigation may not only be misleading but also cause unnecessary expenditure and undue strain on the hospital laboratory. Relative investigations required for various diseases have been discussed in respective chapters.

## TREATMENT

The first and foremost thing a physician must do is to maintain good bedside manners and to assure the patient so that the patient is relieved and becomes fully cooperative. Although false hopes must not be given, careless remarks should always be avoided. The following are the general measures for treatment of infectious diseases:

(a) **Rest:** Bed rest is essential in a febrile patient. In modern times air-conditioned cabins are available but only to those who can afford them. Therefore, it is necessary to ensure that the patient is kept in a room free from direct blast from outside and in a clean comfortable bed and good postures are very important. If the patient has to remain in bed for a very long time he should be looked after with utmost nursing care so that he does not get bedsores or venous thrombosis.

(b) **Care of skin and orifices:** In prolonged bed-ridden patient care of skin is essential and when bath is not possible, daily tepid sponging should be carried out. Skin over the pressure points should be cleaned with surgical spirit and powdered well. Skin may get soiled by urine and faeces, and, if not kept clean, will encourage horrible bedsores which may be worse than the disease.

(c) **Nutrition and fluids:** A patient with fever must not starve. They must be given appropriate diet depending on their ability to digest. Attention to this point is as important as prescribing antibiotics. Fluid and vitamin requirement must be attended to and particularly Vitamin B complex group and Vitamin C should be included daily. In a febrile patient there is additional fluid loss, due to sweating as well as due to excessive respiration and also diarrhoea and vomiting. Excessive sweating may cause water loss up to 1 to 2 litres daily especially in the tropics. If indicated, the doctor may order maintaining a fluid balance chart. If the patient cannot take by mouth or is vomiting or passing loose motions, intravenous fluid therapy to correct fluid and electrolyte balance is essential. In a constipated patient enemas or glycerine suppository should be given when required. Liquid paraffin or magnesium hydroxide emulsion should be given in small doses while drastic purgatives must be avoided. In addition, symptomatic treatment to promote sleep, to relieve pain and to reduce temperature should be carried out depending on the type of the case.

## STREPTOCOCCAL INFECTIONS

### INTRODUCTION

Streptococcal group of organisms is gram-positive cocci, which can be divided into four types:

1) $\alpha$—haemolytic streptococci
2) $\beta$—haemolytic streptococci
3) Anaerobic streptococci
4) Streptococcus or diplococcus pneumonae

Streptococci are non-motile, nonsporing organisms which are mostly aerobic while a few types are anaerobic.

Aerobic streptococci may be haemolytic or non-haemolytic. The haemolytic group has been subclassified into 18 Lancefield groups, according to polysaccharide antigen content. Lancefield group A is also named as streptococcus pyogenes, which are responsible for about 90% of human infections.

Streptococcal sore throat and tonsillitis have been described in the chapter on respiratory diseases. Acute glomerulonephritis and its relation to $\beta$-haemolytic streptococci are discussed in the chapter on renal diseases. Role of $\beta$-haemolytic streptoccocci, in the aetiology of erysipelas, scarlet fever and rheumatic fever is presented in this chapter.

Griffith has classified S. pyogens (Lancefield group A) into M T & R types by virtue of their surface antigens. By this means 51 M types and 30 T types have been isolated. Virulence of streptococci is directly related to M-protein content.

Besides strepto-haemolyticus, other streptococci which cause human infection are as follows:

Str. pneumonae or pneumococcus causes pulmonary infection, known as pneumonia. Str. bovis is an $\alpha$-haemolytic streptococci which is commensal organism of throat but may cause apical and peridonatal infection.

Str. faecalis (enterococcus) are present in the gut, which may cause urinary tract infection. Str. bovis and str. faecalis are also responsible for subacute bacterial endocarditis.

$\beta$-haemolytic streptococci are indirectly responsible for rheumatic fever and acute glomerulonephritis.

The other groups known as group C and group G cause respiratory infections and group D known as streptococcus faecalis or enterococcus, produces gastroenteritis or bowel infection. Streptococci A, C and G can produce endotoxins known as streptolysin O which can be measured in blood and is useful in diagnosis.

## ERYSIPELAS

It is an acute infection of skin due to streptococci of Lancefield group A. The organisms gain access via abrasions in skin and subcutaneous tissue becomes affected due to acute inflammation. Face is the commonest site but any other area may be affected.

### CLINICAL FEATURES

Local skin is erythematous, red and becomes oedematous. Minute vesicles form at the margins and even bullous eruptions may occur. Temperature rises up to 39°C to 40°C (102°F-104°F) associated with headache, rigor and toxaemia.

Infection may spread if not treated promptly and septicaemia may ensue. Complications also causing pneumonia, meningitis and cavernous sinus thrombosis.

### DIAGNOSIS

Inspection of the skin and clinical features should establish the diagnosis. However, β-haemolytic streptococci can be cultured from fluid collected from vesicles.

### TREATMENT

Crystalline or procaine penicillin should be used parenterally, dose depending on severity.

Infection procaine penicillin one mega unit given I.M. twice daily for five to seven days is good enough for cases of average severity. Supportive therapy is essential.

## SCARLET FEVER

### INTRODUCTION

It is characterised by high fever, sore throat, headache, vomiting and appearance of punctionform erythematous rash. This is not so common in the eastern world and may pass unnoticed due to non-recognition of rash in dark-skinned people. In such circumstances, these cases may be diagnosed as sore throat.

### CLINICAL FEATURES

Fever, tonsillitis, rash and lymphadenitis are the characteristic features.

Rash appears on the second day of the disease, in the face, trunk and proximal part of limbs. It usually fades within 48 to 72 hours. Some cases may develop rheumatic fever or acute glomerulonephritis after ten days. The rash should be differentiated from measles, rubella and drug rash.

## SURGICAL COMPLICATIONS

Streptococci may complicate pregnancy, producing severe puerperal sepsis. It may complicate burns, injury and surgical operation. However, due to appropriate antibiotic therapy, these are now rare. Usually anaerobic streptococci, e.g., streptococci aureus are involved in surgical infection.

## TREATMENT

Penicillin therapy as in the case of erysipelas.

**Drug therapy in streptococcal infections:**

Drug of choice is penicillin. Oral penicillin is better avoided. Erythromycin can be used if patient is penicillin sensitive. Cephalexin is also quite effective.

Ampicillin, though effective, has broader spectrum and hence may be used when mixed infection is suspected.

Sulphonamides do not completely eradicate the organisms and are not therefore the drug of choice. Tetracycline-resistant streptococci are known to occur and hence are not recommended.

# RHEUMATIC FEVER

*M. K. Mukherjee*
*G. C. Mookerjee*

## INTRODUCTION

Rheumatic fever is believed to occur as a delayed sequel to infection (mostly pharyngeal) by group-A streptococcus beta-haemolyticus, manifested by migratory polyarthritis subcutaneous nodules, fever, and carditis. In the chronic stage valvular diseases of the heart result in some of these cases. Chorea is a rare complication of rheumatic fever.

## AETIOLOGY

Predisposing factors

a) Age: Between the ages of four and fifteen years, peak years being between six and fourteen years.

b) Sex: Females predominate.

c) Climate: Low temperature, high humidity and high altitude predisposed.

d) Hygienic condition: More in insanitary conditions and in crowded slum areas.

e) Race: No particular race is immune but the disease is more prevalent among the whites.

f) Diet and economic status—More among the poorer section of the community living in slums having multiple dietary deficiencies, especially of Vitamin C.

g)Heredity: Has no specific role, but a Mendelian recessive inheritance has been suggested.

## PATHOGENESIS

a) **Infective:** Infection by group-A streptococcus beta-haemolyticus has been suggested to be the prime criterion in the causation of the disease process. It has been suggested that the hyaluronidase produced by the bacteria, injures the connective tissues and thereby produces the pathological lesions directly affecting mostly the connective tissues.

b) **Allergy:** It has also been suggested that the rheumatic lesions are the outcome of hypersensitivity reactions occurring in the collagenous tissues as a result of specific sensitisation to strepto-beta-haemolyticus. This theory is mostly based on the facts that (a) there always is a latent period of two to six weeks between an overt antecedent infection by strepto-beta haemolyticus, (pharyngitis, tonsillitis etc.) and developemnt of rheumatic fever; (b) high titres of streptococcal antibodies like antistreptolysin "O" antihyaluronidase, antinicotinamide-adenine dinucleotidase, antistreptolinase etc. have been demonstrated in the blood during the acute phase of the infection; (c) isolation of strepto-beta-haemolyticus from rheumatic lesions has never been possible; (d) steroids exert beneficial effects on the course of the disease.This allergic theory has further led to the present-day conception of it being an *Autoimmune Disease* and that the autoimmunity is induced by the streptococcal antigens in the following ways:

(i) The streptococcal prosthetic groups combine with the protein of the host connective tissues to render it antigenic (autoantigen) and the antibodies thus provoked cross-react with the myocardial fibres, arterial smooth muscle cells and connective tissues glycoproteins to elicit the characteristic lesions of the disease.

(ii) Antihyaluronidases are produced by the host against the streptococcal hyaluronidase and the antibodies react with the connective tissues of the host (connective tissues are rich in hyaluronic acid and allied mucopolysaccharides). The ultimate reaction is then an antigen-antibody reaction taking place in the collagenous tissues of the host and hence rheumatic fever is also considered as one of the collagen diseases resulting from autoimmune process.

The manifestations and pathological changes of the disease are basically the result of antoimmunity as a result of preceding infection by group A streptococcus beta-haemolyticus which are also known as streptococcus pyogenes.

The fundamental lesion in rheumatic fever is *Fibrinoid Degeneration* and necrosis. The fibrinoid material is composed of an acid "mucopolysaccharide-protein" complex. This connective tissue damage is the fundamental basis of all allergic reactions inclusive of rheumatic fever. Pathologically the fibrinoid lesions with inflammatory cells accompanying it constitute the rheumatic granuloma seen microscopically as Aschoff's Nodule which is the hallmark of rheumatic fever. In the evolution of *Aschoff's Nodule* four distinct phases are clearly discovered:

(a) **Degenerative phase:** (Fibrinoid degeneration)—Collagen fibres swell up, fragment, lose their typical staining reaction and stain deeply eosinophilic. Histochemically this stage is due to infiltration by some glycoprotein.

(b) **Exudative phase:** After one to four weeks from the previous phase the area becomes infiltrated with neutrophils, eosinophils and monocytes.

(c) **Granulomatous phase:** From the fifth week onward from the beginning, the Aschoff's Cells appear from the typical *Aschoff's Body* (Aschoff 1904) which looks like—

(i) a central zone of necrotic material consisting of swollen and fragmented collagen;

(ii) Around the centre are the *Aschoff's Cells* (Aschoff giant-cells) which are peculiar large endothelial cells with one or more vesicular nuclei and with cytoplasm with characteristic rugged edges. This is the most characteristic feature of the lesions. These are derived from the histiocytes or wandering cells which are members of the reticuloendothelial system.

(iii) The *Anitschkow Myocytes* which are large mesenchymal cells and are probably altered fibroblasts are often found in large numbers in the cardiac lesions. These in fact are cardiac histiocytes. They have an increased cytoplasm, a highly characteristic serrated bar of chromatin in the centre of the nucleus and fibrils radiating from the bar to the periphery.

(iv) Lymphocytes and plasma cells and

(v) the granulation tissue surrounds all these.

(d) **Healing Phase:** There is an increase in the connective tissues, gradual collagenisation, fibrosis and scarring.

The *Aschoff's Body* which is the hallmark in the pathogenesis of this disease is usually submiliary, difficult to visualise macroscopically, paravascular in distribution, bearing a definite relation to the adventitia of the small branches of the arteries. In the heart it is seen in the interstitial tissues of the myocardium, valvular as well as mural endocardium and pericardium. *Aschoff's Bodies,* however, are not always found in rheumatic carditis.

## PATHOLOGICAL LESIONS

The sites of the lesions can be divided into two groups—cardiac and extracardiac. The extracardiac sites are the joints, brain, kidneys, skin, lungs and the arteries.

### Cardiac lesions:

The basic lesion is a *Pancarditis* that is affecting the pericardium, myocardium and the endocardium.

a) **Pericardial lesions:** In the acute stage of the disease there is a serofibrinous pericarditis (bread and butter type) with thick deposition of fibrin and scanty effusion (about four to six ounces). Later on, as the disease process progresses there develops adhesions between the parietal and visceral layers of the pericardium leading to "adhesive pericarditis". Even the pericardium may become calcified but constrictive pericarditis never develops.

b) **Myocardial lesions:** Left side of the myocardium, mostly abundant towards the back of the interventricular septum and the walls of the auricles. When they heal by fibrosis, they leave scattered scars.

c) **Endocardial lesions:** Verrucous valvulitis with vegetation affecting the mitral, aortic and pulmonary (rare) valves are the classical lesions.

The reasons for which the mitral valve is most commonly affected are (a) it is this valve which is most abundantly supplied with blood vessels; (b) it is this valve whose blood vessels extend to the extreme free margin of the valve cusps.

The well-known vegetations are small bead-like bodies, arranged in a straight line along the line where the cusp comes in contact with its fellow (not along the free margin of the valves). The vegetations are situated on the auricular aspect of the A-V valves and on the ventricular aspect of the semilunar valves. They are firm and adherent. The myocardium lining the left auricle as well as that covering the valve may be affected and this lesion in the left auricular endocardium has been classically called as MacCallum's patch. The importance of this MacCallum's patch is that it is in this area that the lesion in subacute bacterial endocarditis occurs.

## EXTRACARDIAC LESIONS

a) **Joints:** Joints, mostly the big joints, show the characteristic exudative reactions rather than proliferative ones and healing of the joint lesions leads to minimum scarring and/or deformity. Focal necrosis with proliferation of endothelial calls and associated vascular changes are prominent microscopic lesions. It is the great vascularity of the joints which account for this exudative type of lesions with other associated features of acute inflammation.

b) **Subcutaneous nodules:** These painless nodules are seen only during the acute phase of the disease process. As the name suggests they are situated subcutaneously in the deep fascia mostly over the bony prominences in association with the tendons and ligaments attached to the prominences. Pathologically they are composed of granulomas with localised areas of fibrinoid degeneration of the subcutaneous collagen nodules with perivascular reaction in the form of collection of large cells with pale nuclei and prominent nucleoli. To be precise, they are merely florid *Aschoff's Bodies* with very little central necrosis.

c) **Erythema marginatum, erythema nodosum, erythema multiforme, petichae, livedo reticularis:** All these are various types of skin involvements associated with the rheumatic fever and are more of importance as clinical findings than pathologically.

d) **Lungs and pleurae:** Non-specific changes of acute serofibrinous pleuritis and acute among the pneumonitis with consolidation very common, particularly among the younger victims. Even pneumonitis with eosinophilic hyaline membrane lining the alveolar ducts with resultant patchy consolidation is common in younger children than among adults suffering from the same disease.

e) **Brain:** A non-specific meningoencephalitis like that found in encephalitis lethargica with perivascular collection of round cells, thrombosis and endothelial proliferation is the only pathological change, seen particularly affecting the corpus striatum, cerebral cortex and the meninges without the formation of the typical *Aschoff's Bodies.*

f) **Kidneys:** Proliferative glomerulitis with capsulitis is the only pathological finding which again is common in older patients.

## CLINICAL FEATURES

The *incubation period* is between one and three weeks, may be longer. This is the period between the infection anywhere in the body with streptococcus beta-haemolyticus and the clinically manifested acute rheumatic fever.

**Onset** is usually acute, may also be insidious, the initial attack occasionally being overlooked and/or ignored. Sometimes some unsuspected cases are diagnosed as acute rheumatic fever during the routine examinations of the children suffering from fever of apparently 'unknown origin'. Even many cases of children suffering recurrently from fever during childhood are treated symptomatically and are diagnosed in the third or fourth decade of life with features which in fact are the hallmarks of the healing processes of previous attacks of acute rheumatic fever.

## MAJOR CLINICAL MANIFESTATIONS

### ARTHRITIS

Acute febrile illness associated with a migratory or "fleeting" joint pain with swelling, mostly affecting the big joints, is a classical picture. Classically big joints of the extremities are mostly involved, but rarely, the small joints of the extremities and even the spinal joints and temporomandibular joints may also be involved. Effusion in the affected joints is as a rule present and this is the cause of swelling of the joints. The swelling is also associated with other features of acute inflammation like redness and extreme pain and gross painful limitation of movements of the joints and also the joints appear tender and warm on palpation. The reason for which it is called a "migratory" is that when pain, swelling and tenderness subsides in one joint, another joint gets involved. But occasionally this typical migratory nature of the joint involvement may be absent. The duration of involvement of each joint is widely variable and may be from one day to about three weeks. The involvement of the joints is associated with high fever, leucocytosis in the form of polycytosis and raised E.S.R. In contrast to rheumatoid arthritis, permanent deformities involving the affected joints never occur. Salicylates and corticosteroids promptly and dramatically reduce symptoms and signs of acute arthritis and is of much diagnostic value and in fact one of the main criteria for the diagnosis of doubtful cases of arthritis.

## CARDITIS

It is the most dreadful manifestation of rheumatic fever as it leads to permanent disability and/or death. Death usually results form cardiac failure during the acute stage of the disease. Although the term 'carditis' indicates some inflammatory involvement of the heart, in many cases there remains no subjective complaints from the sufferer referable to the heart, even during the early stages of active carditis.

In children below 6 years of age, carditis is the presenting symptom, whereas in older children polyarteritis and chorea are more common. Carditis occurs in about 50% of patients during the first attack of the disease.

As mentioned earlier, rheumatic carditis usually means pancarditis. As such clinical features will depend upon the involvement of the three different elements of pancarditis. *Endocarditis* involving the valvular endocardium is predominant when there is appearance of any cardiac murmur and it has to be borne in mind that such murmurs may be functional. Appearance of an apical pansystolic murmur indicates either damage to the mitral valve or a functional mitral regurgitation associated with myocarditis. Appearance of a low-pitched short mid-diastolic murmur in this apical area (Carey Comb's murmur) is strongly suggestive of the rheumatic involvement of the mitral valve. This murmur may disappear in the course of time shortly or it may persist for even years until the typical features of mitral stenosis develop. But a mere presence of an apical short mid-diastolic murmur in rheumatic fever is not necessarily an evidence of mitral stenosis or of subsequent development of mitral stenosis. The mid-diastolic murmur in aortic or pulmonary area is never a diagnostic criterion of cardiac involvement due to the rheumatic process as it is not uncommon among children with any fever but without cardiac involvement, and it usually disappears with the subsidence of fever.

## MYOCARDITIS

It is an important and a common finding in 50% of cases of acute rheumatic fever but it is very difficult to diagnose it with confidence, especially in children. Myocarditis is suspected when there are (i) cardiac enlargement, (ii) tachycardia out of proportion to the fever (iii) persistence of tachycardia even after the fever subsides and (iv) appearance of cardiac failure right-sided or left-sided in the absence of any valvular damage or any other obvious cause for the same. A patient with myocarditis will show dyspnoea, orthopnoea, tachypnoea, precordial discomfort and oedema in various combinations. There may be gallop rhythm because of exaggeration of the 3rd heart sound with diminution in the quality of the lst heart sound in the presence of tachycardia resulting in so-called TIC TAC rhythm. But simply the finding of a gallop rhythm does not necessarily mean involvement of the myocardium as it may occur in any child with fever and tachycardia. Arrhythmias of varying degrees may be present. E.C.G. may reveal the nature of the arrhythmias but the commonest finding is the prolongation of the P.R. interval with or without inversion of the T-waves in two of the three standard leads. But E.C.G. findings in the absence of any suggestive clinical manifestation of carditis have no diagnostic significance.

## PERICARDITIS

Precordial pain in a suspected case of rheumatic fever strongly suggests involvement of the pericardium causing pericarditis, which is further substantiated by the clinical finding of a pericardial friction rub both on palpation and on auscultation, provided pericardial effusion has not yet developed when there will neither be pain nor the rub. When clinical evidence of pericarditis is present, the carditis is usually severe and advanced and has already involved the myocardium as well as the endocardium. Once pericardial effusion develops, pre-existing retrosternal pain and the pericardial rub both disappear. But with the development of effusion there may be some cardiorespiratory embarrassment if large quantity of fluid accumulates rapidly. The distinction between pericardial effusion and cardiac dilatation becomes often difficult both by bedside clinical examination as well as by X-rays, but in pericardial effusion the apical impulse may disappear, the heart sounds become indistinct and muffled but the quality of the pulse remains fair with pulsus paradoxus. The X-ray appearance of the pericardial effusion shows the cardiac shadow more rounded (pitcher-shaped) than that in cardiac dilatation. By ultrasound imaging however, this diagnosis is easy.

## SUBCUTANEOUS NODULES

These are very characteristic findings of rheumatic fever and are not found in association with any other disease except the rheumatoid arthritis. They never give rise to any symptom but are of great diagnostic value. They are better felt than seen and are painless structures attached to the tendon sheaths, joint capsules and deep fascia with the overlying skin remaining movable over them. They occur mostly over the bony prominences like the extension surfaces of the elbows, knuckles, knees, iliac crests, back of the head, spines of the vertebrae. Usually they have a bilaterally symmetrical distribution and also usually do not appear early in the course of the disease and are most abundant in patients suffering from associated carditis who are sick in bed for several weeks.

## CHOREA (Sydenham's chorea. St. Vitus's dance):

The term 'chorea' itself is derived from the Greek word which means 'dance'. In medical profession it denotes and refers to the sudden, widespread, purposeless, involuntary, irregular, arrhythmic movements of a forcible, rapid and jerky type with emotional instability, and muscular weakness due to involvement of the central nervous system. It is in fact a delayed manifestation of the rheumatic fever and by the time it appears, other features of the disease may or may not still be present. It occurs mostly between the ages of seven and fourteen years, with peak incidence at eight years of age and rarely after puberty and never occurs after the age of twenty years. The attacks are recurrent and often prolonged, but eventual recovery is complete. The characteristic thing about it is that such choreic movements are triggered off and increased by effort, excitement and fatigue but cease when the patient is asleep.

The clinical onset is usually gradual. The patient with rheumatic fever, who was previously controlled, becomes increasingly nervous and fidgety, having difficulties in writing and drawing and his speech becomes indistinct with varying types of disturbances and characteristic choreic movements of the legs and the arms develop. Often the patient, usually the child, drops things from hand and starts grimacing and stumbling which might be the early symptoms before the typical choreic movements develop.

Choreic patients are usually afebrile with normal C.S.F. findings. The C-reactive protein (CRP) is often negative with a normal WBC count and a normal ESR. The antistreptolysin 'O' titre in many instances is within normal limits.

The criteria to confirm chorea clinically are:

(i) Choreic movements are exaggerated after periods of direct questioning.

(ii) Speech disturbances may be elicited by asking the patient to count rapidly when the first few numbers are uttered clearly but then suddenly the speech becomes thick with inability to utter the next numbers without a pause for several seconds.

(iii) When the patient is asked to protrude his tongue and to hold it quietly, the tongue shows undulating and jerky movements.

(iv) The patellar reflex is 'hung up'.

## LABORATORY APPRAISALS

In fact there is no definite and specific laboratory test to indicate the presence of rheumatic fever, but the appraisal of rheumatic *Activity* by laboratory findings is of some value, especially when the clinical features are not very specifically apparent.

a) Acute phase reactants like ESR, C-reactive protein, WBC count, serum complement, alpha-2 and gamma globulins.

b) Streptococcal antibody tests to ensure preceding streptococcal infection.

(a) (i) **ESR**—In patients with rheumatic polyarthritis and/or carditis unaccompanied by cardiac failure the ESR is almost always raised. During the stage of cardiac failure, it may be also normal but again rises as soon as the cardiac compensation takes place. ESR also remains normal in uncomplicated cases with rheumatic chorea, but a finding of chorea with a raised ESR suggests cardiac involvement. Again often the ESR remains raised when all the clinical symptoms have subsided; this indicates that the rheumatic process is active at subclinical level and in such cases the patient who is symptom-free should be kept on bed-rest until the ESR shows a tendency to fall. ESR indeed in rheumatic fever has some prognostic value in assessment of the management of a case.

(a) (ii) **C-reactive protein** (**CRP**)—The name comes from the fact that the blood of patients suffering from pneumococcal pneumonia contains a protein which reacts with the carbohydrate (so the symbol "C") of the pneumococcus to form a precipitate long before any antibody to the pneumococcus can be detected. Its presence in the serum is detected by a highly specific precipitation reaction. CRP is always present in the serum of persons suffering from an acute rheumatic fever. It is absolutely negative in normal persons. It, of course, is never a specific test for rheumatic fever. Its value is in doubtful cases of acute rheumatic fever. As the patient with acute rheumatic fever improves, the test becomes normal (negative) as the protein disappears. Its value is again mainly in assessing the activity of the disease process and it also has some prognostic value too.

(a) (iii) **Blood cells**—Leucocytosis is evident during the acute stage of the disease, but it is a less reliable indication of subclinical rheumatic infection than is the ESR The rheumatic process should not be considered inactive when the WBC count is consistently above 10,000 per cubic millimetre, especially when there is a definite shift of the polymorphs to the left.

Persistence of anaemia is also an indication of the activity of the disease process. This anaemia is due to suppression of erythropoiesis which is characteristic of any chronic inflammatory disease.

b) **Streptococcal antibody tests:**

Presence of streptococcal antibodies in the blood is a strong and definite indication of acute rheumatic fever. Commonly, antistreptolysin O (ASO) titre is estimated and a level of 250 Todd units in adults and 333 Todd units in children is diagnostic.

The other recently developed tests are antihyaluronidase test (AHT), antideoxyribonycleotidase B test, antistreptokinase test (ASKT) and a few others. Antistreptozyme test (ASTZ)—a haemagglutination test is also a very sensitive indication of recent streptococcal infection. In fact all patients with acute rheumatic fever show litres above 200 units per millilitre. The value of this test lies in the detection of doubtful and borderline cases of ASO titres and are not routinely carried out.

## DIAGNOSTIC CRITERIA OF RHEUMATIC FEVER

Sometimes it becomes extremely difficult to diagnose a case only on clinical grounds and on many occasions even with the laboratory aids. As such to confirm a case it is often advisable to follow Jones criteria, which shows certain MAJOR manifestations and certain MINOR manifestations of the disease and conclusion is from certain combinations of them along with the help of laboratory appraisal as shown below:

## JONES CRITERIA

| **Major manifestations** | **Minor manifestations** |
|---|---|
| Carditis | Fever |
| Polyarthritis | Arthralgia |
| Chorea | Raised ESR |
| Erythema marginatum | Positive CRP |
| Subcutaneous Rh nodules | Prolonged P-R interval in ECG |

The findings of TWO MAJOR criteria or a combination of ONE MAJOR and TWO MINOR criteria along with a preceding history and/or of supporting evidence of streptococcal infection associated with a high ASO titre or ASTZ titre are diagnostic of rheumatic fever. One of the most important criteria is the prompt and dramatic relief of joint pains with salicylates, sometimes loosely known as therapeutic diagnosis.

## ASSESSMENT OF THE ACTIVITY OF THE DISEASE PROCESS

The following are the criteria upon the combinations of which the activity of the rheumatic process is assessed:

a) Presence of symptoms
b) Persistence of anaemia
c) Persistence of WBC count above 10,000/per cubic mm

d) Presence of CRP
e) Raised ESR
f) Presence of raised ASO litre
g) Presence of subcutaneous rheumatic nodules
h) Presence of erythema marginatum

## DIFFERENTIAL DIAGNOSIS

a) Acute arthritic conditions
b) Conditions with chorea
c) Conditions with erythema
d) Conditions with carditis

## ACUTE ARTHRITIS

a) Gonococcal arthritis
b) Rheumatic arthritis
c) Infective arthritis
    (i) Non-specific
    (ii) Specific
d) Palindromic rheumatism
e) Allergic arthritis
f) Gouty arthritis

a) **Gonococcal Arthritis:**

Usually nonarticular, commonly affecting the knee joint, but may also be polyarticular even involving the small joints, but not typically "migratory" and more painful than that of rheumatic arthritis. Muscular atrophy is a striking feature. Salicylates have no decided effect upon the relief of painful joints. Response to penicillin and sulphonamides is prompt.

b) **Rheumatoid Arthritis:**

More among women in the child-bearing age. Joint affection may be "fleeting" but usually involves the small joints. Rose-Waaler test and latex fixation test are usually positive in nearly 80 per cent of cases.

c) **Specific Infective Arthritis:**

Specific infective arthritis relating to specific diseases like typhoid arthritis, pneumococcal arthritis, tuberculous arthritis, viral arthritis (especially in mumps and O'nyong-nyong in Uganda caused by virus following mosquito bites associated with lymphadenopathy and arthritis) can be diagnosed individually from their respective clinical features and supporting laboratory appraisals.

d) **Non-specific Infective Arthritis:**

Occurs mostly in adults in the 3rd or 4th decade of life. Usually it follows some non-specific septic focus in the body. Response to penicillin and sulphonamides is prompt as in many cases the organism is streptococcus.

e) **Palindromic Rheumatism:**

Occurs in adults. Recurrent afebrile attacks of acute arthritis, periarthritis and para-arthritis of several joints. Attacks are acute, lasting for few hours to few days, then disappears completely just to reappear after regularly spaced intervals.

f) **Allergic Arthritis (Henoch's and Schonlein's arthritis):**

Recurrent with severe synovitis and effusion, especially involving the knee joint. Lasts for few hours to few days. Usually some provocating allergic factor triggers the tissue.

g) **Gouty Arthritis:**

Usually involving small joints. Gouty tophi may be present. High blood uric acid level with classical response to colchicine and classical clinical features confirm the diagnosis.

h) **Conditions with Erythema:**

Erythema may be caused by many internal and external causes and may be localised or generalised and as such may be produced by various causes and disease conditions but erythema marginatum is a distinct clinical entity particularly characteristic of rheumatic fever during the acute stage, along with few other classical features of acute rheumatic fever which differentiates it from other conditions associated with it.

## CONDITIONS WITH CARDITIS

There are many causes of carditis but the carditis of rheumatic aetiology is easy to diagnose as it is usually associated with few other features of rheumatic fever. But it is very difficult to diagnose an isolated carditis where no other feature of rheumatic never is present and in such rare cases the history and the laboratory appraisals help in finding the aetiology.

## COURSE AND PROGNOSIS

The course of rheumatic fever is unpredictable at the onset. In some apparently severely ill patients, complete recovery within a few days is not unusual whereas in others the disease drags on for months. Age is an important factor in the assessment of the course and prognosis of the disease. It is rare for a young child with acute rheumatic fever to escape carditis. The risk of developing chronic rheumatic heart disease with valvular damages after an acute attack diminishes with the age and it is not unusual for an adult to get a first attack without any sequel.

About more than 70% of acute attacks subside within a period of two months, 90% within three months. In about 5 to 10 per cent cases acute phase persists more than three months and they comprise of patients with persistent carditis and chorea.

Recurrence of the disease is not uncommon as explained under the discussion on pathological background and pathogenesis. The evidence of recurrence varies widely in different series and may be as high as 50 per cent and with each attack of recurrence the chances of permanent cardiac damage are greater. The frequency of recurrence depends upon the frequence and severity of the streptococcal infection, the presence or absence of rheumatic heart disease following each attack, the duration of freedom from the last attack, the duration and dosage of chemotherapy and the type of the streptococcus attacking each time as there are about 50 different antigenic types of group A streptococcus beta-haemolyticus.

The course of the chronic phase of the disease is also variable depending upon the degree of chronic rheumatic carditis and its sequel as chronic rheumatic heart disease depends on (1) the duration and severity of the rheumatic process, (2) the amount of scarring of the myocardium and of the valves following the inflammation, (3) the location and severity of the valvular lesion and its effect upon the haemodynamics and on the scarred myocardium, and (4) presence and progress of the valvular sclerosis and calcification.

Although the first attack is seldom fatal, it is claimed that 70 per cent patients develop carditis within the first week of the disease and 85 per cent within the first 12 weeks and almost 100 per cent within the first 6 months of the disease. Carditis during the initial attack is of bad prognosis. Moreover, the prognosis of patients with carditis is more related to the severity of the myocarditis than to the valvular impairment because if the cardiac musculature is healthy and uninvolved and in good condition then it can compensate for the valvular deficiencies for many years to come. But if the myocardium is damaged, the heart dilates and congestive failure may develop.

## PREVENTION:

Rheumatic fever can be prevented by the prophylaxis and prompt energetic treatment of acute streptococcal infections especially among children and young adults. The best means of treating any acute attack is to give a single intramuscular injection of 0.6 to 1.2 mega units of benzathine penicillin (Inj. Penidure LA 6 or LA 12 depending upon requirement). Alternatively potassium salt of penicillin (Penicillin V) may be given orally (Phenoxymethyl Penicillin) for at least 10 days. Those who are hypersensitive to penicillin can be given oral erythromycin also for 10 days.

Every patient who has suffered an attack of acute rheumatic fever should be explained, assured and asked to receive the long-term prophylatic therapy by way of long acting intramuscular injection of Benzathine Penicillin of 1.2 mega units (Inj. Penidure LA 12) once a month, alternatively Phenoxymethyl Penicillin (V) 125 mg twice a day or sulfadiazine 0.5 gm twice a day. The duration of such prophylactic therapy following an initial acute attack should be minimum during the entire period of childhood, preferably up to the age of 25 years.

## TREATMENT

a) **General Measures:** During the acute phase of the disease till the temperature, pulse rate and ESR have returned to normal and till the evidences of acute arthritis and carditis have disappeared, bed-rest is a *must*. Then gradual ambulation and rehabilitation to be instituted. As long as the rheumatic process is active, there remains the possibility of progressive cardiac damage and hence bed-rest in such cases is essential and may be necessary for a long period until clinical and laboratory appraisals suggest absence of the activity of the disease process.

Presence of active carditis specially needs *absolute bed-rest* and even for several weeks and each case has to be assessed separately and on this issue no generalisation of principles can be laid down. Then assessing each individual case, resumption of normal physical activity has to be adjusted and delayed at least to 6 months from the time when the last sign of active carditis has resolved. Nutrition should be maintained adequately with time-to-time reassurance.

b) Specific Drug Therapy:

Drugs like salicylates and corticosteroids are most valuable in controlling the acute and exudative phase of the disease with prompt relief of symptoms, but in spite of that no guarantee can be assured against subsequent development of chronic rheumatic heart disease. Even the full coverage with penicillin over a prolonged period does not prevent the most dreadful complication of the disease—subacute bacterial endocarditis.

The chief targets of the drug regimen are—

i) Prompt symptomatic relief and (ii) prevention of residual cardiac damage.

i) Regarding prompt symptomatic relief, salicylates still remain the first choice with dramatic responses but patients with severe carditis especially those with congestive cardiac failure often improve more rapidly and uniformly with steroids than with salicylates, although there remains the hazards of indiscriminate and injudicious uses of steroids.

ii) So far as the prevention of residual cardiac damage is concerned, there is no agreement as to whether salicylates or the steroids should be preferred. But in patients with carditis steroids should always be preferred as the first choice as they promptly control the acute exudative reactions in the myocardium than the salicylates. But even then it has been found that even steroids used initially and continued for many weeks do not guarantee complete prevention against the development of residual cardiac disease, which as such may develop insidiously but definitely with lesser frequency than without it.

Penicillin is of no value in relieving the manifestations of rheumatic fever, but as the activity of the rheumatic process may be prolonged by the presence of group A streptococci, it is always a *must* to cover all patients with acute rheumatic fever or chorea with a 'therapeutic course' of injectable penicillin for two weeks to eliminate those organisms from the body, followed by the scheduled "prophylactic regime of penicillin" as discussed under the heading "Prevention" earlier.

**An ideal regime for an acute rheumatic fever** is (a) Inj. crystalline penicillin—10 lacs unit (one lac unit is equivalent to 1 mega unit which is equivalent to 600 mgm) by intramuscular injection every 8 hours with or without probenecid (which interferes with the renal tubular excretion of penicillin by competition and thereby increases the penicillin plasma level) along with (b) Prednisolone 60 mgm a day for 2 weeks and then gradually tapered off during the 3rd or 4th week and (c) Salicylates 90 to 120 mgm per kg. body weight a day divided into 4 equal doses for 2 weeks then 60 mgm per kg. body weight a day in divided doses for another 4 weeks.

**Salicylate Therapy:**

Salicylates relieve the acute symptoms of joint pains and fever promptly and dramatically. Aspirin (Acetyl-Salicylic Acid) and Sodium Salicylates—Either of them can be used but aspirin is the drug of choice between the two because (i) the children prefer aspirin, (ii) aspirin is a better inhibitor of prostaglandins than sodium salicylates and as such has a quicker and more definite result, (iii) aspirin is available as enteric coated and as dispersible tablets which cause less gastric irritations and (iv) aspirin is less protein-bound after absorption than sodium salicylate.

**Dosage:** Dosage of salicylates, to start with in acute cases, should be 90 to 120 mgm per kg. body weight, in divided doses to be continued for two weeks, then reduced to 60 mgm per kg. body weight, for further 3 to 4 weeks. Then it can be discontinued provided the symptoms and other criteria of the activity of the disease as discussed earlier subside. But if the symptoms recur then a second course in the same regime has to be continued. Oral dosage should be divided with 6 hourly schedule as 6 hours is the half-life of the drug in normals although this can vary widely with the urine pH.

**Side Effects:** Certain side effects do appear with a high dosage, which subside as soon as the dosage is also reduced and they include—

1) Gastric irritation in the form of gastritic vomiting, headache, tinnitus and even gastric haemorrhages manifested clincially by a positive occult blood test for the stool.
2) Salicylate allergy manifested clinically by asthma, urticaria, rashes, angioneurotic oedema and rhinorrhoea. Aspirin may also aggravate chronic urticaria.
3) Bleeding manifestation in the form of purpuric rashes, echymoses and even frank haemorrhages. This is due to hypoprothrombinaemia (due to interference with prothrombin synthesis) and also due to inhibition of platelet aggregation.

These reactions are reversible by Inj. Vitamin $K_1$.

**Overdosage:**

The typical clinical picture of "moderate over dosage" consists of nauseas and vomiting, tinnitus, headache, deafness, hypernoea, sweating, restlessness and mental confusion along with varying degrees of haemorrhagic manifestations. With a "severe overdosage" the previous symptoms are followed by paradoxical hyperpyrexia, convulsion and coma with severe dehydration and ketosis.

In children with overdosage the picture resembles metabolic acidosis whereas in adults it resembles respiratory alkalosis.

The treatment of salicylate overdosage is "Forced Alkaline Diuresis (FAD), exactly the similar as done in case of Barbiturate overdosage.

**Points to remember in salicylate therapy are:**

a) Aspirin should be preferred to sodium salicylate as explained earlier.
b) Although enteric-coated tablets of aspirin cause less gastric irritation, they should be avoided in acute rheumatic fever because absorption of such tablets is delayed for 4 to 6 hours or even more and as such onset of action is delayed as also is the clinical efficacy so far as the prompt relief is concerned.
c) Aspirin tablets should contain aspirin, citric acid and calcium carbonate. When such a tablet is put into water, the citric acid reacts with the calcium carbonate to form calcium citrate solution and this dissolves the aspirin to form calcium acetyl salicylate and this pharmacologically effective compound is almost the same as sodium salicylate and as such less efficacious than plain aspirin.
d) The simultaneous administration of sodium bicarbonate along with either aspirin or with sodium salicylate with the idea of reducing gastric irritation is not desirable in treating a case with acute rheumatic fever as this combination decreases the absorption of salicylates thus decreasing the serum level which has the same effect as lowering the dose.
e) The mode of action of salicylates is due to blockade of biosynthesis of prostaglandins from arachidonic acid whereas the steroids act by blocking their release and not their biosynthesis.

**Other analgesic, antipyretic and anti-inflammatory drugs:**

They are less efficacious than time-honoured salicylates, but on rare occasions, especially when someone is allergic to salicylates, they are useful. They include phenylbutazone, indomethacin, etc., all of which act by blockade of prostaglandins biosynthesis but less efficiently than salicylates. Moreover, they all do possess many untoward effects in therapeutically effective doses and as such they are not discussed at length here.

## STEROID THERAPY

Steroids in the form of plain prednisolone is the drug of choice. Steroids as discussed earlier should get initial choice along with salicylates or individually in cases with active carditis especially in those with congestive failure.

Since steroids mask symptoms of all kinds, children kept on steroid therapy should be observed closely for serious complications and intercurrent infections.

Regarding the dosage and duration of therapy, discussion at length has been made earlier. The important points to remember are to watch closely for the side effects of systemic glucocorticoid therapy which are—

i) Cushing's syndrome with acne, moon-face, hirsutism, hyperpigmentation, striae, buffalo-humps etc.
ii) Adrenal suppression and atrophy
iii) Salt retention and hypertension
iv) Hyperglycaemia
v) Infections especially tuberculosis, viral and fungal
vi) Osteoporosis
vii) Growth retardation in children
viii) "Withdrawal Phenomenon" with vomiting, hypercalcaemia panniculitis, and
ix) "Rebound Phenomenon" of the disease on reduction of the dosage.

Points to be remembered during steroid therapy are:

1. Its usage should be optimally justified.
2. Dosage varies with the severity and tempo of disease process.
3. Dosage should be gradually tailed off to prevent 'Rebound phenomenon'.
4. Close observations should be made on possible hazards of steroid therapy as discussed earlier.
5. The steroids act by preventing the release of prostaglandins in the blood and not by blocking their biosynthesis from arachnidonic acid.

## COMPLICATIONS

The only complication, rather it is better to name it as 'sequel' than 'complication', of rheumatic fever is chronic rheumatic heart disease. Its classical involvements with or without superadded subacute bacterial endocarditis. In fact chronic rheumatic heart disease as discussed earlier is the result of damage produced by recurrent attacks of acute rheumatic carditis and the subsequent healing process. The valvular deformities may take many years to develop. These deformities of the cardiac valves result from thickening and distortion of the cusps at the time of acute rheumatic carditis and contracture of the valve structures, fusion of the commissures, shortening of the chordae tendinae and finally calcification during the stage of healing. Stenosis of a valve occurs if the fusion of the cusps takes place and incompetence of a valve occurs if shortening of the chordae tendinae and contracture of the valve leaflets take place.

# MENINGITIS

*S. N. Sengupta*

## INTRODUCTION

'Meningitis' means inflammation of the meninges. Inflammation of the dura mater is known as pachymeningitis. It is secondary to infection of the adjacent bones and is never generalised. If unqualified, the term 'meningitis' means leptomeningitis or infective inflammation of the leptomeninges, i.e. the pia-arachnoid system. Once infection sets in, it becomes generalised all round the cerebrospinal axis through the circulation of the cerebrospinal fluid (CSF). When the infective process involves both the meninges and the parenchyma of the brain the condition is called meningoencephalitis. Similarly, inflammation of the meninges and spinal cord is known as meningo-myelitis and when the meninges is affected together with the brain and the spinal cord the condition is described as meningoencephalomyelitis.

Meningism is a term which means a non-inflammatory irritation of the meninges, generally found in some systemic infections without infection of the meninges itself. The irritation of the meninges perhaps results from circulating toxins. Examination of the CSF does not show any abnormality.

Meningitis may be classified into two broad groups according to the nature of the infective organism:

1. Septic : Bacterial-(a) pyogenic,
   (b) tuberculous.
2. Aseptic : (a) Viral
   (b) Spirochaetal-syphilis, leptospirosis
   (c) Fungal and parasitic when organisms like yeast, cryptococcus neoformans, toxoplasma gondii etc. are responsible.

Of these the last two are very rare and will be discussed later on in this volume.

## PYOGENIC MENINGITIS

### AETIOLOGY

Though the disease is well under control in advanced countries it is still prevalent in the underdeveloped and developing countries. Of the different pyogenic forms meningococcal meningitis is the commonest. It not only occurs sporadically throughout the year but sometimes as epidemic in closed communities. The other organisms often responsible for pyogenic meningitis are D. pneumoniae, H. influenzae, streptococcus, staphylococcus, N. gonorrhoea and E. coli, B. anthracis etc.

Meningococcal meningitis occurs more commonly among the infants and small children. Adolescents and young adults are less commonly affected. Males are more commonly affected than females. The incidence is more among commonly affected than females. The incidence is more among males than females. Poverty and malnourishment are common predisposing factors.

Meningococcal infection appears to occur through droplets, the organism reaching the meninges through blood stream from the nasopharynx. Asymptomatic carriers are often responsible for transmission of the organisms. Infection by other pyogenic organisms like streptococcus, staphylococcus, pneumococcus, H. influenzae etc. is generally secondary to infections elsewhere like lung, heart, bones etc. There may, however, be direct spread from contiguous areas like the middle ear, mastoid and air sinuses or the pyogenic organisms can also be introduced through fractures involving air sinuses and penetrating open injuries of the skull. Lumbar or cistern puncture for diagnostic or therapeutic purposes may be responsible for iatrogenic infection of the meninges if sufficient aseptic care is not taken. Rarely a brain abscess may drain into the subarachnoid space causing infection of the meninges.

## PATHOLOGY

There is severe congestion and oedema of the leptomeninges over the brain and the spinal cord. The cerebral convolutions are often partly obscured by collection of greenish yellow exudate in the sulci and around the surface of the brain. Localised collection of pus may be found if there is a source of primary infection in the neighbourhood. The convolutions are flattened as a result of raised pressure of CSF both in the subarachnoid space as well as inside the ventricles which are distended.

There is infiltration of the meninges predominantly with polymorphonuclear cells. Lymphocytes and plasma cells may appear at a later stage. The brain tissue shows little evidence of infection, though areas of necrosis are sometimes found as a result of thrombosis of cortical veins. In case of a brain abscess draining into the subarachnoid space, however, appropriate pathological changes are evident in the brain.

In acute stage the cranial and spinal nerves passing through the subarachnoid space may be inflamed and their functions interfered with. In neglected survivors the exudate may undergo organisation causing entrapment of these nerves and sealing of the interventricular foramina and the communicating openings between the fourth ventricle and the subarachnoid space. This may result in permanent damage of the nerves and in hydrocephalus. The vascular endothelium may be damaged, causing intravascular thrombosis and local haemorrhage which may bring about necrosis of the surrounding tissues. In severe meningococcaemia there may be haemorrhage in the suprarenal cortex. This together with the effect of the endotoxin on the myocardium and vascular endothelium is responsible for the state of collapse found in Waterhouse-Friderichsen syndrome. There may also be inflammation in the joints and mild degenerative changes in the kidneys.

## CLINICAL PICTURE

All cases of pyogenic meningitis, irrespective of the cause, present with similar clinical picture and their clinical distinction is often difficult unless a primary infection is evident elsewhere. Since N. meningitidis is the commonest causative agent of pyogenic meningitis, meningococcal meningitis should serve as a model for the description of the general clinical features of all of them

There is a sudden rise of temperature, often with chill and rigor. The fever is accompanied with bodyache and headache which are persistant and severe. There may be vomiting, often projectile in nature. Epileptiform convulsion is common in children. The patient is irritable and soon becomes confused and delirious. Deep coma is not very common. Generally there is constipation and retention of urine, but in later stages there may be incontinence.

The patient lies huddled up in bed and resists interference. Photophobia is a prominent feature. The patient prefers to lie with his back towards the light, covering the head with bed clothes. Later, there may be progressive head retraction and arching of the back leading to opisthotonic decubitus. The temperature is usually between 39° and 40°C of irregular remittent type. Hyperpyrexia may occur. There may be a relative bradycardia which is replaced by tachycardia and irregular pulse at a later stage. Tachypnoea and irregular breathing may also be seen towards the end. In some cases a scanty morbiliform or papular rash is seen scattered over different parts of the body including the mucous membrane, on the second or third day of illness. These spots may turn into petechial or echymotic areas which may later undergo necrosis. Emaciation is a late feature. The abdomen is retracted and the abdominal muscles are taut. The urinary bladder may be distended. Liver and spleen are not palpable. The heart sounds remain essentially normal, but pericardial friction sound may rarely be audible. There is no significant abnormality in respiratory sounds except when secondary infection sets in. Herpes labialis is of common occurrence.

In infants the anterior fontanelle may bulge, indicating intracranial hypertension. But this sign may not be prominent in the presence of dehydration as a result of vomiting. Obvious signs of hydrocephalus may appear gradually if the disease becomes chronic. Neck stiffness is an important sign. This is caused by spasm of the neck muscles as a result of stretching of the inflamed nerves supplying them. Similar spasm of the trunk muscle may cause arching of the back leading to opisthotonos. The stretching of the nerves supplying the hamstring muscles is responsible for Kernig's and Brudzinski's signs.

Kernig's sign is the strong resistance felt during an attempt to extend the knee with the thigh flexed at right angle at the hip. Brudzinski's sign consists of flexion of both the lower limbs during bending of the head forward and flexion of one lower limb when Kernig's sign is elicited on the other.

An internal squint may appear early as a result of overstretching and inflammation of the 6th cranial nerve from intracranial hypertension. The oculomotor, facial and cochlear nerves are also sometimes affected, resulting in temporary loss of functions. There may be bilateral dilatation of the pupils or they may be unequal. The light reflex may be sluggish or absent on one or both sides. The ocular fundi generally show little abnormality though mild papilloedema may occasionally be present. In chronic stage, however, optic atrophy may occur, resulting in blindness. The tendon jerks are sluggish or absent and the plantar reflex, though generally flexor, may be unilaterally or bilaterally extensor.

## DIAGNOSIS

The best way to diagnose meningitis is to collect a clean sample of CSF for physical, chemical and bacteriological examination (see Table 7.1).For this a lumber or cistern puncture is obligatory. It must, however, be remembered that in a partially treated case the CSF picture may be confusing, as the cell count may be comparatively low with the predominance of lymphocytes and the organisms may not be demonstrable. In pyogenic meningitis a smear examination is generally more helpful in demonstrating the organisms than culture which is frequently sterile.

In the peripheral blood there is a polymorphonuclear leucocytosis. Blood culture is not positive except in bacteraemic stage, but the organisms can be isolated from the petichial spots in the skin.

There may be mild albuminuria and transient glycosuria with hyperglycaemia. The glycosuria is a non-specific effect of raised intraventricular pressure on the hypothalamus.

*Meningococcal meningitis* is to be differentiated from the following clinical conditions:

1) *Other forms of pyogenic meningitis*—The nature of the primary lesions and their bacteriological identity help in the diagnosis. However, there is no substantial difference in the line of treatment of the different types of pyogenic meningitis.

2) *Tuberculous meningitis*—The onset is much more insidious and the temperature is comparatively low. Study of the CSF is the most helpful way to differentiate. But there may be confusion in partially treated cases of meningococcal meningitis. Radiological evidence of an active primary lesion and miliary tuberculosis in the lungs and presence of choroidal tubercles in the eyes are strongly presumptive of tuberculous meningitis. The peripheral blood count is normal.

3) *Aseptic meningitis*—It is of less acute and much shorter course. Neurological deficits are rare and permanent disabilities do not occur. Cerebrospinal fluid picture is distinctive and peripheral blood count is within normal limits.

4) *Encephalitis*—Sign of meningial irritation is not prominent, but involvement of the parenchyma of the nervous system is more in evidence in the form of coma and nerve deficits. The CSF picture is much unlike the different forms of meningitis.

5) *Cerebral type of falciparum malaria*—The acute onset of fever with headache, delirium, confusion and convulsion may simulate pyogenic meningitis. A palpable spleen, presence of malaria parasite in the peripheral blood and a normal CSF picture help in the correct diagnosis.

6) *Primary subarachnoid haemorrhage*—Abrupt onset with severe headache, ptosis and squint and without total loss of consciousness is the common mode of presentation. The temperature is generally normal. A frankly haemorrhagic CSF with xanthochromia of the supernatent fluid on standing, is diagnostic.

7) *Meningism*—This condition is often associated with some systemic infections like typhoid fever, pneumonia and acute tonsillitis in children. Such febrile illnesses when accompanied with neck stiffness may be confused with meningitis. But detection of the primary disease and a normal CSF picture should easily point to correct diagnosis.

## COMPLICATIONS AND SEQUELAE

If pyogenic meningitis is diagnosed early and treated properly complications will rarely arise. However, some possible complications require particular mention.

1) *Hydrocephalus*—If early and effective treatment is not instituted or if the treatment is inadequate the condition may pass into a chronic stage and the organising exudate may block the circulation of the CSF as has been explained. The resulting hydrocephalus can be easily detected in infants and children. But in adults separation of sutures does not occur and the diagnosis is not so apparent. Its possibility should be considered if the signs of intracranial hypertension persist.

2) *Neurological complications*—Paralysis of 3rd, 6th and 7th cranial nerves is somewhat common in the early course of the disease, but complete recovery is the rule when properly treated. The recovery may, however, be only partial in untreated or partially treated cases. Irreversible optic atrophy may be responsible for permanent blindness in neglected cases and destruction of the cochlear nerve may render the patient patially or completely deaf. Peripheral neuropathy is generally not a serious problem.

Rarely parts of the brain may be damaged. In such cases hemiplegia, monoplegia, aphasia and impairment of intellectual functions may occur. But recovery is the usual rule.

3) *Pyogenic arthritis of multiple joints* can be a rare complication. This may be overlooked in acute stage of meningitis, but becomes evident during convalescence.

4) *Secondary infections,* especially of the respiratory tract, was a common complication in the past, but is rare at present, thanks to antibiotics.

5) *Bedsore* may develop if proper nursing care is not ensured. Emaciation, urinary incontinence and gangrene of the echymotic areas are contributory factors.

6) *Waterhouse*—Friderichsen syndrome is manifested by sudden collapse and severe prostration with cyanosis and extensive haemorrhage in the skin and mucous membrane.

## COURSE AND PROGNOSIS

While some fulminant cases may die within a short time before there is enough opportunity for diagnosis and treatment, the common sporadic cases are amenable to treatment and the mortality now stands at 5 to 10 per cent in well-equipped hospitals. The death rate is the highest among the infants and children and also among the elderly. Hyperpyrexia is often a terminal event.

The fever usually subsides and the patient recovers generally without any residual defects within three weeks. In some cases, however, minor residual disabilities are seen. Major neurological deficits are very rare. If recovery does not occur in this period or if there is relapse of symptoms after initial improvement, the condition may pass into a chronic stage. Hydrocephalus and opisthotonos develop, sometimes with other neurological deficits. Subdural effusion which may occur in small children may resolve with repeated aspiration.

## TREATMENT

While the need for general nursing care cannot be too strongly emphasised, specific treatment must be instituted without loss of time. Where facilities exist, the patient should be admitted to an infectious diseases hospital or infectious diseases ward of a general hospital. The patient should be laid on a soft comfortable bed in a dark quiet room with feeding ensured through a naso-gastric tube if the patient is unable to take feeds through mouth. Attention to the oral hygiene, pressure points, bladder and bowels must be thorough and the patient should be turned sides frequently.

Sulphonamide is still the drug of choice in the treatment of meningococcal meningits. Sulphadimidine or sulphadiazine may be given in an initial dose of 4 gm followed by 1 gm every four hours till the temperature settles to normal and the toxaemia abates. It may then be continued in a dose of 0.5 gm every four hours for 4 or 5 days more. Average duration of the course is seven days. When the patient is unable to swallow, the tablets may be crushed and given with feeds through the naso-gastric tube. If this is not possible or if the patient be vomiting 5% solution of sodium salt of sulphadiazine may be given i.v. in a dose of 2 gm repeated every 12 hours, till oral administration is possible. Though the injectable preparation of sulphonamide can be used intramuscularly, its strong alkalinity may cause severe pain and muscle necrosis. It must never be used intrathecally. A child below 3 years of age should be given 3 gm per day in divided doses 4 hourly and after 2 to 3 days dose should be reduced to 2 gm per day.

The use of a penicillin with sulphonamides should be obligatory in view of the emergence of sulphonamide resistant strains in increasing number. Though the blood brain-barrier against penicillin is high, the drug can reach adequate concentration in CSF through the inflamed meninges. It can be given intramuscularly in four divided doses of 5 million units each, in 24 hours, or intravenously with dextrose or isotonic sodium chloride solutions in a dose of 10 million units in 24 hours. Intrathecal injection of 10,000 units is justified after the diagnostic lumbar puncture if the fluid appears turbid. Repeated lumbar puncture is not desirable.

Other antibiotics like chloramphenicol and ampicillin can be used in H. influenzae meningitis, but are seldom necessary in meningococcal meningitis. Principles of antibiotic therapy have been discussed in a separate chapter.

Symptomatic treatment like analgesics and infusion of 20% mannitol solution for headache, injection of diazepam 10 mg or phenobarbitone 60 mg for repeated convulsions, i.v. fluid therapy for dehydration etc. must be instituted as required. Care should be taken to prevent complications. Nonetheless some of them are often unavoidable. Those which may occur should be detected and treated promptly. Corticosteroids are not indicated except in Waterhouse-Friderichsen syndrome.

# TUBERCULOUS MENINGITIS

*S. N. Sengupta*

## AETIOLOGY

Tuberculous meningitis is much more common among children and young adults than among the elderly. During the process of development of primary tuberculosis blood stream dissemination occurs in distant organs, including the brain. Metastatic sub-pial cortical foci may form and extend to involve the meninges either directly or on reactivation after the lapse of many years of latency, or there may be direct dissemination in the meninges as in acute miliary tuberculosis.

## PATHOLOGY

As a result of tuberculous infection of the meninges a yellowish gelatinous exudate forms round the base of the brain and it spreads along the blood vessels in the sulci. Seedlings of small tubercules may be seen scattered in the meninges. The fibrin rich exudate produces early adhesion between the layers of meninges and may entangle the cranial and spinal nerves. The blood vessels may also be constricted and this together with an endarteritic change may cause occlusion of some of the arteries at the base of the brain, leading to cerebral infraction. Meningeal adhesions leading to occlusion of interventricular and ventriculo-cisternal communication of the CSF pathway may lead to hydrocephalus. Histologically the picture of tubercle is easily recognisable, though giant cells are inconspicuous.

## CLINICAL PICTURE

The onset is insidious. Generally the child becomes listless and apathetic and complains of headache, vomiting, anorexia and constipation. Convulsion is rare and the temperature is not generally high, though in some cases it may be 38°C or above. This condition may persist for 2 or 3 weeks and, if not recognised early, the patient becomes drowsy, confused and delirious. Signs of meningeal irritation, raised intracranial tension and nerve deficits gradually appear. There may be diplopia, squint and 7th and 8th cranial nerve palsy. The pupils may be dilated. Papilloedema is not uncommon and detection of choroidal tubercles is diagnostic. Monoplegia and hemiplegia may occur in a few cases. Neck stiffness is often marked, but Kernig's and Babinski's signs may not be always positive. The jerks may be sluggish or absent and the plantar reflex may be flexor or extensor.

### TABLE : 7.1

**Laboratory Investigations**

| Cerebrospinal fluid | Pyogenic meningitis | Tuberculous meningitis | Aseptic meningitis | Encephalitis |
|---|---|---|---|---|

| | | | | |
|---|---|---|---|---|
| Pressure | High | High | High | Slightly raised or normal |
| Colour | Yellowish or greenish | Colourless | Colourless | Colourless |
| Transparency | Turbid | Clear or faintly hazy | Clear | Clear |
| Coagulum | Absent | Fine coagulum may form | Absent | Absent |
| Protein | 100-400 mg% | 100 mg% or less | $>500$ mg% | $<100$ mg% |
| Sugar | Very low | Low $<50$ mg% | Normal | Normal or slightly raised |
| Chloride | Low | Low | Normal | Normal |
| Cytology | High polymorphonuclear pleocytosis. May be 1000 per mm$^3$ | Predominantly lymphocytic pleocytosis, rarely exceeding 500 per mm$^3$ | Predominantly mononuclear, pleocytosis may be 100-1000 per mm$^3$ | Count normal or slight mononuclear pleocytosis, rarely exceeding 200 per mm$^3$ |
| Organisms | Demonstrable by gram stain of the deposit | Acid fast bacilli may be demonstrated by Ziehl Neelsen stain of clot or deposit | Not demonstrable in stained smear | Not demonstrable in stained smear |
| | Culture may be positive | Ordinary culture negative. Guineapig inoculation and culture in Lowenstein-Jensen medium may help in isolating tubercle bacilli | Culture negative in ordinary media | Culture negative in ordinary media |
| Blood Count | High polymorphonuclear leucocytosis | Normal leucocyte count | Normal leucocyte count | Normal to moderately raised leucocyte count |
| Blood Culture | Culture may be positive in septicaemic stage | Culture negative | Culture negative | Culture negative |
| Serology | Serological tests required | No useful serological test | Rising antibody titre in paired sera very helpful in diagnosis but time-consuming | Rising antibody titre in paired sera very helpful but time-consuming |

## DIAGNOSIS

Tuberculous meningitis is to be distinguished from other diseases with features of infection and intracranial hypertension with or without neurological deficits (*see* pyogenic meningitis). The difficulty in diagnosis is experienced particularly in infants and small children who cannot give a history and who may develop meningism with fever convulsion and squint in diseases like pneumonia, typhoid fever, tonsillitis etc. These diseases should be carefully excluded. The CSF picture is the most distinctive diagnostic charter (table). The fluid is clear or faintly hazy but a fine flocculent coagulum may form in it on standing. If acid fast bacilli are not demonstrable in the smear of the coagulum or in the centrifugalised deposit, guineapig inoculation and culture for tubercle bacilli are advisable. However, it should be remembered that these investigations are time-consuming and that the treatment can never be deferred till the diagnosis is confirmed by bacterial culture. The leucocyte count of the peripheral blood is normal. A radiograph of the chest may demonstrate active primary lesion or miliary tuberculosis and tuberculin test may be positive in children.

## COMPLICATIONS

The neurological complications are similar to those of pyogenic meningitis but the chances are greater, because the disease may remain unrecognised in the initial stage and effective treatment may be delayed.

## COURSE AND PROGNOSIS

Early recognition and proper treatment ensure complete recovery. In neglected or partially treated cases the patient may be crippled with different neurological complications, chronic hydrocephalus and epilepsy. Ultimate death is almost inevitable in such cases and in untreated cases.

## TREATMENT

The general treatment consists of proper nursing and feeding as has been mentioned under pyogenic meningitis. As soon as a reasonable diagnosis is made from clinical examination and the laboratory findings of the CSF specific antituberculous treatment must be instituted immediately without waiting for the report of the culture. The usual treatment with streptomycin, rifampicin, INAH, PAS, thiacetazone and the other available drugs in suitable combinations should be used and continued for a total period of at least 18 months. It must be emphasised that three drugs should be used at the onset and be continued till culture and sensitivity report of the organisms CSF is available. Subsequently two drugs may be continued for a minimum of 18 months.

Streptomycin 25-50 mg or INAH 25-50 mg diluted with 10 ml of sterile water may be injected intrathecally daily for a week or two in addition to systemic antituberculous treatment. Intrathecal treatment is usually recommended in seriously ill patients and in these cases systemic corticosteroids also should be used (*vide* Chapter on Tuberculosis).

Corticosteroids are sometimes helpful in reducing toxaemia and in preventing complications resulting from plastic exudate. It also gives a sense of well-being. Prednisolone can be given orally in a dose of 40 mg daily. When there is evidence of subarachnoid block, like fall in CSF tension and rise in its protein content, hydrocortisone hemisuccinate 50 mg may be given intrathecally daily for a period of a week.

# VIRUS MENINGITIS

## AETIOLOGY

In the advanced countries, with the effective control of most of the pyogenic and tuberculous infections the predominant infection of the meninges occurs due to the viruses. Non-bacterial meningitis of viral, spirochaetal and fungal origin is termed as aseptic meningitis. But since the spirochaetal and fungal meningitis are extremely rare the term has almost come to be synonymous with virus meningitis.

All age groups except the elderly are susceptible. Aseptic meningitis generally occurs sporadically, but sometimes small epidemics may occur. Some known viruses may primarily be responsible for meningitis or meningoencephalitis, like the viruses of infectious mononucleosis, lymphocytic choriomeningitis, mumps, coxsackie, ECHO, herpes simplex etc. But in many cases a virus has not been demonstrated.

## PATHOLOGY

There is congestion and infiltration of the meninges with mononuclear cells, although in early stage plenty of polymorphonuclear cells may be seen. The underlying parenchyma of the brain may also show signs of inflammation in some cases. The CSF is increased in amount. There is no adhesion between the layers of the meninges and damage of the nerves does not generally occur.

## CLINICAL PICTURE

The disease starts usually, but not invariably with fever, headache and bodyache. Drowsiness, confusion, stupor etc. may occur, but are not generally very prominent features. Convulsions may rarely occur in children. There may be diplopia, squint and mild papilloedema, but significant neurological abnormality is rare. Neck stiffness is present, though Kernig's and Brudzinski's signs are generally absent. The jerks are sluggish or absent and the plantar response is variable.

## DIAGNOSIS

Though the clinical picture is not characteristic, the CSF findings are sufficiently diagnostic of aseptic meningitis. The ordinary culture of the CSF is negative and only an elaborate and time-consuming series of investigations in a well-equipped virus laboratory can give a positive diagnosis. In infectious mononucleosis the peripheral blood picture together with the other systemic manifestations of the disease is of great diagnostic importance. In other cases also specific clinical features of the particular virus infection should be carefully looked for.

## COURSE AND PROGNOSIS

Complete recovery within a couple of weeks without any residual effects is the rule. But in the presence of associated encephalitis or myelitis neurological deficits may occur.

## TREATMENT

Since there is no specific drug effective against these viruses the treatment of virus meningitis consists essentially of general management and symptomatic treatment as in other forms of meningitis.

# ENCEPHALITIS

*S. N. Sengupta*

Encephalitis means an inflammation of the brain. When the brain is primarily inflamed it is reasonable to expect that the covering meninges may also be inflamed secondarily. While in most of the cases of meningoencephalitis the cause of the inflammation is direct infection, in many other clinically indistinguishable conditions the abnormalities in the brain are due to some toxins. The latter conditions are regarded as encephalopathy rather than encephalitis.

Infective and non-infective diseases causing inflammation, congestion, oedema and degenerative lesions of the brain can be acute, subacute or chronic in nature.

## A. ACUTE ENCEPHALOPATHY AND ENCEPHALITIS

### 1.TOXIC ENCEPHALOPATHY

The brain and the meninges may be affected by bacterial or metabolic toxins in the course of some severe systemic infection elsewhere or some metabolic crisis. Although there may not be much pathological changes except, perhaps, diffuse congestion and oedema of the brain and meninges, there may be considerable functional disturbances. Confusion, delirium, stupor, coma and convulsion are common features. Since it is always a secondary condition the primary disease invites serious attention.

### 2. ACUTE ENCEPHALITIS

In the matter of diffuse infection of the brain tissue the bacteria do not usually play a significant role, though localised bacterial infection may produce brain abscesses. Parasites like plasmodium falciparum, toxoplasma gondii etc. may sometimes affect the brain. Spirochaetal and fungal infections are extremely rare causes of encephalitis. The principal agents responsible for primary infection of the brain are the viruses. Many of them have been identified, but many still remain anonymous. Detection of inclusion bodies in the neurones and glial cells, as in acute inclusion body encephalitis, suggests a virus aetiology. Herpes simplex virus has been isolated from such cases, though this may not be the only virus causing such lesions. Even when a positive proof of the presence of a virus is not forthcoming the eliminaton of the other possible infections and circumstantial evidences strongly point towards a virus as the culprit. This also applies to encephalitis lethergica. The status of benign myalgic encephalomyelitis is not very clear. Its epidemic nature, febrile onset, neurological involvement etc., all point to a virus aetiology although no virus has been demonstrated.

### 3. ACUTE DISSEMINATED ENCEPHALOMYELITIS AND ACUTE NECROTISING HAEMORRHAGIC ENCEPHALOMYELITIS

These are acute inflammatory and degenerative lesions which occur probably as an immunological reaction to some virus infection. The close association between this type of neuropathology and some antecedent virus infection or inoculation of smallpox or anti-rabies vaccine suggests a causal relationship with the virus though no virus has been demonstrated in the lesion itself.

## B. SUBACUTE ENCEPHALITIS

### SUBACUTE INCLUSION BODY ENCEPHALITIS AND SUBACUTE SCLEROSING PANENCEPHALITIS

This is a group of diseases with a protracted pathological course which is a slow degeneration and gliosis of the parenchymal tissue of the nervous system, sometimes without conspicuous inflammatory reaction. Subacute inclusion body encephalitis, which belongs to this group and in which eosinophilic inclusion bodies have been demonstrated in the cytoplasm and the nucleus of the nerve cells, is undoubtedly due to the measles virus. But some other viruses may also be responsible.

## C. CHRONIC 'SLOW VIRUS' ENCEPHALITIS

Certain acute and subacute forms of encephalitis are followed by a slow degeneration and gliosis of the nerve parenchyma over many years. The demonstration of inclusion bodies in some of these cases and the similarity of the degenerative process with that seen in scrapie which is a proved virus disease among the sheep suggest that there is a slow degenerative form of virus encephalitis. These conditions have been grouped as 'slow virus encephalitis'.

It must be admitted that the existing knowledge of virus diseases of the nervous system is far from satisfactory. It permits a concept that virus encephalitis may start as an acute inflammatory process or a subacute inflammatory degenerative process, both of which may ultimately proceed to a slow degeneration and sclerosis of the nerve parenchyma over many years though many of them may recover with or without minor damage. The role and behaviour of an individual virus in the matter of the type of lesion it may produce is not very clear. In many cases a virus has not even been identified and the assumption of a virus as being responsible is supported only by indirect evidences.

## ACUTE ENCEPHALITIS

As explained the unqualified term of acute encephalitis means acute virus encephalitis.

### AETIOLOGY

Certain well-recognised types of encephalitis are prevalent in different parts of the world. Many viruses have been identified as their causative agents, like those of Russian Spring-Summer, Murray Valley, West Nile, Japanese B encephalitis etc. Many other viruses are still to be identified. Sometimes the viruses which normally produce systemic diseases elsewhere or different other neurological diseases may produce encephalitis, e.g., mumps, measles, herpes simplex, poliomyelitis etc. The prevalence of Japanese encephalitis (J.E.) has been recognised from time to time in South India since 1952. It was in 1973 that the first authenticated epidemic occurred in West Bengal. Since then periodic epidemics have occurred in several parts of North India.

Japanese encephalitis occurs predominantly in children in those places where the disease is normally prevalent. But all ages are equally susceptible in places where the virus is newly introduced. This is because subclinical infection in an affected community provides immunity to the adult population and protects them from further infection. In virus diseases there are a large number of subclinical infections for each clinical case. It has been stated that in case of J.E. for each clinical case there are 500-1000 subclinical cases who develop immunity without suffering from manifest disease. People of lowest economic strata are particularly vulnerable and the incidence is more common in males.

Japanese encephalitis virus is a group B, ARBO-virus (arthropod-borne virus) and is transmitted by mosquitoes. Pigs and some birds are the main amplifiers or living hosts in whom the virus multiplies freely without producing manifest disease. The mosquitoes maintain a transmission cycle among the animals and birds and man is only an incidental victim.

The mosquito vector of J.E. belongs to the culex family 'C vishnuii complex' comprising of C vishnuii, C pseudovishnuii and C tritaeniorrhyncus and is recognised as the principal group. Though the virus has been detected in some other species and some anophiline mosquitoes, their capacity for transmission has not yet been fully assessed. The mosquitoes of 'C vishnuii complex' are rice field breeders. Epidemics of J.E. reported from different parts of India have occurred during the rains which is the season for rice cultivation.

## PATHOLOGY

Except for some specific types, the morbid anatomy of acute infection of the nervous system conforms to a given pattern. There is congestion and oedema of the brain and sometimes of the spinal cord. The overlying meninges is also inflamed in most cases. There is cellular infiltration, initially with polymorphonuclear and latter with mononuclear cells. Perivascular cuffing is seen inside the brain substance. Many parenchymal cells undergo degeneration and disappear. These changes may be most marked in the cerebral or cerebellar cortex or in the basal ganglia according to the type of the disease. Proliferation of the microglial cells occurs for the repair of the damaged areas.

## CLINICAL PICTURE

The clinical picture of the different types of acute encephalitis follows more or less the same pattern. Japanese encephalitis is the most prevalent type in India and is clinically well studied.

The disease starts with sudden onset of fever, headache and often bodyache. There may be vomiting and convulsion, especially in children. Drowsiness, confusion and delirium may soon set in and later there may be stupor and coma.

The temperature generally varies between 37.5°C and 39°C, though hyperpyrexia may occur, generally as a terminal event. The convulsion may be generalised or focal in type. Bizarre types of movements of the limbs and side to side rolling movement of the head are often seen in the acute stage. Neck stiffness is common, but Kernig's sign is less frequently positive. Pupillary size and light reaction are generally normal, but may be different on the two sides. Ocular fundi are generally normal though papilloedema may rarely occur. There may be signs of paralysis of 3rd, 6th and 7th cranial nerves. Monoplegia, hemiplegia and diplegia may occur, but are not very common. The jerks are generally sluggish or absent and the plantar reflex is either extensor or flexor on one or both sides.

The acute febrile stage usually lasts for a week or ten days, but sometimes a low grade fever may persist or recurrent bouts of fever may occur for several weeks.

## DIAGNOSIS

It is not difficult to suspect encephalitis on clinical ground, but examination of blood and CSF gives a more clear picture. Encephalitis is to be differentiated from meningitis and other toxic febrile illness with neurological involvement (*see* under pyogenic meningitis). It should be noted that neither tl peripheral blood picture nor the CSF picture singly helps in arriving at a diagnosis. Both taken togeth along with the clinical manifestations, however, are of considerable importance in eliminating the oth possibilities and lead to an indirect diagnosis. The peripheral blood may show mild to moderat leucocytosis with some relative increase in neutrophils. The CSF tension may or may not be increased. It clear. Some rise in protein content is common but sugar and chloride remain normal. In a few cases of J.E sugar may be slightly increased. There is some mononuclear pleocytosis which rarely exceeds 250 per $mm^3$.

For a specific diagnosis elaborate virological investigations are necessary. In India facilities for such studies are available at the National Institute of Virology, Pune, and certain other regional laboratories like the Calcutta School of Tropical Medicine. Isolation of the virus from the blood and CSF is the surest method of diagnosis, but is hardly ever successful. But brain biopsy with a Vim-Silverman needle introduced through the nostril and ethmoid bone is a practical possibility. Post-mortem diagnosis by this method is always possible and should be attempted virus during an epidemic. The material thus collected can be processed for culture or demonstration of the virus by fluorescent antibody technique and a good bite may also help in the histopathological study. However, the investigation generally done is the search for specific antibodies and their rising titre in paired samples of serum drawn in the acute and convalescent states with an interval of 7 to 10 days between them. It should be remembered that there is cross-immunity among some of the ARBO-viruses and that the serological studies are too time-consuming to be of any practical help during the acute phase of the disease.

## COURSE AND PROGNOSIS

The death rate has been between 40% and 60% in epidemics reported from different parts of the world. The patient generally dies in a week or ten days. Hyperpyrexia and pulmonary oedema are the common terminal events. The mortality is higher in the non-endemic areas than in the endemic areas and is higher among the elderly than among children. In the survivors the disease may follow a protracted course often with progressive emaciation and bedsores. Even after the return of consciousness noticeable changes are evident in the patient's personality and emotional behaviour. An akynetic mutism and loss of initiative is often striking. Involuntary movements like athetosis and tremor may persist. Parkinsonism and cerebellar ataxia may also occur. Residual paralysis of cranial and spinal nerves, monoplegia and hemiplegia are not very common.

## TREATMENT

Since there is no specific treatment against most of the viruses the treatment of encephalitis consists essentially of general care and symptomatic treatment as well as prevention and treatment of complications.

The patient should be provided with a soft dry and comfortable bed. Proper attention should be given to the bladder and bowels and soiled bed lines should be replaced promptly. If the patient is unconscious he should be nursed semiprone with the foot-end slightly raised and the sides should be turned frequently. Proper feeding should be ensured through a nasogastric tube if oral feeding is not possible.

Analgesics may be used for headache and convulsions should be controlled with phenobarbitone or diazepam. If there is evidence of raised intracranial pressure, infusion of 20% mannitol is helpful, but repeated lumbar puncture should be avoided. Antibiotics have no role to play except in the presence of secondary bacterial infection. Corticosteroids are of little benefit.

During convalescence the patient should be given adequate diet with supplements of vitamins. Physiotherapy and proper measures for psychological rehabilitation should be arranged for those who remain physically and mentally handicapped.

## ENCEPHALITIS LETHERGICA

The acute form of encephalitis lethergica occurred as pandemic during the First World War but is not seen at present, though some of the cases of Parkinson's syndrome may be the sequel of encephalitis lethergica which may have occurred many years back.

The acute stage of encephalitis lethergica conforms to the general clinical pattern of other forms of acute encephalitis, except that severe asthenia, reversal of sleep rhythm and oculogyric crisis are the notable features. A virus has never been isolated. The sugar content of CSF is generally raised. Parkinson's syndrome may be a 'slow virus' effect.

## ACUTE BENIGN MYALGIC ENCEPHALOMYELITIS

This disease occurs in epidemics and females are more affected than males. The pathology is unknown, as no autopsy report is available. Clinically, the disease is characterised by low temperature, severe bodyache, widespread paralysis, emotional liability and insomnia with altered sleep rhythm. The paralysis of the cranial and spinal nerves is generally partial and may be accompanied with sensory disturbance. The muscle tone is increased and the jerks are brisk, though the plantar reflex is flexor. Recovery is generally complete, but may take a long time. Parkinson's syndrome or persistent athetoid movements may be rare sequelae.

# TETANUS

*T. P. Mukherjee*

### DEFINITION

It is an acute infectious disease clinically characterised by lockjaw, general muscular rigidity with or without convulsive seizures.

### AETIOLOGY

Causative organism—Clostridium tetani (cl. tetani) is an obligatory anaerobe, which produces two powerful exotoxins; one of these known as tetanospasmin, a neurotoxin, is responsible for manifestations of the disease but the other called tetanolysin, which is a haemolysin, has very little clinical significance.

### PATHOGENESIS

Tetanus spores remain localised at the site of injury but under suitable conditions they germinate producing bacilli. The bacterial exotoxin reaches the C.N.S. through perineural lymphatic sheath. From there it spreads to the central nervous system.

It is further observed that these exotoxins chiefly affect the motor nerves. But while analysing the clinical aspect of the patients, it is observed that some symptoms like constriction of pupils, salivation and lacrimation could not be explained without involvement of autonomic nervous system (A.N.S.). Therefore, it is presumed that Cl. tetani might have some action on A.N.S., in addition to motor nerve endings or anterior horn cells.

## CLINICAL FEATURES

Formerly the tetanus was divided into two types:

a) Localised tetanus

b) Generalised tetanus

But as a matter of fact the localised tetanus is also a manifestation of generalised tetanus. Lastly, the author has observed a few cases of cephalic tetanus, which may be a variety of local tetanus.

**Incubation period:** Two to fifty-six days.

**Prodromal symptoms** are characterised by vague symptoms like malaise etc. but the only early diagnostic point is heaviness of the limbs proximal to the injury.

**Stage of rigidity** is first proclaimed by lock-jaw. Lock-jaw is painless contraction of the masseter group of muscles. This can be better shown with the help of a tongue spatula known as "spatula test" (discovered and practised at the Infectious Diseases Hospital, Calcutta).

**Spatula test:** With the help of spatula we try to negotiate inside the mouth, giving a sudden jerk at lower jaw or touch the posterior pharyngeal wall. If it is a case of tetanus, latent or obvious, there will be a bitting of the spatula and it will be difficult to negotiate it out.

Rigidity of all the skeletal muscles of the trunk is usual but peculiarly sparing the limbs. There is cardboard-like rigidity of the trunk muscles. There may be neck rigidity.

**Convulsive seizures:** Over the rigid condition of the body the patient will have convulsive seizures due to contraction of antagonist and protagonist group of muscles, clinically characterised by extension of the four limbs, dorsiflexion of the feet and bending of neck either to one side or back side. Froth may or may not accumulate. Later on patients may get rid of convulsions but rigidity will be there or sometimes convulsions may go on repeatedly (status form). In this stage the patient may develop apnoea; the author has observed sudden death occurring from this type of convulsions. The patient however retains consciousness till the time of death.

**Stage of rigidity:**

**Risus sardonicus:** All the muscles of face supplied by the motor branch of facial nerve remain in tonically contracted condition, clinically characterised by peculiar appearance of the face. constricted pupillary orifice, oral orifice, contracted muscles of forehead known Satan's facies or risus sardonicus. Due to tonic contraction of the muscles of the back, which is more powerful than the muscles of the front of torso, peculiar shape of the patient occurs known as opisthotonus or pleurosthotonus.

## DIFFERENTIAL DIAGNOSIS

Clinical features of tetanus are so obvious that it does not require differential diagnosis. However, symptom-wise if neck rigidity be the presenting feature, meningitis or meningoencephalitis will come into differential diagnosis for which lumbar puncture is to be done.

If lockjaw is the presenting feature, conditions like impacted tooth, tonsillitis, suppurative parotitis, will come into differential diagnosis. If convulsion is the presenting feature, hysteria, epilepsy, strychnine poisoning will come into differential diagnosis but in tetanus muscles of the patient will remain tonicially contracted all the time, in contrast to other cases.

## PROGNOSIS

Onset time—It is the time taken by an individual to develop convulsive seizures over and above rigid condition of the body. It is divided into 3 groups.

| | |
|---|---|
| Very severe | Within 72 hours |
| Severe | 72 hours-6 days |
| Moderately severe | 6 days-12 days |

Nowadays prognosis of the patient entirely depends on the onset time. Formerly the following points were considered:

(i) Age of the patient
(ii) Weight
(iii) Site of injury
(iv) Nature of injury
(v) General nutrition of the patient

## TREATMENT

(i) It is observed that if anyhow the patient can remain alive for 10 days, the patient will usually survive.

(ii) In autopsy cases of tetanus, it is observed that there is no tissue change in a patient dying from tetanus except congestion of viscera and local septic area through which infection entered.

(iii) Statistical data show that the maximum number of deaths occur within 10 days. Keeping these points in view modern treatment has been designed which if properly done will reduce mortality to minimum.

Treatment consists of complete anaesthetisation of the patient, to perform a tracheostomy, to give oxygen through positive pressure apparatus, to maintain electrolyte balance and to feed the patient through gastrostomy tube. If this can be achieved and the patient kept alive for 10 days chances of recovery are almost certain.

## TETANUS NEONATORUM

Due to its high mortality rate, neonates have snatched a separate name. It occurs within 12-28 days of the birth of the baby; clinically it is characterised by peculiar grimacing of the face, inability to suck, lock-jaw and convulsive seizures characterised by extension of the four limbs, dorsiflexion of the feet, clinching hands, opisthotonus and pleurosthotonus. It may go on continuing and the baby may pass to stage of status epilepticus.

## PROGNOSIS

Very bad, but if properly taken care of, prognosis may be good.

Patient requires intensive care and respiratory support as in the case of adult tetanus.

(a) General treatment—

Careful expert nursing is a *must*. The patient should be kept from all sorts of external stimuli as far as practicable. Unnecessary medical manoeuvre is avoided.

(b) **Specific treatment—**

It is further observed that when a tetanus develops the exotoxin has already become fixed to anterior horn cells. Hence antiserum will have little specific effect. Two types of antiserum are available.

Antiserum is derived from human source known as T.I.G., the prophylactic dose is 300 I.U., half life period is 21 days. Now it is available in India but too costly for mass use.

ATS derived from animal sources is of two types. One type is prepared from horse, the other from sheep. Preventive dose is 3000 I.U.; curative 20,000 I.U. irrespective of age. Serum is to be given after skin test. Positive reactors are to be given by rapid desensitisation method.

**Serum reaction:** It is known as acute anaphylactic shock clinically characterised by profound shock, cyanosis, bronchospasm etc. and should be tackled immediately with adrenaline, parenteral steroids and intravenous fluids etc.

Delayed serum reaction is characterised by urticaria, skin rash, scleritis, fever, joint pain etc. and can be treated with antithistaminics, aspirin and steroids.

**Antibiotics**—Cl. tetani is sensitive to all types of antibiotics, but we generally recommend benzyl penicillin 5 lacs units I.M. daily for 7 days to prevent super infection.

Ganglion blocking agents and muscle relaxants like curare preparations are used but it has got a drawback of falling back of tongue. Expert respiratory support with positive pressure respirator should be available. In the absence of these, cocktail of anticonvulsants has been used, e.g., mephenesine hydrochloride (mynesin), diazepam and chlorpromazine hydrochloride. Mephenesine hydrochloride, however, has been abandoned by the manufacturers.

**Hyperbaric oxygen** has been used in some cases. It is found to be superior but requires elaborate apparatus. Tracheostomy has been practised as a routine in some centres. It claims a little better result.

**Steroids** are contraindicated in infectious diseases but can be carefully used as a life-saving measure in special circumstances.

## PREVENTION

Majority of the cases follow street accidents. But in our country we have noted special groups of tetanus, following abortion, (spontaneous or induced), puerperium and even following menstruation. Hence prevention and mass education will be more important in our country. In antenatal clinic mother should be given at least 2 doses of toxoid before childbirth. In school health programme, ample care should be taken to detect and treat otitis media cases. To adults proper hygienic care should be taught.

Deep and lacerated wounds should be particularly treated by proper surgical toilet carefully. All street accidents are dangerous. Soil contamination needs careful management. Triple antigen should be given to all children. In developing countries all children do not yet have facilities to go to school. Hence health centres should do this job through health workers at village level.

# DIPHTHERIA

*P. K. Talukdar*

## INTRODUCTION

An acute infectious disease caused by Coryne bacterium diphtheriae (Klebs-Loffler bacillus) which produces membranous exudate on the fauces, pharynx, larynx, and rarely in nasal mucosa, genitalia and open wounds. Infection causes constitutional symptoms, e.g., fever, malaise and toxaemia and sometimes serious circulatory failure.

**Incubation period: Two to six days.**

In developed countries the disease is now rarely reported but still occurs in developing countries and mass immunisation is yet to be perfect.

As the disease is now becoming future doctors are likely to miss it or diagnose it in late stage. Early diagnosis is vital for recovery.

**Type of organism:**

C. diphtheriae may occur in three strains, e.g., gravis, intermediate and mitis types, in order of virulence.

Most commonly diphtheria affects the upper respiratory tract, i.e., tonsillar areas, pharyngeal mucosa, larynx and nasal mucous membrane.

Rarely it may occur elsewhere, e.g., tongue, oesophagus, ocular conjunctiva, ears, cutaneous wounds, valva, vagina and penis.

Hence these are clinicially recognised as follows.

1. **Tonsillar type**—Most common.
2. **Pharyngeal type**—Most dangerous as toxins are quickly absorbed in this site.
3. **Laryngeal type**—Causes acute respiratory distress and requires urgent tracheostomy.
4. **Nasal type**—Mild symptoms but mucopurulant discharge with bleeding may occur.
5. **Extra-respiratory tract types**—Have already been mentioned which are mild indolent affections.

## PATHOLOGY

Local mucous membrane becomes acutely inflamed at the site of leison.

There is outpouring of exudate which coagulates to form the classical false membrane containing fibrin, leucocytes, red blood cells and desquamated epithelium. In the inflamed area KLB multiplies and produces exotoxin, which is absorbed to produce toxic effects in distant tissues and organs.

The membrane so produced can be stripped off by a pair of forceps, baring raw areas which may bleed.

The toxin is particularly neurotoxic, as also causes degenerative changes in myocardium, liver, kidneys cervical glands and even skeletal muscles; peripheral circulatory failure is due to toxic capillary damage, bronchopneumonia and segmental collapse of lungs are also possible associated changes.

## CLINICAL PRESENTATION

Prevalent in infancy and early childhood, rarely an older child or even an adult may be affected. Very young infants have protection by transferred immunity from the mother, provided the mother was properly immunised.

Sore throat and salivation are the initial markers of the disease. Fever is not very marked. Examination of the throat reveals pearl-white patch on the tonsils and the fauces, may extend to the palate and the pillars of the tonsils. The cervical glands are enlarged. In severe cases along with the hugely enlarged glands there may be associated subcutaneous oedema which gives the patient the so-called bull-neck appearance. General condition of the patient may be very low because of toxaemia and cardiac involvement. The blood pressure falls. Pulse is weak and feeble at times with irregularity due to arrhythmia. Lower motor neurone type of paralysis may involve any muscles, particularly eye, neck and limb muscles. Involvement of eye muscles may cause squint and loss of accommodation. Cardiac and voluntary muscular involvements are reversible but may be so severe as to threaten life. Secondary infection producing bronchopneumonia may complicate the picture.

List of various complications is shown in Table 7.2.

LIST OF COMPLICATIONS

TABLE 7.2

a) **Peripheral circulatory failure—(1st week):**
Low BP cold and clammy extremities, rapid thready pulse.

b) **Myocarditis—(2nd week):**
Tachycardia, arrhythmias and heart block may occur, ECG changes are obvious showing type arrhythmias, grades of heart block, and ST-T changes.

c) **Neurological complications:**

i) **Palatal palsy—(3rd week):**
Nasal regurgitation with nasal twang in voice.

ii) **Ocular muscle palsy—(3rd to 5th week):**
Blurred vision paralysis of accommodation ptosis or squint.

iii) **Facial palsy—(5th to 6th week):**
Usually unilateral but rarely both sides.

iv) **Cervical and trunk muscles:**
Inability to balance the head.

v) **Bulbar centre—(7th week):**

Causes serious complications, e.g., paralysis of pharyngeal muscles, laryngeal muscles, diaphragm, vagus nerve and respiratory paralysis.

vi) **Limb muscles—(7th to 9th week):**

Weakness due to lower motor neurone paralysis (note muscular wasting).

Diagnosis of faucial diphtheria can be made on clinical grounds. Nasal diphtheria has typical serosanguinous nasal discharge with little constitutional symptom and has to be differentiated from foreign body and congenital syphilis.

Though serum therapy is important patients should be given penicillin in high doses, e.g., one mega units 4-6 hourly. Erythromycin can be used if patient is allergic to penicillin.

## DIAGNOSIS

Though the diagnosis is to be confirmed by swab test from the lesion by smear and culture of organisms, yet clinical diagnosis is essential.

On clinical grounds alone, serum (ADS) should be given, and throat swabs should be sent to the laboratory. Therapeutic test is also an indirect proof of the disease.

The appearance of diphtheritic membrane is typical. It is soft, yellowish or greyish and appears membrane-like. It cannot be wiped out by a swab but has to pinched out with forceps as it is very adherent.

A rapid swab test or gram staining will show Chinese letter-like disposition of organisms under microscope. Culture also confirms it.

## TREATMENT

Antidiphtheretic serum (ADS) in adequate doses will only counteract the circulating toxin but has no effect on the fixed toxin in the tissues. ADS is to be given in a single dosage 10,000 to 100,000 units intramuscularly or in severe cases intravenously after a proper test dose to detect sensitivity; usually dosage is 8000 units for mild cases while 16,000 to 32,000 units for moderate cases. Immediate treatment is essential for severe or late cases with large dose .In case of any allergic reaction inject 0.5 ml of 1 in 1000 **dilution of adrenaline and hydrocortisone.** The serum should be given then in diluted form with gradually increasing concentration and amount till the total dose has been introduced, closely observing the patient for any sensitivity reaction and treating that accordingly. In severe cases with cardiac complications steroids can be used. Laryngeal diphtheria with obstruction needs urgent **tracheostomy** with bigger doses of serum and steroid. Respiratory paralysis needs mechanical ventilatory support.

# WHOOPING COUGH
(Syn : Pertussis)

*P. K. Talukdar*

## INTRODUCTION

Whooping cough is a highly infectious disease spread by droplet infection, caused by haemophilus pertussis bacillus. The classical clinical picture is characterised by spasmodic cough followed by typical whoop. H. pertussis are gram-negative, non-motile ovoid bacilli, frequently taking bipolar staining.

## EPIDEMIOLOGY

It is a global disease, especially affecting children, but becomes rare in adolescence. Infection spreads via contacts, fomites and droplet infection.
Incubation period—Three to twenty-one days.

The disease has three typical stages. In the pre-whoop stage there are signs of upper respiratory tract catarrh, mild fever and cough. In a typical spasm of coughing bout, the child goes on coughing incessantly until almost exhausted. The face gets congested even cyanosed, eyes protrude and in desperate effort to breath in, the typical whoop may be produced. Any interference, even emotional upsets, may precipitate a spasm. The paroxysm often ends up in vomiting or bleeding from the nose. Subconjunctival haemorrhage may occur. In severe cases there may be convulsions, due to central anoxia or from intracranial haemorrhage. In between spasms there may be little or no abnormal findings in the system. This paroxysmal stage may vary a lot but usually lasts for 3 to 4 weeks, then the frequency of cough diminishes, general condition improves and the child goes into convalescent stage. He may take weeks before being totally normal and during this stage relapse may also occur.

## COMPLICATIONS

**Haemorrhages :** Subconjunctival, epistaxis and haemoptysis are quite common. Whooping cough is perhaps the commonest cause of haemoptysis in children.
**Pulmonary complication:** Pneumothorax, mediastinal and subcutaneous emplysema may be quite serious as to cause death. Secondary bacterial infection causes bronchopneumonia which may end up in bronchiectasis. Activation of arrested primary complex to progressive primary tuberculosis may sometimes occur.
**Encephalopathy:** Whether this is due to actual bacterial invasion or due to anoxic damage or haemorrhagic encephalitis, is not exactly known.

## DIAGNOSIS

In the catarrhal stage it may be difficult to diagnose but typical paroxysms of cough proclaim the diagnosis.

Tracheobronchitis, primary tuberculosis with enlarged hilar glands irritate the air tubes and respiratory involvement in mucoviscidosis may simulate whooping cough spasm.

## TREATMENT

Antibiotics particularly chloramphenicol may be helpful, if used in the catarrhal stage, but by the time the spasm is established antibiotics have little role to play.

Skilled nursing care is most important during spasm and for prevention of frequent spasm. Here sedation definitely plays a good role. Severe cases may require nursing in hospital in oxygen tent.

Syrup codeine is recommended. Antihistaminic syrups may be used sparingly, especially at night.

Complications, e.g., bronchopneumonia may be severe in small children and infants; this should be treated vigorously with appropriate antibiotics, depending on the secondary invaders involved.

Vomiting may be really troublesome and hence i.v. nourishment may occasionally be required.

Encephalitis may very rarely lead to post-encephalitic mental retardation, convulsions and chorioathetosis. These should be symptomatically treated.

Prevention by active immunisation in time must be ensured. Strict isolation of the cases avoiding contact with non-immunised kids should be tried.

# BACTERIAL FOOD POISONING

*G. C. Mookerjee*

Food poisoning can be caused by taking eatables contaminated with bacteria, bacterial toxins or chemical poisons. The following types of poisoning may be encountered:

(1) **Salmonella Food Poisoning:**

Due to salmonella group of organisms such as S. typhimurium and S. enteritidis. Occasionally other forms of salmonella may be encountered.

(2) **Staphylococcal Food Poisoning:**

Usually staphylococci contaminate the foodstuff and multiply in it, producing exotoxins which actually causes gastroenteritis.

(3) **Botulism:**

The term 'botulus' actually means sausage. The poisoning is due to eating food contaminated by exotoxins of clostridium botulinum. The sources usually are infected food in which these spore-bearing anaerobic organisms grow and produce exotoxins. Tinned food is often a rich source. Rancid taste and odour are often a pointer but this toxin is thermolabile and hence easily destroyed by heat but staphylococcal toxin is relatively thermostable.

(4) **Chemical Food Poisoning:**

Chemical poisoning is usually due to suicidal or homicidal purposes rarely accidental. Arsenic, mercury, antimony and copper salts cause dangerous poisoning. Details about chemical poisoning are discussed in a separate chapter.

Gastro-enteritis due to cholera may also be mistaken for food-poisoning and it must be admitted that cholera is also transmitted via eatables and contaminated water. Ice cream and sweets are often common causes.

## CLINICAL FEATURES

Food poisoning is suspected whenever there is a sudden onset of vomiting and diarrhoea with abdominal pain. In cholera however, abdominal pain is lacking and the stool is rice water in colour. In staphylococcal food poisoning the incubation period is very short and the symptoms start within 3 to 4 hours. In salmonella food poisoning it may be a few hours that salmonella may be transmitted through milk of infected animals and via under boiled or raw eggs. Cattle, sheep, dogs, cats and horses, may be carriers. The clostridial food poisoning occurs due to injection of infected poultry or meat products. Botulism is often traceable to sausages or meat products.

## DIAGNOSIS

All cases of gastro-enteritis have to be differentiated but it must be remembered that usually food poisoning can be suspected when more than one member of the family or a group sharing the same food are affected. However, several people eating the same food from the same container may not be equally affected because some portion of the food may be harbouring more toxin than the remaining portion. Therefore it is a great health problem for medical officers to investigate any occurence of food poisoning so that the source can be traced out. Food poisoning commonly occurs in community eating, hotels, melas, army camps, camping in a strange and new environment or in religious congregations where community eating is a common practice.

### Treatment :

Prophylaxis is the best treatment which means good hygienic measures and avoidance of food sold in open areas and where there is fly menace.

## CLINICAL TREATMENT

In most cases the supportive treatment to control dehydration and collapse is essential. Mild cases of dehydration may be treated oral fluids too; in severe cases intravenous fluids should be given. Initially it is normal saline followed by glucose saline and glucose as indicated. Details of fluids and electrolyte therapy have been discussed in a seperate chapter. Antibiotics and anti-bacterial drugs have practically no role to play excepting in case of salmonella infection. In salmonella food poisoning the combination of streptomycin and chloromycetin should be given. Most cases will require 0.5 gm of chloramphenicol I.M, 12 hourly as oral administration is futile due to vomiting. When the patient is able to take by mouth, oral therapy can be resumed.

# RICKETTSIAL DISEASES

**(Rickettsial fever, the Rickettsiosis)**

## INTRODUCTION

The term Rickettsia was introduced to honour the name of Dr. H. T. Ricketts, who was the pioneer investigator to establish the cause of epidemic typhus fever and rocky mountain spotted fever (RMSF) but unfortunately he died due to the same disease. Rickettsias are organisms which form a group between virus and bacteria. They usually exist in coccoid or rhomboid form. They are gram-negative organisms and can infect most animals including man. Rickettsial infections are transmitted via various arthropods such as louse, mite, flea and tick. It is on this basis that the rickettsial infections are termed as:

i) Louse borne typhus fever,
ii) Mite borne typhus fever,
iii) Flea borne typhus fever, and
iv) Tick borne typhus fever.

## LOUSE BORNE TYPHUS FEVER

(Epidemic typhus)

This is an acute infectious fever due to R. Prowazeki. It is transmitted by human louse known as pedicellus humanus. Therefore, it does not cause infection to other animals. Both humans corporeal (body louse) and louse commonly humanus capitis (head louse) are vectors. Bad hygienic living condition is therefore the predisposing factor.

## CLINICAL FEATURES

The clinical feature is characterised by sudden rise of temperature with chill and rigor associated with musculoskeletal pain and restlessness. Usually there is a prodromal phase of milder symptoms often resembling skeletal pain and restlessness. Usually there is a prodromal phase of milder systems often resembling flu. With the onset of high temperature around 39° to 40° the patient becomes mentally confused with a cloudy mental state. The term "typhus" meaning cloud is therefore justified. Usually on the 5th day rose spot-like macular rash appears and these change into papules or even purpuric rash. Sometimes subcutaneous mottling may be noted.

Patients therefore look acutely ill with fever, toxaemia and may even become comatose. The clinical picture resembles typhoid fever during its 2nd or 3rd week. Blood pressure may fall, with toxaemia, rapid pulse and oliguria. Complications include bronchopneumonia, myocarditis and nephritis leading to renal failure. Sometimes hematemesis, melaena or haematuria may occur.

## PATHOLOGY

The chief pathological feature is damage to the endothelium of small blood vessels by the organism. It may occur anywhere in the body, especially heart muscle, skeletal muscle, liver, spleen, skin and brain. Clumps of round cells and mononuclear macrophages form around the damaged capillaries associated with local thrombosis haemorrhage.

## DIAGNOSIS

The disease may have to be differentiated from other types of typhus fevers, typhoid fever, exanthematous fevers as well as meningitis. The ideal laboratory tests, however, are not possible to do everywhere as these require highly specialised laboratory facilities. Guineapig inoculation test (Neill-Mooser) reaction may be useful. Agglutination tests are also of some value. Complement fixation tests using rickettsial extracts are also quite specific.

## LABORATORY DIAGNOSIS

Commonly Weil-Felix reactions are carried out though it is to some extent non-specific. Rising titre of 1/160 or greater is strongly suggestive (Table 7.3).

| | OX19 | OXK | OX2 |
|---|---|---|---|
| Louse & Flea borne | +++ | Negative | + |
| Mite borne | Negative | +++ | Negative |
| Tick borne | ++/- | + | +++ |

TABLE 7.3 : Weil-Felix reaction in serum of typhus fevers

## TREATMENT

Chloramphenicol is the drug of choice although oxytetracylines are also quite effective. Any one of these may be prescribed with a loading dose of 50 mg per kg of body weight followed by 0.5 gm six hourly for 2 to 3 days. The temperature should come down to normal within three days and then the dose may be reduced for further 3 to 4 days. Occasionally there is relapse when further therapy may be required. In severe cases, corticosteroids may be added for a few days.

In addition, supportive therapy as in the case of typhoid fever will be necessary.

It is also essential to disinfect the patients and their clothes properly.

# MITE BORNE TYPHUS

## INTRODUCTION

This has several names such as Tsutsugamushi fever, scrub typhus and Japanese river fever; this type of typhus fever is due to R. orientatis and was discovered in the Far East areas. This type of typhus fever occurs in the case of wild animals, generally rodents.

The infection is transmitted by mites, commonly 6-legged trombicula. The larval mites have their first and the last blood meal of their lives during which they suck the organisms to become infected. The female trombicula passes the organisms into their ovaries and finally to the human host during their only feed.

## PATHOLOGY

The pathological changes are similar to louse borne typhus infection but the lesions are less extensive and clinical picture is usually not so serious.

## CLINICAL FEATURES

Incubation period is from 6 to 18 days.

The disease resembles epidemic typhus but less severe in its form and usually settles down within 10 to 14 days. However, mortality may be high in the untreated cases. The clinical diagnosis can be easily made due to presence of a small necrotic ulcer with a black scab indicating the site at which the bite of the mite took place. Regional lymph nodes are inflamed. The macular rash also occurs during the later part of the first week.

## LABORATORY DIAGNOSIS

Weil-Felix reaction is again commonly carried out although it is not highly reliable. Other tests also mentioned are more specific.

## TREATMENT

It is similar as in case of louse borne typhus but no de-lousing is necessary.

# TICK BORNE TYPHUS

## INTRODUCTION

It is a disease of wild animals but man is involved when accidentally tick bite takes place. The disease is not common in this part of the world, but is found in rocky mountains of North America, South America, Africa and North Australia. It is also known as rocky mountain spotted fever when it is due to R. rickettsiae. There is another variety which occurs in African coast due to R. conori.

## PATHOLOGICAL AND CLINICAL FEATURES

Pathological and clinical features are not much different from other variety and diagnosis is made as in the case of other typhus fevers.

The treatment is also carried out on similar lines.

# FLEA BORNE TYPHUS

(Syn: Murine typhus; Rat typhus)

## INTRODUCTION

This variety of typhus fever is caused by R. Mooseri which is transmitted from infected rats through rat-fleas known as xenopsylla cheopis. Human infection may occur by inhalation of dusts infected with faeces of infected rats, lice or fleas. Urine of rats may also contain the organism, thus food may be infected.

## DIAGNOSIS

Clinical features are similar to other varieties but the disease runs a milder course. Method of diagnosis and treatment are similar to louse borne typhus fever.

## TREATMENT

Similar to louse borne typhus.

# QUERY FEVER
(Syn: Q-Fever)

The disease is due to Rickettsia burneti (coxiella burneti). Chiefly disease of wild or sometimes large domestic animals. Tick bite conveys the infection but human infection may also occur by inhalation of contaminated dust, or ingesting milk, infected urine contaminating food. Laboratory workers and animal handlers, and butchers may be affected.

## CLINICAL FEATURES

Fever 39° C to 41° C with respiratory symptoms and toxaemia are usual presenting features. Pulse is slow, occasional rash may be seen. Fever may continue over 7 to 10 days up to 2 weeks and haemoptysis may occur. X-rayed chest shows patchy ground glass areas of opacities in both lung fields, more marked in bases and midzones.

Complications include hepatitis, endocarditis, myocarditis and encephalitis.

## TREATMENT

Chloramphenicol or tetracyclines as in the case of typhus fevers.

# RELAPSING FEVERS

*G. C. Mookerjee*

Three are two types of relapsing fevers (RF):

a) **Louse borne:** Transmitted by human body lice (Pediculus humanus). The organism is a spirochaete, Borrelia recurrentis.
b) **Tick borne:** Transmitted by ticks is also a spirochaete, Borrelia duttoni.

Bad hygienic condition, refugee camps and famine usually favour outbreaks. Louse borne R.F. is internationally quarantinable.

## CLINICAL FEATURES

The special features of these two diseases are as follows:

| Louse borne R.F. | Tick borne R.F. |
|---|---|
| Incubation period two to twelve days.<br>High fever with profound toxaemia, myalgic pain, rigor, nausea and vomiting.<br>Macular eruption all over or petechae may occur.<br>Fever may settle after 5 to 10 days, then relapses after an afebrile period of 5 to 15 days.<br>Rarely there is a third relapse.<br>Iritis, facial palsy, and paraplegia may occur. | Usually occurs as sporadic disease in Mediterranean zones, Central Asia, some parts of U.S.A., Africa and North India.<br>The clinical features initially are similar to louse borne RF but febrile paroxysms are of shorter duration while relapses are more up to five or six times.<br>Tendency to haemorrhage is greater. |

## DIAGNOSIS

Organisms can be seen in stained blood films if collected during paroxysms. Giemsa, Leishman or D.G. examination should be made.

Animal inoculation also confirms.

## TREATMENT

Tetracyclines and chloramphenicol are both effective in all types of typhus fevers. Therefore tetracyclines should be the drug of choice in most cases. Dose—500 mg four times daily for first three days, subsequently 250 mg four times daily for another three to five days. In severe cases parenteral route may be necessary.

Symptomatic and supportive treatment is similar to any acute febrile condition.

# RAT-BITE FEVERS

*G. C. Mookerjee*

## INTRODUCTION

Rat bite fevers are due to spirillus minus or actinobacillus muris (streptobacillus monilliformis) through rodents or mammals.

## CLINICAL FEATURES

The disease is caused due to accidental bite by an infected animal. It is followed by local inflammatory reaction, regional adenitis within two to ten days of the bite. There are some clinical differences between the two types of infection as follows.

| Sp. Minus | Act. Muris |
|---|---|
| Onset abrupt with high fever and shivering. | Fever not so regular bouts of relapsing cycles but is usually intermittent. |
| Local lymphangitis with ulcer at the bite. Fever subsides in 3 to 4 days but bouts of relapses occur every 3 to 7 days. Several cycles may occur. | Arthritis involving several large joints as feature. |

In both there are skin rashes with fever; liver and spleen may also enlarge.

## DIAGNOSIS

Blood film is rarely positive. Organisms may be demonstrated from local ulcer juice. The fluid should be stained with Leishman, Giemsa or examined under D.G. illumination.

Animal inoculation (mice) is ideal method to confirm.

## TREATMENT

Inj. penicillin in doses of one to two mega units daily for two or three days rapidly controls the infection.

Inj. streptomycin 1.0 g daily for 10 days may be given, if penicillin cannot given.

# BRUCELLOSIS

(Syn:Undulent fever; Abortus fever; Malta fever.)

*G. C. Mookerjee*

## INTRODUCTION

Brucellosis is primarily a disease which affects the cattle. The humans are also affected by drinking milk which is not adequately pasteurized. In this country it is not so common as milk is usually boiled. Cheese is also a very probable source. The cows and goats are the common sources and the animals are most infective soon after delivery and for succeeding weeks. The organisms are found in the udder and milk is contaminated as long as the infection of udder persists.

## PATHOLOGY

The brucellosis species causing infection consists of Br. abortus, Br. malitensis, and Br. suis. Br. malitensis usually affects goats and Br. suis infects pigs. The organisms affect these cells, especially the RE cells, and get widely disseminated affecting various organs. Because the organisms thrive intracellularly high doses of antibiotics may be required to destroy the organisms. Possibly the immune mechanism is more important in controlling the infection.

## CLINICAL PICTURE

The clinical picture depends on whether the person is a non-immune individual, in which case there will be constitutional symptoms such as high fever, headache, rigor, severe muscle pain, profuse sweating and great weakness. Initially this may be confused with an episode of influenza but when the temperature continues the possibility of brucellosis should be thought of. Temperature may continue for weeks and months and there may be periods of remission in between.

On the other hand, brucellosis among farm workers and veterinary surgeons may sometimes take a mild course and in many persons the disease may pass off as minor illness. Antibodies, however, will be present in the blood even a few years after the initial infection. In acute stage of infection spleen becomes usually enlarged and other organs such as heart and liver may become affected. There may be evidence of osteitis, arthritis and even osteomyelitis. Mild jaundice may be present. Long-standing cases may show narrowing of intravertebral spaces in the spine, which can be mistaken for spinal tuberculosis.

## DIAGNOSIS

Diagnosis of the brucellosis may sometimes be difficult when the patient runs low-grade temperature without much serious joint pains. Blood culture is not always positive because the cultures are often done in later stages. Commonly, brucella agglutination tests are carried out and rising titre is highly suggestive. However, farm workers and contacts may show positive serology even without active disease. Special tests include Coomb's test and complement fixation test.

Intradermal brucellin skin test is another way of establishing the diagnosis in patients suffering from active disease.

## DIFFERENTIAL DIAGNOSIS

All causes of prolonged pyrexia will have to be considered in the differential diagnosis particularly tuberculosis, kala-azar, chronic malaria, rheumatic fever and rheumatoid type of arthritis.

## TREATMENT

A combination of tetracycline 0.5 gm, six hourly by oral route for three to four weeks along with inj. streptomycin 1 gm daily for the same period should be given.

Co-trimoxazole in doses of 1 gm twice a day or even in double doses have been used in certain cases for six to eight weeks. However, there is risk of bone marrow depression when Co-trimoxazole is used in such high doses for long periods. However, it is claimed that these changes can be normalised by folic acid administrations.

# LESS COMMON BACTERIAL INFECTIONS

*G. C. Mookerjee*

## LISTERIOSIS

L. monocytogenes is a gram positive, nonsporing, motile organism easily confused with diptheroids. It usually affects animals but contacts of animals may sometimes be affected. Intrauterine and perinatal infections have been recorded. Septicaemia, meningitis and oculo-glandular infection may occur.

These infections are amenable to tetracyclines and chloramphenicol therapy, usually recommended for ten days.

## BERTONELLOSIS

(Syn: Oroya fever; Carrion's disease & Verruga peruana)

This infection is due to Bartonella bacilliformis which is transmitted by female phlebotomus (sand-fly). The disease is limited to Andes, Columbia, Ecuador and Peru, i.e., in the continent of South America.

It is a small gram negative organism which causes toxic fever and anaemia as well as a distinct skin condition known as verrucs peruana, producing haemangiomatus formation in the skin.

The organisms invade red cells and RE cells. Haemolysis causes anaemia; involvement of RE cells results in hepatosplenomegaly and lymphadenopathy.

### TREATMENT

No antibacterial agents are known to be specific for Bartonellosis but associated super-infection with salmonella group of organisms is really cause of mortality.

This should be treated early with chloramphenicol. Combat anaemia with blood transfusion. Otherwise treatment is symptomatic.

## GLANDERS

It is an infectious disease due to Gram-negative organism, pfeifferella mallei or actinobacillus mallei. Usually it affects horse, mules and asses but cattle are immune. Human infection is rarely obtained from nasal discharges and pus from cutaneous sores.

### CLINICAL FEATURES

There are two forms, acute and chronic, distinguished as follows :

| Acute Glanders | Chronic Glanders |
|---|---|
| Incubation period—Four to eight days.<br>Onset sudden with fever, nasal discharge with necrotic ulcers in nose and eruptions may occur with pustule formation.<br>Multiple abscesses may form. | Incubation period up to ten days.<br>Multiple abscesses and ulcers may form associated with mucopurulent nasal discharge. |
| Bronchitis, pneumonitis and septicaemia may occur.<br>Typhoid-like picture with high mortality may occur. | Spreading ulcers, recurrent abscess and lymphangitis proclaim chronicity. But sometimes acute exacerbation may occur after apparent cure. |

## DIAGNOSIS

Organisms are demonstrable in discharges, seen in smear preparations and culture. Sometimes blood culture is positive. Intraperitoneal injection in guineapigs causes suppurative orchitis and peritonitis.

Mallein skin test is used to determine infected animals.

## TREATMENT

Chloramphenicol and tetracyclines are both effective in both acute and chronic forms.

# MELIOIDOSIS

It is also a disease of animals due to pseudomonas pseudomallei which affects horses and rarely stable-workers.

The disease occurs in the Far East, Africa and Australia.

It also has an acute or chronic form. Acute type is characterised by fever, toxaemia, pneumonitis, hepatosplenomegaly and dysentery. X-ray chest may be mistaken for tuberculosis.

Chronic form is characterised by multiple abscess formation in subcutaneous tissues.

## DIAGNOSIS

Blood culture, sputum culture and pus from abscess will reveal the organisms.

## TREATMENT

Tetracyclines or carbenicillin very useful. Abscess should be drained.

## TULARAEMIA

This is an infectious disease caused by yersinia tularensis and is transmitted to birds and mammals by blood sucking flies and ticks through bites. Humans may be accidentally infected, usually by infected animal source.

The disease occurs in U.S.A., Europe, U.S.S.R. and is also reported from Japan.

### CLINICAL FEATURES

Incubation period : One to ten days.

High fever, toxaemia, lymphadenitis and hepatosplenomegaly may occur. Focal suppuration is noted in multiple organs. Cutaneous, conjunctival and oral lesions may also occur. The fever continues up to three or four weeks. Lymph glands remain for longer periods.

### DIAGNOSIS

Organisms may be recovered by blood culture or guinea-pig inoculation.

Intradermal test is also done by using killed tularensis vaccine.

### TREATMENT

Tetracyclines are effective or inj. streptomycin 1.0 g daily I.M. for a week may also be given.

## AMOEBIASIS

*G. C. Mookerjee*

### INTRODUCTION

Amoebiasis means invasion of entamoeba histolytica (E.H.) of the large intestine with or without clinical manifestations. E.H. can remain in the large gut for days and weeks without invading the mucosa of the gut; therefore this stage may be called amoebic infection. When however invasion causes colitis and ulcer formation in the gut it should be called amoebic disease or colonic amoebiasis. The disease can be divided into intestinal and extraintestinal amoebiasis. The colonic amoebiasis includes acute amoebic dysentery, subacute or chronic amoebic dysentery, amoebic typhilitis and colonic amoeboma and colonic amoebiasis with extra-colonic complications. Extraintestinal amoebiasis involves liver, lungs, pericardium, brain, spleen, skin etc.

### AETIOLOGY

E.H. is a unicellular organism belonging to the animal phyllus protozoa and class sarcodina. The parasite has trophozoite and cystic forms. The trophozoite is the invasive form and it contains erythrocytes, food particles etc. Its shape is not fixed because of its constantly changing position and its size averages between 25 and 50$\mu$. The cyst, the non-invasive form, measures between 10 and 15$\mu$ and does not contain erythrocytes and food particles. (see Fig. 7.1). There are a few other forms of amoeba which are nonpathogenic.

## EPIDEMIOLOGY

Man is the selective host. Houseflies and sometimes cockroaches are the vectors, and faecal contamination of food and drink is the cause of the disease. The infection is known to occur in every part of the world but it occurs more commonly where there are poor environmental sanitation, lack of sanitary awakening among the people and bad customs.

A man acquires the infection by ingestion of the cysts. Excystation occurs in the lower part of the small intestine and the upper part of the large intestine and each viable cyst liberates a 4-nucleated amoeba which subsequently splits into single nucleated entamoeba. The trophozoites live in the mucous and submucous layers of the large intestine and multiply by simple binary fission. Excystation occurs in the lumen of the intestine and the cysts are passed in faeces and they contaminate food and drink.

## PATHOLOGY

After excystation the trophozoites enter through the crypts of Leiberkhun in the large intestine and penetrate directly through the columnar epithelium of the mucous membrane. They then burrow their way deeper to reach the submucosa where the amoebae rapidly multiply and destroy the tissues undermining the mucous membrane above, resulting in coagulative necrosis and the formation of small pea-sized abscesses strictly confined to the large intestine and they may involve the whole length of it, as far down as the internal anal sphincter or they may be localised so as to involve the ileocaecal region and sigmoidorectal region. The ulcers have characteristic ragged and undermined edges. Into the depth, the abscess is larger than the opening into mucosal surface, giving flask-shaped anatomy. Several mucosal ulcers may ultimately coalesce to form larger areas of ulcers covered with sloughs but in between mucosa has normal appearance.

Healing occurs by fibrosis. Strictures do not form as these ulcers tend to spread along the long axis and not around the large gut.

Amoebic granuloma may form (rare nowadays due to effective therapy) in any part of large intestines but usually in caecum, sigmoid and flexures are involved. These masses are granulation tissues and may cause signs of obstruction and may be mistaken for carcinoma.

Sometimes the trophozoites of E.H. are carried as emboli by the radicles of the portal vein from the base of an amoebic ulcer in the large gut, causing obstruction to the circulation and produce thrombosis of portal venules resulting in necrosis of the surrounding liver cells. The centre of necrotic material liquefies later and a fairly big-sized abscess is formed by coalescence of the several abscesses. Typically amoebic abscess is usually a large single abscess, may be as large as a pingpong to a cricket ball. Sometimes more than one abscess may be present. Amoebic abscess may be very chronic and long standing with thick abscess wall.

Hepatic abscess may rupture in pleural cavity, lungs, pericardium and peritoneal sac. It may also disseminate to brain causing brain abscess. Genital or cutaneous involvement is rare.

## MANIFESTATIONS

The incubation period is generally one or two weeks but in case of massive infection it may be shorter. The onset is usually insidious.

*In acute amoebic dysentery* several motions, copious in amount, may occur in a day with grumbling pain and tenesmus in the abdomen. The stools are loose and of offensive odour and many mucus-rich stools are passed, sometimes with streaks of blood. Fever, if at all present, is only of low grade type. Fishy odour is characteristic. On palpation tenderness is present along the line of the colon which is marked over caecum and pelvic colon. The "amoebic point", as described by Sir Philip Manson Bahr, in the left iliac fossa may show maximum tenderness thus mimicking appendicitis.

Acute amoebic dysentery may sometimes be quite severe and mixed amoebic and bacillary infections may also occur. Careful inspection and microscopic examination of stool should settle the diagnosis.

*In subacute or chronic* cases the number of motions is less frequent and they are manifested as indigestion, flatulence, abdominal pain which subside only to recur at invervals for months or years, if not properly treated. These people are also cyst passers and spread the infection. Amoebic diarrhoea may occur without much systemic manifestations. There may be bouts of bowel upsets, associated with flatulence, indigestion and chronic ill health. Sometimes one or two large semiformed stools are passed with mucus without any obvious dysenteric character. Abdominal gripes and colics occur off and on, especially after dietary indiscretion.

*In hepatic amoebiasis* pain and tenderness in the right hypochondrium are the earliest manifestations, the pain being sometimes referred to the right shoulder due to irritation of the phrenic nerve which supplies the undersurface of the diaphragm. A slight rise of temperature or a low remittent temperature, later becoming hectic in character may be present.

On examination the lower border of the liver is palpable below the costal margin and is tender. Liver dullness may extend upwards. A right-sided pleural effusion may occasionally be present due to collapse of the lung caused by growing liver abscess.

Intercostal fullness and tenderness is often a definite pointer.

Heavy percussion over the chest wall over hepatic area causes severe discomfort. As commonly amoebic abscesses occur in the right lobe of the liver, deep tenderness on percussion is a very reliable sign but congestive heart failure should be excluded. Jaundice may rarely be present due to intrahepatic obstruction close to porta hepatis by large abscess. It is rare.

*Pulmonary amoebiasis* may present as right-sided pneumonitis, lung abscess, pleural effusion or empyema thoracis.

*Cerebral amoebiasis* presents as space-occupying lesion with signs of focal neurological deficit, while ruptures of such abscess may cause fulminant meningitis.

*Splenic abscess* is found in association with hepatic abscess and cutaneous amoebiasis may present as extensive area of necrosis and sloughing adjoining the visceral lesions.

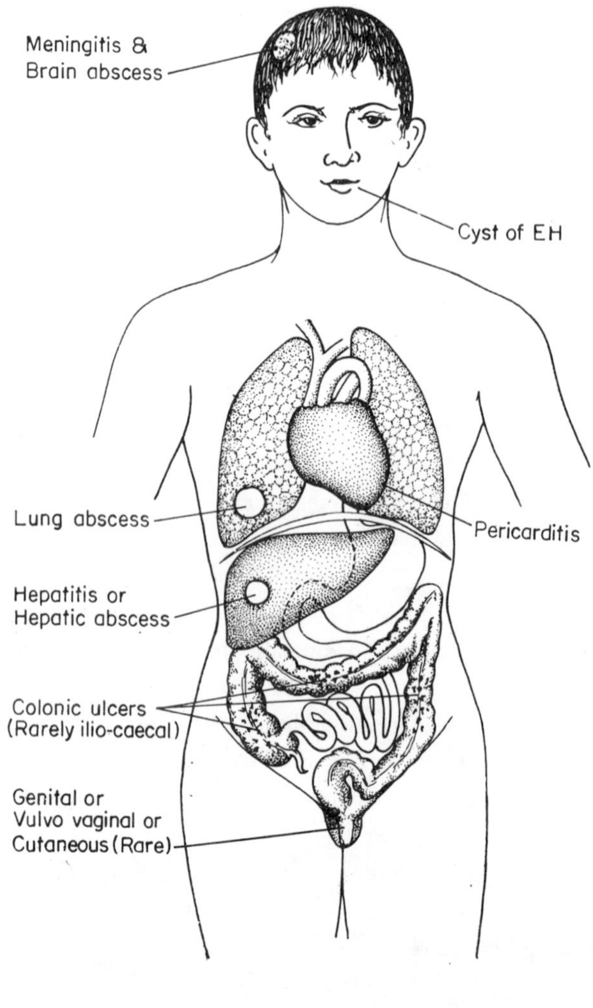


Fig. 7.1 Complications of Amoebic Dysentery

## DIAGNOSIS

Attempts should be made to demonstrate E.H. in the material obtained from any particular lesion, such as stool, 'pus' of liver abscess and sputum.

*Symptomatic group*—Cases of acute amoebic dysentery.

Inspection and microscopic examination of stool reveal trophozoites of E.H. reddish-yellow erythrocytes in clumps, scanty pus cells and sometimes Charcot-Leyden crystals.

Examination of blood may show moderate leucocytosis, though it is not the rule.

*Asymptomatic group*—Cyst passers or cyst-carriers will show presence of E.H. cysts.

Repeated examination of stool is sometimes necessary to demonstrate E.H. cysts by microscopical examination of a formed stool; samples of stool may be examined by concentration method or stool obtained after a saline cathartic may be positive. Rectal swab through a proctoscope or samples obtained through a sigmoidoscope are often useful. I have many times obtained positive result in stool by obtaining a small sample of faeces through P.R. examination with gloved fingers followed by microscopic examination.

*Serological test*—This is an indirect method and not very useful, as it can be positive when active infection is not present.

*Hepatic amoebiasis*—Diagnostic aspiration is done to demonstrate typical pus known as anchovy sauce pus, although it may not always be so. Yellowish and greenish pus is also obtained.

*Examination of blood*—Acute liver abscess will show polymorphonuclear leucocytosis but long-standing cases may not show any rise.

*Intradermal test*—In an infected individual injection of 0.1 ml of an antigen prepared from cultures of E.H. produces at the site of injection an erythema which manifests after 3 hours, reaching a maximum (9-10 cm. in diameter) after 20-24 hours and disappearing in another 24-48 hours.

*Radiological examination*—The right dome of the diaphragm is usually found to be elevated at a higher level. Sometimes there may be tenting of the diaphragm (signifying basal pleurisy).

*Liver-scan*—This is the most dependable and non-invasive test for locating a liver abscess. A radio-isotope, e.g., $I^{132}$ Rose Bengal may be used for scanning and the area is scanned by Gamma camera. Ultrasonic technique is also equally good but both these techniques are expensive.

## PROGNOSIS

Intestinal amoebiasis usually responds well to appropriate drugs. But visceral amoebiasis may be accompanied by mortality, when diagnosis is made too late.

## TREATMENT

### Intestinal Amoebiasis

*Acute attacks*—Metronidazole 400 mg. thrice daily orally for 7 days or Tinidazole 300-600 mg. twice daily orally for 7 days or combination of metronidazole and diloxanide furoate can be given. Tetracycline or oxytetracycline 250 mg. four times daily for 7 days is to be combined with one of the above drugs so as to break the vicious cycle of 'amoeba-bacteria' symbiosis. In severe amoebic dysentery dose of metronidazole may be increased to 800 mg. three times daily.

Emetine is nowadays avoided due to its toxic effects. However, dehydroemetine is less toxic and efficient. Adequate fluids and electrolytes and vitamins should be given.

*Chronic cases*—Metronidazole 400 mg. twice daily orally or combination of two drugs is sometimes necessary, e.g., metronidazole and diloxanide furoate or metronidazole and di-iodoquinoline group of drugs. A list of anti-amoebic drugs is given in Table 7.4.

### Extra Intestinal Amoebiasis

Oral treatment as for acute amoebic dysentery, along with broad spectrum antibiotic is recommended. I.V. metronidazole is now available and may be used in severe cases.

Alternatively dehydroemetine or chloroquine can be used. Emetine is more toxic than dehydroemetine but both these drugs, though effective anti-amoebic agents, should be avoided in cardiac patients. Even when it is used, ECG check and follow-up is advisable.

### Amoebic Liver Abscess

In addition to intensive antiamoebic therapy, surgical drainage of pus may have to be considered. Small abscesses are usually absorbed. In severe cases chloroquine may be combined but is rarely necessary if early treatment has been started with metronidazole. Emetine, though a very effective drug, is not the first choice now due to its toxicity.

### Follow-up

Follow-up consists of rechecking stool for EH-cysts. Repeated examination of stool monthly for three months and three-monthly for one year is an ideal method, but rarely followed.

TABLE 7.4 : DRUGS USED IN AMOEBIASIS

| Drug | Mode of administration | Dosage |
|---|---|---|
| I Emetine derivatives: | | |
| a) Emetine Hydrochloride. | I.M. | 30-60 mg. daily for 6-10 days. |
| b) Dehydroemetine. | I.M. | 30-60 mg. I.M. daily for 6-10 days. |
| c) Emetine Bismuth Iodide | Orally as enteric coated capsules. | 60 mg.—1st day at night; 120 mg.—from 2nd night for 10-12 days (if tolerated). Rarely used now. |
| II Halogenated Oxyquinolines: | (Not for amoebic hepatitis) orally or retention enema. | Orally 250 mg. thrice daily for 10 days. |
| a) Chiniofen or Yatren. | | |
| b) Iodochlorhydroxyquin | Oral. | 250-500 mg. thrice daily for 10 days. |
| c) Diiodihydroxyquinoline | Oral. | 650 mg. thrice daily for 3 weeks. |
| d) Broxyquinoline + Brobenzoxaldine | Oral. | 600 mg. four times a day for 7-10 days. |
| III Aminoquinolines—Chloroquin: 150 mgm. base = 250 mgm. of Chloroquine phosphate | Oral, parenteral and local instillation into cavities. | Oral 300 mg. of base twice daily for 2 days, 150 mg. twice daily for next 12-18 days. I.M. 200-300 mg. daily during acute phase till patient can tolerate oral medication. |
| IV Organic Arsenicals: | | |
| a) Carbarsone | Oral. | 250 mg. thrice daily for 10 days. |
| b) Glycobiarsol | Oral. | 500 mg. thrice daily for 10 days. |
| V Antibiotics Paromomycin | Oral. | 250 mg. × 4 hourly for 5 days. |

| Drug | Mode of administration | Dosage |
|---|---|---|
| | | VI Miscellaneous: |
| a) Diloxanide Furoate | Oral. | 500 mg. thrice daily for 7-10 days. |
| b) Biahylamical | Oral. | 500 mg. thrice daily for 10-12 days. |
| c) Chlorphenoxamide | Oral. | 250 mg. thrice daily for 10 days. |
| d) Metronidazole | Oral. | 400 mg. thrice daily for 7 to 10 days. |

## FILARIASIS

### INTRODUCTION

It is a disease caused by one or more of several genera and species of nematodes of the family Filaridae are transmitted by mosquitoes. In India filariasis denotes diseases caused by Wucheria bancrofti and Brugia malayi.

Man is the definitive host and mosquito the intermediate one. The adult parasites are usually found in the lymphatic system of man. The males are about 40 mm. long and the females about 50-100 mm. The females are viviparous and following copulation they give off microfilariae which find their way into the blood stream. Periodic nocturnal form occurs in India and the maximum density of microfilariae in blood is reported between 10 p.m. and 2 a.m. Female mosquitoes ingest the microfilariae along with the blood meal from infected persons and then the microfilariae develop into infective stage in the thorax of the mosquitoes. A healthy person acquires the infection through the bite of the infective mosquito.

### CLINICAL FEATURES

The disease is characterised by periodic attacks of fever with chill and rigor associated with lymphadenitis and lymphangitis. Associated streptococcal super infection usually occurs. Lymphangitis mainly involves the lymphatics of the testes and epidydimis whereas lymphadenitis affects mainly groin, sometimes axilla. Then occurs dilatation of lymphatics which may rupture giving rise to lymph scrotum, lymphocele, lymphuria. Obstruction in the chyle-bearing vessels may lead to chylocele and chyluria. Hyperplasia of skin and connective tissue causes elephantiasis of various parts and secondary bacterial infection with streptococcus pyogenes or staphylococcus may lead to septic lymphangitis or abscess formation.

*Presenting features are:*

*A) High fever, toxaemia followed by remission or further complications mentioned below.*

*B) Acute lymphangitis: Onset with high fever, rigors. Toxic manifestations followed by acute lymphangitis. Local, regional glands enlarged and tender.*

*Lymphangitis may occur anywhere but testicles and epididymis most vulnerable.*

*C) Late complications:*

*I) Obstruction to lymphatic drainage results in obstructive signs, e.g., lymph-scrotum, hydrocoele ascitis and pleural effusion chyluria may also occur.*

*Dilated lymph channels result in varicosity of lymphatics and result in chyle leakage, e.g., chyluria, chylous diarrhoea, chylous pleural effusion or ascitis.*

*II) Elephantiasis: One or both lower limbs may be swollen progressively, long after active filarial infection. Skin and subcutaneous tissues are thickened due to hyperplasia. This is the end stage of filariasis.*

## DIAGNOSIS

Diagnosis includes a search for microfilariae in the peripheral blood or in the chylous urine or hydrocoele fluid or demonstration of adult worms in the biopsied lymph node. Blood examination reveals eosinophilia (8-15% or more).

a) Examine peripheral blood at about midnight and wet preparation can be made on a slide, which may show live-microfilariae under microscope. Organisms may also be demonstrated in hydrocoele fluid, pleural or peritonial fluid or chyle.
b) Dead filaria (adult tissue round worm) may be calcified and seen in X-ray film.
c) Gland biopsy may also be useful.
d) Intradermal test may show positive reaction in 90% cases with filarial extracts used for skin test.
e) Complement fixation test may be positive, indicating past or present infection.

## TREATMENT

Diethylcarbamazine is the drug used. The dose is 4-6 mg/kg. orally daily for 14-21 days. The drug is effective against microfilariae and probably against adult worms. Anti-allergic drugs may be combined with diethylcarbamazine. When secondary bacterial invasion is suspected, a full course of antibiotics is necessary. Application of elastic pressure bandage during an early stage of lymphoedema can be of great help by forcing the lymph out of the affected parts.

Acute lymphangitis should be treated with inj. penicillin or erythromycin to combat associated secondary infection usually due to streptococci.

For elephantiasis, crepe bandage, elevation of limbs and surgical treatment especially for hydrocoele may be necessary. Reconstructive surgical treatment may also be considered in form of skin grafting.

Rare manifestations of filariasis include occult filariasis where there is massive eosinophilia (30-80%), generalised lymph node enlargement, hepatosplenomegaly, pulmonary symptoms without microfilaremia and tropical pulmonary eosinophilia which is characterised by low fever, loss of weight, paroxysmal cough with scanty blood tinged sputum, inspiratory dyspnoea and splenomegaly. X-ray chest may show diffuse miliary mottling and increased bronchovascular marking microfilariae may be demonstrated in tissues obtained by lung biopsy, but not in the peripheral blood.

(See special chapter on Pulmonary Eosinophilia)

Prevention of filariasis includes destruction of mosquitoes, control of infection amongst insect vectors, treatment of carriers and protection against mosquito bites.

# TRYPANOSOMIASIS

These are conditions caused by the protozoal organisms trypanosoma. Trypanosoma gambiense and Trypanosoma rhodesiense cause African trypanosomias, being transmitted by the Glossina or tsetse fly. Trypanosoma cruzi causes American trypanosomiasis, the vector being certain large bugs.

T. gambiense and T. rhodesiense are morphologically identical and are found in the blood and tissue fluid measuring 10-30$\mu$ with a pointed anterior end and blunt posterior. The undulating membrane projects beyond the anterior end of the body as a free flagellum. T. cruzi measures 15-20$\mu$ in length with the usual undulating membrane and anteriorly placed flagellum.

African trypanosomiasis is characterised by infection of the blood stream, enlargement of lymph nodes and eventually invasion of the central nervous system. The early symptoms include fever (high and fluctuating in "rhodesian" type), severe headache, loss of nocturnal sleep. The lymph node enlargement is a feature of "gambian" form whereas the invasion of the central nervous system is rapid in "rhodesian" type, eventually leading to the development of classical sleeping sickness.

T. cruzi infection may be acute or chronic. The acute form occurs in children and infants and is characterised by fever, conjunctivitis, unilateral oedema of the face, splenic and lymph node enlargement whereas the chronic form seen in adults is chiefly notable for venous cardiac disturbances.

Diagnosis is established by demonstration of the parasites in blood, bone-marrow, lymph gland juice and cerebrospinal fluid.

Drugs used in African trypanosomiasis are Suramin, Pentamidine Berenil and Melarsoprol. American trypanosomiasis is treated with Nifurtimox (a nitrofurantoin).

## SCHISTOSOMIASIS

These are caused by infection with the blood fluke schistosoma. Three major species of this trematode infect men, schistosoma japonicum causes Asian schistosomiasis, Schistosoma mansoni causes intestinal schistosomiasis and schistosoma haematobium leads to genitourinary schistosomiasis.

The fluke passes its life cycle in men and fresh-water snails.

Schistosoma mansoni and schistosoma japonicum infection are characterised by dysentery, hepatomegaly, portal hypertension and cor pulmonare whereas schistosoma haematobium causes general anaphylactic reaction characterised by fever, enlarged tender liver, palpable spleen and painless haematuria.

Diagnosis is based on the demonstration of eggs of schistosoma in urine and faeces or in materials removed by cystoscopic biopsy and rectal biopsy.

Sodium antimony tartrate and stibocaptute drugs are used in schistosomiasis.

## LEISHMANIASIS

### INTRODUCTION

Leishmaniasis is caused by Leishmania donovani and transmitted from animal to man or from man to man by female species of the sandfly of the genus phlebotomus argentipes.

The disease may be generalised or localised. General infection is caused by Leishmania donovani (Donovan bodies) giving rise to visceral Leishmaniasis or kala-azar whereas localised infection involves the skin or mucous membrane.

The parasites assume flagellate form in laboratory culture media but during tissue invasion the organisms have no flagella. In tissues they are ovoid, two to four microns in size, have a large macronucleus peripherally situated and a small micronucleus (kinetoplast). When cultured in blood-agar, they develop flagella (leptomonad form).

Human Leishmaniasis occurs in three clinical types:—

a) Visceral
b) Mucocutaneous
c) Cutaneous

Visceral Leishmaniasis is due to Leishmania donovani.

Mucocutaneous Leishmaniasis is due to Leishmania braziliensis, cutaneous form is due to Leishmania tropica (major), Leishmania tropica, (minor), Leishmania braziliensis and Leishmania mexicana.

## KALA-AZAR

(Visceral Leishmaniasis)

*G. C. Mookerjee*

Kala-azar is known to occur in various parts of India such as West Bengal, Bihar, Assam, Tamil Nadu, other parts of South India as well in Burma, Mediterranean areas including Iraq, Iran, Arabian Peninsula, as also in southern Russia, Africa, South and Central America.

In India, man is the only reservoir of the infection but in other countries animals also act as reservoirs of infection.

Kala-azar was once upon a time an epidemic disease in eastern and southern parts of India, but later on it appeared to have been extinct round about World War II. It has shown its presence at least in sporadic form in recent years. Since 1970, National Institute of Communicable Diseases (NICD) has reported about 70,000 cases up to 1977. The disease is confined to rural districts, especially in alluvial plains.

There are two main types of the disease, the Mediterranean and the Indian. The former is found most commonly in infants and young children and does not occur in epidemics whereas the latter form is seen in older children and young adults occurring in epidemics. However, the organism is the same for all forms of the disease wherever it occurs. In the Indian disease the reservoir is man and in the Mediterranean it is commonly the domestic dog.

### PATHOLOGY

The parasites reside in the cells of the reticuloendothelial system, lymphatics, bone-marrow and multiply by binary fission causing ultimately rupture of the host-cells to liberate the parasites. They are then either taken up by R.E. cells or invade other cells afresh. In this way the whole of the reticuloendothelial system becomes infected which causes hepatosplenomegaly. Some of the free parasites are phagocytosed by the macrophages in the circulation and the vector, the female sandfly, sucks them during its blood-meal, inside which the parasites develop into flagellate form and multiply by binary fission and when the heavily infected sandfly bites the host transmission is effected.

Proliferation of the parasite occurs in the reticuloendothelial system and hence they are distributed all over the body and are particularly found in tissues rich in reticuloendothelial cells like liver, spleen, bone-marrow and lymph nodes. The liver and spleen enlarge rapidly. The lymph nodes are also enlarged throughout the body. The bone marrow is depressed resulting in pancytopenia. Serum albumin concentration falls but serum globulin concentration rises, the albumin-globulin ratio is thus reversed.

### CLINICAL FEATURES

The incubation period generally varies from a few weeks to 18 months but it may exceed even two years. The onset is more frequently insidious.

Fever is often an early symptom and it may be continuous or remittent in type, becoming intermittent at a later stage. In about 40% cases, four hourly temperature chart may show double or triple rise in 24 hours. Splenic enlargement is progressive and it extends several inches below the costal margin, often filling up the entire abdomen. The liver is also enlarged but not as much as the spleen. Lymphadenopathy may as well be there. The tongue is clean, emaciation and anaemia are noticeable in a fully developed case.

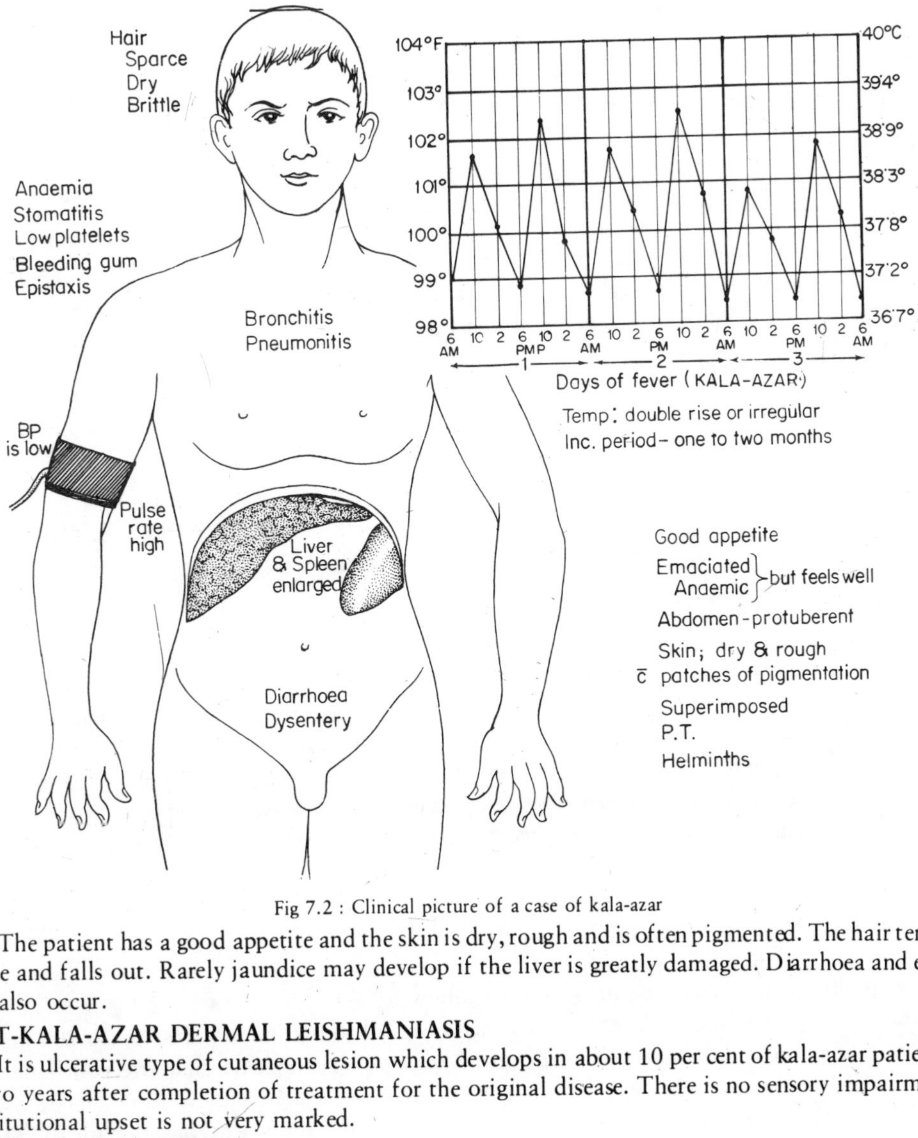


Fig 7.2 : Clinical picture of a case of kala-azar

The patient has a good appetite and the skin is dry, rough and is often pigmented. The hair tends to be brittle and falls out. Rarely jaundice may develop if the liver is greatly damaged. Diarrhoea and epistaxis may also occur.

## POST-KALA-AZAR DERMAL LEISHMANIASIS

It is ulcerative type of cutaneous lesion which develops in about 10 per cent of kala-azar patients, one or two years after completion of treatment for the original disease. There is no sensory impairment and constitutional upset is not very marked.

## LABORATORY DIAGNOSIS

*Direct evidences:*

Microscopical examination of a stained film—material being blood, bone-marrow or splenic pulp tissue.

Cultural examination of blood in NNN medium produces flagellate forms.

*Indirect evidences:*

Blood count reveals progressive leucopenia.

There is marked diminution of polymorphonuclear leucocytes with a relative increase of lymphocytes and monocytes. Eosinophils are reduced or absent. Erythrocytes are also decreased in number with fall of haemoglobin level.

**Serological tests :**

*Aldehyde Test: (Formal gel test of Napier)*

It is not positive till the disease is of at least three months' duration. The test depends upon an increase of serum globulin and is also positive in multiple myeloma, cirrhosis of liver and African trypanosomiasis.

The test can be done at bedside. One ml of clear serum is taken in a test tube and one drop of 30% formaldehyde is added. After shaking well, it is kept at room temperature and within 15 to 20 minutes the serum coagulates to a solid white mass like hard boiled egg-white. Jellification of serum may occur without opaque appearance in early cases and in chronic malaria, leprosy and trypanosomiasis.

*Antimony Test (Chopra's test) :*

Solution of urea stibamine is used to coagulate the serum instead of formaldehyde. It is also helpful.

*Complement fixation* test with W.K.K. antigen.

It is positive within three weeks of the infection. The test is also positive in cases of pulmonary tuberculosis, tropical pulmonary eosinophilia and leprosy.

*Immunological reactions:*

Gamma globulin is greatly increased. Increase in IgG fraction can be demonstrated by starch electrophoresis.

In kala-azar complement fixing haemagglutination and fluorescent antibodies also become positive.

## DIFFERENTIAL DIAGNOSIS

D.D. should be made chiefly from any condition presenting with fever and splenomegaly, e.g., chronic malaria, tuberculosis (sometimes splenomegaly occurs) cirrhosis of liver, chronic leukaemias (myeloid especially), Hodgkin's disease, splenic anaemia, Bengal splenomegaly, Egyptian splenomegaly, bacterial endocarditis, chronic brucellosis, sarcoidosis, histoplasmosis and schistosoma Japonicum. The patients of K.A. usually have good appetite and general well-being in spite of fevers, however cases of acute kala-azar may rarely occur and have to be differentiated from acute fevers with enlarged spleen.

## TREATMENT

The specific chemotherapeutic drugs are the following:—

*Urea stibamine* starting with 50 mg. and increasing by 50 mg. in each dose up to 200 mg. given intravenously daily or on alternate days, till total 2 to 3 gm. is completed. Side effects include nausea, vomiting, abdominal pains, diarrhoea and joint pains. It is not available at present.

*Sodium stibogluconate (Pentostam 100 mg/ml)*—Give 6 ml. daily by I.M. injection for 10 to 14 days. If required the course may be repeated after intervals of 14 days. Side effects include fever, urticaria, spasmodic cough and a sense of constriction in the chest.

*Pentamidine Isethionate*—Ten daily injections of 3 to 4 mg. of the base per kg. body weight (maximum single dose being 300 mg) given I.M. Side effects include hypoglycaemia and hypotension.

*2-hydroxystilbamidine isethionate*—250 mg. daily given intravenously by slow infusion in 5 per cent dextrose for 10 days. Side effects include fever, rigor, headache.

*Supportive therapy*—Nutritious diet, vitamins, haematinics.

It should be borne in mind that cure of visceral leishmaniasis can only be accepted when the patient remains afebrile, the leucocyte count returns to normal, the hepatosplenomegaly subsides and when this state is maintained for a period of at least one year.

The treatment of post-kala-azar dermal leishmaniasis is the same as for visceral leishmaniasis. Response to treatment is usually slow but some respond well to pentamidine.

### CUTANEOUS LEISHMANIASIS

It is a condition due to infection of reticuloendothelial cells of the skin and in some cases also of mucosa with leishmania tropica. It produces a cutaneons lesion over the exposed parts of the body. The lesion starts as a raised nodule eventually ulcerating which heals slowly but spontaneously leaving a depressed scar.

Clinical differentiation should be made from blastomycosis, yaws, syphilis, lupus vulgaris.

Blood picture shows a normal leucocyte count. Serum aldehyde test is negative. Pyrimethamine has also been used with success in dosage of 25 mg. daily for two weeks. Further repeat course may be necessary after 7-10 days.

Inj. Sodium Stibogluconate (BP): Pentostam 600 mg. in 5 ml. sterile 5% dextrose is often successful when infiltrated into the surroundings 3-4 times daily or on alternate days. Dehydroemetine 100 mg. orally daily for 10-12 days may also be useful.

### MUCOCUTANEOUS LEISHMANIASIS

It is a condition due to infection of reticuloendothelial cells initially of the skin and subsequently of the mucosa of the mouth and nose with Leishmania. Variety of skin lesions is seen. These are commonly papular, becoming nodular and then ulcerating giving rise to development of metastatic lesions later on, in the mucosa which extensively erode the adjacent tissues.

The demonstration of the parasite in smear taken from lesions or its recovery by culture clinches the diagnosis.

Antimony sodium tartrate 100 mg. intravenously given on alternate days for 15 days may give good results.

Pyrimethamine 25 mg. daily orally for 2 weeks with folic acid and vitamins may also prove useful.

### PREVENTION

It includes elimination of the reservoir hosts, control of sandflies and individual protection from sandfly bites.

## PLAGUE

### INTRODUCTION

Plague is a serious disease with high mortality due to Gram-negative bacilli, *Pasteurella Pestis.* It is now rarely reported in India but sporadically occurs in tropical and subtropical zones especially in some parts of Africa, Middle East, South America, Iraq, Iran, Sri Lanka, Burma, China, Mongolia, eastern Russia etc.

Rodents harbour the infection and it is transferred from rodent to rodent by fleas. The common vector is rat flea, known as Xenopsylla Cheopis. Other varieties of rat fleas may also be responsible.

Plague exists as enzootic form in wild rodents but may be transmitted by rat fleas to urban dwelling rats, Rattus Norvegicus. When these rats die, infected fleas transmit plague to humans.

In pneumonic plague droplet infection is a possibility.

*Incubation period* is two to four days.

## CLINICAL FEATURES

Three clinical types are recognised :

a) *Bubonic*
b) *Pneumonic*
c) *Septicaemic.*

*Bubonic Plague:*

Recognised by painful glandular swelling in the groins, later on other glands may also be affected sometimes. Mostly localised in groin glands are bogy, painful and tender, with varying grades of fever usually high for two to four days, then gradually falls, while buboes enlarge and may go to suppuration. The temperature usually relapses at this time.

Red congested eyes, flushed face, rapid pulse and delirium are common. The patient may get convulsions and go to comatose state. Death may occur within five to seven days.

*Pneumonic plague:*

Patients develop respiratory symptoms in the beginning with bronchopneumonic signs. Haemorrhagic sputum and severe toxaemia suggest the diagnosis. Sputum will show typical organisms microscopically.

*Septicaemic plague:*

Initial presentation is with high temperature, toxaemia, suffused conjunctiva, mental confusion and delirium. Buboes then appear and follow similar course as for bubonic plague.

## LABORATORY DIAGNOSIS

Smear of gland material, blood (septicaemic type) and sputum examination (pneumonic type) will show the organisms. It may also be cultured in the laboratory in blood agar.

Animal inoculation in guinea-pigs can be done. Animal dies within five days when its blood and tissues will show the organisms.

During possible outbreaks dead rats or live trapped rats should be examined.

## TREATMENT

a) Good nursing care, fluids, analgesics and care of hyperpyrexia.
b) Local treatment of buboes with glycerine-belladonna application, dressings and surgical incision when required. Chloramphenicol cream may be applied.
c) Specific therapy:
Inj. streptomycin I.M. 0.5 g × four hourly till fever subsides followed by 1.0 g daily to a total of 15 to 20 g.

Inj. streptomycin sulphate should be combined with chloramphenicol 0.5 g × six hourly for seven to ten days.

If there is any contraindication, tetracyclines can be used.

In early bubonic plague streptomycin alone is also effective.

*Plague vaccine:*

Vaccination is given to those who are at risk and according to travel regulations.

# ANTHRAX

**(Syn: Woolsorter's disease, malignant pustule, Siberian plague)**

## INTRODUCTION

Anthrax is an acute infectious disease typically presenting with a local angry looking skin ulcer, known as malignant pustule. It also presents as septicaemia, pneumonia or intestinal disorder.

## AETIOLOGY

The causative agent is a gram-positive organism known as bacillus anthracis, which develops a characteristic filamentous form in culture media. Organisms produce spores in contact with oxygen but not in the tissues.

It is endemic all over the world but is a rare disease in humans. It usually affects animals, especially cattle, goats, sheep and horses. It affects butchers, farmers, tanners, veterinary people, stable-workers, hence is classified as occupational disease.

The source of human infection is infected animals. Woolsorters used to get pneumonia in olden days but now preventive measures have eliminated it.

## PATHOLOGY

There is local inflammation, coagulation-necrosis and haemorrhagic pneumonitis, quickly becomes fatal in most cases.

Intestinal anthrax causes gastroenteritis due to contaminated milk.

## CLINICAL FEATURES

Malignant pustule is usually noted in exposed parts, e.g., face, neck and limbs. The typical lesion has diagnostic appearance. The central angry looking area of inflammation and necrosis is surrounded by ring of small vesicles like a chain round the lesion. Finally a black scab or eschar forms. There is local lymphangitis and adenitis of regional lymph node. There are usually mild constitutional symptoms with low grade fever but toxaemia is severe with high fever if septicaemia occurs. Pneumonic form presents with high fever, dyspnoea, toxaemia and haemoptysis.

## DIAGNOSIS

In cutaneous form, diagnosis should not be difficult, especially if occupational history is taken.

In septicaemic form, blood-culture gives the clue.

A single circumscribed inflamed skin lesion and without much pain, should arouse suspicion.

In pneumonic form it may be rapidly fatal before diagnosis is confirmed by sputum examination or culture.

## TREATMENT

Patients should be isolated with precaution enforced for medical paramedical persons; masks and gloves should be used.

Combined therapy with inj. penicillin ten-lac units I.M. 4 to 8 hourly and inj. streptomycin gm 1.0 to 2.0 I.M. daily for 10 days should be used. If contraindicated, chloramphenicol or tetracyclines are also effective. Local treatment of pustule and symptomatic treatment should be carried out as usual.

*Preventive therapy:*

a) Control of infected animals
b) Immunisation of animals
c) Proper disposal of carcasses and skin of animals
d) Proper pre-treatment of wool
e) Vaccine for occupationally exposed people (now used in Western countries)
f) International regulation for control and notification.

# CHOLERA

*T. P. Mukherjee*

## HISTORY

Cholera was a dreaded disease in India in the past but its incidence has declined considerably in the present century.

The pandemic of cholera caused by biotype, El-tor Vibrio, invaded India in 1964 and the classical V. cholera is replaced.

Classical V. cholera is found in some areas in Bangladesh and was detected in some refugee camps in India in 1971. 80 per cent of the cases are reported from Bengal, Bihar and Orissa and 20 per cent from Tamil Nadu, Karnataka, Andhra Pradesh etc. (Srivastava, J.B., 405-426, *Cholera*—edited by Barua and Burrows).

## INTRODUCTION

The incidence of cholera is going down every year. In 1980, there was not a single death from cholera reported from Calcutta Metropolitan area.

## BACTERIOLOGY

The causative organism V. cholera is a Gram-negative organism with a single polar flagellum. It has got two antigens, O and H.

Classical V. cholera as well as the El-tor variety has got 3 sub-types, e.g., Inaba, Ogawa and Hicojima.

## PATHOGENESIS

Once V. cholera organisms enter the small intestine, they multiply in astronomical number and produces enterotoxin. It has got a molecular wt. of 84,000 and stimulates adenyl-cyclase that increases in turn the permeability living endothelium and capillaries, causing copious drainage of water and electrolytes. In recent studies conducted at Infectious Diseases (I.D.) Hospital at Calcutta by the workers of Tropical School of Medicine, Johns Hopkins University and workers of I.D. Hospital, it is observed that fluid lost in the gut by the patients of cholera, are isotonic to plasma with increased amount of base. Serial observations of jejunal biopsy specimens microscopically reveal normal mucosal pattern of jejunum. On the other hand, stools of patients suffering from cholera seen under microscope show astronomical number of V. cholera, mucus and crystals of electrocytes.

It is clear that all pathophysiological changes in cholera result from the interaction of this single enterotoxin with the epithelial cells in small bowel, which results in stimulation of cell bound adenyl-cyclase, which in turn leads to increased level of cyclic AMP in epithelial cells. The cyclic AMP is responsible for pouring of isotonic fluid in intestinal lumen (Carpenter).

## CLINICAL FEATURES

Clinically for the purpose of treatment patients are divided into three groups—mild, moderate and severe.

*Incubation period*—16 to 48 hours :

Severity of the disease depends upon the amount of vibrio being ingested and how many of them bypass the gastric juice.

Malnourishment, debility, extremes of age, adversely affect the course of the illness.

*Very severe (8-11%):*

There is profuse vomiting and diarrhoea, stool becomes rice-water-like but evacuations are painless. Patient is completely prostrated with old washer-woman-like fingers developing and fontanellae becomes depressed in children. Patient may or may not be conscious. Pulse-thready—if perceptible it is above 120 per minute. Blood pressure unrecordable. Skin turgor totally lost. PSG (measured by an instrument devised by an Americal optical company) 1036 and above.

*Moderately severe (6-8%) of body weight loss:*

In this condition patient is conscious, prostrated, with cold limbs, washer-woman-like fingers, pulse above 120 mm. per minute, skin turgor lost; patient complains of muscle cramps; PSG 1036 to 1030.

*Mild (less than 5%):*

Patient is conscious, pulse 90-120 per minute, B.P. 90 mm and above (systolic), skin turgor(±), no muscular cramps; PSG 1030 and less.

## PROGNOSIS

Before 1967, cholera patients had very bad prognosis but with more knowledge about pathophysiology of cholera the prognosis is very good now. If properly treated there is very little chance of death.

## TREATMENT

Recently the treatment of cholera has been revolutionised and the treatment also has been directed according to the clinical grading of the patient. It is observed and accepted by WHO and other authorities that electrolyte-glucose combination (oral fluid) is a standard mode of treatment in majority of cases. This method of treatment is also inexpensive and large number of cases can be treated without too much load to the nursing and medical staff.

Rest is very essential.

*Segregation of patient:*

It is recently observed that segregation is not essential because carriers outnumber actual patients, hence it is not really hopeful.

*Antibiotics:*

Our choice in I.D. Hospital, Calcutta, is tetracyclines 2 gm in divided doses for two days or till the patient becomes vibrio-negative. However, it is observed, that the patients can be treated without antibiotics. If no improvement occurs within 48 hours, antibiotics may be started. Some of the antibiotics previously used in cholera are also nephrotoxic. Hence, when it is not essential, they should not be given in early stage, at least for acute watery diarrhoea cases. When, however, it is suspected that the diarrhoea may be due to bacterial origin suitable antibiotics should be given.

*Fluid therapy:*

Rehydration and control of acidosis are the sheet anchor of treatment. In an epidemic when large number of cases have to be tackled, classification of cases should be rapidly carried out. Mild cases will usually respond well to oral fluids (*vide infra*). Some of the moderately severe cases may also respond to oral fluids. The remaining cases will require intensive I.V. fluid therapy. If Ringer's lactate is available it can be given to correct acidosis. Previously in epidemics a special fluid called "Dacca solution" was in vogue containing sod. chlor. 5.0 g, sod. bicarb. 4.0 g, pot. chlor. 1.0 g and sterile water one litre. However, in our experience of epidemics, two bottles of normal saline alternating with one bottle of M/6 molar lactate usually change the clinical picture; when patients can drink orally they quickly recover. Wide bore needles should be used so that fluid may flow initially pretty rapidly. Delay and hesitancy may be dangerous.

In mild cases, oral fluids must be tried.

*Oral Fluids:*

During the Bangladesh movement, when large number of diarrhoea cases had to be managed in a short time, scientists like Macferson et al, needed a quicker and cheaper substitute for parenteral fluid.

It was observed by the physiologist Dr. Taylor that inflamed gut in the presence of fixed percentage of glucose can absorb water and electrolytes. This led to the discovery that oral fluid can be used in treatment of cholera. Composition of oral fluid is as follows:

| | |
|---|---|
| Sodium chloride | — 3.5% Gm |
| Sodium bicarbonate | — 2.5% Gm |
| Potassium chloride | — 1.5% Gm |
| Glucose | — 20% Gm. |

It is to be mixed in a litre of drinking water.

*Advantages:*

This fluid is easy to store, administer and to transport, as also very cheap. Plus there is no deterioration on storage.

*Stimulants and vasopressor agents:*

Generally there is doubt regarding their role in the treatment and management of cholera cases. From the author's experience from observations made in I.D. Hospital, Calcutta, where large number of cholera cases are treated for years together, it is felt that initially vasopressor agents like mephentermine sulphate along with parenteral steroids have some beneficial role in severe cases.

*Disposal of excreta:*

As already discussed the number of carriers outnumber the sufferers; therefore no extraordinary measures are necessary but we should ensure that the excreta do not get in contact with fomites, food and drinking water. Fly menace must be avoided at all costs; use of phenol type of disinfectants in bedpans, however, is recommended.

*Cholera vaccine:*

There are two types:

a) Parenteral

b) Oral vaccine

Oral vaccine is still in the experimental stage. In our country, parenteral vaccine is given as follows:

| | |
|---|---|
| Up to 12 years | 0.5 ml at weekly interval (two doses) |
| 12 years | 1.0 ml at weekly interval (two doses) |

In emergency condition one injection is sufficient for adults for mass vaccination programme but one second dose may be of considerable importance for the cholera in patients under 5 years of age.

## COMPLICATIONS

a) Renal failure—Due to acidosis and potassium deficit and hypovolaemia.

b) Acute pulmonary oedema—Rare.

*Cardiac arrhythmias:*

Inadequate replacement of potassium is responsible and hypokalaemia is the likely cause.

*Paralytic Ileus:*

More in children due to hypokalaemia. Usually not found in adults.

*Seizures:*

Children with cholera may develop grandmal seizures not associated with hypoglycaemia and these have very bad prognosis.

*Abortion:*

Acidosis and hypovolaemia are responsible for abortion with 50 per cent risk of foetal mortality in third trimester.

*Carbohydrate intolerance and malabsorption:* May follow.

Profound and prolonged milk intolerance has been noted in children convalescing from cholera. Supportive fluid therapy with 5 per cent dextrose is suggested.

*Tetany:* Disappears after dehydration.

Atherosclerosis and cholera may sustain stroke and myocardial infarction (Nalin and Cash).

D.D. : Enterotoxic variety of E. coli may sometimes give rise to cholera-like dramatic syndromes in Indian subcontinent in 12-24 hours. Acute gastroenteritis due to salmonella, viral gastroenteritis or food poisoning may produce similar picture but rice-water stool is diagnostic of cholera and painless evacuations are also characteristic.

## PREVENTION

There is no standard full-proof method for prevention of cholera but it is observed that vaccine prepared from dead cholera vibrio may give the patient short lasting immunity. That should be given in two divided doses after an interval of 1 week; during epidemic time it is given in one shot. Besides, few directions should be given to the patients during epidemics :

a) They should not keep the stomach empty

b) They should not take food-material unhygienically stored

c) Pure drinking water should be supplied as far as practicable.

# MALARIA

*G. C. Mookerjee*

## INTRODUCTION

Though Hippocrates described association of bad health and bad air with periodic fevers and splenomegaly, Lavaran (1880) first established genus plasmodium as the causative organism of malaria. Ronald Ross (1897) in Calcutta associated its transmission by mosquitoes in sparrows. Syndenham in the 17th Century used cinchona bark in treatment of malaria. Malaria is prevalent in tropics and subtropics between latitudes 60°N to 40°S, in humid and warm climate.

It is most common in India, Bangladesh, Burma, Malaysia, Thailand, Indonesia, Middle East, Central and East Africa, and Central and South America.

Malaria which was once a great hazard all over the eastern India, Burma and adjoining countries during the period prior to World War II and caused havoc during World War II, was more or less eradicated by the extensive malaria eradication programme launched by WHO.

However it is unfortunate that malaria has again raised its head, possibly due to development of DDT-resistant anopheles mosquitoes and drug-resistant parasites.

Malaria is caused by sporozoal organisms of the genus plasmodium. These parasites cannot directly enter the human tissues unless introduced through the bite of its vector mosquito, the female of anopheles. These parasites have their own peculiarities in causing symptoms like fever, rigor, nausea, vomiting etc. due to their metabolism in the human blood and tissues. The four parasites which are important in human malaria are:

1) **Plasmodium vivax (benign tertian malaria or vivax malaria).**
Most common and extensive distribution, not only in tropics and subtropics but also in temperate zones. It responds to anti-malarials promptly but relapses are common. Intracorpuscular cycle is 48 hours. Widely prevalent in tropics and subtropics.

2) **Plasmodium falciparum (subtertian or falciparum or malignant tertian or M.T. malaria)**
It is found all over the globe in warm climate and is a most dangerous disease. Mortality is high, if not promptly treated. May occur in epidemics during war. Cycle: 48 hours.

3) **Plasmodium malariae** (quartan or Q.T. malaria)
Not very common. Difficult to eradicte due to relapses. Cycle: 72 hours. Occurs widely in tropics, especially in India, Sri Lanka and Africa.

4) **Plasmodium ovale malaria**
Occurs usually in Central, East and West Africa. Attacks mostly mild. Cycle : 48 hours.

Before we go into the characteristics or symptomatology of these infections, it is essential to understand their life cycle in the mosquito as well as human tissues.

**TABLE 7.5 : Mosquitoes & Malaria**

VECTOR OF MALARIA IS FEMALE ANOPHELES MOSQUITO

a) It has several species which act as transmitter in various countries. Each geographical area has its own type of vector.
b) These mosquitoes feed only at night or dusk, breed in tanks, water collection around houses and *nullas*.
c) The mosquito is definitive host.
d) Man is intermediate host where both sexual forms (gametocytes) and repeated asexual cycles occur.

## LIFE CYCLE OF THE PARASITES

Their life cycle consists of two phases:

a) The life cycle in humans (schizogony)

b) The life cycle in the mosquito (sporogony).

*Schizogony*—The parasitic agents, which are introduced by the bite of the infectious female anophelene mosquito, are known as *sporozoites.* After sporozoites are introduced into the bloodstream, these reach the polygonal liver cells within two hours, where they undergo development for about 5 to 10 days. It is about six days for M.T. and longer for others. In the liver, a large number of schizonts are formed from sporozoites and subsequently these produce thousands of merozoites. Merozoites enter the red blood cells and they undergo modifications to produce ring-form and trophozoites. Within the red blood cells, these trophozoites are further sub-divided into schizonts. These schizonts continue by asexual division again and provide numerous merozoites which can infect the new red blood cells and the process is repeated, if not controlled by treatment (for reference see Pg 53 Plate IV).

As these processes take some time, the parasites are liberated at more or less the same regular intervals. Each of these four parasites has their own time-constants.

In case of plasmodium falciparum, the cycle takes 48 hours. In case of plasmodium vivax and p. ovale, the time interval is also 48 hours, while in the case of p. malariae the cycle takes 72 hours.

As the fever and rigor depends on the time, when these parasites are released into circulation, the patient gets fever every 48 hours or 72 hours depending on the nature of infecting parasites.

The phase of development in the liver cells is known as PE-cycle (PE = pre-erythrocytic) while the phase of blood cell invasion and asexual cell-division is known as E-cycle (erythrocytic).

In plasmodium falciparum (M.T. malaria), there may be more serious complications because these have special capacity to occlude the cerebral capillaries resulting in malignant malarial granuloma.

Except P. falciparum, other three parasites re-enter the liver and continue repeating the cycle once again and hence there is possibility of relapses, without fresh mosquito bite.

*Sporogony:* In human cycle some of the merozoites mature into sexual forms and are named as gametocytes. These gametocytes mature into male and female forms. The male gametocytes develop flagellae, while the female gametocytes remain spherical. These gametocytes are picked up during the process of blood sucking by the female mosquitoes and fertilisation takes place to form new cell named *Ookinete*. The *Ookinete* finally penetrates into the stomach wall of the mosquito, and develops into *oocysts* and these when matured liberate *sporozoites* which reach the salivary glands of the mosquito. These *sporozoites* are injected into humans during a mosquito bite as already described (see Table 7.5).

## PATHOGENESIS

In all malarial infections, there is destruction of red blood cells during the liberation of sporozoites. Hence the haematin pigment is liberated from haemoglobin and deposited in the tissues, especially in the R. E. cells as haemozoin pigment. It may also result in anaemia due to destruction of too many red cells. The most significant pathological changes occur due to P. falciparum infection.

In endemic areas, recurrent episodes may cause lack of cellular maturation of RBCs in the host due to chronic anaemic anoxia.

Susceptibility, acquired resistance and severity of attack depend on nutritional, racial, genetic as well as not-so-well-understood immunological factors. Individuals with Hb-S are resistant to M.T. malaria. Glucose 6-PD deficiency also offers similar protection.

In case of M.T. infection, the destruction of red cells may be extensive and may block the capillaries of various organisms and especially in the cerebral tissues. The RBCs containing parasites are sticky and form clumps due to agglutination. The freshly liberated merozoites are also sticky and these may form clumping and ultimately may block the lumen of capillaries, leading to ischaemic infarction. Petechial haemorrhage and granuloma formation may occur in the white matter of the brain, brain stem and even cerebellum. Liver and spleen get congested and enlarged and mild jaundice may be produced. Liver is affected in M.T. malaria and mild jaundice may occur. Transaminase levels may be raised and liver function tests also may become abnormal. Kidneys also may be affected leading to anoxic renal damage and acute nephritic changes. In the case of M. T. infection the serious catastrophy may occur in form of medical shock and even free haemoglobin may escape in the urine when the condition is known as *black water fever.*

When brain tissues are affected, neurological complications like convulsions and coma may occur. Even renal, suprarenal, cardiac and pulmonary vessels may be affected.

Other complications may include hyperpyrexia, cholera-like syndrome, algid malaria and even acute abdominal symptoms.

## CLINICAL PICTURE

Pictures vary considerably depending on the type of plasmodium. M.T. malaria carries highest mortality, if not timely treated. P. ovale and P. malariae also may cause serious outcome if inadequately treated. B.T. malaria, however, runs a recurrent and chronic course leading to ill health, recurrent fever, rigor, anaemia and splenomegaly.

Incubation period is one to two weeks. The symptoms start with malaise, headache, feverish chill for a few days before the actual attack. Generally three clear-cut stages are recognised:

1) **Cold stage**—Onset with shivering from head to limbs all over. Teeth may clatter and several blankets may be necessary to combat the subjective feeling of cold. This stage lasts for a half to one hour during which temperature starts rising.

2) **Febrile—hot stage**—Once fever is established, the patient no more feels cold. He throws out the blankets and feels hot. He has headache and may even have bilious vomit. In M.T. malaria symptoms are severe (Table 7.6). In all types temperature is high and usually above 40° C and tendency to hyperpyrexia lasts for about four to five hours, rarely up to eight hours.

3) **Sweating stage**—Hot stage is followed by profuse sweating and within a half to one hour temperature subsides to normal with profound subjective relief.

The picture repeats itself in characteristic manner in different types of plasmodial infections (Table 7.6).

TABLE 7.6: Types of fever in different types of malaria

| | |
|---|---|
| B.T. Malaria | — Alternate day fever. |
| Ovale Malaria | — Fever every 3rd day. |
| M. T. Malaria | — Temperature continues for 24 to 36 hours with remission for a few hours to rise again. Pernicious forms of M.T. malaria are dangerous (Table 7.7) and may cause fatality if treatment is inadequate. |

In case of M.T. malaria there may be severe complications. (Table 7.7)

TABLE 7.7: Pernicious complications of M.T. malaria

| | |
|---|---|
| 1) HYPERPYREXIA | — Temperature is above 40°C and may lead to coma and death. Clinical picture may be mistaken for heatstroke in tropics. |
| 2) CEREBRAL | — Headache, vomiting, high fever, delirium, mental confusion, acute psychiatric symptoms, meningism, convulsions, coma are presenting symptoms. High fever with any two or three of these symptoms is suspicious. The clinical picture may be mistaken for acute alcoholism, acute liver failure or meningoencephalitis. L.P. should be done. |
| 3) ALGID TYPE | — Picture of medical shock with collapse; cold clammy skin, low grade or absent fever, with vomiting, diarrhoea, muscular cramps is mistaken for cholera or food poisoning. |
| 4) RENAL FAILURE | — Due to acute nephritic damage. It may also rarely occur in P. malariae. |
| 5) BLACK WATER FEVER | — Due to intravascular haemolysis, this may also lead to severe anaemia and renal failure. |
| 6) MISCELLANEOUS COMPLICATIONS | — These include mild jaundice, dysenteric stool, typhoid-like picture and hyperpyrexia. Cardiac failure and pulmonary oedema may rarely be presenting features. |

## CHRONIC MALARIA

If B.T. malaria is not treated or inadequately treated, there will be relapse of fever with anaemia and gradual enlargement of liver and spleen. The period of free interval between the acute attack of initial malarial episode and relapse of paroxysms of fever varies considerably but usually six to eight weeks.

The patients gradualy develop moderate enlargement of liver and considerable splenomegaly with anaemia and signs of malnutrition. These cases are rare today as the patients are treated earlier in most cases, in village health centres.

During febrile stage, malaria parasites are detected microscopically in stained blood films; leucopenia with low granulocytes is often present and very rarely serum bilirubin may be slightly elevated.

### Malaria in Children:

Both infants and children are prone to malarial infection and it becomes particularly dangerous when pernicious forms of malaria affect this age group.

Even B.T. and Q.T. forms of malaria may produce serious attacks. The clinical picture is somewhat different from the adults in that it may present symptoms of gastroenteritis, abdominal colic or hyperpyrexia. Temperature usually ranges between 38.0°C & 40.5°C (100.4°F & 104.9°F). The classical pattern of temperature is not seen and the fever usually may be continuous, remittent or intermittent. Instead of rigors, convulsions are most common and signs of meningitis may be noted.

In endemic areas if the child has had repeated attacks, the pattern later on becomes less acute and the child appears to be a malnourished individual with retarded growth. Fever may be periodic or intermittent with periods of remissions in recurrent episodes. Anaemia is very common and spleen is moderately enlarged.

Chronic malaria in children is not difficult to diagnose but if acute cases are not recognised, especially in infants, it may end in fatality.

### Malaria in Pregnancy:

Malaria is a common cause of complications in pregnancy resulting in abortion and miscarriage. This is more common in rural areas of developing countries where malaria is endemic. Besides periodic fever, the patient looks particularly anaemic and complains of rigors even with low grade pyrexia. In later months of pregnancy it is often mistaken for B. Coli infection particularly because the spleen is not palpable and the possibility of malaria is not considered.

### Diagnosis of Malaria:

The diagnosis is confirmed by microscopic examination of thick and thin blood film after staining by Giemsa's method or Leishman's stain. Presence of trophozoites and similar growing forms of asexual parasites are noted within the red cells. Plate IV Pg 53, shows the various patterns commonly seen microscopically in a stained slide.

In developing countries even facilities for microscopic diagnosis may not be available for millions of patients and therefore the clinicians must be more careful to suspect the disease in all cases of fever particularly in endemic areas or especially those who have travelled recently in endemic zones. Clinically periodic paroxysms of fever with fever-free periods and enlarged spleen may be highly suspect in endemic areas. However, an enlarged spleen with fever may also be found in enteric group of fevers, brucellosis, septicaemias, SBE especially in cases of chronic rheumatic or congenital heart diseases and kala-azar, Hodgkin's disease etc. (*see* chapter on P.U.O.)

It should not be forgotten that malaria and tuberculosis may also co-exist, especially in undernourished individuals. Mixed infections with both B.T. and M.T. forms are also recognised. Hence clinical picture should be taken into account.

## TREATMENT

Treatment of malaria consists not only of drug therapy to cure a clinical attack, but prevention and control of malaria is also extremely important. The malarial infection may be present in human body in two forms, i.e., 'E' phase and 'EE' phase. Drugs which kill E forms of parasites are called schizonticides. These drugs are 4-aminoquinolines, quinine, mepacrine, proguanil, pyrimethamine.

For the treatment of EE phase, 8-aminoquinolines such as primaquine are used.

### Choice of Drugs:

In treatment of malaria the choice of drugs depends on the severity of the infection and also on the types of parasites concerned. Quinine which is the most effective anti-malarial is not used routinely because chloroquine and amodiaquine are effective and less toxic. Mepacrine, though quite effective, is seldom used nowadays because of its side effects. Proguanil and pyrimethamine are used when the other drugs are not tolerated. These two drugs are less effective than chloroquine and amodiaquine.

In P. falciparum infections the E phase requires urgent treatment but there is no need to follow up as there is no EE phase in this type of infection. But in P. vivax, P. malariae and P. ovale, both E phase and EE phase must be treated to prevent relapsing malaria. For individuals visiting endemic areas or who are resident in endemic areas it may be necessary to suppress rather than eradicate malarial infection as the possibility of reinfection is always present. In modern times it is also necessary to carefully watch for the possibility of drug resistance, especially for 4-aminoquinolines, proguanil, pyrimethamine and mepacrine. In such cases quinine and 8-aminoquinolines should be used as resistance to these two drugs is very rare.

Drug treatment of malaria consists of :

(A) **Prophylactic therapy by drugs**

(B) **Curative therapy.**

Mosquito control, however, is most important.

A) **Prophylactic drug therapy** means prevention of infection in people exposed to bites of infective mosquitoes, either by regularly taking drugs producing suppression of erythrocytic infection or destroying EE cycle by drugs which are schizonticides. The following drugs are used for people who are likely to be exposed from non-endemic areas to malarial zone.

i) *Tab. Proguanil*—Usually 100 mg. daily.
In intensely affected M.T. zones, the dose may be double, for children up to 1 year—25 mg. to 50 mg. daily, for children from 1 to 5 years—50 mg. to 100 mg. daily. The drugs should be started at the time of entering the endemic area and should be continued for one month after leaving the endemic zone.

ii) *Tab. Chloroquine (150 mg. base) or other 4-aminoquinolines*
Adults—2 tablets (300 mg) once a week.
Children—1/4 to 1/3 tab. weekly up to 1 year old.
From 1 to 3 years—1/2 to 2/3 tab. weekly.
From 4 to 6 years—2/3 to 1 tab. weekly.
From 6 to 10 years—one tab. weekly.
From 10 to 12 years—1½ tabs. once a week.
Over 12 years—adult dose.

Amodiaquine tablets (200 mg) (Camoquine, Basoquine or Flavoquine) may be also used instead of chloroquine. Basoquine suspension contains 150 mg. of amodiaquine per 5 ml.

However, it should be remembered that drug resistance of parasites is a very important factor and requires close supervision so that the drug is not misused. Irregular drug intake and irrelevant administration may be major factors in developing such resistance. Parasites become resistant more easily by proguanil and pyrimethamine as these drugs block folic acid and folinic acid of the parasites, while 4-aminoquinolines block the glycolytic cycle.

In chloroquine resistant areas it is best to use a combination of pyrimethamine 25 mg and sulphamethopyrazine 500 mg (Metakelfin); two tablets single dose, to be repeated after a week.

B) **Treatment of uncomplicated cases**—Complications of M. T. malaria and to less extent other forms of malaria may sometimes be serious. If uncomplicated cases are treated properly from the beginning, further problems are not likely to occur.

**M. T. Malaria :**

*Tab. Chloroquine (4-aminoquinoline)*—Give 4 tablets (600 mg. base) stat., then repeat two tablets (300 mg. base) after six hours, same day and subsequently two tablets (300 mg. base) once daily for 3 days.

Alternatively give tablet quinine 650 mg. b.i.d. or t.d.s. for 10 days.

As M. T. malaria has no E. E. cycle, further treatment is unnecessary.

**Other forms of malaria :**

In all other forms of malaria also same treatment will be followed but if no drug is given to eradicate E. E. forms of malaria, relapses will tend to occur. Therefore, in these cases, chloroquine is combined with primaquine (15 mg.) daily for 10 days concurrently. It is better to give two doses of primaquine 7.5 mg. daily for two weeks.

Primaquine can also be combined with quinine if chloroquine cannot be used. Precaution must be taken to watch for possible toxic effects of primaquine and advise patients to rest in bed during treatment and take plenty of fluids to avoid dehydration. Some individuals may possess glucose-6-phosphate dehydrogenase deficiency (6-GPDD) in erythrocytes and these people are susceptible to develop haemolysis while taking this drug. Jews and dark races are particularly susceptible.

**Complicated M. T. malaria and cerebral malaria :**

Complications of M. T. malaria have been discussed. Table 7.7 gives the salient points briefly. These cases must be urgently treated. In comatose cases or if there is convulsive fit L. P. must be done to examine the C. S. F.

Nowadays chloroquine is commonly used but in resistant cases quinine dihydrochlor is still the drug of choice.

*Chloroquine*—Dose 200-300 mg. (base) I. M. or I. V. (very slowly) and subsequently 200 mg. repeated eight hourly till oral dose can be administered.

In comatose cases or if shock is profound give chloroquine in 5% glucose drip 20 to 30 drops per minute along with I. V. hydrocortisone or dexamethasone to combat shock.

Severe anaemia needs fresh blood transfusion.

If resistance to 4-aminoquinoline is suspected, quinine-dihydrochlor should be used. Dose: Quinine-dihydrochlor 600 mg. in 10 ml. of sterile normal saline (600 mg.) given slowly in five minutes, followed by another ampoule of quinine (600 mg.) by slow I. V. drip in 5% glucose drip (30-40 drops per min). Three doses of 600 mg. of quinine may be parenterally given via I. V. route in 24 hours.

I.M. quinine injection should be avoided as it is likely to suppurate or form permanent tender nodule.

I. V. quinine therapy is usually required for 24 to 48 hours, then it should be followed by oral quinine or chloroquine as required. Daily monitoring of blood film may be rewarding even if the patient is improving and temperature subsiding.

In young children chloroquine may cause toxic encephalitis; hence quinine is the drug of choice. Here again it should be given by I. V. route in 5% glucose solution to avoid I.M. injection.

## BLACK WATER FEVER

It is rare nowadays. It is due to sudden intravascular haemolysis in some cases of M. T. forms of malarial infection. It used to occur due to quinine or primaquine in susceptible subjects. It should be treated as medical emergency.

Corticosteroids should be used parenterally along with fresh blood transfusion. If further antimalarial drugs are required, quinine and primaquine (8-aminoquinoline) should be avoided.

As these patients may develop recurrence in future, preventive antimalarial measures are essential.

### Malaria & HB-S :

HB-S is protective against malaria, especially M. T. variety. In endemic zones children with normal HB may die due to untreated malaria, while those with HB-S may survive.

# TYPHOID FEVER

**(Syn: Enteric fever, Typhus abdominalis, Autumnal fever)**

*T. P. Mukherjee*

## INTRODUCTION

It is an acute infectious disease clinically characterised by continuous temperature of step-ladder pattern, with headache, somnolence, splenomegaly, abdominal discomfort, diarrhoea, bradycardia, leukopenia caused by salmonella typhi (Bacterium typhosum).

## PREVALENCE

Mostly prevalent in tropical and sub-tropical countries.

It is usually more common during rains and peak incidence is during autumn. It is common among young adults of both sexes between 12 and 35 years, less common in smaller children, rarely in infants. New incumbents in the tropics are more susceptible.

## MODE OF INFECTION

a) Carrier: Patients during illness and convalescence may spread the organism through faeces and sometimes healthy people too are carriers. Organisms may remain in chronically inflamed gallbladder and are discharged in bile for many months.

b) Water supply can be contaminated with sewage in urban areas. Ponds and wells may be contaminated with infected clothes, stool or urine in villages, which serve as only source of drinking water. Flies, utensils and fomites used by the patients may contaminate food and drinks and are sources of infection.

c) Ice creams, milk products, canned meat, raw vegetables, oysters and mussels are specially liable.

**TABLE 7.8 : Pathology of typhoid fever**
**Organism : Salmonella Typhi**

(Previously called Eberthela Typhi)

INFECTION VIA ← Excretion by stool & urine

↓

Oral route via food & water

↓

Small intestine

↓

Lymphatics & Lymph nodes & Glands of mesentry (Multiplication of Organisms)

↓

Dissemination via thoracic duct to all tissues. →

↑ Further multiplication in RE cells allover

↑ Bacteremia & Excretion by liver via Gall bladder

↑ Proclaimed by onset of symptoms

↑ Payer's patches formed

↑ Tissues & Organs affected by endotoxin

↑ Excretion by stool & urine

**Intestinal lesions:**

a) *Stage of hyperaemia and swelling*—Endotoxin is liberated by the bacteria producing hyperplasia and hyperaemia of the lymphoid tissues and produce proliferation of large mononuclear cells producing lesions, reddish grey in colour, swollen and raised above the surrounding surface.

b) *State of necrosis and slough formation*—In second week greyish necrosed areas appear in the inflamed lymphoid tissue which ruptures and yellowish brown sloughs are formed.

c) *Stage of ulceration*—Slough separates in the third and early part of fourth week. Haemorrhage may occur due to erosion of blood vessels; gut perforation and peritonitis may result. The ulcer has got the following characteristic features:

i) Situated in the long axis of the gut, opposite to the attachment of the mesentery.

ii) Most abundant in the lower third of the ilium and iliocaecal valve.

iii) Oval in shape, edges are raised and floor is moderately undermined showing worm-eaten appearance.

d) *Stage of Healing*—By the middle of fourth week, ulcers heal without forming scar tissue. There is slaty pigmentation with depression at the site of healed ulcer.

*Mesenteric lymph glands*—These may be considerably congested, swollen, sometimes up to the size of hen's egg due to proliferation of large mononuclear cells.

*Spleen :*

Spleen is found to be enlarged in almost all the cases (80%) and returns to normal size during fourth week.

*Liver :*

Focal necrosis, accumulation of mononuclear cells, cloudy swelling, hepatic abscess and pyelephlebitis may occur.

*Gallbladder :*

Cholecystitis may occur and persist harbouring the bacilli in chronically inflamed mucosa.

*Respiratory organs :*

Bronchopneumonia, lobar pneumonia, pleurisy.

*Heart & Blood vesels :*

Pericarditis, endocarditis, valvulitis, myocarditis, femoral and saphenous vein thrombosis.

*Brain & Meninges :*

Hyperaemia and oedema of brain.

*Kidneys*—Focal nephritis.

*Voluntary muscles :*

Zenker's degeneration.

*Bones & joints*—Osteomyelitis, arthritis, synovitis, periostitis of tibia, lower end of radius are mostly affected.

## CLINICAL MANIFESTATION

*Mode of onset*—Insidious; disease may be mild for 10 to 15 days. But usually three to four weeks or even longer with gradually increasing toxaemia and high fever.

*1st week* : i) Gradual rise of temperature (step-ladder rise), toxaemia mild, tongue is coated with fur in the middle, tip and the margins are red and clear.
*Spleen*—Palpable in 80% cases.
*Liver*—Palpable in 50% cases.
*Pulse*—Relative bradycardia and dicrotic pulse.

ii) Bronchitis common, bronchopneumonia especially in children. Patient in untreatd case may become stuporose by the end of first week.

iii) *Skin*—Rose spot-like rashes may appear in 20% cases around 6th or 7th day, maculopapular in nature, 2 to 3 mm. in diameter, lasting for 3 to 4 days. may reappear in some cases between 19th and 34th day. They are distributed over buttocks, thigh, forearms, arms and face in some cases, found mostly in Indians.

iv) *Urine*—Shows presence of albumin and hyaline cast. Stool culture may be positive on 5th to 7th day.

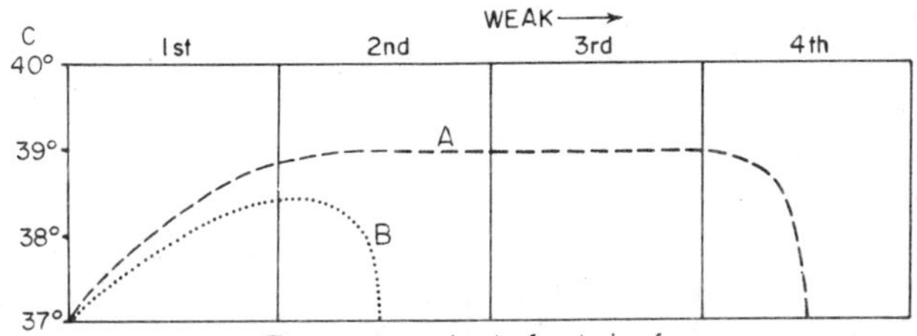


Temperature chart of enteries fever

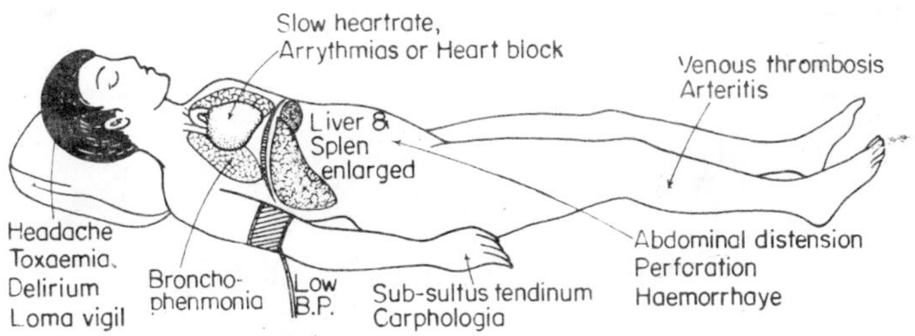


Fig. 7.3 : Clinical picture of Enteric fever

*2nd week* —Patient stuporoses and does not respond to questions. Temperature reaches the fastigium, i.e., about 39.5-41°C (103-106°F).

Tongue is coated, yellowish fur in the middle, margins are deep red. Lips, teeth gums are dry; covered with sores which consist of food, micro-organism and food materials.

Abdomen is tympanitic, with distension. Patient passes pea-soup stools, several times in 24 hours.

Spleen enlarges gradually which is soft, on palpation. Pulse is usually slow but later on may become rapid, 120-140/min. Gallop rhythm may be present, soft systolic murmur may appear, B. P. may beocme low.

Bronchopneumonia may occur, producing respiratory distress.

*Untreated cases*—Haemorrhage and perforation of gut may occur. Relapses may occur in 10% cases, especially if not adequately treated.

Anaemia, granulopenia, lymphocytosis, monocytosis, in some cases leukocytosis of 25% have been also observed in second to third week.

*3rd week*—Mild cases recover, but in serious untreated cases, the patients pass in to *typhoid state* characterised by—

(a) High fever and delirium.

(b) Dorsal decubitus and unable to turn on the sides; tend to sink in the centre of bed.

c) Coma vigil (wide open eyes), pupil slightly dilated with dull expression. Sometimes stuporose or comatose.

d) Finger tremor, muscular twitching present (sub-sultus tendinum).

e) Carphologia.

f) Tongue-dry tremulous; thick brown fur in the centre; periphery red and protrusion is difficult.

g) Lips, gums and teeth are dry and covered with sordes.

h) Occasional gum bleeding.

i) No control of bladder bowel but sometimes there may be retention of urine.

Pulse may rise to 140-145 per minute, may be irregular. Auricular fibrillation and various grades of heart block may occur. Cold, livid extremities, 1st sound weak; bronchopneumonia, hoarseness, dysphagia, are noted. Marked tympanitis, haemorrhage and perforation of gut may supervene.
Pyelonephritis or focal (toxic) nephritis may occur.

*4th week*—Aggravation of all signs and symptoms described in 3rd week, may occur or convalescence begins. Temperature comes down to normal or subnormal. Tongue becomes clear. Spleen regresses gradually. Appetite improves and feeling of well-being proclaims way to recovery.

*5th & 6th week*—In favourable cases patients progress to recovery. In severe cases marked toxaemia persists. Fatal termination is rare though it may cause extreme anxiety.
It should be emphasised that the clinical picture depicted above will vary widely in different cases, and also different age groups as also in adults and children and pregnant women.

*Atypical mode of onset :*

1. Sudden onset with chill and rigor.
   Pneumotyphoid—When the onset is like that of lobar pneumonia.
   Pleurotyphoid—When the onset in like that of pleurisy.
   Meningotyphoid—When the onset in like that of meningitis.
   Nephrotyphoid in features of acute focal nephritis.
2. Besides, patient may present with features of acute gastritis, acute appendicitis, opposite are hepatitis and cholecystitis, and haemorrhagic manifestation.

*Atypical variation in course :*

1. Abortive form—Fever is slight. Lysis occurs in 2nd week or early.
2. Ambulatory form (mild disease)—In this group patient remains ambulatory in 1st week but has stormy course in 2nd week. Occasionally patient remains ambulatory throughout the illness.
3. Paediatric typhoid—Has got the extra characteristic features like:
   Vomiting is more; so also diarrhoea; meningism to start with and bronchopneumonia is a common complication.
   Haemorrhage and perforation are rare in paediatric cases.
   Moderately, though less comprising in untreated cases, the course may be prolonged 5 to 6 weeks.
5. *Geriatric typhoid*—Rare variety—Fever is slightly irregular—Hypostatic congestion of lungs and heart failure occur. Mortality is high, convalescence is prolonged.
6. *Typhoid in pregnancy*—60% cases end in abortion and premature delivery.

*Complications of Typhoid Fever :*

a) Digestive system—Parotitis, Duguet's ulcer :
   Appear as superficial ulcer in anterior pillars of fauces, soft palate and pharyngeal wall found in 1st week.
   Tympanitis, diarrhoea, intestinal haemorrhage, perforation with peritonitis, non-perforative peritonitis.
b) Liver, gallbladder—Acute cholecystitis, cholangitis, jaundice, perforation of gallbladder.
c) Spleen—Multiple splenic abscess, spontaneous rupture in some very rare cases.

d) Respiratory system—Bronchitis, lobar pneumonia, bronchopneumonia, fibrinous pleurisy or pleural effusion, very rarely empyema, lung abscess, infarcts and spontaneous pneumothorax may occur.
e) Circulatory system—Acute myocarditis and peripheral circulatory failure are common complications in severe cases. Pericarditis, endocarditis are rare. Arteritis, arterial thrombosis, venous thrombosis and gangrene are also rare.
f) Nervous system—Meningism may occur either at onset or later especially in children, may turn to meningitis or encephalitis. Delirium tremens found in later part of the disease. Rarely convulsions, cerebral thrombosis, hemiplegia etc.
g) Special sense—Eyes, conjunctivitis, iritis, optic neuritis and retinal haemorrhages are rare. Ear—Temporary deafness is a common complication; otitis media is rare.
h) Urinary system—Acute haemorrhagic nephritis, cystitis, pyelitis, pyelonephritis may rarely occur.
i) Generative system—Orchitis, prostatitis and ovaritis are rare.
j) Locomotor system—Periostitis and osteomyelitis of clavicle, tibia etc. may develop during convalescence or many months after the attack.
k) Arthritis—Of one or more large joints.
l) Typhoid spine—Rare complication found during convalesence.
m) Skin—Sudaminal eruption over abdomen and axilla, bedsore in neglected cases, so also abscess and boils.

Of all these the following complications are common :

(1) Tympanites, (2) Diarrhoea, (3) Marked bronchitis, bronchopneumonia or hypostatic pneumonia, (4) Acute circulatory failure, (5) Coma with low muttering, (6) Infection of urinary tract, (7) Haemorrhage from bowels, (8) Bedsores, (9) Parotitis, (10) Perforation and peritonitis.

## RELAPSE

10 to 15% cases may relapse, especially due to inadequate therapy. Resistance of organisms to chloramphenicol is also rarely noted. More than one relapse may occur, possibly due to organisms remaining in R. E. system. Probable course is reinvasion of blood by typhoid bacilli from gallbladder.

However in modern times, most cases do not have these complications because of specific therapy and early diagnosis.

## DIAGNOSIS

i) History of continued fever with toxaemia and bradycardia lasting for more than 5 to 6 days, is very suspect of enteric fever, especially in tropics where the disease is too much prevalent. Blood examination reveals leucopenia with relative lymphocytosis. Blood culture is positive during 5th to 10th day.

Culture of stool and urine—positive in second or third week but it may be positive in carriers.

*Agglutination test (widal 1 reaction) :*

Widal test becomes positive in early second week and titre gradually rises becoming maximum in the third or fourth week. Rising titre is only significant. Enteric fever will cause rise in the titre of H & O antigen. H-agglutinins are non-specific, and anemnestic reaction may occur due to other infections. Rising titre of O-agglutinin is specific indication of disease. In uninoculated people, rise of titre from 1/40 to 1/80 is suggestive of infection, but this is not a diagnostic test like positive culture of organisms.

## DIFFERENTIAL DIAGNOSIS

*Malignant tertian Malaria*—Onset acute, early splenic and hepatic enlargement and presence of malarial parasite in blood smear settles the diagnosis. Response to antimalarial drugs is prompt.

*Acute Kala-azar*—Double rise of temperature. Absence of toxaemia, enlargement of spleen, leucopenia with neutropenia. Positive complement fixation test for K. A. Demonstration of L. D. bodies in bone-marrow.

*Paratyphoid*—Toxaemia is less; positive blood culture. Clinical course similar but milder. Agglutination test for paratyphoid A or B positive.

*Tuberculosis*—X-ray chest, Mantaux test, and C.S.F. findings in case of meningitis may be useful.

*Influenza*—Sudden onset with headache, bodyache, presence of occulonasopharyngeal catarrh. Short course lasts for one week.

*Meningitis*—Sudden onset with headache, signs of meningeal irritation, and leucocytosis; C.S.F. shows evidence of pyogenic meningitis. *Note* meningism may occur in typhoid fever.

*Subacute bacterial endocarditis*—Evidence of valvular heart disease, frequent rigors, anaemia, embolic signs and positive blood culture.

## PROGNOSIS

Mortality varies from 2-5%. Prognosis used to depend on the following factors before the days of antibiotics, e.g., hypostatic pneumonia, persistent diarrhoea, repeated haemorrhage, perforation of gut etc. Now prognosis is good if diagnosis is not delayed.

## MANAGEMENT

*Supportive therapy*—Patient needs complete bed-rest and symptomatic treatment as in the case of toxic fevers. Before chloramphenicol era, it was only this method which saved many lives. Care of orifices, skin and bowel is most important. Do not give purgatives. Food should be light, low residue-type and easily digestible. Watch for complications, especially haemorrhage and perforation. Haemorrhage needs fresh blood transfusion. If intestinal perforation is suspected, surgical consultation should not be delayed.

*Specific chemotherapy :*

Treatment of enteric group of fevers has been revolutionised since the introduction of chloramphenicol.

*Dose:* Oral dose is 50 mg/kg of body weight, i.e., 60 kg patient will receive 3.0 gm per day in four divided doses.

The temperature settles within three to four days, unless there is some other complication. Once temperature is normal, reduce the dose to 2 gm daily for a total period of 10 to 14 days.

Milder cases need smaller dose and sometimes seven to ten days course is good enough. Parenteral dose should be 0.5 gm chloramphenicol hemisuccinate 0.5 gm, I. M. given 8 hourly. It can also be given I. V., if required, as in the case of intestinal haemorrhage or perforation. Best course is to give a suitable preparation in the I. V. drip continuously. Total dose is 1.5 gm to 2.0 gm in 24 hours.

If the organisms are not sensitive to the drug, co-trimoxazole tablets containing 80 mg of trimethoprim and 40 mg of sulphamethoxazole are given orally. (2 tablets x 3 times daily). Parenteral preparation is also now available, or Furaxone also appears to be useful and may be used where other drugs cannot be used. Dose: Furazolidine (Furaxone) 200 mg t.i.d.

The risk of aplastic anaemia is not usually great but must be closely watched for. It is wise to monitor blood picture every four days or if patient feels unwell, too weak or develops oral ulcers.

If the patient has glucose-6-phosphate deficiency (glucose-6 PD) chloramphenicol may cause severe haemolysis and be best avoided.

Steroids in short course may have to be used in very toxic cases. Be careful about intestinal haemorrhage and perforation.

## PREVENTIVE MEASURES

Two doses of typhoid vaccine should be given at one week's interval. Immunity lasts for about 12 to 18 months.

Chronic carriers should be treated with co-trimoxazole or amoxycillin. Cholecystectomy may be necessary if gall bladder is pathological.

# PARATYPHOID FEVER

It is caused by paratyphoid bacilli A, B and C. Of these paratyphoid A infection is common in India. Mode of infection age and sex incidence of paratyphoid fever is the same like that of typhoid fever but the course is milder than typhoid fever.

## PATHOLOGY

Large intestine is more frequently involved. There is catarrhal inflammation without ulceration. There may not be much intestinal involvement at all.

## CLINICAL PICTURE

Clinical course is the same as that of typhoid fever but milder and shorter in duration. Occasionally it presents with moderately severe toxic manifestation. It has got sudden onset with prodromal symptom-like nausea, vomiting, epigastric pain, initial diarrhoea, upper resipratory catarrh, herpes labialis with temperature-intermittent type, terminates by rapid lysis. Liver, gall bladder may be palpable and tender; jaundice may be present, rash occurs more in paratyphoid than typhoid fever.

## COMPLICATIONS

Pyelonephritis, jaundice, chlolecystitis are common complications but rare complications are

*[Contd. on p.233]*

## INTESTINAL HELMINTHIASIS

### TABLE 7.9 : Showing in brief the clinical features, life cycle and treatment of common intestinal helminths of man.

| HELMINTHIASIS | INTRODUCTION | LIFE-CYCLE |
|---|---|---|
| 1. Ascariasis | This is infection with Ascaris lumbricoides which is the largest intestinal nematode, parasitising man. It has a world-wide distribution being specially prevalent in the tropics like China, India and South-East Asia. The disease is common in persons with unhygienic haibts. The adult worm resembles an ordinary earthworm. The male is about 15-25 cm. in length with the tail end curved ventrally like a pointed hook. The female worm is neither curved nor pointed. | Man is the only defintive host. The worms reside in the small intestines. A fertilised female liberates eggs which escape in faeces and undergo development in faeces and further development in soil so as to infect food, drink or raw vegetables. Now the man ingests eggs containing larvae which bore through intestinal mucosa and are carried by portal circulation to liver and via right heart to lungs. Therefrom larvae break out of pulmonary capillaries and enter lung alveoli to grow and eventually crawl up the bronchi and trachea into the larynx and pharynx to be swallowed again to localise in the upper part of the small intestine to develop into adult worms. |
| 2. Ancylostomiasis | This is infection with ancylostoma doudenale. It occurs in temperate climates in Europe, in the Middle East, North Africa and in certain areas of the Far East. The adult worms measure 1 cm. in length, the female is a little larger than the male, the body is slightly curved and tapered at both ends. | Man is the only definitive host. Eggs escape in faeces and develop in soil so as to cause hatching out of rhabditiform larvae and filariform larvae, the latter being infective enter the body penetrating the skin and pass through the lymphvascular system into the venous circulation to be carried to the right heart into the pulmonary capillaries. Therefrom through the alveolar spaces they migrate on to the bronchi trachea, larynx and crawl over the epiglottis to be swallowed to develop into adult worms in the intestine. |
| 3. Enterobiasis | This is the infection with Enterobius Vermicularis. It has world-wide distribution and is not influenced by climate. The worm is small thread-like. The males have coiled tails and are about half the size of the females which may reach about 1 cm. in length. | The gravid femaleworms creep out of anus and lay eggs which adhere to the skin or the clothing and are transferred therefrom to fingers and towels. The embryonated eggs rapidly develop and become infective when swallowed, larvae escape in the intestine and male and female worms develop. |
| 4. Trichuriasis | This is infection with trichuris trichura. It is especially found in the tropics.<br>The worm measures about 5 cm. in length. The female is larger than the male. The anterior part thread-like, the posterior thicker and cylindrical. | The eggs come out of the human host with faeces and develop in soil to produce embryonated eggs which when swallowed larvae are liberated and each larva becomes an adult worm. |
| 5. Strongyloidiasis | This is infection with strongyloides stercoralis. It occurs in many parts of the world, particularly in the East, South America and Africa. This worms are hardly visible to the naked eye. | The eggs hatch in the human host and larvae are passed in the faeces which usually develop into free living adults and this cycle may be repeated, ultimately, however, filariform larvae are formed which penetrate the human skin to reach via heart, the pulmonary vessels and alveoli and then the intestine. |

| CLINICAL FEATURES | DIAGNOSIS | TREATMENT |
|---|---|---|
| Pain abdomen, abdominal distension, anorexia, malnutrition, urticaria, and diarrhoea. Occasionally intestinal obstruction is encountered. Migration of larvae may cause ascaris pneumonia (Loeffler's syndrome), hepatomegaly or encephalopathy. | Discovery of the adult worms or the eggs in the faeces. | (i) Piperazine salts give a maximum of 3-4 gm, as single dose in adults for two days. For children dose is 75 mg/kg.<br>(ii) L-tetramisole 5 mg/kg given in a single dose.<br>(iii) Mebendazole tablet given in a dosage of 100 mg, twice daily for 3 days. |
| Pain abdomen, malnutrition, progressive anaemia, anorexia, oedema and diarrhoea alternating with constipation. Larvae can cause ground itch at their site of penetration. | Discovery of the eggs in the faeces. | (i) Bephenium hydroxynaphthoate—5 gm daily to be taken for 3 consecutive days in stomach. For children dosage in 20 mg/kg. It is the drug of choice and is also useful for mixed HW & RW infestations. |
| Itching round the anus and perineum, nocturnal enuresis, rarely appendicitis, pruritus vulvae may occur in young girls. | Demonstration of the worms or of the eggs in the stool or in the scrappings from the perianal skin. | (i) Piperazine 50-75 mg/kg daily (maximum 2 g) orally for 7 days.<br>(ii) L-tetramisole 2.5 mg/kg in a single dose.<br>(iii) Mebendazole—as in ascariasis.<br>(iv) Other effective drugs are viprynium embonate and pyrantel embonate. |
| Abdominal pain, dysentery often with blood-stained stool occurs in heavy infection. Appendicitis may also develop if vermiform appendix is infected. | Discovery of the characteristic eggs by a microscopical examination of a saline emulsion of the faeces. | (i) Thiabendazole—50 mg/kg orally for 2 days.<br>(ii) Mebendazole—as in ascaris. |
| Abdominal discomfort, pain abdomen, diarrhoea, urticaria. | Demonstration of the typical rhabditiform larvae in freshly passed stool. | (i) Thiabendazole 25 mg/kg twice daily for 3 days. |

N.B. Intestinal tapeworms have been separately discussed.

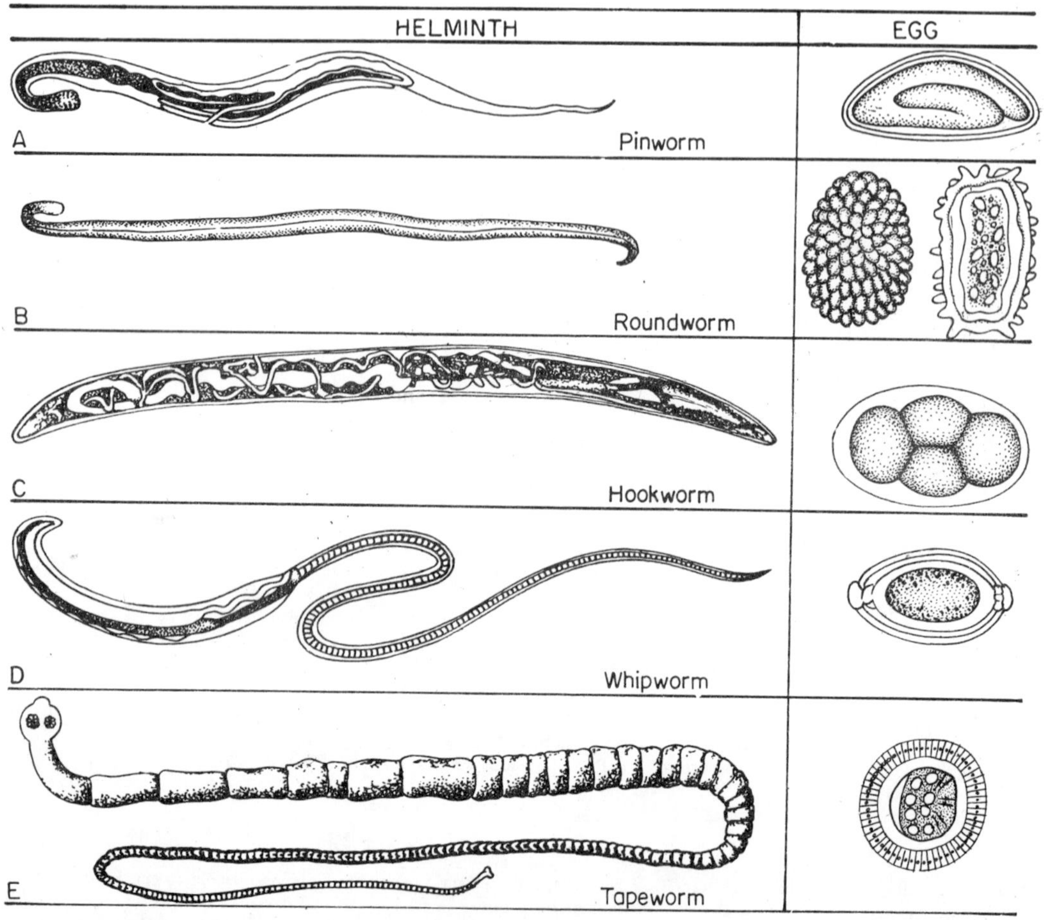


Fig. 7.4 : Common Helminths

[Contd. from p. 229]
intestinal haemorrhage, perforation, cardiovascular, pulmonary, neurological disorders as described under typhoid fever. Prognosis—good; mortality less than typhoid.

## TREATMENT

On similar lines as in the case of typhoid fever but co-trimoxazole is also very effective, particularly in paratyphoid fever.

[See Table 7.9 at p. 230]

# HELMINTHIC INFECTIONS

*G. C. Mookerjee*

These are due to :

**A) Nematodes**

1) *Ascariasis* (ascaris lumbricoides)
2) *Ancylostomiasis* : Two varieties, e.g., A.duodenale and Necator americanus
3) *Enterobiasis* (oxyuris vermicularis—old name; now called enterobius vermicularis); also called pinworm or thread worm
4) *Trichuris trichura* : Whipworm
5) *Strongyloidiasis* (strongyloidis stercoralis)
6) *Trichniasis* (trichnia spiralis), a viviparous worm
7) *Dracontiasis* (Dracunculus medinensis or guinea worm)

All the above except guinea worm and T.spiralis inhabit small intestines of human beings.

**B) Cestodes** (Taeniasis)

1) *T. solium*
2) *T. saginata*
3) *Echinococcus granulosis (T. Echinococcus)*
4) *Hymenolepis Nana (H. Nana)*
5) *Diphillobothrium latum (fish tape worm)*

**C) Trematodes**

These are called flukes.

1) *Fasciola hepatica*—(Liver flukes) causes cholangitis and liver abscess
2) *Clonorchis sinensis*—Affects biliary passages of the liver
3) *Paragominiasis* (Distoma westermani or lung fluke)
4) *Schistosomiasis* (Bilharziasis)

Three types are known :

1) Schistosoma haematobium,
2) Schistosoma mansoni, and
3) Schistosoma japonicum.

Various helminths are transmitted by different modes, to infect human beings. Some of them are faeces borne and transmitted by soil contamination, e.g., ascaris, ancylostoma, trichuris, strongyloides. Faecal oral transmission occurs in enterobiasis. Dracanculosis and filariasis are arthropod transmitted.

Schistosomiasis is due to snails.

Teniasis by animal meat or fish.

## HYDATID DISEASE

Humans are infected by larvae of T. echinococcus, from dog's faeces. Jackals and wolves may also harbour the worms and act as source. A terminal segment of the worm, conveyed via dog's faeces reaches the stomach of a dog-lover. Ova contained in the segment liberate a 6-hooked embryo (oncosphere) which penetrates the mucosa of upper small intestines and reaches liver by portal vein radicles. Some of these may escape the liver and reach lungs or other tissues including brain.

These form hydatid cysts in tissue.

Hydatid cyst has two layers :

1) *Laminated external layer* called ectocyst which is chitinous.

2) *Germinal or internal layer* called endocyst.

Surrounding the cyst wall there is fibrous tissue reaction attempting to form a barrier layer.

From the germinal layer daughter or secondary cysts are formed and the cysts may grow into large size (cricket ball to football size a or even larger).

*Cyst fluid*—Clear; sp-gr. 1005-1010 containing sodium chloride, daughter scolices, hooklets.

*Effect of cysts*

1) Pressure effect

2) Suppuration

3) Rupture

4) Inspissated

5) Calcified

Cysts commonly form in the liver and less commonly in lungs and pleura, brain, stomach, kidneys, uterus, omental areas or anywhere in the body.

Unless suppurating it will behave as a space occupying tumour producing local pressure effects.

Rupture causes symptoms of visceral rupture. Bleeding may occur. Associated urticaria is often a pointer.

Although radiology may help in the diagnosis of pulmonary hydatid cyst, ultrasonic scan is very helpful in diagnosis.

### TREATMENT

1. Surgical removal where possible.
2. Do not aspirate for diagnostic purposes.

## CYSTICERCOSIS
(Syn : Cysticercus cellulosae)

It is due to larval form of T. solium (pork tapeworm), causing cysticercus form in human. Usually the adult worms inhabit the human intestines and intermediate host in pig. But, if the eggs are regurgitated in the stomach, shells are digested.

Auto-infection may also cause similar effect. Therefore be very careful in treating T. solium.

Proglottides of the worm is digested and ova are liberated and subsequently cysticerci form in muscles, subcutaneous tissues, viscera, nervous system and even in vitreous humour. Cerebral cysticercosis is recognised cause of epilepsy. Sometimes the cyst may block the fourth ventricle and cause internal hydrocephalus. The cysts may become calcified after a few years and are then seen as multiple calcified spots in X-ray films of skull (especially lateral view) and the long bones, e.g., muscles around femur.

## DRACONTIASIS

This is infection with the nematode Dracunculus medinensis. It is found in India, Burma, Arabia, Iran, eastern regions of the U.S.S.R., East, West and Central Africa, West Indies and South America. The clinical effects are produced by female worms only and they measure up to 3 feet in length.

### LIFE CYCLE

The gravid female reaches the surface of skin of the host and local vesicle formation and ulceration occurs. Now larvae in large number are ejected wherever the lesion comes into contact with water. The larvae escaping from the female enter the crustacean cyclops and man becomes infected by swallowing water containing infected cyclops. In the duodenum the larvae escape and they penetrate the wall of the small intestine.

Afterwards development continues in the connective tissue of the host.

### CLINICAL FEATURES

Allergic manifestations, fever, giddiness, cutaneous blister formation and secondary bacterial infection of the ulcer may occur.

Anaphylactic shock may be produced if the worm bursts in the tissue.

### DIAGNOSIS

Detection of the adult worm at the surface of the skin or detection of embryos in the fluid obtained from the affected part.

### TREATMENT

Gradual mechanical extraction of the worm by rotating it round a stick. Niridazole 25 mg/kg. orally for 10 days or thiabendozole 50-100 mg/kg. for 1-3 days orally or metronidazole 25 mg/kg. orally for 10-15 days may be given which may act as anti-inflammatory agent and help emerging worm to be taken out easily. Antibiotic therapy and prophylaxis for tetanus may be required in presence of secondary infection.

## TAENIASIS
### (Intestinal tapeworms)

There are many varieties of tapeworms (cestodes) which affect animals but humans are affected by the following types :

1. Taenia Solium (Pork tapeworm)
2. Taenia Saginata (Beef tapeworm)
3. Hymenolepis nana or (Dwarf tapeworm)
4. Diphyllobothrium Latum (Fish tapeworm)

*Definitive host*—Humans are infected by eating undercooked meat or fish, containing cysticercoid form. These develop into adult worms and inhabit small intestines. Ova and cysts are discharged in faeces.

*Intermediate host*—Animals; they ingest ova and then larval forms are produced; finally larval cysts are deposited in muscles and solid viscera.

*Cysticercoid forms in humans*—Sometimes larval cystic forms occur in humans which are very dangerous complications :

1) *Hydatid cysts*—Due to T. echinococcus. Humans commonly get infected from dogs.
2) *Cysticercus cellulosae*—From larval forms of T. solium

Tape worms vary in length, shape and size :

The common anatomy being presence of a small head and a narrow neck (= Scolex) and a few to numerous segments or proglottides.

These segments grow and larger distal segments being more mature discharge eggs, and are discharged in faeces, subsequently these are swallowed by intermediate hosts and cycle is completed. T.saginata, the beef tapeworm is about 5-10 metres in length whereas T. solium, the pork tapeworm measures about 2-3 metres in length. H. nana is one of the smallest intestinal cestodes infecting man and measures 1-4 cm.

## LIFE CYCLE

The eggs or segments are passed out of the intestine of man in the faeces on the ground and while grazing the animals (cow or pig) swallow the eggs. In their alimentary canal, the eggs rupture liberating oncospheres and they penetrate the gut wall to gain entry into the portal vessels or mesenteric lymphatics to reach the systemic circulation. From the circulating blood the oncospheres are filtered into the muscular tissues where they undergo further development to produce cysticercus. Human beings are infected due to eating undercooked beef or pork containing the cysticerca and in the intestine of man adult worms develop.

Embryonated egg of H. nana when ingested burrows into the villi of the small intestine and produce larvae which re-enter the small intestine rupturing the villi and develop into adult worms.

## CLINICAL FEATURES

Passage of segments of worms in stools, abdominal distension, pain abdomen, diarrhoea, voracious appetite, calcified nodules in the muscles. If brain is involved, convulsions may occur.

H. nana infection is associated with pain abdomen, loss of appetite. chronic diarrhoea and malnutrition.

## DIAGNOSIS

Naked eye examination of stool for adult worms and microscopical examination for the eggs in stool.

## TREATMENT

(i) Niclosamide 2 gm. orally in divided doses for 2 days.
(ii) Mebendazole 300 mg. twice daily for 3 days.
(iii) Mepacrine 15 mg./kg. in a single dose or in divided doses to be followed by a saline purgative in H. nana infection. Niclosamide is 60-80 mg./kg. for 5 days.

# PYREXIA OF UNKNOWN ORIGIN

(Syn: Pyrexia of undetermined origin or P.U.O.)

*G. C. Mookerjee*
*Subir Kumar Dutta*

Unexplained fevers can be a difficult clinical problem. Fevers of less than a week's duration are usually due to viral infection or other infective fevers, the nature of which is usually revealed due to typical symptoms, appearance of skin-rash or localising physical signs. However, in some cases, fever may continue over two or three weeks or even longer without any obvious clue to the diagnosis.

*However the term P.U.O. or pyrexia of undetermined origin is used when any febrile condition is continued for over ten days, without any obvious physical signs or aetiological diagnosis.*

Sometime diagnosis may be missed due to faulty clinical approach or inadequate experience in choosing correct investigations in proper time. In such cases it is wise to discuss the problem with the pathologist before ordering a score of tests which may be really be of no use.

The clinician should know about the significance of laboratory tests he is going to order. He should also provide adequate clinical data to the pathologist and should not utilise the laboratory as a mechanical aid to get reports. There is a tendency among some clinicians to order a proforma of investigations and then to review the patient for treatment on the basis of reports. Such wrong method should be condemned, as most important clinical clues may be lost, while the doctor was waiting to get the diagnosis through laboratory tests and X-ray reports.

Malingering is sometimes a rare cause of P.U.O. Taking of temperature is made by sucking the thermometer or warming by bedside electric bulb or rubbing between fingers. Thermometers can occasionally be erratic and should be checked carefully.

It is difficult to classify all causes of P.U.O. but one should try to enumerate the causes in a logical manner. P.U.O. is most often due to a common disease, presenting in an unusual manner or the diagnosis is missed due to use of inadequate doses of antibiotics or drugs. Sometimes rare diseases are responsible, which should be excluded by appropriate tests or investigations. The following conditions may present as P.U.O.

1) **Tropical diseases, e.g.:**

a) Malaria—B.T. type, especially in endemic areas in patients taking antimalarials irregularly. Spleen is usually enlarged. If repeated blood examination is negative, therapeutic trial is justified.
b) Kala-azar—Sternal marrow examination usually gives the clue.

2) **Respiratory diseases:**

Viral or atypical pneumonias, deep-seated lung abscess, interlobar or small basal pleural effusions may be missed. X-ray chest usually diagnostic.

3) **Cardiac condition:**

a) Presence of chronic valvular disease with prolonged pyrexia should draw attention to subacute bacterial endocarditis. Repeated blood culture reveals the causative bacterial organism.

b) Rheumatic fever may occasionally be responsible when typical peripheral signs are missing. Careful auscultation of heart, presence of C-reactive proteins and high ASO titre should help.

4) **Abdominal causes:**

a) *Liver abscess*—If it is deep-seated its local signs may be obscured.

b) *Kidney*—Pyelonephritis and perinephric abscess are often missed.

c) *Prostate*—Infection of prostate or even prostatic carcinoma may be responsible.

d) *Chronic gallbladder* and biliary tract infection or pancreatitis.

e) *Pelvic abscess and* parametritis can be determined by PV examination.

5) **Neoplasms, Reticulosis & Hodgkin's disease :**

All these conditions may produce unexplained temperature. Especially in old people if no cause of fever is found, neoplastic possibility should be excluded. Similarly in young-age group Hodgkin's reticulosis is often difficult to exclude; especially deep-seated glands are involved in the initial phase.

6) **Infections diseases:**

a) *Tuberculosis*—Usually has some clue but sometimes it can present as P.U.O.

b) *Brucellosis*—Arthralgia, sweating and agglutination tests will give the clue.

c) *Glandular fever*—Paul Bunnel tests should be done.

d) *Undulant fevers or relapsing fevers*—May often be difficult to exclude.

7) **Deep-seated suppuration :**

Brain abscess, deep-seated stitch abscess, subdiaphragmatic abscess may often cause difficulty.

8) **Collagen diseases :**

Usually these conditions present protein clinical features and can be diagnosed by careful investigations.

9) **Miscellaneous conditions, e.g. :**

Deep mycoses, cytomegalovirus infection, psittacosis, cirrhosis of liver, chronic acute hepatitis and thrombophlebitis usually have some clues and should not cause confusion.

Foreigners or unacclimatised hill-dwellers coming to hot and humid tropics may suffer from low grade fever.

Malingeering is sometimes encountered especially among recruits during war.

History of previous drug intake is important. Drug fevers, especially due to methyldopa, warferin and antibiotics are well known but often not remembered.

## INVESTIGATION

The first step is to take a good history, carry out a sound clinical examination and order only a few tests like the TLC, DLC, haemoglobin level and a urine examination.

Subsequent steps should be decided on the result of initial screening reports.

*Diagnostic methods:*

It is very difficult to formulate a standard procedure for diagnosis of bewildering varieties of clinical conditions responsible for pyrexia of unknown origin. The elucidation of this type of problem requires skilful application of all diagnostic methods—a careful history, detailed clinical examination, rational laboratory tests and roentgenograms.

*Clinical investigations:*

*History :*

i) *Age*—Obscure temperature in elderly may be due to hidden carcinoma though cancer and tuberculosis is no respecter of age.

ii) *Sex*—In females pelvic organs are often seat of chronic infection. Attempted abortion may be a reason.

iii) Place of residence, history of recent visit to other places or history of contact with persons recently arrived from other parts of the world, may give a clue.

iv) Occupation, hobby, animal pets: Brucellosis, psittacosis-ornithosis etc.

v) History of contact with tuberculous patient.

vi) Family history of tuberculosis.

vii) Previous history of similar episodes of fever, rheumatic fever, gonorrhoea, congenital heart diseases; recent history of dental extraction, boils or carbuncles.

viii) Onset of present illness—insidious or abrupt lobar pneumonias and typhus fever have acute onset while enteric group of fevers has insidious onset.

ix) Chronology of evolution of symptoms may draw attention to a particular organ.

x) Localising symptoms, if any,should be meticulously searched for.

xi) Study of temperature chart—intermittent, remittent, sustained or relapsing.

Intermittent pyrexias are paroxysmal swinging high fevers associated usually with rigors, which is relieved with profuse sweating. Causes are malaria, pyaemias, acute renal infection, acute cholangitis due to stone and carcinomatous obstruction etc.

Remittent pyrexia denotes fever which remains high throughout the day with variation of 1°C (1.5°F) or more.

Undulant fevers are usually relapsing type of fevers in which there are bouts of fever for a few days, followed by remission and relapses again and again. These are due to spirochaetal or bacterial infections often due to rat or cat or animal bites.

*Clinical examination—a thorough clinical examination is indispensable and this should be repeated frequently :*

i) Examination of skin, closely and on each day, for rashed, petechial haemorrhages, nails for splinter haemorrhages and finger pulp for tender nodules.

ii) Examination of ear, nose and throat for septic foci.

iii) Examination of ocular fundus for any haemorrhagic spots. In miliary tuberculosis, fundi may show tubercles.

iv) Examination of lymph nodes—carefully palpated and special attention put for supraclavicular, axillary, epitrochlear group. Tuberculous glands are matted, malignant glands are hard and fixed, Hodgkin's glands are rubbery.

v) Examination of heart for murmurs or any other abnormality, change in the character of murmurs to be noted.

vi) Examination of lungs—for any change in breath sounds and presence of dullness etc.

*Routine blood count, haemoglobin percentage and ESR:*

i) Leucocytosis with polynucleosis—common in pyogenic infections. Also found in diverse conditions like rheumatic fever, amoebic liver abscess, leptospirosis, following myocardial infarction or in rapidly growing tumours.

ii) Normal count or slight neutropenia only—common in viral diseases, also found in bacterial diseases like enteric fever, tuberculosis or subacute bacterial endocarditis.

iii) Leucopenia with neutropenia—also common S.L.E. and hypoplastic or infiltrative lesions of bone marrow.

iv) Eosinophilia—found in parasitic diseases (helminthiasis and filariasis), polyarteritis nodosa, sometimes in lymphomas and blastomycosis. Eosinopenia occurs in K.A.

v) Leucocytosis with high proportion of atypical lymphocytes found in infectious mononucleosis. Similar but less distinctive pattern found in toxoplasmosis or cytomegalovirus infection.

vi) Leucocytosis with increased monocyte count found in tuberculosis, brucellosis, typhoid fever and subactue bacterial endocarditis.

vii) Presence of leucocyte precursors in peripheral blood film with usually increased leucocyte count found in leukaemias.
Sometimes precursor cells may be scanty in peripheral blood film with leucopenia in subleukaemic form of leukaemia (aleukaemic leukaemia).

viii) Presence of abnormal red blood cells and immature cells of red blood series found in haemolytic states.

ix) Presence of parasites in peripheral blood film may be clue to malaria, filaria, rarely K.A. and trypanosomiasis.

x) Haemoglobin low in anaemia and such anaemia may be marked in prolonged febrile illness.

xi) Erythrocyte sedimentation rate (ESR)—moderately raised in most infections and may also be normal in others.
A significantly high ESR found in tuberculosis, connective tissue diseases, liver abscess, pyogenic infections, malignancies and myelomatosis. A persistently normal ESR, in spite of prolonged fever, indicates abscence of a serious disease process.

*Examination of Urine:*

Routine chemical and microscopical examination of urine is the simplest and most reliable method of establishing the diagnosis of urinary tract infection.

Presence of albumin and microscopical pyuria signifies urinary tract infection. Presence of bile pigments and salts found in hepatic disorders and urobilinogen in haemolytic states. Sp. gr. of urine must be taken. If sp. gr. is persistently below 1010, it suggests poor concentrating power of kidneys.

*Liver function tests:*

Bilurubin level including fractions, totals protein level including A : G ratio, transaminases, alkaline phosphatase, 5 Nucleotidase, LDH, electrophoretic protein fractionation and detection of Australia antigen (hepatitis B-virus infection).

*Microbiological examinations:*

Isolation of pathogenic organisms from blood, internal fluids and urine establishes the diagnosis beyond doubt, provided contraction is excluded during collection.

*Serological examinations:*

i) Widal test to exclude enteric group of fevers, done in the second week of illness.
ii) Weil Felix test and complement fixation test to exclude rickettsial diseases.
iii) Brucella agglutination test to exclude undulant fever.
iv) Paul Bunnell test to exclude infectious mononucleosis.
v) Complement fixation est and cold agglutination test to exclude primary viral atypical pneumonias.
vi) Antistreptolysin O titre in cases of rheumatic fever.
vii) L E cell test, rheumatoid factor, antinuclear factor and serum complement level in cases of connective tissue diseases (collagen diseases).
viii) In viral diseases—a rise in antibody titre is most significant. The viral diseases causing prolonged pyaemia may be diagnosed serologically but diagnosis cannot be made (*vide supra:* section on Virus Diseases).

*Skin sensitivity test:*

Skin test (Mantaux) may be helpful to exclude tuberculosis; other tests sometimes done are Casoni's test (hydatid disease), Brucellin test (brucellosis) or Kveim test (sarcoidosis).

*Biopsy:*

i) Needle biopsy of bone marrow, liver, spleen, kidney, lung, lymph node, pleura, pericardium or peritoneum may provide useful information.
ii) Surgical excision biopsy of lymph node gives more useful information in appropriate cases. Scalene node biopsy may give clue to sarcoidosis.
iii) Biopsy of skin muscle, temporal artery, bone or from other accessible sites with lesion also may be helpful in collagen disorders.

*Radiological investigations:*

i) Chest X-ray and follow-up films may be necessary in severe cases.
ii) X-ray of paranasal sinuses, skull long bones and straight X-ray of the abdomen.
iii) Cholecystogram and pyelogram may be done when necessary.
iv) Lymphangiogram and arteriogram may be rarely necessary.

*Modern non-invasive methods:*

i) Ultrasonography
ii) Radioactive scanning of organs and computerised axial tomography (C.A.T. Scan).

*Conclusion:*

It has been found that in 90-95% of cases of pyrexia of unknown origin a diagnosis can be arrived at. This remaining small group usually recovers spontaneously. Clinicians should patiently watch, observe and correctly investigate instead of prescribing antibiotics one after another, giving steroids without actual indications and ordering indiscriminate tests; a joint consultation, a second opinion or pathologist's view may also be very rewarding.

# CHAPTER – 8
# ENDOCRINOLOGY

## INTRODUCTION TO ENDOCRINOLOGY

*G.C. MOOKERJEE*

An endocrine gland is a specialised group of tissue cells which synthesise hormones. As these hormones are produced in minute quantities and are directly absorbed into venous blood and not secreted via ducts, endocrine glands are also called ductless glands. Even two decades ago, most of these hormones were estimated either by biological assay or by chemical methods while many others were not known or could not be accurately estimated.

Patients with classical symptoms or signs of endocrine disorder can be clinically recognised by any competent physician while borderline cases are difficult to diagnose and it is not correct to treat such patients with hormones, without proper confirmatory laboratory tests.

In recent years advances in newer techniques have been developed, by which almost all hormones in blood and tissue fluids can be estimated by the following tests :

1) Radioimmuno-assay technique
2) Competitive protein binding method
3) Fluorometry
4) Cytochemical methods

By the technique of immunological assay antibodies against pituitary, thyroid and adrenal glands have been detected. The role of autoimmune factors in the aetiology of endocrine diseases has been recognised, which were previously considered idiopathic.

It is due to these modern sophisticated methods, role of hypothalamus as chief whip of endocrine orchestra, has been established. Earlier we thought that it was the anterior pituitary gland which was in supreme control of the other endocrine organs.

The discovery of prolactin as an anterior pituitary hormone is also a great advance in this field. It is now known that hyperprolactinaemia may be related to many gonadal disorders.

Dopamine is now established to be the prolactin releasing hormone of hypothalamus. Pharmacology of bromocriptine has been realised, as a real dopamine agonist. Bromocriptine is a semi-synthetic alkaloid obtained from ergot, its chemical structure being 2-bromergokryptine. This compound has no cardiovascular or oxytocic action of ergot alkaloids but is a compound which is true long acting dopamine receptor agonist. It has direct action on hypothalamus to lower serum prolactin. It also causes a little elevation of GH in normal subjects while fall of GH in patients with acromegaly.

Today this wonder drug is available for suppression of puerpereal lactation and for treating patients with hyper-prolactinaemia and acromegaly. High blood level of prolactin may cause amenorrhoea and gonadal dysfunction, probably by blocking action of gonadotrophic hormones.

Clinical eye alone is not therefore always adequate in recognising borderline cases of endocrine disorders. Moreover, to start treating these cases without proper laboratory tests is not justified.

The problem becomes more acute, especially in developing countries, due to limited laboratory facilities, as these tests can only be done by specially trained laboratory technicians in highly sophisticated laboratories. The normal values of these tests are also not so absolute and comparable, as in case of chemical tests.

In radio-immunological or competitive protein binding tests, the techniques of preparing reagents are not so well standardised, hence each laboratory must prepare their own reagents, to establish normal levels of their own centre.

*These factors have made tremendously difficult impact in our practice in developing countries, where limited facilities are only available in the vast areas, due to lack of such specialised laboratories. Hence clinical recognition will still remain a major diagnostic factor atleast for selection of cases for referral to specialised centres.*

Genetic, familial, racial and environmental factors have also to be kept in mind, as many of these factors may produce syndromes mimicking dwarfism, hirsutism, anorexia nervosa and obesity. None of these may have any specific endocrine basis.

It is, however, well established now, that hypothalamus situated above the midbrain and below the optic thalamus is really the band-master of most endocrinologic functions. The pituitary gland and hypothalamus are intimately related. The pituitary gland has two lobes, anterior and posterior. The posterior lobe is really a projected bundle of neural tissues containing axons from paraventricular and supraoptic nuclei of hypothalamus. There are a tuft of blood vessels around the pituitary stalk extending from hypothalamus to the pituitary known as hypothalamo-hypophyseal portal system, carrying the transmitters or hypothalamic hormones. Besides its endocrine function, hypothalamus is the highest centre for autonomic nervous system, and controls sleep, thirst, body temperature and appetite.

**Origin of Endocrine Cells**

Most polypeptide hormone secreting cells arise from neural crests of the embryo. These cells later on migrate to their ultimate sites where the endocrine gland is formed to secrete specific hormones.

Many of these hormones are polypeptides having specific sequences of aminoacids of varying lengths of chain-like structure or configuration. Some hormones like steroids and sex hormones have cyclo-pentano-phenanthrine ringed structure, related to cholesterol chemically.

It is now well established that two messengers collaborate for action of many polypeptide hormones.

The first messenger, i.e. the hormone acts on the second messenger located on the surface of cell-membrane. Nucleotide cyclic AMP (the second messenger) on the cells surface, is then responsible to mediate the hormonal action on the enzymes within the cell.

Steroid hormones however act more directly and enter into the cells to be attached to the receptors within cytoplasm.

The secretion of anterior pituitary hormones is controlled by the hypothalamus, through releasing and inhibiting factors as follows :

| Hypothalamic Hormones | Pituitary Hormones |
|---|---|
| Corticotrophin — Releasing factor (CRF) | Growth Hormone (GH) |
| Luteinising hormone/follicle stimulating hormone-releasing hormone (LH/FSH-RH) | Thyrotrophin (TSH) |
| Growth Hormone-Releasing factor (GHRF) | Luteinising hormone and follicle-stimulating hormone (LH & FSH) |
| Thyrotrophin-releasing hormone (TRH) | Corticotrophin (ACTH) |
| Prolactin-release inhibiting factor (PRIF) | Prolactin (PRO) |

The interaction of hormones of hypothalamus and anterior pituitary gland and their functional relationship are presented in Table 8.1 and enumerated as follows :

**Table 8.1 : Hypothalamic Hormones**

1) Somatotrophin releasing factor (SRF) or growth hormone releasing factor (GH — RE) — Stimulates growth hormones (Somatotrophin of anterior pituitary gland).
2) Somatotrophin release inhibiting factor (SRIF) — Has opposite affect to SRF.
3) Corticotrophin-releasing factor (CEF or CRH) controls ACTH (corticotrophin secretion).
4) Thyrotrophin-releasing hormone (TRH) controls TSH secretion of anterior pituitary gland
5) Gonadotrophic releasing hormone (Gonadotrophin) controls both follicle stimulating hormone as well as leutinising hormone.
6) Prolactin-releasing hormone (PRH) and prolactin releases-inhibiting hormone (PRIH) controls prolactin (mamotrophin) secretion from the anterior pituitary gland.
7) Melanocyte-stimulating hormone (MSH) releasing factor (MRIF) and MSH release-inhibiting factor (MRIF). The last two hormones (6 and 7) have not yet been chemically identified and can better be called factors. The remaining hormones have been identified and synthesised.

However, therapeutic use of these hormones is still in the realm of experimental medicine.

**Dopaminergic mechanism of Hypothalamus :**

Recent researches have shown that certain neurones in the hypothalamus release, adrenaline, dopamine, and hydroxytryptamine. Of these, dopamine is the most potent factor influencing prolactin and growth hormone secretion, through the cells which secrete the neurotransmitters from the hypothalamus.

Bromocriptine can increase growth hormone secretion and decreases prolactin secretion in normal individuals. Bromocriptine is now used in the treatment of hyperprolactinaemia, which is often associated with amenorrhoea in females.

Bromocriptine have also been found paradoxically to reduce the level of growth hormone in acromegaly and is useful in the treatment of acromegaly. This action is possibly mediated through the abnormal receptor sites of the pituitary tumour cells.

Some drugs block dopamine receptors e.g. phenothiazines, reserpine and oestrogen. These drugs can raise the prolactin level in blood causing galactorrhoea.

## PITUITARY GLAND

*S. KUMAR*

The pituitary gland has two lobes, anterior and posterior. Posterior pituitary gland is developed from a diverticulum arising from the floor of the 3rd ventricle. The anterior pituitary is developed from an outgrowth arising from the roof of oropharynx. (Rathke's pouch), i.e. both are ectodermal in origin.

**Anatomy and Physiology :**

The pituitary gland is situated in the pituitary fossa called (sella turcica) in the body of sphenoid bone. It is roofed over by a tough membrane of dura mater called the diaphragm sellae. It related to cavernous sinus as well as 3rd, 4th, 6th cranial nerves and it lies below the optic chiasma. It is supplied by direct branches of internal carotid artery and the veins drain into the carvernous sinus. The posterior pituitary is connected to the hypothalamus via the pituitary stalk. Around the stalk a tuft of blood vessels runs downwards from the median eminence of the hypothalamus to anterior pituitary. This is called hypothalamo-hypophyseal portal system. It conveys the neurohormones from the hypothalamic nuclei to the anterior pituitary. In severe post-partum haemorrhage or in any forms of severe shock if the blood pressure suddenly falls below critical level, there is a spasm of arterioles specially affecting sensitive areas of hypothalamus; this in turn leads to infarction of the anterior pituitary gland but post-pituitary is rarely affected.

The anterior lobe of the pituitary gland contains chromophobe, eosinophil and basophil cells. Chromophobe cells are the precursors of chromophil cells, which produce active hormones. The anterior pituitary gland secretes several hormones but are released through hypothalamic hormonal influences. Posterior lobe is called pars nervosa which contains nerve cells (pituicytes) and nerve fibres.

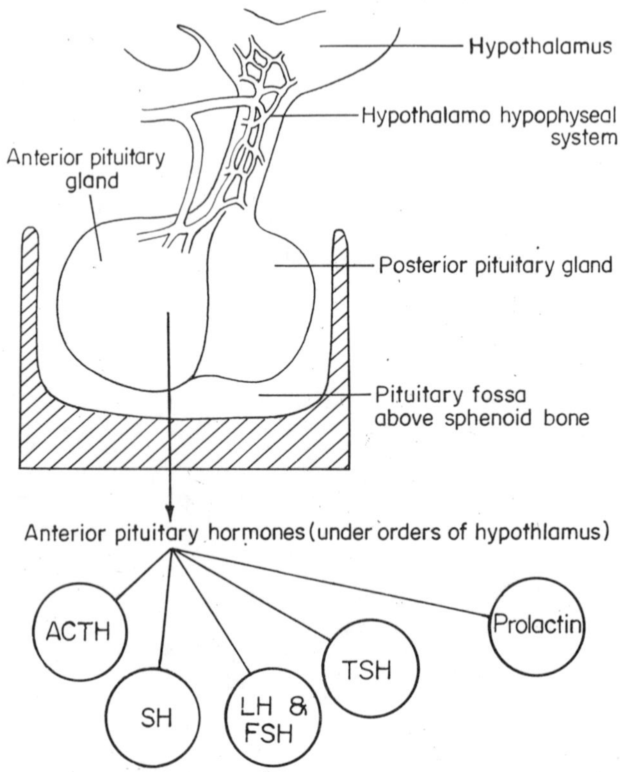


Fig.8.1 : PITUITARY HORMONES — Note posterior pituitary hormones are prepared in hypothalamus and come via hypothalamico-hypophyseal system to the posterior pituitary gland.

Anterior pituitary hormones control growth, metabolism, development and function of sex organs, lactation and skin pigmentation. Posterior pituitary is chiefly concerned with water and electrolyte balance. It has two hormones, oxytocin and vasopressin; oxytocin stimulates contraction of gravid uterus and vasopressin stimulates smooth muscle contraction and promotes water absorption through distal renal tubules.

**Hormones of the Anterior Pituitary Gland**

1) Thyrotrophic hormones (T.S.H) : The thyroid stimulating hormone is glycoprotein in nature and stimulates the synthesis of thyroxine. It is not related to exophthalmos. In thyrotoxicosis, the TSH level is low and in primary hypothyroid state the reverse occurs.

2) **Gonadotrophins :** These are also glycoprotein in nature.

(a) **Follicle stimulating hormone (F.S.H.) :** Stimulates the ovarian follicle in females and spermatogenesis in males.

(b) **Leutinising hormone (L.H.)** : It stimulates the corpus luteum to produce progesterone and in the male it stimulates the interstitial cells of the testis (Leydig Cells).

**3) Adreno-corticotrophic hormone (ACTH)** : It is a polypeptide comprising of 39 amino -acids. The first 13 amino-acid sequence in ACTH and MSH is same and the melanin forming activity is dependent on this sequence. It stimulates the cells of adrenal cortex to synthesise the cortisol and to some extent the corticosterone. Adrenal androgens are also synthesised by ACTH stimulation.

**4) Growth hormone (GH)** : It is a polypeptide comprising of 191 amino acids with two disulfide bridges. It has got anabolic action and stimulates protein synthesis. It also causes lipolysis and increases NEFA (non-esterified fatty acids) in the blood. It has got considerable influence in carbohydrate metabolism producing insulin resistance and stimulating neoglucogenesis. Thus it is diabetogenic in nature. It has specific action on the epiphyseal cartilage, stimulating growth of the long bones. It is believed that the action of the growth hormone is mediated by somato median synthesised by the liver.

**5) Prolactin (mammotrophin)** : Causes enlargement of breasts during pregnancy and controls lactation.

**(6) Melanocyte stimulating hormone (M.S.H.)** : Concerned with skin pigmentation by its melanocyte stimulating effect.

**Hormones of the posterior pituitary gland :**

Posterior pituitary gland is actually a storage organ for vasopressin and oxytocin. Hormones of the hypothalamus are carried through the neural stalk, through the axons, to reach the posterior pituitary gland. The release of vasopressin is controlled by the osmolality and tonicity of the plasma which stimulates the osmoreceptors of the hypothalamus. Structurally the vasopressin and oxytocin are similar with five amino acids arranged in a circular manner and a chain of three amino acids attached at one point.

## TUMOURS OF THE PITUITARY GLAND

Tumours of the pituitary gland accounts for 10% of all intracranial tumours while 85% of pituitary tumours arising from the chromophobe cells are non-secretory.

Tumours may be :

(1) **Macroadenoma** — Causing enlargement of pituitary gland and pressure effects. Sometimes it may cause symptoms of hypopituitarism due to pressure atrophy of secretory cells.

(2) **Micro-adenoma** — Causing no pressure effects or enlargement of pituitary fossa.

Excess pituitary hormone may also occur due to lack of hypothalamic imbalance. Excess of hypothalamic releasing hormone or deficient inhibitory hormone may be responsible.

Acidophil cell tumour causes acromegaly and gigantism. Micro-adenoma of the acidophil cells secreting prolactin is not uncommon. Basophilic tumours are rare and when present causes Cushing's syndrome.

Occasionally tumours arising from the remnants of Rathke's pouch are called craniopharyngiomas. It is commonly suprasellar and causes pressure on the optic tract and pituitary gland. These tumours may occur in children and are liable to undergo frequent calcification.

**Clinical features :**

Clinical features are due to pressure effects and hormonal deficiency or excessive hormone secretions.

**Pressure-effects :**

Pressure effects are due to macro-adenomas causing enlargement of pituitary fossa or encroachment of adjacent structures.

- **Headache —** It often may be a prominent symptom. It is central in type and occasionally associated with nausea and vomiting due to stretching of the dura mater.
- **Visual symptoms —** Are due to pressure on the optic chiasma leading to characteristically bitemporal hemianopia involving both the superior quadrants in the beginning.
- **Perimetry** is useful in localising the lesion. Other cranial nerves may be involved in 20% of cases and the patient complains of diplopia, squint and ophthalmoplegia.
- **Pressure on the hypothalamus** any cause disturbance in sleep, appetite and emotional behaviour and there may be fits of the uncinate type.

**Destruction of the anterior pituitary cells :**

More than 75% of the pituitary cells have to be destroyed before producing any signs due to hormonal deficiency. The earliest hormonal deficiency is lack of gonadotrophins followed by lack of growth hormone, ACTH and lastly TSH.

Deficiency of prolactin is not manifested except in Seehan's syndrome. ACTH reserve may be normal at rest but is unable to cope under conditions of stress.

Occasionally diabetes insipidus may be produced. This condition may be readily diagnosed by a skiagram of the skull (lateral view), tomography and, if required, by CT scan.

Skiagram of the lateral view of the skull shows widening of the floor of the pituitary fossa due to erosion of the bony wall and disappearance of the anterior and posterior clinoid processes due to osteoporosis. Normally adult pituitary fossa measures 15 mm. horizontally and 12 mm. vertically.

**Treatment :**

Radiotherapy or surgery depending on the merit of each case and the size of the tumour.

## PITUITARY APOPLEXY

This is a serious complication due to haemorrhage within the tumour leading to sudden blindness, shock and hypothermia and progressive drowsiness, associated with headache and vomiting due to increased intracranial pressure.

**TREATMENT :**

Neuro-surgical approach to control the bleeding, may be necessary. However, emergency treatment with diuretics, glucocorticoid and resuscitative procedure may be life saving.

**Empty Sella Syndrome**

Occasionally routine radiograph of the skull reveals enlarged pituitary fossa without visual field defect or clinical manifestations of pituitary disorder. In these rare cases the normally functioning pituitary gland is situated at the periphery and the central part appears empty. This may possibly be due to leakage of CSF from the diaphragma sellae or due to a pituitary cyst which bursts into the subarachnoid space.

**Hyperfunction of the pituitary gland :**

Hyperfunction of anterior pituitary gland may be due to tumours or hyperplasia of the hormone secreting cells.

**Hyperfunction Anterior Pituitary Gland :**

Gigantism and acromegaly due to over-production of growth hormone by acidophilic cells (microadenoma or hyperplasia).

Microadenoma or hyperplasia of the lactophil cells (a type of acidophil) causes excessive secretion of prolactin. This causes hirsutism, galactorrhoea, amenorrhoea in females and impotence in males.

This syndrome of lactation in non-puerperial women often associated with obesity is described as Forbes-Albright syndrome. This condition can now be readily diagnosed by CT—scan and by estimating serum prolactin levels which is invariably increased.

It can be treated by bromocriptine or microsurgery. The latter is becoming popular than to remove a microadenoma of the pituitary.

**Other causes of galactorrhoea :**

1) Chiari Frommel syndrome causing amenorrhoea, gonadal atrophy, psychological disorder and persistent lactation possibly due to hypothalamic disorder.
2) Hypothalamic disorders resulting from cranio-pharyngioma, sarcoidosis, metastatic or inflammatory disorders of hypothalamus.
3) Drugs, e.g. phenothiazines, reserpine and methyldopa.
4) Miscellaneous : Hypothyroid state (excessive TRH secretion), prolonged mechanical stimulation of the nipples, and acromegaly.

## HYPERFUNCTION OF BASOPHIL CELLS

This condition is rare and occasionally produces Cushing's syndrome due to bilateral adrenal hyperplasia.

Occasionally after bilateral total adrenalectomy, the microadenoma increases in size and produces pressure effect (Nelson's syndrome) and hyperpigmentation.

## GIGANTISM AND ACROMEGALY

**Medical history :** In 1866 Pierre Marrie described two cases of skeletal enlargement which later on came to be known as acromegaly. Later on, it was realised that acromegaly and gigantism are both due to excessive growth hormones of the anterior pituitary gland.

**Onset :** Acromegaly usually starts between third and fourth decades and has a slow insidious progression so the condition is likely to be missed.

**Progress of the diseases :**

The excessive growth may be arrested spontaneously at any phase. Usually the growth ceases after a period of years.

Sometimes the pressure effect of the tumour may cause hypopituitarism with features of hypogonadism, thyroid and adrenal insufficiency.

**Clinical Features :**

(A) Pressure effect

(B) Excess hormone effect.

(a) Pressure effect — Discussed before

(b) Excess hormone

1) **Facies :** Progressive coarsening of the facial features is obvious and scrutiny of old photographs may be quite useful in early diagnosis.

Bony changes include progressive enlargement of the mandible which in pushed forward resulting in prognathism. There is overgrowth of the maxilla and the frontal and nasal bones with enlargement of the sinuses.

There is also excessive growth of soft tissue with thick lips, enlarged nose, thick eyes and macroglossia.

2) **Hands appear enlarged as well as the feet.** Enlargement of feet necessitates change of shoes quite frequently. Similarly, due to enlargement of the hands, the gold rings (if any worn) become tighter and are difficult to be taken out.

In women, the bangles appear to become tighter. The hands look like spades with fingers becoming wider and thicker. Gain in weight is also seen in all the patients.

X-Ray of hands show tufting of the tips of the terminal phalanges and metacarpal bones, formation with cortical thickening of all the metacarpal bones. Due to pressure effect on the median nerve in the carpal tunnel — carpal tunnel syndrome may be produced often associated kyphosis is found with other bony changes.

3) **Visceromegaly :** All the viscera of the body are increased, cardiomegaly is found invariably in all the cases. This may lead to cardiac failure. However, hypertension is seldom found in these patients.

4) **Other endocrinal manifestations :**

(a) Thyroid — Thyroid gland is enlarged and palpable. But the thyroid function is usually normal.

(b) Gonads — In case of males, there may be enlargement of testes. In the early stage, sex urge may be increased. Later impotency and loss of libido are common.

In females amenorrhoea is usually present.

(c) GTT is impaired in 1/3rd of cases. In 10% of cases, glycosuria and frank diabetes may develop.

5) **Skin changes :** Skin becomes thickened and leather-like due to proliferation of fibrous tissue.

Shiny due to excess sweating and sebum production.

Hirsutism and fibrosum mollusacum are common associated findings.

**Diagnosis :**

(1) Clinical history and radiological examination of hands and skull are useful.

(2) Serum phosphorus is elevated in 1/3rd of cases.

(3) GH measurement :

Fasting level usually remains above long/ml.

After administration of 100 g. of glucose the level remains persistently high. In normal individual it usually remains below 5 ng/ml.

**Treatment :**

Depends on the stage of acromegaly.

1) Active acromegaly — This would be manifested by persistent pressure symptoms, sweating, hirsutism and greasy skin. The GH level would be high and GTT may also be abnormal.

2) Burnt out acromegaly or spontaneously arrested acromegaly is usually not associated with pressure symptoms or excessive hair growth.

Joint symptoms may be present but frequently there would be features of thyroid insufficiency, general weakness, dry skin and hypotension.

GH level would be normal. So to decide the treatment of acromegaly it is essential to assess the clinical manifestations, the growth hormone level, and other endocrine manifestation, especially adrenal and thyroid function.

If it is active acromegaly,proper treatment followed by substitution therapy is required.

Active treatment includes careful radiotherapy.

Surgical removal of the tumour by transphenoidal microsurgery or by transfrontal route is usually employed.

Bromocriptine, a dopamine antagonist is now recommended for treatment of acromegaly in dosage of 2.5 mg/3—4 times daily and the dose is increased as required. This may be useful if there is no visual defect or any other pressure symptoms.

**Complications :** Blindness, CCF, diabetes mellitus, pituitary apoplexy and intercurrent infection. Later hypopituitarism.

## HYPOPITUITARISM

Hypofunction of the anterior pituitary can affect all the trophic hormones and this condition is called Simmond's disease, the commonest cause of hypopituitarism. When it develops in children there is dwarfism and delayed puberty along with other features of hypopituitarism. In this group craniopharyngioma may be detected in some cases. Occasionally this can involve a single hormone, i.e. monotrophic deficiency as for example — Isolated growth hormone deficiency causes dwarfism, gonadotrophic deficiency causing hypogonadism and combined growth hormone and gonadotrophin deficiency causing infantilism. Sometimes hypopituitarism in varying degrees can result from deficiency of hypothalamic releasing factors.

### Dwarfism

When the height of an individual lies below the 3rd percentile with shortness of skeletal growth it is called dwarfism. This means, if height of 1000 children aged 12 years is measured, the level below which height of 30 children will fall, is defined as 3rd percentile.

### Types of Dwarfism

**1) Genetic dwarfism or familial short stature :**

Here there is history of dwarfism in the family bone age and teeth age are normal. Growth hormone response is normal. There is no specific treatment.

**2) Slow growth with delayed puberty :**

There is slight retardation of bone age and teeth age. Growth hormone response is normal. Sexual development is characteristically delayed. These cases may be treated with very low dose of androgen or estrogen but eventually they develop normal stature in due course. This is possibly due to delayed maturation of hypothalamopituitary gonadal axis. It is a constitutional delay.

**3) Primordial dwarf :**

This may be associated with or without congenital anomalies. They may have low birth weight and may have other physical abnormalities. (Ptosis, deformity of little finger, craniofacial disproportion known as Seckles syndrome bird headed dwarfism).

Bone age and teeth age are normal and GH response is normal.

Aetiology is unknown but placental insufficiency and intrauterine infection as in rubella, syphilis and toxoplasmosis. Occasionally growth hormone treatment is beneficial.

**4) Chromosomal disorder :** (Turner syndrome)

Here the appearance is short stature with webbing of the neck and increased carrying angle. There is primary amenorrhoea and infantile gonads and no secondary sex characteristics. Bone age, teeth age and growth hormone response are all normal. Occasionally the bone age may be slightly retarded and estrogen treatment has been found in some cases to produce the pubertal stimulus and promote skeletal growth.

The treatment should be started at the expected age of puberty.

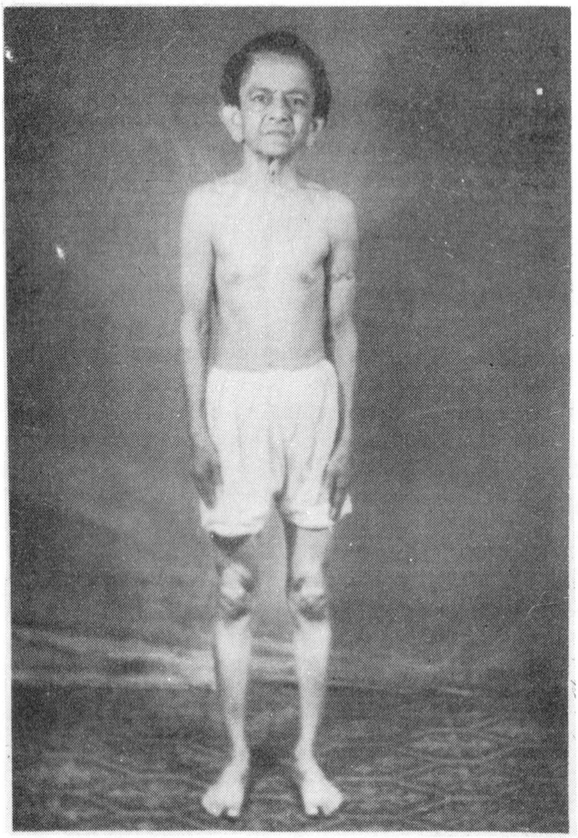

Fig.8.2 : GENETIC DWARF — (Mentally normal. Occupation: stage acting; Aged 52 — Editor's Case)

**5) Systemic disorders :**

This includes malnutrition, malabsorption syndrome, cyanotic congenital heart disease, chronic renal failure, renal rickets, bronchial asthma particularly if they are treated for a long time with corticosteroids which depresses the growth hormone secretion.

**6) Skeletal disorders :**

These conditions primarily affect the growth of long bones and the trunk is usually of normal length while the legs are shorter typical examples are seen in cases of achondroplasia. Other causes include epiphyseal dysplasias, metaphyseal dysplasia and pseudo hypoparathyroidism.

**7) Endocrine disorders :**

(a) Thyroid deficiency which includes cretinism and juvenile myxoedema.

(b) Hypopituitarism : Any causes producing pan-hypopituitarism before puberty will result in dwarfism along with other features (Fig.14.1).

**Selective growth hormones deficiency :** Occurs in about 10% of cases of dwarfism and is observed in early years of life. Bone-age and teeth-age are considerably retarded and growth hormone response is poor (less than 5 mg/ml. after stimulation with insulin 0.1 unit per kg. of body weight or levodopa 10 mg/kg of body weight).

(c) **Excessive androgen or estrogen production** or exogenous administration which promotes early epiphyseal fusion. This can be observed in cases of adrenogenital syndrome and certain testicular and ovarian tumours. It causes precocious sexual development and early epiphyseal fusion.

**Psychosocial dwarfism :** Here there is emotional disturbance frequently due to maternal deprivation characterised by low growth hormone response. This condition can be successfully treated by removing the child to suitable environment. It is suggested that it is a hypothalamic disorder — (functional hypopituitarism).

When glucocorticoids are administered in growing children in large doses for a long period dwarfism is common. This can be seen in Cushing's syndrome in children and long term steroid therapy in children producing shortness of stature.

In 50% of such cases abnormalities of other hormones can be demonstrated. This condition can be treated with administration of growth hormone 2.5 mg/twice a week and the growth rate is about six inches within the first year. This has to be continued for a few years.

**Frohlich's syndrome :** This is a condition first described by Alfred Frohlich in 1901 and really a secondary hypopituitarism. It is hypothalamic disorder characterised by subnormal height, (growth hormone releasing factor — GHRF deficiency) hypogonadism (gonadotrophic release hormone, i.e. G.N.R.H. deficiency) pituitary tumour. The hypothalamic lesion may be idiopathic or due to an inflammatory lesion of the hypothalamus or compression from pituitary tumour or cysts arising out of the third ventricle. Obesity is common.

## SIMMOND'S DISEASE

In 1914 Morris Simmonds described a condition characterised by weakness, wasting and failure of sex organs. There was fatal termination and after autopsy atrophy fibrosis of the pituitary gland was found.

**Causes of Hypopituitarism :**

1) Injury — traumatic, surgical removal of tumour or irradiation to the pituitary.

(2) Infection — Following meningitis, encephalitis, chronic tuberculosis and rarely syphilis.

3) Vascular — (a) Post partum haemmorrhage causing hypotension, thrombosis and spasm of the vessels leading to ischaemia and necrosis of the anterior pituitary gland (Sheehan's syndrome)
- (b) Diabetic atherosclerosis
- (c) Sickle cell anaemia
- (d) Cavernous sinus thrombosis
- (e) Temporal arteritis.

These are rare causes except Sheehan's syndrome.

4) Infiltration (very rare) —
- (a) Hands Schuller Christian Disease
- (b) Sarcoidosis
- (c) Haemochromatosis

5) Tumour : chromophobe adenoma and acromegaly in late stages.

6) Occasionally it can be secondary to hypothalamic disorder.

Among the causes of hypopituitarism — Sheehan's syndrome and pituitary tumours are common.

**Clinical features :** Clinical picture of hypopituitarism usually develops when more than 75% of gland is affected — the clinical manifestation of hormonal deficiencies occurs in the following order :

(1) Gonadotrophin — deficiency

(2) Growth hormone deficiency, e.g. dwarfism in children

(3) TSH deficiency

(4) ACTH deficiency

(5) Prolactin deficiency which is readily recognised in Sheehan's syndrome by failure of lactation.

Total ablation of the pituitary gland without replacement therapy is incompatible with human survival.

With partial deficiency the onset is gradual :

(1) Gonadotrophin deficiency — There is progressive atrophy of breast and areola with depigmentation of the nipple (ACTH) deficiency there is diminished libido and atrophy of the gonads. The testes become soft and small and there is atrophy of uterus and vagina. In women there is amenorrhoea and in males there is azoospermia.

There is loss of axillary and pubic hairs which may be totally absent, which is an important diagnostic clue particularly in cases of missed Sheehan's syndrome which may remain undiagnosed for several years.

Typical features of myxoedema are usually absent. Occasionally myxoedematous facies with weight gain may be seen. The common features include lethargy, lassitude, intolerance to cold, psychomotor retardation, dry skin, sparse hair, waxy pallor, delayed ankle jerk and normocytic normochromic anaemia.

These clinical features may take 5—10 years to develop or in severe cases may be obvious within six months after PPH. But in patients who have their pituitaries removed and operated upon and are replacement therapy, it takes 6—8 weeks for the symptoms to develop.

(2) **ACTH deficiency —** Without suitable replacement therapy there is danger to life. The earliest features include :

(a) Muscular asthenia with weakness and lassitude and atrophy of the muscles;

(b) Vascular asthenia – small thready pulse, hypotension with systolic B.P. around 90 mm Hg; and

(c) G.I. symptoms including sweating, nausea and occasional cases of vomiting and weight loss.

In Sheehan's syndrome, the onset is more gradual. Skin pigmentation often decreases specially absence of tanning after exposure to sunlight is a diagnostic feature of this disease.

(3) **Prolactin deficiency :** Failure of lactation in Sheehan's syndrome.

**Anorexia nervosa :** This clinical condition has to be differentiated from hypopituitarism which occurs in young women with a history of psychological disturbances. There is severe loss of appetite which leads to emaciation and amenorrhoea. The axillary and pubic hairs are present. The thyroid and adrenal function tests are within normal range. The gonadotrophin secretion is normal or low normal and growth normal response is normal.

**Diagnosis of Hypopituitarism :**

(A) Evidence of possible cause of hypofunction of pituitary.

(B) Demonstration of hormonal deficiencies.

(a) As already discussed common causes include Sheehan's syndrome and pituitary tumour history of post partum haemorrhage is always present in Sheehan's syndrome and may take several years before this condition is suspected.

Similarly persistent headache, visual field defect and X-ray of this skull reveals an enlarged sella turcica in pituitary tumours.

(b) **Laboratory tests :**

(i) Adrenal function — Urinary 17-hydroxysteroid excretion and plasma cortisol level is low after administration of ACTH 40 units daily for 3 days. Synthetic ACTH (tetracosactrin) can be used to demonstrate the rise in plasma cortisol level within a few hours.

**Metyrapone tests :** This substance inhibits synthesis of cortisol by blocking the action of 11B — hydroxylation. In normal persons after administration of metyrapone 500 mg every 6 hours for 48 hours there is a rise of 17-hydroxysteroid excretion (more than 50% above control level).

(ii) The plasma TSH level, T3T4 and $I^{131}$ uptake is low. After administration of 10 units of TSH daily for 3 days the $I^{131}$ uptake is normal.

(iii) FSH and LH level in the plasma are abnormally low or absent. Even after administration of (GNRH) gonadotrophin releasing hormone the level of gonadotrophin would be low.

(iv) GH response : After injection of insulin 0.1 unit per kg. of body weight or L-Dopa 500 mg. in a single dose there is no rise of GH level.

If the level is below 5 mg/ml. this is diagnostic and between 5mg/ml. it is borderline.

**Treatment :** Replacement therapy should be instituted so that the patient can lead a normal life. Cortisol therapy is mandatory and should be given in dosage of 20 mg. in the morning and 10mg. in the evening. The dose of gluco-corticoids may have to be increased in conditions of stress.

Thyroxine (Eltroxin) should be given 0.1 mg tablet half to one tablet daily, the dosage may be adjusted according to the patient's need.

Oestrogen or testosterone may be given to restore normal sexual function. Ethinyl oestradiol 50 mg daily or methyl testosterone 40 mg twice daily may be given orally. Alternatively Testosterone propionate may be given I.M. (25 ml.g per week). Prednisolone in daily dose of 5—10 mg daily may be given instead of cortisol.

## DIABETES INSIPIDUS

*S. KUMAR*

Diabetes insipidus (D.I.) is a clinical condition characterised by profuse urination usually between 5—20 litres per day of low specific gravity due to deficiency of A.D.H. from the posterior pituitary gland. J.P. Frank in 1794 first described this clinical entity.

**Cause**

(1) In 50% cases no cause is detectable (Idiopathic)

(2) **Injury :**

This may follow trauma, neurosurgical procedures and irradiation to the pituitary gland. The D.I. in these cases may be transient and may improve with time. Care need be taken in instituting treatment in this group.

(3) **Tumour :** Pituitary tumour, craniopharyngioma and rarely metastatic tumour from Ca-Breast, Ca-Bronchus can produce D.I. by damaging the post-pituitary gland.

(4) **Infection :** Meningitis, encephalitis and tuberculosis and syphilitic affection of the brain may cause D.I.

(5) **Infiltration :** Hand Schuller Christian disease and Sarcoidosis.

**Nephrogenic D.I.** In this type the renal tubules are unresponsive to the ADH. Long acting thiazides like chlorthiazide acts dramatically in such cases. It is a hereditory defect and appears in children. In some cases the unresponsiveness of the tubules may be secondary to kidney disease like pyelo-nephritis or glomerulonephritis causing tubular damages.

**Clinical features :**

The onset is rapid. There is polyurea and urinary volume varies from 5-20 litres with specific gravity around 1005. There is intense thirst for water. With excessive loss of water there is rapid dehydration weakness and constipation.

**Diagnosis :** Wherever possible the aetiology should be determined. Past history of meningitis, tuberculosis, presence of visual field defect, abnormal sella turcica etc. may be helpful. Tubular reabsorption failure can be assessed by —

(1) **Water deprivation test :**

The patient is not allowed to drink water for 12 hours and this produces 3—5% loss of weight. In normal persons it produces rise in urinary specific gravity to 1020 or more and urinary osmolality rise above 800 mmol/litre.

In D.I. urinary specific gravity remains around 1005 and urinary osmolality around 200 mmol/litre. Occasionally the response may be better but it never reaches normal level. In case of compulsive water drinking the response is excellent and may go up to normal or near normal level.

(2) **Hypertonic saline test :**

2.5% of hypertonic saline is given I.V. at the rate of 15 drop a minute for 45 minutes and the urine output is measured every 15 minutes. In normal person there is sharp antidiuresis with rise of urinary specific gravity. In D.I. there is poor response.

(3) **Nicotine test :**

The test consists of injection of nicotine I.M. one mg of Nicotine is given to non-smokers and three mg to smokers. In normal persons it induces fall in urinary output which raises the specific gravity. D.I. shows poor response. However, side-effects like nausea, dizziness, salivation and flushing may be troublesome.

(4) **Vasopressin test :**

Vasopressin can be used as a nasal spray. Administration of 20 mgm causes rapid antidiuresis with improvement of symptoms in case of D.I.

Alternatively 5 units of pitressin tannate in oil can be given I.M. at 7 A.M. which produces significant improvement next morning when hourly output of urine is measured.

In cases of compulsive water drinking, the response is poor as the patient continues to drink water and develops water intoxication with headache, nausea, vomiting, drowsiness and may have epileptic fits.

(5) **Plasma osmolality :**

| | |
|---|---|
| Normal level | 280 ± 6 mmol/litre |
| In D.I. it is high | (295 ± 15 mosmol/lit) |
| In C W D it is low | (265 ± 10 mosmol/lit) |

As the normal values vary widely, in some cases diagnosis may be difficult.

**Causes of Polyurea :**

(1) **Diabetes Mellitus :**

Produces osmotic diuresis because of high glucose content in the urine; other features of diabetes and determination of blood sugar and urinary sugar establishes the diagnosis.

(2) **Chronic Nephritis :**

Polyurea is due to tubular atrophy and dilute interstitial fluid into renal tissue. The urine volume varies between 2 and 3 litres and there is history of renal disease with presence of albumen, high blood urea and granular caste in the urea. Hypertension and eye changes may be clinical associations.

(3) **Hypercalcaemia :**

It produces renal damage due to deposition of $CA^+$ in the renal tubules, and $Ca^+$ level is always high.

(4) **Hypokalaemic :**

It produces tubular damage causing diuresis. The cause of hypokalaemia can be usually established and serum $K^+$ is always low. ECG may show flat or inverted T waves.

(5) **Compulsive water drinking (CWD) :**

In this group there are invariably some psychological disturbances and in clinical practice, the differentiation from D.I. is essential. The tests described above would be sufficient for diagnosis. In CWD, response to water deprivation test (WDT) is excellent and response to VT is poor with feature of CWI which may supervene in CWD. Contrary to this in D.I. response to VT is excellent and response to WDT is poor.

**Treatment :**

Vasopressin tannate inj. or snuff along with fluid restriction is sufficient to control the disease. In mild cases, chlorthiazide, chlorpropamide and clofibrate may be useful. These drugs promote ADH release and potentiate the action of tubular reabsorption of water. Chlorthiazide reduces the GFR by causing $Na^+$ depletion. (Refer to Appendix).

## SYNDROME OF INAPPROPRIATE ADH

**Causes :**

(1) Malignant disease : Oat-cell carcinoma of the bronchus, Ca-pancreas, lymphosarcoma and other neoplastic disorders.

(2) Pulmonary causes : Tuberculosis, lung abscess, injury to chest.

(3) CNS : Trauma, cerebral strokes.

(3) Sedatives : General anaesthetics, narcotics, barbiturates

(5) Hypothyroidism : In these cases there is dilutional hyponatraemia with feature of water intoxication, e.g. headache, nausea, vomiting and drowsiness. The urinary $Na^+$ excretion is high and urine osmolarity is high. After water load for patient, shows poor diuresis and the urine osmolarity fails to reduce.

**Treatment :**

(i) Fluid should be restricted.

(ii) Hypertonic saline (5%) may be given with Frusemide.

(iii) Fludro-cortisone 0.3 — 0.4 mg daily may be useful.

(iv) Demethyl chlortetracycline is effective as it interferes with renal tubular reabsorption; daily dose is 900-1200 g. lastly, whatever drug is used, the underlying cases should be treated whenever possible.

# THYROID GLAND

*S KUMAR*

## Anatomy.

The thyroid gland has two lobes joined by an isthmus. It is situated in front of the neck, the isthmus lying just below the cricoid cartilage. The two lobes are closely affixed to the anterior and lateral aspects of trachea by loose connective tissue. Average weight of adult gland is about 20 mg.

**Blood supply :** Chiefly by two pairs of arteries : Superior thyroid arteries arising from the external carotids and inferior thyroid arteries from the thyrocervical trunk enter the respective poles.

Average blood flow to the gland ranges from 4—6 ml/min/g.

## Microscopic Structure :

Through light microscope the gland is found to be made up of numerous tiny follicles or acini (200 $\mu$ in diameter) which are lined by a single layer of cuboidal epithelium and containing in its interior a clear proteinaceous colloid. The size of the acinar epithelium varies with the degree of glandular activity, becoming columnar when active, and flat when inactive.

In addition to the follicular cells, the thyroid gland contains parafollicular cells, which are the source of the calcium lowering hormone, calcitonin.

## Physiology of the Thyroid Gland :

The thyroid gland plays a very important role in physical and mental well-being of an individual from the very beginning of life, its function is to synthesize, store and secrete two thyroid hormones, thyroxine ($T_4$) and Tri-iodothyronine ($T_3$). An essential constituent of these hormones is iodine. Normal daily requirement of iodine is 100-200 $\mu$ g and is derived from natural water, vegetables grown in iodine containing soil, fish, meat, cow's milk and iodinated table salt.

## Synthesis of Thyroid Hormones :

Step—1 : Iodide uptake from the plasma by the thyroid gland is an active transport requiring energy for the process. This step is stimulated by the thyroid-stimulating hormone (TSH) and inhibited by thiocyanates and perchlorates.

Step—2 : Oxidation of iodide to iodine, meditated by an enzyme — iodide peroxidase. However, the iodine never appears as such in the free state, but is immediately organified.

Step—3 : Organic iodination, which involves binding of iodine to tyrosine-residues in the glandular protein to form monoiodotyrosine (MIT) and di-iodo-tyrosine (DIT).

Step—4 : Oxidative coupling, again through mediation of peroxidase, thyroxine being produced from two molecules of DIT, while tri-iodo-thyroxine results from coupling between a MIT and DIT. Both Step 3 and Step 4, primarily the former, are inhibited by thiouracil and carbimazole. These are stored in combination with a glycoprotein — thyroglobulin in colloid state within the acini of the gland.

## Release of thyroid hormones

The release of hormones involves initial pinocytosis of follicular colloid into the follicular cell and subsequent fusion with thyroid lysosomes to form phagolysosomes, hydrolysis by proteases and peptidases to produce free iodo-thyronines including $T_4$ and $T_3$ — a step stimulated by TSH. Finally, release of $T_4$ and $T_3$ into blood, while inactive iodotyrosines are stripped of their iodine by an intrathyroidal enzyme, iodotyrosine dehalogenase, so that iodine is retained within the gland for future use.

## Transport of thyroid hormones

In plasma, $T_3$ and $T_4$ are bound to thyroid binding proteins. Minute quantities of free hormones are adequate for metabolic purposes and induction of feed-back effect. In plasma 99% of the T3 and T4 are bound to thyroid hormone-binding proteins.

In the peripheral blood, most of the hormonal iodine is thyroxine and a very small proportion is tri-iodothyroxine. However, an occasional normal subject may be predominantly T3 secretor. About 60% of T4 is bound to a specific thyroxine binding globulin (TBG), 30% to a pre-albumin (TBPA) and 10% to albumin. Normally less than 0.05% of T4 is in the 'free' or, non-protein bound state. This free hormone, which is in reversible equilibrium with the bound form, is the metabolically active form. Homeostatic regulation of thyroid function is aimed at maintaining a normal concentration of the free rather than total hormone.

**Regulation of thyroid hormone secretion**

This is dependent upon a reciprocal 'feed-back' mechanism. The immediate regulator of thyroid function is thyrotropin or TSH, a glycoprotein secreted by basophilic cells of the anterior pituitary gland. TSH stimulates hypertrophy and hyperplasia of the thyroid and augments all steps in iodide metabolism in the gland leading to synthesis and secretion of thyroid hormones. These actions are thought to be mediated, at least in part by cyclic 3′5′ adenosine monophosphate (CAMP).

TSH secretion, in turn, is controlled by two opposing influences :

— A stimulatory effect of thyrotropin releasing hormone (TRH) a tripeptide secreted from the hypothalamus and an inhibitory negative feed-back effect of the level of free thyroid hormones in blood, thyroid hormones may have direct effect on secretion of TRH also.

**Physiological effects of thyroid hormones**

Thyroid hormones have widespread physiological effects which are mediated through influence on cellular metabolism in most tissues.

Many intracellular enzymes are increased following administration of thyroxine and one of these is alpha glycerophosphate dehydrogenase which is important in degradation of carbohydrates.

Skeletal growth, sexual maturation and mental development, all require normal thyroid function.

An important aspect is its calorigenic action, which was initally thought to be caused by uncoupling of oxidative phosphorylation; but later workers have suggested that this caused by specific synthesis of proteins involved in oxidative phosphorylation.

## THYROID FUNCTION TESTS

Thyroid function tests are carried out to determine the functional status of the thyroid gland, whether hypo-hyper euthyroid. In case of hypothyroidism these are also useful to determine whether it is primary or secondary.

(1) Total serum T4 : Normal range is 4—11 μg/100 ml, though it may vary slightly from laboratory to laboratory.

Total serum T4 measures both the bound and free forms of T4. It has the advantage that its value is not unduly influenced by exogenous iodides. But the value will be altered by changes in the level of TBG.

In thyrotoxicosis, total serum T4 is high. But falsely high values may also be found due to elevation of TBG values as in pregnancy, oestrogen therapy, including oral contraceptive pills, drugs like clofibrate and phenothiazine.

In hypothyroidism, T4 level is low. But falsely low values may again be met in conditions associated with true or, apparent low values of TBG, as in androgen therapy nephrotic syndrome, hepatocellular failure, corticosteroid administration in high dosage, active acromegaly or congenital abnormality.

**Note :** Certain drugs like salicylates, phenylbutazone, sulphonylureas and phenytoin compete for the binding sites on TBG and cause falsely low values for T4.

(2) **Total serum T3 (Tri-iodothyronine)**

Normal level is 70—170ng/100ml. The limitations are similar to total serum T4 in relation to level of TBG, although to a lesser extent. Particular importance is in diagnosis of T3-thyrotoxicosis, where T3 is elevated, while T4 is normal. Serum T4 and T3 may decrease with ageing particularly after 65 years.

(3) **T3 resin uptake**

This test measures the degree of saturation of the binding sites on the thyroid hormone binding proteins (TBP). It is carried out by adding radioactive T3 to patient's serum *in vitro*. Some of the added T3 will be taken up by the unbound sites of the patient's TBP. The remaining unabsorbed T3 is the absorbed in a resin and amount of T3 uptake by the resin is measured.

In thyrotoxic patients, most of the binding sites on the TBP are already saturated, so on addition of radioactive T3 very little of it gets absorbed on patient's TBP or, in other words a large fraction of added T3 is taken up by the resin, hence it gives a higher than normal value for T3 resin uptake.

With a similar reasoning it can be shown that T3 resin uptake will be low in hypothyroidism.

However conditions that alter TBP concentration will also affect T3 resin uptake value but in a direction opposite to that found in estimation of total serum T4.

(4) **Serum free thyroxine and free thyroxine index :**

Normal value of free T4 is about 2ng/100ml.

Ideally, serum free T4 should be measured to get an accurate idea of the metabolic state as it is the free from which is metabolically active. However, this direct measurement is difficult. Hence, an indirect approach is used — in the form of **Free thyroxine index (FTI).** It is calculated as : Total serum T4 × T3 resin uptake. This value is independent of the concentration of TBP and correlates well with the amount of free-non-protein bound T4 as measured by the more difficult procedure.

In clinical practice this is the single most reliable indicator of thyroid secretory function.

(5) **Serum rT3 (Reversed T3)**

T3 is mostly obtained from T3 and differs from it only by a different positional attachment of the 3 iodine atoms. Measurement of serum rT3 may be useful in selected clinical conditions. Normal level ranges from 20 to 40ng/100 ml.

(6) **Radioactive iodine uptake (RAIU)**

This is an important test for assessing thyroid function. Physiologically speaking, it measures the iodine concentration ability of the thyroid and is only indirectly related to thyroid hormone synthesis or, release. The usual radioisotope to be used is $I^{131}$ with a half life of 8 days and the uptake is usually measured after 24 hours with the help of a suitable counter over the thyroid. The normal range of 24 hours uptake is 15—45% of the administered dose (however, the range should be determined by each laboratory).

Increased RAIU occurs classically in

(a) Hyperthyroidism; it may, however, be seen in certain other conditions also, eg. :
(b) Iodine deficiency
(c) Dyshormonogenesis
(d) Recent stoppage of antithyroid drugs
(e) Recovery from subacute thyroiditis.

Low RAI occurs in :

(a) Hypothyroidism, primary or secondary

(b) Iodine excess, either from ingestion of iodine containing medications, e.g. iodochlorhydroxy-quinoline (a common antiamoebic drug), cough mixtures etc. or from use of contrast agents for special radiographic studies, e.g. cholecystography or pyelography.

(c) Cardiac or renal insufficiency.

(e) Low RAIU may also be associated with certain thyrotoxic states, namely, thyrotoxicosis factitial and iodine induced hyperthyroidism.

Apart from measuring the radioactivity over the thyroid gland, renal clearance of radioiodine can also be measured — these values vary in inverse proportion to the RAIU, i.e., are high in hypothyroidism and low in hyperthyroidism.

(7) **Thyroid suppression test**

In a normal person exogenous thyroid hormone (in this test, usually given as $T_3$ 20 $\mu$g thrice daily for 7 days) suppresses pituitary TSH and hence the RAIU falls below 50% of previous level. If the thyroid gland is functioning as an autonomous entity, e.g., in Graves' disease, autonomous thyroid nodule etc., exogenous $T_3$ fails to supress RAIU. Apart from helping in diagnosis of Graves' disease, this test is also useful in guiding when antithyroid drugs may be stopped in Graves' disease (for return of $T_3$ suppressibility usually indicates that there will be no relapse on stopping antithyroid drugs).

(8) **Serum TSH level**

In myxoedema (primary thyroid failure) it is significantly raised, while in thyrotoxic states the level is undetectable the radioimmunoassay techniques currently available.

This test is especially useful for diagnosing primary hypothyroidism.

(9) **TRH stimulation test**

This is of particular use when diagnosis of hyperthyroidism is in doubt. The principle of the test is that in Graves' disease because of autonomous $T_3$ and $T_4$ secretion. TSH response to TRH administration is suppressed. The test consists of determining serum TSH levels before and 30 minutes after administration of a standard intravenous dose of TRH (usually 200 ng.). In a normal case, TSH rises by at least 15 units/kl. and the peak response is at 20—30 min. In primary hyperthyroidism (even if mild and serum $T_4$ and/or $T_3$ levels are equivocal) there will be no TSH response to TRH, and this is the main value of the test.

In primary hypothyroidism there is a high basal level of TSH and an exaggerated response to TRH.

In hypothyroidism due to pituitary disease, the TSH response is absent or impaired; when the cause of thyroid failure lies in the hypothalamus the TSH level shows a slower rise and the highest level is seen at 60 minutes.

(10) **Thyroid scan**

This involves scintiscan or, gammascan with Radioiodine ($I^{131}$) or, technetium (Tc 99m) and is useful for defining areas of increased or decreased function within the thyroid; it also helps in detecting retrosternal goitre, ectopic thyroid tissue and functioning metastatic thyroid carcinoma.

In Graves' disease there is uniform increased radioactivity over the thyroid; in case of single or, multiple autonomous toxic nodules, the nodules show up as 'hot' areas on the scan, surrounded inactive thyroid tissue. A 'cold' nodule (i.e. an area of very low radioactivity surrounded by normal thyroid tissue) raises the suspicion of thyroid malignancy; however, a cyst or, benign adenoma can also have a similar appearance.

# THYROTOXICOSIS

*S KUMAR*

The term 'thyrotoxicosis' refers to the clinical condition resulting from the presence of excessive amounts of thyroid hormones in the circulation. The various conditions that could lead to such clinical state are listed below :

(1) Graves' disease — By far the commonest cause of thyrotoxicosis and characterised by thyrotoxicosis, diffuse goitre, ophthalmopathy and sometimes dermopathy. As the toxic symptoms are noticed at the same time as the thyroid becomes enlarged, it is also known as primary thyrotoxicosis.

(2) Toxic multinodular goitre, also termed secondary thyrotoxicosis as features of thyrotoxicosis supervene on a goitre that is present for quite some years.

(3) Toxic adenoma.

(4) Thyrotoxicosis factitial— Due to self-administration of thyroid hormone, for a long time.

(5) Ectopic thyroid tissue producing thyrotoxicosis

(a) most commonly located in the ovary — Struma ovarii

(b) metastatic functioning thyroid carcinoma. As a whole, however, this is a rare cause.

(6) Thyrotoxicosis due to excessive production of TSH or TSH—like peptides.

(a) Production of TSH-like peptides by trophoblastic tumours, e.g. hydatidiform mole or choriocarcinoma of testis.

(b) Production of excessive amounts of TSH itself — by a very rare TSH, a secreting tumour of the pituitary.

It is important to recognise from the above list that the conditions (4) and (5) are not associated with any hyperfunctioning of the thyroid gland itself; on the contrary the anatomical thyroid gland is suppressed and the gland is not palpable in these disorders.

There may be some justification in calling these conditions thyrotoxicosis without hyperthyroidism.

We shall now discuss these above conditions in some detail, the maximum stress being given to Graves' disease.

## GRAVES' DISEASE (Basedow's disease)

**Medicial History :** The three major manifestations of Graves' disease are : (i) Diffuse toxic goitre (ii) Ophthalmopathy, and (iii) Dermopathy.

However, all these three manifestations may not be present in a given patient, dermopathy being the one which is most often absent; moreover, the three tend to run a course largely independent of one another.

### Incidence

**Age :** Though no age is immune, it is most common in the third and fourth decades of life. In general, males tend to develop the disease at an older age than females.

**Sex :** There is a marked female preponderance — a ratio of affected females to affected males being about 7:1.

### Familial incidence

There is a distinct familial predisposition to Graves' disease. In addition, family members of patients with Graves' disease may have various other thyroid disorders — some clinical, some only biochemical.

### Aetiopathogenesis

With respect to the thyrotoxic aspect of Graves' disease, it is obvious that there is a disruption of homeostatic mechanisms that normally control thyroid hormone secretion. The basis of this disruption is now believed to be an immunologic disturbance leading to development of auto-immunity. The autoimmune basis is supported by (a) the association of Graves' disease. Hashimoto's thyroiditis and primary thyroprivic hypothyroidism, with other disorders known to have autoimmune basis, for example pernicious anaemia, myasthenia gravis, primary adrenocortical failure and rheumatoid arthritis.

(b) Various immunoglobulins of the IgG class have been identified in Graves' disease, which have specific actions on different regions of thyroid cell membrane.

These include LATS, LATS protector, TBII, TSI etc.

LATS (Long Acting Thyroid Stimulator)

It was Adams and Purves who first demonstrated that serum from patients with Graves disease, when injected into mice, produce a sustained increase in radio-iodine uptake by the thyroid. This was later identified as an IgG immunoglobulin and described as Long Acting Thyroid Stimulator (LATS) as its action was more prolonged than that of TSH. This is generally said to be present in only about 50% of patients with Graves' disease.

LATS Protector :

Serum from about 90% of patients with active Graves' disease contains another IgG which is stimulatory for human, but not mouse, thyroid tissue. Since this material is capable of preventing the binding of LATS with thyroid tissue in vitro, it is called **LATS protector.**

T.B.I.I. (TSH binding inhibitory immunoglobulin)

By radio-receptor technique it is now possible to demonstrate an immunoglobulin from serum of active Graves' disease which binds to human thyroid cell membrane and thus prevents the binding of $I^{125}$ labelled TSH to its receptor site. This binding inhibitory immunoglobulin (TBII) or TSH displacing activity (TDH) is demonstrable in about 60% of cases.

**T.S.I. (Thyroid Stimulating Immunoglobulin)**

An immunoglobulin has been detected in the serum of 80% of patients with active Graves' disease which is capable of stimulating adenylate cyclase activity of human thyroid tissue. This is known as thyroid stimulating immunoglobulin (TSI) or, human thyroid adenylate cyclase stimulator (HTACS). Another IgG has been demonstrated, which increases colloid droplet formation in human thyroid tissue, this being termed **Human Thyroid Stimulator (HTS).**

The exact role of these various humoral antibodies is yet to be clarified.

The aetiopathogenesis of the ophthalmopathic component of Graves' disease is still obscure. In many patients with progressive infiltrative ophthalmopathy, the serum contains an immunoglobulin, distinct from LATS, which can cause exophthalmos in various animals.

A recent theory suggests that there is retrograde lymphatic transport of thyroglobulin to the retrobulbar tissues and this sets up an immune reaction, which in turn causes an inflammatory infiltrate consisting of lymphocytes, plasma cells and mast cells and also deposition of mucopoly-saccharides.

The aetiology of dermopathy of Graves' disease is not known.

### Pathology

**Thyroid gland** is diffusely enlarged and vascular. The enlargement is cause by parenchymatous hypertrophy and hyperplasia, characterised by increased height of the epithelium and is associated with lymphocytic infiltration. The **ophthalmopathy** of Graves' disease is characterised pathologically by infiltration with lymphocytes, plasma cells, mast cells and also deposition of a mucopolysaccharide complex in retro bulbar space. The extrinsic eye muscles in the orbit are mainly involved and are often oedematous. The muscle fibres show degenerative changes with loss of striations and eventual fibrosis.

**Dermopathy** consists of a thickening of the dermis due to deposition of mucopolysaccharides and infiltration by lymphocytes.

**Clinical Features**

The clinical picture in a full blown case of Graves' disease includes –

(A) Features of thyrotoxicosis
(B) Diffuse goitre
(C) Infiltrative ophthalmopathy
(D) Infiltrative dermopathy.

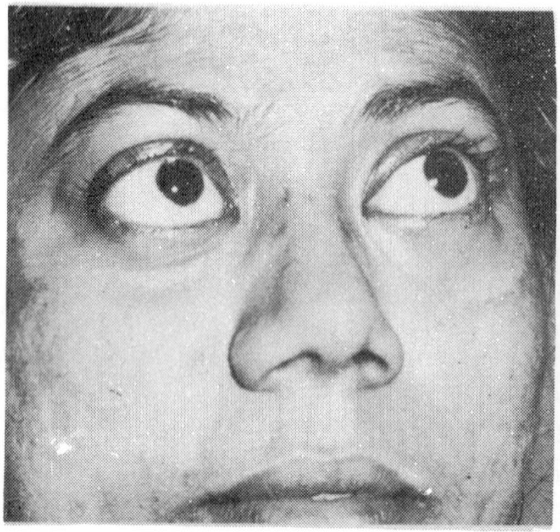

Fig.8.3 : Early thyrotoxicosis (Editor's Case)

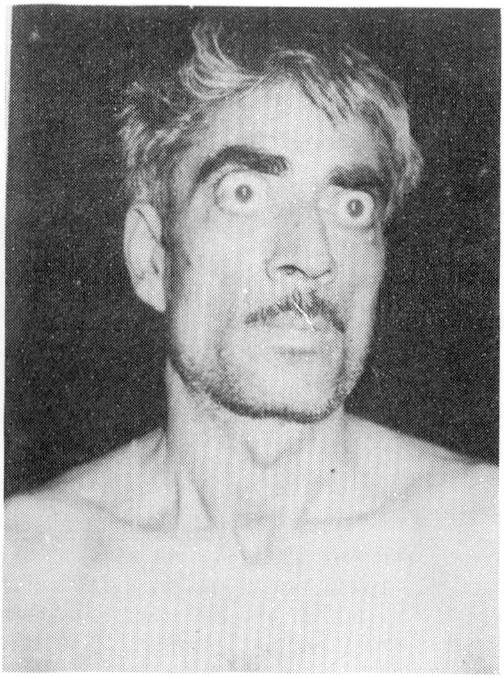

Fig.8.4 : Florid thyrotoxicosis (Editor's Case)

**(A) Features of thyrotoxicosis**

The common manifestations are tachycardia and palpitation, fine tremor, nervousness, emotional lability and hyperkinesis, heat intolerance and excessive sweating, weight-loss despite an increased appetite and the characteristic staring look with widened palpebral fissures and infrequent blinking.

The details are described below :

**(1) Cardiovascular system :**

These changes are mediated by direct stimulatory effect of thyroid hormone on the heart, as also by adrenergic stimulation, most probably by increasing the number of $\beta$-adrenergic receptors.

(a) Palpitation : This may be the subjective complaint of the patient due to tachycardia and is present at rest as well as on exertion.

(b) Tachycardia : The heart rate and pulse rate are almost invariably raised and persists during sleep. In fact, sleeping pulse rate about 90/mm. is one of the cornerstones in the clinical diagnosis of thyrotoxicosis. (Rarely thyrotoxicosis has been reported with normal pulse rate).

(c) Blood pressure : There may be gross peripheral vasodilatation which causes an increase in systolic and considerable decrease in diastolic pressure leading to wide pulse pressure and **Water-Hammer pulse,** an increased capillary pulsation.

(d) Apex beat and heart sounds : Apex beat may be forceful and displaced due to cardiac enlargement. Increased intensity of first heart sound, (fybctuibak systolic murmur), and high pitched second heart sound in the pulmonic area are all evidences of hyperkinetic state.

(e) Cardiac arrhythmias – These are almost invariably supraventricular and include paroxysmal supraventricular tachycardia and paroxysmal or persistent atrial fibrillation. About 10% of patients with Graves' disease have atrial fibrillation. These arrhythmias are more common in the elderly.

(f) Cardiac failure : This may occur in thyrotoxicosis and is an example of high-output failure. However, heart failure is uncommon without underlying heart disease or, cardiac arrhythmia. The response to digitalis is poor and dose requirement is high, probably due to rapid metabolism of the drug. However, one should remember that mild pedal oedema may occur in thyrotoxicosis even without heart failure.

(2) **Nervous system :**

(a) Behaviour and emotion :

Characteristically, the patient is irritable, restless, hyperkinetic and unable to concentrate; there is also marked emotional lability and the patient may sometimes cry out without reason. Rarely, there may be frank psychosis.

(b) Tremor :

There is fine tremor of the hands, well demonstrated by asking the patients to hold out the hands with the fingers separated. Tremor of the tongue and lightly closely upper eyelids, are also seen. This is an expression of increased adrenergic activity.

(c) Thyrotoxic myopathy : This is clinically manifested by gross wasting and weakness of the limb-girdle musculature and shoulder muscles are worst affected. An early clinical indicator is difficulty in climbing up stairs. Thyrotoxic myopathy is more common in males than in females.

E.M.G. may show polyphasic potentials, but myopathic pattern is absent.

These changes are mostly reversible with successful control of thyrotoxicosis. Rarely, ocular muscles may also be affected and the condition may mimic myasthenia gravis.

In this context, it should be remembered that true myasthenia gravis may co-exist with Graves' disease and this is more common in femles.

Muscle weakness in a patient with Graves' disease may also be due to associated hypokalaemic familial periodic paralysis. This is mostly seen in Chinese and Japanese.

**(3) Gastrointestinal system**

**Increased appetite,** both at meal times and in between meals, is commonly present. However, because of a hypermetabolic state, there is commonly **weight-loss** in spite of the increased appetite.

In severe cases and particularly in the elderly, anorexia may be seen.

There is commonly **increased frequency** of bowel movement; the stool is less well-formed, but frank diarrhoea is rare.

Symptoms like nausea, vomiting and abdominal pain may herald the onset of thyrotoxic crisis.

Gastric achlorhydria is often associated with thyrotoxicosis, secretion usually returning with control of thyrotoxicosis.

Hepatic dysfunction may be seen in severe thyrotoxicosis and will be manifested by hypoalbuminaemia and raised transaminase levels in serum.

**(4) Ocular signs of thyrotoxicosis**

These are supposedly caused by sympathetic overstimulation causing contraction of Mueller's palpebral muscle and usually subside when thyrotoxicosis is corrected.

There are a number of classical clinical signs, descriptive of the ocular abnormalities of thyrotoxicosis, which are of historical and examination interest :

(a) Retraction of the upper eyelid, due to contraction of Mueller's muscle, leading to widened palpebral fissure — DALRYMPLE'S SIGN.

(b) On asking the patient to look down slowly, the upper eyelid lags behind the eyeball (lid lag), so that the while sclera becomes visible above the iris. — VON GRAEFE'S SIGN.

(c) Infrequency of blinking — STELLWAG'S SIGN.

(d) On looking upwards, there is no wrinkling of the forehead — JOFFROY'S SIGN.

(e) Inability to converge or sustain convergence — MOBIUS' SIGN.

The above manifestations may be asymmetrical or, even completely unilateral for a period. At this stage, it is important to realise that these changes characteristic of thyrotoxicosis are not due to infiltrative ophthalmopathy.

**(5) Skin and its adnexa**

(a) The skin is characteristically warm and moist reflecting a high basal metabolic rate.

(b) Palmar erythema, indistinguishable from that seen in hepatocellular failure, is often found and is a manifestation of perpiheral vasodilatation.

(c) Telangiectasia in various parts may also occur.

(d) Diffuse pigmentation of skin, somewhat like Addison's disease, rarely be seen. However, in uncomplicated cases buccal pigmentation is not present. Rarely, patchy vitiligo may also be seen.

(e) Hair : It is fine and friable and there may be undue loss of hair, particularly from temporal aspects of the scalp.

(f) Nail : Nails may be soft and friable. Plummer's nails may be seen, due to separation of distal margin of nail from the nail bed.

**(6) Reproductive system**

Thyrotoxicosis beginning in early life may cause delay in sexual maturation, though physical growth may be normal or even accelerated. Thyrotoxicosis starting after puberty may cause menstrual disturbances — oligomenorrhoea or amenorrhoea being seen in more than 50% of patients with severe thyrotoxicosis. Menorrhagia may rarely occur. A return to normal menstruation after control of thyrotoxicosis is usual. Impotence in males may be seen. Incidence of infertility and abortion is more in thyrotoxic females.

However, when pregnancy occurs in a thyrotoxic patient, the thyrotoxicosis may not change in severity or, may even be ameliorated.

**(7) Metabolism**

The essential action of thyroid hormones is an acceleration of metabolism.

(a) This is manifest by increased heat production, causing increased body temperature and *intolerance of heat.*

(b) Protein metabolism : Both synthesis and degradation of proteins are increased, but the degradation outweighs synthesis. This is reflected in the *loss body weight* and negative nitrogen balance.

(c) Carbohydrate metabolism : Oral glucose tolerance test is mildly abnormal and pre-existing diabetes mellitus is made worse, due to increased glycogenolysis and probably also due to increased degradation of insulin.

(d) Lipid metabolism : There is increased lipolysis, causing disappearance of fat-depots of the body. This is also manifested by rise in plasma free fatty acids and fall in serum cholesterol and triglycerides.

(e) Tendency to ketosis is increased.

(f) Calcium and phosphorus metabolism : Hypercalcaemia may be seen in 25% of cases; radiologically demonstrable rarefaction of bone and a negative calcium balance may be seen. These may be due to a direct effect of thyroid hormones causing net bone resorption; however, in a few cases there may be coexisting primary hyperparathyroidism.

(8) **Kidneys**

There is increased renal blood flow and increased glomerular filtration rare (GFR).

There may also be mild polyuria.

(9) **Haemopoietic system**

(a) There may be splenomegaly in 10% of cases and there may occasionally be lymphadenopathy and thymic enlargement as well.

(b) There is increased red cell mass either due to a direct stimulatory effect of thyroid hormones on bone marrow or, secondary to increased production of erythropoietin. But plasma volume also increases, so that haematocrit remains normal.

(c) Due to increase of 2,3-DPG in erythrocytes oxygen-haemoglobin dissociation curve shifts to the right, thus facilitating oxygen release from haemoglobin.

(d) Total leucocyte count may be low due to reduction in neutrophils.

(10) **Respiratory system :**

Dyspnoea is not uncommon in overt thyrotoxicosis and does not necessarily imply congestive cardiac failure.

It is partly explained by the increased ventilatory effort due to increased metabolic demands on one hand and a weakness of the respiratory muscles due to protein catabolism on the other.

## THYROTOXIC CRISIS OR THYROID STORM

Both these terms refer to a very serious complication of thyrotoxicosis which may supervene due to thyroidectomy, or any other surgery, or an acute infection, or any other stress, or sudden withdrawal of antithyroid drugs in a patient with uncontrolled thyrotoxicosis. The clinical manifestations include.

(a) Hyperpyrexia
(b) Cardiovascular : Extreme tachycardia and peripheral circulatory collapse
(c) Cerebral : Mental confusion, acute mania and delirium
(d) Gastrointestinal : Nausea, vomiting, diarrhoea and abdominal pain.

## APATHETIC THYROTOXICOSIS

This condition, seen more often in toxic multinodular goitre than in Graves' disease, may cause diagnostic difficulty. The patient is usually elderly; in contrast to the usual hyperkinesia, the patient is prostrated and depressed; rather than an increase in appetite, there is anorexia; the skin is cool, dry and wrinkled instead of the classical warm and moist skin; in addition ocular signs of thyrotoxicosis are absent or minimal; but the myopathic element is pronounced and cardiovascular changes like tachycardia, atrial fibrillation, or intractable heart failure are often prominent.

**Masked Thyrotoxicosis :** This is also seen in the elderly and the manifestations are unexplained diarrhoea, myopathy and atrial fibrillation.

The above description more or less covers the varied manifestations of thyrotoxicosis. We now turn our attention to the other components of Graves' disease.

**(B) Goitre :**

Goitre, i.e. enlargement of the thyroid gland is present in most cases of Graves' disease; however, in about 3% of cases, especially in the older age group, thyroid size is normal.

The goitre is in the form of a diffuse and usually symmetrical enlargement of both lobes, though occasionally one lobe may enlarge more than the other. Consistency of the thyroid varies from soft to firm. Occasionally, the goitre may reach such a huge size as to cause pressure symptoms like dyspnoea, or dysphonia or dysphagia. Often a thrill is palpable and a bruit heard over the gland; the bruit is usually continuous, but occasionally is only systolic. A bruit usually signifies that the patient is thyrotoxic, but rarely it may be heard in other conditions where the thyroid is markedly hyperplastic. It is important to distinguish a bruit arising from the thyroid, from a murmur arising from the heart.

**(C) Infiltrative Ophthalmopathy**

This condition, unlike the ocular changes of thyrotoxicosis, commonly follows a largely independent course and hence little influenced by control of thyrotoxicosis. Infiltrative ophthalmopathy is clinically obvious in about 50% of cases of Graves' disease. In an occasional patient there may occur infiltrative ophthalmopathy without goitre or thyrotoxicosis — this condition is termed Euthyroid ophthalmic Graves' disease.

The major manifestations of infiltrative ophthalmopathy are : (1) Exophthalmos or Proptosis of varying degree, (2) Congestive oculopathy, and (3) Ophthalmoplegia.

**(1) Exophthalmos or Proptosis :**

Clinically, exophthalmos is usually said to be present, if on looking straight ahead, the upper bulbar conjunctiva is visible. According to another view a strip of at least 2 mm width of sclera is visible between the lower margin of the iris and the lower eyelid. It is usually bilateral, though often asymmetrical.

It may be accompanied by periorbital oedema, which, in fact, tends to obscure the degree of exophthalmos.

The degree can be measured by various forms of exophthalmometer, which measure the anterior projection of the eyeball from the lateral angle of the bony orbit — the upper limit of normal being 20 mm. When the exophthalmos is severe it is known as malignant exophthalmos and there is inability to oppose the eyelids to panophthalmitis and corneal ulceration and infection. If unchecked, it may lead to panophthalmitis and blindness.

In this context, it may help to remember other causes of exophthalmos.

(a) Orbital neoplasms which may arise (i) from the eyeball, e.g. retinoblastoma or malignant melanoma, (ii) from the boundary walls of the orbit, (iii) from other soft-tissue structures in the orbit, or (iv) as secondary malignant deposits in any of the above structures from outside.

(b) Cavernous sinus thrombosis

(c) Internal carotid artery aneurysm and carotico-cavernous fistula

(d) Craniostenosis

(e) Hand-Schüller-Christian disease

(f) Idiopathic.

**(2) Congestive oculopathy**

It is manifested by (a) congestion, (b) oedema, and eventually (c) frank chemosis of conjunctiva, and (d) periorbital swelling. There may also be (e) subconjunctival haemorrhage. The early symptoms are gritty sensation in the eyes and increased watering. Ophthalmoscopy may reveal (f) congestion of the retinal veins and even (g) papilledema. If left unchecked these may progress to (h) optic atrophy.

**(d) Ophthalmoplegia**

This refers to the weakness of ocular muscles and most commonly manifests as (a) weakness of upward and lateral gaze. It gives rise to (b) squint or strabismus and (c) diplopia.

**(d) Infiltrative Dermopathy**

This is the most uncommon component of Graves' disease, being present in only 5—10% of cases. It is almost always associated with infiltrative ophthalmopathy.

The lesions are most commonly seen over the shins and *dorsum* of feet and are known as **pretibial myxedema** or localised myxedema. The nomenclature is confusing as it is not a feature of hypothyroidism *per se*. About half of the cases occur during the active stage of thyrotoxicosis; in the remainder the lesions develop after treatment. The lesions usually present as symmetrical, well-demarcated, raised and indurated shiny area, which do not pit on pressure. The surface usually has a *peau* d' orange appearance and may be hyperpigmented. These may be pruritic.

**Thyroid acropathy**

This refers to clubbing of fingers and toes together with hypertrophic osteoarthropathy which may accompany the infiltrative dermopathy.

**Natural history and course of Graves' disease**

The natural course is unpredictable. In some patients the thyrotoxicosis may persist and may even progress downhill; in others there may be waves of remissions and exacerbations. However, over a period of several years, the thyrotoxicosis may subside even without any specific treatment and the patient may even become hypothyroid.

Ophthalmopathy and dermopathy usually run independent and often self-limiting courses.

**Diagnosis of Grave's disease**

This has two components :

**A. Clinical —** Based on the various manifestations as described already. In a florid case, the clinical picture itself is diagnostic, in mild and typical cases laboratory tests would be valuable.

**B. Laboratory tests :**

The abnormalities seen in the various laboratory tests, which are of diagnostic or prognostic value, are as follows :

(1) Increased radioactive iodine uptake (RAIU) by the thyroid.

(2) Increased serum levels of $T_4$ and $T_3$.
However, in an occasional case only $T_3$ or $T_4$ may be increased.

(3) Increased free thyroxine index.

(4) Low serum TSH level.

(5) Impairment of $T_3$—Induced suppression of RAIU.

(6) Impairment of TRH-induced rise of TSH.

(7) Detection and measurement of thyroid stimulating immunoglobulins in serum. This is important in prognosticating the outcome is appearance of TSI from serum after antithyroid drug treatment generally suggests a lasting remission.

**Differential diagnosis :**

**(A) Anxiety state :**

This is the most common differential diagnosis. In anxiety state, the palms are cold and moist, while in Graves' disease, these are warm and moist. Moreover, in anxiety states, tachycardia does not persist during sleep.

**(B) Phaeochromocytoma**

Because of sympathetic overactivity and a hypermetabolic state, phaeochromocytoma may present with weight loss, tremor, tachycardia, sweating, neuro-psychiatric manifestations etc.

The most important clinical distinction is diastolic hypertension in phaeochromocytoma. Further differentiation is by finding elevated levels of vanillyl mandelic acid (VMA) in urine and normal levels of $T_3$ and $T_4$ in serum.

Other conditions which may occasionally cause diagnostic difficulty include cirrhosis, chronic obstructive airway disease, myeloproliferative diseases etc.

## TREATMENT OF GRAVES' DISEASE

Though our knowledge about pathophysiology has increased tremendously in recent years, treatment, in whatever form, cannot yet be aimed at the basic cause and so cannot be claimed to be curative. However, in some cases, the disease may enter a latent phase or it may run its natural course and go into remission during treatment.

Broadly, the treatment plan is divided into two parts :

I. General management
II. Specific therapy

**I. General Management :**

**1. Rest**

Except in mild cases an initial period of restricted physical activity is advocated. In severe cases, particularly with cardiac failure, rest in bed is essential especially for a week or two at the outset. However, most patients can be managed as outpatients.

**2. Sedation**

Mental rest should be achieved with the help of sedatives and tranquilizers, e.g. Diazepam 5 mg TDS, or Phenobarbitone 30-60, TDS, to start with.

**3. Diet**

High-caloric diet should be preferred.

**4. Adrenergic antagonists, e.g. $\beta$-blockers**

Because of the pronounced adrenergic component in thyrotoxicosis, various adrenergic antagonists have been used in this disorder; moreover, these may reduce conversion of $T_4$ to $T_3$. Of these, propranolol is the most popular.

Propranolol helps to control such manifestations as tachycardia and palpitation, nervousness, anxiety, excessive sweating, tremor, increased bowel activity and lid retraction. $\beta$-blockers are useful as (a) an adjunct to more specific forms of therapy, particularly in the initial stages when the response to conventional antithyroid drugs, or to radio-iodine is being awaited; (b) these are also extremely useful in the management of thyrotoxic crisis. (c) Some rely on $\beta$-blockers only for preparing the patient for surgery.

**Dosage**

In an average case, propranolol is used in a dosage of 20—40 mg 6—8 hourly.

**5. Thyrotoxicosis with atrial fibrillation**

Attempts to convert atrial fibrillation to regular rhythm by quinidine, or cardioversion with D.C. shock should be postponed until some weeks after hyperthyroidism has been controlled; in fact, in some patients sinus rhythm returns automatically after control of hyperthyroidism.

**6. Thyrotoxicosis and Surgery**

Surgical operations such as tonsillectomy, or appendicectomy in the thyrotoxic patient can carry the same risk of post-operative thyroid crisis as thyroidectomy in the uncontrolled thyrotoxic. If possible, such operation should be deferred until the patient has been rendered euthyroid.

**II. Specific treatment**

The main forms : 1. Conventional anti-thyroid drugs
2. Radio-iodine
3. Surgery

## 1. ANTITHYROID DRUGS

**Indications :**

(a) Initial form of treatment for children and young women with primary hyperthyroidism, particularly when thyroid enlargement is unobtrusive.
(b) Treatment of hyperthyroidism in pregnancy. The smallest effective dose should be used, otherwise the foetal thyroid will be depressed and the baby will be born with a goitre.
(c) In any patient with thyrotoxicosis where surgery is decided upon as the definitive form of treatment, antithyroid drugs have to be used initially to make the patient euthyroid and thus eliminate risks of post-operative thyroid crisis. However, some authorities rely solely upon adrenergic antagonists in the pre-operative preparation of patients.

Also, where radiotherapy is contemplated, if there is severe thyrocardiac disease, antithyroid drugs are also given initially for rapid control of symptoms.

**Drugs used :**

(a) **Perchlorates and thiocyanates**

These act by blocking the iodide uptake by the thyroid gland. However, because of serious side-effects like hypoplastic anaemia, these drugs have practically been discarded.

(b) **Thiourea derivatives**

These are the drugs currently in use, of which the commonly used ones are carbimazole, methimazole (a metabolic product of carbimazole) and Propylthiouracil.

Of these, only carbimazole (NEOMERCAZOLE)® is available here.

**Mechanisms of action**

Sequential inhibition of the following steps in thyroid hormone synthesis :

(a) Oxidation of iodide to iodine.
(b) Organic binding of iodine to tyrosine residues.
(c) Coupling of iodotyrosines to produce iodothyronines ($T_3$ and $T_4$) — this is believed to be the principal site of action.
(d) Propylthiouracil also inhibits peripheral conversion of $T_4$ to $T_3$ and may be the preferred drug where rapid control is needed.

**Dose schedule**

Usual starting dose of carbimazole is 40-60 mg daily, which is to be given at 8 hrs. intervals, and not merely thrice daily. However, in patients with severe thyrotoxic manifestations and very large goitre much larger starting dose may be needed — for the latent period for development of effect would be shortened by larger dose.

As these drugs inhibit the synthesis of hormones, but do not inhibit the release or peripheral action of already synthesised hormones, clinical response is felt after a latent period, usually about a week. Early response occurs in the form of a decrease in nervousness, palpitation, sweating and diarrhoea. Usually, normal metabolic state can be restored within 6 weeks. At this stage, the dose is usually reduced to one-third and continued. If thyroid gland enlarges in size during treatment, then small doses of thyroxine may be added.

**Features that may be aggravated following treatment :**

(a) Gland size may enlarge further in some. This may be due either to intensification of the disease process in its natural course, or due to induction of incipient hypothyroidism leading to excessive TSH stimulation by negative feedback.

(b) Pre-existing bruit over the thyroid may be accentuated.

(c) Ophthalmopathy may also get worse.

**Side-effects of drugs**

Probably the commonest is skin-rash; others include drug-fever, gastrointestinal disturbance, arthritis, hepatitis, lymphadenopathy and most important of all, agranulocytosis. Agranulocytosis usually presents with a sore throat and is usually seen in the first few weeks or months of starting therapy. Treatment involves prompt withdrawal of the drug and the condition is usually reversible. Some patients would also need antibiotics, steroids and isolation.

Every patient put on antithyroid drugs must be told to stop the drug immediately if sore throat develops and report for a leucocyte count. In this context, it is useful to recognise that granulopenia may be a forerunner of agranulocytosis. But at the same time it should be known that mild granulopenia may only be manifestation of thyrotoxicosis. So, if granulopenia is found in a thyrotoxic patient taking antithyroid agent, the WBC count should be repeated and if it continues to fall, then only should be drug be stopped.

If hypersensitivity reaction in the form of agranulocytosis is seen with one agent (e.g. Carbimazole), then some other agent (e.g. Perchlorate or propylthiouracil) has to be used for that patient in future. If these other drugs are not available then there are 2 alternatives.

(a) Symptoms controlled with propranolol with or, without steroids and the patient given radio-iodine.

(b) Patient subjected to surgery after preparation with propranolol and iodine.

**Duration of medical treatment**

The appropriate duration of treatment is matter of current discussion, but generally treatment is continued for at least 12 months and in many cases for 18-24 months. The withdrawal of the drug should always be gradual and never abrupt.

Incidence of fasting emission after the conventional duration of treatment is roughly 50% in females; in males, however, the success rate is lower.

There is no sure criterion to predict which patient will remain in remission, but there are two important guidelines :

(1) Decrease in size of the gland with treatment

(2) Return of $T_3$ suppressibility of the thyroid.

Certain newer tests like return of TRH responsiveness, or disappearance of thyroid stimulating immunoglobulins may also herald a favourable outcome.

In any case, most relapses occur within 6 months of stopping treatment and if the patient remains well 6 months after stopping drugs permanent remission may be hoped.

**Other durgs**

**Iodide**

In the past iodine in large doses was used in the treatment of thyrotoxicosis, before the use of antithyroid drugs prior to 1944.

**Mechanism of action**

(a) Inhibition of organic binding of iodine — Wolff-chaikoff effect. The effect is transient.

(b) Inhibition of hormone release.

**Drawbacks of using Iodine or iodides :**

(a) Loss of effect with time — "Iodine escape".

(b) It causes iodine enrichment of the gland, so that response to subsequent administration of antithyroid drugs is impaired.

(c) As it suppresses radioactive iodine uptake, radio-iodine cannot be given for several weeks after stopping iodine.

**Present-day uses of Iodine in thyrotoxicosis**

1. Thyroid crisis
2. Severe thyrocardiac disease
3. Preparation for subtotal thyroidectomy.

**Glucocorticoids**

**Mechanism** — (a) Inhibition of hormone release
b) Inhibition of peripheral conversion of $T_4$ to $T_3$.

**Use :** In thyroid crisis, along with iodine and antithyroid drugs.

**Lithium :** It also has got antithyroid action but has no advantage over the conventional agents.

**Radioactive Iodine**

It affords a relatively simple, effective and economic means of treating thyrotoxicosis.

**Indication :** A—Thyrotoxicosis above 40 years of age and now a days even for younger patients, who for some reason appear to have a short life-expectancy or, who have been sterilised. B—Recurrence of thyrotoxicosis after surgery.

**Disadvantages and contraindications :**

(A) Previous fears about radio-iodine were the risks of

(a) Leukaemia
(b) Thyroid malignancy
(c) Gonadal damage causing genetic defect in off spring.

However, the first two have not been substantiated; about the radiation risk to the gonads, one can say that the radiation dose delivered to the gonads is similar to that given during an intravenous urogram or barium enema and is probably negligible.

(B) However, because of potential teratogenic effects, a definite contraindication to its use is the presence, or, even contemplation of pregnancy.

(C) Another difficulty is its slow onset of action — response may not be maximal for 2-3 months.

(D) Another problems is an occasional radiation thyroiditis, appearing 10-14 days after administering radio-iodine. This is associated with excessive release of hormone into the blood. So patients with severe hyperthyroidism, or underlying heart disease should be rendered eumetabolic with antithyroid drugs before giving radio-iodine. Interruption of antithyroid drugs for at least 2 days before and after radioiodine will suffice to permit adequate accumulation and retention of administered radioiodine. Some authorities depend on propranolol only for the control of thyrotoxicosis.

(E) However, the major disadvantage with radio-iodine has been the onset of hypothyroidism, either early or late — after 10 years its incidence may approach 40-70%.

**Mechanism of action**

There is an initial inflammatory reaction, to be followed by (a) fibrosis and (b) progressive vascular narrowing; moreover, there appears to be some amount of (c) autoimmune destruction following radioiodine. These are responsible for the control of thyrotoxicosis and in some cases eventual hypothyroidism.

**Type of radioisotope used**

Conventionally, $I^{131}$ is used. $I^{125}$ showed some promise for it was expected that the lower energy and shorter path length of its $\beta$ emission would cause less permanent damage to the thyroid follicles — so theoretically incidence of hypothyroidism should be less. However, long-term trials have failed to establish its improved efficacy.

**Dosage** : It is difficult to standardise the dose as the susceptibility, or radio-sensitivity varies from patient to patient. The treatment is carried out in special centres.

About one-third of patients require a second dose of radioiodine — the dose has to be judged on clinical evaluation of the patient.

3. **SURGERY**

**Aim** — Removal of sufficient thyroid tissue so that remaining gland cannot secrete toxic amounts of thyroid hormones — thus aiming at permanent cure. This is in contrast to the temporary effect of antithyroid drugs.

**Indications**

(1) Graves' disease with large goitre because :
   (a) Such a case is less amenable to medical treatment.
   (b) The large goitre may be producing obstructive symptoms like dyspnoea, dysphagia, or hoarseness of voice.
   (c) Cosmetic reasons
   (d) A large goitre may also indicate callousness and apathy on the part of the patient in availing of medical facilities earlier. Such a patient cannot be depended upon to follow medical treatment for 1—2 yrs. and so surgery may be preferable.

(2) Recurrence of thyrotoxicosis in the younger age group (below 40 years) after medical treatment, especially if more than once.

(3) Patients who are unwilling, or cannot afford to continue medical treatment over a long period.

(4) Relatively young patients who show intolerance to antithyroid drugs.

(5) Secondary thyrotoxicosis in the younger age group.

**Pre-operative management**

This is very important because of the ever-looming danger of thyrotoxic crisis in the post-operative period.

The usual practice is to bring the patient to euthyroid state with antithyroid drug, with or without β-blocker. Then, for the last 10–14 days before operation Lugol's iodine 5–10 drops TDS or Potassium iodide tablet 60 mg OD is given to reduce the vascularity of the gland and to make it firmer, thus making surgery easier. Some authorities advise continuation of antithyroid drugs even while iodine is being given.

Pre-operative management may also be done with the help of β-blockers only, when propranolol may have to be given at 40 mg QDS or more. After the thyrotoxic symptoms and tachycardia are controlled, iodine is given as before; but propranolol is continued even on the morning of operation and also for 7–10 days after operation, until $T_3$ and $T_4$ levels return to normal.

**Nature of Surgery**

Subtotal thyroidectomy where about seven-eights of the gland is removed.

**Complications**

1) Haemorrhage at the operation site – An early complication, which may cause respiratory obstruction and requires urgent reopening of skin sutures to drain out the blood and ligation of the bleeder.

2) Thyrotoxic crisis – This dreaded complication is fortunately rare nowadays because of better pre-operative preparation.

3) Damage to recurrent laryngeal nerve – If damage (incidence 0-5%) is bilateral, then severe stridor due to airway obstruction occurs soon after operation and the treatment is emergency tracheostomy.

If damage is unilateral there is only some hoarseness of voice, which, too, recovers with time in most cases.

4) **Hypoparathyroidism**

Incidence 0–4%, may arise due to

(a) accidental removal of all 4 glands, or

(b) damage to their vascular supply. This is usually manifest within a week of surgery. Treatment is with calcium preparation and sometimes Vitamin D. In milder cases, it is possible to withdraw these after sometime, while in severe cases, treatment should be continued indefinitely.

7) Recurrence of thyrotoxicosis

Usually less than 10% and manifested within one year. It is best treated with radio-iodine.

6) **Hypothyroidism**

Usually develops within a year of operation. However, today it is believed that the incidence rises progressively with time, as is observed after radio-iodine. This may be explained by the contention that Graves' disease, in its natural evolution, eventually ends in hypothyroidism, due to autoimmune destruction. Incidence of hypothyroidism after surgery varies from series to series and also on the period of follow-up and may vary from 5-30%.

## SUMMARY OF TREATMENT

For patients above 40yrs, radio-iodine is the treatment of choice. If symptoms are severe, then initially antithyroid drugs are also given. For younger patients,if the goitre is small, antithyroid drugs should always be tried first.

Surgery is primarily indicated if the goitre is too big and causing obstructive symptoms, or is cosmetically unacceptable; moreover, surgery may be need if there are two recurrences after antithyroid drugs, or if the patient shows hypersensitivity to the available antithyroid agents. Before surgery, the patient is prepared with antithyroid drugs with or without propranolol and iodine is given for the last 10 days before surgery.

**Treatment of Thyrotoxic crisis**

Thyrotoxic crisis is grave complication of Graves' disease and it should be treated as an emergency. The treatment aims at controlling the severe thyrotoxicosis and the precipitating illness, if any, apart from providing general supporting measures. The actual management consists of the following :

1. Rest in bed and sedation with 60mg of phenobarbitone given IM is useful.
2. I.V. drip with glucose and saline of correct dehydration that is always present and also to provide some calories in the hypermetabolic state.
3. Iodine, given as IV sodium iodide acts rapidly by inhibiting release of hormones from the thyroid. Subsequently Lugol's iodine (1 mgm). may be given by Ryle's tube.
4. Steroids in large doses, e.g. hydrocortisone 200mg stat I.V. and then 100-200 mg every 6 hrs. for the first 48 hours.

   Apart from providing glucocorticoid support, these help by inhibiting hormone release from the gland and also inhibiting peripheral conversion of $T_4$ to $T_3$.
5. Provided there is no cardiac failure, propranolol 40 mg 6 hrly, is given orally or, better still 2 mg. IV.
6. Hyperpyrexia is treated with aspirin, cold sponge, ice-packs and inj. chlorpromazine to prevent shivering.
7. Large doses of antithyroid drug by mouth or by Ryle's tube. Here propylthiouracil is preferred to carbimazole because the former also inhibits peripheral conversion of $T_4$ to $T_3$. Propylthiouracil is given 4-6 hourly. The role of antithyroid drug is to initiate therapy for the post — crisis period and also to prevent iodine enrichment of the thyroid.
8. If heart failure of pulmonary congestion is present, digitalis and diuretics are to be used.

When treatment is successful, improvement occurs in 1-2 days and $T_4$, $T_3$ values quickly return to normal and recovery occurs within a week. At this time, iodine and steroids are gradually withdrawn and plans for long-term management made. As the condition improves, adequate nutrition should be maintained.

**Thyrotoxicosis in Pregnancy**

Pregnancy may occur in thyrotoxic women and also some women may develop thyrotoxicosis during pregnancy. Both these conditions produce hyperdynamic circulation and thyroid enlargement.

So, there may be diagnostic. The investigations of use are :

1. Plasma $T_4$ (corrected for pregnancy) only if it is more than 12 $\mu$g/100 ml, then thyrotoxicosis can be diagnosed.
2. Free thyroxine index.
3. TRH stimulation test which will show absent or poor response in thyrotoxicosis. This is probably the most useful test.

Thyrotoxicosis in pregnancy is usually treated medically. The requirement of antithyroid drug is less in pregnancy because of a decline in titre of thyroid stimulating immunoglobulin.

It is essential to know that antithyroid drugs cross the placenta and may cause goitrous hypothyroidism in the foetus whereas maternal Thyroxine does not cross the placenta. So, the dose should be kept to a minimum, even mild thyrotoxicosis in the mother may have to be accepted; in general, the daily dose of carbimazole should not exceed 20 mg. Treatment should be monitored so as to keep plasma $T_4$ within 12 $\mu$g/100 ml.

Iodine and propranolol are not used in the management, for the former may cause foetal goitre and the latter affects foetal growth.

Surgery is indicated only in the more severe cases (where requirement of antithyroid drugs is high) and is done only in the middle trimester.

The mother on antithyroid drugs should not breastfeed her baby, as the drugs are excreted in breast milk. Neonatal Thyrotoxicosis may be present which is self — arresting.

**Thyrotoxicosis in childhood and adolescence**

This almost invariably due to Graves' disease. Treatment is initially by antithyroid drugs for 1-2 years, though remission rate is lower in this age group than in adults. After the first course if there is relapse, or recrudescence, a second course of drugs is routinely employed. Some authorities recommend regular supplementation of thyroxine in this age group to ensure adequate growth. Surgery is done only if the second course of antithyroid drugs also fails.

## THYROTOXICOSIS FROM OTHER CAUSES

**Toxic Multinodular Goitre**

This refers to thyrotoxicosis developing in a case of multinodular goitre, usually long-standing. Many of these show low TSH levels and subnormal TSH response to TRH, even before, thyrotoxicosis appears, thereby suggesting some degree of pre-existing thyroid autonomy. However, unlike Graves' disease various thyroid stimulating immunoglobulins cannot be detected in these cases; and what causes the toxicosis to supervene is yet to be understood.

Overproduction of $T_3$ and $T_4$ is less in this condition compared to Graves' disease.

**Clinical features**

Usually seen in the elderly age group, above 50 years, who have multinodular goitre for several years; it is more common in females.

It is never associated with infiltrative ophthalmopathy and dermopathy.

In these patients, cardiovascular manifestations and myopathy predominate; obstructive symptoms may be seen due to restrosternal prolongation of goitre.

**Diagnosis**

Radio-active iodine uptake, $T_3$ and $T_4$ values may be only slightly raised.

$T_3$ suppression test and TRH stimulation test are useful in diagnosing the condition.

**Treatment**

Radioactive iodine is the treatment of choice. However, the dose required may be higher and in some a second course may be needed. The usual procedure is to make the patient euthyroid first with antithyroid drugs and then give radioiodine.

In patients with obstructive symptoms, surgery and proper preparation is the preferred form of treatment.

## TOXIC ADENOMA

Usually caused by a single adenoma which has been present for a long time and is distinctly less common than Graves' disease and toxic multinodular goitre. Histologically it is a follicular adenoma.

Thyroid scan demonstrates the adenoma as a "hot" nodule, i.e., the uptake of radioiodine is practically solely in the adenoma and the rest of the thyroid is suppressed. Usually seen in the age group 30-50 years. The thyrotoxicosis is usually milder than Graves' disease and infiltrative ophthalmopathy is never seen. Cardiovascular and myopathic manifestations are common. Occasionally, there may be spontaneous infarction in the adenoma and thyrotoxicosis becomes selfarrested. Characteristically, no bruit is audible over the adenoma.

Diagnosis made from raised RAIU, $T_3$, and $T_4$ and impaired response to TRH stimulation. Occasionally, $T_4$ is normal and $T_3$ alone is raised as per condition being known as $T_3$ toxicosis.

**Treatment**

Surgery is the treatment of choice. Alternatively radioactive iodine may be used, if surgery is contraindicated. Preoperative preparation with antithyroid drugs alone is sufficient, and iodine is not needed as such an adenoma is not very much vascular.

**Special aspects of Thyrotoxicosis**

T3 Toxicosis :

This is a state of thyrotoxicosis resulting from a predominant hypersecretion of T3, with normal T4, such a condition may precede the more common picture of elevation of both T3 and T4, but may rarely persist as such. This may be seen in all the main causes of thyrotoxicosis, e.g., Graves' disease, toxic multinodular goitre and toxic adenoma, but is particularly common in the elderly patient with a toxic adenoma. It is important to realise that a normal T4 level does not exclude thyrotoxicosis and T3, TSH levels and TRH stimulation tests may also have to be done.

**T4 Toxicosis**

This, as the name suggests, is a condition where thyrotoxicosis results from a rise in serum T4 only, while T3 is normal or low. This may be seen in iodine induced thyrotoxicosis and in thyrotoxicosis associated with severe inter-current illness (where peripheral conversion of T4 to T3 is impaired).

## THYROIDITIS

Thyroiditis is a generic term embracing several disorders of differing aetiology. There are four general types :

1. Hashimoto's thyroiditis
2. Subacute thyroiditis (de Quervain's thyroiditis)
3. Riedel's thyroiditis
4. Infective thyroiditis due to pyogenic or tuberculous aetiology

1. HASHIMOTO'S THYROIDITIS

This is a chronic inflammatory disease of the thyroid in which autoimmune factors are thought to play a prominent role and is a common cause of goitrous hypothyroidism.

**Pathogenesis**

Evidence of an autoimmune basis in this disease includes lymphocytic infiltration of the gland, as well as the presence in the serum of increased concentrations of immunoglobulins and very characteristically, of antibodies directed aganist several components of thyroid tissue. There is also association with other diseases in which autoimmune component is prominent, for example, pernicious anaemia, primary adrenocortical failure, S.L.E., rheumatoid arthritis, diabetes mellitus and Graves' disease.

It appears that either, or both of humoral and cell-mediated immune reactions may be involved in destruction of the gland. There is increasing evidence that these manifestations of autoimmunity result from a genetic defect in immune surveillance causing deficiency of suppressor cells.

Recently, a significant correlation with HLA—DRW 3 has been noted.

**Clinical picture**

It is seen most commonly in women around 40 years of age. A familial predisposition to various thyroid disorders is seen in this condition.

The commonest finding is firm enlargement of the entire thyroid gland, though one lobe may enlarge more. There is no nodularity. Pain and tenderness are rare except in the early stages, when differentiation from subacute thyroiditis becomes important. Compression of adjacent structures occurs only rarely.

Early in the disease, the patient is usually euthyroid, though rarely there may be mild thyrotoxicosis in the initial stages. With passage of time, hypothyroidism of increasing severity supervenes, owing to progressive replacement of thyroid parenchyma by lymphocytes or fibrous tissue.

As already mentioned there may be clinical features of other autoimmune disorders.

**Diagnosis**

The results of thyroid function tests are variable, depending on the stage of the disease. Initially, serum TSH and radio-active iodine uptake (RAIU) are often increased, but with normal serum $T_3$ and $T_4$. With the passage of time, however, radioiodine uptake (RAIU), $T_4$ and last of all, $T_3$ progressively fall to subnormal values.

The diagnosis is confirmed by the demonstration of various **thyroid auto-antibodies** in high titre. Four types of antithyroid antibody have been demonstrated in Hashimoto's thyroiditis.

(a) Antithyroglobulin antibody
(b) Antimicrosomal antibody
(c) Antibody against a colloid antigen distinct from thyroglobulin.
(d) Antibody against a nuclear component.

Of these antibodies, the first two are most important in clinical practice and the various techniques for their demonstration include tanned red-cell-agglutination, complement fixation, fluorescent antibody and radioimmuno assay. Because of simplicity and specificity, tanned red cell agglutination is the preferred technique. The antimicrosomal antibody is — more important as it is more frequently positive and usually in higher titre. This is particularly important in young patients (under 20 years) when antithyroglobulin antibody may not be detectable in half of the patients.

Rarely, (usually in the younger age group where antibody titres tend to be lower) thyroid biopsy (usually a needle biopsy) is needed for confirmation of the diagnosis and it demonstrates the diffuse lymphocytic infiltration, fibrosis and the characteristic oxyphil Ashkenazy cells.

**Treatment**

No treatment is usually necessary as long as the patient is euthyroid and the gland is not enlarging. Careful follow-up is essential. But later, as hypothyroidism develops, replacement with thyroid hormone is needed with $T_4$ usually in a dosage of 0.1 to 0.2 mg daily and this may have to be continued life-long.

Surgery is contraindicated except where pressure symptoms are present, or the goitre is too big and unsightly.

2. SUB-ACUTE THYROIDITS

(de Quervain's thyroiditis; Giant cell thyroiditis)

This disease, which often follows an upper respiratory infection, appears to be viral in origin; the mumps, coxsackie, ECHO, and influenza virus have all been implicated in its aetiology.

**Histopathology**

There is patchy infiltration with chronic inflammatory cells and varying degrees of degeneration of thyroid cells. A characteristic finding is follicles with colloid at the centre surrounded by multinucleate giant cells.

**Clinical picture**

Women are far more frequently affected than men and maximum incidence is in the fourth and fifth decades.

The disease usually starts with constitutional disturbances like fever, malaise and lassitude. There is associated pain and tenderness over the thyroid gland. The pain is aggravated by movements of the neck, or swallowing and may be radiated to the ear, lower jaw or back of the neck. Pressure symptoms like hoarseness or dysphagia may occasionally be seen. In some, tachycardia and palpitation may be important initially.

Physical examination reveals enlarged thyroid gland which is firm and tender on palpation; occasionally one lobe is more enlarged and occasionally tenderness may shift from one part of the gland to another.

The usual course is that the disease subsides on its own after a few months, leaving no sequelae. Rarely, it may persist longer and hypothyroidism ultimately develops.

**Diagnosis**

Typically there is a high E.S.R.

RAIU is invariably depressed during the active phase of the disease and gradually returns to normal as the disease subsides.

Initially, $T_3$ and $T_4$ values may be high because of leakage from damaged thyroid epithelium, while TSH is low. At an intermediate stage, $T_3$ and $T_4$ values may be lower than normal as stores of pre-formed hormone are depleted. But eventually, $T_3$, $T_4$ and TSH all return to normal.

**Differential diagnosis**

A. Haemorrhage into a pre-existing nodular goitre. In such cases :

(i) Tenderness is confined to the haemorrhagic nodule only, rest of the gland being non-tender.
(ii) ESR is usually normal
(iii) There is always history of pre-existing goitre

B. **Hashimoto's thyroiditis**

It is differentiated by :

(i) presence of high titre thyroid autoantibodies
(ii) different histopathological picture on biopsy (however biopsy is rarely needed)
(iii) tenderness is absent or minimal

C. **Acute pyogenic thyroiditis**

It is characterised by

(i) greater constitutional disturbance
(ii) marked leucocytosis
(iii) usually identifiable pyogenic focus
(iv) usually normal RAIU

**Treatment**

In mild cases, aspirin only is needed for control of symptoms.

In more severe cases, glucocorticoids, e.g. prednisolone 20—40 mg/day, are given and cause rapid improvement of clinical manifestations. Return of RAIU values to normal indicates the time at which steroids may be withdrawn without recurrence of symptoms.

Thyroxine (0.1 mg/day) is sometimes prescribed.

However, none of these influence the underlying disease process, which usually subsides on its own.

## RIEDEL'S THYROIDITIS

This is a very rare disorder seen in middle aged women and characterised by intense fibrosis of the thyroid and surrounding structures leading to induration of the tissues of the neck; it may be associated with mediastinal and retroperitoneal fibrosis. It was once thought to represent an extreme form of Hashimoto's thyroiditis but is now known to be a separate entity of unknown aetiology.

The thyroid is moderately enlarged, often stony hard in consistency and usually fixed to surrounding structures. Pressure symptoms are not uncommon. These features sometimes make it difficult to differentiate clinically from carcinoma; in such cases biopsy is needed.

RAIU is normal, or low. Hypothyroidism may be present in later stages. In some anti-microsomal and antithyroglobulin antibodies are demonstrable, but in low titres.

**Treatment**

If there are pressure symptoms, then surgery is needed. If hypothyroidism develops then replacement with thyroxine is obviously needed.

## HYPOTHYROIDISM

It is a clinical condition where there is deficiency or lack of thyroid hormone. The deficiency may be manifested in the newborn or in early infancy, when it is known as cretinism. When it starts around puberty, it is called juvenile myxedema and in adult life it is called myxedema.

**Aetiology**

On aetiological basis, the disease may be in the thyroid gland itself, i.e. thyroprivic hypothyroidism. But in some cases thyroid may be normal but the defect is in the hypothalamus or pituitary gland (i.e. trophoprivic type). Third variety is associated with goitre.

(a) **Thyroprivic hypothyroidism :**

Here there is progressive atrophy of thyroid tissue and the cause is unknown. It can also be due to thyroidectomy, antithyroid drug therapy, X-ray-radiation, or after $I^{131}$ therapy where insufficient or no functioning thyroid tissue may be present. Rarely in children there is thyroid aplasia and the child is born with cretinism (congenital defect).

(b) **Trophoprivic hypothyroidism** (secondary hypothyroidism)

Here the thyroid gland is normal but there is deficiency of TSH. This may be due to fault either in hypothalamus or in pituitary.

(c) **Goiterous hypothyroidism –**

Here hypothyroidism is associated with goitre. This could be due to :

(i) Auto-immune thyroid disorder (Hashimoto's thyroiditis)
(ii) Defective hormone synthesis due to enzyme deficiency (dys-hormonogenesis)
(iii) Iodine deficiency in certain endemic areas
(iv) Administration of antithyroid agent as PAS, phenylbutazone, lithium; excessive administration of iodine can rarely induce hypothyroidism. Cabbage can also induce goitre.

Common causes include atrophy of the thyroid gland, following surgical or medical treatment of thyrotoxicosis, Hashimoto's disease and iodine deficiency in endemic areas.

Atrophy of thyroid gland is more common in women around 40 years, with insidious onset. About 70-80% of these cases show circulating thyroid antibodies and some of them are a part of polyglandular atrophy with involvement of gonads, adrenals, parathyroid glands, and pancreas. Parietal cell antibodies are detected as in (juvenile-onset diabetes) in the blood in some cases.

Atrophy of the thyroid gland, Hashimoto's thyroiditis, and Graves' disease are grouped together as autoimmune disorders. The natural course of all the three conditions end in hypothyroidism.

## MYXEDEMA

*(Adult hypothyroidism)*

*Clinical Features :*

**Facial appearance**

More than 70% of the patients have characteristic facial appearance. The face appears pale (due to anaemia) and puffy (due to mucinous infiltration of skin). Mucinous material consists of hyaluronic acid and chondroitin β sulphate.

The hair becomes lustreless and dry. There is fall of hair of the eyebrows, especially over the lateral halves. The patient presents a lethargic and tired look which is often characteristic. The tongue is enlarged in size (macroglossia) and the lips often become thick. In some cases xanthomatous deposits may be found around the eyelids due to hypercholesterolaemia. In fair complexion persons a yellowish tinge may be seen due to hypercarotenaemia. In early cases, the diagnosis is suspected from the look of the patient and advanced cases, the diagnosis is too obvious.

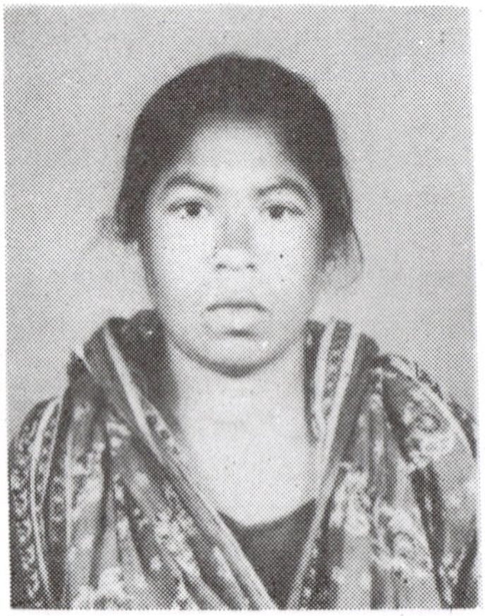

Fig.8.5 : Myxedema
(Dr.S. Kumar's case)

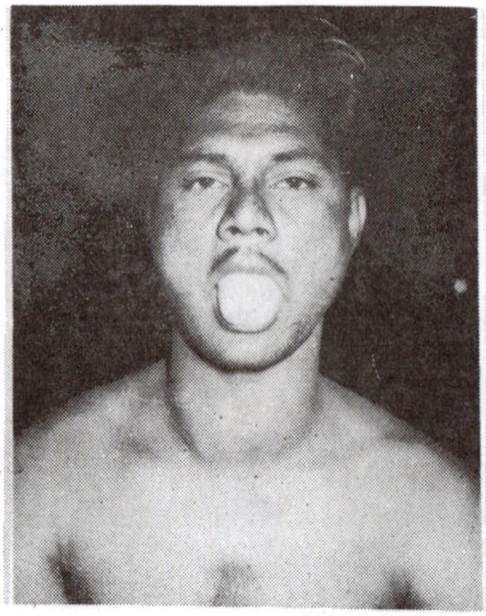

Fig.8.6 : Hypothyroidism
(Dr.S. Kumar's Case)

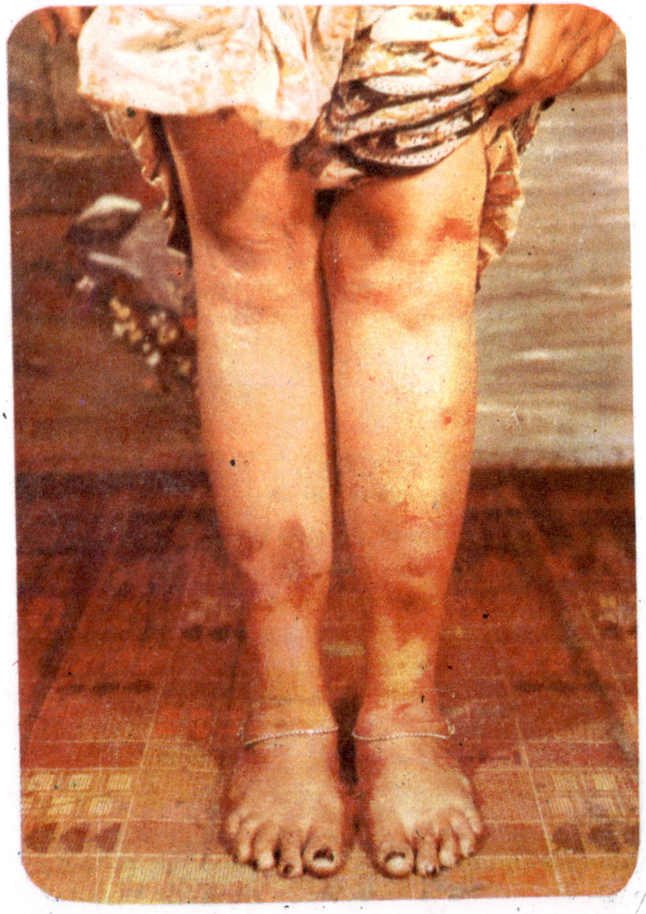

Fig.8.7 : Pretibial myxedema
(By Courtesy of Dr.S.Jain)

The skin becomes thick due to myxedematous deposit. It is pale, dry (due to decreased sweat secretion), coarse and rough with sparse hair. This characteristic appearance is seen in only cases of primary hypothyroidism.

In secondary hypothyroidism, the skin is pale and dry but other features are often absent. Similarly features due to myxedematous deposit such as hoarseness of voice, puffy face, tingling and numbness of fingers are rarely present in secondary hypothyroidism.

(ii) **Cardio-vascular changes**

Hypercholesterolaemia is common, which often is associated with atherosclerosis. This explains frequent anginal pain which is noted in long-standing cases of myxedema. In some cases following treatment the pain may be increased. Due to slow metabolism, the heart rate slows down to around 60/min. Heart sounds are muffled and the size of the heart is increased due to myxedematous cardiomyopathy (deposition of myxedematous tissue in between the cardiac muscles) which is reversible after treatment. Pericardial effusion is common but usually minimal. ECG shows bradycardia associated with low voltage and flattened T waves and small QRS complexes. The haemodynamic effect of reduced stroke volume leads to small pulse, prolonged circulation time and reduced blood flow to the tissues that may account for some of the symptoms. Serum enzymes especially CPK, SGOT and LDH are increased and the evidence suggests that there is leakage of these enzymes from the cardiac muscle.

**(iii) Effect on C.N.S**

(1) Disturbances of higher functions may be an early manifestation. Impairment of memory, sluggish mental reactions and lack of interest in day to day work are frequently noticed by an intelligent patient or the relatives.

There is progressive slowness of physical and mental activities (psychomotor retardation). In severe cases progressive dementia and depression supervene and in some cases the patient becomes frankly psychiatric (myxedema madness).

(2) **Deafness :** Conductive type of deafness occurs due to deposits of myxedematous tissue in the middle ear. This is frequently present and occasionally brings the patient to ENT clinic.

(3) Tingling and numbness of the fingers are also seen (due to compression of the median nerve in the carpal tunnel). This is frequently confused with rheumatism or arthritis of wrist joint.

(4) Hoarseness of voice : The voice becomes husky due to involvement of larynx by the myxoedematous tissue.

(5) Muscles are hypotonic. Delayed nerve conduction results in delayed contraction and relaxation-time of deep reflexes while relaxation time is more affected. This is best demonstrated by delayed relaxation time of the ankle jerk. It is an important physical sign for diagnosis.

(iv) **Affection of G.I. Tract**

Appetite is frequently poor and thirst for water is decreased. In spite of poor appetite the patient complains of weight gain and the rings may become tighter and become difficult to take out. Obstinate constipation due to reduced peristalsis is also an important feature. Occasionally the patients have motion every 2 or 3 days.

Vague symptoms such as flatulence, anorexia, especially for fatty food are usually associated.

On clinical examination, the abdomen becomes distended and the colon appears palpable.

Rare features include faecal impaction with subacute intestinal obstruction, malabsorption, cholelithiasis, ascites etc.

**(v) Features of slow metabolism :**

Hypersensitivity to cold is commonly seen. Sterility and loss of sexual interest may also develop. In untreated cases, body temperature may be subnormal (hypothermia), even coma may supervene (**myxedema** coma), especially in old people.

**(vi) Affection of Locomotor system**

Commonly vague ache and pains with stiffness of joints all over the body are present in most cases. This may be due to involvement of joints, muscles and periarticular tissues by myxedematous deposit. Particularly knee, ankle, wrist and small joints of hands are affected, simulating rheumatism. Due to deposition of glycoprotein in between the muscle fibres, the size of the muscles is increased. This is most commonly seen in the muscles of lower limbs and one muscle may be more affected than others, e.g. quadriceps, hamstrings, or glutei but frequently the cuff muscles are particularly increased in size disproportionately to other muscles. This is known as Hoffman syndrome. With treatment the size returns to normal and there is no weakness of muscle and EMG is normal.

**(vii) Reproductive system**

In females menorrhagia is usually seen but amenorrhoea can also develop. In males sterility and loss of libido may develop.

**(viii) Blood picture**

Anaemia is commonly present. Normally normocytic normochromic anaemia develops due to depression of bone marrow. Occasionally the anaemia is microcytic hypochromic due to loss of appetite and poor absorption of iron. If there is associated pernicious anaemia, as mostly seen in Western countries the anaemia becomes macrocytic hypochromic. According to some reports about 50% cases show achlorhydria often after histamine stimulation. Parietal cell antibodies have also been demonstrated in hypothyroidism in about 30% cases. Frank pernicious anaemia is only seen in 10% cases of primary hypothyroidism.

**(ix) Respiratory system**

Usually there are no symptoms but in severe cases, there may be myxedematous deposit in respiratory muscles which may lead to hypoventilation aggravated by reduced ventilatory drive. In severe cases carbon dioxide retention occurs and is regarded as a contributory factor for the development of myxedema coma. Small collection of myxedematous fluid in the pleural sac is not uncommon and only detected in radiological examination.

## CRETINISM

The first account of goitrous cretinism was given by Paracelsus a Swiss physician in 1516.

The earlier signs are obstinate constipation, feeding problem as the child refuses feeds, hoarse cry and the child appears lethargic and readily falls asleep. If undetected, the condition gradually progresses and there is delayed physical and mental development.

The normal milestones of development such as sitting, crawling, walking and talking are delayed. Another important feature includes delayed appearance of deciduous death. The full blown picture of cretinism includes the following :

(1) Cretinous facies — Child has flat nose with widely set eyes, puffiness of face, macroglossia, thick lips and dull appearance. (Fig.13.3 — A Typical Cretin).

(2) Skin is dry, thick, rough with loss of hairs.

(3) Trunk is characteristic : There is deposition of supraclavicular fat, protruberant abdomen and an umbilical hernia.

(4) Physical and mental retardation : Mental deficiency may be severe; I.Q. is definitely subnormal. There is also retardation of physical growth leading to dwarfism. Bone and teeth age are retarded. The centres of ossification appears late or may not appear at all in some places. A genesis of femoral head may be seen and the child may have deformity of the legs and delayed closure of fontanelle.

**Diagnosis** — The condition when suspected should be diagnosed as early as possible with measurement of $T_3$, $T_4$ and TSH.

**Radiological examination**

As already explained that epiphysial centres of ossification appears late or occasionally may be absent. Instead of a single centre, multiple centres appear within the epiphysis and this gives an irregular stippled, appearance (Epiphyseal dysgenesis).

This is best seen in the long bones, especially in the ends of the long bones and navicular bone of the foot. It must be clearly understood that epiphysial dysgenesis can be observed only in those bones where centres of ossification appear after the onset of hypothyroidism. If this condition can be treated early, normal development can be expected in those centres which are due to appear at a later age.

Skull X-ray shows delayed closure of fontanelle.

## JUVENILE MYXEDEMA

This term is used when hypothyroidism appears around puberty. The salient features are the same as in adult hypothyroidism with dwarfism and hypogonadism. Mental deficiency as seen in cretinism is characteristically absent. Bone and teeth age are delayed and epiphysial dysgenesis may be present or absent.

INVESTIGATIONS

1) **Blood** — Anaemia is usually present and serum cholesterol level is above 300 mg%, cholesterol may not rise.
2) **Serum PBI** — Is lower than 3 μg% but this test has many fallacies, hence not reliable.
3) **Basal metabolic rate (BMR)** — BMR is less than minus 20% but nowadays not done for clinical work, because it is difficult to measure it correctly in the out-patients and is non-specific.
4) **ECG** — Shows low voltage complexes and T-waves are flattened and may be mistaken for I.H.D. Bradycardia is often present.
5) **Photomotogram** — It reveals delayed relaxation time of ankle jerk.
6) **Thyroid hormone tests** : The diagnostic tests are radio-immunological measurement of TSH $T_3$ and $T_4$. In primary hypothyroidism TSH is raised. Even in mild cases of primary hypothyroidism, TSH level will be increased and there will be increased TSH response to TRH stimulation. This test is valuable in the early diagnosis of hypothyroidism.

**Serum $T_3$ and $T_4$** level — Plasma thyroxine level is diminished in the early phase. Serum $T_3$ level may be normal initially but later on $T_3$ level will also be subnormal. However, in the diagnosis of hypothyroidism $T_4$ value is more important than $T_3$ as because under increased TSH stimulation the thyroid gland synthesises more $T_3$ than $T_4$ in the early phase of primary hypothyroidism.

**$T_3$ resin uptake test** — Free thyroxine index also shows subnormal values. Radioactive iodine uptake is low in case of primary hypothyroidism. The differentiation from primary and secondary hypothyroidism rests upon the measurement of TSH which is invariably depressed in pituitary or hypothalamic failure. The TRH response is impaired in pituitary hypofunction.

Radiological survey of bones has been discussed and is a valuable aid in cretins and juvenile myxedema.

Mongolism sometimes has to be differentiated from cretinism as both have retardation of mental development and dwarfism but the mongol child is usually cheerful, has normal texture of skin and shows specific features such as oblique eyes, presence of epicanthic fold, shortness of the middle phalanx of the little finger and abnormal palmar crease. These children unlike lazy cretins are playful and found of music. Karyotyping reveals presence of trisomy — 21.

**Treatment**

The treatment of hypothyroidism is usually very satisfactory and rewarding. The drugs used are L-thyroxine or sodium levothyroxine, ($T_4$) tri-iodothyroxine or sodium liothyronine ($T_3$), thyroid-extract and thyroglobulin (proloid) (1 mgm of Eltroxin is equivalent to 20 μgm of $T_3$ and 60 mgm of thyroid extract. The commonest drug used in Eltroxin or Roxin (0.1 mgm tablet). A daily dose of one to two tablets is usually sufficient to depress the TSH to normal value and the patient remains euthyroid.

It helps to maintain sufficient peripheral thyroxine pool and its conversion to $T_3$ in the tissue. Omission of a few doses not affect the pool.

In elderly subjects and long-standing undiagnosed cases, the initial dose should be small (usually 0.05 mg daily to be increased every two weeks until a normal metabolic status is achieved. (Within a week there is diuresis with loss of weight and puffiness of the face improves. Gradually the pulse rate increases, appetite improves and bowel habit returns to normal. Psychomotor retardation and delayed ankle jerk also gradually disappear. Cutaneous changes take longer time to disappear. The criteria of adequate thyroid replacement are :

(i) Clinical well being of the patient and clinical assessment

(ii) Plasma $T_4$ and TSH values should become normal.

**Treatment of juvenile myxedema and cretinism :**

Juvenile myxedema also requires thyroid replacement like adult hypothyroidism; however treatment should be more energetic to ensure normal physical and sexual development.

In cretinism the most important aspect of treatment is attainment of normal intellectual development and that is possible only if treatment is started as early as possible but definitely within six months of birth. If treatment is started after the age of 2 years response is often unsatisfactory. Usual starting dose is 25μ g of 1-thyroxine (i.e. ¼th tablet of Eltroxin) daily, which is to be increased by 25μ g day every week to reach a maintenance dose of 100μ g/day (i.e. tablet 0.1 mg or one of Eltroxin). Plasma $T_4$ level should be monitored and maintained in the upper normal range. Clinical response should be carefully observed and if necessary the dose may be increased further. In the early stage of treatment appetite improves, constipation disappears and the child becomes playful and milestones of development become gradually normalised.

In the management of older children skeletal and dental age should serve as guidelines in therapy.

Daily requirement of thyroxine in hypothyroid children is found by recent studies to be higher (about 3.5μg/kg/day) than in adults (about 2.5μg/kg/day). Lastly it may be remembered that it is better to err on the higher side, in deciding the dose of thyroxine in treating hypothyroidism in infancy and childhood.

## HYPOTHYROIDISM

How to assess whether a patient receiving Eltroxin genuinely requires permanent replacement therapy ?

Eltroxin should be stopped and plasma $T_3$, $T_4$, TSH and TSH response to TRH should be assessed after four to six weeks. If the hypothalamic-pituitary-thyroid axis is essentially normal, then all the above tests should show normal values by this time. $I^{131}$ uptake after TSH stimulation is also useful.

**Subclincial hypothyroidism**

This term refers to minimal clinical evidence of hypothyroidism and even normal $T_3$ and $T_4$

levels but with high TSH level. It is probably useful to give these patients replacement doses of thyroxine to bring TSH level to normal.

## MYXEDEMA COMA

It is a grave emergency associated with high mortality rate. It is more common in elderly patients in very cold climate. The precipitating factors include :

(1) Injury or surgical operation

(2) Severe infection

(3) Administration of sedatives and anaesthetics as these patients are unduly sensitive to these drugs.

(4) Sudden withdrawal of therapy over a long period.

Clinical manifestations include :

(1) Drowsiness which may be associated with epileptic fits; occasionally it is due to hypoventilation with $CO_2$ retention and dilutional hyponatremia.

(2) Bradycardia with feeble pulse and hypotension

(3) Hypothermia

(4) External manifestations of myxedema (absent if the patient has suddenly stopped the drug.)

Occasionally the diagnosis becomes difficult in elderly subjects with cerebro-vascular lesions.

**Treatment**

Ideally the patient should be treated in intensive care unit. Active measures to be taken include :

(1) $O_2$ inhalation and artificial respiration if required to combat $CO_2$ retention and hypoventilation.

(2) Gentle warming of the patient by wrapping with blankets. External heat application may cause sudden peripheral vasodilatation and further fall of B.P.

(3) Administration of glucocorticoid to prevent adrenal crisis. Adrenal glands may fail to cope with the sudden metabolic stimulation following intravenous use of $T_3$.

It would also circumvent the danger of associated adrenal insufficiency.

Hydrocortisone 300-400 mg, should be given I.V. initially followed by 100 mgm I.M. every 8 hours for the first two or three days and it should be tapered off judiciously.

(4) $T_3$, Tri-iodo-thyronine or sodium liothyronine should be given I.V. in a dosage of 10$\mu$g. every 8 hours.

(5) Fluids should be given with close monitoring of the electrolyte level. Hypertonic saline may be useful to combat dilutional hyponatremia.

(6) I.V. Hypertonic glucose should be given as hypoglycaemia is usually present.

## THYROID – CARCINOMA

*GC. MOOKERJEE*

### INTRODUCTION

Thyroid carcinoma is a surgical problem and surgical textbooks should be consulted for details. The essentials of the problem are being discussed here because general practitioners should remember the important features for its early diagnosis.

The most important point to remember is that thyroid-carcinoma is usually not associated with hormonal abnormalities. Initially there may be painless enlargement of the gland or there may be palpable nodule. Thyroid function tests are normal. There may be past history of thyroiditis or local radiation therapy. Goitrous gland may sometimes become malignant.

The progress of the case and prognosis depend upon the histopathological nature of the growth.

**Types of thyroid carcinoma :**

Anaplastic type is most dangerous but fortunately the rarest type.

Papillary and follicular types of carcinoma have better prognosis after treatment, provided diagnosis is not late. Familial occurance has been recorded and its association with multiple endocrine neoplasia is well known.

CLINICAL FEATURES :

Most commonly it presents as a nodule, painless but hard swelling or it may present as enlarged gland in one side, later the tumour enlarges to a big mass in the neck (Fig.8.8).

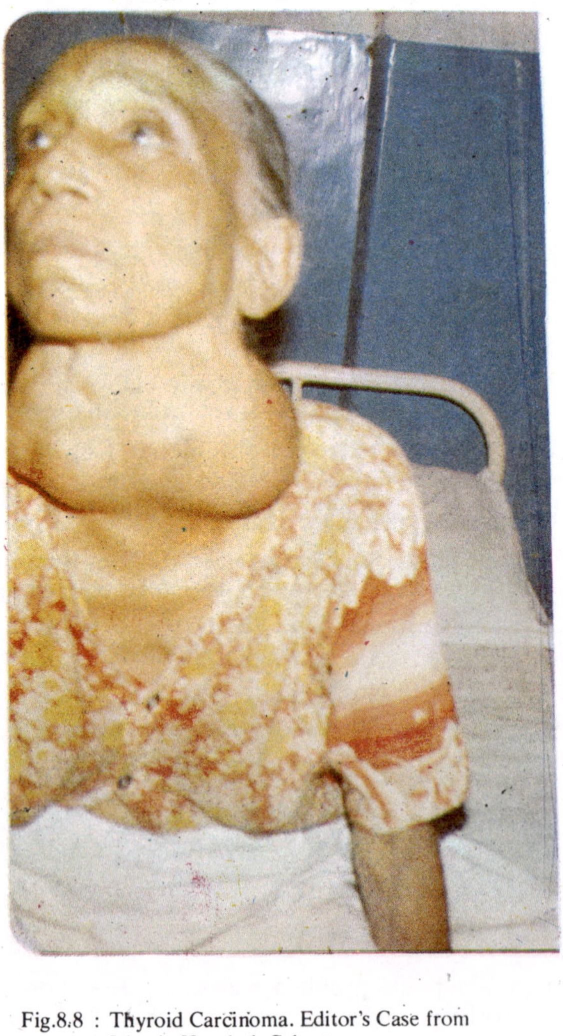

Fig.8.8 : Thyroid Carcinoma. Editor's Case from Islamia Hospital, Calcutta

Thus the enlarged gland may cause pressure symptoms in the neck. A small nodule is often a problem as it apparently looks small, benign and symptomless. It is difficult to convince the patient and submit him to an array of expensive investigations.

It is also true that non-malignant enlargements are more common than malignant ones.

Anaplastic carcinoma is most invasive locally as well as it produces distant metastasis. Papillary tumours are invasive locally while follicular tumours usually metastasize via blood stream.

The clinical manifestations of metastasis will depend on the nature of organs involved. Local complications will lead to dysphagia, hoarseness and respiratory embarassment.

(1) Adenoma — usually multiple, well encapsulated and fairly common (D.D. — multinodular gotire). Some colloid containing adenomas may produce hyperthyroidism.

(2) Carcinoma Thyroid — rare. Histological diagnosis is essential to determine types.
   (a) Papillary cystadenocarcinoma — well differentiated form. Locally spreading type.
   (b) Follicular — encapsulated type, usually metastasis occurs via blood vessels commonly to lungs and bones. The original growth may be small solitary nodule.
   (c) Anaplastic type is highly malignant. Local compression is due to growth and distant metastasis.
   (d) Medullary carcinoma — occur from the calcitonin producing cells of the thyroid gland.
   (e) In familial type other endocrine glands are involved due to multiple endocrine tumours.

INVESTIGATIONS :

(1) Thyroid function tests are mostly normal
(2) Thyroid gland scintiscan may reveal a cold nodule
(3) Thyroid auto-antibodies may sometimes be detected in serum
(4) Thyroglobulin level may be elevated in papillary and follicular tumours with metastasis.
(5) Calcitonin assay is a very reliable test for medullary carcinoma. Calcitonin level in serum is invariably raised.
(6) Ultrasound (echo) scanning will differentiate cystic from solid tumours. This is help as cystic swellings are usually not malignant. Multinodular goitres are usually not malignant.
(7) Thyroxine therapy for three months shows regression in non-malignant goitres.
(8) X-ray studies may reveal metastasis in bone and soft tissues.

TREATMENT :

Surgical removal as far as possible should be attempted but depends on the stage.

External irradiation is also an alternative or an adjunct to surgical excision.

Radioiodine therapy has some role in follicular tumours or in metastatic masses after thyroidectomy.

Chemotherapy in inoperable cases is also being done specially with doxoruibcin, which however is a toxic drug.

After thyroidectomy or irradiation of the gland, life long thyroid — therapy is necessary.

## PARATHYROIDS

*G.C. MOOKERJEE*
*S. KUMAR*

In 1880, a Swedish Physician, Sandstorm recognised four independant structures, situated by the side of thyroid gland and named them as parathyroid glands. It was frequently observed that removal of thyroid gland produces hypothyroidism as well as intractable tetany. In 1923, Collip et al demonstrated the existence of the parathyroid hormone and proved that parathyroid gland extracts can prevent tetany.

### Anatomy & Physiology

The parathyroid glands, usually four in number and about 5 mm in length, are arranged in pairs abong the posterior borders of lobes of the thyroid gland. Occasionally however, the glands are embedded in the substance of the thyroid gland or may be found lower in the neck or even in the thorax. These glands secrete parathyroid hormone called parathormone (PTH) and also small amounts of Calcitonin (however main source of calcitonin are the 'C' cells of the thyroid gland).

### Parathyroid hormone

It is a 84 — amino acid peptide-hormone whose physiological action is regulation of extracellular fluid calcium and phosphorus concentration. The secretion of parathormone is controlled by the level of ionised serum calcium level, by a negative biofeedback mechanism i.e., a fall of ionised calcium stimulates parathormone secretion and vice versa.

The main action of parathormone is to increase serum calcium; this is achieved by its action on three organs,bone and kidney by a direct and intestine by an indirect effect.

(1) **Effect on bone**

It causes mobilisation of calcium from bone by increasing the dissolution of calcium phosphate bone.

(2) **Effect on kidney**

On one hand it reduces renal tubular reabsorption of phosphate, thereby increasing phosphate excretion, and on the other hand it increases the reabsorption of filtered calcium thus conserving body calcium.

(3) **Effect on intestine**

Through its stimulating effect on the synthesis of 1, 25 — dihydroxy vitamin D (which is the most active form of vitamin D), it enhances intestinal absorption of calcium.

## HYPERPARATHYROIDISM

Hyperparathyroidism is due to excessive secretion of parathyroid hormone (parathormone) causing hypercalcaemia and excessive loss of calcium and phosphorus in urine.

Hyperparathyroidism may be

(1) Primary.
(2) Secondary.
(3) Tertiary.
(4) Pseudo hyperparathyroidism.

Primary hyperparathyroidism may chiefly be due to adenoma or hypertrophy (95%) while 5% cases are due to carcinoma.

Sometimes it is familial. Secondary hyperparathyroidism may be complication of chronic renal failure, osteomalacia, pseudo hypoparathyroidism and acromegaly.

Tertiary hyperparathyroidism may be due to flank hyperplasia or autonomous tumour. Pseudohyperparathyroidism is however a nonparathyroid syndrome which resembles hyperparathyroidism.

### Primary Hyperparathyroidism

Medical history — The first recorded case, was described by **Courtial** in 1700. Much later in 1926, Mandl removed a parathyroid tumour and produced considerable improvement in a case with generalised osteitis fibrosa. In 1934, Albright & Bloomberg emphasised the frequent occurrence of renal calculi in hyperparathyroidism which may be the only clinical manifestations.

## CLINICAL FEATURES -

The onset is usually gradual but occasionally sudden with renal colic or a pathological fracture. Sometimes the condition may be asymptomatic and detected on routine biochemical examination. The common clinical features are :

Fatigue, muscular weakness, anorexia, nausea, vomiting,diarrhoea and constipation are common. Psychiatric symptoms and peptic ulcers may occur. Hypotonia of muscles even weakness and atrophy of muscles may occur (hypercalcaemic myopathy). These may be mistaken for rheumatism.

Skeletal changes are usually generalised and marked :

(1) There is demineralisation of the bones, rarefaction and softening of the bones which results in skeletal deformity.

(2) The lower limbs become bowed inwards and may result in waddling gait.

(3) Due to increased osteoclastic activity there may be formation of Osteoclastoma (Brown tumour) in the jaw.

(4) The vertebrae tend to become soft due to loss of calcium and may collapse with resultant kyphosis and loss of height.

(5) Pathological fractures may be seen with slight trauma and union is delayed.

(6) Radiological findings are very characteristic :

(a) There is generalised rarefaction of the bones.

(b) Cyst formation may be detected due to excessive osteoclastic activity and proliferation of fibrotic tissue.

(c) Subperiosteal erosion of the terminal phalanges and loss of the lamina dura are classical signs of hyperparathyroidism.

(d) X-ray of skull may show granular appearance — "pepper pot skull". Renal and tissue calcification are characteristic features :

(1) Hypercalcaemia, hypercalciuria and secondary tubular atrophy leads to polyuria and polydypsia in some cases.

(2) The incidence of renal stone is high. There may be multiple stones or a single large stone in the renal pelvis. This leads to haematuria and renal colic.

As in all soft tissues, calcium may be also deposited in the renal parenchyma as small particles known as renal calcinosis. This leads to progressive hyaline degeneration and fibrosis, resulting in hypertension and azotaemia due to chronic interstitial fibrosis. Once the disease is advanced, the removal of adenoma may not be useful to the patient.

Rare features include deposition of calcium in the heart and lungs resulting in dyspnoea and cyanosis. Mental confusion, anaemia due to excessive destruction of the bone marrow may occur. Band keratopathy due to calcium deposition at the corneal margins fast demonstrated by slit lamp examination has also been reported.

**Diagnosis :**

The condition should be remembered in all cases of renal colic and bone tenderness, unexplained myopathy pathological fractures, vague gastrointestinal symptoms not responding to treatment.

Estimation of urinary calcium by Sulkowvitch's test is simple screening test. If urinary calcium is more than 200 mg in 24 hours diagnosis should be suspected.

High serum calcium above 11 mgm% and low phosphorus below 3 mgm% are diagnostic. Occasionally repeated estimation may be required. Radioimmunoassay (RIM) of parathormone shows high value.

Prednisolone in a dose of 30 mgm daily for 10 days brings down the Calcium level significantly in most cases by hypercalcaemia other than hyperparathyroidism.

Radiological examination of bones is also helpful as already described.

**Acute Hyperparathyroidism :**

This rare presentation includes, acute pain in the abdomen with vomiting, dehydration, vascular collapse and mental confusion due to sudden elevation of serum calcium.

**Differential diagnosis** — This condition may have to be differentiated from Albright's syndrome, characterised by segemented pigmentation, precocious puberty with features with osteitis fibrosa cystica and other causes producing hypercalcaemia and hypercalcuria.

**Treatment** — Surgery is the treatment of choice. Removal of adenoma produces considerable improvement except in cases with long standing renal involvement. Occasionally there is difficulty in locating the adenoma situated in the mediastinum or behind the oesophagus. In rare E.C.G. shows short Q—T interval. Post-operatively tetany may occur.

**Secondary Hyperparathyroidism** — It compensatory increases in parathormone secretion along with hyperplasia of the parathyroid glands in response to any primary disease that tends to lower serum calcium level. This may be seen in :

(1) Chronic renal failure
(2) Malabsorption states
(3) Rickets and osteomalacia from dietary deficiency.
(4) Acromegaly.

In secondary hyperparathyroidism the serum calcium level is not high.

The clinical manifestations may be that of the underlying disease or may be due to hyperparathyroid bone disease. Treatment is that of the underlying cause, whenever possible. In cases of chronic renal failure use of phosphate buffer, aluminium hydroxide, vitamin D and particularly 25-dihydroxycholecalciferol is beneficial.

**Tertiary hyperparathyroidism :**

This occurs in long standing cases of secondary hyperparathyroidism and is due to development of autonomous adenoma in the previously hyperplastic glands. In this condition serum calcium level is elevated. This condition is treated by surgical removal of the autonomous adenoma.

## HYPERCALCAEMIA

**Causes :**

(1) Primary hyperparathyroidism.
(2) Malignant disorders with metastasis as in multiple myeloma, lymphoma, breast carcinoma etc.
(3) Malignancy without metastasis as in hypernephroma, carcinoma of lungs, cervix, oesophagus etc. Where ectopic parathormone of prostaglandin secretion has also been observed.
(4) Thyrotoxicosis — Thyroxine leads to increased resorption of calcium from bones and may lead to mild degree of hypercalcaemia which should return to normal after antithyroid drug therapy. If there is coexistant hyperparathyroidism, serum calcium level remains high and RIA of parathormone would reveal high level.
(5) Vit D intoxication — Excessive of Vit D for the treatment of hypoparathyroidism or if taken inadvertantly for too long period may result in hypercalcaemia, nephro-calcinosis and ectopic calcification. Careful history is often diagnostic. In suspected cases estimation of serum 1,25 $(OH)_2D$ the principal metabolite responsible shows increased concentration.
(6) Sarcoidosis — Due to increased formation of serum 1,25 $(OH)_2D$. There is hypercalcaemia in sarcoidosis.
(7) Milk-alkali syndrome — Milk and sodium bicarbonate used in the treatment of peptic ulcer

may produce hypercalcaemia and ectopic calcification (Burnett). It is rarely seen at present as absorbable alkali is not used nowadays.

(8) Thiazide diuretics — These may produce hypercalcaemia by increased reabsorbtion of calcium from the renal tubules and potentiates the action of parathormone.

(9) Immobilisation — There is increased resorption of calcium from the bone but the mechanism has not been clearly established.

## AETIOLOGY :

Hypoparathyroidism causes fall in tonic serum calcium level due to deficient secretion of P.T.H. and leads to neuromuscular irritability. Usually this may be due to Autoimmune disease, accidental surgical removal or congenital deficiency.

Clinically the following types may be observed :

1. Idiopathic hypoparathyroidism
2. Secondary hypoparathyroidism
3. Pseudohypoparathyroidism
4. Pseudo-pseudo hypoparathyroidism
5. Pseudo hypoparathyroidism with secondary hyperparathyroidism

## CLINICAL FEATURES

The presenting symptoms of acute hypoparathyroidism may be tetany, epileptic fits, laryngeal spasm, convulsions. Carpopedal spasms are characteristic. Dyspnoea with wheezing and stridor as well as diplopia may occur.

In mild cases only night cramps of the calf muscles, tingling and numbness of the fingers and forearm or only a burning sensation is present.

Due to tonic contraction of the facial muscles there may be wrinkling of the forehead or the face may assume a mask-like appearance.

Chronic cases may show mental changes, lethargy, blurred vision due to cataracts and recurrent abdominal pain.

Muscle spasm and pain may commonly affect the bands and feet (Carpopedal spasm) lasting for several minutes. There is flexion at the metacarpo phalangeal joint with extension at the inter phalangeal joint and the thumb is adducted (accoucherouer's hand). In latent tetany the above changes may be brought about by inflating the sphygmomanometer cuff to a little above systolic pressure for a few minutes (Trousseau's sign). Latent tetany may also be revealed by tapping the facial nerve in front of the parotid gland, which causes contraction of the facial muscles (Chvostek's sign).

Flexion of the wrist and elbow are also associated. In the lower limb the ankle is extended, toes are flexed and the foot is inverted. Fibrillary twitching may be observed in different muscles at the same time. The above abnormality is due to increased neuro-muscular irritability.

Irritability of the intestinal muscles is increased resulting in acute colicky pain and vomiting. It frequently stimulates biliary and appendicular colic.

The laryngeal spasm with stridor may be seen specially in children with features of rickets. Bronchial spasm is not uncommon. The smooth muscle spasm is due to increased neuromuscular irritability.

Higher function are frequently disturbed. Irritability, impairment of memory, anxiety state and dementia may all be found. Petitmal or Grand-mal fits associated with migraine may be observed in some cases E.E.G. changes.

In rare instance, hallucination, depression, mania, psychosis and schizoid personality may develop. Clinical findings may reveal papilloedema, cerebellar ataxia, and calcification in the brain, cerebral tumour needs differentiation in such cases.

Skin is usually dry, rough and scaly. Various skin disorders such as psoriasis and dermatitis herpetiform is may occur. Moniliasis is also common. Hairs may fall off, eyebrows, pubic and axillary hairs may be affected. Nails become brittle, grooved and may undergo necrosis even detachment.

Teeth are often defective and dental caries is common. Cataract may be seen in 10% of the cases at an early or late stage. The cause is unexplained.

TREATMENT :

In acute cases 10-20 c.c. of 10% calcium gluconate should be given slowly I.V. In severe cases additional 20 ml. of 10% calcium salt may be mixed with 5% glucose or glucose-saline to be given as a slow drip.

In most cases crisis can be controlled in this way and subsequently.

Calcium lactate may be given orally in a dose of 1 to 2 g thrice daily for the next 3-4 days. Maintainance therapy should be carried out with calciferol in dose of 50,000 to 1 lac unit or 1-2 mgm daily. Serum calcium level should be monitored, because over treatment may lead to multiple tissue calcification. Dehydro-tachysterol or synthetic Vit. D. analogue therapy should be given along with oral calcium.

Dihydrotachyferol tablets are available in 0.125, 0.2 and 0.4 mg strengths and initially 1 to 2 mg per day may be prescribed.

Alternatively calciferol 80,000 to 160,000 units (1 mg = 40,000 units) can be given daily.

In chronic cases, high calcium and low phosphate diet is advised. Diet should be rich in calcium and low in phosphates. Hence cheese should be avoided. Too much milk is also not desirable. Aluminium hydroxide helps in reducing serum phosphate level; calciferol 40,000 to 80,000 units daily is adequate.

Treatment of tetany from other causes — Treatment of the underlying cause such as malabosorption syndrome, renal failure should be carried out along with administration of Vit. D and calcium. In cases of alkalosis due to vomiting isotonic saline is the treatment of choice. Excessive administration of alkalies should be stopped and ammonium chloride may be given by mouth. In hyperventilation syndrome psychotherapy is sufficient.

Phenothiazine drugs should be avoided as these may cause dystonia. Furosemide may also lead to loss of calcium.

## TETANY

**Definition :**

This is a condition of increased neuromuscular excitability leading to prolonged muscular spasm, first described in 1950 by Clarke John.

It is caused by a low plasma ionised calcium fraction. This in turn, may be due to depletion of plasma calcium as a whole or due to alkalosis which cause increased protein binding of plasma calcium, thus lowering the free ionised fraction, though total plasma calcium may be normal.

Low magnesium level may also cause tetany.

**Aetiology :**

(1) Hypoparathyroidism of different causes.

(2) Intestinal malabsorption syndrome.

(3) Inadequate dietary intake of calcium or vitamin D.

(4) Chronic renal failure, particularly if the acidosis is corrected alkali therapy.

(5) Pregnancy and lactation — due to increased demands for calcium.

(6) Alkalosis, which may occur in —

(a) Excessive vomiting or gastric lavage.

(b) Hysterical hyperventilation.

(c) Administration of large amounts of absorbable alkali e.g. for treating peptic ulcer.

(d) Primary aldosteronism.

**Pseudo-hypoparathyroidism :**

The condition is often inherited and present at birth. All the biochemical and clinical features of hypo-parathyroidism are present. In addition, there is pronounced mental deficiency with dwarfism and short metacarpal bones. The plasma parathormone level is usually raised. The aetiology is probably due to renal tubular and skeletal resistance to the action of parathormone.

**Infantile hypoparathyroidism :**

This may be due to hyperparathyroidism in the mother or it may be due to a developmental defect and associated with thymic aplasia as in Di Geores's syndrome. In the former condition it is transient.

## ADRENAL GLANDS

*GC. MOOKERJEE*
*S. KUMAR*

**INTRODUCTION :**

Two small adrenal glands situated at the upper pole of the kidneys, are also known as suprarenal glands. Each gland approximately weighs 5 to 6 g. and has a distinct outer layer, the cortex and the inner core medulla. The cortex is mesodermal origin while medulla is ectodermal. Richly supplied by blood the arterial supply comes from branches of aorta, renal artery and phrenic arteries and the venous drainage is via single adrenal vein. The right adrenal vein drains into inferior vena cava, while the left into left renal vein.

Nerve supply comes from celiac sympathetics and the branches enter into adrenal medullary cells.

The adrenal cortex has three layers :

(a) Zona glomerulosa — the outer layers

(b) Zona fasciculata, the middle layers

(c) Zone reticularis, the inner layers

Medulla, the deepest core consists of chromaffin cells like cell of sympathic ganglia.

Z. glomerulosa secretes mineralo-corticoid hormones e.g. aldosterone, corticosterone and desoxy-corticosterone (DOCA) while other two layers produce glucocorticoids (cortisone & hydrocortisone) as well as androgens and oestrogens (sex-steroids) in varying proportions. These anabolic sex steroids include androstenedione and other $C_{19}$ steroids, having protein building (anabolic) properties and are also androgenic and virilising.

The mineralocorticoids chiefly affect the water sodium and potassium metabolism while glucocorticoids chiefly control, protein, carbohydrate and fat metabolism but has minor effect on electrolyte metabolism in addition.

(Depressing signs of inflammation). Glucocorticoids are the real anti-stress hormones and are vital hormones for survival.

Their functions are generally catabolic as follows :

(1) Increased protein break down leading to elevated aminoacid level in blood (negative nitrogen balance).

(2) Increased glycogen break down as well as neoglucogenesis (anti-insulin effect).

(3) Anti-inflammatory properties.

(4) Lymphopenia and eosinopenia altering immune-response.

The chief mineralo corticoid hormone is aldosterone which regulates electrolyte balance. Aldosterone helps sodium retention and potassium excretion and thus regulates water balance as well as blood pressure.

All steroids are synthesised from cholesterol. Steps of biosynthesis are presented in Table 8.1 (Simplified).

**TABLE 8.1 : BIOSYNTHESIS OF STEROIDS**

CHOLESTEROL

PREGNENOLONE

| | | |
|---|---|---|
| Progesterone | Hydroxy-Progesterone | Hydroxy-Pregnenolone |
| Doca | Deoxycortisol | Androsterone |
| Corticosterone | | Testosterone |
| Aldosterone | Cortisol | Oestradiol |
| (Mineralo-Corticoid-hormones) | (Glucocorticoids : Hydrocortisone) | (Androgens) |

Secretion of glucocorticoids is controlled by "feed back mechanism" through the hypothalamus, (corticotrophin releasing factor — CRF) and also by anterior pituitary gland 'corticotrophin — ACTH). Mineralo-corticoids however are not under hypothalamic control but regulated through renin-angiotensin system. After release from the adrenal glands glucocorticoids-circulate in free as well as bound form with plasma globulin (cortisol binding globulin = CBG).

Steroids are catabolised in liver and are excreted in urine as glucuronides and sulphates in inactive form but traces of active hormones are also excreted in urine.

Estimation of steroids in urine is useful for assessment of adrenocortical function. These can now be accurately measured by labelled radioisotope method (radio-immunoassay). Older chemical or biological methods have been abandoned.

## ADDISON'S DISEASE

Thomas Addison physician in Guy's Hospital described the clinical condition in a meeting of the London Medical Society (1849). The clinical monograph was published in 1889.

DEFINITION :

Dysfunction of adrenal cortex with deficiency of cortisol, aldosterone and adrenal androgen, irrespective of the aetiology, is called Addison's disease. The cardinal features are pigmentation, gastrointestinal symptoms with nausea, vomiting, loss of appetite and constipation, weakness of the muscles and generalised asthenia, hypotension with dehydration and emaciation. Hypofunction of the adrenal cortex may be chronic (Addison's disease or acute adrenal crisis).

## AETIOLOGY :

It affects young adults of both sexes between 3rd and 4th decade. It is not common in children and old age but, rarely it may be congenital. Aplasia of the zona glomerulosa and zona reticularis may be associated with diffuse demyelination of the CNS in children.

(1) Tuberculosis — Until recently it was the commonest cause of Addison's disease but with modern chemotherapy tuberculosis can be controlled and Addison's disease due to tuberculosis is now quite uncommon. Histologically the lesion resembles tuberculosis anywhere else.

(2) Idiopathic atrophy of the adrenal : This is the commonest cause today. The autoantibodies detected in these cases also cross react with thyroid, islet cells of pancreas, ovary and parietal cells of the gastric mucosa. There is little doubt that it is an auto-immune process. Histologically there is dehydration of the cells with lymphocytic infiltration and presence of histiocytes.

(3) Haemorrhage in adrenal cortex may occur in fulminant infections particularly in children. Meningococcal infection is notable cause. (Waterhouse - Friderichsen syndrome). It may occur spontaneously in neonates or also due to anti-coagulant therapy.

(4) Rare causes include metastatic carcinoma, amyloidosis, leukaemia, granulomatosis, haemachromatosis, amyloid, torulosis and histoplasmosis.

(5) Bilateral adrenalectomy — performed for adrenal hyperplasia or ovarian tumours or for any other disease.

**Clinical Features**

Onset is insidious with fatigue and malaise persisting for years before the full blown clinical picture appears. More than 90% of the adrenal has to be destroyed before the symptoms arise.

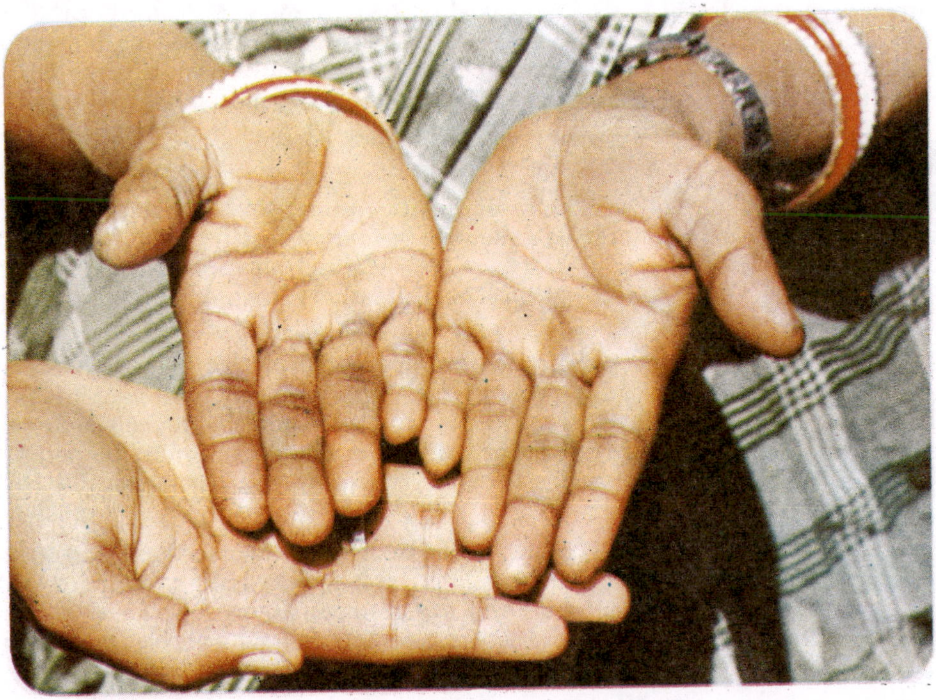

Fig.8.9 : Addison's disease — Note pigmentation Compared with normal hand.
(By Courtesy of Dr.S.Jain)

In the initial phase compensatory rise of ACTH level may bring the cortisol and aldosterone level to near normal in the resting phase. When affected individuals are subjected to trauma infection or stress of any form, adrenal crisis may be precipitated.

(1) **Skin changes**

(a) The skin is dry and shrivelled due to diminished extracellular volume and subcutaneous fat is depleted leading to emaciation and weight loss. The dehydration is due mainly to aldosterone deficiency while the emaciated appearance is due to lack of cortisol.

(h) Pigmentation – There is progressive darkening of the skin with brownish pigmentation. The skin becomes darker, due to melanin deposition in the basal layer of the skin. The pigmentation is most commonly seen in areas exposed to light and pressure. The palm and sole escape except the creases. The parts most affected are face, neck, arms, axillae, nipple, waist line and medial aspects of the thigh.

Pigmentation of the mucous membrane of the mouth, lips, palate and gum is pathognomonic of the disease.

(c) Leukoderma – Occasionally patches of vitiligo are seen in the face, neck, arms and trunk possibly related to autoimmune process. In case of idiopathic leukoderma with Addison's disease, the pigmented areas become darker while the vitiligo remains unaltered. The severity of pigmentation do not always correlate with the severity of the disease and may be present for years before other features develop. Similarly in white people, who show little pigmentation when exposed to sun, pigmentation may be minimal or absent. It is wise to remember that absence of pigmentation does not exclude the diagnosis of Addison's disease.

(2) **G.I. system** – Anorexia specially for fatty food with nausea, vomiting with weight loss is common. Constipation is usual and sudden onset of diarrhoea should be regarded as a warning sign for adrenal crisis. Occasionally it may be due to steatorrhoea. Sometimes abdominal pain simulating peptic ulcer or biliary or renal colic may be present. Gastric analysis may show hypochlorhydria or achlorhydria. Loss of weight is partly due to poor appetite and low extracellular volume, giving an emaciated appearance.

(3) **Respiratory system** – It is always important to look possibly for tuberculous focus in the lungs or else where.

(4) **Myopathy** – Weakness of the muscles sets in with wasting, which is generalised. The patient is unable to do any normal work and sometimes lies curled up in bed. This is due to (i) loss of sodium, (ii) Depleted glycogen reserve in the liver and muscles. Lassitude and apathy, confused state and psychosis may be present. This is due to cortisol deficiency and hypoglycemia.

(5) **Cardiovascular changes** – Hypotension with systolic BP around 100 mm Hg is a common finding, hypotension may lead to postural syncope. This is due to (i) Lack of cortisol (ii) Deficiency of aldosterone leading to $H^+$ loss and a diminished extracellular volume and hypovolemia. The cardiac size is reduced and there is diminished cardiac output. The renal blood flow is diminished and there may be prerenal azotaemia. There may also be cardiac asystole due to hyperkalaemia.

Plasma volume and electrolyte. There is retention of $K^+$ with loss of $Na^+$ and there is mild acidosis. The depletion of extracellular volume leads to dehydration evidenced by dry and shrivelled skin with collapsed veins and low intraocular tension. There is peripheral vasoconstriction and the extremities become cold. Intermittent fever is uncommon without any cause.

(6) **Renal function**

Diminished renal flow and abnormal sodium loss may lead to renal tubular damage with raised blood urea.

Genital system — Impotence and amenorrhoea with sterility is common. Loss of axillary hair in women is due to adrenal androgen deficiency.

(7) **Carbohydrate metabolism** — Blood sugar and GTT is impaired. This partly accounts for the mental change and muscular weakness.

(8) **Blood picture** shows leukopenia with lymphocytosis, **eosinophilia** and microcytic hypochromic anaemia.

CLINICAL FEATURES OF ADRENAL CRISIS

(1) Acute abdominal pain with vomiting or diarrhoea
(2) Sweating with dizziness and drowsiness
(3) Hypotension — Systolic below 100 mm with marked tachycardia and cold sweats.
(4) Features of dehydration with or without high fever (ACUTE ADRENAL INSUFFICIENCY)
(5) Low serum sodium and raised potassium
(6) Low cortisol level
(7) High blood urea and eosinophilia
(8) ECG shows low voltage

Acute adrenal crisis may occur in a patient of established Addison's disease due to lack of treatment severe superimposed infection, trauma or stress, anticoagulant therapy. It may also occur in normal individual due to bilateral adrenalectomy, destruction of anterior pituitary gland or administration of insulin in case of panhypopituitarism. Severe infection e.g. meningococcal septicaemia may be the cause (known as Waterhouse — Friderichsen syndrome).

TREATMENT —

Prompt antishock treatment is life-saving and marked improvement occurs within 24 hours. In advanced cases with peripheral circulatory failure the mortality is high.

(1) **Intravenous hydrocortisone** — 200 mg stat and can be repeated every 4—6 hours of 24 hours. Subsequent dose can be adjusted according to response of the patient. After 2—3 days oral cortisol can be given or prednisolone can be used as substitute, along with flurocortisone.

(2) **I.V. 5% dextrose** — Saline should be given very rapidly (3—4 litres in 6 hours) to correct dehydration, $Na^+$ loss and hypoglycemia. Once the clinical condition improves, oral fluids may be started.

(3) Careful monitoring of the patient's temperature, pulse, B.P. and respiration are necessary. Oxygen inhalation is helpful. Attention to oro-pharyngeal air way and urine flow should be given.

(4) **Control infection :** Appropriate antibiotics should be used.

DIFFERENTIAL DIAGNOSIS

(i) Pigmentation of the skin
(ii) Pellagra with hyperkeratosis of the skin
(iii) Cirrhosis
(iv) Crohn's disease
(v) Chronic renal failure

Pigmentation of mucous membrane :

(i) Arsenic poisoning
(ii) Abdominal carcinoma
(iii) Haemochromatosis

## INVESTIGATION OF ADDISON'S DISEASE

(1) Metabolic effect — Routine blood test reveals microcytic hypochromic anaemia with low $Na^+$ and high $K^+$.

(2) X-Ray chest and abdomen may show calcification in the lungs or adrenals. Blood sugar is usually low with flat GTT due to absence of insulin antagonism by cortisol. Water load test (Kepler's test) was used in the past demonstrating inability to excrete water load.

(3) **Cortisol and 17 hydroxysteroid level —**
Diurnal rhythm of the cortisol is usually absent. The cortisol value seldom goes above 7 microgram %. Presence of diurnal variation with low normal values suggest the hypothalamus — pituitary — adrenal axis is still present but in times of stress, there would be cortisol insufficiency.

(4) **Tetracosactrin,** a potent analogue of ACTH can be given in a dose of 1 ngm IM and blood samples can be drawn 4 and 6 hours after, normally there would be more than 100% rise in cortisol level while poor response is obtained in adrenal deficiency.

(5) **ACTH injection** in dose of 40 units daily × 3 days shows similar impaired cortisol response, 17 hydroxy steroid excretion is also impaired, rising rarely to 10 ngm in 24 hours while in normal individuals values up to 20 to 30 ngm or more found. In severe cases, dexamethasone can be given I.V. (2 mgm) before tetracosactrin.

(6) **ACTH level —** normal 60 picogram/cc in primary adrenal insufficiency it goes to 200—1000 picogram/ml.

## TREATMENT :

Cortisol should be given by mouth in dosage of 20 mgm in the morning and 10 mgm in the evening. This should be checked with cortisol value in the blood frequently. In time of stress the daily dose may be increased to 80 — 100 mgm.

Alternatively prednisolone can be used in a daily dose of 10 mg twice daily. Later a maintenance dose is adjusted usually 7.5 to 10 mg per day and increasing the dose if required.

**Flurocortisone** can be added in a daily dose of 0.05 mg to 2 mg if required. Development of oedema, increased IVP or hypertension with headache and muscular weakness suggest overdosage with mineralocorticoid and the dose should be reduced. Plasma electrolyte should serve as a useful guide.

Rarely it may be necessary to use desoxycorticosterone acetate (DOCA) instead of Flurocortisone when the latter is not tolerated. DOCA however has to be given by I.M. injection. Dose usually varies between 1 to 4 mg I.M. daily.

# CUSHING'S SYNDROME

## DEFINITION

Cushing's syndrome is a clinical syndrome due to persistent excess of cortisol production, with some degree of adrenal androgenic excess by the zone fasciculata and zona reticularis of the adrenal cortex.

It occurs in the middle aged and females are more affected than male. However in the ectopic ACTH producing tumour (commonly carcinoma bronchus), the incidence is higher in elderly males.

The clinical entity of "Fat bearded diabetic women" was known for a long time. Harvey Cushing in 1932 first described the clinical condition in detail and his paper "Basophil Adenoma of the Pituitary Body" was published subsequently.

## AETIOLOGY

(1) **Hypothalamic :** Disorder of the hypothalamus and higher centres has been found to be associated with increased production of ACTH realeasing factor CRF and resulting in Cushing's syndrome.

(2) **Pituitary :** Basophilic or chromophobe adenoma of the pituitary may secrete increased ACTH causing Cushing's syndrome, due to bilateral adrenal hyperplasia. This occurs in 70% of cases of Cushing's syndrome.

(3) **Adrenal :** Adrenocortical adenoma or carcinoma are mostly unilateral but may be rarely bilateral. They secrete excessive glucocorticoids along with significant amount of androgens.

(4) **Ectopic ACTH producing tumour :** Common cause is bronchogenic carcinoma though carcinoma of prostate, liver, ovary, thymus also can secrete ACTH.

(5) **Iatrogenic :** Due to exogenous administration of ACTH or steroid for a long time. Today this is the commonest cause of Cushingoid features met with in clinical practice.

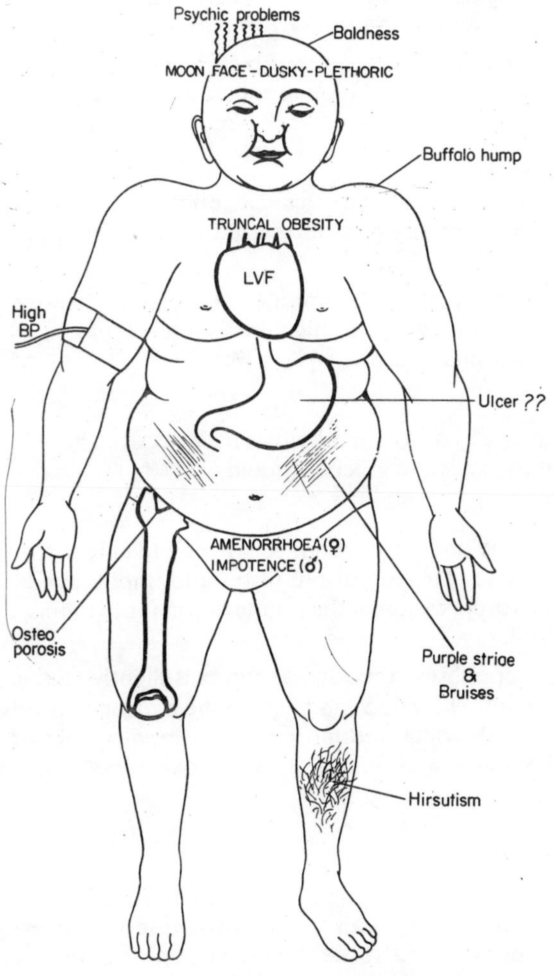


Fig.8.10 : CUSHING'S SYNDROME — Showing Classical features

(1) **Adiposity :**

There is centripetal deposition of fat involving the face,trunk, supraclavicular region, breast, abdomen, and buttocks.

The limbs are less affected but in children,forearms and legs may not be spared. Weight gain is significant. It is probably due to increased appetite and conversion of protein and carbohydrate to fat.

(2) **Facies :**

The face becomes rounded in appearance (moon facies) with plethora and facial hair becomes quite prominent in females.

(3) **Skin changes :**

Changes of the skin are extensive. Due to protein catabolism it becomes thin. Plethoric appearance of the skin may be due to thinning associated with polycythaemia. Patchy areas of cyanosis and telangiectasia often seen are due to local vascular dilatation.

Acne and hirsutism specially observed in the face are due to cortisol effect. Bruising on slight trauma is specially seen in the forearm and is due to increased fragility of the capillary wall and tissues of the skin.

Most characteristic finding is the presence of purple striae in the lower abdomen, buttocks and loin. This is due to accumulation of subcutaneous fat stretching the overlying skin and the underlying capillary venous network becomes visible.

(4) **Hypertension :**

Hypertension in a patient with truncal obesity should draw attention to Cushing's syndrome. There may be angina pectoris, left ventricular hypertrophy and left ventricular failure.

High BP, e.g. systolic above 200 mmHg and diastolic above 120 mmHg is common in Cushing's syndrome and is due to high cortisol level and Na+ retention. Blood pressure falls rapidly after adrenalectomy.

(5) **Diabetes Mellitus :**

Hyperglycaemia, glycosuria and ketosis may occur. There is no shortage of insulin but the effect is due to excessive glucocorticoids.

(6) **Gonads :**

In females genitalia undergo atrophic changes and amenorrhoea or scanty period is very common. In the males atrophy of the testes and impotence is invariably present. These changes are due to suppression of the pituitary gonadotrophins, due to excessive amount of circulating cortisol.

Androgen production from the adrenal cortex is slightly increased. This may play a role in hirsutism mostly confined to face and legs. If the androgen production is significantly high as seen in adrenal adenoma and more so in adrenal carcinoma, the hirsutism becomes generalised with recession of temporal hairs, hoarseness of the voice and enlargement of clitoris in female.

(7) **Skeletal changes :**

Protein catabolism as already described leads to rarefaction and softening of the bones. Compression of the vertebrae may lead to kyphosis; fractures of ribs or long bones may also occur. In children growth may be arrested unless prompt treatment is undertaken.

(8) **Kidney :**

There is hypercalciuria with normal calcium and phosphorous levels in plasma. Alkaline phosphatase is usually within normal limits. Polyuria, polydipsia may sometimes be a manifestation due to hypercalciuria.

Similarly, renal calculus, nephrocalcinosis with secondary nephrolithiasis has been observed. Renal damage with impaired function has occasionally been found.

(9) **Psychoneurotic features :**

Depression, mania, personality change, behavioural disorders are quite common though the mechanism is not clearly understood.

(10) **Endocrine and metabolic change :**

Thyroid gland may show diffuse enlargement and its function is usually normal or depressed. Cortisol has a direct depressant action on thyroid. Similarly, gonads and pituitary may also be depressed.

(11) **Myopathy :**

Steroid myopathy due to protein catabolism and hypokalaemia has now been well recognised specially affecting the proximal limb muscles. The muscles become weak and wasted. In advanced cases the patient cannot get up and remains confined to bed.

(12) **Pigmentation :**

This is seen in cases of basophil adenoma or malignant tumours with ectopic ACTH secretion and the sites affected are face and neck.

Occasionally, after bilateral adrenalectomy, the ACTH output rapidly increases even with steroid replacement commonly from the pituitary microadenoma resulting in extreme pigmentation (Nelson's syndrome).

INVESTIGATIONS FOR DIAGNOSIS

It is essential to find out if Cushing's syndrome is due to :

(1) Hypothalamic lesion
(2) Pituitary basophil adenoma
(3) Hyperplasia of adrenal cortices
(4) Adenoma in one of the adrenal glands
(5) Adrenal carcinoma
(6) Bronchial carcinoma, ovarian tumours etc.
(7) Iatrogenic-prolonged steroid or ACTH therapy.

The following investigations are relevant :

(1) **Haemogram**

Polycythaemia is common but WBC count may also be raised. Eosinophils and lymphocytes are reduced.

(2) **Biochemistry**

(a) Blood sugar level is raised indicating a diabetic state.
(b) Bicarbonate may be elevated and serum $K^+$ and $Cl^-$ may be reduced.
(c) Hormone profile

(1) **Urinary 17 ketosteroids excretion**
Adenoma — low or normal
Hyperplasia — normal or high
Carcinoma — very high
(2) Diurnal variation of plasma cortisol is absent.
(3) Urinary free cortisol is elevated.

(d) **ACTH — stimulation test** — Administration of Inj. ACTH causes increased secretion of cortisol in plasma and urinary 17-hydroxy-corticosteroids and 17-ketosteroids in Cushing's disease and in most cases of adenoma but not in carcinoma.

(e) **Plasma cortisol** — In Cushing's syndrome the diurnal variation in plasma cortisol level is abolished and the cortisol level is permanently high. Obesity, stress and hypertension also diminish the diurnal rhythm. Plasma cortisol below 7 μg% in the evening rules out Cushing's syndrome and above 15 μg% confirms the diagnosis (normal 5—8 μgm% at 8 p.m.).

**17 hydroxy-steroid** — 24-hour excretion of 17 hydroxy reflects the cortisol output and the usual value is 8—22 mg% values above 30 mg% is diagnostic (more than 80% cortisol is excreted as 17-hydroxy steroid after being metabolised).

(f) **Dexamethasone suppression test** — Dexamethasone is a potent synthetic analogue of cortisol and has the advantage of depressing the pituitary ACTH and not interfering with fluorometric measurement of cortisol in the blood or with the measurement of 17-hydroxy steroid in the urine by Zimmermann's reaction.

Dexamethasone given in dosage of 0.5 mg six hourly over 48 hours, will depress the 24-hour urinary 17-hydroxy-steroid excretion and the cortisol level in the blood by 50% in normal individual.

In Cushing's syndrome there will be no suppression.

(g) The normal urinary excretion of free cortisol in 24 hours is about 140—150 μmg. Values above 200 μgm support the diagnosis.

(h) Cortisol secretion rate using C 14 labelled cortisol can be accurately measured for 24 hours. In Cushing's syndrome this is high (normal : 12—30 mgm/24 hours).

(i) **ACTH level** — In pituitary tumour or ectopic ACTH secreting tumour, this is significantly high (more than 200 picogram/ml).

(3) **ECG** — LVH is common due to hypertension; T—waves may be flattened or inverted or low voltage due to hypokalaemia.

(4) **Radiology :**

(a) X-ray skull should be taken for sella turcica, which may be enlarged due to adenoma but usually a small basophil adenoma does not reveal any enlargement. Tomogram may be useful in some cases.

(b) X-ray of the chest may be useful to detect bronchogenic carcinoma.

(c) Plain X-ray abdomen may reveal outline but IVP is more useful in showing displaced or deformed kidney. Air insufflation will demonstrate tumour or enlargement of adrenal retroperitoneal quite clearly but is rarely done nowadays.

(d) Renal scan is another useful method by using radio-isotopes to assess the renal size and position.

(e) Angiography is rarely necessary nowadays as non-invasive methods are available.

(f) CT-Scan, if available, makes the diagnosis easy and any tumour may be discovered with great ease.

TREATMENT :

It depends on the aetiology. If there is basophil adenoma of the pituitary gland, pituitary irradiation or pituitary microsurgery should be done with excision of the adenoma. Radiation therapy is given either by external radiation delivering 5000 rads over a three-week period. Local injury to other tissues is a possible danger.

Alternatively, proton beam (alpha particle) may be used and even 12000 rads can be given without much local damage. Follow-up measurements of pituitary hormones are essential for subsequent replacement therapy.

**Adrenal tumour** – Removal of the tumour with steroid replacement is essential. The healthy gland is usually atrophied and cannot take up the function but ACTH stimulation should be tried. Even after successful surgery patients with carcinoma die within 2 to 3 years of surgery due to metastasis commonly in liver and lungs.

In case of ectopic ACTH secreting tumour the metyrapone and aminoglutethimide may be tried.

In cases of adrenal hyperplasia causing Cushing's syndrome chemical adrenalectomy may be tried. This can be successful by giving OP/DDD and/or aminoglutethimide and metyrapone in appropriate dosage.

PROGNOSIS

In untreated cases cardiovascular accident or infection may prove fatal. The outcome of surgery after benign adrenal adenoma or bilateral hyperplasia is good. In malignant tumour the outlook is poor with metastasis developing early.

## CONN'S SYNDROME

This occurs due to excess production of aldosterone, usually from a solitary adrenal adenoma arising from the zona glomerulosa; rarely there are multiple adenomas. The production of excess aldosterone causes sodium retention and increased potassium excretion by the kidneys and also by the gastrointestinal tract, sweat glands and salivary glands.

CLINICAL FEATURES

(a) Due to excess sodium retention, there is expansion of the extracellular fluid volume and hypertension. If left untreated, it produces hypertensive complications.

(b) Hypokalaemia leading to alkalosis and tentany with muscle-cramps, twitching.

(c) Muscular aesthenia – There is weakness of the muscles and the patient is unable to carry on his usual occupation.

(d) Hypokalaemic nephropathy – Due to damage of the renal tubules, there would be polyuria, polydypsia and the urine may show albumin.

(d) ECG changes; there is depression of S-T segment and flattening of T-Wave and appearance of U-Wave. The most dangerous complication is ventricular extrasystole and ventricular tachycardia and ventricular fibrillation. Q-T interval is prolonged.

This symptoms are manifested when the serum potassium level is below 3.0 mEq. per litre.

DIAGNOSIS

The condition should be suspected whenever there is hypertension with unexplained hypokalaemia. The diagnosis is confirmed by :

(1) Serum potassium level below 3.0 mEq. per litre.

(2) 24-hour potassium excretion in the urine is increased (more than 25 millimoles).

(3) Depressed plasma renin activity (less than 300 ngm per 100 c.c.).

(4) Increased aldosterone excretion – The patient is given a diet containing more than 100 mEq of sodium per day for several days and no medicines and diuretics are given which might alter aldosterone production. Under such condition, if the aldosterone excretion in the 24-hour urine exceeds 20 microgrammes, then the diagnosis is confirmed.

(5) Location of the tumour can be confirmed by I.V.P. with renal tomogram and CAT scan.

TREATMENT

The treatment is surgical removal of the tumour and the blood pressure comes down to a normal level after a few weeks. If the patient cannot be operated, spironolactone can be given to control the hypertension and hypokalaemia. But the side – effects include weakness and lassitude, impotence, menstrual irregularities and gynaecomastia.

## SECONDARY ALDOSTERONISM

This occurs in disorders which induce increased renin secretion, which causes increased production of angiotensin, which, in turn stimulates the zona glomerulosa to produce increased aldosterone. This can occur with :

(i) reduction of extra volume

(ii) reduction of the plasma volume, or

(iii) pooling of blood on the venous side of circulation.

It commonly occurs in congestive cardiac failure, nephrotic syndrome and hepatic cirrhosis. The other causes include congenital adrenal hyperplasia, sodium loosing nephritis, renal artery-stenosis and increased renin secretion from hyperplasia of the juxtaglomerular cells.

This condition may have to be differentiated from hypokalaemia induced by thiazide diuretics, Cushing's syndrome, and certain cases of severe hypertension, potassium loosing nephritis usually associated with pyelonephritis etc.

**Adreno-genital syndrome in children**

## CONGENTIAL ADRENAL HYPERPLASIA :

The principal hormones synthesized by the adrenal cortex include cortisol, corticosterone, aldosterone and sex-steroids. Synthesis of these hormones takes place through successive steps, each step being controlled by a specific enzyme. This has already been discussed. Now, if there is a deficiency of particular enzyme then the synthesis of one or more hormones would be impaired and the precursors would be synthesized in excess due to increased ACTH stimulation. Clinical manifestations would depend upon the degree of deficiency of cortisol and aldosterone and pharmacological action of the excessive steroid synthesized due to increased ACTH stimulus.

Up-till now, six varieties of enzymatic deficiencies have been detected :-

(a) Deficiency of 21-hydroxylase : This is the most common type (90%) of congenital adrenal hyperplasia. This results in deficient secretion of cortisol and aldosterone and due to increased ACTH stimulus, there is increased synthesis of dehydroepiandosterone and testosterone and pregnanetriol. This condition can be easily diagnosed by detecting increased urinary excretion of 17-ketosteroids and pregnanetriol.

CLINICAL FEATURES

This disorder may be present in certain families. In severe cases early virilization becomes evident when the child is born. In a female child, there is clitoral hypertrophy, partial fusion of labioscrotal folds and frequently urogenital sinus is found and this condition is known as female pseudohermaphrodite. Genetically, the child is female as can be proved by karyotyping. This is also marked sodium depletion leading to dehydration and hypotension. The diagnosis can be quickly confirmed by 17-ketosteroid and pregnanetriol estimation.

In a male child, the diagnosis becomes difficult as the external genitalia are more or less normal but the salt depletion and associated dehydration and hypotension become clinically evident. The condition may be fatal unless quickly diagnosed and should be treated with glucocorticoids, mineralocorticoids and sodium-chloride in a similar fashion as in Addison's disease. In milder form, the child may grow up to 5 to 10 years of age when suspicion arises due to premature precocious puberty. There is rapid linear growth causing increase in height which soon ceases due to closure of the epiphyses. Early appearance of axillary and pubic hairs, hoarsening of the voice, hirsutism and acne. In females, even after reaching puberty, there is amenorrhoea, failure of development of the breasts and secondary sex characters. Hypertrophy of the clitoris is also evident in females. The treatment is same as before with glucocorticoids and sodium-chloride. In a male child, in addition to hirsutism, acne, hoarsening of the voice, there would be increased size of penis and testes with increased sexual drive. But spermatogenesis would be depressed.

(b) Deficiency of 11 beta ($\beta$) hydroxylase :

This results in impairment of cortisol, aldosterone and corticosterone production. Due to feedback mechanism there is increased production of ACTH resulting in overproduction of desoxycorticosterone and desoxycortisol and dehydroepiandosterone. The condition is diagnosed by subnormal level of plasma cortisol with increased 17-hydroxy and 17-ketosteroids excretion in the urine. Clinically, there is virilization due to increased androgen effect and hypertension due to increased production of DOCA. This condition may sometimes simulate Cushing's syndrome but there is no obesity, plethoric appearance and purple striae and the plasma cortisol level is invariably low. The condition can be successfully treated with glucocorticoids to suppress the ACTH production which further suppresses the increased production of androgen and DOCA.

(c) Deficiency of 3 beta ($\beta$) hydroxysteroid-dehydrogenase :

This prevents the conversion of pregnenolone to progesterone. So there is deficient secretion of cortisol, aldosterone but increased secretion of D.H.E.A. Clinical features include masculine features of the external genitalia with aldosterone and cortisol deficiency. Treatment is the same as in 21-hydroxylase deficiency.

(d) Deficiency of 17 alpha ($\alpha$) hydroxylase :

This results in impairment of the synthesis of cortisol and sex-steroids like D.H.E.A. androstenedione and oestrogens. Aldosterone secretion remains normal. Due to increased A.C.T.H. stimulus, the adrenal synthesizes large quantities of corticosterone and DOCA. Because of the deficiency of the gonadal hormones from the adrenals as well as from the gonads, there is hypogonadism in both sexes. Biochemical data include low level of plasma cortisol and urinary 17-hydroxy and 17-ketosteroids with high level of A.C.T.H. and corticosterone. The oestrogen and testosterone levels are also reduced with increased level of pituitary gonadotropins. The important clinical features include hypertension with retardation of sexual growth. The treatment include the administration of glucocorticoids and sex-steroids.

(e) Deficiency of 20-hydroxylase :

This blocks the synthesis of all adrenal and gonadal steroids as conversion of cholesterol to pregnenolone does not take place. Infants with this disorder have a poor survival rate and they are usually born with female external genitalia. If the early diagnosis can be made treatment should be the same as in Addison's disease.

(f) Deficiency of 18-hydroxysteroid-dehydrogenase :

This enzyme is only present in zonal glomerulosa and its deficiency results in aldosterone deficiency. This further results in sodium depletion with hyperkalaemia, dehydration and hypotension. The treatment consists of substitution therapy with mineralocorticoids.

## ADRENOGENITAL SYNDROME IN ADOLESCENTS AND ADULTS

This is due to virilizing tumours in adolescents or in adults. The clinical features include progressive virilization, i.e. hirsutism, acne, amenorrhoea, atrophy of the breasts, enlargement of the clitoris and masculine voice. The condition can be diagnosed by normal plasma-cortisol level but increased 17-ketosteroid level which is not suppressed with high dosage of dexamethasone. The adrenal tumour can be detected as mentioned before with I.V.P. with renal tomography, arteriography and CAT scan. The ovarian tumour rarely secreting excessive androgen should be excluded by Culdoscopy examination. Feminizing adrenal tumours and extremely uncommon. This is characterized by progressive feminization in an adult male and high level of urinary oestrogen and detection of an adrenal mass.

Rarely adrenal tumours can be found in children and the features include progressive virilization and the detection of the adrenal mass.

## PHEOCHROMOCYTOMA

*S. KUMAR*

Pheochromocytomas are new growths of chromaffin tissue, arising anywhere from the sympathetic nervous system though 95% occur in the abdomen and 80% from suprarenal medulla. The tumour secretes excessive amount of catecholamines.

The first classical case was described in 1922 by Ghabbe, Tinel and Dower (Paris).

### Aetiology

Usually, there is a benign adenoma affecting one gland, but it may be bilateral (10%) and sometimes it may undergo malignant changes. Occasionally, the tumour may arise from para--aortic-medullary tissue extending from the thorax down to pelvis. The tumour secretes both adrenaline and noradrenaline in varying proportions. It can occur with neurofibromatosis, familial hyperparathyroidism, Von-Hippel-Lindau's disease and medullary carcinoma of the thyroid.

### Clinical features

The most important features is hypertension which may be sustained or paroxysmal and the blood pressure in between the paroxysmal attacks may be normal. These paroxysmal attacks may occur several times a day or at intervals of weeks and duration may vary from a few minutes to a few hours. During an attack, the patient feels a sense of apprehension with severe headache and dizziness.

The important features include dyspnoea and a feeling of suffocation, palpitation with painful constriction of the chest or angina-like pain, tremor, perspiration and painful cramps of the calf muscles. The skin becomes pale and cold. The blood pressure sharply rises (e.g. 280/ mm of Hg.) The pulse rate in considerably accelerated during the attack, but if nor-adrenaline secretion is more than adrenaline, tachycardia is not so evident. As a result of these repeated attacks, the heart may be enlarged and there may be left ventricular failure with pulmonary oedema. Rarely, there may be phases of hypotension possibly due to vasodilation caused by increased adrenaline or the picture may be one of progressive hypertension without any super-imposed paroxysm. The kidneys and the fundi may be affected in some cases. Retinal haemorrhage or papilloedema also rarely occurs.

Associated features include fever with leucocytosis and diabetes mellitus. Occasionally, there may be abdominal pain with diarrhoea. The attacks may be precipitated by physical or emotional exertion or operative procedure or due to palpation of the adenoma during abdominal examination or even by micturition (in some of the rare cases where the tumour is in the bladder).

### DIAGNOSIS

The diagnosis of pheochromocytoma should be suspected when there is severe and persistent high rise of blood pressure and this has to be differentiated from essential hypertension and other causes of secondary hypertension. The condition should also be suspected if there are episodes of palpitation, tachycardia and tremor. The diagnosis may be difficult if there are episodes of hypotension and circulatory collapse without any other clinical disorder and the clinical has to keep the possibility in mind.

The following disorders may have to be differentiated from phaeochromocytoma :

1. Anxiety state due to psychological disturbances with tremor, sweating and apprehension.
2. Diabetes mellitus because of polyuria and increased blood sugar level (I.G.G.T.).
3. Thyrotoxicosis due to presence of tachycardia, palpitation psychosis, increased respiratory rate, tremor and increased B.M.R.

4. Carcinoid syndrome due to attacks of flushing with sweating and abdominal pain.
5. Hirschsprung's disease due to decreased intestinal motility and constipation.
6. Sudden elevation of intracranial pressure as may be seen in cerebellar tumour may have paroxysmal hypertension.

Features for other associated conditions like presence of multiple neurofibroma or 'cafe-au-lait' spots or presence of a goitre should be looked for.

The condition can be diagnosed with certainty by the following investigations.

**(1) Estimation of V.M.A. (Vanillyl mandelic acid)**

This is the major metabolite from adrenaline and nor-adrenaline excreted in urine and is measured in urine and is measured in the 24 hours sample. It is a useful diagnostic test because in pheochromocytoma the VMA level in urine is considerably increased though false-negative results may occur in up to 25% of cases. VMA excretion of more than 7 mg/24 hour or 500 mcg/hour is generally considered abnormal (though value differs from laboratory to laboratory). The patient should not take coffee, cocoa, chocolates, vanilla, citrus fruits, some vegetables and monoamineoxydase (MAO) inhibitors for a few days before the estimation is done. The treatment for hypertension may be continued with $\beta$-blockers, reserpine, guanethidine, hydrallazine or even hydrochlorthiazide but all other drugs should be stopped.

**(2) Urinary catecholamines including epinephrine and non-epinephrine estimation**

Estimation of urinary catecholamines like epinephrine and non-epinephrine and also useful tests. In pheochromocytoma, the level would be high (normal range 100-200g/24 hours). Before collection of the urine vasopressor agents, tetracycline and alpha ($\alpha$)-methyl dopa should not be used.

Both V.M.A. and catecholamines should be measured as in some cases, only V.M.A. level is high. About 90% cases can be diagnosed by these measurements. In normotensive subjects with paroxysmal rise of blood pressure, the urine should be collected after the episode for 24 hours or the urine may be collected for the next two hours and the V.M.A. and catecholamines, epinephrine, nor-epinephrine can be measured and expressed in microgram per hour which would be high in case of pheochromocytoma.

Catecholamine excretion exceeding 10 mcg/hour is abnormal. If the epinephrine excretion is higher, the tumour is located in the adrenal and when nor-epinephrine excretion alone is high, the tumour is extra-adrenal.

**(3) Phentolamine test**

This test is rarely used and may be required only 10% of cases. The usual recommended dose in 5 mg. intravenously but it may cause severe fall of blood pressure. It would be safer to use one mg. I.V. and a fall of blood pressure of 35/25 mm. of Hg. lasting five minutes in indicative of pheochromocytoma. False positive results may be obtained in uraemia or patients being treated for hypertension or taking hypnotics.

**(4) Provocative tests with histamine, tyrosine or glucagon**

In normotensive subjects, hypertensive attacks may be provoked by using histamine, tyrosine or glucagon and the urinary excretion of V.M.A. and catecholamines may be measured subsequently as described before. Alpha ($\alpha$)-blocking agents such as phentolamine or phenoxybenzamine hydrochloride (dibenziline) may be used. This test is rarely necessary.

**(5) Localisation of the tumour**

(a) Radiography of the chest is useful to detect the paravertebral tumour both P.A. and lateral views should be taken. Similarly X-ray of the abdomen is also useful.

(b) I.V.P. with renal tomography will show the adrenal mass, if present, in about 50% of cases.

(c) Retroperitoneal infusion of air to produce a perirenal insufflation is useful but it may produce hypertensive crisis.

(d) Arteriography and venography can also be done to locate the tumour mass.

(e) Introduction of sonography radio-isotope studies with renal scan are useful to locate the tumour.

(f) CT-Scan easily locates the tumour but an expensive test. At present it is the investigation of first choice and without any hazard.

## TREATMENT

Surgical removal of the tumour is the treatment of choice. Medical treatment is necessary for preparation of the patient for surgery or for malignant pheochromocytoma where the patient is unable to undergo surgery. The effective control of blood pressure can be obtained by alpha-adrenergic blocking agents which inhibit the effect of catecholamines but do not alter their synthesis. Phentolamine and phenoxybenzamine hydrochloride (Dibenzylene) are the drugs used. Usually phenoxy-benzamine is used in an oral dose varying from 40 mg to 100 mg. twice daily. This effectively controls the blood pressure. If cardiac arrhythmia is present because of catecholamine-action on the beta-receptors, propranolol can be used in a dosage of 40 mg. three times daily.

Alpha-methyl-tyrosine, which inhibits the synthesis of catecholamines, has been found quite effective in controlling the hypertension in cases of pheochromocytoma and can be used preoperatively.

After seven to ten days of medical therapy, the patient becomes fit for surgery. Premedication should be done with hyoscine and atropine should be avoided which would induce tachycardia. Thiopental sodium and nitrous oxide are usually used as anaesthetics as they do not release catecholamines.

During the surgical procedure, the blood pressure and E.C.G. monitoring should be routinely done and any rise in blood pressure should be controlled with intravenous phentolamine and tachycardia should be controlled with propranolol. Postoperative hypotension can be prevented by adequate blood transfusion and maintenance of the blood volume. It is rarely necessary to use nor adrenaline infusion. After removal of the tumour, the V.M.A. and catecholamine excretion in the urine returns to normal. The estimation should be carried out at frequent intervals to exclude any recurrence. Particularly if there is a familial incidence.

# CONTRAINDICATIONS & COMPLICATIONS OF STEROID THERAPY

*S KUMAR*

## CONTRAINDICATIONS

There is no absolute contraindication for the use of steroids and whenever it is needed as a life saving measure it has to be used by parenteral route. The other side-effects which may be produced are discussed below.

The incidence of complications largely depends upon the dose of the steroids used and on the duration of treatment and on tolerance of the patient.

The commonest side-effects are appearance of moon-face, development of acne and hirsutism; trunkal obesity is characteristic. The following points are important.

1. **Steroid and infection :** Patients having large dose of steroids may develop inter-current staphylococcal or pneumococcal infections and even septicaemia without much systemic disturbances and the diagnosis may be difficult. Sometimes, latent tuberculous focus may flare up during steroid therapy.

2. **Growth in children :** In children prolonged steroid therapy will depress the growth hormone and may produce dwarfism. This condition may be successfully treated with growth hormone therapy. Some authorities believe that A.C.T.H. causes less suppression of growth hormone and may be useful for treatment in children.

   A.C.T.H. and its synthetic analogue tetracosactrin may produce allergic reactions and in those cases, steroids have to be used either as cortisol or its derivatives. It may be mentioned in this connection that A.C.T.H. has no definite added beneficial effect over steroid therapy.

3. **Steroids and hypothalamopituitary Adrenal (HPA) suppression :** Steroids when used for a short period over a few weeks does not cause suppression of the HPA axis and can be quickly reduced without any fear of adrenal suppression. Similarly, prednisolone when used in a daily dosage of 5-10 mg does not cause adrenal suppression and therefore can be quickly reduced. When cortisol or prednisolone or its synthetic analogues are used in large doses for several months it would produce depression of HPA axis. Sudden withdrawal in these cases could produce adrenal failure. In such cases the dose has to be reduced by 2.5 mg of prednisolone per month or 20 mg of cortisol per month. This would produce gradual adrenal recovery within 6-9 months. Serial measurement of A.C.T.H. and plasma cortisol level should be useful. Both would gradually rise and return to normal level and diurnal rhythm would surely be established. Clinical well-being of the patient, regular measurement of blood pressure are also useful. After one year, stress test should be done by inducing hypoglycaemia with insulin or after pyrogen injection and measuring the rise in the plasma cortisol level. This would give an idea whether the patient would need steroid supplements during conditions of stress such as major operations, or high fever or severe gastrointestinal disturbances.

   It is recommended that for patients who had received steroid therapy within one year, adequate cover should be given at the time of stress. This can be given by a dose of 100 mg of cortisol parenterally, every 6 hours for the first 2-3 days and then gradually reduce it depending on response of the patient. here again the guideline would be serial measurement of the blood pressure and clinical well – being of the patient. Any symptoms suggestive of adrenal insufficiency should promptly be treated by increasing the dose of steroids.

   Long-term A.C.T.H. therapy would produce hypertrophy of the adrenals but would depress CRF (corticotrophin releasing factor) and A.C.T.H. secretion. Hence it has no advantage over steroid therapy.

4. **Steroid and ulcer :** Glucocorticoids do not produce peptic ulcer because in Cushing's syndrome when the steroid level in the blood is quite high, increased incidence of peptic ulcer has not been reported. When given by mouth it is debatable whether it produces peptic ulcer. Recent reports indicate that the incidence of ulcers in subjects on steroid therapy, is not significantly higher than in those not receiving steroids.

   Another interesting aspect is that only patients with rheumatoid arthritis receiving steroid have been reported to develop ulcer by some workers and this may be due to the effect of other analgesics such as aspirin or phenylbutazone. Neverthless steroids may produce gastric irritation and in cases of pre-existing ulcers it can cause haemorrhage, and perforation which is often silent and may delay the healing. It can also delay the healing of an active ulcer. Thus in patients who develop gastric symptoms like nausea or pain or discomfort in the epigastrium it would be wise to add antacids along with steroids and if necessary to switch over to parenteral therapy. In case of pre-existing ulcers, steroids should only be given if it is urgently needed and by parenteral therapy.

5. **Steroid and Osteoporosis :** Osteoporosis is a common feature in Cushing's syndrome. Patients with sustained steroid therapy may develop osteoporosis and fracture of various bones, especially collapse of the vertebrae or fracture of the long bones or ribs. As there is

no warning symptom of an impending fracture, it would be wise to assume that osteoporosis is slowly developing in all patients taking steroids for a long period. Aseptic necrosis of head of femur has also been rarely report.

Usually the fractures heal up reasonably well. Role of calcium supplements of vitamin D therapy or anabolic hormones is of doubtful value. If a patient develops fracture, when steroid therapy is essential as a life-saving measure, it would be imperative to continue steroids in minimum possible low dose despite the fractures.

6. **Steroid and diabetes :** The glucocorticoids cause neoglucogenesis and peripheral resistance to insulin action. Thus these have a diabetogenic role. In normal persons there may be mild impairment of glucose tolerance which returns to normal after stopping steroid therapy; but those patients who are liable to develop diabetes later on show marked impairment of glucose tolerance with glycosuria and clinical features of diabetes mellitus. The incidence of diabetes developing after steroid therapy is small.
7. **Steroid and Hypertension :** Steroid therapy causes mild degree of hypertension in some causes which returns to normal after stoppage of therapy. The rise of blood pressure is primarily due to sodium retention.
8. **Steroid and Psychosis :** Steroid should be given with caution in patients with history of psychological disturbances. It produces a sense of euphoria even in normal subjects. Occasionally depression, mania and psychotic state may develop.
9. **Steroid and Myopathies :** Glucocorticoids are catabolic in nature and may cause negative nitrogen balance. When used for a considerable period in large doses, there may produce wasting of the muscles, especially of the pelvic and shoulder girdle and triceps are also frequently affected. In most cases, it is of mild degree but in some the extent is considerable and produces symptoms. Triamcinolone has the worst effect. Triamcinolone produces much higher degree of myopathies than others.

## CRYPTORCHIDISM

*S KUMAR*

Cryptorchidism or undescended testes on one or both sides may occur in 3% of fully term males and in 30% of preterm males children at birth. However, descent of testes can continue till puberty, so that postpubertally less than 1% of males have unilateral or bilateral undescended tests. Cryptorchidism may occur in otherwise normal boys or may be a part of hypogonadotrophic hypogonadism. True cryptorchidism needs to be differentiated clinically from pseudocryptorchidism or retractile testes, which is not uncommon in children. The two main problems associated with cryptorchidism are :

(1) Spermatogenesis does not occur in the undescended testis and if the condition is bilateral there will be sterility. This is conventionally ascribed to failure of development of the seminiferous tubules due to high intra-abdominal temperature. Another view suggests that the basic defect is in the testis itself, which causes both the maldescent and the infertility.

(2) Undescended testis has increased risk of undergoing malignant changes. It is also probable that even if the undescended testis is surgically brought down into the scrotum, it retains some increased chance of becoming malignant.

TREATMENT :

A course of human chorionic gonadotrophin (HCG) is usually given in dosage of 4000 I.U. three times a week for 3 weeks at about 6 years of age, this causes testicular descent in many patients; however, in the majority of such cases the descent is temporary and the testes may return to nonscrotal position when treatment is stopped. However, even if there is temporary descent with HCG, it can reasonably be hoped that permanent descent will occur at puberty and surgery may not be necessary. In those children who fail to respond to HCG, surgery should be done at the beginning of puberty to allow spermatogenesis to occur and also for easier clinical examination of the testes, thus allowing early detection of possible malignancy. It is suggested that if the repositioned testis does not demonstrate normal spermatogenesis within a reasonable time, then that testis should be removed (if the affection is unilateral).

## IMPOTENCE

*S KUMAR*

**Definition**

Impotence is a type of male sexual dysfunction characterised by inability to achieve an erection.

**Causes :** **I. Psychological,** e.g. anxiety, depression, mental discord, disinterest in sexual partner etc. — this is by far the commonest cause of impotence.

**II. Organic causes**

A. **Endocrine**

i) Testicular failure, either primary or secondary to pituitary or hypothalamic defect.

ii) Hyperprolactinaemia, e.g. due to pituitary microadenoma — as prolactin suppresses luteinising hormone releasing hormone (LHRH) production.

B. **Neurologic**

i) Autonomic neuropathy, e.g. in diabetes mellitus

ii) Tabes dorsalis

iii) Multiple sclerosis

iv) Damage to nerves during surgery, e.g. prostatectomy, rectosigmoid operation etc.

C. **Vascular**

i) Leriche's syndrome due to thromboembolic obstruction of abdominal aorta at its bifurcation.

D. **Drug induced**

i) Antihypertensives, e.g. clonidine, methyldopa, propranolol.

ii) Antidepressants, e.g. amitryptiline.

iii) Antipsychotics, e.g. chlorpromazine, haloperidol.

iv) Antihistaminics, e.g. diphenhydramine, cimetidine.

E. **Local penile disease**

i) Peyronie's disease

ii) Previous priapism

**Management**

The primary task is to identify whether the cause is organic or psychological. This involves meticulous elucidation of history and physical examination including neurologic and vascular assessment and genital and gonadal examination.

In the larger group of psychologic causes, removal of the cause whenever possible, together with psychotherapy and sexual counselling usually helps. Where organic causes are responsible treatment may involve withdrawal of an offending drug, treatment with androgens in definite causes of hypogonadism, treatment of hyperprolactinaemia either medically by bromocriptine or surgically by removal of pituitary tumour, surgical treatment for aortic occlusion. In refractory cases mechanical help may be provided by implanting a suitable penile prosthesis.

## INFERTILITY

*S. KUMAR*

Infertility or failure of conception may be due to a defect in the husband (in about 1/3rd of cases) or, in the wife (in about 1/3rd of cases) or in both (in the remaining 1/3rd of cases). Female infertility is primarily in the gynaecologist's jurisdiction and we shall consider here some aspects of male infertility.

**Causes of infertility :**

(A) Hypothalamic — pituitary disorders.

(i) Panhypopituitarism due to tumours, chronic granulomatous diseases, trauma etc.

(ii) Selective deficiency of gonadotrophin e.g. Kallman's syndrome

(iii) Hyperprolactinaemia

(B) **Testicular disorders**

(i) **Developmental**

(a) Klinefelter's syndrome

(b) Cryptorchidism especially if bilateral; even in unilateral cryptorchidism there may be infertility.

(ii) **Acquired**

(a) Viral orchitis, probably the commonest cause of acquired testicular failure and is most commonly due to mumps but may also be due to echo virus, lymphocytic chorio-meningitis virus etc.

(b) Varicocele due to dilatation of the peritesticular pampiniform plexus of veins associated with increased scrotal temperature. This is probably the most common treatable cause of male infertility.

(c) Trauma, either mechanical or thermal.

(d) Chronic infections e.g. lepromatous leprosy, tuberculosis.

(e) Radiation and drugs i.e. Iatrogenic.

Excessive exposure to X-rays or, irradiation of one testis for treatment of seminoma without adequate protection of the other testis can cause infertility. Cytotoxic drugs, most notably cyclophosphamide, used for malignant diseases can cause infertility.

(f) Autoimmune diseases

Testicular failure may occur as part of Schmidt's syndrome, where there are multiple endocrine deficiencies of autoimmune basis or there may be selective autoantibodies against spermatozoa only.

(g) Testicular abnormalities associated with systemic disease

(h) Testicular abnormalities associated with systemic disease, e.g. chronic liver disease, chronic renal failure, myotonic dystrophy etc.

(i) Idiopathic

There is asplasia of the germinal cells of testes for unknown reasons.

(j) Post testicular defect

(i) Structural, e.g. atresia of the vasa deferentia either congenital or post inflammatory.

(ii) Functional, e.g. androgen receptor resistance, which causes infertility as well as under androgenisation.

**Management**

History should be taken about pubertal development and also about various systemic diseases. The patient should be examined especially for gonadal development, external genitalia, and secondary sex characteristics.

Seminal analysis should be done on at least two occasions for detection of low sperm counts or presence of abnormal or immotile forms.

Testicular biopsy may be needed to know the degree of maturation of germinal epithelium.

A simple buccal smear examination of Barr body or better, a full Karyotype of chromosomes can detect chromosomal anomalies. Further, estimation of gonadotrophin levels will help to determine whether the defect is primarily of the testis (where gonadotrophins are high) or it is secondary to hypothalamic — pituitary defect (where gonadotrophins are low).

Treatment includes surgical intervention for varicocele, some cases of obstruction of vasa deferentia or for cryptorchidism (for the last condition surgery should be done before puberty). In patients with hypogonadotrophic hypogonadal infertility, both androgen secretion and spermatogenesis may be restored to normal by injections of FSH and LH or clomiphene or FSH/LH-RH. FSH/LH-RH.

Where hyperprolactinaemia is the cause, bromocriptine is often useful. It should be remembered that up to 25% of cases of idiopathic infertility show spontaneous resolution.

## HERMAPHRODITISM

*S KUMAR*

**Hermes (the messenger of Gods) + Aphrodite (the Goddess of Love)**

Hermaphroditism is a condition where there is varying degree of ambiguity regarding the sex of an individual. The word literally means combination of character of both sexes. It is important to recognise that sex of an individual should be considered from several points of view.

(1) **Chromosomal or genetic sex,** determined from the karyotype : males having 46 XY and females 46 XX.

(2) **Chromatin sex** depends on the presence or absence of chromatin dot or Barr-body in the nucleus of cells from buccal smear or polymorphonuclear leucocyte. Normal males are chromatin negative and normal females are chromatin positive.

(3) **Gonadal sex** depending on presence of testes or ovaries.

(4) **Genital sex** or phenotypic sex — depending mainly on the anatomy the external genitalia, as well as the development of secondary sexual characteristics after puberty.

(5) **Psychological sex** depending on psychosexual orientation or 'gender role' of an individual.

Hermaphrodites may be true hermaphrodites where both testicular and ovarian tissue are found in the same individual or **pseudo,** hermaphrodites where gonad is of one type only, but genital development shows some contradiction to gonadal or — chromosomal sex.

### A. True Hermaphroditism

There may be an ovary on one side and a testis on the other or an ovotestis on one side and ovary or testis on the other or an ovotestis on both sides.

About 33% of these cases show a 46 XX karyotype, about 10% have a 46 XX karyotype and the remainder are chromosomal mosaics. In those cases of 46 XX karyotype it is assumed that sufficiently chromosomal material is present, either by translocation nondysfunction or mutation to cause testicular development.

Clinically, the external genitalia have various grades of male to female characters. About 2/3rds have sufficient masculine appearance to be reared as males, however most have hypospadias, often with perineal urethral opening and many have incomplete labioscrotal fusion. At puberty, varying degrees of feminisation and virilisation develop. Ovulation may occur in up to 25% cases and is more common than spermatogenesis.

B. **Pseudohermaphroditism**

This may be :

(1) Female pseudohermaphrodites where gonads are ovaries but genitalia show maleness.

Causes : (a) Congenital adrenal hyperplasia most commonly due to 21-hydroxylase deficiency.

(b) Administration of progestogens with androgenic side, effects to pregnant women carrying female foetus, e.g. to prevent abortion.

(c) Virilising tumour, e.g. arrhenoblastoma of the mother pregnancy.

(d) Rarely no aetiology can be determined.

(2) **Male pseudohermaphroditism**

Where there is varying degree of feminisation of genitalia in a chromosomally XY male with testes.

Causes : (a) Disorders in androgen synthesis due to various enzymatic defects.

(b) Disorders in androgen action — this acounts for 80% cases.

This may be due to end organ insensitivity as in testicular feminisation syndrome which may be complete, where the individual is phenotypically a normal female who presents with primary amenorrhoea, or incomplete where some virilisation of external genitalia is also present.

(c) **Presistent mullerian duct syndrome :**

Here the individual is externally male but has, in addition, fallopian tubes, uterus and upper vagina due to failure of regression of mullerian duct.

(d) **Unknown aetiology**

## HYPOGONADISM

*S.KUMAR*

**Definition**

Hypogonadism, as the term suggests, refers to deficiency of one or both of the main functions of the gonads, namely the production of germ cells, i.e. spermatozoa from testes and ova from ovaries and the secretion of sex hormones.

**Clinical features**

A. If onset is before puberty, then manifestation is in the form of poor development of external genitalia and secondary sex characteristics.

In females, there is, addition, failure of onset of menstruation known as primary amenorrhoea.

B. If onset is after puberty, then there is regression rather than lack of secondary sex characteristics. Moreover, infertility is an important presentation. In females, there is also secondary amenorrhoea.

**Aetiology**

1. **Hypothalamic disorders**

These may be acquired; e.g. inflammatory, neoplastic etc. or congenital e.g. Kallmann syndrome, which is hypogonadism due to deficient FSH/LH-RH secretion from the hypothalamus associated with anosmia due to agenesis of the olfactory bulbs.

2. **Pituitary disorders**

These may be of diverse aetiology and deficient gonadotrophin secretion is usually associated with deficient secretion of other trophic hormones; but rarely it may exist as a monotrophic deficiency.

3. **Primary gonadal disorders**

   A. Congenital e.g. Klinefelter's syndrome in males and Turner's syndrome in females.

   B. Acquired, e.g. infections like tuberculosis, mumps, leprosy; surgical removal etc.

4. **Non-endocrine disorders**

   In males particularly haemochromatosis, dystrophia myotonica, and cirrhosis of liver and any severe systemic illness in either sex, e.g. malabsorption states, chronic renal disease etc.

**General Plan of Treatment of Hypogonadism**

The hormonal deficiency can be corrected by replacement therapy. The sex hormones themselves can be used e.g. the androgens for male hypogonadism and oestrogen or oestrogen and progestogen combination for females hypogonadism. For androgen replacement long acting preparations like testosterone enanthate may be used intramuscularly every 1-2 weeks initially and then every 2-3 weeks for maintenance or unconjugated testosterone pellets may be implanted subcutaneously every 4-6 months or sublingual methyl testosterone or oral fluoxymesterone may be used daily.

For female hypogonadism, commonly oestrogen-progestogen combinations like the oral contraceptive pills are used cyclically. Needless to say, sex hormone replacement causes development of secondary sex characteristics, but cannot lead to spermatogenesis or oogenesis. When germ cell production is also desired, pituitary gonadotrophin may be used. More recently hypothalamic gonadotrophin releasing hormones are also available.

## GONADS AND SEX

*S KUMAR*

**Introduction**

Among the gonadal disorder, we shall consider hermaphroditism hypogonadism in both sexes, cryptorchidism and impotence in males, the problem of infertility as relevant to the physician and also sexual precocity in both sexes. We shall discuss the problem of hirsutism. Oral contraceptives especially their side effects, will also be discussed, disorders of breasts, particularly galactorrhoea and gynaecomastia will also be discussed.

## FEMALE SEXUAL PRECOCITY

**DEFINITION**

Precocious puberty (P.P.) girls is defined as sexual maturity and/or menarche before the age of 9 years. Another sign is early appearance of breast buds before the age of nine. P.P. is more common in girls than in boys.

**CLASSIFICATION AND AETIOLOGY**

Broadly, it may be of two types : True P.P. or pseudoprecocity.

**True precocious puberty :** True P.P. is characterised by premature development of an otherwise normal puberty including ovulation and menstruation.

**CAUSES**

1. **Idiopathic or constitutional P.P.**

   Most cases (about 90%) are of idiopathic type.

2. **Organic brain disorders,** e.g. brain tumours, encephalitis, meningitis, hydrocephalus, head injury, tuberous sclerosis etc.

3. **Hyperthyroidism**

4. **Congenital adrenal hyperplasia** (21-hydroxylase deficiency in girls), where glucocorticoid replacement therapy is delayed until 4 to 8 years of age.

Congenital adrenocortical hyperplasia also leads to heterosexual precocious pseudopuberty. McCune Albright syndrome characterised by polycystic fibrous dysplasia, is associated with precocious pseudopuberty.

## PRECOCIOUS PSEUDOPRECOCITY

Here girls show sexual maturity externally but to not ovulate or develop cyclic menses. There result from premature sex hormone secretions by ovarian or adrenal hyperfunction or teratomas or administration of oestrogen containing medications.

The problem of prepubertal phase of development is quite complex and careful watch is necessary that things are developing in the right direction.

The term isosexual precocity is used where males or females are becoming sexually mature earlier. Heterosexual precocity is more serious as in this variety of sexual maturity, females become masculine (virilisation) while males are feminised. In addition to these, there can be incomplete sexual precocity, i.e. premature development of a single clinical pubertal even, e.g. precocious breast development (thelarche) or premature development of pubic hair (pubarche). These events are due to inordinate end organ sensitivity to the low levels of hormones circulating prior to puberty.

## TURNER'S SYNDROME
### (Ovarian dysgenesis)

This is a rare congenital anomaly due to defective sex chromosomal constitution. The classical and the commonest karyotype in Turner's syndrome is 45, XO with negative Barr body; some others have mosaicism e.g. OX/XX,/XO,/XY, XO/XXX etc.;still others have a structurally abnormal X chromosome with or without mosaicism. In the latter two varieties, Barr body may or may not be negative, depending on the actual chromosomal consitution.

The clinical features of classical Turner's syndrome are short stature (usually less then 5ft. in height), webbing of the neck, cubitus valgus, low posterior hairline, shield-like chest with wider space nipples, primary amenorrhoea and poor development of secondary sexual characters-short 4th metacarpal bone may be present. There is also significant association. With coarcatation of aorta and and congenital lymphoedema. Some of them are mentally retarded.

The ovaries are represented by white fibrous streaks lacking identifiable follicles and ova. Plasma oestradiol level is low, while FSH and LH levels are high.

In Turner's syndrome,due to an abnormality in the second X chromosome or mosaicism, the clinical picture is more variable. In some of these patients with mosaicism, sufficient normal ovarian tissue may be present to allow some menstruation and very rarely pregnancy.

## MANAGEMENT

At the anticipated time of puberty, development of menstruation and secondary sex character should encouraged by cyclical treatment with oestrogen and progesterone. In cases of Tumer's syndrome having virilisation or Y-containing cell line the streak gonads should be removed because of risks of malignancy. Besides, coarctation of aorta might need surgical correction.

## HIRSUTISM

### DEFINITION

It is excessive hair growth in a female resembling pattern characteristic of males.

### AETIOLOGY

Physiological e.g. during pregnancy, at menopause, due to genetic difference in different races.

**Pathological**

(1) **Idiopathic or simple hirsutism :** Where cause is not definitely known. These cases may represent the extreme end of a normal condition and the great majority of hirsutism falls in this group. Cases may be branded idiopathic only when menstruation is normal and there are no stigmata of virilisation; urinary 17-ketosteroids are not elevated, and there is no obvious abnormality of ovaries and adrenals.

This is now thought to result from increased conversion of normal or minimally elevated amounts of androstenedione and testosterone to dihydro-testosterone in the skin.

(2) **Endocrinopathies**

(a) Ovarian androgen excess

(i) Polycystic ovary syndrome — The commonest cause of ovarian hyperandrogenism and may present with amenorrhoea, hirsutism and bilateral polycystic ovaries.

(ii) Virilising ovarian tumours, e.g. arrhenoblastoma and hilar cell tumour.

(b) Adrenal androgen excess

(i) Androgen secreting tumours of adrenal (adenoma or carcinoma)

(ii) Cushing's syndrome

(iii) Congenital adrenal hyperplasia due to enzymatic defect.

(3) Iatrogenic or drug induced hirsutism

It may be an isolated symptom or part of a virilising syndrome.

(a) Drugs causing hirsutism without virilisation :

Diphenylhydantion (for epilepsy), minoxidil (for hypertension), diazoxide (for hypoglycaemia or hypertension), ACTH and prednisolone.

(b) Drugs that can cause both hirsutism and true virilisation :

Androgens and certain progestogens.

**TREATMENT**

A. **Systemic**

(1) Cyclical administration of oestrogen-progestogen combinations (e.g. oral contraceptive pills) for 3-6 months for ovarian androgen suppression in idiopathic hirsutism or polycystic ovary syndrome.

(2) Antiandrogens like

(a) Cyproterone acetate

(b) Spironolactone

(c) Cimetidine

(3) In iatrogenic cases stoppage of the offending drugs is mandatory, but is not always followed by regression of hirsutism or other evidences of virilisation.

(4) Surgery

e.g. removal of tumours of ovary or adrenal; bilateral wedge resection of ovaries in polycystic ovary syndrome.

B. **Local**

(1) Shaving — in contrast to popular belief it does not increase hairiness

(2) Depilatory wax or cream

(3) Plucking or tweezing

(4) Electrolysis

## MALE SEXUAL PRECOCITY

### DEFINITION

It is the onset of puberty or sexual development in a body before the age of 10 years.

### CLASSIFICATION AND AETIOLOGY

**True precocity** — Here complete sexual maturity including spermatogenesis occurs prematurely. The causes are :

1. **Idiopathic or constitutional**
2. **Intracranial lesions,** e.g. brain tumours, meningitis, encephalitis etc.
3. **Endocrinal,** e.g. congenital adrenal hyperlpasia (due to 21 — or 11 — hydroxylase enzyme deficiency) where increased adrenal androgens occasionally trigger gonadotrophin release from anterior pituitary.
4. **Non-endocrine tumours,** e.g. hepatoblastoma that may secrete gonadotrophins.

### PSEUDOPRECOCITY

Here there is development of secondary sex characteristics, but true sexual maturity and spermatogenesis do not occur precociously. In males pseudoprecocity is more common than true precocity. This can also be isosexual or heterosexual.

**The causes are :**

Congenital adrenal hyperplasia

Adrenal tumour

Testicular tumour.

### KLINEFELTER'S SYNDROME

This is a type of male hypogonadism due to the presence of one or more extra X chromosome. The karyotype in the classical case is 47, XXY, in Barr body positive and is due to meiotic non-disjunctions of chromosome. There are several reported variations in karyotypes which include 48 XXXY, 48 XXXY, 49 XXXXY. Occasionally sex chromosome mosaicism is found. The mosaic form may result from mitotic mondisjunction after fertilisation, after fertilisation, or from double non-disjunction, both meiotic and mitotic.

Classical klinefelter's syndrome is characterised by small testes with partial or/complete hyalinisation or seminiferous tubules with absent spermatogenesis, axospermia, infertility, gynaecomastia, varying degrees of androgen deficiency, elevated plasma gonadotrophin levels, some degree of intellectual deficiency and tall stature. These subjects are also prone to developing obesity, varicose veins, diabetes mellitus, breast cancer and chronic pulmonary diseases.

### TREATMENT

Androgen therapy may correct the manifestations of androgen deficiency but such treatment may aggravate the gynaecomastia. Hence gynaecomastia should be treated by plastic surgery. But there is no treatment for the infertility.

## BREAST

### Anatomy & Physiology

The breast consist of numerous lobules made up of clusters of rounded acini or, alveoli which are connected by a duct system to the nipples — all these being embedded in a fatty connective tissue. Beneath the areola, just before it reaches the nipple, each due has a dilatation, the ampulla, which acts as a milk reservoir. The alveoli are surrounded by myoepithelial cells which help in expression of milk.

At birth there may be slight mammary enlargement, and even secretion of so-called 'witch's milk' due to the influence of maternal oestrogens and placental lactogens. This, however, soon subsides and the breasts remain rudimentary in both the sexes until puberty when there is development of the breasts in females.

**Hormonal influence**

Oestrogens, particularly oestradiol, cause growth and division of the ducts, maturation of nipples and also deposition of fat around the ducts.

Proper alveolar development at the end of the ducts requires synergistic action of oestrogen and progesterone at an optimal ratio of 1 : 20 to 1 : 100. Once the anatomical development of the ducts and alveoli is complete, continued action of oestrogens and progesterone is probably not essential for lactation itself.

During pregnancy there is further branching of the terminal ducts and increase in the number and size of the alveoli, due to the high plasma levels of oestrogen and progesterone.

Normal lactation requires specific lactogenic hormones along with appropriate priming by oestrogen and progesterone and joint action of thyroxine, glucocorticoid, growth hormone and insulin.

There are two lactogenic hormones

(a) Human placental lactogen (HPL)

(b) Prolactin.

HPL is produced in large amounts from the placenta in the later phases of pregnancy and prepares the breast for lactation. Prolactin, a peptide hormone of the anterior pituitary, is the most important hormone for the initation and maintenance of both normal and inappropriate lactation. Prolactin secretion is normally under control of prolactin inhibitory factor (P.I.F) of hypothalamus which in turn, is controlled by a dopaminergic pathway. Thyrotrophin releasing hormone (TRH) may have a positive effect on prolactin secretion and thus act as a prolactin releasing factor also. The ejection of milk is dependent upon a neurohumoral reflex initiated by stimulation of the nipple by sucking, which leads to secretion of oxytocin from hypothalamus and posterior pituitary, which stimulates the myoepithelial cells surrounding the terminal ducts and acini; suckling also stimulates prolactin secretion.

## GALACTORRHOEA

The term refers to an inappropriate or non-puerperal secretion of milk.

## AETIOLOGY

Galactorrhoea may occur in a wide variety of conditions and in many cases there is demonstrable hyperprolactinaemia, which may be intermittent.

**Clinical conditions associated with galactorrhoea**

A. Failure of normal hypothalamic inhibition of pituitary prolactin release.

(1) Central nervous system disease

e.g. intracranial tumours, meningitis, encephalitis, hydrocephalus, sarcoidosis.

(2) Drug which inhibit P.I.F. synthesis, e.g. phenothiazines, tricyclic antidepressants. In practice this is the commonest known cause of galactorrhoea.

B. Increased prolactin-releasing factor

e.g. in hypothyroidism due to increased secretion of TRH.

C. Autonomous prolactin release

(1) Pituitary dysfunction e.g.

(a) Chiari-Frommel syndrome — seen following pregnancy, but without radiological evidence of pituitary tumour.

(b) del Castello syndrome-occurs spontaneously in women without pregnancy of X-ray evidence of pituitary tumour.

(c) Forbes Albright-syndrome-galactorrhoea may occur spontaneously or post partum, and associated with enlarged sella turcica on radiology.

(d) Mixed growth hormone and prolactin secreting tumours.

(e) Chromophobe adenomas.

(2) Ectopic production of HPL and/or prolactin, e.g. hydatidiform male and choriocarcinoma or other tumours e.g. bronchogenic carcinoma, hypernephroma.

D. Idiopathic — It is now suggested that these patients probably have undetected pituitary or para pituitary tumours and so should be kept under follow-up. This group probably accounts for 50% of all cases.

E. Miscellaneous causes : Trauma to chest wail, herpes zoster etc.

Galactorrhoea is unusual in men, even in presence of hyperprolactinaemia but when it does occur it is usually upon the background of a feminising state and associated with impotence and infertility. There can be other symptoms depending on the underlying pathology, e.g. those due to hypothyroidism, intracranial tumour etc.

## DIAGNOSIS

Careful history regarding offending drug is essential. Thorough physical examination to detect the underlying pathology, e.g. CNS disease, hypothyroidism, etc. Investigations include : serum prolactin estimation and meticulous search for pituitary or non-pituitary tumours.

### Treatment

A. Treat underlying cause whenever possible, e.g. stop the causative drugs, treatment of hypothyroidism, treatment of pituitary tumour.

B. In idiopathic cases, bromocriptine, a dopamine agonist which stimulates secretion of PRIH, is effective in lowering prolactin levels, stopping galactorrhoea and restoring menstruation. It is usually started with a small dose of 2.5 mg daily, given after dinner to avoid nausea and postural hypotension. Gradually the dose is increased over a few weeks to 2.5 mg. to 5 mg. two or three times daily.

In those patients who develop it after stopping oral contraceptives, clomiphene citrate 50—100 mg. daily for 5—7 days or, longer may be useful.

## GYNAECOMASTIA

Gynaecomastia refers to enlargement of the male breast due to development of its glandular component which may be unilateral or bilateral. Prominence of the breasts due to deposition of fat may be referred to as pseudogynaecomastia where the whole breast is uniformly enlarged. But in true gynaecomastia the hypertrophied glandular component is tender and is felt beneath the nipple as thickened lumps.

## CLINICAL FEATURES

**A. Physiological Gynaecomastia**

(1) **Neonatal :** This is transient, ordinarily disappearing in a few weeks and may be seen up to 70% of male infants. It may be caused by maternal and/or placental oestrogens or, by maternal chorionic gonadotrophin stimulating. Leydig cells of the testes to secrete oestrogen.

(2) **Pubertal :** Some degree of temporary gynaecomastia lasting 1—3 years may occur in many boys at some time during puberty. It may be bilateral or, unilateral. Usually

the gynaecomastia is not very marked, but occasionally may resemble normal adult female breast and may be the cause of much embarrassment. It is very rarely due to a teratoma of the testes. So testes should be examined.

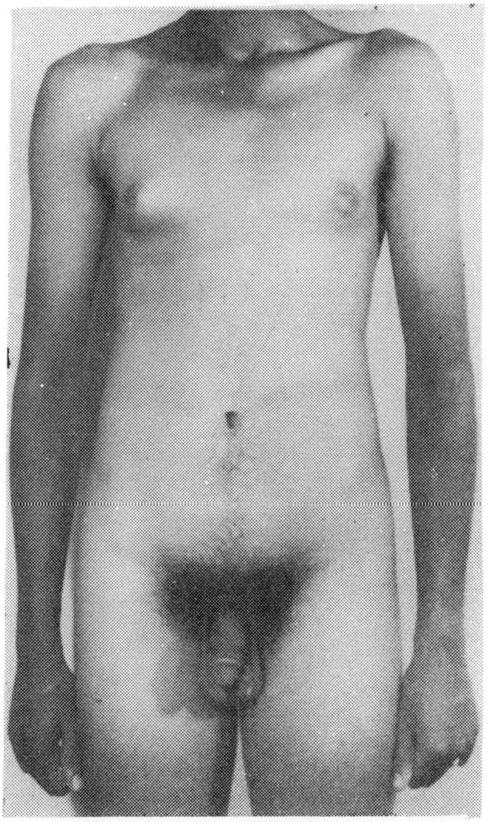

Fig.8.11 : Gynaecomastia in a normal adult aged 18. Semen showed normal sperms.
(Editor's Case)

It is commonly attributed to excessive oestrogen secretion by the Leydig cells of testes, but there is little laboratory evidence in its favour. It may be due to the mammary glands being unduly sensitive to oestrogens.

(3) **Ingolutional :** Gynaecomastia may occur with ageing in otherwise healthy men. A likely explanation is the increase in peripheral conversion of androgen to oestrogens with age.

## B. Pathological Gynaecomastia

(1) **Testicular defect :** Leading to reduced testosterone secretion or sometimes increased oestrogen production.

(i) Congenital absence of testes

(ii) Tumours, e.g. Teratoma, chorion epithelioma, interstitial cell tumour, sertoli cell tumour – the last two being oestrogen secreting tumours chorion epithelioma secretes large amounts of chorionic gonadotrophin, which stimulates the production of oestrogen by the interstitial cells.

(iii) Secondary testicular failure may occur following mumps, orchitis, trauma, lepromatous leprosy, granulomatous diseases, castration and renal failure.

(b) **Disorders of sex**

(i) Testicular feminisation syndrome — due to end-organ insensitivity to testosterone

(ii) True hermaphroditism.

(c) **Adrenal**

(i) Feminising adrenal tumour

(ii) Congenital adrenal hyperplasia.

(d) **Thyroid**

(i) Hyperthyroidism

(e) **Pituitary**

(i) Acromegaly — while galactorrhoea may occur occasionally, gynaecomastia is only very rarely reported.

(ii) Chromophobe adenoma

(f) **Sex chromosomal anomaly**

(i) Klinefelter's syndrome

(2) **Liver disease**

(i) Cirrhosis of liver — due to diminished catabolism of androgen by usual pathways, so that more of it is converted to oestrogen; moreover normal inactivation of oestrogen is also hampered.

In some cases, treatment with spironolactone is contributory.

(3) **Diseases of respiratory system**

(i) Bronchogenic carcinoma (oat-cell type) — due to an ectopic secretion of gonadotrophin and or prolactin.

(4) **Diseases of nervous system**

(i) Paraplegia

(ii) Friedreich's ataxia

(iii) Syringomyelia

(iv) Dystrophia myotonica

(5) **Dermatological disorder**

(i) Exfoliative dermatitis

(6) **Drugs**

(a) Oestrogen e.g. diethylstilbestrol therapy for prostatic cancer.

(b) Chorionic gonadotrophin which may be given for undescended testis.

(c) Oestrogen like side-effects of digoxin

(d) Interference with testosterone synthesis, e.g. Alkylating agents.

(e) Blocking action of androgen by preventing its binding to cytosol receptor protein in target tissues, e.g. spironolactone and cimetidine.

(f) Unknown mechanism — isoniazid, ethionamide, methyldopa, tricyclic antidepressant, d-penicillamine and diazepam.

(7) **Miscellaneous**

(a) Starvation or renutrition

(b) Ulcerative colitis

(c) Immobilisation in a plaster spica

(d) Chronic renal failure

**Diagnostic evaluation**

It should include :

(1) Careful history including particularly exposure to drugs.

(2) Thorough physical examination, which must include examination of the testes.

(3) Haemoglobin and liver function tests, if necessary.

(4) Investigations, e.g. X-ray chest, bronchoscopy, to exclude carcinoma.

(5) Karyotype, if Klinefelter syndrome is suspected.

(6) Urinary gonadotrophins if testicular tumour is suspected.

(7) Endocrine evaluation to include 24 hours urinary 17-ketosteroids, plasma oestradiol, luteinising hormone and testosterone. However, even with these tests,a definite etiologic diagnosis may be difficult in any case.

**Treatment**

(a) Where a primary cause can be identified, treatment of that condition usually suffices, e.g. removal of a hormone-secreting tumour or stopping offending drug.

(b) However, if the gynaecomastia is of long duration, correction of the primary defect may not be followed by improvement of gynaecomastia. In such cases and when primary cause cannot be identified or corrected, plastic surgery may be needed.

The chief indications for surgery are :-

(i) Psychological and/or cosmetic problems

(ii) Suspected malignancy.

(c) A few patients with painful gynaecomastia may respond to anti-estrogens like Tamoxifen.

## ORAL CONTRACEPTIVES

*S. KUMAR*

Oral contraceptives are among the most effective agents for conception control in women and are being increasingly accepted by women of our country too.

**TYPE :**

(1) **Combined** — This is the most common and also the most effective. It contains a synthetic oestrogen (e.g. ethinyl oestradiol or mestranol) and a synthetic progestogen (e.g. norethindrone, norethynorel, ethynodiol diacetate, norgestrel). some common proprietary preparations are :

Ovral; Lyndiol; Noracyclin.

These are administered one table daily for 21 days (usually starting from the 5th day of menstruation) followed by several days rest.

(2) **Sequential** — Here an oestrogen only is given for the first part of menstrual cycle and oestrogen-progestogen combination during the last week or so.

(3) **Progestogen only** — This consists of continuous daily administration of small amounts of progestogen.

## MECHANISM OF ACTION

Most oral contraceptives, particularly the combined type act by :

(1) Inhibition of ovulation by acting at hypothalamopituitary level.

(2) There may be an additional defect on the reproductive tract by (a) altering cervical mucus and thus impairing sperm penetration.

(b) Altering motility and secretions of the fallopian tubes and uterus.

## SIDE-EFFECTS

Deep vein thrombosis, pulmonary embolism, coronary thrombosis, hypertension, thromboembolic and haemorrhagic stroke appear to be more common among regular users of contraceptive pill. The risk are increased by older age, obesity and cigarette smoking; in general it appears that Indian women are less liable to develop deep vein thrombosis and pulmonary embolism.

The vascular complications are generally ascribed to the oestrogen component and are believed to be reduced by decreasing the oestrogen content to 50 g. or less as in most of the present-day preparations. However, today it appears that the progestogen content plays as equally significant role.

Some women taking oral contraceptives develop impaired glucose tolerance and so oral contraceptives are contraindicated in diabetes.

Cholestatic jaundice may be occur in oral contraceptive users, particularly in those predisposed to developing recurrent jaundice of pregnancy.

A rare but potentially fatal complication related to long term use of oral contraceptive is peliosis hepatis. Oral contraceptives also increase the chances of cholelithiasis and cholecystitis.

### Psychological effects

Though in general oral contraceptives may produce a favourable mental state, (partly due to removal of fear of pregnancy) a small proportion of patients develop mental depression. Pyridoxine 50 mg daily may often correct the depression.

### Relation with reproductive neoplasm

There is no convincing evidence that oral contraceptives lead to increased incidence of cancer of the breast, uterus or ovary.

## ENDOCRINE MANIFESTATIONS OF NON-ENDOCRINE DISEASES

*S. KUMAR*

In recent years production of hormones has been recognised in various non-endorcine tissues particularly in some malignant disorders. The neoplasms with which endocrine manifestations are commonly associated are those arising in the bronchus, thymus, thyroid, breast, pancreas, kidney and mesenchymal tissues.

## PATHOGENESIS

Production of hormone by non-endocrine tumours may be due to 'de-differentiation' to an embryonic state with removal of the normal repressors which mask specific segments of the DNA molecule in various differentiated cells. The hormones known to be produced by non-endocrine tumours include ACTH, ADH, para-thormone, thyrotropin, bio-chemicals with insulin-like activity, gonadotrophin growth hormone, erythropoietin.

## ECTOPIC WITH SECRETION

This is most commonly associated with oat cell carcinoma of the lungs, but may be associated with thymoma, pancreatic tumour, bronchial adenoma, bronchial carcinoid, medullary carcinoma of thyroid. Though biochemical evidence of excess ACTH secretion is seen quite commonly, clinical manifestations are not so typical. The manifestations may include, weakness, hyperpigmentation, hypertension, alkalosis, weight gain, centripetal obesity, and abdominal obesity. The features of classical Cushing's syndrome are usually absent. Hypokalaemia and alkalosis may occur.

## ECTOPIC ADH SECRETION

This is most commonly seen with oat cell carcinoma of the lung, carcinoma of pancreas, lymphoma, thymoma etc. it may also be associated with a large number of non-malignant pulmonary and central nervous system disorders and also with different drugs. The clinical manifestations are those of water intoxication, e.g. nausea, vomiting, mental confusion, weakness and lethargy. The characteristic laboratory findings include hyponatraemia, urinary sodium excretion more than 20 mEq/litre and urine hypertonic relative to plasma.

## HYPERCALCAEMIC SYNDROMES

Hypercalcaemia in association with malignant diseases is most commonly due to osteolytic invasion of bone by the tumour; but this may also be due to ectopic secretion of parathormone or parathormone-like substance as in epidermoid carcinoma of the lung, hypernephroma, hepatoma, pancreatic carcinoma etc. Other calcium mobilising substances-like prostaglandin $E_2$, osteoclast activating factor or cyclic AMP stimulating factor may also be secreted by various tumours.

The clinical picture may be dominated by the primary disease or by hypercalcaemia itself, e.g. constipation, anorexia, nausea, polyuria, thirst and mental confusion.

## HYPOGLYCAEMIA SYNDROMES

Malignant tumours not arising from pancreatic islet cells may also cause hypoglycaemia, e.g. large mesenchymal tumours-like fibrosarcomas or hepatoma or lymphoma. Usually insulin is not found in tumour extracts; but circulating non-suppressible insulin-like activity (NSILA), like the somatostatins may be found in some cases.

## ECTOPIC GONADOTROPHIN SECRETION

This may be seen with oat cell carcinoma of the bronchus or chorio-carcinoma of testes, hepatoblastoma. In men, such ectopic gonadotrophin secretion usually manifests as gynaecomastia but in women this is usually asymptomatic.

## ECTOPIC TSH SECRETION

This is principally associated with trophoblastic tumours, e.g. choriocarcinoma of placenta and testes and also hydatidiform mole.

## POLYCYTHAEMIA

Apart from various benign and malignant disorders of the kidney, various extrarenal tumours like cerebellar haemangioblastoma, uterine fibroid, hepatoma, ovarian and adrenal tumours may also produce erythropoietin and cause polycythaemia.

# CHAPTER – 9
# METABOLIC DISORDERS

## INTRODUCTION TO METABOLIC DISORDERS

*G.C. MOOKERJEE*

The living process consists of anabolism and catabolism which constitutes biochemical process, known as metabolism. Numerous enzyme reactions are involved in these biochemical reactions. Genetic faults may occur due to some enzyme deficiencies, leading to metabolic disorders. Some of the metabolic disorders may be acquired while many more are congenital. The disorders may be related to carbohydrate, protein or lipid metabolism.

**Carbohydrate metabolism** – The most important disorder is diabetes mellitus, which will be discussed in great detail in this chapter. There are many rare genetic errors of carbohydrate metabolism, e.g. fructosuria, galactosaemia, glycogen storage disease (von Gêirke's disease) for which reference should be made to textbooks of paediatric medicine.

**Amino acid metabolism** – In-born errors of amino acid metabolism, e.g. phenyl ketonuria, cystinuria and Fanconi's syndrome are also rare diseases encountered in infancy. Cystinuria and Fanconi's syndrome have been discussed in the chapter on renal diseases. Phenyl ketonuria, though rare, is important and can be detected at birth by simple urine test. If not detected in neonatal age it may lead to mental retardation. But if detected in time and the infant is treated with tryptophan-free diet, the mental defect can be avoided.

Gout is another metabolic disorder which affects joints and kidneys in particular and has been included in the chapter on rheumatology, as clinical presentation of the disease is chiefly with joint pains.

Hyperlipidaemia is a major risk factor for I.H.D., discussed in the following pages.

Rickets, Osteomalacia and obesity are also important in clinical practice, which has been discussed in this chapter.

Porphyria is a disorder of porphyrin metabolism.

Porphyria may be primary or secondary.

(1) Primary types are :
- (a) Porphyria erythropoeitica
- (b) Protoporphyria erythropoetica
- (c) Porphyria hepatica.

It has several sub-types :

(2) Secondary type :

This is due to toxic agents and drugs, e.g. arsenic, lead, phosphorus, sulpha drugs, barbiturates, sulphonal, trional, sudormid etc.

Porphyria erythropoetica – Inherited but rare disorder which occurs in infancy. The chief feature is photo-sensitivity. Blisters appear in the skin on exposure to sun. These blisters heal with scar formation. Exposed areas are affected and splenomegaly may occur. Teeth may be coloured with tinge of red-brown or reddish urine and stool contains large quantities of uroporphyrin 1.

In erythropoetic protoporphyria skin may itch and become erythematous but no blister formation takes place.

**Treatment** — No curative treatment is available. Avoiding exposure to sun is only preventive measure.

## ACUTE INTERMITTENT PORPHYRIA

This variety usually presents in adults. There may be vomiting, fever, tachycardia associated with abdominal pain usually colicky in type. When there is obscure abdominal pain without any localising signs, urine should be tested for porphyria. The voided urine also changes to portwine colour on standing in a urine-glass.

Sometimes neurological complications may occur including neuropathy, encephalopathy, paraplegia or hemiplegia.

Psychiatric symptoms are often associated.

Barbiturates often precipitate the attack.

**Treatment** — Steroids, EDTA, BAL and chlorpromazine have been used. Glucose and high carbohydrate diet may be useful.

**Porphyria cutanea tarda** —

Cutaneous symptoms usually start in teenage or adults, before other complications, e.g. abdominal pain or neurological signs, Jaundice and hepatic cirrhosis may occur.

Urine and stool contain large quantities of coproporphyrin and proporphyrin when attacks occur.

**Treatment** — No specific treatment is known, supportive and symptomatic treatment should be done.

### Toxic porphyria

This is associated with alcoholic cirrhosis. These patients develop photo-sensitivity and form blisters due to sunlight and trauma to the skin.

Abdominal colic and neurological complications are absent.

**Lipid metabolism** — It is of great clinical interest and has great significance in atherosclerotic disorders and coronary heart disease.

The subject has been discussed in this chapter.

## CARCINOID SYNDROME

This is a peculiar disorder which is due to excessive formation of vaso-active substances, e.g. histamine, serotonin, dipeptides and catecholamines from argentiffin cells present in bronchus, stomach, ileum and ileocaecal region.

Clinically it causes reddish or violaceous flush associated with respiratory symptoms, abdominal pain and colic, diarrhoea, arthritis or right sided cardiac failure. Some cases may be associated with pulmonary or tricuspid valvular stenosis.

Diagnosis is made by demonstrating 5-hydroxyindole acetic acid (5 HIAA) in urine which is more than 25 mg in 24 hours. Blood serotoxin level is also high.

**Treatment** — Alpha methyl dopa, dibenzyline, regitine and prednisolone may reduce flushing.

If tumour is demonstrated, surgical removal should be attempted. Cyclophosphamide and doxorubicin can be used.

## HYPERLIPIDAEMIA

*YASHPAL*
*K.C. CHUG*
*B.K. SHARMA*

## INTRODUCTION

Hyperlipidaemia is a result of abnormal lipid metabolism. Basically there are four types of circulating lipids, namely, free cholesterol, cholesterol esters, triglycerides and phospholipids. Circulation of lipids occurs as spherical macromolecule complexes termed as lipoproteins (chylomicrons, low density lipoproteins, LDL and high density lipoproteins, HDL).

Hyperlipidaemias are of two types : Primary genetic hyperlipidaemias (type I — type VI) and secondary hyperlipidaemias based upon the genetic concept and modified version from Fredrickson, Levy, *et al* as reflected in Table 9.1.

Primary genetic hyperlipidaemias : inheritance by single gene disorder (dominant or recessive mechanism) or multifactorial type; should be suspected if there is positive family history; age of onset during infancy, childhood or adolescence; absence of associated secondary disease or distribution of xanthomas over the tendons.

Secondary hyperlipidaemias are suspected by associated diseases, such as, diabetes mellitus, nephrotic syndrome, hypothyroidism, acromegaly. Cushing's syndrome, acute intermittent porphyria, or drug induced (oral contraceptives, alcohol and corticosteroids). Family history is non-contributory; age of onset is usually in middle age group and lipoprotein analysis often reveals type 4 (rarely 5), 2a or 2b.

## APPROACH TO THE PROBLEM

It is based on conventional methods of assessment by history, clinical features, laboratory tests and correlation of clinicobiochemical evaluation (Table 9.6).

History of onset of disease, dietary habits, family history of disease, iatrogenic effects, such as, steroids, oral contraceptives, alcohol should be explored.

History, clinical and laboratory tests would be useful to detect associated disease, such as, diabetes mellitus, nephrotic syndrome, pancreatitis, hypothyroid state etc. Course of disease; therapeutic response; distribution pattern of xanthomas should be examined in detail.

## LABORATORY TESTS

These could be of two types, first to identify type of hyperlipidaemia and secondary to establish or exclude associated secondary disease. Important tests are as under :

(1) Lipoprotein electrophoresis in particular for cholesterol and triglycerides are useful to find out the type of abnormality in most of the cases. Samples should be collected in fasting state after at least 12 hours.

(2) Lipaemic plasma should be collected in EDTA. Incubation at 4°C in refrigerator should be done for inspection.

(3) Special tests for lipoprotein analysis may be required in exceptional cases where primary genetic hyperlipidaemia is suspected.

(4) Tests for associated diseases for secondary disorders may be done for proper assessment.

## THERAPEUTIC PRINCIPLES

(1) Long-term treatment and follow-up is mandatory.

(2) Diet therapy (Table 9.3) should be tried first and drugs (Table 9.2) should be the last resort. It is important to identify two emergent situations where energetic treatment is indicated, viz, severe hypertriglyceridemia (more than thousand mg ml) which must be reduced to prevent possible pancreatitis, secondly severe hypercholesterolemia (more than 350 mg per ml) owing to elevated LDL as in familial type where there is grave risk of ischaemic heart disease.

(3) Drugs should always be avoided during pregnancy, before age of six years, for mild attack of hyperlipidaemias (triglycerides less than 500 mg/ml, LDL cholesterol more than 200 mg/dl). Drug should always be considered in younger patients to prevent occlusive lesions, positive family history or in presence of associated risk factors (diabetics, hypertensive and smokers).

(4) Aggravating factors like alcohol, oral contraceptives, steroids, thiazides should be avoided. Beta-adrenergic blocking agents may depress HDL levels, and therefore should not be used.

(5) Treatment of secondary disorders helps to control hyperlipidaemias of secondary type.

(6) Drugs comprise of cholystyramine, nicotinic acid, clofibrate, betasitosterol, neomycin, D-thyroxin, probucol or combined regimens. However, first three drugs are commonly used in dosage as indicated (Table—9.2).

**TABLE — 9.1 : MAJOR CATEGORIES OF PRIMARY HYPERLIPIDAEMIA**

| GENERIC DEFECTS & LIPO PROTEIN ABNORMALITY | Type | Appearance of serum | Triglyceride elevation | Cholesterol elevation | Clinical presentation | Differential diagnosis |
|---|---|---|---|---|---|---|
| Fasting chylomicro-nemia<br>(Rare type) | I | Creamy layer over serum | often 1000-10,000 or more | Elevated to about 10% of triglyceride level | Creamy blood, lipaemic retina, hepatosplenomegaly; recurrent abdominal pain:ERUPTIVE XANTHOMA onset, in childhood | 1.Pancreatitis<br>2.Diabetes mellitus<br>3.Systemic Lupus Erythematosis<br>4.Familial lipoprotein lipase deficiency |
| Hypercholestero-lemia (LDL) | IIA | Clear | No | Usually more than 300—600 | Xanthalesma, tendon Xanthoma, accelerated atherosclerosis detectable in childhood | 1.Hypothyroidism<br>2.Nephrotic syndrome<br>3.Cushing's syndrome<br>4.Acute intermittent porphyria<br>5.Hepatic obstruction<br>6.Familial hyper-cholesterolemia |
| Mixed Lipaemia (LDL + VLDL) | IIB | Turbid | Usually 200—600 | Usually 250—600 | Relatively common like IIA or with diabetes mellitus or obesity | Same as IIA |
| Dys-betalipo-proteinemia | III | —do— | High variable 175-1500 in | Variable from near normal | Relatively uncommon. Hyperglycaemia. hyperuricaemia. Tuberous Xanthoma. | 1.Hepatic disease<br>2.Diabetes mellitus<br>3.Familial type |

*Table : 9.1 .. contd...*

*Table : 9.1 ... contd...*

| | | | | | | |
|---|---|---|---|---|---|---|
| Endogenous hyperlipaemia (VLDL) | IV | —do— | 200—5000 | 300—800 | Most common in adults. Eruptive xanthomas, early atherosclerosis abnormal GTT. uric acid. | 1.Nephrotic syndrome 2.Hypothyroidism 3.Glycogen storage disease 4.Oral contraceptives |
| Mixed lipaemia VLDL + Chylomicrons | V | Creamy layer over Turbid Infranate | Usually 500—10,000 or more | 300—1000 | Adulthood mainly recurrent abdominal pain, eruptive xanthomas, hepatosplenomegaly | 1.Alcoholism 2.Insulin deficient 3.Diabetes mellitus 4.Pancreatitis 5.Familial |
| Mixed | VI | This is rare disorder whereas pre-β-lipoproteins and chylomicrons are present. Onset in adult age with features of acute pancreatitis : Diabetes mellitus : Alcoholism. | | | | |

**Table 9.2 : Types of Hyperlipidaemias Dietary & Drug Therapy**

| Types of hyperlipidaemia | Diet Therapy | Drug Therapy |
|---|---|---|
| TYPE I | 1. Total fat and cholesterol is restricted to 35% of total calories<br>2. Avoid alcohol<br>3. Supplement medium chain triglycerides (unsaturated fat). | — |
| TYPE IIa | 1. Calorie and weight control not important. Rest all same as in type I<br>2. Avoid sucrose and alcohol | —<br>CHOLESTYRAMINE AND CO-LESTOPOL Hydrochloride are the drugs of choice |
| TYPE IIb | 1. Weight reduction is important<br>2. Intake of fat as in type I<br>3. Alcohol is restricted | |
| TYPE III | 1. Weight reduction is required<br>2. Balanced diet (carbohydrate 40%, fat 40%, protein 20% and low cholesterol diet)<br>3. Restriction of alcohol as in type IIb | Drugs in order of priority are :- Cholestyramine 16-326/day Nicotinic acid 3-7 g/day and lastly clofibrate 1.5-2 g/day |
| TYPE IV | 1. Weight reduction to ideal weight<br>2. Carbohydrate restriction to 40% of total calories and avoid sucrose & alcohol<br>3. Substitute poly-unsaturated fat | Nicotinic acid or CLOFIBRATE |
| TYPE V | 1. Weight reduction<br>2. Reduction of fat to 30% of total calories with increased carbohydrates to 50%. Poly-unsaturated fat substituted for saturated type<br>3. Avoid alcohol | |

TABLE 9.3 Distribution of fatty acids in Food Fats

| FATS | FATTY ACIDS (g/100 mg fat) saturated | Polysaturated | P : S ratio |
|---|---|---|---|
| **Vegetable oils** | | | |
| SAFFLOWER | 8 | 72 | 90 |
| SUN FLOWER | 12 | 62 | 5.3 |
| SOYABEANS | 15 | 52 | 3.5 |
| PEANUTS | 18 | 29 | 1.6 |
| **Animal fat** | | | |
| LARD | 38 | 10 | 0.3 |
| BUTTER | 54 | 3 | 0.1 |

## RICKETS AND OSTEOMALACIA

*YASHPAL*
*K.S.CHUG*
*B.K.SHARMA*

### DEFINITION

Osteomalacia is the adult counterpart of rickets. It comprises of a group of metabolic bone diseases in which there is decreased mineralisation of bones and cartilages. Aetiological basis is due to deficiency of vitamin D, calcium or inorganic phosphorus.

### Classification

1. Deficiency of vitamin D
   Low dietary intake
   Low synthesis in skin

II. Malabsorption :
   Gastric surgery (resection)
   Bowel surgery (resection)
   Coeliac disease
   Biliary cirrhosis

III. Renal Disease :
   Renal tubular disorders
   Glomerular disorders
   Nephrotic syndrome
   Transplant kidney
   Dialysis bone disease

IV. Other Conditions :
   Iaterogenic : Anticonvulsant drugs (dilantin, barbiturates)

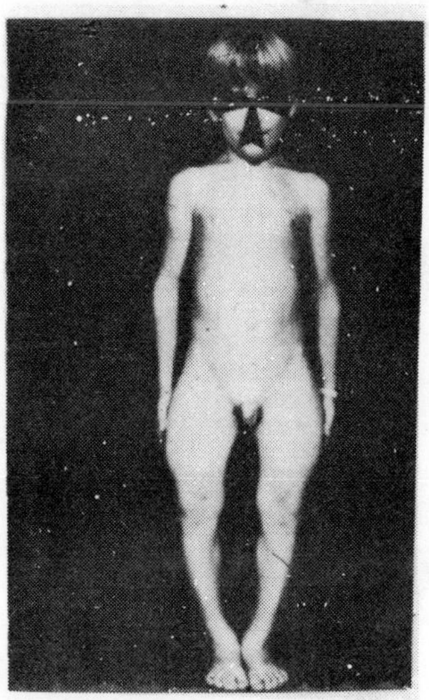

Fig.9.1 : Renal rickets. Note bowing of legs and thighs as well as short stature.

Non-absorbable antacids :
Fluoride treatment
Parentral alimenation
Intoxication Outdated tetracycline
Cadmium
Lead
Vitamin D dependent rickets.

## PATHOPHYSIOLOGY

Due to deficiency of Vitamin 'D' there is reduction in serum calcium. This leads to hyperparathyroid state with adaptation mechanism of increase in phosphorus excretion and increase of serum calcium. Osteoblast activity increases and defective mineralization occurs owing to quantitative inadequate calcium and phosphorus levels.

Thus biochemical and hormonal alterations subsequently form the basis of radiological and clinical spectrum of the diseases.

## CLINICAL FEATURES

**Rickets** — Affects growing long bones and cartilages. Clinical features would vary according to the quantum of deficiency and age of onset.

Infants often are well nourished pale, restless with increased susceptibility for respiratory and gastrointestinal upsets, also epileptic fits and tetany. Earliest features in order of frequency are craniotabes (crackling feeling of membranous bones of skull), rickety rosary (swelling of costochondral junction of ribs), Harrison's sulcus, pigeon breast, bossing of parietal and frontal bones and delayed closure of fontanelle.

Kyphosis, knock knees, bow legs,enlargement of lower ends of radius, ulna, femur, tibia and fibula are features of rickets,if the process continues through second, third and fourth year of life. Features of a case of renal ricket illustrated in Fig. 9.1.

## OSTEOMALACIA

Presentation in osteomalacia is in the form of bone pains and tenderness as the early features. Later on, skeletal deformities, proximal myopathy, waddling gait. Triradiate pelvis, gross kyphosis may develop accompanied by the features of underlying disorder and those of hypocalcaemia.

Anaemia, tiredness, steatorrhoea, pigmentation, thirst, noctures are the usual features of underlying disorders. In chronic renal failure a mixed picture of osteomalacia with secondary hyperparathyroid (renal osteodystrophy) is more common when hypocalcaemia is very pronounced. It is often associated with spontaneous tetany, stridor or carpopedal spasm.

**Biochemical features —**

Relation of aetiology with biochemical features is given under Table 9.4 :

| Aetiology | Biochemical features |
|---|---|
| I. Deficiency of Vit D | 1. Serum calcium is normal (9—10.3 mg/100 ml) or low.<br>2. Serum Phosphorus (2.8—4.5 mg/dl) and 25—OH—D (5 mg.ml) are characteristically low.<br>3. Raised plasma alkaline phosphatase (13KA—U) is the earliest marker of disease.<br>4. Decreased urinary calcium (50—25 mg/day). |

| | |
|---|---|
| II. Malabsorption — | Low urinary calcium. |
| III. Renal disease — | Phosphaturia. |
| (a) Tubular disease | Proteinuria, glycosuria, acidosis and aminoaciduria are present.<br>Even when blood urea, creatinine are normal. |
| (b) Glomerular disease | Blood urea, creatinine and phosphates are elevated.<br>Serum calcium may be normal, low or elevated.<br>Serum alkaline phosphatase is elevated. |
| IV. Hypophosphataemic Rickets | Serum calcium and alkaline phosphatase, both are normal : serum phosphorus low. |

**Radiological features**

Radiological features of rickets and osteomalacia are given in **Table 9.5 :**

| Rickets | Osteomalacia |
|---|---|
| 1. Epiphyseal growth plates are hazy, cupped and increased in thickness. | 1. "Pseudofractures" : Looser's zones often symmetrical at ribs, pubic rami, medial cortex of upper femur, axillary border of scapula. |
| 2. Metaphyses show abnormal trabecular pattern. | 2. Washed out bones appearance on X-rays. |
| 3. Diaphyses cortices are thinned out. | 3. Triradiate pelvis |
| 4. Bowing of shafts of long bones. | 4. Changes of osteomalacia with osteosclerosis and/or subperiosteal resorption of phalanges in renal osteodystrophy. |
| 5. Other features as documented in clinical protocol. | 5. Milkman's syndrome — Special form of osteomalacia — moth eaten epiphysis : pseudofracture may show callus near blood vessels. |

**Bone Scinti-scan**

It may reveal increased uptake of tracer elements and locate lesions not visualized on conventional radiograms, e.g. pseudofractures.

**Bone Biopsy**

It gives early diagnosis even when blood biochemistry and X-rays are normal. Osteoid and osteoblastic overactivity may be ascertained by under-calcified sections with special staining methods.

**Management :** It comprises of the following principles :

1. Specific measures : Vitamin D and calcium
2. Treatment of aetiological basis
3. Prevention of disease by adequate exposure to sunlight, dietary calcium and Vit D and C therapy as prophylactic dosage following bowel surgery, long-term anticonvulsant drugs.
4. Clinical, biochemical; radiological parameters should be checked for cure and follow-up of such cases.

: Treatment Schedule

| Aetiology | Therapeutic Regimen | Remarks |
|---|---|---|
| 1. Dietary Therapy | 1. Vitamin D 50,000 units/day for 2–3 weeks<br>2. Followed by normal diet 400 unit vitamin D. 800 mg calcium/day as maintenance therapy | 1. Till serum calcium and alkaline phosphatase are normal.<br>2. 26 OHD is also normal after cure<br>3. Radiological healing takes 3–6 months for regression to normal state.<br>4. Serum calcium phosphorus & alkaline phosphatase should be done at least once in 15 days. |
| 2. Malabsorption | 1. Sprue syndrome : Glutin free diet : Folic acid and $B_{12}$<br>2. Pancreatic insufficiency. Pancreatic enzymes : High calcium Vit K diet (Ca-1600–2400 mg/day)<br>3. Inj. Vitamin D 1.25 mg daily or I.M. at weekly interval | 1. Once bony mass is restored, long-term alkalisation therapy is continued for life long. |
| 3. Renal tubular<br>(a) Acidosis | 1. Sodii bicarb : Phosphates : citrates replacement therapy<br>2. Calcium 4–10 g/day<br>3. Vitamin D 50,000 – 100,000 units/week or 1 – CH – D analogue .2 – .6 mg 1 – 25 (CH°2 D .5 – 2.0 mg daily) | After six months Calcium 6G/day + Vit D 800-2000 units/day for long term. |
| (b) Glomerular disease | Same dose of calcium & Vitamin D is required besides metabolic and dialysis therapy : Vitamin D 50,000 units/day<br>+<br>Calcium 1–1.5 g/day for 3–6 months | Long term-therapy |
| (c) Isolated Renal phosphate leaks | Phosphorus 1.3 – 2.4 g/day in 3 divided doses + vitamin D 50,000 units/day | Long-term therapy |
| 4. Anticonvulsant drug therapy | Phosphates 1.8 – 2.4 g/day in 3 divided doses + Vitamin D 50,000 units/day. | Long-term therapy |

## Prognosis

Prognosis is usually excellent with early diagnosis and treatment in dietary and malabsorption disorders. Vitamin D resistant rickets take a very long time or may not recover despite large dosage of vitamin D. In renal form, ultimately prognosis depends on basic renal disease. Hypercalcaemia may occur as a complication of Vit D therapy leading on to metastatic calcification. Respiratory paralysis may occur due to relative hypokalaemia leading on to fatality.

# OBESITY

*G.C. MOOKERJEE*

Obesity is a world-wide problem. In clinical practice eye-estimation and record of height and body weight are the best methods to judge the degree of obesity.

Physiologists are still wondering about how to measure fat-content or study the nature of fat-cells and correlating skin fold measurements at different sites to obesity. In very obese it is difficult to even raise a skin fold. In research units density of body and plethysmographic measurements have been carried out and mathematical equations constructed. Even fat cell numbers and their fat-content are being calculated, yet to the practising clinicians, these are still of theoretical value. While intensive research on metabolism of fat cells will continue, clinicians must investigate the causes of obesity.

Obesity among affluent people is mostly due to overeating and excessive alcohol consumption. It is however, interesting that obesity among British people of low socio-economic class is due to too much carbohydrate consumption and beer intake.

For practical purposes if an individual is 10% heavier than his ideal weight as reckoned from LIC data, he is considered obese. This limit may be raised to 20% according to some authorities. The best obesity index formula is :

$W/H^2$ where
W = weight in kg; H = height in metre.

## CAUSES OF OBESITY

### Age

The so-called tendency to get heavier among middle-aged prople is mostly due to overeating and alcohol intake. In poor sections, obesity is low in developing countries. In Western countries diet of poorer sections chiefly consists of plenty of cheap bread, potato and beer. Too much sugar consumption in tea is quite common.

### OCCUPATION

Occupation has some relation to obesity. Cooks, barmen and sedentary workers tend to gain in weight while stage-artists, film-stars, modelling girls and sportsmen usually keep themselves in shape. Diet of soldiers may be around 4000 calories but regular exercise and active habits keep most of them in shape.

It is the high-ranking military officers who sometimes gain weight and develop double-chin due to desk-job and too much alcohol consumption and rich uncontrolled diet.

Thus obesity related to alcohol and overeating is quite common while it is sometimes observed that some people eat and drink well but do not gain weight. These people somehow have higher metabolic rate and they burn out calories without gaining weight. The exact cause is not well understood.

### HEREDITY

Familial tendency in obesity is quite well-known. Eating habit of the family has also considerable contribution. High caloric high fat diet and little physical activity from childhood are important contributory factors. Whether any specific gene has influence on body fat is not yet definitely known.

Babies of very obese mother are not usually large babies at birth, unless mother is prediabetic. These infants born out of obese mothers usually start gaining weight after the age of one year, due to overfeeding.

**Endocrine factors**

(1) Diabetes mellitus — Obesity itself leads to diabetic state in some patients. Excess of insulin in plasma is usually a feature of obesity yet blood sugar is high in obese NIDDM. In USA non-ketotic NIDDM constitutes 90% of the diabetics and 80 to 90% of these people are obese (Harrison — 1983). Even among low and middle socio-economic class of people, obesity is predominant among nonketotic NIDDM. From our data at VIMS, diabetic clinic* (Mookerjee *et al*) among 1000 diabetic patients, 92% were NIDDM and 33% of them were controlled by diet only. Similar data are available all over the world.

**Hypothalamic syndromes**

Hypothalamus has important role to play in contributing to excess appetite and weight gain. Frolich's syndrome may occasionally be due to pituitary tumour (original Frolich's patient had pituitary tumour) but usually it is syndrome associated with gross obesity, hypogonadism (deficiency of gonadotropic hormone) in boys with features of visual defect and mental retardation. Sometimes diabetes insipidus is present.

Laurence-Moon-Biedle syndrome also has obesity, retinitis pigmentosa, mental deformities and poly or syndactyly.

**Cushing's disease**

Obesity here is trunkal in type with thin upper and lower limbs. Face is moon-shaped along with deposition of fat in neck and supra-clavicular regions.

**Hypothyroidism**

Some cases of hypothyroidism may develop obesity. This may be due to low metabolic rate and lazy habits, while food intake continues with excess calories. These lethargic patients are also anaemic and also stuffed with additional nutrition to improve their health, leading to fat accumulation.

**Psychological causes**

Sometimes too much happiness or frustration may lead to over-eating and obesity. The presence of hypothalamic centres which control appetite and satiety has not been proved beyond doubt. There is a lot of scope for research in this area. The cause of anorexia nervosa also remains unclear.

**Energy balance**

There is no doubt that most people gain weight due to intake of high caloric diet and lack of exercise. But there is also no doubt that a few fortunate people may eat too well, yet will not gain a pound of weight.

However, most obese people have low resting metabolic rate. The pathological changes of obesity are, however, unmistakable. There is large adipose tissue deposits everywhere. Not only the skin all over the whole body is infiltrated with adipocytes (cell laden with fat) but all organs are covered with adipose tissue and internal organs are affected. In obese people liver, heart, kidneys and skeletal muscles become enlarged. In younger people adiposites not only become hypertrophied or hyperplastic but they also increase in number. However, the capacity of increasing the number of adiposites decreases in adults and older people.

The exact mechanism of adipose tissue formation leading to obesity still remains unsolved.

**Pathogenesis**

James *et al* (1978) observed that obese people generally have higher resting metabolic rate than normal subjects. There is a lot of controversy also in this area and it is also true that indirect calorimetry may have some limitations about the accuracy of true metabolic rate.

---

* *Vivekananda Institute of Medical Science, Calcutta.*

## Complications

Complications of obesity are well-known and are well-illustrated in the diagram (Fig.9.2).

It is really easier to present obesity than to cure once it has been well established.

Hence practitioners should warn their patients as soon as tendency to obesity is manifesting.

*Treatment*

Diet control and exercise are the two dependable methods. There are no magic-pills which can solve the problem. Some drugs act by depressing appetite, e.g. amphetamine but are potentially harmful due to possible addiction. Other drugs are diethylpropion and phentermine. None of these are recommended.

Phenfluramine possibly acts on satiety centre (does it exist ?) indirectly depressing desire to eat. Dose 20 mg twice daily up to 60 or even 120 mg a day. Some patients develop side-effects, e.g. nausea, diarrhoea, depression as well as allergic symptoms. However, it is better to avoid drugs.

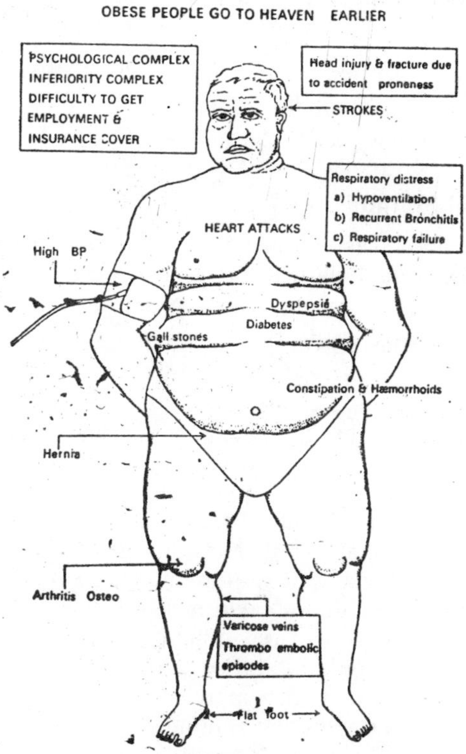

Fig.9.2 : Complications of Obesity

Weight consciousness is an important method to prevent obesity. Every practitioner should have a weighing machine in his clinic and should keep record of all patients during each visit. Thyroid medication for treatment of obesity is only justified if there is evidence of hormonal deficiency. Even human chorionic gonadotrophin injection have been tried but not recommended.

## Diet-Therapy

People who are over-weight by 20 to 30% can be easily treated with diet and proper exercise, if patient has desire to lose weight.

Diet should be rich in fibre and contain minimal fat. For non-vegetarian people 100 mg of lean meat (preferably small chicken) is recommended. Total calories 800 to 1200 calorie per day. Too much restriction ends in non-compliance. Diet therapists may help in preparing menu, which is acceptable to the patients depending on food-fads and type of diet patients used to take. Alcohol also should be discontinued as it has high caloric value (7 cal/gm). 100 ml of whisky or brandy contains about 45 ml of pure alcohol i.e. 315 calories which is equivalent to 35 g of butter. Diet for obesity is presented in the Appendix.

Exercise should be planned according to the individual's occupation and psychological make-up.

An executive who lives in 14th floor in crowded city will do well to practise indoor exercises or still better attend a club or clinics, where he will receive sauna bath, massage as well as intensive physical exercise on tread mill or cycle. Many of the author's patients have been benefited by yogic exercises. Refer to chapter, yoga therapy.

Weight reducing programme is a great challenge and its success depends on doctor's proper guidance and patient's sincerity.

Many obesity clinics are run in big cities and are expensive ways of reducing weight. Restriction of all carbohydrates will lead to ketosis.

However, if patient is grossly obese it is better to hospitalise him for proper weight reduction programme. But if the patient has genuine desire to lose weight family doctor with the help of dietician may succeed.

Well-planned exercise programme may be helpful but cardiovascular fitness should be assessed carefully before any severe exercise programme is prescribed.

**Surgical Methods**

This method is employed when the patient is so grossly over-weight that even movement becomes difficult and cardiovascular function is affected due to hypoventilation and excessive overload.

Over-zealous bowel-shunts (small bowel bypass) results in rapid loss of weight but these may end in post-operative complications.

Some of the likely complications are diarrhoea, vomiting, thirst, fatigue, anaemia and incisional hernia. But in some cases thrombo-embolism, osteoporosis, renal failure and even post-operative deaths have been recorded. Other surgical measures are gastro-jejunal bypass or gastroplasty, dividing the stomach into a smaller upper chamber and a larger lower chamber. This will limit to smaller food intake and delay in emptying. Alternative operations include lipectomy from anterior abdominal wall or more modern technique of suction operations, an ingenious technique of sucking out fat under vacuum-suction. These operations can only be done in special centres at prohibitive cost as well as with limited success. It is felt that family doctor is the best man to warn, his patients in time. The author finds numerous examples among ladies who were about 50 kg and quite slim when they were married but have scored a century around their menopause. How is it that nobody warned them so long ? Or how is it than she did not realise what was happening ?

## DIABETES MELLITUS

*G. C. MOOKERJEE*
*K. KABIR*

### DEFINITION

Diabetes mellitus is not a single disease but a hormone-dependent syndrome which causes complex metabolic changes in the body and is characterised by high blood glucose level with or without glycosuria. There is either absolute or relative lack of insulin or ineffective insulin action, which interferes with the metabolism of not only carbohydrate but also protein and lipids. Other hormones like growth hormones, glucagon and steroid hormones are also directly or indirectly concerned. The most important single pathological lesion is capillary basement membrane changes occurring in multiple organs of the body, detected by electron microscope.

### HISTORY

Earliest description of the disease was noted in 1500 B.C. in the Ebers papyrus of Egypt. In India about 400 B.C. Charak and Susrut for the first time noted the sweetness of urine (madhumeha), its hereditary nature and its relation with obesity. In the first century A.D., Roman physician Arétaeus gave the name diabetes (= Siphon) mellitus (melli = honey or sweet). Some description of the disease was found in Chinese and Japanese literature of the first century. In 1000 A.D. Avicenna, an Arab physician described its relation with gangrene. Dabson (1775) demonstrated that sweetness of urine in diabetes is due to sugar.

Langerhans (1819) described the islet cells of pancreas gland. In 1889 von Mering and Minkowski experimentally produced diabetes by total pancreactomy. In 1901 Opic noted changes in the Islets of Langerhans in patients, who died of diabetes. Finally, in 1921 Banting and Best discovered that alcoholic extract of dog's pancreas has potent hypoglycaemic effect, which was later known as insulin. The discovery of insulin was a great landmark which saved millions of diabetic lives.

In 1938 long-acting insulin preparations were introduced and about 34 years after the discovery of insulin, oral antidiabetic drugs came into use for treatment of adult onset diabetes (non-insulin dependent type).

**Age, sex and race**

It is now known that except juvenile onset diabetes, the incidence of diabetes increases with increasing age. Glucose tolerance also decreases with the increasing age and the highest incidence of maturity-onset diabetes is usually after 40 years of age. In the West, diabetes is more common among females while in India males are more commonly affected.

In India, diabetes is more common among Bengalis, Marwaris and Gujaratis, who are generally fond of rice and sweets, along with high carbohydrate diet. Many tribal Indians, Eskimos and some African races, on the other hand, show lower incidence. Highest incidence (30-50% and above 35 years) has been observed in certain (human leucocyte antigen) type and are more susceptible to juvenile onset diabetes mellitus (JODM), as follows :

$A_1$, $CW_7$, $B_{18}$, $DW_3$, $DRW_3$, HLA types.

The HLA antigen sites may serve as markers with which it will be easier to identify diabetics in future, such as $A_2$, $CW_3$, $B_{15}$, or $B_{40}$, $DW_4$, $DRW_4$. Specific HLA antigents are not yet found with maturity onset diabetes mellitus (MOD).

**Obesity**

We know obesity is one of the important risk factors for maturity onset diabetes (MOD). In Eastern countries 80% of diabetics are obese while in India the percentage varies from 25 to 30. It has been observed that most obese patients become euglycaemic with reduction of weight. This may be the fact that beta cells get exhausted and fail to secrete adequate insulin for metabolism in obese people and eventually there is relative shortage of insulin. This is corrected when weight is lost.

**Effect of diet**

There is an interesting co-relation between eating habit of persons and diabetes. Diabetes is more prevalent amongst rice eaters, e.g. Bengalis, Marwaris and Gujaratis. In Yamerite Jews incidence is very low; they take high protein and low carbohydrate diet. In Western countries when they were exposed to more refined carbohydrate containing food prevalence of diabetes was more. In tribal people of India and Africa, low incidence has been attributed high fibrous content of diet and physically active vigorous life. The exact mechanism is unknown.

**Heredity**

That heredity plays an important role in the causation of diabetes has been known since the time of Charak and Susruta of ancient India (400 B.C.). Diabetes also runs in certain families. If one of the identical twin suffers from diabetes there is every possibility that the other twin is going to suffer from the disease. Thus heredity is transmitted through genes. If both parents are diabetic there is about, 30% chance of children becoming diabetic. The exact genetic make-up is unknown. About 12% of newly diagnosed diabetics have close relatives with diabetes.

Maturity onset diabetes mellitus (MOD) appears to have a set of genes that may be responsible for the familial inheritance. Of course it is influenced by environment, such as stress and obesity. Juvenile onset diabetes mellitus (JODM) may be related to a specific genetic factor.

Genetic influence appears to be stronger in non-insulin dependent diabetes (NIDD adult onset type) and among twins: both are likely to be affected if they are identical twins. But in case of insulin dependent diabetes (IDD), concordance among identical twins is about 50-60%.

Research work on histocompatibility antigens has revealed that diabetic gene of IDD is related to chromosome 6 and antigens $DW_3$, $DW_4$, $B_8$, $BW_{18}$ are at high risk. But in case of NIDD, HLA-linked susceptibility is not evident. In North Indian IDDM patients, HLA $AW_{28}$, $BW_{21}$ or $BW_{35}$ antigens are common.

In case of NIDD, inheritance appears to be poly-factorial. It should be noted that even if the parents are both NIDD, all children are not diabetics. The percentage shows wide variations in different series of available information.

**Auto-immunity**

There is strong evidence available that auto-immunity plays an important role in the aetiopathogenesis of IDD. Diabetes also co-exists with Hasimoto's thyroiditis, hypo or hyperthyroidism, Addison's disease and pernicious anaemia.

**Viruses**

In 1864, a Norwegian scientist reported case of diabetes after mumps infection. Since then scientists are trying to find the possible causative factor of diabetes. Swedish scientists noted the development of diabetes after mumps and in England, coxsackie virus infection has also been implicated. In animal experiments, diabetes has been produced after EMC (encephalomyocarditis) virus inoculation.

Possible mechanism may be that virus infection in beta cells leads to an antigen-antibody reaction in the circulation, which in turn causes damage to beta cells just like auto-immune thyroiditis. Recently antibodies against beta cells have been found in some cases. This theory may uphold the possibility of prevention of diabetes through vaccination which will be discussed later on.

**Stress**

Various types of stress, mental, physical, infection or even pregnancy may act as precipitating factors for diabetes.

**Hormones & Drugs**

Many diabetogenic hormones circulate in body. These are mainly corticosteroids, sex hormones, growth hormones and glucagon; all these hormones try to block the action of insulin whereas somatostatin enhances the action of insulin and inhibits the action of glucagon.

Several drugs such as beta-blockers, sympatho-mimetics may unmask latent diabetes or aggravate the existing diabetes. These drugs should be avoided in treatment of diabetics.

**Pathogenesis**

It is a very difficult job to describe the pathogenesis of diabetes with the present knowledge of aetiological factors of the disease. However, following is an arbitrary hypothetical attempt of explain the pathogenesis of the disease. For this purpose diabetic syndrome has been divided into two groups — namely :

(1) Acute diabetic syndrome and (2) Chronic diabetic syndrome.

**Acute Diabetic Syndrome**

In this entity, the syndrome of the disease has been explained as a consequence of hyperglycaemia which in turn leads to osmotic polyurea when it crosses the normal renal threshold for glucose. Polyurea in turn leads to thirst and hunger and increased production of glucose from sources other than liver such as fat and muscle, thereby mobilising and catabolising protein and fats. This process ultimately results in ketonaemia and ketonurea. If ketone production exceeds peripheral utilisation and excretion, ketoacidosis results which may lead to coma and death. This is the normal course of IDDM provided it is not checked by treatment.

### Chronic Diabetic Syndrome

Chronic diabetic syndrome may remain quite silent in early stages. Symptoms usually start due to complications of diabetes, chiefly due to macro-or micro-vascular angiopathy as well as due to complicated biochemical alterations. Histological changes consist of deposition of material containing glycoprotein, mucopolysaccharide or glycoprotein either within the cells or in cells or in capillary basement membrane. Macroangiopathy leads to deposition of atheromatous plaque in big vessels resulting in CVA or CAD. Microvascular angiopathy leads to retinal and renal involvement of diabetes. The basic fact, however, is absence or deficiency of insulin or defective and antagonistic insulin actions.

Insulin is secreted by beta-cells of islets of Langerhans of pancreas. Each normal contains about 100,000 islets, each islet has about 80-100 beta cells. These cells are sensitive to changes in blood glucose level of two mg within 10 seconds and within 60-90 seconds they can organise themselves to deliver necessary amount of insulin required to metabolise this amount of glucose. Pancreas also contains alpha cells which secrete glucagon and delta cells that secrete somatostatin.

Glucagon raises blood glucose level and its release is stimulated by amino acid level of blood. Glucagon has anti-insulin effect. Normal blood glucose level is dependent on balance insulin-glucagon relationship. Somatostatin mediates between glucagon and insulin.

The beta-cells manufacture proinsulin, which is protein in nature, consisting of a chain of 81 amino acids. This is taken up by golgi complex of the beta cell where maturation of granules takes place and possibly proinsulin is converted into insulin. Release of insulin may occur either by emiocytosis or intracytoplasmic dissolution of granules or by directly discharging it into microvesicles without granule formation. Chemically proinsulin is broken down into units. The part of fifty-one (51) chain becomes insulin and the other part of 30 amino acids is known as C-peptide but has no hypoglycaemic effect, as it is released, along with insulin, it may be a useful marker for the determination of function of beta cells. The beta cells are stimulated by glucose in two stages. After a carbohydrate meal and subsequent intestinal digestion, blood glucose tends to rise and stimulates the release of already stored insulin. With the increase in blood glucose level signals are sent to ribosomes within the beta cells through RNA messenger, so the system gets ready to manufacture more insulin from raw materials. The normal person can produce and release 40-50 units of insulin daily while several hundred units are kept stored in pancreas for future use.

### Function of insulin

Insulin is the chief hormone of the body that can control the storage and mobilisation of carbohydrate, protein and fat. Carbohydrates are broken down chiefly into glucose, protein into amino acids and fats into fatty acids and glycerol.

### Factors influencing insulin secretion

It has been observed both *in vivo* and *in vitro* study that basic alimentary *substrates* such as glucose, amino acids, short-chain fatty acids, ketone bodies are potent stimulants for insulin release. They act via cyclic AMP. Different hormones such as growth hormone, corticosteroids, ACTH, epinephrine and glucagon enhance the release of insulin. Their action is probably mediated by cyclic AMP. Even direct feedback mechanism of insulin secretion is also suggested. Experimentally administration of insulin decreases pancreatic insulin release.

Certain observations suggestive of neuronal control of insulin release have been made. Vagotomy decreases insulin, on the other hand vagal stimulation increases it.

### Mechanism of action of insulin

Insulin secretion at cellular level is preceded or action accompanied by a possibly reversible binding of hormone to the receptors (responding sites). These receptors are inversely proportionate to insulin concentration of blood. High insulin concentration causes the number of receptors to decline so that responsiveness to insulin also declines (insulin resistance). Thus in case of NIDDM with obesity, insulin resistances develop because of hypersecretion due to overeating. Low calorie reducing diet results in return of insulin sensitivity. Exact cellular mode of action is however uncertain.

The process can be summarised as follows :

Insulin reduces blood glucose level by : Step (1) Increasing peripheral glucose uptake and conversion into glycogen,

Step (2) Stimulating peripheral utilisation of glucose (carbohydrate utilisation and energy production).

Step (3) By reducing hepatic output of glucose (diminished glycogenolysis and diminished gluconeogenesis);

Step (4) By enhancing protein synthesis. Along with glucose mobilisation into the cells the transit of amino acids and potassium into the cells is enhanced.

In IDDM the patient is dehydrated due to osmotic diuresis and ketosis due to over-production of ketone bodies.

## TYPES OF DIABETES

The present-day classification is based on clinical behaviour, and newer concept of the aetiology of diabetes. The classification adopted by W.H.O. Expert Committee on Diabetes Mellitus, 1980 and National Diabetes Data Group, 1979.

Diabetes mellitus can be broadly classified under as :

(A) Clinical Classes e.g. Type I & II, secondary types

(B) Statistical Risk Classes e.g. I.G.T., Gestational etc.

**Clinical Classes.**

(1) Insulin dependent diabetes mellitus (IDDM) or Type 1 (previously known as Juvenile diabetes, juvenile-onset diabetes, brittle diabetes or ketosis prone diabetes). This group constitutes about 15% of total diabetes. Usually younger age group below 40 years. The symptoms usually occur with acute onset of disease. It is usually associated with beta-cells damage and there is hardly any insulin production. Islet cell antibodies are frequently found in this group. The patients thus require insulin injection as a therapeutic measure in addition to diet regulation.

(2) Non-insulin-dependent type (NIDDM) or type II (previously known as adult onset diabetes maturity onset diabetes, or stable diabetes or ketosis resistant diabetes).

In this group there may be :

(a) NIDDM — obese type

(b) NIDDM — non-obese type.

Usually the patients are obese and develop the disease after 40 years and about 85% of diabetics belong to this group. There is partial production of insulin. Sulfonylureas are useful in the treatment of this type as these drugs help in release of insulin which were as if locked inside the gland. Drugs act as keys to unlock the door and thus insulin is released. The obese NIDDM usually respond very efficiently by low calorie diet regime. Environmental and genetic factors are also responsible for this type of diabetes.

**Secondary Diabetes**

(a) Pancreatic disease — acute or chronic pancreatitis due to mumps virus, other viruses (%), cystic fibrosis, pancreatic calcification, carcinoma of pancreas.

(b) Endocrine disorders —
Acromegaly (growth hormone excess)
Cushing's syndrome (Glucocorticoid excess)
Conn's syndrome and pheochromocytoma (adrenal cortical influence).

(c) Drug therapy (Iatrogenic)
Prolonged steroid therapy and thiazide diuretics.

(d) Metabolic disorders
Haemochromatosis (Bronze diabetes) and a number of genetic syndromes.

(4) **Gestational Diabetes**

In this type glucose intolerance is only found during pregnancy and is believed to be due to complex metabolic and hormonal changes usually causing insulin resistance. Usually it settles down after child birth but sometimes these women may become diabetic in later years.

(5) **Prediabetes**

This is purely a theoretical conception. In this type both the parents are diabetic or identical twin is diabetic. The individuals have no symptom or sign and their blood or urine sugar remains normal even by provocative method. Actually individuals may never become diabetic but still they are diabetic prone or 'probable' diabetics.

(6) **Impaired Glucose Tolerance (IGT)**

This is a new conception which means that the subjects with IGT are asymptomatic and their blood sugar is within 200 mg%. Previously this group was given various names, e.g. chemical diabetes, sub-clinical diabetes and borderline diabetes. The diagnosis is based on O.G.T.T.

It should be stressed that blood glucose level is not the only criterion of severity of diabetes. Many patients with blood glucose levels of over 400 mg remain symptomless and are accidently diagnosed while others with moderate elevation of blood sugar are quite ill.

The modern classification of diabetes may be presented as follows (based on W.H.O. and Modern Diabetes Data Group).

Modern researches however indicate that the existing W.H.O. classification may have to be updated, as a new class of diabetes known as "malnutrition-related diabetes" is prevalent in tropics. Dietary intake of casava (tapioca, containing cyanogen glycosides) and protein deficiency the chief offenders.

**PRIMARY**

(1) Insulin dependent diabetes mellitus, i.e. IDDM or Type I diabetes mellitus.
(2) Non-insulin dependent diabetes mellitus or NIDDM or Type II DM which may be of three types :
    (a) Non-obese NIDDM
    (b) Obese NIDDM
    (c) Maturity onset type of DM of the young (MODY)

**SECONDARY**

(1) Pancreatic disorders
(2) Endocrine disorders
(3) Drug therapy (Iatrogenic)
(4) Metabolic organic defects including genetic syndrome.

## COMPARISON OF IDDM AND NIDDM

| Features | IDDM | NIDDM |
|---|---|---|
| Age at onset (in years) | Infancy to adult age usually before 40 | Usually over 40 |
| Prevalence | Maximum 10-20 but may occur in 4th decade | Middle age and old people |
| Seasonal trend | Autumn & Winter ? cause | Not known |
| Body weight | Loss of weight | Commonly obese |
| Ketoacidosis | Common | Very rare |
| Plasma insulin | Low | Variable |
| Association with auto-immune disease | Common | Rare |
| Antibodies to islet cells | Present in 60-80% | Less than 5% |
| Immune mechanism | 40-50% | Less than 5% |
| Concordance in identical twin | 50% | 100% |
| HLA association | Positive | None |

### Clinical manifestation

40% of diabetics are asymptomatic; symptoms are present in 60% only. The onset is usually insidious but rarely acute. In JOD the initial presentation is often loss of weight. The child eats voraciously but gains no weight. Failure to gain weight in a child is an indication of ordering a GTT.

In many instance the patients are referred from eye specialists, then neurologists, dermatologists and obstetricians. Rarely they present with renal failure and for the first time the diabetic aetiology is proved. This is more so in developing or poor countries where facilities of medical investigation are limited.

Clinical manifestation of DM can be described in simplified form as : (a) Symptoms due to hyperglycaemia, (b) Symptoms due to altered immune profile, and (c)Symptoms of complications.

### Symptoms due to hyperglycaemia

Classical symptoms of DM, e.g. polyurea, polydypsia, polyphagia and loss of weight which are due to hyperglycaemia as explained earlier. In uncontrolled cases there is increased mobilisation of fatty acids such as hydroxy-butyric acid, aceto-acetic acid and acetone as a result of deficiency of insulin leading to metabolic acidosis. This has serious and adverse effects on the central nervous system leading to coma (hyperglycaemic ketoacidosis). Hyperosmosis may affect eye leading to blurring of vision due to transitory errors of refraction.

### Symptoms due to altered immune response

Due to disturbance of intracellular glycolytic metabolism immune system of body is affected. As a result the patient suffers from recurrent attacks of boils, carbuncles, balanitis, vaginits, pruritis etc.

This group of symptoms is suggestive of diabetes and a post-prandial blood sugar check is mandatory.

### Physical findings

1) Detailed clinical examination with emphasis on certain special points is needed for complete evaluation of patient.

2) Emphasis should be given for the assessment of nutritional status and must include examination of skin, dependent oedema, or parotid swelling.

3) Pulse, particularly peripheral pulsation (posterior tibial and dorsalis pedis) blood pressure, J.V.P. cardiomegaly or any presence of cardiovascular deficit should be noted.

4) Respiratory system is thoroughly examined to exclude any pulmonary tuberculosis or any infection. Tuberculosis often co-exists, especially in developing countries and this should be borne in mind. All lean diabetics should be checked for tuberculosis and *vice versa.*

5) Thorough abdominal examination is necessitated to exclude any possibility of secondary diabetes, e.g. hepatomegaly, signs of portal hypertension (haemochromatosis), pancreatic pathology (calcified pancreatitis).

6) Palpation of kidneys is done to evaluate renal system. Renal angle tenderness is an indication of pyelonephritis.

7) Thorough neurological examination in diabetes is necessary to evaluate the nervous system involvement.

8) Diabetic neuropathy is a predominating sensory though motor and autonomic nervous system are also affected. There is wasting and weakness of quadriceps muscles.

9) Ophthalmoscopic examination must be done in all cases.

10) Lipid profile must also be checked.

**Complications of Diabetes Mellitus**

Complications of diabetes can be divided into two groups :

1) Preventable complications are due to infections, injury, neglect in treatment, indiscreet diet or alcohol.

These factors will produce complications in each diabetic whether he is in early stage or late stage of the disease.

2) **Delayed complications**

These may occur in all diabetics after some years since the onset of the disease. These occur in multiple organs and are due to microangiopathy or macroangiopathy. Non-diabetics may suffer from atherosclerosis in old age but it seems that the process gets accelerated in diabetics. However, the current view is that even these complications can be delayed or even reversed by tight control of diabetics.

**Aetio-pathology of atherosclerosis**

Probable series of events in atherogenesis are as follows :

(1) Endothelial injury
(2) Platelet adherence to the site of injury
(3) Platelet aggregation at the site of injury
(4) Release from platelets material stored intracellularly (mitogen) which can stimulate smooth muscle cell proliferation
(5) Smooth muscle cell proliferation and migration (foam cells) into the subendothelial layer at the area of damage
(6) Accumulation of extracellular matrix (collagen elastic tissue)
(7) Accumulation of lipids and lipoproteins
(8) Thrombosis.

Endothelium may be injured by :

Hypertension, hypercholesterolemia, hyperglycaemia, archidonic acid, homocystine, cigarette smoking, virus, bacteria and immune complexes.

Endothelial injury at the branch points or around atheromata is due to turbulent flow of blood. The same type of mechanical stress can be produced by hypertension. Vascular injury may be due to repeated immunisation leading to development of antigen-antibody complexes.

Platelets interact with collagen at the site of endothelial injury and release ADP and platelet derived growth factor which in turn stimulate smooth muscle cell proliferation (foam cells). This ADP activates phospolipase leading to release of arachidonic acid. Arachidonic acid is converted to prostaglandins and thence to thromboxone, that promotes smooth muscle contraction. Thromboxone and ADP together with thrombin cause further platelet aggregation. The thrombin also causes polymerisationof fibrinogen and generation of a thrombus. The whole process is counter-balanced by prostaclin, which is produced by endothelial cell. Platelets do not aggregate on a healthy endothelium.

In diabetes, there is stable deformity of red blood corpuscles resulting in reduced oxygen transformation. This hypoxia is one of the factors for endothelial injury. Increased glycosylated haemoglobin, hypertriglyceridemia may impair oxygen transport. LDL itself can cause endothelial injury.

In diabetes, there is high concentration of LDL, VLDL and decreased prostocyclin synthesis by endothelium.

Platelet aggregation rises in diabetes and there is increased thromboxone production which may lead to increased adhesiveness of platelets, which then becomes hypersensitive to aggregating agents.

Diabetic serum containing LDL, excess, growth hormone and increased insulin enhance the growth of arterial smooth muscle cells.

Hyperinsulinaemia and hypertriglyceridemia are associated with each other. In presence of excess insulin, hepatic VLDL production increases. Obesity aften accompanies hypertriglyceridemia and obesity is also associated with insulin resistance with hyperinsulinaemia. VLDL itself lowers the insulin-receptors activity. All these factors together enhance the process of atherogenesis.

The accyletated process of atherogenesis is responsible for major part of morbidity and mortality of diabetes and the pathogenesis of long-term complications of diabetes.

**Eye changes**

All parts of eye are susceptible to be affected in diabetes. Hyperglycemia may lead to cataract (snow flake). Microangiopathy of iris leads to rupture and haemorrhage (haemorrhagic glaucoma) or neovascularisation of ciliary body and iris causing open angle glaucoma. Micro-angiopathy of retina produces microaneurysm which may rupture and appear as waxy exudate. So-called cotton-wool exudate is due to extravasation of protein from capillaries.

Macrovascular angiopathy is vulnerable to rupture leading to large haemorrhage. If it is macular the patient becomes blind. If there is haemorrhage anterior to vitreous, resorption may lead to contraction and detachment of retina. There may be neovascularisation of retina (retinitis proliferous). Assessment of early retinopathy is difficult because visual acuity is not affected. Once the patient develops visual loss, treatment becomes difficult. Regular ophthalmoscopic examination and timely treatment may, however, prevent visual loss.

Evaluation of retinopathy is done by direct or indirect ophthalmoscope, fluorescin angiography and slit lamp biomicroscope.

Management consists of tight control of hyperglycaemia. Photocoagulation either by xenon arc or by argon arc method. In the past pituitary ablation either by surgical operation or by transphenoidal implantation of Yttrium-90 (freezing pituitary) was performed. In some cases vitrectomy or retinal surgery may be necessary.

**Coronary Artery Disease**

Diabetes has a higher incidence of atherosclerosis involving coronary and peripheral arteries.

(1) Incidence of hypertension, particularly systolic hypertension is more in diabetes.

(2) In diabetes, there is raised ESR, blood viscosity, higher VIII (factor VIII coagulant activity). Increased B-thromboglobulin levels. Levels of total triglycerides, LDL, VLDL, cholesterol and apolipoprotein B (Apo B) are significantly increased.

In uncontrolled IDDM levels of HDL cholesterol and apolipoprotein $A_1$ (Apo $A_1$) are significantly reduced.

(3) The absence of hyperlipidemia with atherosclerosis does not mean that lipid risk factors are absent.

(4) Mean endosystolic volume of the left ventricle is greater in diabetics as compared to non-diabetics.

(5) Echocardiographic and vectorcardiographic abnormalities are present in some asymptomatic adult diabetics. Diabetic cardiomyopathy can be suspected by study of apexcardiography, calculating systolic time intervals (STI) and by echocardiography. The final verdict, however, in cardiac muscle biopsy is by using a bioptome.

**Diabetic foot**

Diabetic foot is a very difficult problem, once ulcers have developed. Neuropathy and associated vascular complications are the main aggravating factors; trauma and ill-fitting shoes often trigger the situation. Good diabetes control as well as proper supportive treatment may save the limb (Fig.9.3). Otherwise amputation may be necessary. All diabetics must be advised to take proper care of the foot.

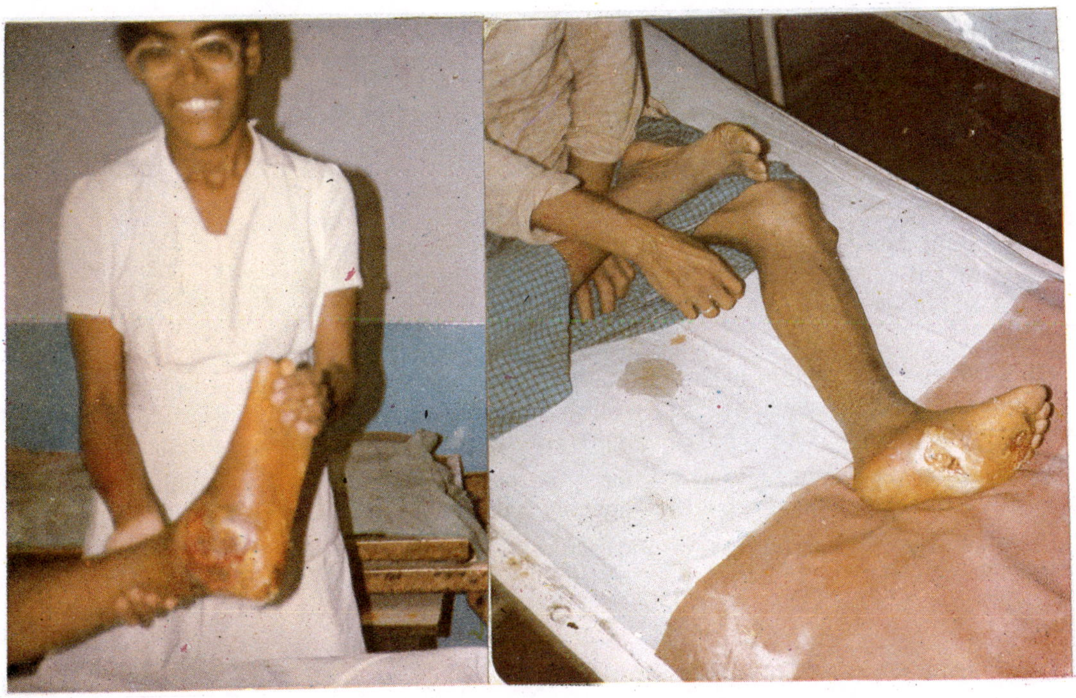

Fig.9.3 : Diabetic foot showing ulcers and gangrene.

**Nephropathy Table 9.11**

Alternations in renal functions and structure are found even at the very one of diabetes. Early detection and tight control of diabetes can prevent and even can reverse the early changes of five years' duration. There is thickening of basement membrane. Biochemical analysis shows that glycoprotein synthesis is increased in renal glomeruli leading to excess deposition of collagen-like substance of abnormal chemical structure containing too many disaccharide radicals.

**Detection of nephropathy**

(1) Proteinurea — Proteinurea has been thought to be as the first sign of serious renal disease. Severity of nephropathy in a particular patient is suggested by clinical picture and amount of proteinurea. It is a fact that poorly controlled diabetics show much higher incidence of nephropathy than those who are well controlled and periodically reviewed.

(2) GRF — In early stages GRF is increased at the rate of 0.1 to 1.5 ml/min depending on duration and severity of the disease.

Early and antihypertensive treatment reduces both proteinurea and rate of decline of GFR in young IDDM.

(3) Ultrasonography provides a non-invasive method to visualise kidneys and urinary tract as I.V. pyelography may lead to acute renal failure. In early stages there is increase in size of kidney.

Retinopathy is always associated with nephropathy. If retinopathy is absent renal biopsy is indicated to detect nephropathy.

A special chapter on diabetic nephropathy has been included.

## MANAGEMENT OF DIABETES MELLITUS

The goal of treatment of diabetics is to restore the patient's functional capacity and his physiological state to as normal as possible. The blood sugar level should be normal or near normal and urine free of sugar. There should not be elevation of plasma lipids and blood biochemistry should remain within normal limits.

The principles of treatment are as follows :

(1) Adjustment of diet
(2) Exercise
(3) Insulin therapy
(4) Oral anti-diabetic drugs
(5) Psychological preparation of the patient and adjustment of life style.

In a survey conducted in Diabetic Clinic of Ramakrishna Seva Pratisthan of Vivekananda Institute of Medical Science, Calcutta, we noted that only 6.8% cases required insulin while 36.5% were controlled by diet only. The remaining were controlled by diet plus oral anti-diabetic drugs.

Many other reports in India and different parts of the world also show similar trend. **JOD patients will require insulin** but there may be occasional **exception** i.e. on MODY types.

Too much of food may increase insulin requirement, less food or vigorous exercise may reduce blood glucose level.

### Diet

Food consists of carbohydrate, protein, fat, minerals and vitamins.

To plan a diet for a diabetic individual, the daily requirement of calories is calculated according to his occupation, build and age. For example, adults in sedentary occupation may only require 1200-1500 calories daily whereas active or growing persons may require 2000-2500 calories. Calculation of daily requirement of calories on the basis of bodyweight per kilogram is as follows :

| Built | Sedentary activity | Moderate activity | Strenuous activity |
|---|---|---|---|
| Heavy | 20 Cal. | 25 Cal. | 30 Cal. |
| Ordinary | 30 Cal. | 35 Cal. | 40 Cal. |
| Thin | 35 Cal. | 40 Cal. | 50 Cal. |

Sedentary diabetic having body weight of 60 kg. the total calories requirement will be 60 × 20 = 1200 Cal. Similarly, for a hardworking diabetic with thin body build and weighing 45 kg. the total calories will be 45 × 50 = 2250 Cal.

For a juvenile diabetic the requirement of calories may be calculated on body weight (B.W.) basis, i.e. B.W. × 50 Cal. If B.W. is 30 kg the calorific need is 30 × 50 = 1500 calories.

Alternative method of calculation is 1000 calories plus 100 cal per year of age up to 16 years.

The need for additional nutrients including iron, calcium and vitamin supplement depends on nutritional status of the patient. In developing countries poor sector of the people is generally malnourished. Hence these women will need additional protein, fat, vitamins and minerals. The best method is to give five or six meals per day instead of two or three large meals, which is normally done by most people. Five meals are usually convenient and the calories can be divided as follows :

Breakfast 1/7; Lunch 2/7; Tea 1/7; Dinner 2/7 and Night cap 1/7. Further adjustment may be required depending on job, duty, hours and availability. Generally 50% of total calories should come from carbohydrate while fat and protein should consist of 25% each, 50% of total protein should be animal protein. Whenever planning a diet, go into the details of the patient's duty hours, his own timings of diet and night duty schedules.

**Insulin therapy**

As already mentioned insulin is synthesised and stored in islet cells($\beta$-cells) of pancreas. Commercially, insulin is prepared either from beef pancreas (bovine) or pc.k pancreas (porcine). Human insulin preparation is a cumbersome procedure and expensive also. Proinsulin has also been made *in vitro* by introducing genetically determined DNA into E Coli which then produce in cuture media.

Insulin cannot be given orally as it is destroyed by digestive enzymes. It is given by injection (S.C., IM or IV); it is absorbed into blood plasma rapidly, half-life of crystalline (insulin) is only 10 min. This is convenient for continuous insulin therapy but much inconvenient for routine replacement in IDDM diabetes. Therefore, slow release preparations have been developed tc provide a nearest approach to natural insulin function. However, these preparations do not come close to accurate replacement of natural system.

Optimal control is generally best achieved by two doses of soluble insulin 30 min. before breakfast and dinner.

Normally most IDDM needs 30—50 units daily as normal pancreas secretes 30—40 units.

Roughly the following schedule may be followed :

Blood sugar 300 mg% : 20 units
Blood sugar 200-300 mg% : 10 units

The dose is then adjusted according to usual blood sugar and/or urine sugar.

The conventional insulins used in our country are presented as follows along with action-duration :

| | Action duration in hours | | |
|---|---|---|---|
| | Onset | Peak | Total |
| Soluble insulin (Regular or crystalline) | 1/2 | 2—3 | 6—8 |
| Protamine zinc insulin (PZI) | 3—6 | 12—24 | 30—36 |
| Isophane insulin (NPH) | 1—2 | 10—12 | 14—30 |
| Globulin zinc insulin suspension | 2—4 | 8—16 | 18—24 |
| Insulin lente | 1—2 | 8—12 | 18—24 |
| Insulin semi lente | 1—2 | 6—10 | 12—18 |
| Insulin ultralente | 4—6 | 8—16 | 18—24 |

Urine sugar +++ (red/brick) 30 units
Urine sugar ++ (yellow) 20 units
Urine sugar + (green ppt) 10 units.

Daily increments of dose should be four units. When the patient is stabilised 2/3rd of total daily dose is generally given before 30 minutes before breakfast and 1/3rd before dinner..

If only lente or NPH insulin is preferred then initial dose should be 10-14 units with breakfast. Daily increments (four units) may be given on alternate days.

If there is a great fluctuation of blood sugar then soluble insulin is to be added with lente insulin and the dose to be adjusted with the patient's response. Sometimes lente or NPH insulin plus soluble insulin may be required twice a day but night dose should be less.

Adverse effects are due to overdose of insulin resulting in hypoglycaemia that may lead to coma, convulsions and even death. Hypoglycaemia may manifest as disturbed sleep and morning headache. Other effects are lipoatrophy or lipomata at the injection site as a result of repeated injection at the same spot. Local reaction such as itching or generalised allergic reactions, though rare, may occur.

The newer insulins are not available in this country and imported drugs are also quite expensive. In the West, most diabetics are now getting the new insulins. In developing countries these older insulins will have to be used for some years till they are freely available with reduced cost. It is also probable that in near future oral insulins may also be available Intranasal insulins are also being used experimentally. However, the newer insulins and modern advances of insulin therapy have been discussed at the end of this chapter. Wherever possible, newer insulins can be used in newly diagnosed cases and also where the older insulins are causing allergic reactions and showing resistance.

**Insulin resistance**

A diabetic requiring more than 200 units/day is regarded as insulin resistant. As already mentioned, it is due to antigenic effect of insulin. Beef insulin being more antigenic, change to purified porcine insulin or human insulin may be beneficial. Sometime corticosteroid (Prednisolone 20-40 mg/day, may restore insulin sensitivity.

**Oral hypoglycaemic drugs**

These are two kinds of oral hypoglycaemic drugs :

(1) Sulphonamide derivatives (Sulfonyl-ureas) and
(2) Guanidine derivative (biguanides).

In 1918 hypoglycaemic effect of guanidine was observed and tried in diabetics in 1926 but abandoned for fear of hepatic toxicity.

In 1930 hypoglycaemic effect of sulphonamide was noticed but the first sulfonylurea (carbutamide) was discovered by German scientists in 1955. Later on, other sulfonylureas such as chlorpropamide, glibenclamide, glipizide were discovered. Biguanides include phenformen and metformen.

Sulfonylureas act primarily by stimulating the β-cells to produce insulin. For successful treatment, 30% cell function must be preserved. It is useful where daily diet has failed to control NIDDM, nonketotic diabetics, irrespective of age where insulin requirements is below 40 units per day.

Biguanides act :

(a) By increasing peripheral glucose utilisation,
(b) By reducing glucose absorption from the gut and
(c) By reducing hepatic neoglucogenesis.

Both the groups are effective only in presence of insulin.

The commonly used oral drugs are presented in Table 9,7.

**Table 9.7 : Preparations of oral antidiabetic drugs**

| Name | Approx. duration of action (hrs.) | Daily frequency | Remarks |
|---|---|---|---|
| **A. Sulfonylurea** | | | |
| Tolbutamide (0.5 – 1 gm) | 8.0 | twice daily | Quite safe and effective. Tolerance occurs. |
| Chlorpropamide (100-250 mg) | 24–36 | once daily | Less safe than Tolbutamide. Dose increment weekly. Potent and prolonged action. |
| Glibenclamide (5 mg) | 8–12 | once to thrice daily | Avoid in hepatic & renal failure. Contraindicated in IDDM, pregnancy infection & surgery, weekly increments. |
| Glipizide (15 mg) | | once to thrice daily | Similar to glibenclamide |
| **B. Biguanides** | | | |
| Phenformin | 8–14 | twice daily | Lactic acidosis may occur. Use with care. |
| Metformin | 12 | once daily | Can be used with insulin or other agents. Gives metallic taste in mouth. Prolonged use leads to vit. $B_{12}$ deficiency due to malabsorption |

Hypoglycaemia may occur with all oral drugs. The drugs should be carefully used in elderly particularly with heart disease. Because of long half life, chlorpropamide is not the drug of first choice in the old. *Biguanides should not be used in patients with hepatic or renal disorder, the risk of lactic acidosis should be remembered.* However, in our country most diabetologists have been using the biguanides cautiously and without much problem. However, dosage schedule is never high.

Drugs failure may be accounted for :

(1) Irregularity in taking drugs
(2) Presence of infection or metabolic disorder
(3) Simultaneous use of antagonistic drugs e.g. steroids, oral contraceptives, diuretics.

**Sulfonylureas and Drug Interactions**

Some of the drugs which are affected by sulfonylureas are listed below

(1) Beta blockers
(2) Diuretics particularly thiazides
(3) Alcohol
(4) Analgesics
(5) Sulphonamides
(6) Monoamine oxidase inhibitors
(7) Coumadin.

Beta blockers mask the most important signs of hypoglycaemia such as tachycardia, tremor, though sweating is not affected.

Alcohol enhances hypoglycaemia due to inhibition of hepatic glucose output and adrenergic effect. Alcohol and tolbutamide together increase the risk of myocardial infarction.

It should also be remembered that advanced diabetics may get little or no pain due to myocardial infarction due to neuropathy. Alcoholic excess may further complicate the matter due to alcoholic cardiomyopathy.

Aspirin interferes with the urinary excretion of chlorpropamide and increases the blood level. Therefore, there is chance of accumulative effect.

**Management of diabetes in renal failure**

The kidney destroys about 40% of endogenous insulin. With renal failure, insulin requirements are greatly reduced in diabetes. Soluble insulin acts like long-acting insulin. 5—10 units of soluble insulin is more than sufficient.Oral agents are better avoided. Lactic acidosis may develop with biguanides.

Excretion is delayed & if hypoglycaemia develops it is prolonged and difficult to control.

Haemodialysis is not as successful as in non-diabetics. There is increased risk of intraocular haemorrhage.

Peritoneal dialysis is better tolerated by diabetics than haemodialysis but again there is risk of infection.

Renal transplantation with related donors is better accepted though diabetic nephropathy develops on biopsy within 2½ years, but clinical nephropathy takes about 5-10 years to develop. (Refer to chapter on Diabetic renal disease).

**Neuropathy**

Numerous nerves related problems of diabetics are termed "diabetic neuritis" or neuropathy. Neuropathy affecting peripheral and autonomic nervous system is common in young IDDM. Broadly, diabetic neuropathy can be classified into (1) more common distal symmetrical polyneuropathies (sensory or sensorimotor with or without autonomic involvement) and (2) less frequent focal and multifocal neuropathies (cranial neuropathy; intercostal neuropathies and asymmetrical proximal motor neuropathy).

Symptoms may appear in a known diabetic or those may be the presenting symptoms of the patient. Enough attention is to be paid to detect autonomic dysfunction which may be asymptomatic.

The cause of diabetic neuropathy is multifactorial with metabolic factors and vascular factors both playing a significant role.

According to one theory, hyperglycaemia results in increased accumulation of sorbitol in the nerves and other tissues. Myo-inositol content of the nerve is reduced which results in slowing of nerve conduction and disturbed nerve function. Micro angiopathy of nerves results in focal neuropathies which in turn causes segmental demyelination and ultimately axonal degeneration.

Schwann cells are affected. Genetic factors also play some role. Glycosylation of protein in the neurons could result in altered nerve function.

**Symptoms of Neuropathy**

Tingling, numbness, pain, paresthesias are the most frequent symptoms the patients complained of. The symptoms are aggravated at night and in winter. The patients are unaware of injury, trauma, blisters when the sensory nerves are involved. Immediate medical care is to be sought even for an innocent looking lesion of foot.

Muscle-wasting (diabetic amyotrophy) is a special form of diabetic neuropathy. There is extreme sensitivity of skin of thighs, pain and tenderness of thigh muscle and wasting of muscle bulk — may be followed by loss of body weight. Motor neuropathy may cause diplopia or foot drop. When the intercostal nerves are involved the patient complains of girdle pain in the chest (radicular pain). It is a sharp, shooting burning pain that is constant and excruciating.

When the autonomic nerves are involved, bladder and bowel movements are disturbed. Digestion is disturbed. The patient experiences nausea, bloating and vomiting of undigested food. There is infrequent but voluminous urination (autonomic bladder) and constipation or diarrhoea.

Besides, the patient may experience gastatory sweating, orthostatic hypotension and impotence.

The management of diabetic neuropathy consists of symptomatic relief and effective control of hyperglycaemia. For pain and paresthesia simple analgesic, diazepam, massage and even in obstinate cases largactil may be helpful. Anti-cholinergic, e.g. neostigmine, metoclopropamide are found to be beneficial in gastatory sweating, For diarrhoea, tetracycline and choline phosphate may be instituted.

In case of autonomic bladder, double or tripple voiding technique and cholinergic drugs, e.g. bethanechol 10-20 mg (T.D.) may be helpful.

HYPOGLYCAEMIA

Hypoglycaemia effect usually occurs in patients due to either over-dose of medicine which may be insulin or oral drugs or when a patient does not take the proper diet. Reaction following soluble insulin usually occurs in 3-4 hours or with lente insulin or chlorpropamide, these appear in 8-10 hours. All the patients or relatives must be told about the symptoms, early treatment may herald the fatal outcome. The symptoms dramatically responded to a lump of sugar or glucose or even a bottle of soft drink. The diabetic should carry a card mentioning that he is a diabetic and if he behaves abnormally he must be given sugar or glucose.

Four types of symptoms in relation to blood glucose level are recognized as follows :

70 mg : Parasympathetic response, e.g. hunger, nausea, eructation etc.

60 mg : Diminished cerebral function such as inability to concentrate or think clear.

50 mg : Sympathetic response, viz. flushing, perspiration, tachycardia, hyperventilation.

30 mg : Generalised convulsion, transient focal deficit, visual disturbances and coma. Hypothermia and cold extremities is common.

Treatment consists of administration of glucose either by oral route or I.V.

If oral glucose can be given, 15 to 20g. is usually adequate. But, if the patient is unable to swallow 25%, I.V. glucose should be given. 25 to 50 ml may be needed. In case of difficulty in giving I.V. glucose 1.0 mg of glucagon can be given by S.C. or I.M. route. Sometimes patient appears to be refractory and in these cases continuous I.V. glucose drip may be required till the patient can take oral feed. If the patient does not respond within 20—30 minutes. I.V. dexamethasone or even I.V. mannitol may be needed.

**Sleep Sentry**

This is a preventive mechanism against insulin hypoglycaemia. It is like a wristwatch and to be worn at the wrist. The watch by its metallic contact with the skin can detect any change in galvanic skin resistance and lowered skin temperature and gives an alarm signal. The sleeping patient can thus wake up and take appropriate action. This is only a sleep sentry which warns the patient against possible hypoglycaemia but does not detect blood glucose level directly. Sweating and fall in skin temperature raise signals which act through thermo-electric mechanism.

**Hyperosmolal Non-ketotic Coma in Diabetic Mellitus**

The syndrome was first described by Samant and Scherartz in 1957. It is characterized by severe dehydration, stupor with ketosis, severe hyperglycaemia (usually 600 mg) and raised serum osmolarity. It is more common in elderly female patients with infection of a stroke. Severe dehydration is due to the fact that the body fails to maintain osmolarity by drinking sufficient water to match with severe hyperglycaemic diuresis.

**CLINICAL FEATURE**

The patient usually presents with severe thirst, polyurea, convulsion and mental confusion. On examination patient is stuporose with signs of severe dehydration, shallow breathing and sometimes signs of neurological deficit.

Laboratory findings show elevated blood glucose usually more than 500mg per 100ml. Serum sodium is either normal or low. Serum potassium may be high, normal or low; serum bicarbonate level may be normal or low. There is usually azotaemia.

Depressed sensorium is directly related to degree of hyperosmolarity. Serum ketone values are usually normal.

**Laboratory Findings in Hyperosmolal diabetic Coma Normal**

| | |
|---|---|
| 1. Glucose | : 600 mg% |
| 2. Sodium | : 135—145 Eq/L |
| 3. Potassium | : 3.5—4.8m Eq/L |
| 4. Bicarbonate | : 17—22m Eq/L |
| 5. Blood urea | : 80±10mg% |
| 6. Creatinine | : 5.5±1.1mg% |
| 7. Osmolarity | : 350 Osm/kg. |

Management of the case depends on quick replacement body fluid by half normal saline 10.45 per cent. Isotonic saline and isotonic glucose administration may cause higher mortality rate.

In addition, attention should be given for supportive therapy of a comatose patient. Possible underlying infection should be treated with proper antibiotics.

## DIABETIC KETOACIDOSIS

Relative insulin deficit may result from (1) excess diet. (2) actual omission or irregular intake of insulin. (3) vomiting and diarrhoea from any cause, and (4) infection. Ketoacidosis may be induced by myocardial infarction, severe urinary tract infection, acute cholecystitis, acute pancreatitis, hyperthyroidism or pregnancy. The condition is aggravated by increased activity of other hormones, such as, adrenaline, corticosteroid, growth hormone and glucagon which are secreted during stress and strain situations.

## PATHOPHYSIOLOGY OF KETOACIDOSIS

As previously mentioned insulin has got five primary actions :

(1) Activation of glucose-6-phosphate so that Kreb's cycle properly functions

(2) Direct influence on glycogen synthesis;

(3) Inhibition of breakdown of neutral fat into fatty acid;

(4) Inhibition of catabolism of protein;

(5) Increased perpiheral uptake of glucose by adipose and muscle tissue.

Therefore, failure of adequate insulin action at the above mentioned sites leads to "hepatic over-production of glucose" and peripheral under-utilisation of glucose". The result is hyperglycaemia, decreased fatty acid synthesis, increased fatty acid catabolism, decreased protein synthesis and increased protein catabolism. The large amounts of FFA released from adipose tissue are followed by increased uptake of FFA by liver.

Normally these are converted into acetyl-CCA to aceto-acetyl-CCA or into fatty acid in presence of insulin, but if there is insulin deficit these are converted into ß-hydroxybutyric acid, ketone bodies or liberated as such aceto-acetic acid.

## CLINICAL FEATURES

If the patient is a known diabetic and if there is a history of omission of insulin dose or infection the diagnosis is not difficult. The patient may present with weakness, excessive thirst, fatigue, somnolence, nausea, vomiting or even abdominal pain. In severe cases, if the patient may come with altered level of consciousness.

On examination : Face is flushed; tachycardia, dehydration, Kussmaul breathing and fruity (acetone) odour in breath may be obvious. In severe cases there may be hypotension and the patient may develop severe shock, and if not treated may end in coma.

### Differential diagnosis

Diabetic ketoacidosis may be differentiated from other causes, such as, alcoholic ketoacidosis, lactic acidosis, hyperosmolal nonketotic coma. Presence of hyperglycaemia, ketonurea and glycosurea is universal in diabetic ketoacidosis. Hyperventilation, low pH, high lactic acid in plasma and low bicarbonate level are clues for diagnosis of lactic acidosis.

The important differentiating points are as follows :

| | Hyperglycaemia | Hypoglycaemia |
|---|---|---|
| History of | Insulin dose omission or infection | Over-dose of insulin or oral drugs. |
| Symptoms : | Thirst, polyurea, muscle cramps, hazy vision, abdominal pain. | Hunger, sweating, palpitation, tremor. |
| Physical Signs : | Dry tongue, soft eye balls. Kussmaul's breathing in severe cases, acetone smell in breath, BP. | Dyspnoea, faintness, dizziness, abnormal behaviour, profuse sweating pulse, tachycardia. |

| | | |
|---|---|---|
| Treatment | Insulin | Oral glucose sugar, I.V. glucose or Inj. glucagon. |

## MANAGEMENT OF KETOACIDOSIS

Once the diagnosis of ketoacidosis is suspected, the patient should be admitted to a hospital. A search for precipitating factors, such as, an infection, an acute surgical illness or myocardial infarction be carried out. Blood sample is drawn for estimation of sugar, sodium, potassium, bicarbonate, pH. ketone, urea, NPN. Urine is collected for sugar, ketone and routine examination. The aim of treatment is to combat :

(1) Ketosis by insulin administration
(2) Electrolyte imbalance by proper fluid therapy
(3) Infection by antibiotics or anti-bacterial drugs
(4) Treatment of any other precipitating factors.

The method of insulin therapy is changing in modern times. Regular or plain insulin is now-a-days given in slow dose regime, against the previous bolus dose therapy. Soluble insulin may be given I.V. with starting dose of 20 units followed by 5-7 units I.M. hourly provided the patient is not in severe shock.

Insulin can be given also via I.V. infusion or by insulin pump. Argument against the bolus dose is that insulin has half life of 4 or 5 minutes and therefore most of the bolus of insulin will disappear quickly. The effects will not be even and this may lead to adverse effect on counter hormones.

However, there are arguments against low dose therapy also. Some patients are resistant to insulin chiefly due to insulin antibodies. It cannot be predicted prospectively who are really insulin resistant. Hence it is possibly better to give at least 25 to 50 units of soluble insulin hourly via I.V. route at least as long as blood sugar is very high and ketoacidosis is present.

Ketoacidosis must be corrected as soon as possible. Fluid deficit is about 3-6 litres and of which about three litres of extracellular deficit can be combated by infusion of isotonic (0.9% NaCI) saline.

Immediate infusion of I.V. normal saline or Ringer's solution should be started. First, one or two bottles should be given rapidly followed by additional fluids depending on state of dehydration and output of urine. Once blood sugar has come down to about 300 mg%, five per cent glucose solution should be started with 5-10 units of insulin per bottle. At this stage careful watch for signs of cerebral oedema should be made. Treatment of cerebral oedema is dexamethasone and hypertonic mannitol.

When bicarbonate level is very low, 12 m. mol/L (severly acidotic) one bottle (500 c.c.) of normal saline is replaced either by isotonic sodium lactate solution (M/6) or isotonic sodium bicarbonate (14%).

Potassium deficit is always present and it will fall further as soon as the treatment is started because of insulin administration and rehydration. Potassium chloride is usually added to each bottle of saline at the rate of 20m.mol/hr. When the potassium level rises to 5 mml/L, it is discontinued.

Gastric suction is done in stuporose or comatose patients. Adequate antibiotics are given to combat infection. The condition should be usually controlled within 24 hours and oral feeding is started with frequent liquid feeds containing mainly carbohydrate such as milk, fruit juice. cane sugar, vegetable soup etc.

**Table 9.8 : Shows differential features between Diabetic Coma and Hypoglycemia**

| | Diabetic coma | Hypoglycaemia |
|---|---|---|
| History : | Insufficient dose or omission of insulin, infection or myocardial infarction. | Insufficient food, excess insulin, too much exercise |
| Onset : | Usually occurs after several hours or days | Abrupt onset after a few hours of injection of short acting-insulin, this case is relatively slower by many hrs. after injection. |
| Course : | Polyurea, polydipsia, anorexia, nausea, vomiting, laboured breathing, weakness, drowsiness sometimes fever, abdominal pain and coma. | Sudden onset of profound weakness, fainting tendency, profuse sweating, hunger, diplopia, incoordination, twitching, convulsions, even coma. |
| Physical findings : | Coated and dry tongue, dry skin, Kussmaul breathing, odour of acetone in breath BP weak, rapid pulse and soft eyeball pressure. | Pale moist skin, fall of BP, rapid pulse but normal breathing, dilated pupil, exaggerated reflexes and patient may appear confused, unable to answer questions, may be mistaken for C.V.A; |
| Laboratory findings : | Urine sugar (+++) present<br>Urinary ketone<br>Blood sugar high<br>Plasma – $HCO_3$ raised<br>Plasma acetone (++).<br>Blood PH is acid.<br>Blood urea may be raised. | Urine<br>Sugar nil and blood sugar low<br>No ketone<br>Normal $HCO_3$ |
| Treatment : | Little or no response to I.V. glucose or glucagon<br>Blood may be raised; unable to answer question; may be mistaken for C.V.A. | Glucose or glucagon |

## Diabetes and Pregnancy

Diabetes mellitus is an important complication to be recognised during pregnancy. Incidence of diabetes during pregnancy varies from 0.3 to 7.9 per cent. During pre-insulin era, maternal mortality used to be 6 to 45% and perinatal mortality was 50-70%. Now it has reduced to about 5% and maternal mortality is rare with adequate insulin therapy.

Pregnant mother with diabetes not only faces the complication of ketoacidosis or hypoglycaemia but other complications, such as, microvascular, renal, occular, neural complications are accelerated if it is associated with hypertension. Tight control of diabetes reduces both maternal and perinatal mortality. It is essential to hospitalise the pregnant mother from 32 weeks until delivery.

## Joslin Clinical Classification of Diabetes in Pregnancy

Class A : Glucose tolerance test abnormal. No symptoms; euglycaemia maintained with treatment by appropriate diet but without insulin.

Class B : Adult onset (age 20 or older) and short duration (less than 10 years).

Class C : Relatively young onset (age 10-19) or relatively long duration (10-19 years).

Class D : Very young onset (age less than 10) or very long duration (20 years or more) or evidence of minimal vascular disease (e.g. background retinopathy).

Class F : Renal disease

Class R : Proliferative retinopathy.

About 10-15% of patients belong to the class B to F and require insulin to maintain euglycaemia. The perinatal mortality is high this class.

**Detection of Diabetes in Pregnancy**

The usual symptoms of diabetes may not be appreciated as those may be passed as normal during pregnancy. Screening is done in those who give the history of previous big baby, recurrent abortion, previous infants with congenital abnormalities unexplained, still births, neonatal death or recurrent attacks of vaginitis or urinary tract infections as well as family history of diabetes.

Post-prandial blood sugar screening should be done in all these patients. If physical examination reveals disproportionate uterus size, excessive weight gain, hypertension, hydramnios or obesity presence of diabetes should be suspected.

Urine for sugar and albumin must be tested for all patients during each antenatal check-up. Fasting and post-prandial blood sugar is done when urine sugar is present. If any of these values is abnormal, oral GTT with 75 gm glucose in 250-300 ml or water should be done. Even if GTT is normal, a repeat GTT is done during 30-34 weeks of pregnancy.

**Effect of Pregnancy of Diabetes Mellitus**

The effect of pregnancy on diabetes mellitus varies with each trimaster.

1st trimaster : GTT improves. Degree of diabetes lessens. Sensitivity to insulin increases. Hypoglycaemia may precipitate.

2nd trimaster : Patient becomes ketosis prone. Insulin requirement increases.

3rd trimaster : More intensfication of diabetes. Tendency for hypoglycaemia and insulin sensitivity increases.

Post partum and lactation period : Remission of diabetes may occur during post-partum period. Insulin requirement may fall during lactation.

**Effect of Diabetes on foetus**

Foetal hypoglycemia, hyperinsulinemia are responsible for foetal mortality and morbidity. Fluctuating blood sugar level, hyaline disease, congenital malformations are important factors for foetal mortality. Neonatal morbidity includes respiratory distress syndrome (six times more common), hypoglycaemia, hypocalcaemia, polycythaemia, hyperbilirubinaemia.

**Management**

During pregnancy insulin is the drug of choice besides good nutritious diet. Patients taking oral drugs are switched over to insulin. Injection of plain or soluble insulin is ideal, but if possible there is no harm if food control can be achieved by long acting insulin. In future mono-component insulins will be more widely used when freely available in this part of the world. Pre-delivery insulin requirement consists of giving 1/3rd of pre-pregnancy requirements of insulin on the morning of induction. Subsequent dose depends on blood sugar level during labour. Slow infusion of insulin at a rate of 0.06 to 0.07 units per hour with 5% dextrose may be given. Flow chart of blood sugar, electrolytes may be useful. Ideally, paediatrician should be present during confinement to look after the baby.

**Delivery**

If euglycaemia is well maintained throughout pregnancy, there is no harm for vaginal delivery at term if there is no other problem. Otherwise earlier induction is indicated depending on foetal maturity.

Medical termination of pregnancy and sterilization is done in patients with proliferative retinopathy, CAD nephropathy.

## DIABETES IN CHILDHOOD (J.O.D.M.)

Diabetes mellitus in childhood needs a special consideration because of their growth, educational problem, activity, emotional disturbance. In Western countries, the prevalence is high as compared to tropical countries. About 4 to 5 per cent of all diabetics belong to childhood diabetes but in India incidence is comparatively much less, possibly two per cent of all diabetics. It is also possible, the authors feel, that many cases are not detected due to lack of facilities. Diabetes may manifest at any age but common age group is 5 to 6 years, and peak incidence rises in 10 to 13 years. First group may be due to exposure to infection in school going children and latter may be due to insulin antagonism of sex hormones, increased rate of growth hormone and increased level of emotions.

IDD are commonly detected in children, of course in some cases NIDD may be observed.

**Metabolic disorders in children**

(1) Insulin dependent Diabetes Mellitus — IDDM (Type I)
(2) Non-insulin dependent Diabetes Mellitus — NIDDM (Type II)
(3) Ketosis-resistant Juvenile Diabetes (J Type)
(4) Transient neonatal hyperglycaemia.
(5) Asymptomatic intermittent hyperglycaemia
(6) Secondary diabetes :
(a) Cushing's syndrome
(b) Pheochromocytoma
(c) Hyperthyroidism
(d) Excessive growth hormone

## CLINICAL FEATURES

Sudden onset of symptoms is one of the characteristic features of diabetes in children, of course in about 20 per cent cases there may be insidious onset. Polyurea, polydipsia, polyphagia failure to thrive, retarded growth are the usual presenting symptoms. Only 10 per cent of cases may present with ketoacidosis with coma.

Unlike adults, OGTT is done with 1.75 mg/kg with a maximum dose of 100 gm of glucose; in children below 3 years 2.5 gm/kg of glucose is used. Diagnosis is established when fasting blood glucose is above 120 mg/dl at 2 hrs. post-prandial level over 160 mg/dl provided other causes of glycosurea and hyperglycaemia, such as, infection, convulsion, starvation.

## MANAGEMENT

Active co-operation of parents and patient are very much needed in the management of diabetes in children. Parents must be taught about insulin adjustment, injection, diet, schooling etc. Children must not be deprived of their schooling, activity under constant supervision is necessary at all stages. Here is a problem which teachers must appreciate. Instances are no record where schools have refused admission or given compulsory transfer certificates to diabetic children. This is deplorable. Diet should be very strict — parents must have an idea of food exchanges. They must be given good nutritious diet.

Total calories are estimated as follows :

| Body weight kg | Total calories |
|---|---|
| Up to 10 | 100 cal. per kg. |
| 10–20 | 1000 cal. plus 50 |
| 20–70 | 1500 cal. plus 20 |

**Formulation of Diet**

| | |
|---|---|
| Carbohydrate | 55–60% |
| Fats | 25–30% |
| Protein | 10–20% |

**Insulin**

Short acting and intermediate acting insulin is preferred in childhood. Wherever possible, mono-component insulin may be started in fresh cases. Dose is calculated according to blood sugar or urine sugar monitoring. Short acting is given in two doses of which two-thirds are given before breakfast and one-third before dinner. If intermediate acting (lente) is used along with short acting, it is given in a ratio of 2 : 1 or 3 : 1.

Usual problems with insulin therapy in children are allergic reaction, insulin resistance, hypoglycaemia, somogyi phenomenon and lipodystropy. In that case pure bovine or porcine insulin or human insulin is recommended. Early symptoms of hypoglycaemia should be explained to parents, teachers, and children. Use of sugar cold drink is advised.

## DIABETES AND SURGERY

Surgical procedure in diabetes demands special considerations as :

(1) Ensuing surgical stress may lead to metabolic changes including raised blood sugar level thereby worsening existing diabetes;

(2) Delayed healing due to raised blood sugar and concomitant impaired leucocyte function (e.g. chemotaxis and phagocytosis);

(3) Reactivation of dormant infection, e.g. UTI or tuberculosis.

(4) Silent diabetes may be diagnosed on routine examination done before any operation.

Objective or management of diabetes in surgery is to ensure stable euglycaemia and prevent ketoacidosis which may occur during operative and post-operative period.

**Management**

The types of diabetes may come for surgical procedure.

(A) Mild NIDDM – controlled by diet.

(B) NIDDM – Controlled with diet and oral drug.

(C) Diabetes controlled with insulin either by long acting or short acting insulin.

Each type may face either minor or major surgery. Accordingly management differs.

Mild NIDDM undergoing either minor or major surgery needs only careful monitoring of blood glucose in pre-and post operative period.

Diabetes on oral drugs or long acting insulin whether undergoing minor or major surgery must be switched over to regular insulin 2-3 days before operation.

Urine sugar monitoring is not dependable. Regular blood sugar monitoring is to be done.

**Minor Surgery:** Morning dose is to be omitted and resumed post-operatively.

**Major Surgery :** On the morning of operation half of the regular dose is given s.c. and infusion with 5% dextrose and 10 U regular insulin at a rate of 30—40 drops per minute continued. Operative and post-operative blood sugar is checked and dose is adjusted. Blood sugar level should be about 150—200 mg/dl so that hypoglycaemia or ketoacidosis does not develop. Oral feeding re-instituted after 24—72 hrs. depending on condition. A flow sheet is maintained.

**Prevention of Diabetes**

An attempt is going on to prevent diabetes all over the world. As a preventive measure of IDDM the following research works are being conducted.

(1) Virus vaccination — for high risk persons.

(2) Autoimmunity suppression — Islet cell antibodies may be suppressed by steroid or eliminated plasmaresis.

The incidence of NIDDM may be reduced by :

(1) Genetic counselling

(2) Reducing bodyweight

(3) Avoiding sweets particularly in person having family history

(4) Taking precautionary measures for pregnant women to prevent over-gestational diabetes.

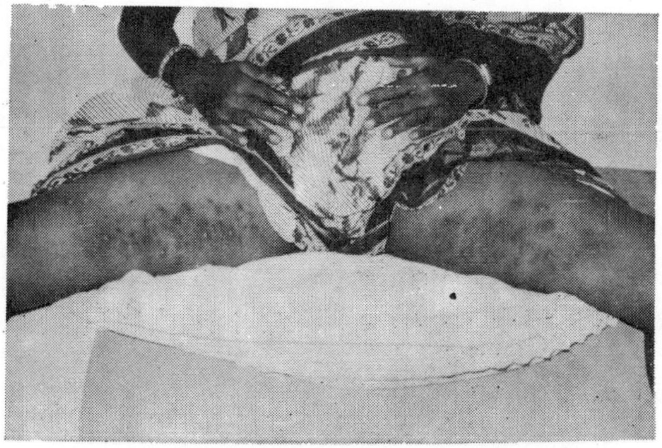

Fig.9.4 : Insulin injections given by unqualified compounder in medial aspect of thighs causing multiple ulcers.

### General Instructions for Diabetics

(1) The diabetics must be strict to the prescribed diet as diet is of supreme importance.

(2) The patients should not take sugar or any food containing sugar — like sweets, cake, pastries, jam, jelly, ice-cream, soft drinks, honey etc.

(3) They must take regular exercise.

(4) The diabetics should never change drugs or dosage of any drug on their own.

(5) The patient should not fast or miss meal after insulin injection or after taking oral antidiabetic drugs.

(6) If hypoglycaemic symptoms develop the patient must take three to four teaspoonfuls of glucose or sugar or a bottle of sweet drink followed by starchy food.

(7) They should not take alcohol or smoke.

(8) They must avoid exposure to infections and take care of skin, feet, fingers and nails.

(9) All diabetes must learn to test urine and blood sugar should be checked up regularly. Nowadays automatic electronic blood sugar testing machines are available which patients can easily operate.

(10) Any fever or painful condition should be reported to doctor.

(11) Insulin injections should be taken in proper sites (Fig : 9.4).

### Six-monthly check-up

All diabetics should undergo a medical check-up as follows at periodic intervals :

(1) Complete medical examination including fundoscopy of the eyes — every six months.

(2) E.C.G. (once or twice a year)

(3) Chest X-ray (once a year if required)

(4) Urine routine examination and culture

(5) Blood cholesterol, lipid profile, urea and creatinine (every six months).

### Newer Insulins

The conventional pork and beef insulins are antigenic because of (1) difference in morphological structure (Table 9.3), (2) presence of impurities, such as, pancreatic glucagon, somatostatin polypeptide, vasoactive substances. Tremendous research to produce pure insulin in the last decade has resulted in production of about 30 varieties of insulin in the market.

**Table 9.9 Morphological Difference in Species**

| Species | Position of amino acids | | |
|---|---|---|---|
| Human | Threonine | Isoleucine | Threonine |
| Porcine | Threonine | Isoleucine | Alanine |
| Bovine | Alanine | Valine | Alanine |

It is evident from that porcine insulin is nearest to human insulin in amino acid composition and it is less antigenic than bovine insulin.

(1) Purified porcine insulin (M.C. Insulin) : Purification is done by gel filtration, thus substantially removing significant amount of peptide and other hormones from the extract. Thus highly purified mono-component insulin (M.C. insulin) is obtained.

(2) Human insulin : is produced commercially :

(a) By replacing alanine of pork insulin with a threonine residue. This is enzymatically modified pork insulin called novo-insulins. Short acting (Actrapid), long acting (Ultratard) and intermediate acting (Monotard) forms are available.

(b) By chemical recombinant biosynthetic process : In this process bacterial organism E. coli is induced by recombinant DNA technology, and thereby A and B chain peptides are produced. These are then chemically linked by S—S bonds and then further purified well. These insulins are known as Humalin. Both short acting (Human S) and intermediate acting types are available (Humalin I).

**Determinants of insulin antigenicity**

It has been observed that insulin antibodies are produced by almost all diabetics receiving conventional insulin. The various factors are operative, such as :

(1) Inter-species structural difference;
(2) Impurities;
(3) Physical state of insulin — precipitated formulation is more antigenic than soluble one;
(4) pH-acidic formulation is more antigenic;
(5) Polymerisation — insulin dimers and polymers are more antigenic than monomer;
(6) Concentration and environment;
(7) Genetic factors.

The indications for using newer insulins are :

(1) Resistance of conventional insulin preparations;
(2) Allergic reaction to conventional insulin;
(3) Pregnancy when conventional insulin is not giving satisfactory results;
(4) Lipodystrophy due to conventional insulin.

**Table 9.10** presents a list of some of the commercial forms of pure insulins available in U.K.

**Table 9.10 New highly purified insulins**

| Preparation | Approximate equivalent in conventional bovine preparation | Action-duration |
|---|---|---|
| Actrapid MC (NOVO) | Soluble insulin (Neutra) | Short |
| Velosulin (Nordisk) | Soluble insulin | Short |
| Semitard MC (NOVO) | Semilente | Intermediate |
| Insulatard (Nordisk) | Isophen (NPH : Hagedorn) | Intermediate |
| Ultratard MC (NOVO) | Ultralente insulin | Long |
| Mixtard 30/70 (Nordisk) | Lente insulin | |
| (30% velosulin and 20% insulatard) | | |
| Monotard MC (NOVO) | | Intermediate |
| Lentard MC (NOVO) | | Intermediate |
| **Human insulins :** | | |
| Humalin I (Lilly) | | Intermediate |
| Humalin S (Lilly) | | Short |
| Protaphane (NOVO) | | Intermediate |
| Human Monotard (NOVO) | | Intermediate |

### Insulin Pump

This is just like a pocket calculator with a syringe for insulin and battery operated pump which continuously delivers insulin. The disadvantage is that it has no glucose sensor, therefore dose should be predetermined. Instrumental failure is rare. The pump can be worn as a belt or kept in hip or side-pocket. A fine needle is to be introduced under the skin. As insulin is continuously delivered, basal level and meal time-dose is to be adjusted. The current cost of a pump is about eight thousand rupees plus ancillary cost of import. It is to be carefully used. Any breakdown may cause trouble. There is chance of hypoglycaemia and rare instances of fatality have been reported due to faulty use.

Velosulin is resistant to bactericidal contamination and is therefore suitable for insulin pumps.

### Artificial Pancreas

It has a computerised glucose sensory system, by which glucose level is continuously monitored and required amount of insulin is delivered into circulation. It is not portable and can be used only for hospitalised patients at present.

### Intranasal insulin snuff

Intranasal installation of insulin snuff has been attempted but only about 15% of insulin is absorbed to produce useful effect, hence there is considerable waste of insulin.

### Surgical transplantation of pancreas

Surgical transplantation of pancreas has also been carried out successfully but still not perfect.

Isolated "islet" cells have also been cultured and then implanted successfully under the skin as such or after packing into tiny special semi-permeable capsules. However, these methods are not available for general use but remain in the field of experimental research in the present decade.

### Modern trend

The modern trend is "how to treat diabetes for ever". Genetic and bio-pharmaceutical research is continued, especially notable contributions are being made by Juvenile Diabetes Foundation (USA).

Attempt to produce oral insulin is another important field of research which however has yet not been successful.

## DIABETIC RENAL DISEASE

*YASHPAL*
*K.C. CHUGH*

### INTRODUCTION

Morphologically the lesion of "Nodular glomerulosclerosis" is diagnostic of diabetes mellitus. Other lesions such as infections (pyelonephritis, papillary necrosis) and vascular disease (renal arteriolosclerosis) are similar to those of nondiabetics, though incidence is significantly higher in diabetics. Kimmel-steil-Wilson's syndrome is nephrotic syndrome associated with nodular diabetic glomerulosclerosis. In a recent review the frequency of this lesion was found to be fifty per cent in autopsy studies and up to eighty-seven per cent in biopsy specimen (Heptinstall, 1966). Its incidence in India varies from 5-7 per cent in different reports.

### Recent developments

The outlook of diabetic renal disease has changed during the last decade with regard to its clinical course and feature prognosis. Important points are as follows :

(1) Earliest feature of diabetic nephropathy is abnormal increase in creatinine clearance (GFR) and kidney size radiologically;)

(2) Microalbuminurea – 30 mg/24 hours occurs very early in diabetic renal disease;

(3) Effective control of diabetic state with insulin may delay the renal damage;

(4) Early detection and treatment of oedema and hypertension may prolong life;

(5) It is essential to start early dialysis in uraemics when serum creatinine is around 5mg% to delay damage to various organs of body;

(6) Renal transplantation should be attempted as perferable mode of therapy for long-term management than long-term dialysis. Survival is prolonged by this regimen.

## GLOMERULOPATHY

### Pathology

These consist of (a) nodular glomerulosclerosis which was originally described by Kimmelsteil and Wilson who designated it as "intercapillary glomerulosclerosis" originating from mesangium or intercapillary tissue. The nodule is along the periphery of glomerulus and away from the lobules. (b) Diffuse glomerulosclerosis comprises of disseminated thickening of the branching mesangial stalk from holes to the peripheral lobules. Thickening of glomerular basement membrane is main change, in addition to mesangium. (c) "Fibrin cap" lesions are found in the loop of capillaries. (d) "Capsular drop lesions" are the hyaline deposits on the inner side of Bowman's capsular lesion (Fig.9.5).

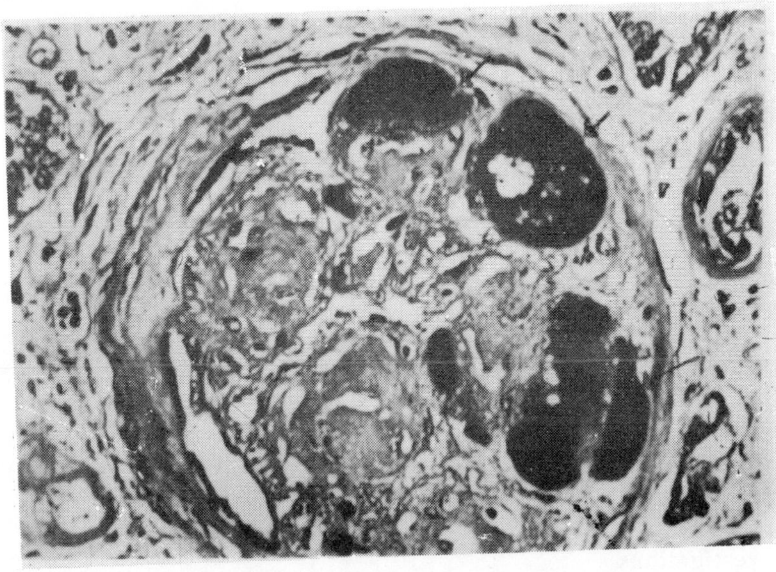

Fig.9.5 : Nodular glomerulo-sclerosis

### Tubular

Glycogen deposition• (Armamm-Ebstein lesion) is rare. It is a feature of diabetic ketoacidosis.

### Predisposing factors

(i) Ultimately 50 per cent of juvenile diabetics ultimately develop nephropathy.

(ii) The development of glomerulosclerosis is thought to correlate well with the overt duration of diabetes that occurs in prediabetes.

(iii) Uncontrolled diabetes and episode of ketoacidosis favour the onset of nephropathy.

(iv) Smoking causes more of vascular damage.

### Pathogenesis

Glomerulosclerosis is an integral part of microangiopathy of diabetes. The pathogenetic mechanism includes : (i) metabolic derangement. This is the most acceptable view. Adequate control of diabetes with insulin helps to delay the onset renal lesion; (ii) genetic predisposition because it has been demonstrated that thickening of basement membrane and muscle capillaries occur even in prediabetics.

## CLINICAL FEATURES

Various clinical features in order of occurrence are :-

(1) Asymptomatic proteinuria
(2) Oedema – nephrotic type
(3) Hypertension
(4) Chronic renal failure
(5) Inter-current urinary tract infection, pyelonephritis urinary tract infections as super added problem. At times there is associated papillary necrosis.

**Table 9.11: Stages of Diabetic Nephropathy ***

| Stage | Time to develop | Presentation | Method of diagnosis | Reversibility or control |
|---|---|---|---|---|
| I | days or weeks | (i) Increase in kidney size (X-ray) | Renal function test X-ray | Reversible |
| | | (ii) GFR creatinine clearance 150 ml/ml. | | |
| II | 2 years | (i) Increases in glo-merular measangium & basement membrane | Renal biopsy | Reversible |
| | | (ii) Microalbuminuria 30 mg 24 hours | Albustix | |
| III | 10–15 years | (i) Intermittent proteinuria | Exercise proteinuria | Can be controlled |
| | | (ii) Hypertension | | |
| IV | 10–20 years | (i) K.W. syndrome | Routine urine bio-chemistry & biopsy | Can be controlled |
| | | (ii) Chronic renal failure | | |

* Adapted from Kidney International (1982)

### Laboratory Investigations

(1) **Urinalysis :** Proteinuria is the first and most important indication for nephropathy. Glycosuria should not be the criteria for control. Acetonuria may or may not be present. Urine sediment shows pus cells, double refractile fat droplets and RBC.

(2) **Glomerular filtration rate (GFR) :** Average value for adult creatinine clearance is 100-120 ml/min. In the initial stages there is increase in GFR possibly due to osmotic load. Later there is progressive decrease in GFR.

(3) Serum proteins are decreased and lipids increased (type IV hyperlipidaemia is most common).

(4) GTT diabetic pattern.

(5) **Fundus** – Diabetic retinopathy.

(6) **X-ray abdomen** — Large size kidneys. Avoid IVP with dehydration prior to the procedure as it may cause failure in decompensated cases. It should be done, however, in a case of suspected renal papillary necrosis or chronic pyelonephritis.

(7) **Renal biopsy** — Confirms the renal disease.

**Approach to therapy**

There has been no promising pharmacological approach. However, the under-mentioned principles are followed :

(1) Adequate metabolic control of diabetes mellitus; Dietary regimen; Insulins are preferred over oral hypoglycaemics.

(2) Mild proteinuria does not require treatment but when it is in nephrotic range, proteins should be adequately replaced as 2 g/kg. body weight. Salt should be restricted when oedema appears to 4 g/day (one teaspoon/day) from average consumption rate of 10 g/day (1 tablespoonful). Diuretics are also indicated.

(3) Control of hypertension helps to prolong life and delay the course of chronic renal failure. Stepped care regimen is followed. Propranolol is not preferred because it may blunt the natural hypoglycaemic features.

(4) Treatment of chronic renal failure is indicated as and when the complication sets in.

(5) Early dialysis is indicated when serum creatinine is around 5 mg/per cent (as against that of chronic renal failure with 10 mg/per cent). This helps to minimize dual target organ damage by uraemia and effects of diabetes mellitus.

(6) Renal transplantation is preferred over long-term dialysis because intercurrent problem of vascular access for haemodialysis and ischaemic heart disease limit the life span more in dialysis cases. Pancreatic islet transplantation is still in experimental stage.

(7) Smoking should be stopped as it increases vasculopathy of diabetics. Intercurrent urinary tract infections would need long-term antibiotic and follow-up therapy for recurrence of the disease.

# CHAPTER – 10
# DISEASES OF KIDNEYS AND URINARY TRACT

## INTRODUCTION TO NEPHROLOGY

*G.C.MOOKERJEE*

In recent years nephrology has advanced with rapid strides, so that many patients in the end stage of renal failure, are now able to survive. Today not only methods of dialysis are available to treat the end stage of renal failure but renal transplantation has become a reality. With these methods in the field of nephrology many nearly dead people have come back to useful lives. The only problem is limited availability of these facilities in developing countries and the high cost involved. Cost of haemodialysis may be about five hundred to one thousand rupees per dialysis in India. In view of the limited facilities and great demand, many centres are not accepting very advanced cases, where transplantation is not likely to succeed. The idea developing in most centres is to keep patients alive till transplantation can be arranged.

Statistics from U.K. and U.S.A. suggest that about 10 to 20 people per million die of renal disease each year, but this data is probably not a correct estimate of renal disease causing human mortality. Because many deaths occur due to diabetic nephropathy, renal failure due to collagen disease and due to congestive heart failure but these are not recorded as deaths due to renal disorders. Hence true incidence of renal failure causing death may be much higher.

Kidney disease often produces very little clinical manifestations and may be mistaken for hypertension anaemia and P.U.O. viral infection or rheumatism. Minor changes in composition of urine is often ignored and therefore presence of renal pathology is often recognised too late.

Disease of the kidney may be due to many causes but the following possibilities should be kept in mind whenever there are some abnormalities of composition in the urine or any urinary symptoms are evident :

(1) Glomerulonephritis acute, subacute and chronic

(2) Nephrotic syndrome

(3) Infections of the urinary tract

(4) Obstructive uropathy especially due to lithiasis and disease of the prostate

(5) Hypertension —essential hypertension, accelerated (malignant) hypertension and special forms of hypertension of endocrine disease, e.g. pheochromocytoma, Conn's and Cushing's syndromes

(6) Reno-vascular hypertension is a special problem

(7) Diabetes Mellitus

(8) Gout

(9) Drug-induced kidney diseases

(10) Congenital renal disorders — especially renal tubular disorders

(11) Severe systemic infection

(12) Plasmodium malariae.

## ANATOMY

The renal system consists of :

Two kidneys are situated retroperitonially in the loin, lying at the levels of $T_{12}$, $L_1$, $L_2$, and $L_3$

vertebrae. Each kidney weighs about 150 to 170g. measuring about 12.5 × 7.5 cm varying according to body weight.

The uterus arise from hilum of the kidneys and end in the urinary bladder where urine is collected till the distended bladder causes evacuation reflex.

The evacuation of bladder is controlled by higher centre in the hypothalamus and may be disturbed in various neurological disorders or due to local causes, e.g. congenital defects of the sphinctres or commonly due to enlarged prostate (often not recognised till too late).

Inadequately treated acute gonorrhoea may produce stricture of the urethra.

**Structure of the Kidneys**

Each kidney has about one million nephrons. Each nephron has a glomerulus and long tubular structure. Tubules have diameter of about 35 mm and the total length of a tubule is about 50 mm (Fig.10.1).

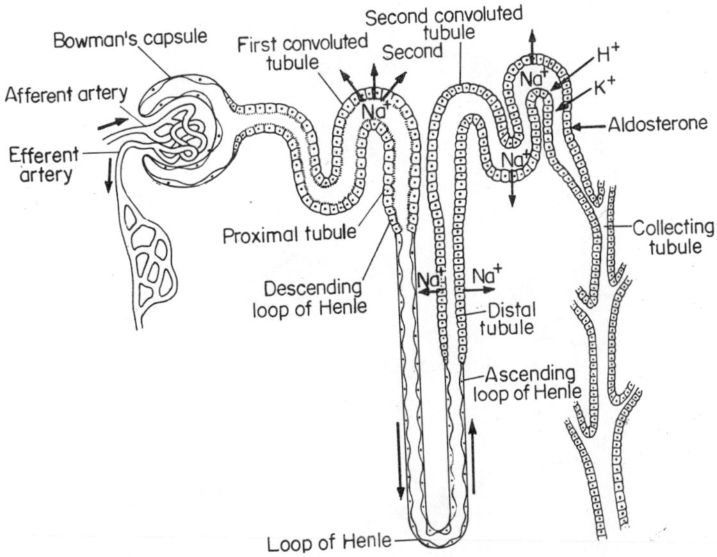


Fig.10.1 · Showing nephronal structures

Glomerulus, the invaginated upper end of the tubule is the most important part of the nephron, which has three types of cells e.g. epithelial, endothelial and mesangial. The glomerular cup receives a tuft of capillaries from the afferent arterioles, through which blood flows and is filtered at the glomerulus. About 25% of the cardiac output flows through the glomeruli per minute, i.e. 1300 ml/min. The blood after passing through glomerular capillaries passes out as afferent arterioles to supply the tubules. The haemodynamic mechanism which maintains 'milieu interior' within the normal range and ensure urine output of about one to three litres of urine to excrete waste products is quite complex (Table 10.1).

*Table 10.1 : Haemodynamic mechanism of Nephrons*

| | | |
|---|---|---|
| *Renal blood flow/min* | = | *1300 ml.* |
| *Hence plasma flow/min.* | = | *700 ml. (PCV 45±)* |
| *Nephronic ultra-filtrate* | = | *120 ml/min.* |
| *Nephronic total ultrafiltration* | = | *180 litres (in 24 hours)* |

The ultrafiltration takes place due to glomerular capillary blood pressure (60mm Hg or 8 K Pa) minus sum of the plasma protein oncotic pressure (25 mm Hg i.e. 3.3 K Pa) and intra capsular hydrostatic pressure (10 mm Hg or 1.3 K Pa). Therefore the actual effective filtration pressure is 26 mm Hg. (3.4 K Pa).

With flów of 180 litres of plasma (which varies according to body weight) about 580g of sodium (or 25,000 m.osmol) is also filtered on at glomerulus in 24 hours. There is equivalent to 1.5kg of NaC1. If the daily output of urine is considered to be 1.5 litres only 4g of sodium is excreted i.e. 580g of sodium and 178.5 litres of water should be absorbed. With the maximum concentrating power of the renal tubules, it is impossible to absorb this quality of sodium, unless at least 500 ml of urine is passed in 24 hours. If the output falls below this level, renal failure is said to be present. Maximum sodium absorption (about 80%) occurs at the proximal tubule. Glucose, potassium and water are also absorbed to a great extent. The sodium water and electrolyte balance is quite complex and has been discussed in earlier chapter.

It is however established that juxtaglomerular apparatus via renin-aldosterone mechanism plays a dominant role (Fig.10.2) in fluid and electrolyte balance.

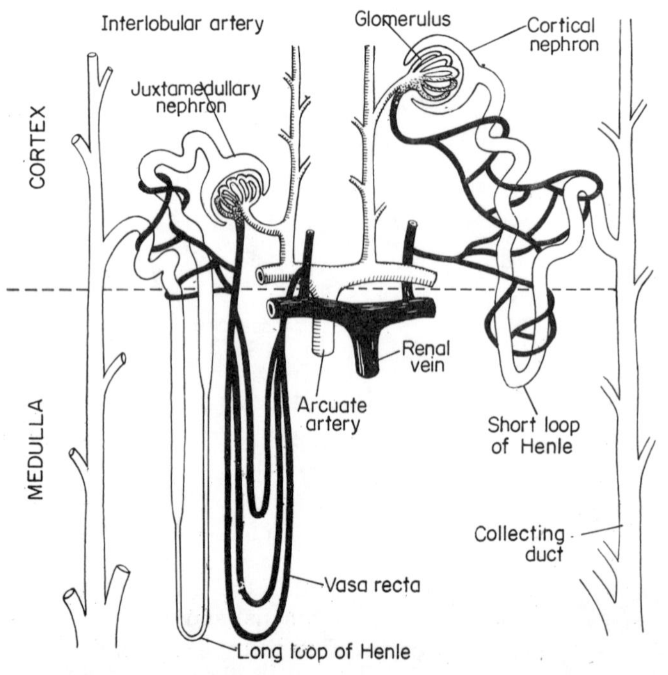


Fig.10.2 : Showing nephronal structure, arteriolar supply and juxtaglomerular apparatus.

Additional controlling factor is antidiuretic hormone ADH of the posterior pituitary gland, which chiefly acts on the loop Henle and collecting ducts, where enormous amount of water and some sodium are also absorbed to produce normal urine. Normal urinary output therefore depends on the following :

(1) Adequate renal blood flow with normal blood pressure.

(2) Proper functional capacity of nephrons and the nephronic health. Having one million nephrons in each kidney, there is plenty of reserve.

(3) Action of juxtaglomerular apparatus and normal renin-aldosterone mechanism.

(4) Appropriate ADH secretion from the posterior pituitary gland, produced by hypothalamic neurons.

(5) Release of ADH (neuro-hormone) by changes in osmolarity of plasma acting on osmoreceptors.

(6) Acid-base changes due to metabolic, gastrointestinal and respiratory causes.

(7) Drug-toxicity.

(8) Allergic assault to kidneys.

(9) Urinary tract infections.

(10) Degree of kidney damage.

Functions of the kidney may be summarised as follows :

(1) Excretion of nitrogenous waste products (Na, K and nitrogenous waste products).

(2) Electrolyte (Na, K and Ca) balance.

(3) Maintenance of blood pH.

(4) Conservation of glucose, aminoacids and phosphates.

(5) Excretion of drugs, poisons and toxins.

(6) Hormonal functions e.g. production of erythropoietin, prostaglandins and renin.

The following hormones are also concerned with kidney function :

| | |
|---|---|
| (1) ADH | (4) Erythropoietin |
| (2) Aldosterone | (5) Parathyroid hormone |
| (3) Prostaglandins | (6) Sex hormones & cortisol |

**Anti-diuretic hormone (ADH)**

ADH due to its action of cyclic AMP in renal tubular cells, allows increased permeability of cells of distal tubules and collecting ducts, so allows increased tubular water reabsorption. ADH secretion increases if osmolarity of serum is raised.

When extracellular osmolarity is low, the ADH secretion is lowered and large volumes of dilute urine will be produced. In different conditions, kidneys may excrete 0.5 ml/min. to 20 ml/min. depending on fluid intake and environmental conditions. Though ADH is chiefly regulated by serum osmolarity yet in conditions of stress, urinary flow may be greatly reduced as in severe haemorrhagic conditions or shock, irrespective of plasma osmolarity.

**Aldosterone, ADH and cortisol**

Aldosterone secretion has profound influence on Na and K metabolism. Aldosterone excess causes more Na-absorption in exchange of K and H-ions. Deficiency of aldosterone causes Na-loss in urine and excess of K in plasma.

Aldosterone secretion is influenced by renin secreted by j.g.a. of the kidneys secreted by muscle cells of the afferent glomerular arterioles.

Renin is an enzyme which is responsible for production of angiotensin II in the following manner :

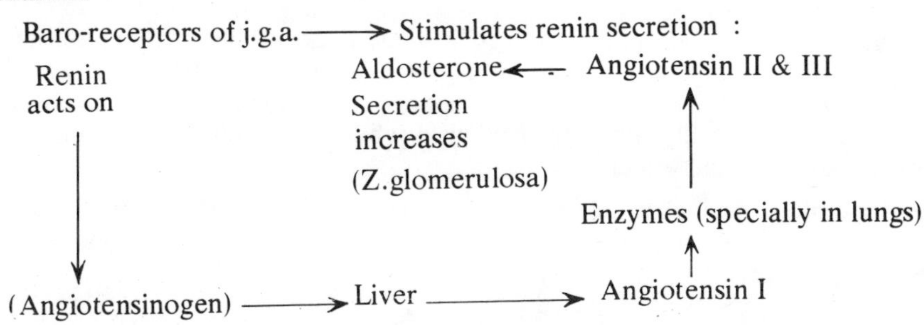

### Prostaglandins

Prostaglandins are produced from arachidonic acid by enzyme action in the renal medulla. There are several prostaglandins out of which PGA, $PGE_2$ and $PGF_2$ appear to be important in regulation of renal circulation. These are still in the realm of experimental research.

### Parathyroid hormone (PTH)

PTH is intimately related to Ca & P metabolism. It increases Ca-reabsorption from tubules and encourages phosphate excretion in urine. Details are discussed in the chapter on Endocrinology.

### Erythropoietin

It is a polypeptide hormone of the kidney which is concerned with anaemia of renal failure.

### Sex hormones & cortisol

Oestrogens cause water retention and increases renal blood flow. Progesterone may cause Na and water excretion to some degree. These are more pronounced during pregnancy. Cortisol also has important role in Na, K & water metabolism. Cortisol excess causes Na retention, K and H-ion loss and vice versa if cortisol is deficient (e.g. Addison's disease).

## IMPORTANT SYMPTOMS AND SIGNS OF RENAL DISEASE

### (1) Disturbances of Micturition

Frequency of micturition is usually abnormal. Normally a healthy man may pass urine four to five times a day and possibly once after midnight. Women may do it three or four times in the day and rarely at night. It however varies with drinking habit, climate and age of the patient.

**Polyuria may be due to the following conditions :**

(1) Diabetes Mellitus — due to loss of glucose
(2) Diabetes Insipidus — due to lack of ADH
(3) Nephrogenic diabetes mellitus — lack of sensitivity to ADH
(4) Chronic renal failure — due to lack of concentrating power of damaged tubules and osmotic diuresis (urea)
(5) Diuretics — due to Na loss.
(6) Psychogenic

Frequency of urine may be associated with burning, scalding or urethral pain. There may be urgency as well as strangury. Frequency at night (nocturia) is usually abnormal except in people who suffer from compulsive water drinking due to emotional problems.

### Oliguria

If total urinary output is less than 500 ml. in 24 hours, it suggests possibility of renal failure. However, in desert conditions urinary output may be as low as 400 to 500 ml. due to water deprivation and very high water loss due to evaporation. In hot and humid jungle-condition, in war times, soldiers with rationed water may also suffer from oliguria, while passing highly concentrated urine. It may even lead to adverse heat effects.

Anuria is a dangerous symptom in which urine output is less than 100 ml per day. When no urine is passed it is called total anuria. If no urine is passed it should be treated as medical emergency.

However, the doctor must be sure that it is not a case of retention of urine which may be due to obstruction at the neck of the bladder e.g. due to enlarged prostate, bladder neck obstruction or neurological complications.

**Pain in bladder and urethra**

Retention of urine may cause pain in bladder unless retention is chronic or due to some neurological complication. Dragging discomfort in the suprapubic region or even severe suprapubic pain may be due to cystitis, stone or new growth in the bladder. Pain of prostatitis may be felt in perineum and urethra. Urethritis may not only cause pain but discharge of pus may be present.

**Pain in the back and renal colic**

Strictly speaking back pain is a very vague term which may be due to musculo-skeletal disorders as well due to renal causes. Distension of renal capsules due to acute nephritis or pyelonephritis may cause bilateral loin pain at the region of $T_{12}$, $L_1$, $L_2$ and $L_3$. Renal colic (really ureteric colic) is due to obstruction of an ureter due to stone, blood clot or fragment of renal tissue. It may be quite often associated with restlessness and shock. It may have to be differentiated from acute abdominal catastrophies.

**Haematuria**

This is a serious symptom of renal disease. Haematuria may be frank or microscopic nature. Even 0.5 ml of blood will be evident microscopically.

Urine may be smoky or blood stained or even may contain frank blood and clots.

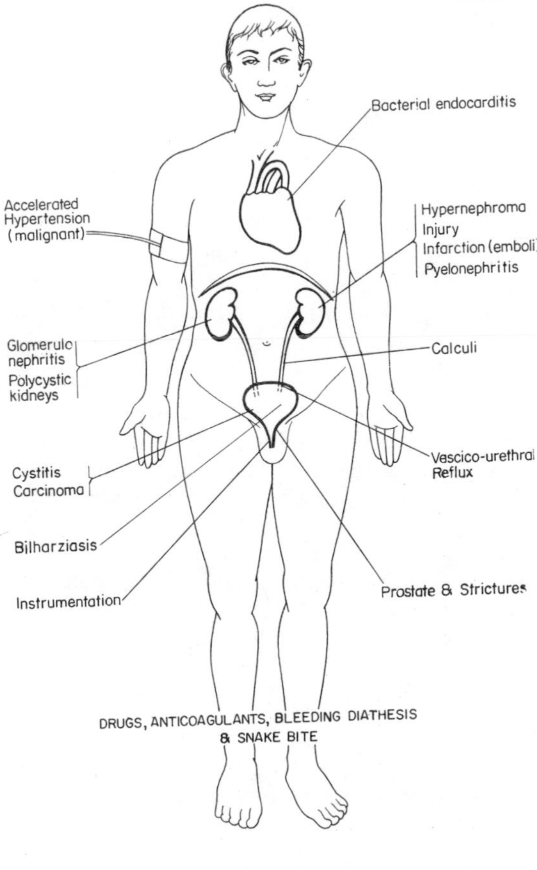


10.3 : Causes of Haematuria.

## DD OF HAEMATURIA

Urine may be coloured due to haematuria, haemoglobinuria metabolites and drugs. The following are the common causes :

(1) Red urine — Haemoglobin, porphyrine, beet root, phenolphthalein, rifamycin

(2) Dark urine — Bile or highly conc. urine (yellowish orange)

(3) Green/bluish-green — Pseudomonas/pyelonephritis, methylene blue and tetracyclines

(4) Black urine — Alkaptonuria (homogentesic acid) methaemoglobinuria and melanin pigments.

### Pneumaturia

Gas may come out with noise from the urethra due to infection by gas-forming organism. Rarely pathological fistula may occur between the gut or vagina causing air to leak into bladder.

## SYSTEMIC EFFECTS OF RENAL DISEASE

Acute or chronic kidney diseases may cause multifarious symptoms, which may not be initially recognised as due to kidney disease. The following complications are commonly met with :

(1) **Hypertension :** Renovascular hypertension may not be recognised if attention is not given to renal aspects. Hypertension in young and especially women of child bearing age may suffer from renovascular hypertension.

(2) **Cardiac failure :** May sometimes be the first manifestation in silently progressing chronic renal disease.

(3) **Oedema :** e.g. Glomerulonephritis or nephrotic syndrome.

(4) **P.U.O. :** Is sometimes due to smouldering pyelonephritis or renal carbuncle.

(5) **Anaemia :** Chronic refractory anaemia is often a chief manifestation of chronic renal disease.

(6) **Fatigue :** Vague ill-beath, tiredness, lack of appetite, inability to go through the day's routine efficiently may be due to long-standing kidney disease, or chronic prostatic infection, without obvious localising signs. Vague backache, myalgia, joint pains possibly nocturia, dilute urine (low sp.gr. and trace of albumin in urine) may be the pointers.

Do not forget to examine the prostate in a man over 40 years whenever there is mildest difficulty in micturition, presence of frequency, nocturia, pain in the perineum. Normal prostate gland has rubbery feel. It is hard in carcinoma. It is better to do a sonogram where facilities are available. One time cost may appear to be high but it will be less than weeks and months of medical investigations and the diagnosis delayed. When sonogram gives the clue, biopsy should be done to exclude carcinoma of the prostate, a major killer of male sex above the age of 40 years.

### Signs of Renal Disease

Renal disease have very few specific signs. Prominent physical signs e.g. cardiac murmurs of heart disease, organ enlargement e.g. hepatosplenomegaly, consolidation and pleural effusion in pulmonary disorders or neurological defects in diseases of CNS, are lacking in most renal disorders.

The physician must be able to see through experienced eyes and may suspect that renal disease may be at the background. When there is chronic refractory anaemia, unexplained hypertension, postural hypotension (low Serum Na), vague ill-health, dyspnoea without obvious respiratory disease, presence of oedema (do not forget to inspect sacrum and back of thighs in a lying patient), ascitis, pleural effusion you must think of the renal problem. Attention to chronic renal failure may brought by non-specific symptoms e.g. unexplained fatigue, anorexia, hiccough, pruritis, loss of memory, dyspnoea and acidotic breathing.

## Investigations of Renal Disorders

### Urine examination

Urinalysis is one of the most important investigations but appears to be neglected nowadays. I have come across patients suffering from diabetes mellitus for many years, who have many blood tests but urinalysis has not been properly done. Even there are many diabetics who are taking oral drugs or insulin but do not bother to do their own sugar test. It seems that their doctors never advised them also.

Most laboratories have now given up chemical tests for urinalysis in favour of "Stix" tests e.g. clinistix, albustix, haemostix etc. These are simple and less time-consuming but may be misleading if date-expired. Bence Jones protein however cannot be done by the "stix" method. Blood test by haemostix cannot be done by holding it in front of the urine stream as RBC's are intact. It detects haemoglobin if RBC's are haemolysed. To determine loss of pathological quantities albumen in the urine (i.e. more than 150mg/24hours), a spot test of urine sample may be misleading. In very dilute urine 'Albustix' will give negative value, while in concentrated urine. 'Albustix' may give positive value even if the loss is less than 150 mg/24hours. It may be simpler at least to collect overnight samples (12 hour collection : 8 pm to 8 am) as 24 hours' collection may be inconvenient for ambulant patients.

Analysis of urinary proteins may be rewarding i.e. to work out ratio of immunoglobulins (large mol. wt. protein) to albumin (small mol. wt.) in cases of albuminuria. If larger mol. wt. protein is minimal or lacking it suggests minimal damage to glomerular basement membrane. Passage of large or larger immunoglobulins suggests more than minimal damage to glomerular basement membrane. In cases of nephrotic syndrome steroid therapy is unlikely to be useful if more than minimal damage is present.

Microscopic examination of urine has very important value. It is customary to centrifuge 10 ml. of fresh urine at 2000 revolution per minute and discard 9 ml from the top of the rest tube. One drop of the remaining urine is examined under microscope. Presence of more than 2 RBC's and/or 5 while cells per high power field is abnormal. Casts should also be searched for in several fields, under the light microscope.

Urine culture for bacteriological studies has great significance. This may lead one by culturing a mid-stream urine. A clean catch sample is usually adequate, if properly done.

Sometime details are not checked and serious mistakes may occur. I remember once a patient who was due to be discharged from the hospital showed presence of pseudomonas organisms in urine culture. Patient had no symptoms and there were no other abnormalities in the urine. On going into the details about method of collection it was found that the 'Ayah' (female attendant — not a nurse) collected the sample from the urinal into the sterile culture tube.

Urine sample for culture should be despatched to laboratory as soon as possible for bed cases or should be collected in the laboratory in ambulant cases. Presence of organisms of $10^5$/ml or urine or more is considered pathological. If urine is left for a few hours before incubation organisms will multiply in urine and erroneous result will occur.

There is another method in which slide glasses are coated with culture media and are available in sterile containers. It should be dipped into the sample of urine collected in a sterile container or wetted with urine directly from the stream of urine. It is then replaced in its container and may even be sent by post to the laboratory.

Catheter specimens are not routinely required and may even be harmful but in cases where in-dwelling catheter has already been placed, serial samples may be collected as required. In these cases $10^5$—rule is not applicable. If the organisms are cultured, the result is considered abnormal. Sometimes supra pubic needling is resorted to, for the young children by the paediatricians to obtain uncontaminated urine. In these cases also colony count is necessary.

**Blood tests**

The following fasting blood samples are usually tested to investigate renal disease :

(1) Urea

(2) Creatinine

(3) Electrolytes

(4) pH and $CO_2$ combining power.

A post prandial blood sugar should always be done at two hours after 75g glucose load to exclude diabetes mellitus, especially in chronic renal disease.

Special tests include endogenous creatinine clearance test to measure GFR. Urea clearance test is not of great value. ETDA (Ethylene-diamine-tetraacetate) labelled with radio-chromium, ($^{51}Cr$) is a very accurate method for which a gamma camera outfit is necessary and not done as routine method.

**Radiology**

Radiological investigations have important role to play in the investigation of chronic renal disease.

**Straight X-ray or plain X-ray** of abdomen for kidneys, ureter and bladder (called KUB) will reveal outline of the kidneys, calcifications and presence of stones in kidneys and urinary tracts. Preparation of the patient is most essential for obtaining a good film for study. Thorough bowel evacuation must be done.

Nephrotomograms sometimes may be helpful for which X-ray films are taken at different depths.

Bone X-ray is also done in some chronic renal diseases.

**Intravenous pyelography (IVP)** may be considered in selected cases, when renal shadows are not well seen. IVP reveals opacification of kidneys, pelvis, calyces, ureters and bladder in serial films.

**Retrograde pyelography**

This method is done when IVP does not give desired information, Antegrade pyelography is also rarely done by nephrostomy tube or canula in obstructed renal out-flow tract.

**Micturating cystogram or cysto urethrogram**

This is done to study vesico-urethral reflux suspected cases.

**Radioisotopic study**

Radioactive-I-labelled hippuran is used intravenously and kidneys are monitored by gamma camera counter which will show the normal and abnormal renograms obtained by this method. It is chiefly used in cases of suspected renovascular hypertension or in other cases of chronic renal disease where IVP is not desirable. Radiation due to radio-isotopes is much less than IVP.

**Ultrasonography**

This is the most valuable non-invasive method today to detect stones, accumulation of fluids and parenchymal cysts or tumours. It can beautifully mark out solid from cystic masses. It is nearly as expensive as IVP but without any radiation or discomfort to the patient.

**Renal biopsy**

Renal biopsy is also a very useful method but has rarely possible hazards due to bleeding. In expert hands this is minimal but it is to be noted that experts are not born but have to gain experience sometimes by making mistakes. Hence this method should be restricted when considered essential. The samples usually obtained by renal biopsy are routinely examined by light microscopy but its value can be enormous if electron microscopy can be done.

Immunofluoresence technique demonstrates glomerular deposits of immunoglobulins.

Human antiserum of IgA, IgG and IgM is added to anti-compliment and antifibrin sera, and these are treated with the biopsy specimen and exposed to fluorescent light. The deposits will cause fluorescence and the deposits of immunoglobulin-type can be studied very well.

## GLOMERULONEPHRITIS

*P.SEN*

The advances made during the past two decades in the understanding of the pathogenesis of glomerular disease with the help of animal models and application of percutaneous renal biopsy study with immunofluorescence and electron microscopy have made it possible to separate, define and classify these disorders far more systematically than was possible in the past.

It is now well established that most forms of glomerular disease are mediated by immunological mechanisms and can be caused by primary glomerular disorder or secondary to disease conditions 98% of these disorders are due to granular immune complex (IC) deposits while 2% are due to smooth deposits of antibody to glomerular basement membrane (anti G B M). This results in a wide spectrum of clinico-pathological entities with considerable overlap in between.

### Definition

Thus glomerulonephritis (GN) may be defined as bilateral diffuse parenchymatous inflammation of kidneys of immunological nature and may be caused by primary and secondary conditions. There are a wide variety of clinicopathological entities with considerable overlap in between them and may be diffuse or focal in nature.

### Clinicopathological classification

This is based on specific morphological characteristics of glomerular change due to primary or secondary conditions which may be proliferative or membranous diffuse or focal, segmental or global in nature. The various clinicopathological types may be classified as follows (Table 10.2).

(A) **Primary glomerular disease :**

1. Diffuse :
   - (a) Proliferative
     - i. Diffuse proliferative (PGN)
     - ii. Membranoproliferative or mesangiocapillary (MPGN)
     - iii. Mesangial (MGN)
     - iv. Rapidly progressive. Extracapillary or crescentic (RPGN).
   - (b) Non-proliferative :
     - i. Membranous epimembranous GN
     - ii. Minimal change nephropathy
2. Focal :
   - (a) Focal and segmental proliferative GN
   - (b) Focal glomerulosclerosis of Hyalinosis.

(B) **Secondary glomerular disease :**

1. With nephritic picture (proliferative changes) e.g.
   - (a) Poly-arteritis nodosa
   - (b) Systemic lupus erythematosis (SLE)
   - (c) Henoch-Schonlein's purpura (H.S.P.)
   - (d) Bacterial endocarditis
   - (e) Wagener's granulomatosis.

2. With nephrotic picture (membranous changes) e.g.
   (a) Diabetes mellitus (KW syndrome)
   (b) Amyloidosis (c) SLE.

**Aetiology**

A wide variety of aetiological agents, infectious or non-infectious in nature have been implicated as the causative factor of glomerulonephritis, depending on the geographical area and prevalent antigen in the environment. They may be classified as follows :

(A) **Immune Complex (IC) Glomerulonephritis**

This may be due to exogenous or endogenous antigens.

1. Exogenous antigens : These are mainly infective in nature. Vary according to geographical area and may be bacterial, viral, rickettsial, protozoal or helminthic.
   (a) Beta-haemolytic streptococci : Nephritigenic strain. Throat infection with group A. Types 4 and 12 or skin infection with Type 49.
   (b) Staphylococcal : Shunt nephropathy, Valve prosthesis.
   (c) Viruses : Measles, $Hb_SAg$, Eb virus, taricella etc.
   (d) Treponema pallidum
   (e) Mycobacterium leprae
   (f) Quartan and falciparum malaria
   (g) Schistosomiasis
   (h) Rickettsial.
2. Endogenous antigens : Usually non-infectious in nature
   (a) SLE : DNA/Anti DNA
   (b) Hashimoto's disease (Thyroglobulin)
   (c) CEA (Tumour antigen)
   (d) Cryoglobulinaemia ($I_gG$)
   (e) Drugs like penicillamine

(B) **Anti-GBM nephritis :**

No known antigen, autoimmune in nature.
e.g. Goodpasture's syndrome

**Pathogenesis :**

This may be discussed under two broad headings. The formation and deposition of antibody immune complexes (IC) on the glomerular tuft and the subsequent train of events leading to glomerular injury and damage.

(A) **Antigen-antibody (immune complex) deposition :**

The various antigens mentioned above evoke as antibody response. Depending on the response three types of immune complexes are formed. When there is antigen excess (Type I response), small soluble complexes form (3-5 dalton size) which easily diffuse through basement membrane with deposits in basement membrane and epimembranous area giving rise of PGN, RPGN and epimembranous glomerulonephritis. On the other hand, when antigen and antibody are produced in balanced proportions (Type II response), poorly soluble medium sized (5 lakh to 10 lakh dalton) complexes are formed which are deposited in endo-membranous area giving rise to MPGN and MGN. But when there is antibody excess which is expected normally, large insoluble complexes (10 lakh dalton) are produced which cannot permeate the glomerulus and hence no glomerular lesion is produced. The pathogenetic mechanisim and its effects are summarised below :

| Antigenic INSULT | Host dependent RESPONSE | Immunological RENAL INJURY | Differing MORPHOLOGICAL PATTERNS | Limited mode of CLINICAL IMPRESSION |
|---|---|---|---|---|

(B) **Mediation of Glomerular Injury**

The immune complex deposits on the glomerulus which occur in a limpy bumpy or granular fashion gives rise to a train of events acting at different levels leading to glomerular injury. The changes are basically due to cellular proliferation, activation of complement system and its effects and activation of coagulation system. The course of events may be summarised as follows :

1. Activation of complement system
   (a) by classical pathway involving $C_1$ or $C_4$, $C_2$
   (b) by alternative pathway involving $C_3$
2. Lytication by complement activation giving rise to lytic or destructive changes.
3. Attraction of polymorphs giving rise to infiltrative and exudative changes.
4. Liberation of lysozomal enzymes and other vasoactive substances giving rise to biological changes.
5. Proliferation of different types of glomerular cells due to irritation and may involve
   (a) Endothelial cells mainly in PGN
   (b) Epithelial Cells with huge crescent formation in RPGN
   (c) Mesangial cells in MPGN and MGN leading to increase in mesangial mass with tabulation of glomerular tuft.
6. Activation of coagulation system : This leads to microthrombi formation, platelet aggregation and fibrin deposition.

The summary of interaction of various factors in the mediation of glomerular injury is given in the diagram below :

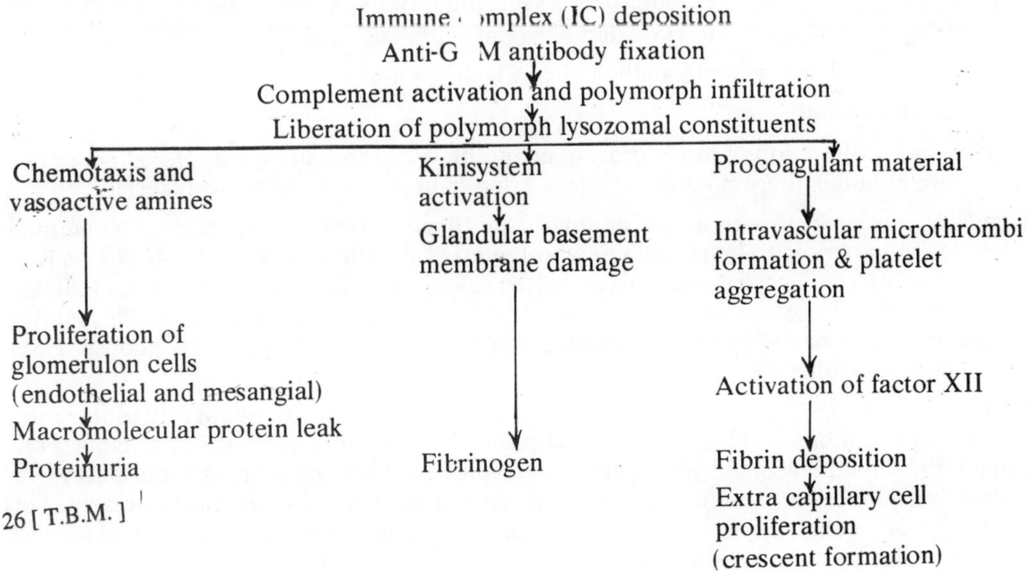

### Histopathological and immunopathological changes

These changes are detected by light microscopy, electron microscopy and immunofluorscent microscopic study of percutaneous renal biopsy specimens. Characteristic changes found in various clinicopathological types are given below :

1. In PGN : Diffuse proliferative changes of endothelial lining with cellular infiltration and exudative changes are prominent, mainly $I_gA$, $C_3$ and fibrinogen deposits detected by immunofluorescence.
2. In MPGN : Most common in adults. There is subendothelial dense deposits giving rise to endothelial proliferation, basement membrane changes and mesangial proliferation. Mainly $C_3$ and $I_gG$ deposits.
3. In MGN : Maximum brunt on mesangial cells which proliferate with increase in mesangial mass giving rise to a lobulated appearance of glomerulon tuft. Mainly $C_3$ and $I_gG$ deposits.
4. In RPGN : The brunt falls mainly on epithelial living with huge epithelial crescent formation and marked necrosis of glomerulon tuft. Mainly fibrinogen and $I_gG$ deposits.
5. In membranous GN : Basement membrane is mainly affected. Smooth deposition of immunoglobulin with spike formation. Minimal proliferation of cells mainly $I_gG$ and $C_3$ deposits.
6. Minimal change nephropathy : An enigma. Adherence of podocytes of glomerulon basement membrane is noticed under electron microscopy. Whether this is a cause or an effect of proteinuria is not known. No deposits seen under immunofluorescence.
7. Focal proliferative GN : Focal proliferation of mesangial cells with $I_gA$ deposits (Burger's disease).
8. Focal glomerulosclerosis or Hyalinosis : Segments of glomerulus hyalinosed. $I_gM$ deposits detected by immunofluorescence.
9. Secondary glomerulonephropathy : Various changes detected in different systemic diseases e.g.

| | |
|---|---|
| (a) Minimal change | : In pollen, bee-sting, lymphoma |
| (b) Membranous | : In diabetes, SLE, $Hb_SAG$ infection |
| (c) MPGN | : In Quartan malaria and SLE |
| (d) RPGN | : Goodpasteur's syndrome, HSO and P. nodosa |
| (e) PGN | : In HSO and P. Nodosa |

[Refer to Table **10.2** under Clinicopathological Classification)]

### Clinical Manifestations

The clinical manifestation of most forms of glomerulonephritis can be considered under two broad groups, although there is considerable overlap in between these two categories :

(1) Some patients present with **acute nephritic picture.** In these cases signs of glomerular inflammation are predominant including proteinuria (normally less than 3.5 g/day). R.B.C. and red cell casts in urinary sediment and often associated with reduction of renal function characterised by hypertension, azotaemia, and retention of sodium and water. This type of picture is usually met with in proliferative glomerulonephritis, polyarteritis nodosa, HSP, infective endocarditis etc.

(2) In the second group of patients the glomerular disease presents with **nephrotic picture** due to basement membrane changes which is characterised by oedema, massive proteinuria (3.5 g/day), hypoalbuminaemia, hyperlipaemia and lipiduria. These patients have normal or near normal renal function when first seen and haematuria and RBC casts are rarely present. This type of picture is characteristically found in membranous glomerulonephropathy and minimal change nephropathy as also in amyloidosis, SLE and diabetic nephropathy.

Besides, the patients with glomerulonephritis may also present with a mixed picture of nephritic and nephrotic syndrome, with recurrent haematuria, asymptomatic proteinuria, renal hypertension, acute and chronic renal failure, as an evidence of glomerular damage. The modes of clinical presentation in various clinicopathological type of glomerulonephritis with relative incidence are given below :

1. Acute nephritic syndrome :
   (PGN, P. Nodosa. HSP. Infective endocarditis)
2. Nephrotic syndrome :
   (Membranous glomerulonephritis, SLE, KW syndrome, focal glomerulosclerosis and minimal change nephropathy)
3. Combined nephritic and nephrotic syndrome :
   (MGN, MPGN,RPGN, etc.)
4. Recurrent haematuria and asymptomatic proteinuria 5-10% :
   (Focal proliferative GN, HSP etc.)
5. Hypertension : 5%
   (PGN, MPGN, P. Nodosa)
6. Acute renal failure : 5%
   (RPGN P. Nodosa, Goodpasture's syndrome)
7. Chronic renal failure :
   Most of the above conditions eventually progress to end-stage renal failure.

**Diagnosis**

This may be considered under the headings of standard baseline investigations for diagnosis and evaluation of a case of glomerulonephritis and the special investigations to assess the degree and nature of glomerulon damage.

(A) **Standard Baseline Investigations :**

1. Blood examination : Blood urea, creatinine, serum albumin (A : G ratio), cholesterol, complement ($C_3$, ASO titre, electrophoresis, haematocrit (PCV and Hb) and electrolytes (serum sodium, potassium, calcium, magnesium).
2. Urine examination for :
   (a) Urinary protein loss (g/day)
   (b) Creatinine clearance (ml/mt)
   (c) Addis count for urinary deposits
   (d) Urine RE including microscopy (RBC, WBC and casts)

(B) **Special investigations :**

1. Differential protein clearance tests : By immuno-electrophoresis and gel filtration methods. In minimal change nephropathy, the glomerular damage is less marked and the protein clearance is highly selective, while in membranous GN the damage is more marked and the protein clearance is non-selective.

$$\text{Protein selectivity ratio} = \frac{\text{Urinary } I_gG \text{ (mg/ml} \div \text{serum } I_g \text{ (mg/ml)}}{\text{urine albumin (or transferin) in mg/ml} \div \text{serum albumin (or transferin) in mg/ml.}}$$

Thus $I_gG$/Transferin ratio in minimal change — 0.15
Proliferative — 0.15-0.4 (selective)
Membranous — 0.4 (non-selective)

2. Urinary fibrinogen degradation products :

   This has been shown to correlate well with protein selectivity and provide simple and useful measurement of selectivity in patients with proteinuria greater than 2g/(normal FDP in urine = 0-8/µ G/ML).

3. Serum complement level :

   Normal C3 (B.C globulin) level = 70170mg%

   Initial low values in most of the GN except minimal change nephropathy, and persistent low level is detected in membranoproliferative (MPGN or MGN) glomerulonephritis and hence it is also known as hypoconglomerular type of GN.

4. Percutaneous Renal Biopsy :

   This establishes not only the clinicopathological entity but also its underlying causes in secondary glomerulonephritis. Percutaneous renal biopsy specimen is studied by :

   (a) Light microscopy
   (b) Electron microscopy — Various appearances been described.
   (c) Fluorescent microscopy.

**Treatment**

The standard treatment of glomerulonephritis is unsatisfactory at present and is mainly symptomatic in nature. As it is the single most important cause of end-stage renal failure research is aimed at possible mode of specific treatment for prevention of glomerular injury which is summarised below :

(A) **Standard symptomatic treatment :**

1. Appropriate antibiotics : For control of underlying infection e.g. penicillin in post-pathological GN.
2. Diuretics : For correction of salt and water retention loop diuretics e.g. Furosemide are most effective.
3. Antihypertensives : To prevent further renal damage. Betablocker and anti-renin substances (captopril), volume depletors in form of loop diuretics and methyldopa and hydralazine alone or in combination are drugs of choice.
4. Protein supplements and salt restriction : High protein salt free diet and salt free albumin in pure nephrotic syndrome.
5. Symptomatic treatment of acute and chronic renal failure : protein restriction, salt and water restriction, maintenance of acid base balance and dialysis — cover as and when necessary.

(B) **Possible modes of specific treatment :**

These methods are still in experimental area, but are promising in prevention and control of glomerular damage.

1. Removal of antigen :
   (a) From environment e.g. P. malarial (eradication).
   (b) From patient e.g. strepto and staphylococcal infection (antibiotics).
   (c) Induction of tolerance e.g. removal of tumour.
2. Loss of immune-balance
   (a) Suppress or remove antibody e.g. cytotoxic drugs like azathioprine or corticosteroids (immunosuppressants)

(b) Increase antibody e.g, Levamisole

(c) Removal of immune complexes e.g. **plasmapheresis.**

3. Inhibit or remove mediators of inflammation :

(a) Inhibition of complement activity e.g. Heparin.

(b) Inhibition of platelet aggregation e.g. platelet deaggregating substance like dipyridamole.

(c) Inhibition of vasoactive substance like histamine Kinins and SRSA e.g. cromoglycates and **diethylcarbamazine.**

(d) Antiprostaglandin substances e.g. indomethacin.

(e) Inhibition and stabilisation of leucocytes e.g. corticosteroids and indomethacin etc.

## FEATURES OF VARIOUS CLINICOPATHOLOGICAL TYPES OF GLOMERULONEPHRITIS

A brief summary of the characteristic features of various clinicopathological types of glomerulonephritis is given below :

### (A) Proliferative Glomerulonephritis (PGN)

This is the common type of GN in children. Peak age between 5 and 12 years. Males predominate over females 2 :1 Betahaemolytic·streptococcus Group A. Types 4.12 and 49 are nephritogenic strain. Type 49 is pyoderma associated and is commonly responsible for PGN in developing countries. Pneumococcus and viruses may also be responsible.

Antigen and antibody response lead to Type I-immune-complexes, which permeate diffusely from endothelium to epithelium and lead to lumpy-bumpy deposits and give rise to intense endothelial proliferation with exudative or infiltrative changes due to polymorph accumulation. As a result endothelial swellings occur, leading to vascular obstruction and damage giving rise to oliguria, proteinuria, salt and water retention and excessive resin liberation and hypotension. $I_gG$, complement and fibrinogen are deposited on glomerulus detected by immunofluorescence. Hypocomplementaemia occurs initially. The condition resolves completely by 3 to 6 weeks and glomerular changes revert to normal. In 5-10% cases persistent leakage of protein and RBC occur which may persist for months to a year.

The child normally presents with classical symptoms of constitutional disturbance like pyrexia along with loin pain, haematuria (smoky urine),oliguria, puffiness of face and oedema feet. This is often associated with azotaemia and hypertension. The diagnosis is confined by examination of urine for proteinuria and microscopy for RBC. WBC and cylindriuria and Addis count. The evidence of streptococcal infection is documented by raised ASO iitre (1 in 333) and DNA-sc antibody.

The condition is usually self-limiting and resolves by 3 to 6 weeks with use of antibiotics like penicillin and dietary restriction of salt, water and protein. However, some children may present with life-threatening complications like acute L.V. failure due to hypertension and hypovolaemia which should be promptly controlled with use of I.V. furosemide, lanoxin and antihypertensive drugs. Others may present with hypertensive encephalopathy and cerebral oedema with headache, vomiting, convulsion, blurring of vision which should be controlled immediately by I.V. furosemide, mannitol and sedatives like phenobarbitone and diazepam. In some rare cases problem of acute renal-failure may arise with persistent oligo-anuria and azotaemia. They are treated conservatively to combat acidosis, hyperkalaemia and induce diuretic by massive furosemide therapy. Sometimes dialysis cover may be necessary.

### (B) Membrano-proliferative or Mesangiocapillary Nephritis (MPGN)

(Mesangial or lobular (MSN) : Dense deposit or hypocomplementaemic type) :

This is the most common type of glomerulonephritis in the adults. Males are more commonly affected than females. It is insidious in onset and not associated with streptococcal sore throat or tonsillitis or skin infection. The aetiological factor or antigen responsible is not exactly known.

Similar picture is found in secondary glomerulonephritis associated with SLE or quartan malaria.

Type II immune complexes are formed which are arrested at lamina propria of basement membrane. Subendothelial deposits of immune-complexes occur with tram-track or dense deposit appearance. Mesangial cell proliferation is intense with increase in mesangial mass and matrix giving rise to characteristic lobular appearance under light microscopy. Immunofluroscent study reveals $I_gG$. $I_gA$ and $C_3$ deposits. Serum complement level is often below 20 mg% and a persistent hypocomplementaemia, lasting for months together. Hence it is also known as hypocomplementaemic type of glomerulonephritis.

The patients usually present with a mixed nephritic and nephrotic picture of insidious onset with generalised oedema and urine examination reveals marked proteinuria (5g/24 hours) with RBC, WBC and casts. It is also associated with hypertension, azotaemia (raised BUN) and hypercholesterolaemia. The fundus oculi may show presence of exudates, haemorrhages and macular star.

The disease is slowly progressive over months or years with persistent glomerular damage leading eventually to end-stage kidney disease. Over 65% patients die of chronic renal failure.

The treatment of the condition is unsatisfactory. They are usually maintained on antibiotics, loop diuretics to deplete salt and water retention, antihypertensives to control hypertension and maintenance dialysis as and when necessary. Immunosuppressive like cyclophosphamides. azathioprine and corticosteroids have been used without much success.

(C) **Rapidly Progressive Glomerulonephritis (RPGN)**

Extracapillary of crescentic nephropathy :

This is fortunately a rare form of GN and occurs usually in adults. It may occur as a primary glomerular disease either immune complex (IC) or anti-GBM disease. In secondary glomerulonephropathy it may be associated with SLE, HSP. Goodpasteur's syndrome, polyarteritis nodosa etc.

Type I immune complexes are formed leading to extra-membranous or subepithelial deposits or anti-GBM antibodies may be deposited leading to huge epithelial crescent formation and hence it is also known as extracapillary or crescentic GN. This leads to widespread basement membrane damage and glomerular necrosis with formation of intravascular thrombi and platelet aggregation. This leads to rapid progression to renal failure.

Immuno-fluorescence study shows deposits of $I_gG$, complement and particularly fibrinogen deposition in abundance, FDP is found in abundant amount in the urine which is a characteristic feature.

The patients usually present with sudden onset of gross nephritic and nephrotic features with massive proteinuria, marked azotaemia, hypertension, papilloedema and acute renal failure. The course is rapidly progressive and patient succumbs within weeks or months, hence it is known as rapidly progressive glomerulonephritis (RPGN).

The treatment of the condition is most unsatisfactory and mortality is high. As it is a desperate situation the patients are treated with immunosuppressive drugs like azathioprine and corticosteroids to suppress the mediators of glomerular injury like anticoagulants (Warferin) platelet deaggregating substance (dipyramole), antiprostaglandin substance (Indomethacin) etc. along with dialysis in the event of acute renal failure.

## MEMBRANOUS OR EPIMEMBRANOUS GLOMERULONEPHRITIS

This is a common cause of nephrotic syndrome in adults usually as primary glomerular disease or secondary to SLE, diabetic nephropathy, $Hb_SA_g$ virus, lymphoma, malignancies and drugs like penicillamine and troxidone etc. Antigen-antibody complexes with complement are deposited in basement membrane and changes are restricted to basement membrane without any proliferation of cellular element. Immunofluorescence study reveals deposits of $I_sG$ and complement in basement membrane but no fibrinogen.

The onset is insidious in adults with features of pure nephrotic syndrome. Azotaemia and hypertension are usually absent in the initial phase; 25% of cases revert to normalcy while another 25% slowly regress over years with periodic exacerbation.

The remaining cases are slowly progressive and renal damage occurs eventually leading to chronic renal failure.

Treatment is mainly symptomatic with high protein diet, diuretics, potassium and protein supplementation and control of infection as necessary. Corticosteroids and immunosuppressives like azothioprines and cyclophosphamide are used to induce remission with some success.

(E) **Minimal change nephropathy**

**("Nil" change under light microscopy)**

This is the commonest cause of nephrotic syndrome in children (over 80%) while 20% of adults may suffer. Common age incidence is between 3 and 8 years. The cause and pathogenic mechanisms are not known. This may occur as a primary glomerular disease or secondary to hypersensitivity (e.g. pollen or besting), lymphoma or malignancy where similar changes are noticed. Under ordinary light microscopy no changes are detected, while under electron microscopy fusion of foot process or podocytes are seen which may be an effect of proteinuria and not a cause. By immunofluorescence no immune deposits are seen.

Clinically they present as pure nephrotic syndrome in children of insidious onset. Facial puffiness progresses to massive anasarca. There is no associated sore throat or pyoderma and absence of consitutional manifestations differentiate it from post-streptococcal GN. Massive hyper-cholesterolaemia (500 to 1000 mg) may be found. There is no azotaemia or hypertension. Despite massive subcutaneous oedema, the patients are hypovolaemic and acute renal failure (ARF) may be precipitated by over-enthusiastic diuretic therapy. Hypogammaglobulinaemia may initiate infection to skin, lungs, urinary tract and peritoneal cavity. Loss of antithrombin factors may lead to intravascular thrombosis and vascular occlusion.

The treatment is supportive with salt-free high protein diet, diuretics and potassium and protein supplements. Antibiotics should be used to control infection. The mainstay of treatment is administration of corticosteroids. This is used in dosage of 20-30 mg (in children) for 3 weeks and the dose is tapered off and total duration is 6 to 8 weeks. The response is 100%. If there is no response in 6 weeks, the diagnosis is assumed to be incorrect.

Among the patients who respond well about 50% cases go into relapse. They respond to further course of steroids till four such courses are given. If the patients are steroid dependent or develop adverse effects due to steroids before or after the 4th course, cyclophosphamide is given in dosage 2-3 mg/kg for 3 months with hope to achieve a permanent remission.

If there is no response after 6 weeks then withdraw steroids and perform a renal biopsy. Often these patients have focal glomerulonephritis or MPGN. They eventually progress to chronic renal failure (CRF).

(F) **Focal Glomerulonephritis**

(1) **Focal proliferative**

This is common in young adults with viral fever-like onset. They present with microscopic haematuria without hypertension or azotaemia. No specific treatment is necessary and prognosis is good. They have to be differentiated from hereditary nephropathy like Alport's disease where mental changes and deafness are associated.

Focal proliferative GN may be primary or secondary to polyarteritis nodosa, SLE, HSP etc. In primary disorder it may be with IgA positive deposits in mesangium, which is known as Burger's disease and have a good prognosis while others are IgA negative where prognosis is worse.

(2) **Focal glomerulosclerosis or hyalinosis**

These patients are usually children presenting with nephrotic syndrome. There is focal and segmental hyalinosis. Histopathologically and by immunofluorescent study IgM deposits in mesangium are detected. They are resistant to treatment by corticosteroids and immunosuppressives and eventually progress to CRF. The diagnosis is suspected when nephrotic syndrome in children is steroid resistant and is confirmed by renal biopsy study.

(G) **Sceondary glomerulonephropathy**

Here the glomeruli are involved by an immunological process secondary to azotaemic disease and they may present with predominant nephritic picture like polyarteritis nodosa. SLE, infective endocarditis, HSP. Goodpasteur's syndrome etc. or it may present with predominant nephrotic picture e.g. SLE diabetic nephropathy, amyloidosis etc. or a mixed picture of nephritic and nephrotic syndromes may be present. They may present with the histopathological picture of various primary types like PGN,MPGN,RPGN, membranous type etc. The prognosis depends upon the underlying cause and the type of glomerular changes they are presenting with. Treatment is of the primary disease with supportive treatment for renal involvement as necessary.

## RENAL AND URINARY TRACT INFECTIONS

*G.C.MOOKERJEE*

### Introduction

Urinary tract infections (UTI) may occur in any part of the urinary tract from renal parenchyma to the urethra, due to micro-organisms. It is a common disease, especially in women and children. Shortness of female urethra makes them more susceptible to lower urinary tract infection, especially after sexual intercourse or due to habit of masturbation by clitoral fingering. Honeymoon cystitis is another example.

Most women experience lower urinary tract infection sometimes in their lives. A few suffer from it repeatedly. Urinary tract infection in males is often due to some obstructive pathology of the urinary tract e.g. enlarged prostate, stones, congenital abnormalities, diabetes mellitus or collagen disease. Pregnancy makes women more susceptible while venereal disease may cause urethritis in both sexes due to sexual intercourse. .

The urinary tract infections may be classified anatomically as follows :

1. Acute pyelonephritis
2. Acute papillary necrosis
3. Chronic pyelonephritis
4. Cystitis
5. Urethritis (urethral syndrome)
6. Prostatitis – acute or chronic
7. Asymptomatic bacteruria.

Combination may also occur, when both renal parenchyma and lower urinary tract are all involved.

### Aetiology

Most urinary tract infections are caused by Gram negative organisms, though rarely Gram positive organisms may also be involved (Table 10.3).

**Table 10.3 Micro-organisms causing renal and urinary tract infections**

| Gram-negative | Gram-positive |
|---|---|
| Esch. Coli | M. Tuberculosis |
| Proteus vulgaris and | Staph. Aurea or albus |
| Mirabilis | Staph. Saprophyticus |
| Klebsiella | Entero-cocci |
| Enterobactor | |
| Serratia | |

Candida albicans and other fungi are known to cause superinfection, especially in diabetics and poorly nourished subjects who are particularly susceptible.

In general practice, E. Coli has been the commonest organism to cause urinary tract infections but in hospitals klebsiella, proteus and pseudomonous are more frequent. Instrumentation e.g. indwelling catheter is a frequent cause.

At the present time exact role of viruses is not clear and it is also not possible to culture viruses in routine practice. Viruses e.g. adenoviruses however have been implicated to cause haemorrhagic cystitis. Distal urethral-end normally may contain streptococci, staphylococci and diphtheroids. These are non-pathogenic but usually infections may enter through urethra due to perineal contamination and proximity of an orifice. In females, sexual intercourse may also be a contributory factor. It appears that patient's own faecal flora has a significant role to play in causing U.R.T. in females. In very cold climate perineum is not always properly cleaned, especially in West due to practice of using toilet papers. Both these factors may lead to faecal contamination of female urethra. Indian practice of ablution, especially with soap and water is definitely helpful.

There has been some controversy in the part regarding the role of faecal strains of Es. Coli in causing urinary tract infections but most modern view is that there are no separate strains e.g. enteropathic or nephropathic Es. Coli. Therefore proper perineal toilet especially in women and during pregnancy is a very important preventive method. Soiled napkins in infants make female children very susceptible. Instrumentation of the lower urinary tract is also another cause.

Unclean tub baths, bubble baths and swimming pool are also additional problems e.g. especially for the female sex. Haematogenous infection is rare. Factors which play defensive role are, presence of urea in the urine, defensive role of mucosal cells, presence of leucocytes in the mucosal wall and for males in additional factor of prostatic secretions which has anti-bacterial property.

However, in both sexes any obstructive pathology e.g. bladder-neck obstruction or stones, vesico-ureteric reflux or congenital defects will encourage urinary tract infection and ultimately pyelonephritis.

**Clinical Features**

Signs and symptoms will depend upon the nature of infection, acute or chronic as well as presence of underlying disease, if any. Symptoms related to pyelonephritis and urinary tract infection may vary widely. Sometimes symptoms are slight and hence presence of disease is missed. Common symptoms of UTI are presented in Table 10.4.

**Table 10.4 : Symptoms of renal and U.T.I.**

| | |
|---|---|
| Dysuria | Rigor (±) |
| Oliguria | Fatigue |
| Haematuria | Loss of weight |
| Back pain (in loins) | Lower abdominal pain |
| Renal colic | Perineal pain |
| Suprapubic pain | Dysparunia |
| Fever—hectic or low grade fever | Enuresis-periodic |
| | Incontinence |

Associated diseases e.g. diabetes, gout, hypertension, collagen diseases, malignant diseases are likely to produce different clinical presentation.

Predisposing factors are : renal cysts, polycystic disease of kidneys, renal calculi, duplex ureter, enlarged prostate or any other causes, obstructing the urinary outflow tract.

Among analgesic drugs. Phenacetin is a well recognised cause of renal damage as well as recurrent urinary tract infection. Uric acid nephropathy is well-known among gout patients.

**Syndromes of renal & U.T.I.**

**Urethral syndromes**

Acute urethritis is sexually transmitted infection due to N. Gonorrhoea and chlamydia trachomatis.

Dysuria, frequency, purulent discharge are signs of acute urethritis. In acute cases burning may be severe.

Microscopic examination of urine will reveal presence of large number of pus cells and plenty of organisms on Gram staining. In women vaginitis may easily occur leading to pain and vaginal discharge. In male epididymis and prostate may be involved.

Besides venereal urethritis many women may sometimes complain of frequency and burning urine but urine examination may not always show any abnormal findings except a few pus cells and epithelial cells. Culture may also be sterile and reveal insignificant growth. Some of these cases may have chronic cystitis with or without cystocoele.

**Cystitis**

It is a very painful infection of the urinary tract in acute stage. There will be signs and symptoms like urethritis, in addition urine may have fishy or foul smell. Suprapubic pain and tenderness may suggest cystitis.

It often occurs after sexual intercourse in females (known also as honeymoon cystitis).

The infection, if not promptly controlled, may travel upwards as causing pyelonephritis.

**Acute Pyelonephritis**

Symptoms of acute pyelonephritis are pain in both loins, fever, rigor, dysuria, frequency of urine. Fever may be very high with too much frequency and severe discomfort while passing small quantity of urine every half to one hour. Urine examination shows albumin, pus cells, RBC's with high specific quantity. In females, it may occur during pregnancy, but pyelonephritis in males is suggestive of some obstructive pathology *(vide infra).*

**Acute Papillary Necrosis**

It is fulminating pyelonephritis in which renal papillae becomes necrotic and may slough off to pass out along the ureters, sometimes causing urinary tract obstruction.

## CHRONIC PYELONEPHRITIS

This can be a very silent disease often discovered too late. It is a slowly progressive renal disease usually sequellae of acute bactérial pyelonephritis or sometimes low grade smouldering infection over many years. The disease can be very silent, till manifestation of chronic renal insufficiency sets in.

Urinary findings may be trace of albumin with a few pus cells and epithelial cells and findings may vary from time to time. Vague ill-health, fatigue, mild anaemia, low back pain, feverish feeling etc. are often present.

### Diagnosis

Chemical and microscopic examination of urine as well as urine culture are the chief methods of diagnosis. Presence of albumin and pus cells confirms the presence of inflammation in urinary passages or kidneys but indefinite findings require more investigations. Culture of urine is essential and presence of more than five pus cells per HPF in a centrifuged urine suggests presence of infection. Urine also should be evaluated for albumin, sugar and casts. Gram stain of centrifuge deposit may show organisms and reveal the nature of organisms present.

Bacterial count is important as sterile urine may be contaminated by organisms of urethra or vulva. If bacterial count is between 10,000 to 100,000 per cu.mm the culture should be repeated. If more than 100,000 bacteria per cu.mm are reported and clinical background is supportive, the diagnosis of UTI is taken to be almost certain. For routine tests catheter specimen should not be taken but a mid-stream catch is enough. Other methods have been discussed at the beginning of this chapter. If the catheter specimen or suprapubic aspirate contains more than $10^2$ organisms, it is strong evidence of urinary tract infection.

If the urine sample is kept for a few hours, cells may degenerate and organisms may multiply in the urine giving a false picture.

For AFB culture the whole of the 24 hours' urine may be collected and a centrifuged specimen is used for AFB culture. Most laboratories prefer 24 hours' collection while three to six successive days' sample should be cultured separately.

## RENAL TUBERCULOSIS

The infection is usually blood borne from focus elswhere in the body and focal lesions usually occur at the junction of cortex and medulla or the apices of the pyramids. The lesion initially may be unilateral affecting right kidney more commonly and ultimately spreads into pelvis,ureter and bladder.

**Pathological types are :**

(1) Ulcerative type — with papillary ulcers extending into pelvis.

(2) Ulcerocavernous type — opening into pelvis.

(3) Caseous type — which may lead to tuberculous pyonephrosis.

(4) Miliary tubercles in both kidneys.

However, these types used to occur before the days when modern anti-tuberculous drugs were available and modern students of medicine are unlikely to see them except in museums. With better diagnostic facilities, renal tuberculosis should diagnosed early with complete chance of cure. While surgical text-book may be consulted for greater details on this subject, only salient and diagnostic points are presented.

### Clinical features

Back pain, low grade fever, anaemia and sterile microscopic pyuria with a few RBCs and acid urine are the pointers. One kidney may be initially affected but may spread into the other kidney as well.

It may affect epididymis, prostate and seminal vesicles. Urine culture for AFB is most important for diagnosis. Mantoux test may be strongly positive.

**Investigation**

Tuberculosis of the genito-urinary tract is often missed as some of the cases may have mild symptoms which are usually of vague ill-health, fatigue and evidence of chronic urinary tract infection. Urine may show acid reaction with pus cells and RBC, routine urine culture is sterile. Only if culture for AFB is specially ordered, the diagnosis can be established; IVP and cystoscopy usually reveal the true nature of the disease.

Renal tuberculosis or genitourinary tuberculosis is usually due to haematogenous spread but the active primary lesion may not be evident. However, it is essential to investigate for the same.

I.V.P. usually shows calyceal deformities e.g. stenosis, obliteration, distortion, moth-eaten appearance and abscess cavities. Calcification of kidney substance may be present.

Cystoscopy may show typical tuberculous lesions of bladder and culture of ureteric catheter specimen for AFB may be useful in establishment of diagnosis. Treatment consists of antituberculosis chemotherapy, as in case of pulmonary tuberculosis. Surgery is rarely required.

## THE PROSTATE & URINARY TRACT

Prostatic disease is a surgical problem usually fully dealt with in surgical text-books. However, it is necessary to remind the practitioners that examination of prostate by P.R. examination is very necessary in all cases of recurrent or chronic urinary tract infection in the males.

Acute prostatitis is not difficult to diagnose as patient has perineal pain, dysuria, urinary frequency, discharge per urethra and possibly fever. Associated cystitis and epididymitis may be present. Even acute urinary retention may occur.

Chronic prostatitis may cause low backache and symptoms of lower urinary tract infection e.g. mild cystitis.

If PR examination is done,prostate will appear enlarged, firm and possibly irregular-shape. Partial obstruction or even chronic urinary retention may be present.

I.V.P. may be helpful while sonography with special gadget to evaluate prostate size may show anatomy of the prostate more clearly.

**Treatment**

In acute stage avoid prostatic massage and get the culture and sensitivity report of urethral discharge to find out appropriate antibiotic. Trimethoprim 400 mg with sulpha-methoxazole or a broad spectrum antibotic amoxycillin or cephaloridin may be started pending culture report. Antibacterial therapy should be continued for about two weeks and follow-up is essential to avoid chronic prostatitis.

Chronic prostatitis is very difficult to treat. Organisms involved are usually gram negative or coliform organisms and drugs which are used to control these infections usually fail to reach the acini of the glandular prostate in sufficient concentration. Regular prostatic massage, prolonged antimicrobic therapy, analgesics and seitz baths are given. Constipation should be avoided. Long follow-up therapy is mandatory as chronic prostatitis may lead to life-long problem.

## RENAL AND URINARY TRACT INFECTION

Infections of urinary tract are common disorders. Bacterial organisms affecting kidneys and urinary tract may produce classical symptoms of acute pyelonephritis, which can be easily diagnosed but chronic and smouldering subacute infection are often difficult to recognise ties considerable damage is done to the kidneys. As mentioned earlier, the following types of urinary tract infection are met with in general practice.

(1) Acute pyelonephritis
(2) Acute papillary necrosis
(3) Chronic pyelonephritis
(4) Cystitis
(5) Urethritis
(6) Asymptomatic bacteriuria
(7) Renal tuberculosis
(8) Prostate and prostatic problems

## ACUTE PYELONEPHRITIS

It is infection of renal pelvis, ureters and adjoining parts of renal parenchyma.

The following organisms are generally involved :

(1) B.Coli is commonest cause.
(2) Klebsiella
(3) Streptococci/Enterococci
(4) Pseudomonas
(5) Proteus

The organisms usually reach this pelvis and renal substance along perineal lymphatics and rarely via haematogenous route. In view of the short urethra in females, they are more often infected due to sexual excess, proximity of anus to this urethral opening, pregnancy causing obstruction to flow of urine (also possible effect of dilated ureters due to progesterone excess).

In children, presence of urethral valves, phimosis and fingering habit may precipitate infection.

In older people prostatic enlargement often insidously leads to obstruction of bladder neck.

Whenever males suffer from urinary tract infection, a possible obstructive lesion should be thought of. Underlying diabetes predisposes UTI.

### Clinical Features

(1) Hectic temperature usually varying between 38° and 40°C (100°C to 104°F).
(2) Frequency of micturition with pain in the loin (stretching of renal capsules).
(3) Urethral burning while passing urine; strangury due to spasm of internal sphincter.
(4) Suprapubic discomfort due to cystitis.
(5) Frequency urine associated may be with oliguria.
(6) Constitutional symptoms e.g. headache, tachycardia, anorexia, nausea, vomiting may be present.
(7) Renal angles and suprapubic region are tender on palpation. Feature of background condition e.g. pregnancy, diabetes, prostatitis, phimosis in children, pin-hole meatus etc, should be taken into account. History of previous renal infection and habit of phenacetin ingestion may be present.
(8) Assess cardiovascular status, presence of hypertension, diabetes mellitus or underlying chronic disease.
(9) Some patients may have evidence of impending renal failure when first seen.
(10) Pyelonephritis and cystitis are common complications of neurogenic bladder present in spinal cord disorders e.g. spastic paraplegia, multiple sclerosis, tabes dorsalis etc.

### Investigations

Urine examination is most valuable for diagnosis. Urine has a fishy or foul odour and the quantity varies considerably. Albumin is present, may be trace or heavy with a plenty of pus cells with variable RBC's and EC'S seen microscopically. If a drop of urine is examined microscopically under cover glass, organisms may be seen and presence of more than 1,00,000 bacteria per ml. of urine is suggestive of infection. Urine should be cultured and colony count should be made wherever possible and sensitivity tests should be done in order to treat the infection properly.

If organisms in colony count show more than 1,00,000 organisms per ml. of urine it is suggestive that the cultured organism is the cause of infection.

For diagnosis of tuberculosis 24 hours samples should be collected and three to six such cultures should be done to exclude tuberculosis.

Other sophisticated tests e.g. immunofluorescence of urinary organisms coated with immunoglobulin are done for research work, which indicates that renal tissues are involved. In this test fluorescein labelled antihuman globulin is used to observe antibody coating of the organism concerned.

The test is negative in cystitis.

Enzyme studies in urine e.g. lactic dehydrogenase and G.O.T. level are also raised but these are not required routinely.

### Management

Treatment of UTI depends on the following important data :

(1) Is the infection acute, chronic or doubtful ?

(2) If it is acute infection, not only it requires prompt treatment but urine culture is mandatory to know about the nature of organism. Routinely a clean mid-stream catch should be adequate. Catheter specimen or still safer suprapubic aspiration may be collected in special circumstances.

(3) If local facilities are not available, a dip-slide sample may be sent by post to the nearest laboratory.

(4) If infection occurs repeatedly, all efforts should be made to find out if any obstructive pathology is present. In males even single episode of urinary tract infection requires careful check-up. Consider IVP if no obvious cause is evident.

(5) IVP or sonogram may be seriously considered if a woman suffers from recurrent pyelonephritis. In men this is more important, as obstructive pathology is likely to occur more often in males, who develop pyelonephritis as a primary disease.

(6) Pregnancy is an additional factor in causing URT. Catheterisation during pregnancy should be rarely done.

(7) Vesicourethral reflux is important cause of UTI in children. Anatomical defects are also to be excluded by IVP. Sometimes cysto-urethrography may be required.

(8) Neurogenic bladder is often a cause of acute or chronic UTI. Constant watch is necessary in patients who have in-dwelling catheter, for sometime.

(9) Hypertension and kidney problems are very much interrelated. Hypertension affects kidney and UTI makes it worse. Proteinuria may be noted in hypertensive cases, which may due to chronic pyelonephritis or effect of hypertensive disease itself.

(10) Diabetes mellitus should be excluded, UTI is often silent or chronic and always makes glycaemic control more difficult. In diabetes as hyperacute type of renal infection may occur leading to necrotizing papillitis.

**Principles of treatment :**

(1) In acute UTI rest in bed and plenty of fluids should be recommended.

(2) After routine urine examination and arrangement for culture is made, appropriate antibacterial drug should be given.

(3) Chemotherapy depends on result of bacterial culture and sensitivity report but it takes a few days. Therefore depending on the clinical background and judgement it is better to start any of the following drugs :

(a) Co-Trimoxazole : one tab twice daily
TMP 160mg @ SMZ 800 mg

OR

(b) Ampicillin 500 mg qid

OR

(c) Amoxycillin 500 mg t.i.d.

When result of culture-sensitivity is available treatment is to be modified. Where such facilities are not available (as in most cases of rural practice), one of the above drugs should be continued at least for 10 to 14 days. When there is no improvement of clinical condition and microscopic urine picture the drug may be changed after 5 to 7 days.

Failure of therapy may be due to insensitive organisms or presence of anatomical defects or obstructive uropathy etc. which should receive serious attention. Rectal and vaginal examination may be useful. A plain X-ray abdomen for KUB study may be used.

IVP is not possible in acute stage but sonography where available may be useful.

(4) Lower UTI infection responds to short course of 5-7 days while upper UTI will require 10 to 14 days' therapy. Recently it has been claimed that single dose therapy can eradicate acute lower UTI. Even single dose of amoxycillin 3.0g or four tablets of Co-Trimoxazole may suffice. This method of single day therapy may be of great value in rural areas, where patient's compliance is often lacking. The patient may be given single dose on the spot and be asked to report after one or two weeks.

Symptoms of the patient and urinary findings (e.g. proteinuria and pus cells) are also be additional guides to continue therapy or change of drug, in such cases.

(5) Acute pyelonephritis however needs longer course of 10 to 14 days but even then follow-up is most essential and in cases of recurrences, not only underlying factors need elucidation but also longer course of therapy for four to six weeks may be required. Possibility of resistance should be considered in these cases.

(6) Acute urethral syndrome in women due to chlamydial infection, should be treated with tetracycline 500 mg × 6 hourly for one week. Tetracyclines however may be harmful to foetus during pregnancy and it should not be used if renal failure is present.

(7) All cases of chronic pyelonephritis require thorough evaluation to exclude obstructive pathology, vesicourethral reflux, diabetes mellitus, hypertensive heart disease and infection due to resistant organisms.

(8) Some cases will benefit by low dose long-term drugs e.g. daily dose of one tablet of Co-Trimoxazole or even one tablet of Trimethoprim (100 mg) or nitrofuradantoin (100 mg) for two to three months or more.

(9) Surgically correctable lesions should be promptly treated. Enlarged prostate or bladder neck obstruction etc. should not be left alone.

(10) All chronic cases should be energetically treated as proper managem nt may prevent chronic renal failure in the long run.

## RENAL CALCULLI

*G.C. MOOKERJEE*

**Aetiology :** The actual cause of stone formation in renal or urinary tract is still largely unsolved. There are several types of stone due to interplay of several factors.

**Types of stones :** Calcium stones are the commonest, existing as calcium oxalate (calcium oxalate monohydrate crystals) and calcium phosphate. They occur in young men in their thirties, while their urine exhibits 'bilfringent' crystals on examination in polarized light. It is a highly familial disease, and usually a stone forms every 2 to 3 years.

Uric acid stones occur mainly in males and are not detectable by radiography. It is also familial disease and over 50% of the patients may be suffering from gout. Cystine stones are about 1% of all stones, These are radio-opaque because they contain sulphur.

Struvite stones are the commonest stones found in women, and they are always associated with infection. The bacteria causing the infection are usually found to possess urease e.g. B-proteus. They are also radio-opaque and may grow sometimes to fill up the renal pelvis producing the "stag-horn" calculus.

**Clinical features :** Small stones may spontaneously travel down all the way through the urinary tract and may pass out without much symptoms. However, if the stone is small enough to enter the ureter and yet large enough to get stuck in its passage typical renal colic supervenes. The pain radiates down into the groin, testes or labia, increasing in intensity in the sensory the distribution of the first lumbar nerve. When the stone gets stuck in the ureter renal colic may be very severe associated with restlessness, pallor, sweating, and often vomiting. The pain may subside even without treatment in 2 or 3 hours or persist for days with varying intensity.

Sometimes acute pain subsides while dull pain continues.

**Investigations :** Urine examination may show albuminuria with pus cells and plenty of RBC's urine. Urine may also be smoky due to blood or frank haematuria may occur.

**Treatment** : Immediate management of renal colic is to assure the patient that no abdominal catastrophy has occurred and immediate surgery is not required. Application of warmth to the area of pain, injection of pethidine (100 mg) I/M stat or morphine (15-30 mg) along with atropine sulphate (8 to 12 mg). These may be repeated in half an hour.

In most cases stones are not large and pass down in due course. Associated infection should be treated. Stones larger than one cm in diameter usually require surgical intervention. According to the cause, treatment may be thiazide for calcium stones, allopurinol and diet control for gouty patients, and alkali replacement for stones caused by distal renal tubular acidosis.

A straight X-ray of abdomen for kidneys and urinary tract (commonly called KUB film) is taken after due preparation of the patient with purgatives and enema. Radio-opaque stones can be seen. If required further investigations e.g. sonograms, intravenous pyelography and rarely C-T scan may be required.

Surgical removal or modern lithotripsy are rarely required.

## MISCELLANEOUS PROBLEMS OF RENAL DISORDERS

*G.C. MOOKERJEE*

**Introduction :**

The kidneys which are responsible to keep the internal environment in order by maintaining acid-base equilibrium, balancing water loss, excreting waste products and poisons, are naturally more susceptible to assault in many extrarenal disorders.

The various systemic disorders which may damage the kidneys have been mentioned already. It should however be stressed that kidneys are often damaged by severe systemic infections e.g.

enteric fever, diphtheria, malaria etc. Gram negative septicaemia and particularly recently discovered legionella pneumophila infection precipitate renal failure more frequently.

Kidneys are also damaged in diabetes and other metabolic diseases, blood disorders, liver failure, collagen diseases, neoplastic diseases, cardiovascular disorders as well as by drugs.

Although most of these conditions have been discussed in various chapters of this book, some special and rare but important conditions are presented in this chapter for practitioners' attention. Congenital defects of the kidneys are rare but have been briefly touched but for further details and rare syndromes larger texts should be consulted.

### Renal Tubular Disorders

There are certain situations where glomerular function remains good while tubular defects are well marked. Renal tubular damage may cause :

(1) Loss of glucose in excess — Renal glycosuria
(2) Loss of amino-acids e.g. Cystinuria
(3) Loss of calcium e.g. Idiopathic hypercalciuria
(4) Defects in acidification leading to renal tubular acidosis.

### Renal Glycosuria

It is a benign disease. There are two types, congenital and acquired. The diagnosis is confirmed by GTT which reveals that blood glucose levels are within normal levels. In acquired type urine shows presence of glucose except in fasting urine sample. In congenital type even fasting sample contains glucose. No treatment is required. Patients should take a normal diet. **Only practitioner should remember that it is dangerous to give insulin depending only on urine sugar test.** Occasionally renal glycosuria may herald true diabetes mellitus, hence follow-up is necessary.

### Cystinuria

It is a rare condition but is responsible for renal lithiasis. **Recurrent urinary infection in childhood, renal colic or haematuria are often the presenting feature.** Diagnosis is made by finding excess of flat hexagonal plate like cystine crystals in urine. **Renal stones may be detected, as they are moderately radio-opaque.**

Treatment consists of high fluid intake to increase urinary output up to 50 to 100%. Acidic and concentrated urine favour stone formation as cystine is less soluble than other aminoacids. Cystine is more soluble in alkaline urine, hence administration of sodium bicarbonate and sodium citrate is helpful especially at bed time. Additional tablet of acetazolamide (Diamox) as well as low methionine diet may also be beneficial. High urine output should be ensured by encouraging excessive fluid-intake during day and night. Treatment with D-penicillamine is helpful which alters cystine crystals into a soluble compound but it is quite expensive and also has side-effects which should be taken into account.

If the stone formation can be prevented by proper management, the prognosis is fairly good.

### Idiopathic Hypercalciuria

There is excessive absorption of calcium which is then excreted via kidneys, hence urinary calcium is high but serum calcium is normal.

Normal urinary calcium output in 24 hours is about 250 mg to 300 mg (6.25 to 7.5 mmol) per day. In I.H. it may be doubled, though serum calcium is normal.

Clinically renal pain, pyelonephritis, haematuria and renal stones are detected. Renal failure may occur.

### Treatment

(1) Low calcium diet i.e. take dairy products minimally
(2) High fluid intake
(3) Sodium cellulose phosphate causes calcium malabsorption and may help.

## FANCONI'S SYNDROME

In Fanconi's syndrome (also called De toni Fanconi's syndrome) there is defect in renal proximal transport mechanism so that aminoacids, glucose, sodium, potassium, calcium, uric acid, phosphates, bicarbonates and proteins are lost in urine.

It may occur as inborn error of metabolism or due to renal tubular damage i.e. acquired type e.g. Wilson's disease, familial nephrosis, myelomatosis, hereditary amyloidosis or in Lowe's syndrome (oculo-cerebro-renal disorder). Diagnosis is made by noticing presence of glycosuria without hyperglycaemia and excess of aminoacids in urine. Phosphates in urine is increased while blood level is low.

In addition to aminoaciduria, glycosuria, there may be hypercalciuria, salt wasting and proteinuria. Blood uric acid is however not raised.

**Histopathology of kidney shows that there is swan neck deformity of the proximal renal tubules, which probably is the cause of absorption defect of essential substances.**

### Clinical features

Fanconi's syndrome in its idiopathic form is diagnosed either during investigation of bone pain or failure to thrive. Urine showing glycosuria without hyperglycaemia in children may also be a pointer.

When it occurs due to renal damage due to systemic disease, there will be no specific features except of the underlying disease.

### Diagnosis

Urine shows presence of sugar while blood sugar is normal. Low potassium level and blood phosphate with high level of phosphates in urine and aminoacid crystals in urine are confirmatory. Aminoacids can be detected in urine by chromatography.

### Prognosis

Renal failure is rare, dwarfism and hypophosphataemic rickets may occur. Prognosis is fairly good if the systemic effects are controlled.

### Treatment

(1) Control of the underlying disease
(2) Vit-D for bone pain
(3) Symptomatic therapy — adequate replacement of Na. K. phosphate and water.

### Renal Tubular Acidosis

Renal tubular acidosis (RTA) is a rare disorder which may be idiopathic or secondary to long-standing chronic pyelonephritis or advanced renal disease. Idiopathic type may occur in infants and young adults but is very rare. *The primary defect is inability of the renal tubules to produce acid urine of/or below pH 5.4, hence acidosis results.* In normal health sodium ions are reabsorbed in distal tubules and hydrogen is excreted as ammonium. In RTA due to lack of excretion of H-ions. Potassium is exchanged for sodium and hypokalaemia results. Anions e.g. phosphates, sulphates and organic acids are lost from blood to buffer urine. The anion-gap, which results is replaced by chloride, resulting in hyperchloraemia. Plasma electrolyte pattern will show low K level, raised chlorides and low $HCO_3$ and $HPO_4$. There are four recognised types of RTA while Types I and II are hereditary : Type III has features of both Type I and II, while Type IV is acquired.

### Uric acid nephropathy and Gout

High blood uric acid may damage renal tissue, leading to interstitial nephritis. Causes of high uric acid in blood are : gout, leukaemia, cytotoxic therapy, myeloma, starvation, prolonged use of thiazides and chronic renal failure.

In gouty arthritis, uric acid calculi as well as tophaceous materials are deposited in the renal tissues which set up inflammatory response.

The ultimate damage stimulates chronic pyelonephritis.

A secondary type of gout develops during treatment of acute or chronic leukaemia with antileukaemia therapy, when numerous neoplastic cells are killed liberating large quantities of uric acid. If allopurinol is used, it inhibits uric acid formation by depressing xanthine oxidase. Thus purine itself is excreted instead of large uric acid load, purine being more soluble in water than xanthine is not harmful. As uric acid is more soluble in alkaline urine, alkaline diuresis and plenty of fluids are helpful. In chronic persistent hyperuricaemia interstitial nephritis may occur leading to renal failure.

**Osteomalacia**

(Also refer to chapter on Metabolic Disorders) :

**Clinical features**

Bone pain is often a typical symptom due to osteomalacia (increased Ca-loss in urine). The typical findings are :

(1) Osteomalacia
(2) Renal calcification
(3) Reduced plasma bicarbonate (acidosis)
(4) Urinary pH is neutral or alkaline or mildly acid
(5) Urinary pH does not become sufficiently acid even after administration of ammonium chloride.

Hypophosphataemia and acidosis are noted. Haematuria may occur. A radiograph of abdomen may reveal renal calcification (nephrocalcinosis). The appearance is characteristic irregular calcification of renal medulla.

**Primary Hyperparathyroidism**

More common in women. Hypercalcaemia is associated with presence of phosphate stones in kidneys. Parathormone level of blood is high. It is important to establish the diagnosis, as treatment is surgical. Refer to chapter on Endocrinology.

**Barter's Disease**

A syndrome characterised by weakness, polyuria and periodic paralysis due to hypokalaemia. There is renal potassium loss associated with elevated aldosterone and plasma renin activity. B.P. is however not raised. Administration of potassium salts and spironolactones may be helpful.

**Nephrogenic Diabetes Insipidus**

This condition is different from posterior pituitary deficiency or damage, where pituitary gland fails to produce ADH.

In this condition injection of posterior pituitary gland (pitressin) is not helpful. Here the urine is dilute because of tubular malfunction and tubules do not respond to endogenous or exogenous ADH.

There are two types — congenital and acquired :

(1) **Congenital Type** — Presents in early childhood. Dilute urine with low sp.gr. and low osmolarity will be present. No response occurs with pitressin. Thiazide diuretics are helpful as they cause sodium excretion in distal tubules but helps proximal tubules to absorb more sodium and water, leading to decreased fluid loss.

(2) **Acquired Type**

It occurs due to chronic pyelonephritis or long-standing hydronephrosis due to obstructive uropathy.

### Diabetic Nephropathy

Proteinuria is the earliest sign of diabetic kidney involvement and the protein losing nephropathy may finally end in nephrotic syndrome. Usually kidneys are involved after about 15 years. It is a bad prognostic sign, once blood urea starts rising. Today it is considered that good control of diabetes will delay or even possibly prevent diabetic nephropathy (Refer to the chapter on Dibetes Mellitus).

### Amyloidosis

Amyloid is an eosinophilic protein-chondroitin sulphate, which is deposited in many organs in patients suffering from long-standing chronic suppuration. Common conditions which may lead to amyloidosis are : chronic osteomyelitis, chronic tuberculosis, multiple myeloma, rheumatoid arthritis or ulcerative colitis.

There is a familial or primary amyloidosis, aetiology of which is not known. Primary amyloid deposits usually occurs in multiple sites e.g. heart, tongue, G.I. tract, even peripheral nerves.

The secondary amyloidosis usually occurs in kidneys, liver and rectal mucosa.

Rectal biopsy is usually positive in 90% of cases. However, in multiple myeloma other organs are involved like primary amyloidosis.

### Anaphylactoid Purpura (Henoch-Schonlein Purpura)

The presenting symptoms are sudden abdominal pain, purpura, arthritis along with G.I. haemorrhage and sometimes haematuria, in large number of cases. The renal lesion is focal proliferative glomerulonephritis. Steroid therapy is useful to relieve cases but some cases may progress to chronic renal failure.

### Haemolytic-uraemic Syndrome (Fig.10.4)

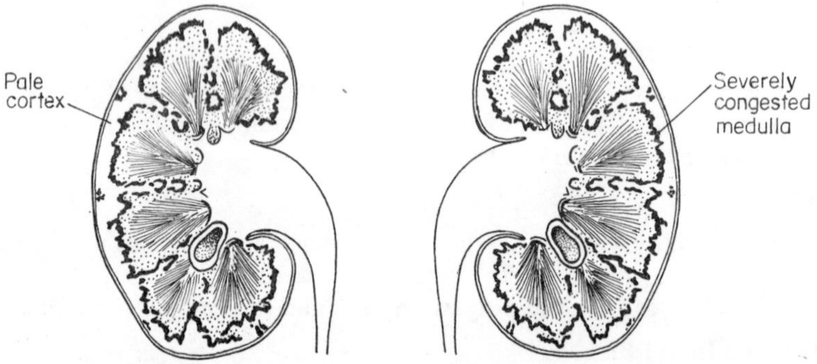


Fig.10.4 : Appearance of kidneys in haemolytic uraemic syndrome.

It is usually a childhood disorder characterised by high fever, vomiting, diarrhoea, followed by severe haemolysis, thrombocytopenia, acute renal failure with oliguria.

In adults, a similar condition associated with thrombotic thrombocytopenic purpura. Besides these conditions, kidneys are also involved in SLE, polyarteritis nodosa, scleroderma, renal-vein thrombosis, Collagen disease has been discussed already.

Renal vein thrombosis may be due to the following :

(1) Severe dehydration especially in infective gastroenteritis
(2) Membranous nephropathy leading to hypovolaemia
(3) Leg vein thrombosis leading to inferior vena cava thrombosis
(4) Secondary deposits (of carcinoma) or amyloidosis

(5) Rejection of renal transplant. Its relation to nephrotic syndrome is not clear. It may be due to hypoalbuminaemia and hypovolaemia as precipitating factors.

Diagnosis is confirmed by selective venography or arteriography.

Treatment is of underlying disease but anticoagulation may prevent extension of thrombotic process and modern fibrolytic agents directly installed may be useful.

## Polycystic Kidneys (Fig.10.5)

Polycystic disease of the kidneys is the commonest congenital renal disease. It usually presents as enlarged bilateral mass which causes hypertension, haematuria and recurrent urinary tract infections after the third decade of life.

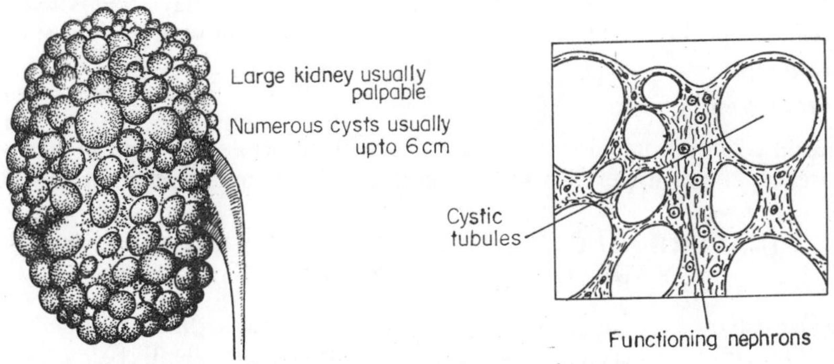


Fig.10.5 : Appearance of kidneys in Polycystic disease

It is often associated with berry aneurysm and cystic liver. S.A.H. may cause death before renal failure occurs.

There are many other congenital disorders of the kidneys which are of surgical interest.

## Nephrocalcinosis

It is a radiological diagnosis, sometimes accidentally discovered during routine abdominal radiography.

Sometimes diffuse calcinosis is noted due to numerous micro-calculi in renal substance, or patchy calcium deposits. The causes of diffuse calcification are :

Patchy calcification may occur in renal tuberculosis or hypernephroma.

**Tramline calcification** – Typically occurs in renal cortex following acute cortical necrosis, if the patient survives at least over a year after the episode.

## Papillary Calcification

It develops due to papillary damage of analgesic nephropathy. Haematuria may occur. Concretions may be passed in urine.

## Treatment

Depends on the underlying disease. Often no treatment is required.

Kidneys are well-known to develop calculi, which sometimes remain silent or at other times cause renal pain of varying degrees. It can produce obstructive uropathy and may cause hydronephrosis.

## Potassium losing nephropathy

There are a number of situations in which the kidney fails to conserve $K^+$ ions, and they may all be termed potassium-losing nephropathies.

Metabolic alkalosis, no matter what the primary cause is, almost always gives rise to potassium depletion. This also happens in osmotic depletions in diabetic keto-acidosis, but this may be masked because acidosis causes a shift of $K^+$ from intracellular to extracellular spaces. The effects of excessive mineralo-corticoids also cause $K^+$ depletion, e.g. primary aldosteronism. Secondary aldosteronism may also cause this, as in malignant hypertension, Barter's syndrome and juxtaglomerular cell tumour. Excessive liquorice ingestion may also cause hypokalemia, as may excess glucocorticoids, as in Cushing's syndrome, ectopic ACTH production of steroid administration, or certain renal tubular diseases as in renal tubular acidosis.

**Liddle's syndrome (or pseudohyperaldosteronism)**

This rare inherited syndrome is associated with hypertension, hypokalaemic alkalosis and negligible aldosterone secretion. There seems to be a peculiar tendency of the distal tubules and collecting ducts, to retain sodium and excrete potassium, although there is a virtual absence of aldosterone secretion. Although no other biochemical abnormalities have been observed, there is an altered rate of transport of sodium in red blood cells. Treatment with 100 mg of triamterene corrects the abnormality.

**Idiopathic hypercalcaemia of Infancy :**

This rare syndrome occurs usually in association with multiple congenital cardiovascular lesions and is characterized by hypercalcaemia. It could be due to hypersensitivity to Vitamin D.

## INAPPROPRIATE ANTI-DIURETIC HORMONE SYNDROME (SIADH SYNDROME)

The syndrome consists of excessive water retention, low plasma sodium, reduced plasma and urine osmolarity. The symptoms are present when plasma sodium level falls below 120 m.mol/L. The syndrome most frequently may occur in carcinoma of bronchus as well as in neurohypophyseal damage, which has been discussed in the chapter on Endocrinology.

**Carcinoma**

In chronic renal disorders question of malignancy should be always kept in mind. Besides carcinoma and nephroblastoma, other new growths may affect the kidneys. The presenting sign may be non-specific e.g. vague back pain, anaemia, low grade fever, arthralgia, high ESR, microscopic haematuria, I.V.P. and sonography may be helpful.

**Myeloma**

This condition though rare should be remembered in all chronic renal disorders. The disease is due to proliferation of plasma cells secreting excessive immunoglobulins. Sometimes excessive proteins of light chain type are produced, which have mol. wt. of 40,000 and are excreted in urine. This is known as Bence-Jone's protein, which dissolves on heating urine at 80°C and precipitates on cooling to 60°C.

Myeloma causes anaemia, bone pains, fever, pathological fractures. Hypercalcaemia nephropathy may occur. There is tubular damage due to precipitation of myeloma proteins and tubular casts are diagnostic. *ESR is always very high.*

**Cardiovascular Disorders**

(1) **Hypertension** causes generalised vascular damage gradually leading to hyaline thickening of afferent renal arterioles. In accelerated (malignant) hypertension there is fibrinoid necrosis of glomerular arterioles and glomeruli which may lead to renal failure.

(2) **Shock** — Any condition causing fall in cardiac output e.g. myocardial infarction, acute fluid losses, toxic states poisoning etc. may lead to acute renal failure.

(3) **Auricular fibrillation** — Clots from felt auricle may cause renal infarcts and haematuria. It can also occur in long-standing auricular fibrillation after cardioversion.

(4) **Subacute bacterial endocarditis**

(Infective endocarditis)

Emboli from vegetations may cause renal infarcts and haematuria but more dangerous complication is due to bacterial organisms causing antigenic response. The organism from the valvular vegetations, produce antigens which form soluble antigen-antibody complexes and ultimately get fixed at the glomerular trap. These immunoglobulin-depositions cause diffuse proliferative changes as discussed in detail in the chapter on Glomerulonephritis.

(5) **Renal vein thrombosis**

Renal vein thrombosis, involving one or both kidneys may occur due to local injury, malignancy (especially hypernephroma), membranous glomerulonephritis causing nephrotic syndrome and in severe dehydration. Rapid thrombosis of both renal veins causes severe low backache and haematuria and severe renal dysfunction.

If the occlusion is gradual, chance of collateral circulation retains renal function to some degree. The clinical picture is typical of nephrotic syndrome with oedema and massive albuminurea.

Diagnosis is made from history, IVP if possible and selective venography. When inferior venacava thrombosis is the cause of renal vein thrombosis, collaterals may show up in anterior abdominal wall. Sonography also may be helpful. Treatment is surgical removal of clots from IVC or anticoagulant or thrombolytic therapy.

**Drugs in renal disease**

Nephrotoxic drugs and poisons are notoriously responsible for renal damage and may also aggravate existing mild renal disease. When toxic drugs are used in existing renal diseases this factor should alwys be remembered.

Drugs which may be nephrotoxic should be carefully prescribed when renal disorders are suspected.

## RENAL FAILURE

*G.C.MOOKERJEE*

### Introduction

Renal failure may be acute or chronic or may be acute on chronic renal disease. However, renal failure may also occur without any kidney disease, due to disturbed fluid-electrolyte balance, acid base disorders as well as abnormal calcium and phosphorous metabolism.

However, physiological oliguria which may occur due to desert condition, water deprivation during military operation or voluntary starvation states, is entirely different from acute renal failure. If physiological oliguria is not properly corrected, acute renal insufficiency may actually set in.

These two conditions should be differentiated by history, clinical findings, blood and urine biochemistry. Urinary findings of physiological oliguria and acute renal failure (ARF) are as follows :

Oliguria

| | Physiological | ARF |
|---|---|---|
| Sp. gr. | 1020 | 1010 |

| | | |
|---|---|---|
| Urea conc. | 1.5g% (250mmol/L) | 1.0g% (160 mmol/L) |
| U/P (urine/plasma) ratio of osmolarity | 1.3 | 1.1 |
| Volume replacement & loop diuretic | Prompt response | Rarely so |

Presence of albumin, casts & RBCs however will always proclaim the presence of renal disease.

If sodium estimation in urine can be made, it will be much lower in physiological oliguria. Facilities of central venous pressure measurement (CVP) are not available everywhere, but if the patient does not respond to 80-120 mg of frusemide and initial fluid replacement, intrinsic renal damage should be suspected i.e. ARF is possibly present.

**Acute renal failure**

Acute renal failure (ARF) is a temporary loss of renal function due to fall in glomerular filtration rate resulting from renal ischaemia, clinically characterised by significant fall in urinary output, even complete anuria. Majority of cases are due to traumatic accidents, burns, surgery, severe dehydration, severe shock, acute hypotension or acute renal tubular injury. Non-steroidal anti-inflammatory drugs can damage renal parenchyma by antagonising vasodilating influence of renal prostaglandins. The biochemical basis responsible for clinical manifestations of renal insufficiency are complex but basically due to alternation in fluid and electrolytes as well as acid-base disturbance. Calcium-phosphorous metabolism is also affected. The hallmark of the syndrome is oliguria and rapidly progressive azotemia. If urine volume is greater than 500 ml. per 24 hrs., this entity is called non-oliguric acute renal failure.

**Causes of acute renal failure**

**Prerenal**

1. Massive haemorrhage e.g. and traumatic bleeding, large haematemesis and malaena post-partum haemorrhage.
2. Severe vomiting e.g. severe gastroenteritis, cholera, hyperemesis gravidarum and pyloric stenosis.
3. Severe fluid loss e.g. intestinal obstruction, perforation, extensive burns, heat stroke,
4. Gram-negative septicaemia.
5. Post-operative shock, myocardial infarction, severe anaphylaxis.

**Renal**

1. Acute tubular necrosis (ATN)
   - (a) Post-operative (Cardiovascular surgery)
   - (b) Nephrotoxins e.g. sulphonamides, aminoglycosides, mercury, arsenic, organic solvents, radiographic contrast agents.
   - (c) Pigment release e.g. incompatible blood transfusion, acute hepatocellular jaundice.
   - (d) Haemolytic crisis, crush injury, and haemolytic uraemic syndrome.
   - (e) Eclampsia, septic abortion, uterine haemorrhage.
   - (f) All conditions of prerenal failure if not treated or relieved.

**Post-renal**

It occurs in all conditions causing obstruction to urinary flow and may lead to acute renal failure :

1. Obstruction to both ureters : Blood clots, papillary necrosis, calculi, extrinsic compression.
2. Bladder-outlet obstruction e.g. prostatic enlargements, carcinoma bladder neck obstruction.
3. Uretheral obstruction — due to any cause.

**Pathophysiology**

Recent experimental studies on animal models suggest that two chief processes either vascular or tubular, may be involved in precipitating acute renal damage leading to ARF. However, exact mechanism is not clear but in some cases one or both factors may be involved.

Severe dehydration or shock may cause renal ischaemia (generalised vasoconstriction), low glomerular capillary pressure, increased capillary permeability, slow tubular flow, sludging effect in tubular pathway due to cellular debris. There may be focal necrosis of tubular or even diffuse necrotic damage of proximal tubular cells is observed. Recovery depends on the ability of regenerationof tubular epithelium which is only possible if there is no diffuse necrosis. Both nephrotoxic and vascular (ischaemic) however present almost similar clinical course.

**Clinical features**

The chief marker of ARF is oliguria or anuria. Urine quantity in 24 hours falls below 400 ml and is usually a few millilitres of 200 ml. The specific gravity is about 1010 to 1016.

However, it has been recently reported that some cases of ARF may have urine output of more than 400 ml per day. This type is specially noted in ARF due to nephrotoxic drugs e.g. aminoglycosides. It is the solute load which causes failure of the kidney to cope with the substances to be cleared i.e. urea and creatinine.

Urine osmolarity of a non-oliguric patient is about 350 mosmol. per kg. of water and this can be cleared with urine output of 1000 ml per day.

In acute renal failure of toxic type the solute load may go up to 1000 mosmol per kg of water, hence even daily output of urine, about 500 ml is not sufficient to clear the solute load and progressive azotaemia will occur. This is called non-oliguric ARF.

However, biochemical abnormalities of non-oliguric ARF are much less profound than the oliguric cases.

**Stage I or oliguric stage**

The clinical features however will depend on severity of metabolic imbalance, degree of azotaemias as well as the background disease, if any.

A healthy individual who received crush injury, trauma, burns or poisoning will present clinical features quite different from those who have pre-existing renal or cardiovascular disease.

Clinical manifestations of progressive renal damage are anorexia, nausea, vomiting, profound weakness, drowsiness, muscular twitching, mental apathy, stupor or even uraemic coma. *Fluid overload, infections* and *potassium intoxication* are three real dangers which should be closely watched for. *Pulmonary oedema* and *uraemic encephalopathy* may lead to fatality.

Early recognition of ARF is most important because proper treatment in this stage is most rewarding. The following aspects are to be carefully watched and treated promptly.

(1) **Infection**

Nephrotoxic drugs should be avoided e.g. aminoglycosides and cephalosporins. Dose of drugs which are excreted through kidney should be modified. This aspect has been discussed elsewhere in this book.

(2) **Cardiovascular problems**

Prompt treatment of LVE, hypertensive crisis, arrhythmias and pericarditis must be properly done. *Fluid overload is most dangerous* which not only causes circulatory congestion and LVF but is contributory to development of hypertension. However hypertension is also due to renin-angiotensin factor in ARF. Arrhythmias may be due to ischaemic myocardium. Anaemia, hyperpotassaemia, digitalis, toxicity, uraemic pericarditis, and fluid overload are all indications of dialysis therapy.

(3) **Anaemia**

Anaemia may develop if the patient of ATN runs a prolonged course but unless the anaemia is severe blood transfusion is not necessary. However, if there is active bleeding packed cell transfusion may be required, as volume overload is undesirable.

Anaemia is usually normochromic normocytic unless there is blood loss and in that case iron deficiency anaemia may occur.

(4) **Convulsions**

Phenobarbital should not be used as renal excretory function is poor. Diazepam without phertosis sodium should be used. Check for presence of acidosis and hypocalcaemia as both these are correctable. Symptomatic hypocalcaemia can be corrected by IV injection of 10–20 ml of 10% calcium gluconate, to be given slowly.

It is however essential that careful assessment should be made to exclude meningitis or intracerebral complications.

**Electrolyte balance**

Acidosis requires careful correction by IV sodium bicarbonate taking proper precaution to avoid overdosage as this may cause cardiovascular overload.

Alkalosis is unusual unless there is severe loss of H-ion due to vomiting, nasogastric suction without proper intake of electrolytes.

In some cases dialysis may be the right treatment in correcting electrolyte imbalance, adjusting pH to normality as well as to avoid fluid overload.

Hyperkalaemia should be also watched for. Faulty diet containing too much fruit juice, may be harmful.

**Management**

(1) For correct management it is essential to determine the cause of ARF. If the cause is due to obstructive aetiology, surgical aid is called for. Cystoscopy and ureteric catheterization may be required.

(2) Heavy metal poisoning (As or Hg) should be treated with Dimercaprol (BAL), unless it is two late and renal damage is already established.

(3) **General Measures**

(1) Bed rest is essential and protects the patients from outside infection by isolating in a cabin and restricting visitors.

(2) Fluid restriction to 400 ml. in 24 hours adding to replace losses due to diarrhoea, sweating and vomits.

(3) Initially 150-200g of glucose per day to reduce protein catabolism orally or I.V. is required. When I.V. route is used. use a large vein to give 25% glucose in 400 ml. of water.

Fats may be given but protein is restricted in oliguric phase. Buttered biscuits, later toasts, puffed rice etc. may be introduced. Vitamin B Complex and Vitamin C supplements should be given.

(4) If the patient has facilities of haemodialysis therapy (or even peritoneal dialysis) aminoacid mixtures glucose and fats can be given with advantage (See chapter on Dialysis).

Daily record of intake and output is essential. In-dwelling catheter should be avoided as far as possible.

**Diuretic Phase**

Once diuresis has started watch for electrolytes carefully, as there may be hypernatraemia, hyperchloraemia, and potassium retention. Hence frequent estimation of plasma electrolytes, urea and creatinine should be made.

Protein restriction should be continued depending on blood urea and serum creatinine levels.

Death may sometimes occur unexpectedly due to congestive heart failure, water intoxication and encephalopathy.

Once these patients recover, renal function becomes almost normal.

## CHRONIC RENAL FAILURE (CRF)

**Introduction**

The clinical syndrome that results from profound loss of renal function is conventionally referred to as "Uraemia" although all its manifestations cannot be explained by retention of urea in the blood alone, mainly because the kidney subserves a host of other endocrine and metabolic functions besides that of excretion.

Normally, the kidneys have fantastic reserve, and it is only when there has been a loss of renal function to about 35% to 50% of normal, the first signs and symptoms of CRF appear. With further loss of renal function azotemia sets in with hypertension and anaemia the two commonest manifestations. While others are hyperuricemia, carbohydrate intolerence, hypertriglyceridemia and inability to concentrate urine leading to polyuria and nocturia.

In early stage no symptoms are present but only stress on the kidney ( e.g. infection, obstruction, dehydration or nephrotoxic drugs) may lead to overt CRF. When the impairment of function is below 20% to 25% of normal, overt uraemia sets in, with metabolic acidosis, fluid overload and G.I. tract, cardiovascular and neurological disturbances. Even now, the ion $K^+$ is still excreted and so hyperkalemia is absent. This end stage of CRF is termed "Uraemia".

Uraemia affects cellular functions so that almost all the organ systems in the body are affected. A brief outline of the pathophysiology and biochemistry and the effects on organ systems is given below.

**Pathophysiology and Biochemistry**

By-products of protein and amino-acid metabolism are urea (which is 80% of the total $N_2$ excreted in the urine), the guanido-compounds which includes guanidinemethyl and dimethyl-guanidine, creatinine and guanidinosuccinic acid urates and other end products of nucleic acid metabolism, aliphatic amines, many peptides and many derivatives of aromatic acids tryptophan, tyrosine and phenyl alanine.

Urea accounts for anorexia, malaise, vomiting and headache.

Guanidinosuccinic acid impairs platelet factor ·III activation by ADP causing abnormal platelet function.

Creatinine may converted to sarcosine and methylguanidine and these together with creatinine may be involved in the pathogenesis of uraemia.

Middle sized polypeptide molecules may be causative of neuropathy since it has been observed that patients maintained on peritoneal dialysis (which removes these large molecules) do not develop neuropathy in spite of high blood urea and creatinine. This is called the "Middle-molecule hypothesis".

The accumulation of these nitrogenous compounds leads to defective iron transport across the cell membrane resulting in increased Na inside the cell and reduced $K^+$ while the reverse takes place in the extracellular space. There is also a decrease in transcellular voltage. All these effects may be to the "uraemic toxins" but parathyroid and natriuretic hormones are also abnormal in uraemia and they may also play some role.

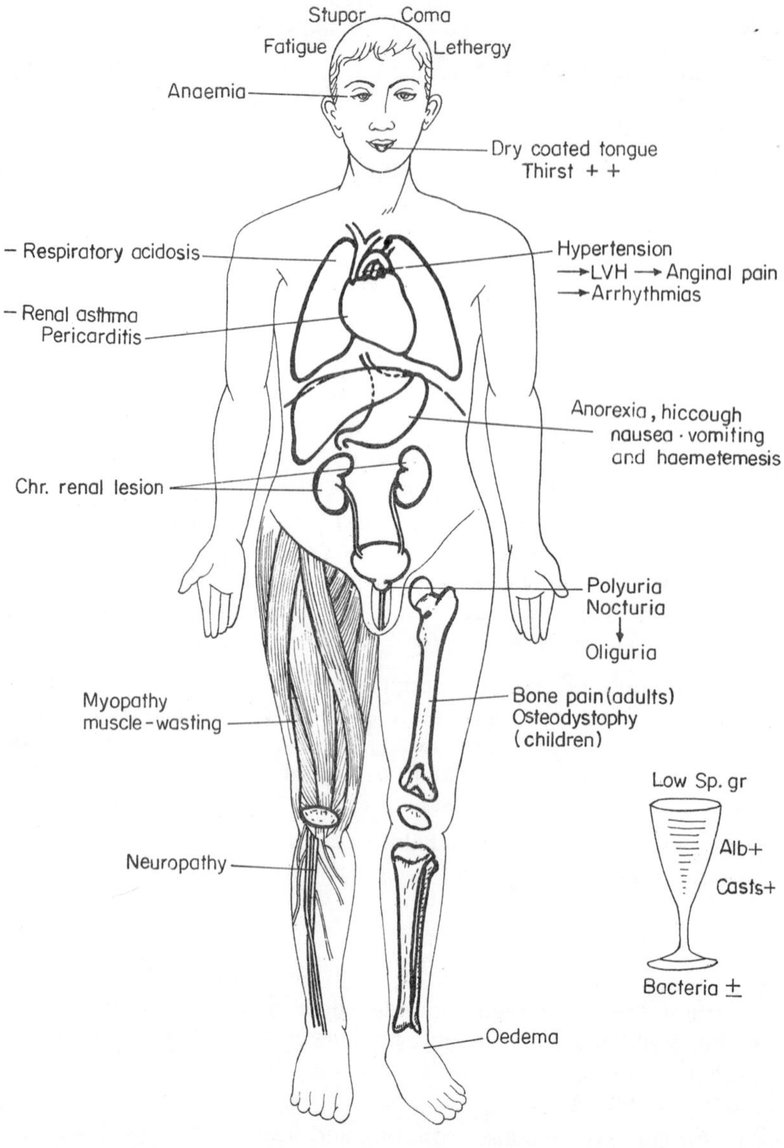


Fig.10.6 : Chronic Renal Failure

Ultimately all these derangements at the cellular levels leads to malaise, anorexia, nausea, vomiting and diarrhoea which may result in classic protein-calorie malnutrition and negative nitrogen balance, with profound loss of Lean Body Mass and fat deposits.

Intracellular $K^+$ defects occur because of defective transport, inadequate intake (poor diet or strict prohibition), excessive losses (vomiting,diarrhoea, diuretics), reduction in $Na^+$ and $K^+$ stimulated ATP ase activity or a combination of all these factors.

**Effects of uraemia on metabolism (carbohydrates, fats and protein) Fluids, Electrolytes and acid base balance**

In uraemia there is usually hypothermia because basal heat production is reduced, due to deficient $Na^+$ transport across cell membranes and this is corrected by dialysis.

**Carbohydrate Metabolism**

There is often a hyperglycaemia or rather a glucose intolerance of CRF which is called "Azotaemia Pseudodiabetes" and does not necessitate treatment. This feature is probably due to the peripheral resistance to the action of insulin. Reduced intracellular $K^+$ and/or raised plasma glucagon levels may also be the reasons for this glucose intolerance.

**Nitrogen and fat metabolism**

Similarly in uraemia, there is protein intolerance, although cholesterol levels in plasma are normal. Hyper-triglyceridemia and high density lipoproteins exists in uraemia as a result of increased triglyceride synthesis by liver or intestine, by the lipogenic effect of hyperinsulaemia and also by the depression of lipoprotein lipase which removes triglycerides from the circulation. This hypertriglyceridemia may be responsible for the increased and premature atherosclerosis seen in uraemia.

In stable CRF there is a modest increase in total body sodium ($Na^+$) and water content, though signs of extracellular fluid (ECF) volume expansion may not be clinically apparent. Excessive ingestion of salt causes or aggravates hyperkinesia, heart failure, ascites and edema formation while excessive ingestion of water leads to hyponatraemia and weight gain.

When there is increased fluid loss due to an extra renal cause such as vomiting, diarrhoea and fever, uraemic patients are prone to develop CCF volume depletion with dry mouth, dizziness syncope, tachycardia, orthostatic hypotension, decreased filling of jugular veins.

Despite progression of renal failure, most patients maintain normal serum $K^+$ until the final stages of uraemia. Oliguria or disruptions of adaptive mechanisms may lead to hyperkalemia and abrupt lowering of blood pH (for every 1 unit, change of pH. serum $K^+$ is reciprocally changed by 0.6 mcg/litre). In some cases, hyporeninemic hypoaldosteronism may be the cause of hyperkalemia. Poor dietary intake of $K^+$ and/or excessive diuretic therapy may lead to hypokalemia. Hypokalemia may also be caused by renal reabsorptive defect as in Fanconi syndrome, renal tubular acidosis or hereditary (acquired tubulointerstitial diseases of the kidney).

Metabolic acidosis also occurs due to fall in total daily acid excretion which can be corrected by 20 to 30 g. of $NaHCO_3$ of sodium nitrate per day.

**Clinical features**

Clinical features will depend on the stage of the renal failure and presence of complications (Fig.10.4).

In chronic renal failure, loss of renal biosynthetic capacity and reduced renal excretory function leads to various complications : (Table 10.5).

**Endocrine & Metabolic :**

(1) Secondary hyperparathyroidism
(2) Carbohydrate intolerance
(3) Renal osteodystrophy
(4) Hyperuricemia
(5) Hypothermia
(6) Hypertriglyceridemia
(7) Protein calorie malnutrition
(8) Impaired growth and development
(9) Amenorrhoea

**Cardiovascular and Pulmonary**

These are : (1) Arterial hypertension

(2) Congestive cardiac failure
(3) Pericarditis due to uraemia
(4) Cardiomyopathy
(5) Uraemic lung
(6) Accelerated atherosclerosis

**Neuromuscular**

(1) Fatigue
(2) Impaired mutation
(3) Headache
(4) Ataxias
(5) Lethargy
(6) Muscular irritability
(7) Peripheral neuropathy
(8) Restless leg syndrome
(9) Paralysis
(10) Myoclonus
(11) Seizures
(12) Coma
(13) Muscle cramps
(14) Dialysis dementia
(15) Dialysis disequilibration syndrome

**Fluid and Electrolyte Disturbances**

(1) Hyper and Hyponatremia
(2) Hyper and Hypokalaemia
(3) Volume expansion and contraction
(4) Metabolic acidosis
(5) Hyperphosphataemia and hypophosphatemia
(6) Hypocalcaemia

**Haematologic and Immunologic**

(1) Bleeding diathesis
(2) Lymphocytopenia
(3) Anaemia (normocytic, normochromic)
(4) Splenomegaly and Hypersplenism
(5) Increased susceptibility to infection
(6) Leukopenia
(7) Hypocomplementaemia

**Dermatological**

(1) Pallor
(2) Pruritus
(3) Hyperpigmentation
(4) Ecchymoses
(5) Uraemic frost

**Gastrointestinal**

(1) Anorexia
(2) Nausea and vomiting
(3) Uraemic fetor
(4) Gastroenteritis
(5) Peptic ulcer
(6) G.I. Bleeding
(7) Ascites (refractory) due to dialysis

**Management**

Chronic renal insufficiency is the last stage of many varieties of renal damage occurring in the past, most of which might have occurred even many years before the renal failure supervenes.

**Important causes may be as follows :**

(1) Chronic pyelonephritis a very important cause, often silently progressing over many years.
(2) Glomerulonephritis (immune complex type)
(3) Renovascular hypertension
(4) Nephrotoxic or analgesic renal disease
(5) Metabolic renal damage e.g. due to diabetes, gout, renal osteodystrophy
(6) Radiation nephritis
(7) Chronic obstructive nephropathy
(8) Congenital renal disorders

(A) **Diet and Fluids**

(1) The most important point is to keep electrolyte balance, reduce azotaemia and prevent acidosis and hyperkalaemia.

(2) Proteins should be restricted to 0.5g/kg of body weight per day as too much restriction is harmful; vitamin supplements are essential.

(3) Additional sodium salt may be required to combat failure of kidney to produce adequate amounts of $NH_4^+$ and $H+$ ions 3 to 6 of NaCl and sodibicarb may be given per day.

Calcium supplements may be required if there is hypocalcaemia. Calcium gluconates (10%) may be given IV (10 to 20ml.) if there is tetany. Aluminium hydroxide gel 15 to 30 ml may be given 3 to 4 times daily to lower raised serum phosphate level. Additional vitamin $D_3$ (cholecalciferol) or still better 1.25 di-hydroxy $D_3$ (calcitrol) may be required for renal osteodystrophy.

(4) Infection should be treated vigorously while choice of antibiotics or antibacterial drugs should be made carefully, avoiding nephrotoxic drugs.

(5) Anaemia — Iron is usually not required as usually serum ferritin level is normal. When anaemia is severe blood transfusion (packed cell) may be given.

If bleeding occurs and bleeding time is prolonged, haemostasis can be achieved by I.V. administration of DDAVP (Desmopressin acetate) to tide over the emergency. The effect is however transient.

(6) Hypertension should be energetically treated (refer to the chapter on Hypertension).

Symptomatic treatment of nausea, vomiting and insomnia should be done avoiding drugs which are nephrotoxic.

Role of renal dialysis and kidney transplantation has been discussed in separate chapters.

## DIET IN ACUTE RENAL FAILURE

The most important principle is restriction of proteins and avoiding water overload. Fluid intake is adjusted to urinary output and obligatory water loss. In first few days if oliguria is severe fluid is usually restricted to 500ml plus previous day's urine output.

If blood urea and creatinine levels are very high proteins are withdrawn and calories should be made with carbohydrates and glucose drinks. This is usually required for 24 to 72 hours.

In oedematous state salt restriction is essential; rice, chapati, bread, bajra, ragi and oatmeal are permitted as soon as improvement starts. Sugar, jaggery, honey, 'murobba', potato, fresh vegetables and salads are allowed in average quantities. "Papad", "chutney" (pickle), dry fruits and nuts are not allowed. Butter and oil can be used in cooking. As long as there is nitrogen retention, fish or meat is not allowed. One egg daily may be helpful. Once the blood urea and creatinine come near normal limits, 0.5 g of protein per kg of body weight can be given. If K-level is rising, fruits and vegetables also need restriction and if hyperpotassaemia cannot be controlled, dialysis may be necessary because diet restriction alone may not be adequate.

**Diet in chronic renal failure**

Diet will depend on the stage of the disease, presence of complication and also the underlying aetiology.

Restriction of proteins is necessary when blood urea and creatinine are rising but proteins of high biological value should be included.

**Specimen diet in chronic Renal failure**

| | |
|---|---|
| Morning tea | : One cup with milk and sugar |
| Breakfast | : One toast with butter, honey or jaggery. One egg, boiled or fried or milk 100 to 150 ml. |
| Mid morning | : Fruit juice 60 to 100 ml with glucose or sugar. |
| Lunch | : Rice 60 to 75 gm. potato and other vegetables average helping, cooked as curry with ghee or cooking oil. |
| Afternoon tea | : With milk and sugar and one or two biscuits. |
| Dinner | : Similar to lunch – suitably adjusted. |

Total milk ratio may be 250 to 300 ml. .

Diet needs constant supervision and should be revised depending on electrolyte picture, urea and creatinine level. *Fluid overload must be avoided.*

The most important additional factor is patient's compliance. Diet is often disliked and unacceptable to some patients and it is only by sympathetic discussion and persuasion that it may be possible to convince the patient. Nausea is often a great problem but judicious use of drugs like metoclorpropamide or chlorpromazine may be useful.

Hypertensive patients will require salt restriction. If plasma lipids are high, butter or ghee will not be permitted.

Diabetic ischaemic and hypertensive patients may develop renal failure and will require sugar restriction also. However, when these patients develop renal failure usually they do not have much hyperglycaemia. Careful insulin therapy will be required but finally these patients will have to go to haemodialysis. Problems of haemodialysis and renal transplantation have been discussed in separate chapters.

Animal protein should be carefully added, depending with degree of nitrogen retention. As long as the blood urea is below 80 mg%, 40 to 50 g of protein may be permitted, provided other parameters are stable but if BUN is rising proteins should be reduced to 20 to 30 g daily to be best provided by milk and one egg per day.

Milk provides both sodium and calcium. Potassium restriction may be necessary when there is hyperkalaemia.

Fluids should be given 2-3 litres daily as long as urine volume is good, as patient has to excrete waste products through the dilute urine, because concentrating power of kidneys is reduced.

Vitamin supplements are required, especially vitamin D, 50,000 units daily or dehydrotachysterol 0.25 mg per day along with calcium supplements. The ultimate requirement will be haemodialysis in most cases. In late stages of renal failure fluid restriction will be necessary.

## RENAL DIALYSIS

*A.R. NANDI*
*SUBHANKAR CHAUDHURY*

### History of Dialysis

As early as 1913 Abel, Rowntres and Turaer performed haemodialysis in dogs with an artificial kidney made of several celloidin tubes. Later, Haas used reed tubes, paper membranes, peritoneal membranes etc. as semipermeable membranes for haemodialysis. With the availability of heparin in 1918, continuous-flow-haemodialysis was attempted. By 1930 most of the basic requirements of modern haemodialysis were available. However, it was not until the mid-1940's that the first successful experiments in human haemodialysis were reported. In 1947 Alwall of Sweden first reported the use of ultrafiltration. Till this period dialysis therapy was limited to acute renal failure. Maintenance haemodialysis for chronic renal failure was made possible only after the problem of vascular access was solved by Quinton and Scribns in 1960 by introduction of arteriovenous shunt. This was further improved by Brescia in 1966 with the development of arteriovenous fistula and the modern era of chronic haemodialysis really started.

The first reported use of peritoneal dialysis comes from Putnam in 1922. However, the first human survivor of the application of peritoneal dialysis for renal failure was reported in 1946 by Irank *et al.* Automatic cycling device for peritoneal dialysis was introduced in 1965 and further improved in 1969; this reduced the risks of peritonitis. It was Tenckhoff in 1968 who gave a boost to chronic peritoneal dialysis by developing the in-dewelling peritoneal catheter. Continuous ambulatory peritoneal dialysis (CAPD) is a significant achievement by such workers as Popovich, Oreopoules and others in the period 1976-1978.

### Introduction

Dialysis is a process by which toxic materials which accumulate in the body due to renal failure may be removed by diffusion across a semipermeable membrane. Dialysis may also be used in some acute poisonings, without any renal failure. On the other hand, patients of acute renal failure with obvious correctable factors like gross fluid electrolyte depletion, obstructive uropathy or due to hepatotoxic drugs can often be managed conservatively.

There are two types of dialysis :

(1) Haemodialysis : where the semipermeable membrane is an artificial membrane e.g. cellulose acetate, amprophan etc.
(2) Peritoneal dialysis : where the patient's peritoneum is utilised as the membrane across which diffusion occurs.

### Indications of Dialysis

Dialysis may be required temporarily in acute reversible renal failure. This method maintains life while the kidneys may recover their function or it may be needed life-long at periodic intervals in chronic irreversible renal failure and in so-called end stage renal disease (ESRD). The indications for dialysis are both clinical and biochemical as follows :

### Biochemical

Blood urea level of 200 mg and creatinine of 10 mg and above are often taken as levels for which dialysis indicated. These usually correspond to creatinine clearances of less than 5 ml/min.

However in general, patients with diabetic nephropathy are started earlier on dialysis.

Hyperkalaemia (serum potassium above 6.5 -7mEq/L is one of the most urgent indications for dialysis.

### Clinical

(1) Intractable pulmonary oedema
(2) Pericarditis
(3) Peripheral neuritis
(4) Gastrointestinal haemorrhage
(5) Refractory hypertension
(6) Uraemic coma

### Haemodialysis

Haemodialysis involves pumping out blood from the patient at a sufficient rate (about 200ml/min), passing it through the dialyser membrane, across the other surface of which is seen the dialysis fluid (at a rate of about 500ml/min), so that diffusion of waste products can occur and then returning the 'purified' blood returns to the body.

The dialyser or artificial kidney may be of different types. The average duration of each haemodialysis is five hours and may have to be repeated two to three times per week. The patient needs to be heparinised (5000-10,000 units of heparin dialysis) during haemodialysis to prevent clotting of blood in the extracorporeal circulation. The most important requirement for haemodialysis is adequate vascular access. In patients likely to require repeated haemodialysis one good forearm vein of at least one side should be spared for intravenous infusions and repeated venepunctures. The various means of vascular access are as follows :

(1) **Arteriovenous fistula :** This is the most important access for long-term use and is most commonly created between the radial artery and the cephalic vein at the wrist. If an artery and adequate vein are not long enough, these may be connected by autologous or homologous vein graft, dacron graft, teflon graft etc. The advantage is that it can be used for several years and frequency of infection and thrombosis is low. Its disadvantage is that it requires a maturing time which may vary from one week to a few months, thus precluding its use for emergency haemodialysis.

(2) **Arteriovenous shunt :** An A-V shunt consists of a silastic tubing with teflon tips inserted between neighbouring artery and vein usually done in lower half of the left forearm. Its advantage is that it is immediately ready for use. For dialysis vessels need not be punctured, only the silastic tubing need to be opened in the middle and the two open ends connected to the tubings of the blood delivery system. Its major disadvantage is its short life because of high incidence of infection, thrombosis and stenosis. It also carries with it risks of serious haemorrhage due to disconnection or snapping of the silastic tubing between arterial and venous tubings.

Both the above access-procedures may be complicated by certain circulatory disorders e.g. :

(i) Distal ischaemia rarely leading even to gangrene through A.V. connection or ligation of the artery.
(ii) Swelling, pain and redness of the extremity due to venous hypertension.
(iii) High output cardiac failure, particularly in elderly individuals with a large promixal A.V. fistula.

(3) **Femoral vein or subclavian vein catheterisation :** Seldinger technique is another means of vascular access for emergency use.

Risks of infection and thrombosis are significant; there has even been fatal pulmonary embolism following thrombosis around the catheter tip. So one catheter should preferably not be kept for more than a few days.

Patients kept on maintenance haemodialysis may have almost a normal diet (especially protein intake needs no restriction); however, restriction of food rich in potassium (mainly fruits, including the dry fruits rich in potassium) should be enforced, except during dialysis itself. Of course, hypertensive patients need some salt restriction. If fluid restriction is needed, depending upon the patient's urine output an average weight gain of 0.5 kg of body weight per day in between dialysis is usually acceptable.

Extra fluid in the body can be removed during haemodialysis by the process of ultrafiltration. Many patients have fluid overload when first put on dialysis. One of the most important jobs of the nephrologist is to determine the ideal or dry weight of each patient.

The drugs that chronic dialysis patients need to take routinely are :

(1) Vitamin B complex including folic acid and iron; these should be taken at least after each dialysis.
(2) Phosphate binders — most commonly aluminium hydroxide gel to be taken with meals.
(3) Some patients also need calcium supplement and active forms of Vitamin D e.g. 1.25 dihydroxycholecalciferol (Rocaltrol).

Many patients on dialysis are also hypertensive and hence will require antihypertensive drugs but the requirements may be reduced once the patient is put on regular dialysis.

Chronic haemodialysis may be done in the following settings :

(1) As 'out patient' treatment in hospital dialysis centres.
(2) Home haemodialysis.
(3) Limited-care haemodialysis.

In our country most dialysis patients have to depend on hospital haemodialysis service but only a few such units are really available in big cities only. Private facilities of haemodialysis are also limited to big cities and very few patients can utilise the facilities due to high cost involved.

**Problems related to haemodialysis**

1. Requirement of adequate vascular access and its complications.
2. Need for heparinisation, with risks of intracranial, gastrointestinal, pericardial and pleural haemorrhage.
3. Cardiovascular instability, particularly hypotension during haemodialysis.
4. Dialysis disequilibrium syndrome manifested by headache, vomiting, confusion and coma most likely due to rapid change in osmolarity owing to haemodialysis.
5. Pyrogenic reaction and other allergic reactions.
6. Abnormal losses of vitamins, aminoacids and blood. During each haemodialysis up to 50 ml of blood may be lost due to deposition of RBC, platelets and fibrin on the dialysis membrane and blood tubings, in spite of use of heparin. Further acute blood loss may infrequently occur from accidental rupture of dialysis membrane.
7. Complement leucocyte induced pulmonary dysfunction.
8. Haemolysis.
9. Dialysis dementia or encephalopathy, which is a long-term problem, is most likely form of aluminium toxicity due to inappropriate high level of aluminium in the water used for preparing the dialysis fluid.
10. Hard water syndrome, manifested by headache, nausea, vomiting and hypertension during dialysis — it is due to acute hypercalcaemia owing to excess calcium in the dialysate. The last two complications call for proper deionisation of the water used for preparing dialysis fluid.

## Peritoneal Dialysis

Peritoneal dialysis, like haemodialysis, may be performed temporarily in acute renal failure or on a long-term basis as chronic peritoneal dialysis.

### Acute peritoneal dialysis

In an acute setting pertioneal dialysis is done by inserting a plastic catheter in the peritoneal cavity under local anaesthesia. Commercially available peritoneal dialysis fluid is run into the peritoneal cavity through the cathether, usually 1.5 to 2 litres at a time and this is retained for about half an hour to allow diffusion across the peritoneal membrane and then allowed to run out. Where excess fluid needs to be removed, hypertonic peritoneal dialysis fluid containing extra glucose is used. Peritoneal dialysis being a slow process, such cycles have to be continued for 24-72 hours in one go, usually the plastic catheter has to be removed after each dialysis. This is a simple procedure requiring sophisticated machine and can be carried out in any general hospital provided the dialysis fluid and the catheter are available.

### Chronic peritoneal dialysis

This requires permanent peritoneal access by surgical implantation of a soft silastic peritoneal catheter, developed by Palmer and modified by Tenckhoff.

Chronic peritoneal dialysis may be of 3 types :

#### (1) Chronic intermittent peritoneal dialysis (CIPD)

This involves 2 litres exchange each hour for 10-14 hours at a time. The process is simplified by the availability of automatic cycler which introduces and drains the peritoneal fluid for patients with some residual renal function. Three such dialyses may be required per week and with the automatic cycler this may be done in the night during sleep. However, with residual GFR falling below 3 ml/min, longer periods are required. This method can be quite useful for short periods in patients waiting for a renal transplant or during maturation of an AV fistula for haemodialysis.

#### (2) Chronic ambulatory peritoneal dialysis (CAPD) :

This is a very significant development introduced by Popovich *et al* in 1976, and promoted by Oreopoules *et al* in 1978. In this method two litres of a commercial peritoneal dialysis fluid contained in soft plastic bag are run into the peritoneal cavity. The empty bag attached to the catheter is rolled up and held under the belt or waist band. The fluid is retained for 4-6 hours during daytime and allowed to remain 10-12 hrs during night and then the fluid is drained back into the empty bag, which is then discarded. A new bag is then connected and fresh dialysate run into the peritoneal cavity. The longer the dwelling time during night, the better is the removal of creatinine; moreover "middle molecule" clearance is better with CAPD. For most patients four exchanges of two litres/day provide adequate dialysis. The special attraction of CAPD for the patient is the minimum interruption of work or recreation as the patients can remain ambulatory throughout.

#### (3) Chronic cyclic peritoneal dialysis (CCPD)

This is a variant of CAPD where dialysis is performed during the night and two litres of fluid are retained in the peritoneal cavity during daytime. The single connection and disconnection in a day is said to reduce the incidence of peritonitis; however the requirement of an automatic cycler device limits the mobility of the patient.

### Advantages of peritoneal dialysis

1. No need for vascular surgery.
2. No need for systemic heparinisation, hence safe for use in presence of bleeding disorders, in a patient with suspected intracranial or pericardial haemorrhage.

3. The slower correction of fluid and electrolyte abnormalities is advantageous for patients with cardiovascular instability and better tolerated by children and the elderly.
4. No need for machines except when automatic cycler is used.
5. Little interference with work or recreation for patients on CAPD.
6. Better biochemical control on CAPD as compared to haemodialysis.
7. Less anaemia on CAPD, possibly because of better removal of middle molecules which are believed to suppress erythropoiesis.
8. Higher levels of high density lipoprotein cholesterol (HDLC) in patients on CAPD, then on haemodialysis — so incidence of vascular disease may be reduced.

**Disadvantages/problems of peritoneal dialysis**

1. Risk of peritonitis is most important. Recurrent peritonitis not only causes impairement of health, and even death from septicaemia but also leads to obliteration of the peritoneal cavity, thus making further peritoneal dialysis impossible.
2. Longer treatment time as it is a slow process; this means that the patient has to be on dialysis for longer periods intermittently, or there has to be continuous involvement.
3. Catheter malfunction.
4. Moderate protein loss (about 5-10 g/day on CAPD).
5. Should not be used in cases of recent abdominal surgery.
6. Should better be avoided in patients with chronic lung diseases or respiratory insufficiency as the large amount of fluid in the peritoneal cavity pushes up the diaphragm causing basal atelectasis and increasing the chance of infection.
7. In presence of certain diseases like systemic sclerosis, vasculitis and malignant hypertension clearance is inadequate.
8. In severe hypercatabolic states clearance with peritoneal dialysis may not be adequate to control hyper potassaemia.

## RENAL TRANSPLANTATION

*A.R. NANDY*
*SUBHANKAR CHAUDHURY*

Renal transplantation is now a standard procedure in the treatment of end stage renal disease. The source of kidney may be from a living donor or from a cadaver. A living healthy donor may be a close blood relation or an unrelated donor. The ideal donor is an identical twin.

The results are however better with properly matched live related donors than with unrelated live donors or from cadaver.

**Indications for Renal Transplantation**

Generally most patients accepted for maintenance haemodialysis are suitable candidates for renal transplantation. The contraindications of transplantation are :

1) Serious extra-renal disease e.g. cerebrovascular disease, coronary artery disease and cancer.
2) Extremes of age is a relative contraindication. Usually accepted age group is 5 years to 55 years.
3) Primary renal diseases are expected to recur in transplants, of which oxalosis is an absolute contraindication. Other disorders e.g. mesangiocapillary glomerulonephritis (particularly dense deposit type), focal glomerulonephritis Ig A nephropathy, anti-GBM antibody nephritis. Cystinosis and amyloidosis also may recur in the transplant, but are considered only relative contraindications.

4) Diabetes mellitus is a relative contraindication because of the problems of widespread vascular disease, blindness and infection.
5) Vesico-urethral abnormalities constitute relative contraindications, renal transplant being possible after creation of an artificial bladder.

**Pre-operative assessment of recipient**

(1) **G.I. System :**

Peptic ulcer is common among patients on haemodialysis.

(2) **Cardiovascular system :**

Blood pressure should be well controlled in all potential transplant recipients.

(3) **Bone disease :**

Metabolic bone disease associated with chronic renal failure should also be properly managed.

(4) **Infections :**

All potential foci of infection e.g. sinuses, tonsils, gums, respiratory tract, urinary tract etc. should be eradicated.

Patients with arrested or healed tuberculosis should receive another course of chemotherapy during transplantation, because of risks of latent infection being opened up due to immunosuppression.

All potential transplant patients should have their serum tested monthly for HBS Ag. because of risks of transmitting hepatitis to other patients and members of the renal unit.

(5) **Psychological factors :**

All patients should be psychologically prepared for the surgery and they should also be warned of the rare possibility of graft failure and need to return to dialysis.

**Selection of Donor :**

The prospective donor should have the following qualities :

1) He should generally be healthy with no structural or functional abnormality of the urinary system.
2) He should preferably be of the same ABO blood goup as the recipient. However, group O kidney may safely be transplanted in A, B or AB recipient. However, the Rh system is not relevant as Rh antigens are not important for the grafts.
3) He should be properly HLA matched.

The best donor is an identical twin. In the absence of an identical twin, the best match from among volunteer siblings or parents should be selected. In cadaver grafts HLA-B locus matching is now found to be more important than HLA-A matching.

Matching for the DR (i.e. D-related) antigen which can be identified quickly by serological tests, is also recognised to be important in cadaver transplant.

**Preparation of recipient for transplantation**

(1) Blood transfusion

Blood transfusions to the recipient prior to transplant are believed to improve graft survival, especially in cases of cadaver transplants. Neither the optimum number nor the optimum time of transfusion is yet settled. But most centres recommend 3-5 units of blood. Some suggest that more than 20 units may be required for maximum effect.

**Post-transplant course**

In almost all living related donor kidneys, the transplant starts functioning immediately. In cadaver transplants only 50-60% show immediate function. This delay varying from a few days to a few weeks may necessitate temporary dialysis.

**Complications following transplantation**

1) Technical e.g. vascular or ureteric problems — mostly seen in the immediate post-operative period.
2) Immunological rejection — this is still the principal factor for graft-loss. The immunological mechanisms for rejection include :
   (a) Cell mediated immune response
   (b) Complement depended antibody-mediated reaction
   (c) Antibody dependent cell mediated cytotoxicity.

**There are 3 categories or rejection :**

(a) **Hyperacute rejection** — Occurs within hours of transplantation and is due to preformed antibodies owing to pre-sensitisation e.g. by blood transfusion, pregnancy or previous allograft to donor HLA antigen. The use of microlymphocytotoxic crossmatch test has resulted in considerable reduction in hyperacute rejection.

(b) **Acute rejection** — Usually occurs within 4-30 days after transplantation, but the term may be used for any rejection with the first three months or even later in a transplant with stable function. Here prompt treatment may salvage the kidney. It is manifested by a drop in urine output or at least a decrease in the rate of fall of urea and creatinine, fever, swelling and tenderness over the graft, and development or aggravation of hypertension. Treatment of acute rejection is usually by 'pulse' steroid therapy with 1.0 gm of methylprednisolone I.V. and three doses given at 12-24 hour intervals. Some nephrologists have claimed benefit with plasmapheresis.

(c) **Malignancy** — Chance of malignancy in the immunosuppressed transplant appears to be as much as 100 times than that in the general population. The malignancies include carcinoma of skin, lips and cervix uteri and lymphomas.

**Immunosuppression in renal transplantation**

Except for transplantation between identical twins immunosuppressives are routinely used.

The most commonly used drugs are steroids and azathioprine; cyclophosphamide may replace azathioprine in presence of hepatic on renal problems. Some centres have also used antilymphocyte globulin. Previously steroids were given in very high dosage e.g. methyl-prednisolone 20 mg/kg/day I.V. for 3 days in the first month after transplant.

Nowadays, steroid dosage has been reduced, (e.g. hydrocortisone 100 I.V. six hourly for first 24 hours, then prednisolone 20 mg/day for first six months, without any reduction in graft survival, but with much less side-effects like G.I. haemorrhage, avascular bone necrosis and infections.

Cyclosporin A, a fungal metabolite, which acts mainly of T-lymphocytes, probably represents a major breakthrough in transplantation. However, problems of nephrotoxicity and hepatotoxicity, high death rate from sepsis and occasional lymphomas were observed after its initial use. Some of these may be related to the high doses initially used, so the dose is now reduced from 25 mg/kg/day to 17 mg/kg/day. More recently one centre has reported high rates of thromboembolic complications following use of cyclosporin.

All these forms of immunosuppression are non-specific and make the patients valuable even to otherwise minor infection. Specific immunosuppression is now being thought of and two types are being experimented.

(1) Active enhancement : (antigen induced immunosuppression). By pre-treatment of recipient with donor cells bearing HLA antigens. In fact blood transfusion (especially donor specific transfusion) may act in this way.
(2) Passive enhancement (antibody induced) by injecting recipient with antibodies to donor HLA antigens.

Result of renal transplantation.

Best is a transplant from an identical twin where there is 94% survival at eight years. For matched living related donors other than identical twins one year survival of graft is 80-90%, while cadaver grafts are successful in about 60%. Survival of second grafts is generally inferior to that of first.

## DRUGS AND KIDNEY DISEASE

*YASHPAL*
*K.S. CHUGH*

### Introduction

Most drugs or their metabolites are eliminated through the kidneys. Toxic drugs or drug allergic response may cause renal damage.

Nephrologic consultations due to drug nephropathy are on the increase and it appears that about 3% cases of end-stage renal disease, on maintaintance haemodialysis in the world are due to analgesic nephropathy.

### Mechanism of Nephropathy

There are multiple factors for Renal vulnerability as under :-

(1) Hemodynamic : Renal blood flow is about 25% of cardiac output.

(2) Metabolic activity : Increased metabolism of drug in the kidney.

(3) Drugs blocking multiple renal enzymes.

(4) Increased concentration of drugs in medulla due to anatomical pecularity of counter current mechanism of blood supply.

(5) Increased concentration of drugs in distal tubule.

(6) Precipitation of drugs due to changes in urinary pH.

(7) Largest surface area of total nephrons of the kidney.

(8) Nephrotoxicity of drugs in normal kidney or acceleration of renal failure in latent renal disease.

### Classification of Drugs

List of important drugs and type of renal damage is reflected in Table 10.6.

**Table 10.6 : List of Common Drugs**

| Type of Renal failure | Aetiological Drugs | Mechanism |
|---|---|---|
| 1. Acute Renal failure (ARF) | G6 PDD due to quinine/ Sulpha drugs etc, | |
| (a) Acute | Heavy metals : organic iodides, amino-glycosides, polymyxin. amphortericin, carbenicillin | Toxic |

| | | |
|---|---|---|
| (b) Acute Interstitial Nephritis | Penicillin, ampicillin, methacillin, rifampicin, phenobarbitone, phenyl-butazone, sulphonamide, thiazide, allo-antipyrine, dilantin phenidiornes | Allergic |
| 2. Glomerulopathy | Penicillamine, gold, captopril, Trimethadione, dilantin, tolbutamide hydralazine, sulpha-drugs | Immunological. |
| 3. Chronic Renal failure (C.R.F.) Chronic Damage | Analgesics (all types) Heavy metals Vitamin 'D' | Toxic |
| 4. Nephrogenic Diabetes insipidus | Lithium, flouride anaesthetic agents | — |
| 5. Obstruction | Crystalluria of sulpha-drugs; methy sergide producing retroperitoneal fibrosis | Precipitation Fibrosis of Ureters |
| 6. Renal tubular disorders | Fanconi syndrome & tetracycline | — |
| 7. Malignancy of Bladder | Cyclophosphamide | Immuno Suppression |
| 8. Toxic Renal Cystic disease | Corticosteroids : stilboesterol, dilantin. | Toxic Type |

**Clinical presentation and therapeutic response**

1. Variable clinical protocol depending upon the nature, duration, dose of offending drug and pre-existing kidney functions.
2. It can be one of the following types e.g.

   ARF : Sudden decrease in urine output (oliguria/anuria) sudden azotemia : Nausea, vomiting, hiccups,oedema, eosinophils may be present in urine.

   C.R.F. : Analgesic nephropathy

   Glomerulopathy : Significant proteinuria 3.5 g/24 hrs.
   Oedema over the body; hypoalbuminemia

   Obstruction : Sulpha group of drugs are common agents

   Renal tubular disorders : Renal rickets nephrocalcinosis.
3. Acute type nephropathy is often reversible whereas chronic can be controlled.
4. Stoppage of offending drug modifies the course of disease. Steroids are useful therapeutic adjuncts in allergic disorders. Symptomatic regimen including early dialysis whenever indicated are very helpful.
5. Avoid furadantin, nalidixic acid, sulpha-drugs terramycin, chlorpropamide, clofibrate, kenamycin, streptomycin and neomycin in renal failure. Penicillin, gentamycin, digoxin failure but monitoring plasma level is very useful.

## ANALGESIC NEPHROPATHY

Zollinger has described significant incidence of chronic interstitial Nephritis — papillary necrosis with abuse of "SARIDON". Its incidence is variable, Australia (20%), Canada (5.5%),

Europe 3.1% and USA 7%. Sporadic case reports are available from India, however its incidence is "rare" this could be due to genetic variations.

**Aetiology**

Aspirin, phenacetin, paracetamol or analgesic mixtures can produce analgesic nephropathy if consumed more than 2 Kg over span of few years duration.

Aspirin interferes with the carboxylation cycle, phenacetin causes exudative damage to all membranes. Thus there is medullary prostaglandin depletion, ischaemia in papillary region resulting in necrosis.

**Histology**

It shows chronic interstitial nephritis (reduced kidney size, mononuclear, plasma cells & eosinophil infiltration, tubular atrophy & fibrosis) with characteristic presence of lipofuschin pigments.

**Clinical Features**

"Analgesic syndrome" comprises of following features :-

A. **Non-renal setting :** of GIT symptoms, peptic ulceration (35%), anaemia (60-90%), splenomegaly, psychiatric disturbances, I.H.D. prematurity.

B. **Renal :** Tubulomedullary dysfunction leading to defects of concentration, salt loosing state, nocturnal polyuria, medullary calcification, acidosis, sterile pyuria (75%), if microscopic haematuria with proteinuria, hypertension and renal papillary necrosis : Urine examination reveals necrotic papillae.

C. **Radiology :** Papillary necrosis in IVP, ring shadows, medullary cavities & calcification : symmetrical reduction of kidney size.

**Prognosis :**

Good, if analgesics are stopped (73.8% five years survival)

**Treatment :**

Symptomatic measures : stoppage of analgesics.

# CHAPTER – 11
# PSYCHOLOGICAL MEDICINE

*BIMAL DE*

## Introduction

The field of psychological medicine ranges from day to day mental expressions to most bizzare forms of abnormal behaviour. Disturbances of mental functioning may be due to :

A. *INTRINSIC FACTORS*

1. Genetic predisposition
2. Personality characteristics
3. Physical states

B. *EXTRINSIC FACTORS*

1. General environment
2. Effects of family interactions
3. Social, religious and occupational milieu

There are constant interactions between these factors and mental illness may result from complex interplay of such forces within the person himself, between him and other individuals and also with society at large. Multiple causation, however, is the rule.

The mechanisms are physical, physiological and psychological and these are brought into operation by the person himself to cope with the causative forces thus bringing about a change of behaviour, which if deviant from normal, results in psychiatric disorders.

## The development of psychiatry

As early as 4th Century B.C., Hippocrates explained some mental symptoms e.g. depression, mania, paranoia, by way of his humoral theory. Plato considered brain as seat of the soul. Aristotle thought that mind is a function of the heart.

By 2nd Century A.D. Galen put forward emotional factors as the cause of mental illness. His work subsequently influenced physicians till 16th Century, when specialised institutions were formed for the mentally ill patients where they were usually confined to restraint by chains etc. and given various types of painful physical tortures.

During the 18th Century more stress was placed on psychological and physical factors as predisposing and precipitating causes. It was Johann Reil in 1808 who first used the term psychiatry and more humane care of the institutionalised patients was developed soon by Philippe Pinel in France and Tuke in England.

By late 19th Century German psychiatrists like Kraepelin and Kahlbaum devoted their attention to the study and classification of psychiatric disorders and tried formulation of a prognostic approach. Since then in various countries, especially in Europe, U.S.A. and Russia various concepts of psychiatric illness developed and contributed to the classification systems. Psychiatry thus gradually developed as an integral part of medicine where its aim remained therapeutic.

## Basic concepts in psychiatry

Mental Health : An individual is mentally healthy when he functions at normal capacity with full use of all the faculties of mind and can enjoy the pleasure of mental well-being. Ability to adjust means forming a meaningful relationship with environment of wide variety and such capability is a sensitive indicator of mental health. Being mentally healthy necessarily indicates absence of diagnosable mental disorders but such healthy person may occasionally seek professional help to booster his positive elements of personality in situations of stress. Of course, there can be degrees of mental health which at its extreme borders into illness.

**Personality Development :** The term personality evolved from the Latin word 'persona' meaning 'mask' i.e. as one appears to others. By popular meaning the word is used in various senses generally signifying specific prominent character aspects of an individual e.g. dominance, imaginativeness, sensitivity, creativity etc.

In psychological sense many definitions have been forwarded of which the following is comprehensive : "It is the dynamicorganisation within the individual of psychophysical systems that determine one's characteristic behaviour and thought."

As the person grows into adulthood his psychological traits (.e.g. attitudes, emotional temperament, habits, intelligence, motivations, social and religious beliefs etc. and his physical development go on integrating, consciously and unconsciously, into a distinctive structure or pattern with specific qualities of behaviour characteristic of the person. It represents a compromise between inner drives and needs of the individual and the controls both internal (i.e. conscience of super-eye) and external (i.e. reality demands) that regulate the behaviour of the person. Because such compromise helps him to avoid tensions and fulfil his potentials, the individual does not entirely recognise his own personality expressions as abnormal, if it be so, unless its repercussions of the people around him urge him to take notice of it or seek professional help. The personality of the individual also determines the nature of mental phenomenon in the occurrence of an illness. The effects may be pathogenic or pathoplastic. Hereditary endowments also determine by way of its interactions with social environment within and outside the family.

Theory regarding human nature was first developed by Ernst Kretchmer (1888-1964) in Germany who attempted to correlate somatotype with personality characteristics as well as illness susceptibility. Subsequently psychoanalytic theories gained foundation by the Austrian psychiatrist Sigmund Freud (1850-1939) who evaluated the concept of psychic apparatus with its components as the Id, Ego and Super-ego as well as the inner processes e.g. libido, regression, transference, oedipus complex and stages of psychosexual development, psychopathology of dreams, etc.

Id — totally unconscious part of the psyche comprising of inner primitive drives governed by pleasure principle requiring immediate gratification.

Ego — that part of the psychic apparatus which mediates between the inner drives and the external reality to help adaptation to the environment.

Super-ego — an unconscious portion of the psyche which judges ego's actions.

**Stages of psychosexual (psychosocial) development**

These are described as :

1. Oral stage — from birth to 18 months of age
2. Anal stage — 18 months to 3 years of age
3. Phallic stage — 3 to 7 years of age
4. Latency period — 7 years of puberty
5. Genital stage or adulthood.

Various forms of abnormal mental phenomenon have been explained specially in neurotics and persons with disorder of personality development, on the basis of abnormalities in different stages of psychosexual development.

During late 19th Century Freudian School of Psychoanalytical psychology found criticisms and contributions came from other schools of thought.

Carl Jung (1875-1961), a Swiss psychiatrist who put forward the theory of analytical psychology describing a collective unconscious which forms the background of human thoughts and emotions.

Adolf Meyer (1866-1950) — An American psychiatrist who proposed the term 'psychobiology' where not only biological but also social, psychological and multiple forces operate to mould personality.

Alfred Adler (1870-1937) — An Austrian psychiatrist who founded School of Individual Psychology and formulated the ideas of inferiority complex, masculine protest, organ inferiority etc. Otto Rank (1884-1939) described anxiety of birth trauma (i.e. separation from mother) as key factor in the development of neurosis.

H.S. Sullivan (1892-1949) proposed the Dynamic-Cultural School of Psychoanalysis which emphasizes sociologic events i.e. more present day contacts with people than past experiences.

Besides Euro-American contribution the Pavlovian theories of development of personality propounded that early training based upon a balance of excitation and inhibition of neural systems and strength and mobility of conditioning processes determines the behaviour of a person.

**Ego Defence Mechanisms**

A group of mental processes go into operation beyond the level of consciousness in order to protect the person from anxiety and are means of controlling the impulses which cause conflict between Id drives and demands of reality. The common mechanisms are :

1. Repression
2. Denial
3. Projection
4. Rationalisation
5. Reaction formation
6. Sublimation
7. Displacement
8. Symbolisation
9. Identification
10. Introjection
11. Condensation
12. Isolation
13. Compensation
14. Undoing
15. Conversion
16. Phantasy.

**Neurosis Vs. Psychosis**

**Neurosis** — The term is synonymous with psychoneurosis. Anxiety is regarded as its dynamic source which may be directly felt or result in ego defences. The form of neurosis is determined largely by the type of defence mechanisms used to control anxiety and there is usually no sharply defined line between various types of neurosis.

**Psychosis** — The term was loosely used originally for any form of mental disorders causing grossly, disordered behaviour and had synonymous meaning with phrases like insanity, madness, lunacy. At present the term 'psychosis' is specifically used to refer to a particular group of mental disorders which includes the following :

A Organic psychosis (organic brain syndrome) where there is evidence of pathophysiologic changes in the nervous system.

B. Functional psychosis e.g.

1. Schizophrenia
2. Manic depressive psychosis
3. Involutional melancholia
4. Paranoid psychosis

In addition, the term is also used in a qualitative sense applicable to other mental disorders when the behaviour shows :

1. Inability to maintain meaningful relationship with external world.
2. Involvement of all areas at personality functioning.
3. Involvement of intellectual functions with distorted thinking and judgement.
4. Behaviour pattern falls back to that of earlier life and even to primitive level (regression).

**Differentiation between neurosis and psychosis**

| Neurosis | Psychosis |
|---|---|
| 1. Manifested by anxiety and its derivatives. | 1. None |
| 2. Does not involve total personality (part reaction). | 2. Involves total personality (whole reaction) |
| 3. Personality remains socially organised. | 3. Social functioning disrupted. |
| 4. Reality is not denied or changed qualitatively but may be altered quantitatively. | 4. Appreciation of reality distorted and may create own subjective form of reality. |
| 5. Inner experiences do not markedly upset external behaviour. | 5. External behaviour abnormal being governed by inner experiences. |
| 6. Thinking is not dereistic. Overvalued ideas may be present but not delusions. | 6. Dereistic thoughts and delusions occur. |
| 7. Conation slightly disturbed. | 7. Markedly disturbed. |
| 8. Environmental factor more evident as causative. | 8. Much less so. |
| 9. Regression rare. | 9. Common may be extreme, causing excretory soiling |
| 10. Greater degree of insight, realises his subjective suffering and there is desire to get well. | 10. Does not recognise that he is ill. Insight impaired or lost. |
| 11. Result of conflict between ego and Id. | 11. Id takes over. |

## Classification of Psychiatric Disorders

Classification of psychiatric disorders into rigid compartments is difficult. Major research studies on a multinational basis has been done to find out the connotations of terms used by psychiatrist to label diagnosis in order to make it understandable both within and outside national boundary. The need for such understanding has to be critical because the criteria of normal also may vary in different geographical places, countries and cultures.

The purpose for a nomenclature with standard terminology was first felt in U.S.A. in 1952 when a Diagnostic and Statistics Manual was devised (DSM–I). This was subsequently revised in 1968 (DSM–II) to conform more closely to the International Classification of Diseases (ICD) developed by W.H.O. and also to the British glossary of mental disorders, both of which have been widely used. Recently a draft glossary of definitions of psychiatric disorders has been proposed by W.H.O. to provide a uniform set of definitions of diagnostic terms for international use.

## Approaches in Psychological Medicine

School of psychiatric practice, research and training in different countries approach the psychiatric illness with different kinds of concepts of illness. There is a psychodynamic approach. In this the origin and development of mental phenomenon are explored in terms of personality development and a cause and effect relationship is sought after both as regards understanding of the nature of illness and its management.

**B. Psychobiologic approach**

This is also known as Meyerian approach after Adolf Meyer's theory of personality development. Here the illness is called a 'reaction pattern' — like schizophrenic reaction, depressive reaction etc.

**C. Multidimensional approach**

It is based with emphasis upon all probable *modus operandi* for the occurrence of illness and includes genetic and physical factors, family and social factors and a study of personality.

## CLASSIFICATION OF PSYCHIATRIC DISORDERS

I. **Psychosis (Functional)**
   1. Schizophrenia
   2. Affective psychosis
      (a) Manic depressive psychosis
         (i) Manic phase, (ii) Depressed phase
      (b) Involutional depressive psychosis
   3. Paranoid states
   4. Other psychoses, viz. reactive psychosis, those accompanying systemic illness, unspecified psychosis.

II. **Organic Brain Syndromes :**
   A. Psychotic (Organic psychosis)
      (a) Acute
      (b) Chronic (also called Dementias)
         (i) Senile type
         (ii) Atretic sclerotic type
         (iii) Presenile type
   B. Non-psychotic
      With brain tumours, cerebrovascular accidents, epilepsy, head injury etc.

III. **Neurosis**
   1. Anxiety neurosis
   2. Depressive neurosis
   3. Obsessive compulsive neurosis
   4. Phobic neurosis
   5. Hysterical neurosis
   6. Hypochondriacal neurosis
   7. Neuresthenic neurosis
   8. Depersonalisation syndrome

IV. **Psychosomatic Diseases :** (Psychophysiologic Disorders)

V. **Personality Disorders**
   1. Psychopathic personality
   2. Other types of personality disorders e.g. paranoid, anankastic, aggressive, passive-aggressive etc.
   3. Sexual deviations viz. homosexuality, transvestism, trans-sexualism etc.

VI. **Mental Retardation**

VII. **Disorders of childhood and adolescence**

1. Childhood psychosis
2. Hyperkinetic syndrome
3. Behaviour disorder e.g. delinquency, truancy, stealing, pathological lying etc.
4. Isolated symptoms (including habit disorders) i.e. enuresis, stammering, tics, eating disorders etc.
5. Miscellaneous e.g. minimal brain syndrome etc.

VIII. **Miscellaneous**

1. Drug and alcohol dependence
2. Post partum mental disorders
3. Transient situational reaction
4. Grief reaction
5. Non-psychotic symptoms associated with systemic illness
6. Adjustment problems
7. Special symptoms e.g. Sexual dysfunction like impotence, ejaculatory disorders, frigidity anorexia nervosa etc.

## Method of Examination of Psychiatric Patients

The techniques of interview and clinical examination of psychiatrically ill persons are yet to be standardised for clinical practice. The practice varies with different teaching centres which influence the acute clinical methods employed by different doctors. As a consequence differences arise in diagnostic process between psychiatrists trained by different academic centres which can influence the communicative value of the diagnostic label used. Standardised techniques e.g. structured interviews, computer generated methods have been evolved which are useful only as research tools as they are impractical for everyday clinical use.

The role of doctor-patient relationship in management of a patient : This may be the result of his own frustrations, ambitions, emotional reactions to his personal experience with mental illness and the like. It is possible that the doctor may begin to react about the patient even before the meeting happens and may become unable to modify it realistically as the exchange occurs. Also in spite of training the doctor may harbour biased attitude towards mental illness.

### A Method of Clinical Examination

1. Personal data

   Name, age, sex, marital status, occupation, source of referral
2. Information by accompanying persons
3. History of present illness

   Mode of onset, progress

   Description of own symptoms by patient, changes in life and adaptations.
4. Past illnesses
   - (a) Mental — date, nature of symptoms, course, number of times occurred, mental condition in the intervening periods
   - (b) Medical history
5. Personal history
   - (a) Birth and childhood development
   - (b) Academic records
   - (c) Social and occupational adjustments
   - (d) Hobbies and habits

(e) Marital history

6. Family history

Description of the family, history of mental illness, adjustment between parents, sibs and other members themselves and in relation to the patient.

**The Role of the Doctor-Patient Relationship**

The relationship which occurs like any exchange between two human beings, is an intergral part of psychological medicine and more so of importance than in any other branch of medicine. The relationship starts to operate as soon as the meeting happens. To form an approach towards the patient's illness, the doctor should have the mind to listen to the patient's own account of what is happening in his or her mental world. The physician should always listen to the version of the relatives and people living with himso as to form an idea of the objective changes of behaviour. It would be a wrong approach to minimise importance of behavioural changes, by forming a bias e.g. it is absurd or wilful, or by using false reassurances. The doctor-patient relationship can also take the form of a therapeutic tool quite useful sometimes in crucial role to determine the outcome of treatment.

The patient's attitude and emotional responses to his own illness are the result of a combined impact of interactions with his own family, social surroundings, previous experiences with other doctors and other significant persons. It is very important to try to understand the personality of the person behind the facade of the illness.

The physician's own attitude may affect the relationship and consequently influence the issue.

**Mental state :**

1. General appearance, gestures, manners, speech
2. Attitude and behaviour
3. Activity — normal/abnormal hyper or hypo
4. Orientation
5. Affect (Emotional tone)
6. Thought process — form, progress, content
7. Perception, pro-hallucinations, illusions
8. Memory — short-term, ultra-short term, remote
9. Intelligence
10. Judgement
11. Insight-ability to understand own behaviour
12. Personality

In suspected organic brain syndromes it is necessary to look for .

(a) Aphasias

(b) Apraxias

(c) Agnosias

(d) A complete neurological examination

In all cases, a good systemic physical examination is mandatory.

## SCHIZOPHRENIA

**Definition**

It is a generic name for a group of disorders manifested chiefly by disorders of thought process, anomalies of emotions, withdrawal from reality and disturbances of interpersonal relationships.

## CONCEPT

The cluster of symptoms that constitutes this disorder of mind has been recognised as early as 18th Century. It was a Belgian psychiatrist who first used the term Dementia Praecox for this illness under the impression that deterioration of mental functions is essential part of the process. In 1906 Adolf Meyer viewed the opinion that such group of symptoms does not constitute a disease entity but is a kind of personality reaction in certain individuals. Eugene Bleuler in 1911 coined the term Schizophrenia meaning thereby "splitting of mind" because disharmony of normal synthesis of thought, feeling and activity are characteristic of it. Bleuler also added that the outcome is not necessarily one of deterioration. It does not give rise to Jekyll and Hyde character of literature who are actually psychopathic personalities with surprising combinations of good and bad qualities.

## AETIOLOGY

The causes leading to development of schizophrenia are not unitary. In fact the illness results from complex interplay of various factors.

## GENETIC FACTORS

The influence of inheritance has been impressive in different statistical research data. However, still there is no unanimity as to the extant mode of transmission. Frequency of occurrence of such illness is greater in families of patients. Twin studies where the offspring have been reared together and in separate environments has also shown high concordance rate which is higher in monozygotic than dizygotic. The transmission is most probably heterogenous and at present polygenic theory is mostly believed.

## BIOLOGICAL FACTORS

The biochemical factors actively investigated are —

**I. Carbohydrate metabolism**

(a) Defects in Embden-Meyerhof pathway resulting in abnormal capacity to utilise glucose.

(b) A possible anti-insulin factor in plasma leading to abnormal production of pyruvate.

(c) A toxic substance in plasma has been found to disturb carbohydrate metabolism in chicken RBC.

**II. Protein metabolism**

(a) An abnormal serum protein, an alpha-2 globulin (S-protein) has been found.

**III. Cerebral amine metabolism**

(a) Defective transmethylation in dopamine adrenaline pathway.

(b) Abnormal serotonin metabolism (e.g. excessive methylation) producing a hallucinogenic substance.

(c) Excessive production of adenochrome and adrenaline-like substance having psychotomimetic effect.

(d) Formation of a mescaline-like derivative.

**IV. Endrocrine abnormality**

Commonly observed marked rise in urine 17-OHCS in acute phase. Physiological changes found are minor in degree and inconstant in nature. These include :

(a) Disturbed head control

(b) Slow circulation time

(c) Abnormalities of $O_2$ consumption

(d) Diminished capacity of autonomic action.

## SOCIAL FACTORS

A wide spectrum of pathological family and social interactions has been postulated.

A. Changes in mother-child relationship and family transactions e.g. :

(a) Double blind communications involving incompatible opposites both of which get disapproved.

(b) Family communication may be hostile or fragmented or overdependent on opposite sex parent. A schizophrenogenic mother is close, engulfing overprotective and ambivalent preventing maturation of the child about his identity.

B. Common in lower socio-economic groups :

It has been observed that though environment plays a clear-cut role there is no definite prophylactic means.

## CLINICAL PICTURE

**Incidence :** 0.5 to 1% between 15 and 45 years of age.

**Prodromal symptoms** present for weeks or months before major symptoms appear. They may be distrustful, isolated form social life, indulges in fantasies and ruminates about unusual problems for him e.g. religion, universe, etc. They become careless about personal appearance, nervous, make vague somatic complaints but is guarded in discussions. Some may complain of perplexity and lack of connection.

**Onset** is commonest in early adult life and usual in asthenic habitus, sometimes head injury, febrile illness, childbirth may precipitate.

The onset is often gradual or insidious except sudden in catatonic type and in acute form. In early case an outsider may detect behaviour abnormality where relatives do not see these because of slow progression of symptoms.

There is disorder of thinking, feeling, disrupted contact with reality and conduct abnormality. Bleulor described fundamental symptoms as --

(a) Disorder of affect
(b) Disturbances of association or thinking
(c) Autism (turning away from reality)
(d) Ambivalence.

Schinder described first rank symptoms as :

(a) Thought progression disorder
(b) Passivity feeling for ideas of influence
(c) Audible thoughts
(d) Delusional perception (i.e. abnormal significance attached to some normal perception) Diagnosis is, however made with total picture presented by the patient and sub-classification is based on most prominent symptoms.

**Thought disturbances**

(1) Disorder of thought form

(a) Concrete thinking
The patient is unable to make abstraction of an idea or a concept. The interpretation is limited to his own senses of perception.

(b) Autistic thinking
The nature of thinking is not influenced by the reality around him. The thought and behaviour is governed by own subjective ideations and experiences.

(2) **Progression of thought**

Many show many different types of abnormalities singly or in combination. The more commonly observed are —

(a) Blocking — Sudden interruption of thought

(b) Asyndetic thinking — There is lack of causal link between successive themes

(c) Overinclusive thinking — There is lack of boundaries of his ideations where the concept of the theme is blurred by impact of his surroundings.

(d) Thought broadcasting — Belief that others know about his own thoughts.

**Perception disturbances**

(1) Hallucinations —

Seen in about 65% cases and are commonly auditory e.g. voice talking to him or about him which can be threatening or commanding or praising or derogatory. Besides these, the sounds may be noises or sound which the patient may hear having special meaning. Hallucinations may also be of other senses, viz. olfactory or tactile or somatic or senses from internal organs. Visual hallucinations are uncommon.

(2) Illusions may also occur in accordance with the ideational content.

**Thought content abnormalities :** Include delusions which are seen in about 75% of cases. They may be :

(a) **Primary** — Occurs in early cases. Sudden onset and is not understandable in terms of previous mental experience. Usually bizarre and fantastic in type.

(b) **Secondary** — Arises out of some other morbid experience e.g. hallucinations, passivity feeling.

Delusions are commonly paranoid or grandiose but it may also be erotic, somatic, litigatory, religious etc. It can influence the behaviour greatly.

**Mood abnormalities**

Emotional expression may be quite inappropriate e.g. smiling or weeping without reasons apparent to people around; there may be flat or shallow affect or sudden violent outburst without any evident cause.

**Behaviour**

Obliviousness of manners and disregard for social behaviour seen in cases of severe degree. A withdrawal into fantasy causing absent-mindedness also common. Chronic untreated or inadequately treated cases shows behaviour deterioration like dirty habits, inattentive towards own dressing and appearance, inability to conform to norms of social customs.

**Volitional disturbances**

Manifested by a reduction of will to productive activity, lack of desire to do any work or participate with surroundings without any explanation for it.

**Sub-types**

Common forms :

1. Simple
2. Hebephrenic
3. Catatonic
4. Paranoid
5. Acute schizophrenic episode

Other rarer types are —

1. Pseudoneurotic

2. Residual
3. Schizo-affective
4. Latent
5. Chronic undifferentiated.

The following are characteristic features of some of the sub-varieties

**Simple type**

Affects young adults. Most marked disturbances are of emotions, interests and activity which are all greatly reduced. They look callous and show absence of drive. Thought disorders are not so prominent and delusions uncommon. Hallucinations are rare.

The onset is usually insidious and the illness slowly progresses over the years to deterioration of personality and social behaviour. It is difficult to diagnose especially in early stages due to lack of florid productive symptoms. Some may develop into hebephrenic or catatonic type.

**Hebephrenic type** (Hebe = puberty)

Onset is usually in adolescence or early adult life. A careful history shows steady progressive deterioration of school work and isolation from peers. Thought disorder is a prominent feature with incoherence of speech which may be totally disjointed and incomprehensible. Neologism seen in advanced cases. Delusions are quite bizarre, unsystematised and even fantastic. Disorder of volition occurs with outburst of motor actions. Affect is capricious and inappropriate e.g. giggling, smiling or laughter with reason.

**Catatonic type**

Motor disorder mostly seen. Other symptoms are perplexity, hallucinations, primary delusions. Acute onset with either excitement or stupor which may alternate or each may be present for a long time. Negative and automatism prominently seen. Not so much commonly seen presently due to early treatment.

Excitement form — Unorganised aggressive motor overactivity which are purposeless, repetitive and without accompanying emotions. Speech varies from mutism to flight of ideas. The patient may remain without sleep for days to weeks and may refuse food leading to dehydration and collapse.

Stupor form — Mute, mask-like facies, uncommunicative, blank stare, almost immobile, flexibilities cerea or automatic obedience. Urine and stool may be retained or may develop soiling. May recover to normality slowly or suddenly.

**Paranoid type**

Later age of onset than other forms, Idea of reference often first symptoms as also misinterpretations. Many are irritable and suspicious. Delusions common as persecutory or grandiose or erotic and are at first localised to one or more ideas but later become numerous, unrelated and changeable. Hypochondriacal delusions are not uncommon. Hallucinations are usually auditary but rarely may be of other senses. There is display of emotions preserved and it is in accordance with ideas. Depression may occur as secondary phenomenon.

**Diagnosis**

Based on total clinical picture, evaluation of premorbid personality and absence of organic brain syndrome.

Frequency of diagnosis varies in different countries and depends on the prevailing concept.

**Prognosis**

Spontaneous recovery in 5%. Prognosis is good if onset acute, obvious precipitating stress, good premorbid personality, strong affective component.

Prognosis is poor if onset is below 20, previous schizoid personality, insidious onset, hebephrenic type, disturbed home atmosphere and persistent hallucination.

**Treatment**

*CHEMOTHERAPY*

Treatment of choice. Antipsychotic agents commonly used are phenothiazines and haloperidol to control active productive symptoms.

Ancillary drugs such as benzodiazepines, barbiturates and antidepressants are used as appropriate for secondary symptoms e.g. anxiety, insomnia etc.

E.C.T. — Not superior to drug therapy but may be combined for a rapid improvement. Useful if depressive features, acute onset and in younger persons.

*ENVIRONMENT AND SOCIAL CARE*

Relapse less likely if home atmosphere has low emotional tension. Institutional care helps in acute phase but long-term custodial care has adverse effects.

Appropriate social stimulation important for rehabilitation. Remotivation useful in some cases.

*PSYCHOTHERAPY*

Simple supportive psychotherapy may be used to encourage establishment of contact with reality. The plan of therapy should be compatible with clinical condition.

*PSYCHOSURGERY*

Cignulectomy and bi-medial leucotomy has been advocated in some chronic drug resistant cases and in those with very much destructive behaviour.

## MANIC DEPRESSIVE PSYCHOSIS

(Syn : Affective psychosis)

It is a disorder of affect characterised by periodic alteration of mood as its cardinal symptoms.

The mood alterations may be recurrent depression or recurrent mania when it is called Uni-polar illness or there may be alternating depression and mania when it is termed bi-polar or circular illness. The latter form usually follows a more malignant course. Population incidence is about 0.3%.

**Aetiology**

The illness frequently commences in 3rd decade and is more common in females. A cyclothymic personality and a pyknic habitus usually predispose. A familial tendency of developing the illness has been observed. It is common in upper social class and within families concerned with their social status and high expectations of achievement. A positive correlation with gout has been noticed.

**Genetic factors**

Transmission by single dominant autosomal gene with incomplete penetration is observed. Concordance rate high in monozygotic pairs with evidence of some degree of X-linkage e.g. Xg-blood system.

Bicohemical theories —

1. Non-adrenalin and serotonin level at receptor site in brain deficient in depression and excess in mania.
2. C.S.F. level of 5-SHIAA is reduced in depression.
3. Increased tryptophan pyrrolase activity in brain leads to reduction of availability of tryptophan for serotonin synthesis.

4. It has been hypothesized that depression is due to a deficiency of excitant type (Type A) of receptor in brain.
5. Brain intracellular $Na^+$ retention occurs in depression.
6. Adrenocortical steroid level is raised in plasma both in depression and mania, possibly due to non-specific stress.

**Organic Theories**

Lesions of orbital part of frontal lobe has been found to cause manic symptoms.

**Clinical Features**

According to severity of occurrence of symptoms it has been graded from least to most severe as follows :

(a) Hypomania
(b) Acute mania
(c) Delirious mania
(d) Manic stupor

The manic phase may be an acute short-lasting episode or pursue a chronic course.

**Hypomania**

The symptoms evolve gradually and in early stages, it may be difficult to comprehend that it is an illness.

Usually begins with a lack of control of own behaviour where the person is unable to restrain his own physical and mental activities. The person becomes boastful, busy, dashing, carelessly gay, buyoant, socially aggressive and sometimes arrogant and whimsical. She may become full of ambitious schemes and may indulge in indiscriminate spending leading to financial ruin. There is lack of sustained interest and newer enterprises are started but soon abandoned. The mood is one of expensiveness and elation but in reality it is more of excitement than enjoyment. There is pressure of thought and activity, distractibility and lack of insight. To diagnose such a state, premorbid level of normal needs careful appraisal.

**Acute Mania**

It might be a progression from the hypomania stage or may develop *per se.*

The mood is of joy, excitement, exhilaration to exaltation. It may lead to noisiness, aggressiveness in which the patient may take delight. She may shout, sing and dance and is overactive. There is, however, chaos of activity which are non-productive. There may be lack of moral and sexual restraints, impaired judgement and self-neglect. The speech shows pressure of talk, flight of ideas, clang association of words (similar in sound but not related in meaning). Delusions when present are inline with mood and may be of grandiose, paranoid or erotic type. Orientation is preserved and so also is memory. The appetite increases but continuous overactivity may lead to loss of weight and exhaustion.

The duration of an attack varies, it may be weeks to months. There is no deterioration of personality. Intervals between attacks tend to be shorter with subsequent relapses and attacks tend to be longer especially in advancing age. Spontaneous recovery may occur but in some persons a chronic maniacal condition may develop. A long interval of normality has better outlook. Restoration of sleep may be first sign of recovery.

**Manic Stupor**

The mind is filled with constant turmoil of ideas so that the patient becomes speechless, quiet (akinetic mania), cannot react with surroundings and hence inaccessible with facial expression of elation or ecstasy.

## ENDOGENOUS DEPRESSION

Also called depressive phase of manic depressive psychosis. Psychotic depression.

### Precipitating factors

It develops with inadequate or remote causative events or may appear out of the blue. Seen commonly in persons with hypothymic or cyclothymic personality. A family history of such illness or of suicides may be obtained. There may be past history of depression as mania.

The intensity of the illness may produce the following grades of clinical features –

(a) mild
(b) severe
(c) depressive stupor.

The nature of symptoms may again be classified into the following types of depression : depression,:

1. Retarded depression
2. Agitated depression
3. Atypical (or masked) depression

### Mild Depression

It develops gradually with general inhibition of behaviour, self-absorption, fatigue, covered initiative, reduced appetite, feeling of inadequacy, lack of confidence, indecisiveness. The mood may vary from downheartedness to gloominess. It is constant and less reactive. There is diurnal mood change which is worse in the morning. Irritability, stubbornness, reduced self-esteem and ideas of unworthiness and self-blame for trivial things. There may be multiple somatic complaints which may mark depression.

Thinking may be difficult causing perplexed expression. There is mental slowing with poverty of ideas. Misinterpretation of people's behaviour occurs with ideas of reference delusion of guilt, ruin and of persecution may also be seen. Concentration is poor, sleeping is disturbed with early waking. Appetite is reduced and body weight is lost. There may also be self-neglect and loss of sexual desire.

### Severe depression

It is an intensification of the symptoms. Delusions are common. Hallucinations, usually auditory, may occur. Suicidal thoughts occur along with ideas of worthlessness or due to it may be delusions. Homicide may occur which is usually found in women and is associated with delusion of disaster and may be followed by suicide afterwards.

### Retarded depression

Gross reduction of psychomotor activity with perplexity, withdrawal of activity, slow and low tone of speech and thought inhibition.

### Agitated Depression

Manifested by motor overactivity like packing, wringing of hands, restlessness. Anxiety and vague apprehension prominent, causing marked indecisiveness in behaviour and even while holding a conversation.

Orientation may be impaired due to inattention. Common in middle or later life.

### Depressive Stupor

The patient may lie down or sit still with practically no spontaneous motor activity. Facies is rigidly anxious or masked. The patient may be mute. There is intense preoccupation with depressive ideas. Marked refusal of food may lead to constipation. Bladder and bowel may also be incontinent.

**A typical Depression**

Usually seen as overconcern with bodily symptoms which may be single or multiple. The symptoms complained of are, however, persistent and ill-defined without physical signs. There may not be any depressive mood.

**Involutional Melancholia**

It is depressive illness occurring for the first time in involutional period (between 45 and 65 years) of life. Precipitating factors are common e.g. systematic illness, financial stress.

Onset usually gradual.

There is special tendency towards agitation, apprehension, irritability. Delusions occur of guilt, of financial ruin or of disease. Hypochondriacal ideas may be of bizarre kind and may reach delusional intensity e.g. bowels not cleaned enough, having malignant illness or part or whole of body is non-existent (nihilistic ideas). Lowered appetite, reduced interest, interrupted sleep with early waking occur. Loss of weight may be rapid. Hallucination may develop and is commonly auditory as threatening or critical voices.

There is a special danger of suicide. Spontaneous remission may sometimes occur.

## PARANOID STATES

Paranoid symptoms occur in many types of conditions and when it includes delusion, it is called paranoid psychosis. Paranoid states include —

(a) Paranoia
(b) Acute paranoid reaction
(c) Involutional paraphrenia.

**Paranoia**

A rare condition. Common in men and usually between ages of 30 and 50. Seen in persons who are stubborn, sensitive, egoistic, isolated and suspicious.

Insidious onset is usual.

Characterised by fixed delusional ideas which are systematically reasoned. The delusions are most commonly persecutory but may also be grandiose, erotic, religious, litigious. There is preservation of clean orderly thinking and actions except those in relation to delusional materials. Some may hide their delusions but may act on these overtly or in a surreptitous way.

**Acute paranoid reaction**

Commonly develops in vulnerable persons who are under considerable mental stress involving alien situations e.g. prisoners, persons living away in unfamiliar surroundings. The patient becomes anxious, excited, overactive and develops delusion of persecution or of jealousy or become suspicious to a psychotic degree. The illness is short-lasting and recovery may be spontaneous especially when shifted from the stressful situation.

## MENTAL SUBNORMALITY

*(Syn : Mental retardation, Mental deficiency, Amnetia)*

**Definition**

It is a state of arrested or incomplete development of mind which includes subnormality of intelligence and is of nature or degree which requires or is susceptible to medical treatment and other special care or training of the patient. (British Glossary of Mental Disorders).

Mental subnormality is to be distinguished from dementia which denotes intellectual defect occurring for the first time after adolescence.

**Aetiology**

It is important to appreciate that subnormality of intelligence is not a clinical entity by itself but is a manifestation of some underlying cause which adversely influences the development and growth of mind. Hereditary transmission plays little role but parental mental defect may be instrumental in providing deficient intellectual and social influences. The causative factors can be grouped as follows :

(A) **Before birth**

Idiopathic — about 50% of the cases.

Maternal infections — Mumps, rubella, toxoplasmosis, cytomegalic inclusion body disease

Foetal causes — These include :

(1) Chromosomal abnormalities e.g. Mongolism, trisomy 13-15, trisomy 18. Turner's syndrome, Klinefelter's syndrome, Cri-du-chat syndrome.

(2) Endocrine disorders e.g. hypothyroidism, pseudohypoparathyroidism.

(3) Metabolic anomalies e.g. galactosemia, fructosuria, porphyria, phenylketonuria, Hartnup disease, maple syrup urine disease, homocysteinuria, gargoylism, amaurotic familial idiocy, Niemann Pick disease, leukodystrophies.

(4) Rh incompatibility.

(5) Neurological disorders e.g. epiloia, Hand-Schuller-Christian disease, Schilder's disease, ataxic telengiectasia, hydrocephalus, dystrophia myotonica.

(6) Cranial developmental abnormalities e.g. microcephaly, hyperteleorism, acrocephaly.

(7) Toxic and conditions due to any process.

(B) **At birth**

(1) Prematurity with low birth weight

(2) Injuries to head causing meningeal tear, intracranial haemorrhage or cerebral palsy.

(3) Anoxaemia produced during delivery.

(C) **After birth**

(1) Cerebral infections like encephalitis, meningitis, cerebral abscess.

(2) Toxic and metabolic causes e.g. bilirubin encephalopathy, lead encephalopathy, chemical intoxication.

(3) Head injury.

(4) Nutritional deficiency.

(5) Social deprivation.

**Clinical features**

A detailed and careful history is essential to detect any slow or incomplete development of mental function during the entire period from birth to adolescence. All milestones of development should be noted in this sphere of psychological, social, emotional and motor functions. The upper limit of development of general intellectual functioning has been arbitrarily set at 16 years of age. In the assessment of development the factors like racial, cultural and ethnic as well as family and social environment should be taken into consideration besides the often-present effects of significant physical handicaps like deafness, blindness, mutism, spasticity, dyslexias.

A mentally defective person shows inability to establish for himself independent social existence. There is limited capacity of learning, thinking, reasoning, comprehension and use of language. They tend to think on the concrete level instead of forming abstracts. Educational performance is poor which may cause inability to adjust to normal schools. This may be first detected as inability to acquire and retain knowledge. Such intellectual handicap may also lead to secondary behavioural problems e.g. delinquency, truancy, lying, stealing and other anti-social activities. Various forms of emotional disturbances of childhood and adolescence may also occur which may be at the forefront of the presenting symptoms. It is important to keep in mind that mental disorder of all forms may develop in an intellectually subnormal person and such a combination may modify the presenting features.

**Degrees of retardation**

Customarily, the levels of mental retardation are determined by the use of psychological tests. Many tests for intellectual functioning are employed of which *Terman-Merril modification of Standford-Binet test,* form M is implied in the classification of mental retardation. Assessment of mental age is the most reliable indicator of the level of intellectual functioning. It should be appreciated that the tests derive their application in a mind with developing intelligence and hence the scores are unreliable in adults.

**The following clinical types are recognised**

The tests for measuring handicap should aim at measuring social behaviour, vocational aptitude as also the secondary emotional disturbance besides measuring intellectual functioning. The tests should be carefully designed according to the age of the child. It is important to know that the level of one's intelligence should not be solely determined by psychological tests, but the entire educational, social and adaptation behaviour needs to be assessed.

(1) **Borderline intelligence** — I.Q. range 68 to 85. Considered as lower most range of normal intelligence.

(2) **Mild retardation** — I.Q. range 52 to 67. They may develop good social adjustment and responsible work habits with training. It is possible for them to live independently. They benefit from specialised remedial education.

(3) **Moderate retardation** — I.Q. range 36 to 51. Depending on the degree of intelligence deficit they can be trained to care for their personal needs. With training some may also learn unskilled work but would require supervision.

(4) **Severe retardation** — I.Q. range 20 to 35. It is possible for them to take care of their personal hygiene and look after the basic needs. Some of them can be useful to do simple household tasks.

(5) **Profound retardation** — I.Q. below 20. They remain totally dependent on others, even for their basic needs like eating, dressing, toilet habits.

**Treatment**

The total management of a mentally retarded individual requires good co-ordination of the services of the psychiatrist, psychologist, social worker and properly trained nurse who will work in close liason with the patient and his family and also his school and/or work atmosphere. Whatever be the degree of handicap it is always rewarding to take the beneficial effects of training, education and rehabilitation. The aim should be to improve the social functioning and adaptation with environment. Management in the patient's own home environment is preferable then putting him in an institution. Hospitalised care when indicated is required for severe retardation, disturbed or aggresive tendencies, anti-social behaviour, superimposed psychotic or neurotic illness and if there is marked reaction or rejection from his own family.

Counselling of parents and family members should be directed to help them accept the reality of mental retardation and its implications, to support and guide them and to help them cope with their own emotional reactions towards the child. The parents may need education as to how to behave with the child, cope with his behaviour problems and to impart from education. In no case life-long prediction of outcome should be made.

The role of a psychologist for educating a defective child is immense. The child should not be sent to a normal school which may produce feelings of inferiority, insecurity and aggressiveness. To try educating a defective child with lessons beyond his ability is highly damaging to his self-esteem and may lead to refusal to study. Special remedial methods are available and should be tailored for him by the psychologists. Similar systematic techniques based on principles of behaviour modification should be applied for vocational training. Psychotropic drugs have their limited use for controlling overactivity, aggressiveness, noisiness and impulsive behaviour.

Simultaneous identification and treatment of associated malady should be done. Physiotherapy and other relevant treatments are given for bodily handicaps in order to facilitate rehabilitation. Genetic counselling may be required where the aetiology has hereditary basis.

## DRUG DEPENDENCE

The term 'drug dependence' was recommended by World Health Organisation instead of older terms like drug addiction and drug habituation.

It is defined as a state of psychic or physical dependence or both on a drug arising in a person following repeated administration of that drug on a periodic or a continuous basis. The characteristics of drug dependence are :

(a) Compulsion to continue the drug and to obtain it by any means.

(b) Tendency to increase the dose.

(c) A psychic and physical dependence on the effects of the drug.

(d) Deteriorating effects on the individual and on the society.

Physical dependence is an altered physiological state caused by repeated ingestion of a drug which has to be continued in order to prevent appearance of characteristic symptoms called the Abstinence Syndrome'. It is a self-limiting process which appears after a time interval, reaches a peak and after a certain period declines at a definite rate.

### Psychopathology

The exact mode of causation is not yet clear. Physiological or constitutional factors and abnormality of personality functioning are of major importance. Adverse social and family environment contributes in many cases and helps to begin the addictive habit and in its perpetuation. The effects of the drug on the body systems also have a role.

Personality imbalance is the core underlying disturbance and choice of a drug depends upon its pharmacological effects acceptable to the person. Drug taking is the result of attempt to cope with adjustment problem and results in personality reaction in the form of inferiority feeling, hostility, frustration, social inhibition etc. Drug habit leads to further secondary educational and occupational deterioration coupled with rejection from family and society causing further involvement with drugs. It may also lead to problem with the law and financial and moral deterioration.

In young adults, drug taking often begins as adventurism in order to seek newer sensations which in people with vulnerable predisposition leads to drug dependence. In elderly, the drug habit is often triggered off by iatrogenic means to alleviate bodily sufferings. Less commonly, drug habit may be secondary to other psychiatric illness, viz. affective illness, schizophrenia, mental retardation.

### Clinical features

Multiple drug intake is common especially, in those with long period of drug habit. However, addictive drugs are sometimes grouped as (i) soft drugs e.g. amphetamines, cannabis, LSD and (ii) hard drugs e.g. opium and its derivatives, barbiturates, pethidine. Many newer drugs and chemicals are now being reported as having addictive effects e.g. pain killers, petroleum products etc. Chronic drug takers are found to prefer certain specific drug combinations like opiates with amphetamines or with cocaine; usually one is a CNS depressant and the other being a stimulant; both are taken to counterbalance each other's side-effects.

The characteristics of the clinically manifested symptoms depend on the drugs used and are grouped as follows :

(a) Cannabis type, (b) Cocaine type, (c) Amphetamine type, (d) Barbiturate type, (e) Opiate (morphine) type, and (f) Hallucinogen type.

Most drugs produce both psychological and physical dependence but some of the drugs produce only psychological dependence i.e. no abstinence symptoms on their abrupt stoppage e.g. cannabis, amphetamines, cocaine, methaqualone, LSD. Prolonged drug habit reduces life expectancy by way of fatal overdose, hepatitis, malnutrition, lowered resistance to infection.

**Treatment**

It must be realised that drug dependence is a complex problem of multi-factorial origin. It requires a team of personnel to handle the various aspects of management. Early detection is important for favourable results and for this alertness of family physician is of utmost importance.

**Care of withdrawal symptoms**

Some drugs can be withdrawn suddenly e.g. LSD, cannabis, amphetamines, cocaine, bromides. There are very little physiological manifestations of drug withdrawal. Narcotics e.g. barbiturates, opium, pethidine, etc. are usually tapered off with adequate doses of suitable substitutes to prevent withdrawal effects until stabilisation is reached. The substitute drugs are then withdrawn gradually. Hospitalisation is essential in the initial stages while the patient goes through the withdrawal phases. Sufficient rest with attention to personal care and nutrition is required. Tranquilizers may be needed for restlessness, aggressiveness and irritability. Sometimes anti-depressant drugs are required for distressing mood variation.

**Psychological care**

Supportive measures should aim at both social and physical rehabilitation. Close involvement with the addict is required to gain his confidence, to provide vocational guidance and to combat unemployment. Because isolation from family and friends causes relapse he is encouraged to participate in and is provided with good social atmosphere and substitute sources of pleasure to keep him away from his addicted associates.

Analytic oriented psychotherapy is indicated with its aim towards correction of personality disorders and to develop motivation and insight. Group psychotherapy is becoming the choice recently. Addicts are often immature, inadequate persons, with low frustration tolerance and the ultimate prognosis depends upon the severity of personality disorder. As they are unreliable and unpredictable by their nature the dropout rate and consequent relapse rate is high in the follow-up.

## HYSTERIA

**Introduction**

It is neurotic disorder with the following conglomeration of symptoms :

(1) Hysterical reactions, which comprises of
 (a) Conversion reaction
 (b) Dissociation reaction

(2) Acute hysterical psychosis

(3) Hysterical personality disorder

(4) Other hysterical syndromes.

The term 'hysteria' has been in use for several centuries. Its nature has always provoked debate in various countries. It is only since past few decades that scientific methods are being applied to the study of hysteria in an attempt to define the abnormality and demonstrate its association with various physical, psychological and social factors.

Psychoanalytic understanding of symptoms has been contributed mainly by Freud, Janet and Dejerine. It is postulated that the symptoms arise from unresolved oedepal and preoedipal conflicts and has symbolic meaning to the patient. Symptoms are thought of to provide self-protective effects from anxiety, thus giving a solution to the problem; the mechanism of this is beyond the conscious awareness of the patient. The symptoms also enable the patient to maintain self-respect, to draw attention of others and to avoid scrutiny of reality. The anxiety manifests itself or is aggravated if attempts are made to disclose to her consciousness the cause of her symptoms and hence, she welcomes physical explanation. Dramatisation or exaggeration of symptoms and manipulation of the environment are efforts to seek relief from consciously felt anxiety. Gestures of deliberate self-harm are meant to attract attention or are appeals for help; these are not usually intended to be serious which may be so only by accident.

Hysterical gain — The aim is always conscious. Primary gain is the relief from anxiety caused by intolerable intrapsychic conflict due to failure of repression of factors causing it. Secondary gain arises from symptoms and may not always be material but emotional. Such secondary gain may be explained by principles of learning theory i.e. what is rewarded with sympathy when a person uses his sickness to avoid demands of life, is perpetuated by the person taking a sick role.

Recently long-term follow-up of patients with hysteria has brought to light that in many cases either organic illness or other forms of psychiatric illness have been the underlying process.

**Clinical features**

It is one of the few psychiatric illnesses that is most commonly diagnosed by non-psychiatrists. One should remember that the term 'hysteria' should not be applied loosely when the physician finds that the patient exaggerates the symptoms or is determined to maintain them or just because she irritates and manipulates her relatives or the doctor.

The incidence is more in early adult life of females but it may occur at all ages and in both sexes. Many have their intelligence in borderline range. The presentation of symptoms whether they are of the nature of conversion or dissociation remains constant. Sometimes admixture with symptoms of other associated psychiatric and physical illness may alter the clinical picture. Some form of abnormal personality traits are not uncommon amongst close relatives.

**Conversion hysteria**

In this state the somatic symptoms are explained by psychoanalytic theories as the expression of unconscious anxiety generated by intra-psychic libidinal conflicts. It can affect any of the motor, sensory and visceral systems.

*Motor symptoms are :*

(1) Paresis or paralysis of limbs e.g. monoplegia, paraplegia, hemiplegia, ptosis, dysphagia, dysphonia or aphonia.

(2) Spasmodic manifestations e.g. torticollis, tics, trismus, blepharospasm, nystagmus, conjugate ocular spasm, glossolabial spasm, gagging, hiccup, limb tremor and cramps.

(3) Others, viz. epileptiform fits, hyperventilation and mutism.

*Sensory symptoms are :*

Deafness, blindness, diplopia (especially monoocular), tubular vision, globus hystericus, pseudo-hallucinations (commonly visual and auditory).

Anaesthesia and paraesthesia at various places, ill-defined pains, headache, dermographia.

*Visceral symptoms include :*

Gastro-intestinal — anorexia, vomiting, aerophagy, bulimia, abdominal fullness, Munchausen syndrome.

Genito-urinary — dyspareunia, amenorrhoea, pseudocyesis, urinary retention.

Others — vertigo

**Dissociation states**

In this situation certain functions of mind or part of personality becomes dissociated from the rest of the mind in presence of overwhelming anxiety. It leads to qualitative changes in the state of consciousness and personal identity. The clinical expression may be any of the following :

Hysterical twilight and trance states
Fugue state
Somnabulism
Hysterical amnesia and agnosia
Automatisms e.g. hysterical mimicing, automatic speech, automatic writing
Hysterical puerilistic behaviour
Multiple personality

## ACUTE HYSTERICAL PSYCHOSIS

Seen commonly in women. The onset is sudden after an episode of marked mental stress. A hysterical personality may act as predisposing factor.

There is panic with overactivity which may lead to violent behaviour towards others or self. Various kinds of delusion, visual and auditory hallucination and depersonalisation may occur. The character of the clinical picture may be determined by culture and race e.g. Amok and Latah in south-east Asia, Imu in the Japanese. Symptoms seldom last more ,than 3-4 weeks and resolve quickly. Relapse may occur.

## HYSTERICAL PERSONALITY DISORDER

It consists of a cluster of personality traits characterised by exhibitionistic and demanding behaviour seeking attention and approval from others. There are egocentricity and emotional dependence with avoidance of closeness in relationship. The temperament is labile and capricious. They may show sexually provocative behaviour but avoid forming a stable relationship. Their marriage usually ends up with marked discord. Some of them tend to attempt suicide impulsively in the face of emotional conflict and also abuse alcohol and drugs. Such personality characteristic is seen more in women.

## OTHER HYSTERICAL SYNDROMES

*St. Louis Hysteria*

**Briquet' Syndrome**

The person exhibits multiple intractable somatic symptoms involving different systems for which no organic cause could be detected. They are mainly young women in their 3rd and 4th decade. Menstrual disorder and frigidity are almost invariable. They dramatise the symptoms and try to manipulate the attending physician. There is usually history of many admissions in hospitals with no significant improvement in their condition. A family occurrence of similar illness is not uncommon.

**Mass Hysteria**

It is an epidemic phenomenon commonly seen in hostels of young women. A predisposing state of apprehension with high emotionality among the inmates having its onset with some incident is observed. Commonly it begins with one girl developing some symptoms such as fainting or falling sick with abdominal pain or exhibiting disturbed behaviour. Sooner similar symptoms rapidly develop in many others. Such state is thought of to result from the combined effect of suggestion and emotional tension.

## MANAGEMENT

The main strategy is to minimise the advantages of sick role. As soon as it is detected, a carefully planned regime of care is needed involving counselling of the relatives and environmental manipulation besides specific attention to the patient. Acute cases respond well to the removal from the stressful situation. Trance and twilight states can be brought to full awareness by powerful sensory stimuli e.g. smell of ammonia. Amnesic patients can be helped by circumstantial talk to lead her into the forgotten period.

Physical examination and laboratory investigations should be completed as fast as possible and thereafter the symptoms are to be ignored if findings are not supportive. Difficulty arises with those having powerful conscious motives for using symptoms. It is wise to avoid discussion of the causation of the symptoms and discourage preoccupation with them, because the patient is very sensitive to doubts of her genuineness. She should not be accused of her lack of desire to get well and instead a firm suggestion of prediction of recovery is desirable. Sometimes it is impossible to distinguish between conscious motivation i.e. malingering and true subconscious motivation to be sick, as the patient's degree of awareness varies from time to time. In resistant cases, the patient should be left with her symptoms if it is found that she has reached some adjustment between it and her life activities. It should also be noted that removal of one symptom may be replaced by another due to not solving the basic anxiety.

*Psychotherapy* — A detailed therapeutic interview is needed to enquire into the nature of the personality stress which causes the patient to take a sick role. The therapy aims at helping the patient to gain insight into her symptoms and her behaviour and to understand the source of anxiety. Individual therapy with classical psychoanalysis or analytic-oriented methods is treatment of choice and may be needed to go on for prolonged period. In some resistant cases having conversion symptom hypnotic suggestion may help.

## ANXIETY STATES

*(Syn : Anxiety Neurosis)*

It is a state of painful uneasiness of mind marked by anticipation and apprehension in absence of an adequate cause. It is the simplest form of neurosis and occupies a central position in psychoneurosis.

### Aetiology

The development may be :

(1) Primary i.e. occurring by itself

(2) Secondary i.e. developing as a reaction to another illness, physical or mental. Although any illness may act as a causative factor, certain systemic diseases are particularly associated, viz. hyperthyroidism, adrenal medullary tumour, rheumatic chorea, organic brain syndrome, premenstrual syndrome.

It is common in persons who are timid, worrysome, dependent, ambitious, sensitive especially to criticism and who are poorly adjusted to social environment. A family history of neurosis or personality disorder may be present. Often the childhood shows neurotic traits like thumb-sucking, nail-biting, fear of darkness, bed-wetting etc.

Psychosocial precipitating factors may be mental stress arising from occupational, financial or family sources or may be triggered by any fearful incidents or by a debilitating illness.

### Clinical features

The onset is usually abrupt. The precipitating cause may not be obvious even to the patient who often focusses on to his symptoms. The manifestations may be grouped as Psychic Anxiety and Somatic Anxiety, but frequently both are present.

### Psychic anxiety

The anxiety is usually vague and free-floating (i.e. not attached to any ideational content). The patient gets feelings of sustained tension, cannot relax and suffers from generalised apprehension worrying almost over everything. He is unable to concentrate, has a feeling of daze or perplexity and is afraid to be alone. The anxious mood is relatively persistent. There is a lack of pleasure in everything he does including his own hobbies. He may find it hard to remember recent events and even immediate recall may be difficult. Sexual desire is inhibited. The patient finds difficulty in falling asleep and gets frightening dreams.

More advanced cases show attacks of weeping, restlessness, aggressive outbursts and syncopal episodes. Acute panic attacks may occur.

## SOMATIC ANXIETY

The anxiety reaction is expressed by way of changes in bodily systems.

**Neuromuscular symptoms** — There is increased tension of voluntary muscles causing aches especially in the muscles of neck, scalp, lower back, legs. Praecordial discomfort may occur due to intercostal muscular tension. The palpebral fissure looks wide, pupils are dilated, fine finger tremor and wringing of hands occur. Tendon reflexes are overactive. Palm is cold and sweaty; speech may be rapid or hesitant or may even show frank stuttering.

**Cardiovascular symptoms** — palpitation, throbbing of neck and head, dyspnoea on effort, pallor and giddiness are commonly seen. The heart rate is increased and blood pressure raised.

**Gastrointestinal symptoms** — includes nausea, vomiting, dysphagia, dyspepsia, epigastric fullness, dry mouth and burning sensation behind sternum. Autonomic responses become brisk, loose or irregular bowel movements occur due to intestinal hypermobility. There is gastric hypersecretion.

**Genitourinary symptoms** — Women may develop amenorrhoea, oligomenorrhoea, dysmenorrhoea. In men, ejaculation praecox or retarda occurs, some may develop erectile disturbances.

### Acute anxiety attack

It may develop *de novo* or as an exacerbation of chronic anxiety. Manifested by abrupt onset of terrifying anxiety lasting minutes to hours accompanied by restlessness, sense of weakness, fainting, dizziness, hyperventilation or choked feeling, palpitation, praecordial discomfort, nausea, vomiting, diarrhoea, tremulousness all over and paresthesias of limbs. A stressful situation commonly predisposes. There is marked activation of autonomic nervous system and adrenal medulla.

### Course and Prognosis

The course may be short-lasting or prolonged. Sometimes the patient may use his symptoms in a purposive way being genuinely unaware of his own motive (hysterical development). In middle and later life depression may superimpose.

Chronic anxiety may result in a state of established tension and if long standing ends up in a state of exhaustion with irritability, weight loss, lack of drive and initiative. Some may develop organ neurosis.

**Treatment**

Cases of anxiety neurosis show a tending for spontaneous recovery, it continues for several months. Analytical psychotherapy is required for recurrent and chronic cases especially if associated personality difficulties are present.

Acute anxiety state and patients with moderate to gross somatic and psychic symptoms will need drug therapy for relief. Drugs reduce the degree of physiological arousal, thereby interrupting the vicious circle of feedback on mental state. Drugs used are as follows :

(a) Barbiturates e.g. amylobarbitone, pentobarbitone, quinalbarbitone.

Medium and short-acting barbiturates can be very effective but in some individuals these become quickly addictive.

(b) Non-barbiturates sedatives e.g. diazepam, lorazepam, nitrazepam, oxazepam, chlordiazepoxide, meprobamate, hydroxyzine (Atarax), chloral hydrate.

Such drugs are generally non-addictive if not used for long periods.

(c) Neuroleptics in lower dosage may be effective singly or alongside other group of drugs. There are trifluperazine, fluphenazine, prochlorperazine, thioridazine, haloperidal.

Acute severe panic attacks respond to diazepam 10—20 mg or amylobarbitone given by parenteral route.

Drugs may also be needed for superimposed depression. Muscle pain and aches are treated by physiotherapy.

Psychological management includes simple confident reassurance that the symptoms are not results of any underlying physical illness. Discussion of problem related to precipitating causes may be helpful to allay excessive anxiety. Some patients may be advised removal from adverse circumstances temporarily. Less severe cases should be advised to continue work unless it is a factor contributing to the anxiety. Physical exercise and recreation are useful. Sometimes abreaction under pentothal is useful if traumatic psychological events precipitate or if there are pent-up emotions.

## PHOBIC NEUROSIS

A phobia is a special form of fear where the anxiety is out of proportion to the demands of the situation, is beyond voluntary control and cannot be reasoned away leading to avoidance behaviour (Marks). The feared situation or object is usually limited to one but may extend to many. A history of past similar frightening experience is common. The fact that normal persons do not develop anxiety with such objects or situations adds to the anxiety, though the patient maintains recognition of no actual danger. The illness is always disabling as many such phobic objects and situations are of common occurrence. A family history of phobia may be present.

Psychoanalytic theories suggest that a phobia is symbolic of some idea or object ,or situation which is displaced by unconscious mechanisms to the phobic content.

**Clinical features**

Phobias are classified as :

1. Agoraphobia (phobic anxiety)
2. Specific phobia of animals or objects
3. Specific situational phobia
4. Hypochondriacal phobia.

**Agoraphobia**

Seen commonly in females in their 2nd and 3rd decade. A neurotic trait is common is childhood.

The onset is sudden with the fear developing in a specific situation which is perpetuated. The situation may be excessive anxiety in going out of the house or to open spaces or to crowded places or to closed spaces like cinema halls. Any attempt to face the situation leads to panic which is relieved within minutes or leaving the feared situation.

During acute anxiety, there may be dizziness, hyperventilation, fainting, tachycardia and such other somatic symptoms of anxiety. In the intervening period, a state of mild to moderate generalised tension may prevail. The illness may perpetuate for years with a fluctuating course and occasionally may go into complete remission.

**Specific Animal Phobia**

It commonly begins in childhood and early adolescence.

The onset is sudden, usually in relation to a specific event in which fear is involved. The phobic object is limited to some animals of commonly place e.g. dog, cat, lizard, cow, etc. or insects e.g. spiders, cockroaches etc. or even their body parts viz. horns of cow, teeth of dog, legs of spider etc. Most children recover spontaneously as they grow older but in some it may persist into adult life.

**Specific situational phobia**

This type of illness may make its appearance any time during late childhood and early adult life.

The anxiety provoking experience is restricted to some specific situations or places e.g. heights, water pools, darkness, thunderstorm etc. There is manifestation of anxiety when the patient is away from the feared situation but sometimes incapacity by way of anticipation of facing the situation may occur. The illness may persist for many years.

**Social phobia**

It is common in males and develops during adolescence. In some situations there is occurrence of anticipating anxiety or excessive sensitivity with the thought that people will watch his behaviour critically or discuss about him e.g. in parties, in resturants, while participating in games. The anxiety is relieved quickly as soon as the person avoids the situation.

**Hypochondriacal phobia**

It is also known as illness phobia. There is anticipatory fear of developing dysfunction or disease of bodily organs or even mental functions e.g. of blindness, of losing consciousness, of dying in sleep, loss of memory, of going mad, of constipation, of impotence, of pain in intercourse in women, of unwanted pregnancy, of having a deformed baby etc. All such fears lead to behavioural changes in the person which may cause problems of adaptation.

**Treatment of phobic neurosis**

The treatment of choice is behaviour therapy along with psychotherapy. Relaxation and desensitisation methods are useful. Psychotherapy helps if there are intrapsychic conflicts and adjustment problems.

Tranquilizers and sedatives help to minimise generalised anxiety especially if interfering with daily life.

## OBSESSIONAL NEUROSIS

It is a type of neurotic illness where there is persistent appearance in the mind of an idea or impulse or feeling and/or an irresistible urge to do an act with subjective sense of compulsion (i.e. against own wish) overriding an internal resistance. The affected person recognises the idea or the act as illogical and any effort by him to resist these leads to anxiety. The greater the endeavour to dispel the thought or action, more stubbornly it comes back.

The sense of compulsion distinguishes it from preoccupation.

### Aetiology

A familial incidence is common. The personality of the individual is usually characterised by lack of flexibility, perfectionistic tendencies, social introversion. The intelligence is generally average or somewhat superior.

Not uncommonly the illness may develop as an early manifestation of an underlying depressive illness, schizophrenia, dementia, brain injury.

### Psychopathology

Psychoanalytic views regard the illness, as a result of fixation in anal stage of psychosexual development. The ideas and impulses are symbolic expression of unconscious aggressive or sexual desire. The compulsive acts are promoted by the unconscious mechanism to counteract such wishes which one recognises as undesirable. The repetitive acts are designed by the person privately in fashion not understandable by others. When such acts are done is a set order it is called ritualistic. Such acts are done to a standard of righteousness to achieve relief from anxiety. The resistance is from the healthy part of the personality where the symptoms are recognised as abnormal.

### Clinical features

The illness is common in 15-40 age group and the incidence decreases with age. It is frequent in women.

The symptoms may take the form of :

A. **Obsessive thinking** — This may occur as ideas, or ruminations or impulses or doubts or fears.

B. **Obsessive acts** — Occur as organised behaviour with or without associated ideas.

**Obsessive ideas** — It is persistent occurrence in one's mind of an unwelcome and distressing thought which may be related to any topic but commonly obscene or aggressive or religious or philosophical in nature. The inability to free himself from such thoughts may lead a person to commit suicide.

**Obsessive impulses** — This is based on ideation leading to irresistible urge to do or actual performance of some acts which may be aggressive, sexual or self-punitive in form.

**Obsessive ruminations** — There are inconclusive circling of certain thoughts with marked exclusion of other interests. The topic may relate to reality matters or it may consist of bizarre ideas e.g. of creation, of religion, of scientific matters, of some numbers or phrases etc.

**Obsessive doubts** — May relate to some ideas or actions which are done and undone in repeated fashion. The patient cannot away from the anxiety situation and carries on the ideas or acts until she makes her own decision to stop when her own standard of rightness is reached.

**Obsessive phobias** — In such condition the fear is not of any object or situation but of the presumed consequences of facing it, viz possible use of sharp instruments against somebody.

**Obsessive compulsive acts** — This state is characterised by compulsion to perform some repetitive acts with or without associated mental activity. The latter may consist of some ideas which may be aggressive or sexual in nature or some phrases or numbers which have some special meaning to the person. The compulsive motor behaviour is an irresistible urge to do certain repetitive acts which reduce the anxiety experienced by the patient. The acts may look simple and meaningless e.g. counting numbers, repeating steps, doing and undoing like bolting door or handwashing. As the patient recognises the irrationality of such acts which is of mild degree may be done in privacy. If questioned the patient may admit the purposelessness of such acts or may offer some irrational excuse to cover up embarrassment. If on marked degree, he may show irritability and even hostile reaction if questioned or teased about his obsessional behaviour due to his own helplessness in the face of overpowering compulsion.

A large percentage of patients become chronic especially those with personality predisposition. If the symptoms are of mild degree, they manage to adapt socially and occupationally though with reduced efficiency. Spontaneous episodic remission occurs, complete recovery is seen usually in symptomatic cases with treatment of underlying malady.

In *de novo* cases, the prognosis is unfavourable if onset in young age and early adults and introverted personality, if the person is unmarried, history of neurotic traits in childhood, if symptoms develop after organic brain disease, if associated mood disorder, it severely disturbed clinical manifestations, if symptoms used for hysterical gain and if there is reluctance to accept help. Generally prognosis is better if the illness is of short duration and if there is precipitation by mental stress.

**Treatment of Obsessional Neurosis**

The outcome of treatment of obsessive neurosis depends greatly on how early the patient comes to the doctor. Obsessive symptoms when they develop without any obvious precipitating causes may have poor prognosis. Obsession when it is manifestation of underlying an mental illness, should be searched for and treated. Some patients respond well to antidepressant drugs even when evidence of depressive illness is not present. ECT may be used if there is suicidal risk. If there is much anxiety minor tranquilizers are helpful.

**Psychotherapy** — Many cases are benefited by simple supportive measures. Discussion helps if symptoms are related to emotional conflict. At times a period of complete environmental change breaks the compulsive rituals and increases the resistance to symptoms.

Formal psychoanalysis is done in deep-seated personality problems; aided by the therapist the fears and complexes take a new meaning and reduce indecision and guilt.

**Behaviour therapy** — It helps to reduce rituals and anxiety where the symptoms are not so pervasive. Various methods used are relaxation, deconditioning and implosion.

**Prefrontal leucotomy** — Indicated in refractory cases where conservative treatment produces no effect resulting in chronic incapacity

## PSYCHOSOMATIC ILLNESS

It is an approach to illnesses where psychological factors are found to contribute significantly and demonstrably to an organic illness either in its causation (psychosomatic sequence) or in its perpetuation (somatopsychic sequence). It can be possible that any illness can have psychosomatic aspects which provide a basic link between psychiatry and other branches of medical sciences.

**Pathogenesis**

The inappropiate propagation of psychophysiologic abnormalities in certain body organs or systems to stress is aimed at adaptation to or protection from stress. However, there is failure to maintain homeostasis with resultant illness. In most instance, the stress is internal being caused by an inner conflict which is interpreted on the basis of personality and relevant past life experiences. An external stress may also be associated in some cases.

**Neurohumoral mechanisms**

The cerebral areas like the hypothalamus, limbic system and reticular activating systems are shown to have a role in the physiologic expression of emotion. The peripheral pathways are, however, not clearly understood. An excess production of anti-diuretic hormone and corticosteroids has been demonstrated.

**Psychopathologic views**

Various theories have been forwarded to explain the development of pathology in body organs. Those commonly believed include :

(i) Specific body organ or system is sensitised in early life by physical trauma along with certain accompanying emotions;

(ii) Certain kinds of mental conflict cause disturbed function of specific organs;

(iii) Some types of personality profile, e.g. ambitious, competitive, conscientious, perfectionistic etc. are particularly vulnerable;

(iv) Constitutional susceptibility of some body organs e.g. stomach, lungs, to stress;

(v) An inherent tendency to respond somatically to stress.

Thus, even though genetic or constitutional predisposition is evident, multiple forces like heredity, biologic, emotional and social factors operate at a given time to produce and perpetuate the illness.

**Clinical manifestations**

The onset may be sudden but commonly there is a gradual build-up. Sometimes a temporal relationship can be observed between an overt external stress and the beginning of the illness.

The illness involves organs which have no voluntary control. There is no associated symptom of psychoneurosis but a psychosomatic illness may be replaced by a frank neurosis or psychosis spontaneously or during treatment.

The malady commonly runs a phasic course. In some cases a phenomenon of syndrome shift occurs, i.e., replacement of one form of illness by another, viz. bronchial asthma is improved, followed by development of eczema. A list of commonly recognised psychosomatic diseases is presented below :

| | | |
|---|---|---|
| Gastrointestinal | — | Peptic ulcer, ulcerative colitis |
| Respiratory | — | Bronchial asthma, hyperventilation syndrome |
| Cardivoascular | — | Effort syndrome, paroxysmal sinus tachycardia, some cases of benign hypertension and ischaemic heart disease. Raynaud's disease. |
| Genitourinary | — | Dysmenorrhoea, amenorrhoea, dysparunia, impotence |
| Neurological | — | Migraine, recurrent vertigo, |
| Dermatological | | Atopic eczema, neurodermatitis, psoriasis, rosacea, urticaria, alopecia areata, |
| Metabolic | — | Obesity (some cases). |

**Diagnosis**

It is mandatory to carry out proper physical investigations to determine the nature and degree of the pathological process of the affected organ or system.

Psychiatric and psychological assessment should then follow with a view to correlate evolution of the physical disease with factors. Serial psychiatric interviews to elucidate personality functioning and development, ways of adaptation to life situations, stress handling, interpersonal relationships etc. are necessary. Psychological study includes psychometric measurements of personality, degree of neuroticism etc.

**Treatment of psychosomatic illness**

The key factor influencing the management of psychosomatic disorders is a well-meaning doctor/patient relationship. This will enable the physician to have a full understanding of the psychological factors by virtue of getting the confidence of the patient with frank discussion and exploration of emotional problems. The patients with psychosomatic illness are often reluctant to consider that their physical symptoms could be of psychological origin. The doctor should be interested, get the trust of the patient and be not unduly sympathetic but provide an image of assurance. With such behaviour he should encourage the patient to express freely stresses and problems which will enable him to accept the probable underlying psychological causative factors.

It is important that treatment must follow complete physical investigation and necessary medical treatment for symptomatic relief. If psychotherapy becomes successful. it will be possible to reduce or even discontinue the drugs.

Psychotherapeutic approach is aimed at tackling the basic anxiety. The form of psychotherapy depends on the nature of the psychological factors causing the psychopathology and the type of disorder. Ventilation aimed at releasing aggression may benefit the hypertensives and asthmatics. Cases of ulcerative colitis benefit from abreactive sessions under narcotic drug. In some cases hypnosis may be useful. Cases with marked personality disorder will need formal analytical psychotherapy. Any concomitant depression or anxiety may need drug treatment. Discussion with relatives and taking care of environmental factors are essential especially if there are inter-personal difficulties with other members of the family. Prolonged psychotherapy may be needed to prevent relapse.

## ALCOHOLISM

The term is applied to excessive drinkers whose dependence on alcohol is of such degree as to show noticeable impairment of bodily and mental health, social and economic functioning and thus requires treatment.

The illness is symptomatic of personality disturbance, the major cause of which is unclear parental role during growing up period causing ego functions to develop inadequately. Most patients have inadequate or sometimes aggressive personality. There is lack of development of a stable superego as a consequence of poor identification process during personality development. The person has a strong need to boost ego for whichhe uses alcohol. A latent homosexuality may also contribute leading to poor heterosexual adjustment. Alcoholic drinking has also been explained on the basis of learning theories where the pleasant sensation caused by alcohol reinforces the drinking habit.

### Characteristics of manifestations

The peak incidence is in the 3rd and 4th decade. Recently, however, some younger alcoholics are coming into prominence. The illness is common in males. The development of alcoholism is also influenced by the culture, race, availability and the society's attitude to drinking.

### Pathological drinking patterns

Various drinking characteristics have been identified and were grouped with the object of identifying alcoholic behaviour and for **prognostic application. Alcoholic drinking** can be primary or secondary. Lellinek has grouped primary alcoholic drinking as follows :

- alpha type — Characterised by sustained psychological dependence on alcohol, ability of tolerance of alcohol is usually high and there is no loss of control of the amount consumed at one episode of drinking, ability to abstain remains.
- beta type — they show no dependence physical or psychological but existence of physical complications is common.
- gamma type — loss of control over drinking is the predominant feature although they may exhibit periods of abstinence. Common in spirit drinkers.
- delta type — they can exercise control over the quantity consumed but cannot abstain because of physical dependence. They show no socially disruptive behaviour.
- epsilon type — also called dipsomaniacs or periodical or bout drinkers. The characteristics are phases of marked drinking of sudden onset without any precipitating cause alternating with periods of total abstinence or normal social drinking.

### Secondary or symptomatic alcoholism

The behaviour becomes oriented around alcohol intake and arises out of some mental stress. It can also be a symptom manifestation of mental illness, viz. :

Neurotic — seen in depression, anxiety states and phobic neurosis

Psychotic — manic-depressive psychosis, schizophrenia, organic brain syndrome.

Other types of mental illness like pathological grief reaction and personality disorder may be manifested by abnormal drinking behaviour.

**Acute Alcohol Intoxication**

Psychological changes — show disinhibited social behaviour, occasional angry outbursts or easily irritated. Some shows withdrawal behaviour, others may do deliberate self-harm (DSH) or genuine suicidal attempts.

**Pathological intoxication**

It is seen following a bout of considerable alcohol intake. The person exhibits profound emotional disturbance like rage or despair with dramatic suddenness and may behave in an aggressive fashion or shows destructiveness or make suicidal attempts. He is not amenable to reasons, looks dazed or confused and has total amnesia for the period which may last from few minutes to hours followed by a phase of prolonged sleep. Such state is presumed to be due to a direct toxic action of alcohol on the brain in individual with probable underlying cerebral damage or dysfunction. A possibility of its being a form of psychomotor epilepsy triggered by alcohol has been forwarded. Such alcoholic behaviour is also common in psychopathic and emotionally unstable personality.

**Alcohol withdrawal effects**

There are a conglomeration of bodily symptoms resulting from sudden stoppage of alcohol intake. The onset is usually between 4 and 8 hours and reaches peak by 24 to 36 hours. Seen in sensors with strong physical dependence. The manifestations are :

A. Physical e.g. :

Neurological — Tremulousness of limbs, ataxia, general asthenia, sweating

G.I. — anorexia, nausea

C.V. — tachycardia.

B. Psychological e.g. :

Anxiety reaction, insomnia, confusional state which may proceed to delirium, craving for alcohol, hallucinations, epileptiform seizures.

**Complications of alcoholism**

Psychiatric —

Acute alcoholic intoxication
Pathological intoxication
Alcoholic coma
Alcohol withdrawal syndrome
Chronic alcoholic hallucinosis
Alcoholic deterioration of dementia (Alcoholic pseudo-paresis)

Korsakoff psychosis
Alcoholic paranoia

Physical —

A. Neurological — Peripheral neuropathy
Hepatic encephalopathy
Alcoholic myopathy
Cranial neuropathy

Marchiafava Bignami disease
Cerebellar cortical degeneration
Central pontine myelinolysis
Wernicke's encephalopathy

B. G.I. Acute hepatic necrosis
Cirrhosis of liver and portal hypertension
Chronic gastritis
Pancreatitis

C. Cardiovascular – Alcoholic cardiomyopathy

The term 'chronic alcoholism' is applied to persons with final stage of damage both physical and mental with effects of alcohol.

## TREATMENT OF ALCOHOLISM

The initiation of an alcoholic into treatment regime includes two segmental parts. The first job is effective abstinence and detoxification of the body systems of alcohol. Once this is achieved, which usually requires 3 to 5 weeks, the management proper of the disease process begins.

**Detoxification or 'drying out'** –

Institutionalisation is essential for efficient medical management and also to enable the patient to save himself succumbing to further drinking which happens due to an increased craving for alcohol. Stoppage of drinking is total and sudden and withdrawal symptoms needs to be controlled. Intensive care is necessary to combat fluid and electrolyte imbalance, for adequate nutrition and vitamin therapy mainly with B-complex group. Neurological symptoms of abstinence are tackled with properly judged doses of non-barbiturate hypnotics. Barbiturates are used for severe symptoms as it is of the same group as alcohol so far as addiction is concerned. Anticonvulsants are used for epileptic fits. Adequate sedation is necessary.

**Management of alcohol dependence**

The aim is to give up all addictive compounds besides alcohol itself. The most difficult part of therapy is to enable the patient to accept that he is unable to control his drinking. To moralise him may induce self-reproach and increases risk of suicide or may provoke hostile reactions. Total abstinence for the rest of his life is imperative, once the established stage is reached.

Alcoholism can also be symptomatic of a background illness, neurotic or psychotic or it is sometimes a reaction to situational stress, all these need to be excluded or treated.

**Psychotherapy** – Supportive form of treatment with analytic orientation helps in many cases. Discussion is done about his anxieties, personality functioning and inter-personal difficulties. Explanation and clarification is given to make the patient understand his reactions to life situation and use of alcohol. Practical guidance may be required to widen activities and interests. Counselling of spouse and immediate relatives helps to reduce family tension. Orthodox psychoanalysis not often practicable because of patient's inherent instability. Recently group psychotherapy is becoming popular as it gives greater degree of insight and motivation.

Voluntary bodies like Alcoholics Anonymous help recovered alcoholics to avoid relapses by providing psychological assistance at times of emotional crisis and/or impending drinking. It also gives a feeling of belonging to people of similar difficulties.

**Behaviour therapy**

Aversion treatment with apomorphine or emetine produces a conditional aversion mechanism so that the experience of vomiting produces aversion to alcohol. Use of antialcohol drugs, e.g. disulfirum acts as a deterrent and is used useful in suitably motivated patients as an adjunct form of treatment.

# ORGANIC BRAIN SYNDROMES

## *Acute Organic Brain Syndrome*

This is a clinical condition arising from dysfunction of brain developing rapidly and is potentially reversible.

The cardinal manifestation is disturbances of the state of consciousness. The term 'consciousness' is defined as a state of full awareness with intact functioning of sensorium whereby the person is able to comprehend his environment and reflect upon it. The malfunctioning in acute brain syndrome extends from diminished alertness to a state of coma. It involves all mental functions in both receptive and effector side. The grades of such disturbances in order of severity are as follows :-

(1) Confusional states
 (a) Twilight states
 (b) Fugue states
 (c) Trance states
(2) Delirious states
 (a) Subacute
 (b) Acute
(3) Stupor
(4) Coma

Distinction between earlier grades may be qualitative and may not be distinct.

## AETIOLOGY

A host of conditions have a causative role. These can be grouped as follows :-

(1) **Infective**
 (a) Cerebral infections – encephalitis, meningitis
 (b) Systemic infections causing bacteraemia or toxaemia
(2) Chemical intoxications, viz, with lead, carbon monoxide, alcohol, cannabis, narcotic drugs.
(3) Head injury
(4) Metabolic causes – uraemia, hypoglycaemia, diabetes mellitus, vitamin $B_{12}$ deficiency, porphyria, hepatic failure, hypothalassaemia.
(5) Circulatory disturbances in the brain, viz., transient ischaemic attack, cerebral thrombosis, vertebro-basilar insufficiency.
(6) Cerebral space occupying lesions.
(7) Miscellaneous – after child birth, after major surgical operation, after epileptic fit.

### Clinical features

### Confusional states

The patient looks anxious, bewildered, irritable and displays emotional liability. Stimuli from outside do not create normal perception. Inaccurate and incomplete attention causes lack of elimination of irrelevant sensory experiences causing illusionary and hallucinatory phenomenon. There is reduced capacity of thinking with customary pace. Secondary delusions may occur as a result of abnormal sensory experiences.

### Twilight states

It is a dreamy state caused by altered consciousness. In such a condition a person can do a normal conversation or perform acts of varying complexity about which there is no subsequent recollection. The condition is usually short-lasting.

**Fugue state**

The person may behave as completely normal. If of recent onset, he may be agitated and disoriented. Characteristically, there is impulse to wander off with no apparent relation to previous activities. Subsequent amnesia is usual. It is commonly seen in epileptics.

**Trance state**

It is a mental state where there is narrowing of the field of consciousness with all attention focussed on some phenomenon of one's own mind. In cases of lesser intensity interaction with environment occurs like that of an absent-minded person.

**Subacute Delirious State**

The features of confusional state are present in this condition with the difference that there is fluctuation in the level of awareness with short intervening periods of lucidity and accessibility. There is fragmentation of perception and actions. Thought incoherence is less bizarre. The patient may realise his own disturbances at times. The condition may go on for days to weeks.

**Delirium**

There is rapid onset of confusion and bewilderment with motor restlessness. The patient exhibits fluctuating emotions ranging from apprehension to panic. Phases of calmness may develop spontaneously. There are tremor and stereotype preservation movements. Repetitive talks may occur as a result of thoughts. Sleep rhythm is altered.

## CHRONIC ORGANIC BRAIN SYNDROME (Dementia)

The term denotes deterioration of intellectual, cognitive, affective and memory functions, the severity of all of which may vary in proportion and degree being caused by brain tissue dysfunction. Some structural changes in brain are always present but there are no necessarily irreversible.

## AETIOLOGY

1. Infective — G.P.I., post-encephalitis changes.
2. Chemical — Lead encephalopathy, chronic alcoholism.
3. Metabolic — Myxoedema, pernicious anaemia, recurrent hypoglycaemia. Wilson's disease.
4. Traumatic — After head injury, punch drunkenness (in boxers).
5. Degenerative — Presenile dementias, viz. Pick disease, Alzheimer's disease, Huntington's chorea, senile dementia, Parkinsonism, cerebellar atrophy, Friederick's ataxia, normal pressure hydrocephalus.
6. Neoplastic — Cerebral space — occupying lesions especially of frontal lobe, corpus callosum and third ventricle, carcinomatous encephalopathy.
7. Vascular — Arteriosclerotic dementia (also called multi-infarct dementia).
8. Miscellaneous — Epilepsy of long duration.

**Clinical description**

It varies according to premorbid personality.

**Memory disturbances**

It is usually the earliest manifestation of dementing process. Memory for recent events is most affected and such disability may cause considerable anxiety. Some persons may effectively adjust to it by keeping diary etc. or may use compensatory ways to cover up.

**Cognitive impairment**

Disorientation as regards to time, place and person results from both memory impairment and reduced sensory perception. In several cases personal orientation may also be impaired or lost.

**Intellectual deterioration**

Early cases show weakening of intellectual grasp, subjective feeling or not being able to think clearly, difficulty in formulating abstracts, difficulty in concentration and diminished learning ability. Later on, slow, and ill-defined thinking becomes apparent in speech incoherence. Judgement becomes impaired causing inability to make even small decisions and tendency to commit social indiscretions.

**Affective charges**

Disproportionate emotional reactions may be prominent. Such capricious emotions may add to social maladjustment or contribute to character changes. Advanced cases show shallow or unresponsive emotions or fatuous euphoria.

All the above changes lead to behaviour disorder the nature of which is determined by degree of diminished cortical control and by the nature of premorbid personality. Development of new kind of abnormal behaviour pattern, e.g. alcohol abuse, promiscuity, aggressive behaviour, lying, stealing etc. in an elderly should always arouse suspicion of an underlying dementing process.

In some, psychotic symptoms may develop as delusions and hallucinations.

Individual cases may include some characteristic mental and physical features of underlying disease process, e.g. brain tumour, G.P.I.

**Special Investigations**

These include — EEG, computerised tomography (C/T) scan and biochemical investigations, all of which have a relevant role in finding the cause of dementia.

**Treatment of acute organic illness**

Success of management depends upon quick and vigorous investigation of underlying physical illness, its detection and correction. In elderly cases, urinary tract infection and vitamin deficiency are to be searched for. In suspected head injury appropriate emergency surgical procedure brings quick recovery. If the physical malady is reversible, mental improvement is rapid and complete.

Intensive nursing is required during delirious states with attention to feeding, dressing, toilet care. Patient is to be nursed in a separate room. Medical management may be needed for dehydration, to restore electrolyte balance and to combat vitamin deficiency and infection. Specific treatment should be given for underlying physical illness. Contact with surroundings by way of allowing relatives to visit and by means of radio. Television will ensure necessary sensory stimulation.

Disturbed and overactive patients will need tranquilizers and sedatives which may help to administer medical aid. Chlorpromazine is the drug of choice; other drugs like thioridazine, prochlorperazine are also used. In very severe cases, e.g. those with frightening hallucinations, short acting barbiturates and benzadiazepines by I.M. route may be needed. Long acting barbiturates, e.g. phenobarbitone are best avoided as they often aggravate confession.

**Treatment of chronic organic brain syndrome**

Though a dementing illness is a progressive condition, the social and intellectual usefulness of the patient should be tried to be kept at best functioning condition. Environmental therapy should include meaningful activity in daily behaviours with rapport with surroundings. Nursing care is aimed to help the patient develop own feeding, dressing and toilet habits, participation with environmental and family activities, viz. listening to radio, watching T.V., talking to family members and relations. Guidance and explanation of patient's behaviour helpful to family members in this matter. Encouragement of previous intellectual habits, e.g. looking up the newspaper, reading magazines is necessary. Physical activities like taking a stroll, care for garden help to keep the patient healthy. In hospitals this is done by occupational and recreational therapy.

There is no specific drug therapy for dementia. Certain cerebral metabolic activators, e.g. hydergine (Sandoz) piracetam has been claimed recently as beneficial in such conditions. Cerebral vasodilators are of dubious value. High doses vitamin B is thought of to ensure nutrition to existing functioning neurones. Use tranquilizers e.g. phenothiazines, haloperidol for disturbed social and moral behaviour or to control irritability and aggressiveness but be careful not to oversedate the person. Associated depression may need appropriate medication. Underlying process may sometimes need treatment to help the progress of the disease and control intercurrent infection, metabolic abnormalities like diabetes and hypertension, if any.

# CHAPTER – 12
# NEUROLOGY

## INTRODUCTION TO NEUROLOGY

*G.C. MOOKERJEE*

Neurology has greatly advanced during the last two decades due to newer methods of investigations and development of newer neurosurgical techniques. It is no more an anatomical and physical jigsaw puzzle in making a diagnosis but today much can be done for the patient who is neurologically affected due to acute subacute or chronic disorders.

However, good knowledge of anatomy and physiology still remains very important, without which correct diagnosis is not possible. No doubt, neurology is a highly specialised branch of medicine like cardiology yet general practitioners must have reasonable knowledge of common neurological disorders like cerebro-vascular accidents (CVA), meningitis, head injury, epilepsy, migraine, Parkinsonism, peripheral neuritis and demyelinating diseases. In many situations, neuro-physicians' or neuro-surgeons' help will be necessary, while multidisciplinary approach will be required for cerebral palsy, muscular dystrophies and chronically disabled subjects. Neurosurgeon, Neuro-physician, reconstructive surgeon, physiotherapists, occupational therapist and psychiatrists will often be necessary to help the neurologically crippled subjects. It is the general practitioner who should be the family consultant for co-ordination and proper economy.

There is no point for an epileptic to go to a neurologist just to repeat the prescription of phenobarbitone, dilantin sodium or even valproate. The initial investigations and diagnosis of a case of convulsion may be required by a specialist in neurology. Similarly a case of CVA during the acute stage needs advice of a specialist but the after-care and rehabilitation is the job of the family doctor with the help of a physical medicine unit. Diagnosis of poliomyelitis does not require even to be confirmed by a neurologist but its after-care, i.e. rehabilitation requires efficient co-ordination of physiotherapist, physical medicine specialist and orthopaedic surgeon. Once the diagnosis of migraine is settled, it is the family doctor who should continue the case from youth to middle age, possibly by then migraine may gradually disappear on its own. It is the so-called G.P. (of good old days) or basic doctor (family physicians modern times) who is the single most important person for these problems.

Therefore, students and practitioners must try to learn the principles of neurology and not shun the chapter being difficult and complicated, hence leave it for the neurologist.

Brain and its peripheral connections constitute the nervous system, which consists of millions of neurons with multimillion connections like complex electronic circuits.

Function of these complex circuits as well as the master organ "Brain" itself easily suffers damage due to anoxia, hypoxia, metabolic damage, lack of blood supply, toxic agents, tissue poisons and various infective processes which may be intracranial or extracranial. For example coma may be due to C.V.A., cerebral oedema, brain tumour, renal failure, organophosphorus poisoning, typhoid fever, endocrine failure (e.g. myxoedema or Sheehan's syndrome) or post-epileptic states.

On the other hand, myocardial infarction or respiratory failure may produce similar disturbances of consciousness.

Organic brain disorders may lead to psychiatric symptoms and if not carefully evaluated the patient may be stamped as 'mental disorder' whereas an organic lesion may be missed.

Before the patient is examined it is necessary to take the full present and past history of the case. Family history is also very important in neurology as genetic faults may run in families.

Neurological examination of a patient demands thorough knowledge of anatomy and physiology of the nervous system. Laboratory tests and special investigations e.g. **radiography**, E.E.G., radioisotopic scanning or C—T scan (computerised tomography) have not replaced clinical examination but some or all of these tests are required in some cases. In most cases, history taking and clinical examination, blood tests and CSF studies will settle the diagnosis.

All headaches or attacks of syncope and fits do not require C—T scan, so it is stressed that chief diagnostic method in neurology is good history taking and meticulous clinical examination. Methodical approach and meticulous history taking of the patient presenting with neurological problem is most important in arriving at a **clinical diagnosis.**

Central nervous system controls higher functions such as **emotion**, desire, memory, orientation and speech, besides controlling volitional action, and involuntary movements. All voluntary movements are carried out by 'prime movers' assisted by **synergists**, co-ordinated by antagonists on a background of proper tone and posture of particular group of muscles. To the physiologists, tone is synonymous with the stretch reaction of stretch reflex but to the physician tone means the resistance offered by the muscle to passive movement.

Tone and posture depends on monosynaptic reflex arc. It consists of afferent and efferent pathways with the synapses at posterior horn cells. The afferent fibres enter the cord by a posterior nerve root and communicates directly or via a chain of neurons to the anterior horn cells. Efferent fibres arise from anterior horn cells. A lesion anywhere along this path will cause loss of the reflex and thus helps in localisation of lesion. The common monosynaptic tendon reflexes are :

Supinator jerk ($C_5$); the biceps jerk ($C_6$), triceps jerk ($C_{6\text{-}7}$); the knee jerk ($L_{3\text{-}4}$); the ankle jerk ($S_1$).

Polysynaptic reflexes are superficial reflexes and the important reflexes are abdominals ($T_{7\text{-}12}$) cremasteric, ($L_{1\text{-}2}$); the anal reflex ($S_{4\text{-}5}$).

The corneal reflex is important, for which **afferent** is trigeminal (V nerve) and the efferent path is facial nerve (VII nerve).

## Nervous control of Bladder and Rectum

Bladder is controlled by sympathetic ($L_{1\text{-}2}$) via inferior hypogastric plexus and hypogastric nerves. Sympathetic nerves act by relaxing the bladder wall while the sphincter is contracted. Parasympathetic supply ($S_{2\text{-}4}$) comes via the pelvic nerve which contracts the bladder wall and relaxes the internal sphincter. Somatic nerve supply ($S_{2\text{-}4}$) enters via the pudendal nerve which contracts external sphincter of the urethra. Sacral reflex arc for bladder consists of afferent path from the bladder wall (pelvic nerves) and efferent path via parasympathetic fibres. **Distended** bladder empties automatically when distension reaches a certain level. This mechanism operates in the **newborn** and infants. Similar mechanism comes to play when the sacral afferent path is destroyed as in tabes dorsalis. It leads to loss of bladder sensation, resulting in overflow incontinence. Damage to efferent path (anterior sacral nerve roots) causes atonic bladder without loss of sensations (lower motor **neuron type**).

Similarly, rectum is also supplied both by sympathetic and parasympathetic fibres arising from higher sacral segments. Acute lesions particularly of sacral segments results in incontinence of stool. In adults as well as in children both bladder and rectum come under the influence of inhibitory and **facilitatory** fibres from higher centres in the cerebral cortex.

Cerebral control inhibits the automatic reflex mechanism of infancy. Both evacuation of rectum and micturition process become a voluntary act.

Spinal cord lesion above 2,3,4 damaging inhibitory fibres cause urgency, precipitancy or incontinence of urine, while damage to facilitatory fibres may result in hesitancy or retention.

In cerebral lesion, there may be retention or incontinence at the beginning but urinary symptoms recover with the recovery of cerebral lesion. Bladder sensation is usually normal but the capacity is reduced and there is precipitancy. With frontal lobe lesions there may be evacuation problems or incontinence of bowel and bladder associated with the intellectual disturbance.

Higher spinal lesions or chronic pontine lesions of chronic type causes tonic contraction of rectal sphincter and result in constipation.

**Extrapyramidal system :**

The extrapyramidal system consists of masses of grey matter scattered from cortex to medulla, which send down descending tracts to influence function of lower motor neurons and lower interneurons. These masses of grey matter are :

(1) Basal ganglia including corpus striatum (putamen and caudate nucleus), globus pallidus (pallidum)

(2) Substantia nigra (pigmented area)

(3) Subthalamic nucleus (reticular formation)

These scattered masses of grey matter are scattered in the white matter and are richly interconnected with optic thalamus and with the spinal motor cells through extrapyramidal tracts. Proper function of the extrapyramidal tract is not clearly understood. However, the extrapyramidal system may be regarded as a functional system with three layers of integration.

1) Cortical.

2) Striatal (basal ganglia)

3) Tegmental (brain stem reticular formation)

Descending spinal pathways (both inhibitory and facilitatory) receive fibres from cortical areas, basal ganglia, anterior cerebellum and vestibular nuclei. The exact anatomy of these tracts is still not clearly established.

Increased excitability of excitatory (facilitatory) fibres leads to increased excitability of the post-synaptic cells on which the fibres terminate and that of latter leads to a decreased excitability.

The extrapyramidal system requires an adequate inflow of information mostly from brainstem, reticular formation for proper control over spinal segments for stretch reflexes. It is dominantly from this region that descending tracts take origin. Brainstem and reticular formation also receive collateral branches from ascending sensory pathways.

Afferent fibres to the basal ganglia come from motor cortex, parietal lobe, auditory, visual cortex, cerebellum and also from vestibular and posterior columns.

As already mentioned volitional act (willed movement) is carried out by activation of prime-mover muscles (LMN). Large or small anterior horn cells lead to activation of these muscles. This is under direct control of pyramidal system, i.e. Upper Motor Neuron (UMN).

Fully co-ordinated movements of any limb or part of a limb or a group of muscles depend on :

(1) Normal cerebral function i.e. initiating process of willed organised action.

(2) Intact pyramidal tracts

(3) The basal ganglia and extrapyramidal system with its scattered grey matters.

(4) Sensory impulses sending continuous flow of information about orientation, posture and position of body and limbs.

(5) Cerebellar non-sensory **afferent** input.

The pyramidal tract has its contribution but extrapyramidal out-flow-tracts e.g. reticulospinal **and rubrospinal tracts have their important contribution in performing co-ordinated as well as** complicated motor activities.(Fig. 12.1)

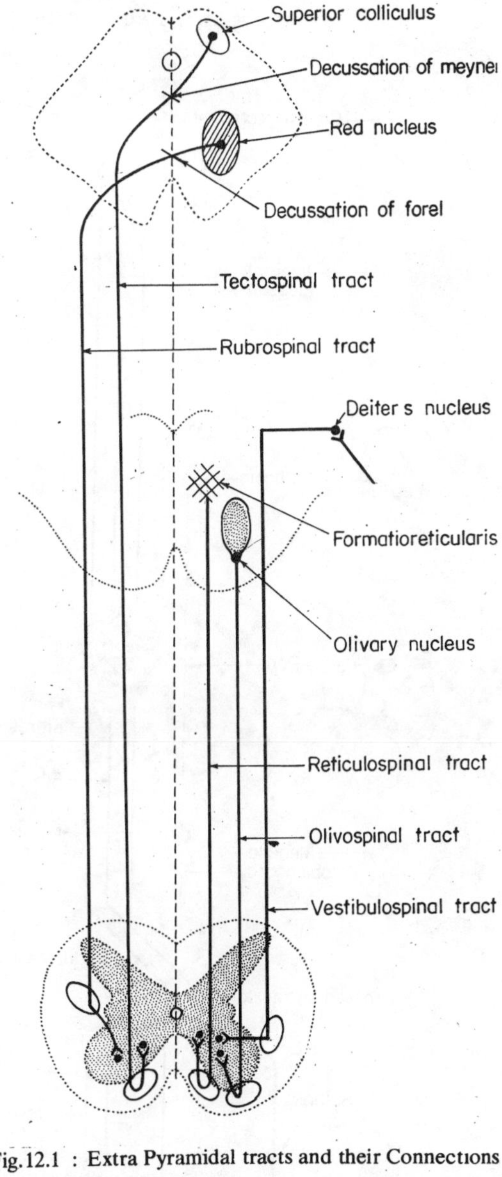


Fig. 12.1 : Extra Pyramidal tracts and their Connections

## Upper Motor Neuron

The pyramidal tract and its nerve cells **constitute upper motor** neurons. The **pyramidal tract** fibres originate in motor areas of the brain and pass downward via midbrain, pons and medulla to the anterior horn cells of the spinal cord.

The pyramidal tract fibres are the axons of pyramidal cells of mainly of 5th layer of precentral gyrus of cortex (area 4.6). They control the voluntary movement of the opposite side of the body except the external ocular muscles.

**The pyramidal tract converges from the motor cortex to form corona radiata and reach internal** capsule. This is mass of white fibres lying between the basal ganglia, the ventricular nucleus (putamen and globus pallidus) laterally and caudate nucleus and thalamus medially (Fig 12.2).

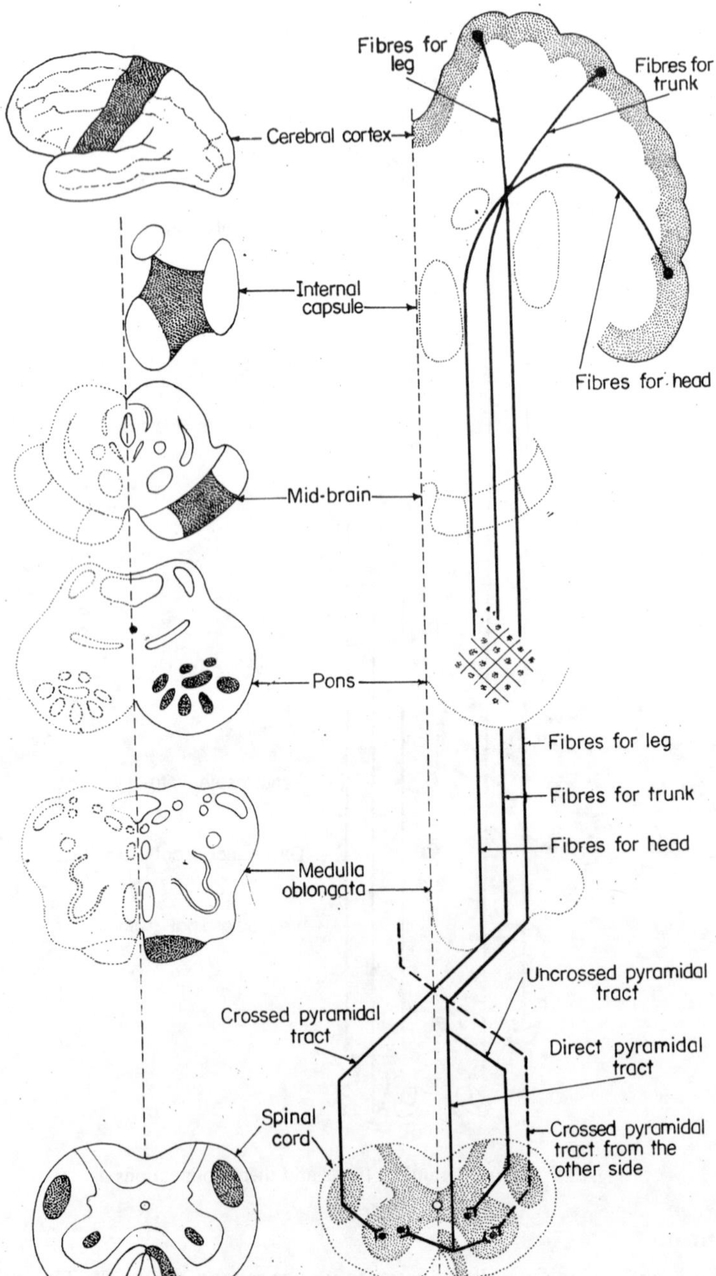


**Fig.12.2 : Pyramidal tract pathways**

The pyramidal tract occupies the genu and the anterior two-thirds of the posterior limb. Immediately behind the pyramidal tract is the sensory path and visual pathway and further behind is the auditory path.

In the midbrain, the fibres occupy the middle three-fifths of the peduncles and passing through these tract fibres, are broken down into scattered bundles by nuclei pontis and the crossing fibres of brachium pontis. Throughout the brainstem, the corticobulbar fibres are crossing to reach the motor cranial nerve nuclei of the opposite side.

In the medulla corticospinal fibres reunite to form a compact mass, the pyramid (form where the pyramidal tract arises). In the lower part of medulla, most of the fibres decussate, cross over to the opposite side to come to the lateral side of spinal cord to form lateral cortico-spinal tract. About 15 per cent of fibres remain uncrossed and constitute anterior cortico-spinal tract. The crossed fibres ultimately connect directly or via inter-neurons to anterior horn cells of the spinal cord. The direct pyramidal fibres do not extend beyond midthoracic region and may be responsible partly to the recovery of function after injury of crossed pyramidal fibres.

**The pyramidal tract :**

(1) In cerebral cortex : As already mentioned upside down major part occupied by tongue, jaws, face.

(2) In internal capsule : From before backwards. Face, shoulder, elbow, hand, trunk and lower limbs.

(3) In midbrain : The order remains the same.

(4) In pons : From without inwards, the order of fibres is foot, foot and leg, thighs and hip and knees, abdomen, chest, upper limbs, face and tongue.

**Lower Motor Neuron :**

The spinal and cranial motor neurons constitute lower motor neurons. Axons from these neurons come out through the anterior nerve roots to enter a mixed peripheral nerve which ultimately branch to supply the motor end-plates of a group of muscle fibres. Anterior horn cells, their, axons and a group of muscle fibres, supplied by that particular cell form a motor unit. Lower motor neuron is the part of spinal reflex arc and is the final common pathway for all motor impulses. Nutrition of the muscle cells also seems to depend on its contact with the spinal cord through the lower motor neuron.

**Signs of lesions of UMN & LMN**

| UMN | LMN |
|---|---|
| (1) Weakness or paralysis of movement of part of one side of the body | (1) Weakness of paralysis of individual muscles or groups of muscles. |
| (2) Increased tone of spastic type (clasp-knife) | (2) Loss of tone on passive movement (flaccidity). |
| (3) Exaggerated tendon reflexes; clonus may be present. | (3) Absence of reflexes supplied by the affected neuron. |
| (4) Superficial reflexes diminished or altered, e.g. absent abdominal reflexes and positive Babinski's reflex, Hoffman reflex; exaggerated jaw jerk. | (4) Superficial reflexes often unaltered unless sensation is also lost or when appropriate LMN is interrupted. |
| (5) Disuse atrophy of the muscle present. | (5) Gross atrophy of muscle within 2 or 3 weeks of an acute episode. |

| | |
|---|---|
| (6) Associated movements **viz. mass** reflexes may be sometimes present. | (6) No associated movements. Fasciculations and myotatic irritability often present. |

**Sensory system**

The modalities of sensation can be stated as **follows** :

(a) Exteroceptive sensations (derived from sources outside the body) e.g. pain, light touch and temperature.

(b) Proprioceptive sensations (derived from body itself) are sense of position, passive movement, vibration and deep pain.

(c) Combined and cortical sensations are **two-point** discrimination, **stereognosis** and graphaesthesia.

(d) Visceral or enteroceptive sensation e.g. nausea, distension, colic and abnormal sensation inside the abdomen which are only felt in diseased process.

**Essential features of the Sensory System**

(1) All forms of sensation must pass through a peripheral nerve and posterior (sensory) root to the spinal cord or brain stem (for cranial nerve).

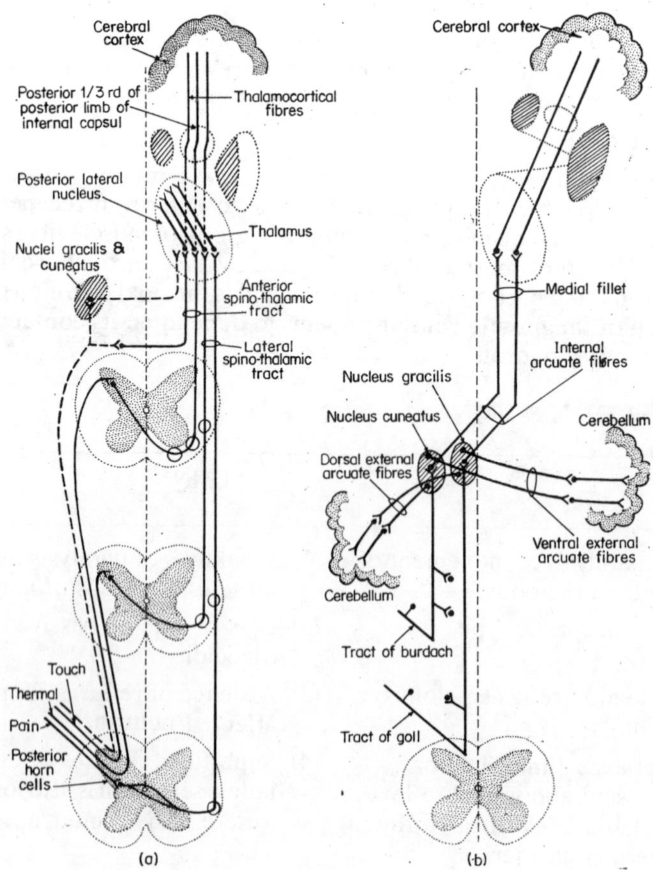


Fig.12.3 : Sensory pathways to the Cerebral Cortex (a) Spinothalamic pathways (b) Tracts of Gall and Burdach

(2) Fibres carrying pain, crude touch and temperature sensation, enter the postero-lateral part of the spinal cord, ascend a few segments and then cross to the opposite antero-lateral part of spinal cord and ascend up to the thalamus as spinothalamic tract. In the brainstem it lied lateral to medial fillet and is joined by the quinto-thalamic tract in the pons. From the thalamus, the third order neurons pass through the posterior limbs of internal capsule and the thalamoparietal radiations to the cerebral cortex (Fig.12.3).

(3) Fibres carrying proprioceptive cortical sensations enter the spinal cord through posterior root, ascend the posterior column on the same side as far as the nucleus gracilis and cuneatus of medulla. From there, the second order neuron crosses to the other side, ascends in the medial fillet to the main sensory nucleus of the thalamus and on to the post-central cortex.

**Arrangement of the sensory fibres**

(1) In posterior column : Fibres from the lower part of the body are displaced medially as more fibres enter.

(2) In spinothalamic tract : Fibres from lower part of the body are displaced superficially to those from the upper part.

(3) In thalamus : Fibres from lower part of the body lie lateral to those of trunk, arms and face.

(4) In sensory cortex : Representation is more or less as that of motor cortex. Spinal cord with its spinal nerves are divided into segments called "dermatome". Each dermatome is supplied by each spinal segment. There is always some overlapping of nerve supply.

The following facts should be remembered for diagnosis of segmental lesions **supply**

Segment $C_1$ has no supply to the skin.

$C_2$ supplies the occiput.

$C_5$ supplies the outer aspect of the shoulder tip.

$C_7$ supplies the middle finger.

$T_3$ lies in the axilla.

$T_5$ supplies a band at nipple level.

$T_8$,$T_{10}$, $T_{12}$ sypply rib margin, the umbilicus and pubes respectively.

$L_3$ supplies knee.

$L_5$ runs diagonally from outer side of tibia to the inner side of foot.

$S_1$ supplies the little toe.

**$S_{3,4,5}$ supplies the anus in concentric form. Proper sensory evaluation is necessary to assess which modalities of sensation are affected and thereby to locate the anatomical basis of lesion.**

## SPEECH

Speech spoken and written needs skilled and elaborate voluntary efforts. As already mentioned like any voluntary movement, speech mechanism also depends on the integrity of the afferent, efferent and central mechanism in the highest brain centres. Spoken speech i.e. expression of language necessitates an intact auditory speech centre in the brain for proper interpretation. It is the mode of human communication of information and emotion. Similarly for written speech, an intact visual pathway, 'visual speech centre' is needed. The final articulation of speech needs bilateral coordination of muscles of tongue , larynx, palate, lips and respiration, influenced by cerebellum and extrapyramidal system, including normal functioning upper limb and the finger.

Normal speech function depends on motor speech centre, auditory and visual speech centres and sensory speech centre. Motor speech centre is Broca's area (area 44) situated on left parietal lobe in a right-handed person.

**Pathways of communication by speech**

(1) Some lesion in may produce word blindness (inability to understand written speech) or,

(2) May lead to inability to understand spoken words (receptive dysphasia).

(3) In others the patient understands but cannot formulate his own speech (expressive or Broca's dysphasia).

(4) Lesions in upper motor neuron, cerebellum, extrapyramidal system, lower motor neurons result in dysarthria.

**Types of speech defects :**

(1) Bilateral upper motor neuron — tongue is small and spastic — spastic dysarthria e.g. pseudobulbar palsy, motor neuron disease, upper brain stem tumours.

(2) Cerebellar lesion — incoordination of muscles of speech — slurred and drunken speech e.g. cerebellar and cerebellopontine angle tumour, disseminated sclerosis.

(3) Extrapyramidal lesion —– rigidity of face of tongue muscle — monotonous speech e.g. Parkinsonism.

(4) Lesions due to L.M.N. and muscle — speech as a whole may be well preserved, individual words and sounds are affected depending on the distribution and extent of muscular weakness.

For diagnosis of disorders of speech the following points should be remembered :

(1) Aphasia or dysphasia — Defect on cerebral integration to produce speech or appreciate to communicate language.

(2) Dysarthria — Defective articulation but cerebral function of appreciation of language is intact.

The defective pronunciation of words is due to disordered function of the muscles of articulation caused by weakness or spasticity of muscles due to neuromuscular disease.

(3) Aphonia or dysphonia — This is entirely caused by local disorder of the larynx either due to laryngitis or new growth or defective innervation of laryngeal muscles.

**Types of Aphasia or dysphasia**

The cerebral speech centres are supplied by the middle cerebral artery. Defects in vascular supply will cause speech defects depending on areas involved. As most people are normally right-handed, the left cerebral lesions are responsible for aphasia. Besides vascular causes, neoplastic lesions or degenerative disorders are also less common causes.

When the aphasia is complete patient cannot speak, understand, read or write. Some patients may understand a little bit of other's speech or greetings and respond by a smile.

These patients are usually hemiphagic who have developed aphasia due to large infarct in their left cerebral hemisphere.

When there is only motor aphasia, patient cannot speak, read or write. The lesion is in Broca's area (area 44), supplied by upper division of left middle cerebral artery in right-handed persons. This is called global aphasia. The area approximately consists of frontal and superior Sylvian fissure and the insula.

There may be variations of the syndrome depending on severity and extent of lesions. Lacunar or focal infarcts produce minor motor aphasia. They also improve more quickly than more extensive global aphasia.

When lower division of middle cerebral artery area is involved, appreciation of language is lost. This is so-called sensory aphasia (Wernicke's aphasia).

There are other variants of speech defects e.g. pure word deafness or pure word blindness, defects in recalling names or recognising close relatives etc. Some degenerative disorders like Alzheimer's disease may show some aphasic manifestations.

## DISORDERS OF CRANIAL NERVES

*AMBAR CHAKRAVARTY*

---

## THE OLFACTORY NERVE

### Anatomy and Physiology

The smell receptors are situated in the olfactory area of the superior meatus of a nasal cavity. The filaments of the olfactory nerve originate from there and pass through the numerous small foramina of the cribriform plate of the ethmoid to the anterior cranial fossa and terminate in the olfactory bulbs. From these, the sensation passes via the two olfactory tracts lying on the under-surface of the frontal lobes. The tracts are inserted in the brain in the region of the anterior perforated substance and the sensation passes via the lateral olfactory stria to terminate in the olfactory area of the cortex in the neighbourhood of the uncus of the temporal lobe.

### Disorders of Olfactory Pathway

Lesions anywhere in the olfactory pathway would cause loss of smell sensation (anosmia) which may be unilateral or bilateral. Smell sensation is tested with essences of familiar odours like coffee, almonds, chocolate, oil of lemon and peppermint. It is inadvisable to use pungent smells like that of Liquor Ammonia which will stimulate the terminations of the trigeminal nerve (general sensory) rather than the olfactory receptors. This agent, may however be necessary to differentiate between organic and non-organic (hysterical) anosmia.

Common causes of anosmia include —

1. Local acute or chronic allergic diseases of the nasal mucosa.
2. Head Injury — by causing damage to the fragile olfactory nerves as they pass through the cribriform plate.
3. Intracranial tumours compressing the olfactory bulbs or tract. A common example is an *olfactory groove meningioma* which in addition to causing **ipsilateral anosmia** would also cause *ipsilateral blindness* due to compression of the optic nerve and *contralateral papilloedema* due to raised intracranial pressure **(Foster-Kennedy syndrome).**
4. Chronic basal (anterior cranial fossa) meningitis e.g. syphilis.
5. Hysteria.

A distorted sense of smell *(parosmia)* may rarely occur following head injury, but is usually a feature of a depressive illness. In this condition the patient may complain of continuous smell of bad or putrid nature *(cacosmia).*

## THE OPTIC NERVE AND DISORDERS OF THE VISUAL PATHWAY

### Anatomical considerations :

The end organs for perception of vision are the rods and the cones situated in the retina. Unmyelinated nerve fibres carrying sensation of vision originate from these receptors and converge to the optic disc where they penetrate the globe at the lamina cribrosa and acquire a myelin sheath. As the eye can be compared with a pin-hole camera, the nasal half of the retina in each eye sees the temporal half of the field of vision and the temporal half sees the nasal half of the field. An understanding of this basic concept is essential for proper appraisal of the disorders of visual pathway described later in this chapter. The macula is the most sensitive part of the retina accounting for central and colour vision. This is situated a little to the temporal side of the disc and hence the fibres from this part (papillo-macular bundle) tend to crowd into the temporal half of the disc.

The two optic nerves, emerging from the orbits through the optic foramina, converge to the optic chiasma. The *macular fibres tend to shift to the centre of the optic nerve* as the latter reaches the chiasma (Fig.12.4).

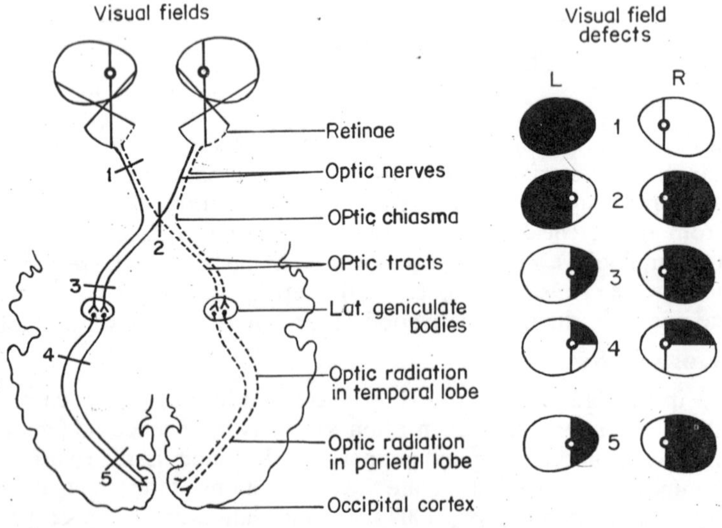


**Fig.12.4 : Optic nerves and its connections. Lesions at different sites produce typical field defects**

At the optic chiasma, the lateral fibres (temporal retinal) go straight back into the optic tract of the same side but the medial fibres (nasal retinal) decussate and pass to the opposite optic tract. Before decussation, they often form a loop projecting into the opposite optic nerve. The lower nasal fibres (upper temporal visual fields) cross low and anteriorly in the chiasma and are damaged by lesions arising in the pituitary fossa. The upper nasal (lower temporal visual fields) cross high in the chiasma and are damaged by lesions involving the chiasma from above and behind — e.g. a craniopharyngioma. The central papillo-macular bundle, because of its position, is affected only later in the course of chiasmal compression.

**The optic tracts form at the caudal end of the chiasma and carry impulses from the temporal half of the retina of the same side and nasal half of the retina of the opposite side. This order of arrangement is maintained till the termination of the visual pathway in the occipital cortex — and subserves the anatomical basis of binocular vision.**

The optic tract fibers terminate in the six layers of the lateral geniculate body of each side. The macular **fibres** occupy a big central wedge of the geniculate body with the lower fields (upper retinal) represented medially and upper fields (lower retinal) laterally.

**The next relay is the optic radiation which fans out from the geniculate body, and passing through the posterior limb of the internal capsule terminates around the lips of calcarine sulcus in the occipital lobe (visual cortex). The upper fibres of radiation (lower field fibres) terminate on the superior lip of the sulcus and the lower fibres of radiation (upper field fibres) end on the inferior lip. The macular fibres terminate at the extreme tip.**

## PARAMETERS FOR ASSESSING DISORDERS OF VISUAL PATHWAY

1. **Visual acuity** — The standard Snellen's Type charts are used for testing distant vision and the Jaegar Type cards for near vision. Loss of visual acuity may be due to defect in the media of the eye, the retina or anywhere in the rest of the visual pathway.

2. **Visual fields** — Confrontation is a fairly accurate bedside method for assessing any gross defect of a field of vision. More subtle defects, can only be picked up by a perimeter or by plotting the field on a Bjerrum's screen. Quantitative perimetry, i.e. testing field with objects of various sizes, is essential in picking up early sectorial field cuts. Assessment of colour fields (using coloured and white objects) may also supplement quantitative perimetric results.

   As central vision is primarily a function of the macula, involvement of the papillo-macular bundle in various disease processes, produce **blind** areas (scotomas) in the central field of vision (the peripheral part being unaffected). Such defects often lie close to the normal blind spot which corresponds to the position of the optic nerve head in the retina which does not contain any photoreceptors. Such defects in the central fields can sometimes be picked up by careful confrontation charting with a pin head but are best assessed with a Central Field Analyser.

3. **Ophthalmoscopy** — Direct examination of the retina, the macula and the optic nerve head appearance is an integral part of the assessment of visual pathway. This will be discussed later on in the chapter.

4. **Visual Evoked Responses (VER)** — This new technique involves subjecting the eye to a flickering chequer board pattern on an illuminated screen while recording the activity of the visual cortex with occipital surface electrodes (as employed in recording EEG). The method has been standardised and differences in latency, size and shape of the potentials recorded indicate damage to one or other optic nerve.

## LESIONS OF THE VISUAL PATHWAY

A. **Retinal Lesions :** Retinal lesions always cause unilateral visual problem. A common cause is interference with the circulation — usually resulting from an embolus occluding the central artery of the retina or one of its branches. A transient blindness might result (amaurosis fugax) or the defect may be long lasting if the artery remains occluded for long. As the central retinal artery divides into upper and lower branches supplying the retina above and below the horizontal meridian, a branch occlusion normally causes a field defect limited by the horizontal meridian.

   The *papillo-macular bundle*, subserving central vision, may be damaged by a variety of toxins, either as it runs in the nerve fibre layer of the retina or in the optic nerve. A caeco-central scotoma (which involves the physiological blind spot) results.

   Choroido-retinitis, due to local patches of inflammation of the retina, causes scotomas of shape and size corresponding to the area of damage.

B. **Optic nerve head lesion** — The two common forms are glaucomatous damage and swelling of the disc (papilloedema). In the former arcuate scotomas radiating from the blind spot usually occur, which may extend upwards (Seidel scotoma) or at a later stage may go round below the blind spot completing a circle (Bjerrum scotoma). Papilloedema or swelling of the optic nerve head commonly signifies raised intracranial pressure. Classically, it produces an enlargement of the size of the physiological blind spot and a peripheral constriction of the visual field. The underlying CNS disease causing raised intracranial pressure may also produce field cuts, depending upon the site of lesion, which may be superimposed on such changes.

C. **Optic Nerve** (See Fig.12.7)

1. **Optic neuritis** — Acute optic or retrobulbar neuritis is commonly unilateral and a manifestation of demyelinating disease, but may also result from toxins such as tobacco, alcohol, vitamin deficiency and ingestion of clioquinol (as a part of *subacute myelooptic neuropathy or SMON).* As the papillo-macular bundle is most sensitive to such injury, loss of central vision with a sharp fall of visual acuity results. The patient normally complains of seeing a black hole in the centre of vision in one eye. The classical field defect is a central scotoma most marked to a red object. However, as described earlier, a Caeco-central scotoma may also result due to involvement of the papillo-macular bundle alone.

2. **Optic nerve compression :** The optic nerve may be compressed by a tumour (usually a meningioma) at any point from its exit from orbit to the chiasma. Again the *papillo-macular bundle being most sensitive to pressure, central field defects are early* (contrary to the anticipated peripheral defects on anatomical grounds). Any case of supposed optic neuritis where the central field defect remains persistent, should be investigated for optic nerve compression. A vital clue is provided by the finding of a temporal field cut on the oposite eye if the compression is at the junction of the optic nerve and chiasma (anterior chiasmal syndrome of Traqnir).

   This is due to the involvement of the decussating nasal fibres from the opposite eye which loop forward into the optic nerve of the other eye before passing into the chiasma (vide *supra* in the section on anatomy).

D. **Optic nerve gliomas :** Gliomas are malignant tumours of the optic nerve, usually seen in children and inthose with neurofibromatosis. These normally produce 'holes' in the field of one eye the situation of which may vary.

E. **Chiasmal lesions :** The classical example of a chiasmal lesion is that produced by a pituitary tumour growing upwards from the sella and pressing on the central part of the chiasma from below. Due to the lamination of the fibres in the chiasma and as the nasal fibres from both eyes cross at the central part, the earliest field defect is an *upper bitemporal quadranopia.* With progression of the disease and further compression, a classical *bitemporal hemianopia* will result. The end result, of course, of an expanding pituitary mass, is bilateral blindness and optic atrophy due to involvement of the whole chiasma and distal portion of the optic nerves.

   Craniopharyngioma (arising from remnants of Rathke's pouch) on the other hand commonly press on the chiasma from above and behind and cause field defects involving the lower fields initially. These tumours often produce suprasellar calcification on skull X-rays and in children cause growth retardation and delayed sexual maturation.

   Lateral chiasmal compression is rare. It may be caused by an aneurysm of the internal carotid artery (supraclinoid position). The field defect is usually a unilateral nasal field loss.

F. **Optic Tract Lesions :** The optic tract conveys the temporal fibres from ipsilateral retina and the nasal fibres of the contralateral retina. In addition it contains fibres from the macula and those concerned with pupillary light reflex (vide *infra*). A lesion of the therefore produces a homonymous (corresponding halves) hemianopia to the opposite side which is usually complete and incongruous (shape of the defect different in two half fields). Macular vision is also affected and pupillary light reflex lost only when light is shown from the lost half field of vision (hemianopic pupillary reaction). Common causes include pressure from adjacent tumours like craniopharyngioma and even a pituitary tumour growing upwards, backward and laterally.

G. **Optic radiation lesions :** On purely anatomical grounds, optic radiation lesions would produce homonymous hemianopias to the opposite side. These are usually incomplete and congruous; macular vision is involved and pupillary light reflex remains intact (the fibres for light reflex having left the optic tract and lateral geniculate body to pass to the midbrain). Vascular lesions are the commonest cause; the blood supply being derived from the posterior cerebral artery and anterior choroidal branch of the internal carotid artery. Hence in a typical case of internal capsular hemiplegia due to middle cerebral artery occlusion, hemianopia should not occur, unless there is simultaneous involvement of the anterior choroidal artery or the radiation fibres are involved due to cerebral oedema. An isolated homonymous hemianopia of sudden onset is the result of occlusion of posterior cerebral artery.

Mass lesions in temporal and parietal lobes involve corresponding parts of the optic radiation. A parietal lesion classically produces a lower homonymous quadranopia and a temporal lesion, an upper homonymous quadrantic defect.

Inattention hemianopias (defect recognised when both half fields are stimulated simultaneously but not when done individually) occasionally occur in more peripheral parietal lobe lesions as part of the inattention phenomenon of such lesions (e.g. sensory inattention or perceptual rivalry).

H. **Lesions of the visual cortex :** The peripheral visual fields are represented in the anterior part of the calcarine cortex and the macular area in the most posterior part. The anterior part receives its blood supply from the posterior cerebral artery and the macular area appears to receive its supply from a branch of the middle cerebral artery. An occlusive lesion of one posterior cerebral artery causing occipital infarction would therefore cause a homonymous hemianopia to the opposite side but the macular area will be spared. Bilateral occlusion (due to occlusion at the tip of the basilar artery or the point of origin of the posterior cerebrals) would cause bilateral occipital lobe infarcts with total blindness sparing the macular but the optic discs and pupillary reflexes would remain normal. The patient would be able to see an object in direct line with the eyes but would be unable to see its periphery (tubular vision). Such a defect needs to be differentiated from non-organic field defect (hysterical) which might also cause tubular vision. In the former the extent of the tubular vision will increase as examiner moves farther away from the eyes but in the latter the diameter of the tubular field will remain constant even if the field is tested at varying distances from the eyes.

Isolated lesions of the macular cortex only, causing hemianopic central scotomas, are extremely rare.

## OPHTHALMOSCOPY

Examination of the optic fundi is an essential part of clinical examination; no matter whether the problem is neurological or not. Vital clues to general systemic diseases (e.g. infective endocarditis, blood dyscrasias, miliary tuberculosis) are often obtained by this simple test. The room need to be darkened and the patient asked to fix his vision at a distance to obtain maximum dilatation of the pupils necessary for good visibility of the fundus. It is not advisable to use mydriatics routinely as these would mask a very important neurological sign i.e. pupillary reflex, in a critically ill patient (e.g. following head-injury) where close observation of pupillary size is essential.

**Important features to be studied are :**

1. The disc
2. The macula
3. The blood vessels
4. The retina as a whole
5. The pupillary response.

**The optic disc :**

Acquaintance with the normal appearance and variations in the appearance of the disc is essential for interpretation of abnormal findings. Normally, it is slightly pinkish in colour, with the temporal side a bit pale and nasal margin slightly blurred.

**The common abnormalities include –**

1. **Papilloedema :** This means swelling of the optic disc. In the earliest stage the retinal veins look congested and venous pulsation is lost. Next there is blurring of the nasal margin of the disc which gradually spreads to the temporal side and the physiological cup is filled up. Later on, the disc itself is lifted up from the surface of the retina as a result of the swelling. In advanced cases flame shaped haemorrhages and white exudates appear. Peripheral constriction of the visual field occurs with enlargement of the blind spot. But visual acuity is only minimally affected until the swelling is very gross (Fig.12.5).

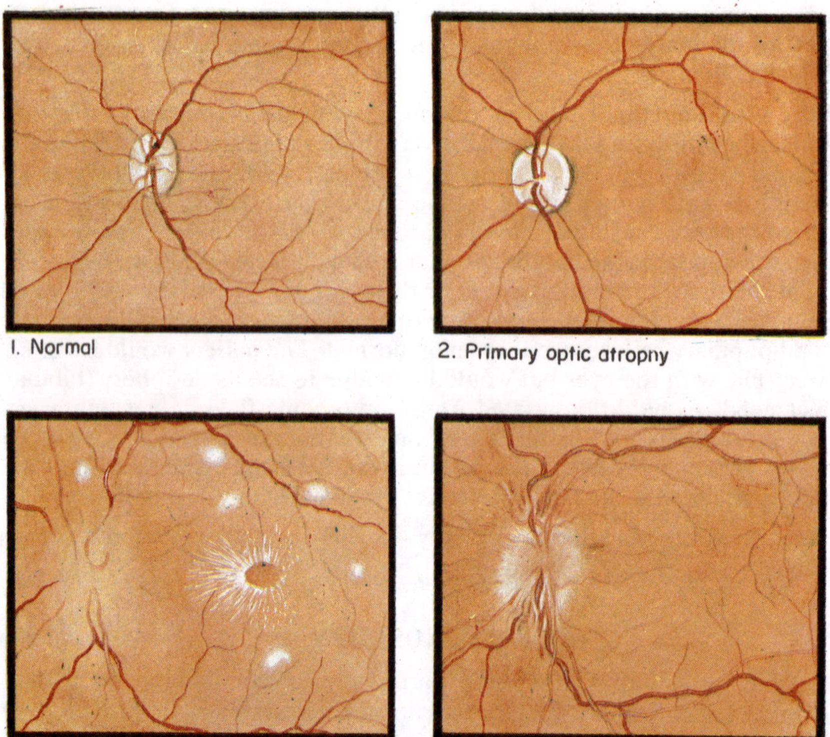


Fig.12.5 : OPTIC DISC NORMAL AND ABNORMAL –

*Primary Optic atrophy* : Sharp, clearcut, margin with fine vessels.

*Chronic nephritis* : Uraemic eye — shows swollen disc with blurred margin, Macular region — radiating whitish dots and lines (Star of India appearance white woolly exudates and flame-shaped haemorrhages here and there.

*Papilloedema* : Swollen disc with blurred margin, engorged retinal veins; haemorrhage may occur in patches.

The commonest cause of papilloedema is raised intracranial tension which causes obstruction to the venous return from the retina by the raised pressure of CSF in the sheath of the optic nerve. Common causes include intracranial tumour, brain abscess, benign intracranial hypertension and meningitis.

Papilloedema may also occur in the malignant phase of arterial hypertension when it is associated with arterial thickening and tortuosity, arterio-venous nipping, flame-shaped haemorrhages and cotton wool exudates.

Thrombosis of the central vein of retina also causes papilloedema and in addition shows gross congestion and dilatation of the retinal veins with widespread perivascular haemorrhages. Inflammation of the optic nerve (optic neuritis — a demyelinating condition) involving the optic nerve head (papillitis) may stimulate early papilloedema. In papillitis, however, the disc looks much pinker and there is disproportionate fall in visual acuity compared to swelling of the disc.

2. **Secondary optic atrophy** : This is the end result of long-standing unrelieved papilloedema. The swelling of the disc diminishes and the disc becomes pale. Visual acquity is grossly reduced. The disc margin remains blurred and the veins congested for a considerable time, distinguishing secondary from primary optic atrophy.

3. **Primary optic atrophy** : This is an optic disc which has become atrophic without having undergone any preliminary visible change. The disc appears very pale with a clear cut margin and the physiological cup is preserved. The vessels remain normal unless optic atrophy is secondary to central retinal artery occlusion when the arteries become thread-like.

Important causes of primary optic atrophy include optic nerve compression by tumours (commonly pituitary tumours), multiple sclerosis, neurosyphilis, hereditary optic atrophy and toxic agents (tobacco, methanol, vitamin deficiency).

Consecutive optic atrophy is a term used to designate cases with primary looking optic atrophy associated with retinal diseases like retinitis pigmentosa and choroidoretinitis.

**The Macula**

The macula is situated on the temporal side of the disc about two disc diameter away when looked through an ophthalmoscope. Normally it has a shiny red appearance (macular reflex). Macular diseases are mainly of interest to the ophthalmologists. Two conditions deserve special mention. The first is the formation of the *macular star* in the malignant phase of arterial hypertension. The star is formed by the folds of oedematous retina spreading from the macular region. The second condition of importance is the appearance of the *cherry red spot* in the macula in cerebral lipidosis like *Tay-Sach's disease* and in central retinal artery occlusion.

Ophthalmoscopic abnormalities in the appearance of the blood vessels and the retina itself which are of interest to the general physician are usually associated with systemic medical disorders like diabetes, hypertension, blood dyscrasias and collagen vascular diseases. These will be discussed in the appropriate sections of the book.

## THE THIRD, FOURTH AND SIXTH CRANIAL NERVES AND DISORDERS OF OCULAR MOVEMENTS

Under normal circumstances the two eyes move together with their axes lying parallel to each other. This causes images of objects seen to form on identical positions of the retina which tend to fuse when interpreted by the brain as a single image. If the axes of the eyes fail to lie parallel, image of a single object falls on non-identical portions of the two retinae which the brain fails to fuse while interpreting — the result being diplopia or double vision. As the parallel position of the eyes is maintained only by a perfect balancing action of the external ocular muscles, paralysis of any one of these would lead to diplopia.

Each eyeball is moved by the action of six external ocular muscles — four recti (superior, inferior, medial and lateral) and two obliques (superior and inferior). Apart from the medial and lateral recti (which only move the eye horizontally inwards and onwards respectively), all ocular muscles have principal and subsidiary actions and these tend to act in pairs (e.g. Superior Rectus

**and Inferior Oblique causing elevation and Inferior Rectus and Superior Oblique causing** depression). The details of these actions are complex and hence a simplified form is given below which is sufficient for clinical evaluation of ocular movements and diplopia.

A. The Superior and Inferior Recti cause **Pure** elevation and depression of the eye respectively **only in full adducted position.**

B. The Inferior and Superior Obliques cause **Pure** elevation and depression of the eye respectively **only in fully adducted position.**

The actions of the Medial and Lateral recti are simple and have been already mentioned.

All recti are supplied by the third cranial nerve except the lateral rectus which is supplied by the sixth cranial nerve. The third nerve also supplies the inferior oblique and Levator palpebrae superioris (which elevates the upper eyelid) and the fourth nerve has a solitary supply to the Superior Oblique.

The nuclei of origin of the third nerve lie in the midbrain and consist of several parts, each corresponding to one muscle supplied by the nerve. The two nerves emerge together between the cerebral peduncles and immediately pass between the posterior cerebral and superior cerebellar arteries and then come in close proximity with the posterior communicating artery. It then enters the cavernous sinus, in the lateral wall of which it lies along with the fourth and sixth nerves and **the first division of the fifth nerve. It enters the orbit along with the other nerves mentioned above** through the superior orbital fissure and divides into branches supplying the various external **ocular muscles. The third nerve also carries in its trunk the pupilloconstrictor fibres mediating the light reflex** (Fig.12.6).

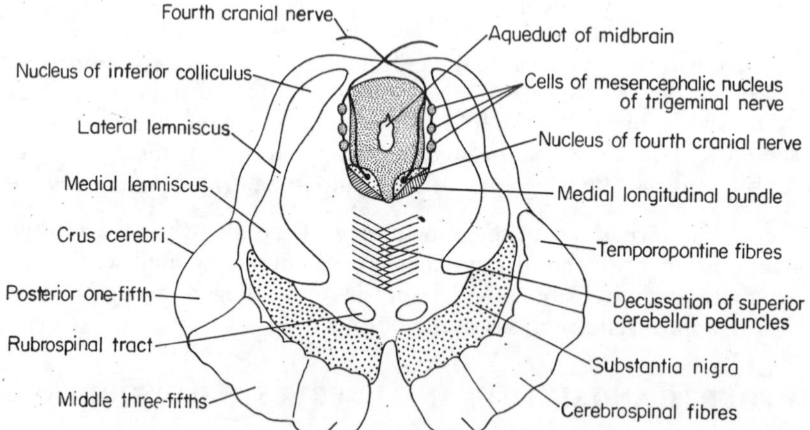


**Fig.12.6 : Origin of the third nerve and periaquidacted grey matter with structures at the level of mid brain.**

**The fourth nerve also originates in the midbrain, but passes backwards and before emerging from the brain at the dorsal aspect of brain stem, decussates to the opposite side. It then turns** forwards on the lateral aspect of the cerebral peduncle and follows the third nerve to enter the cavernous sinus.

The sixth nerve nucleus lies in the pons, very close to the intrinsic fibres from the facial nerve nucleus. The nerve emerges at the ponto-medullary junction and crosses over the petrous tip (in close proximity of the Gasserian ganglion) to enter the cavernous sinus. It has a very long intracranial course and hence is commonly involved by stretching when there is a raised intracranial pressure.

Paralysis of external ocular muscles would give rise to two important features —

A. An altered resting position of eye : due to unopposed action of the antagonistic muscle. A lateral rectus palsy would cause an adducted eye and a medial rectus palsy the reverse. In paralysis of the third nerve as a whole, the eye is not only adducted but will not move vertically. There will be accompanying ptosis and pupillary dilatation.

B. Diplopia : Its physiology has already been mentioned. Of the two images seen, the one from the defective eye is usually less bright and is referred to as the false image. From an analysis of the position of the false image, the defective muscle causing diplopia can be picked up. This is helped by the following principles :

1. Displacement of the false image may be horizontal, vertical or both.
2. Separation of the images is greatest in the direction in which the weak muscle has the purest action.
3. The false image is displaced farthest in the direction in which the weak muscle should move the eye.

Such analysis is helped by the use of coloured spectacles or more accurately by using a Hess chart.

In third nerve palsy diplopia occurs in all directions of gaze except laterally to the side of the eye affected. However, such diplopia is often masked by the associated ptosis.

In fourth nerve lesion, diplopia occurs when the patient looks down and away from the side of the affected eye, e.g. while walking downstairs or while reading a book.

Sixth nerve palsy causes gross diplopia on lateral gaze to the side of the affected eye.

## COMMON CAUSES AND SITES OF OCULOMOTOR PARALYSIS

A. **Nuclear Lesions :** These occur in the brain stem and common causes include vascular infarctions, demyelination and brain stem tumours, like gliomas. Commonly neighbouring structures in the brain stem are also involved e.g. third nerve palsy with contralateral hemiplegia *(Weber's syndrome)*, third nerve palsy with contralateral tremor due to involvement of Red nucleus *(Benedikt's syndrome)* and ipsilateral sixth and seventh nerve palsy with contralateral hemiplegia *(Millard-Gubler syndrome)*. It is important to remember that owing to the multiplicity of the nuclei, nuclear third nerve palsies are often incomplete.

**Infranuclear Lesions :**

1. Unilateral or bilateral sixth nerve palsy results due to nerve stretching from raised intracranial pressure usually due to a posterior fossa space occupying lesion (false localising sign).
2. During cerebral herniation from a space occupying lesion in one hemisphere, the ipsilateral third nerve may be compressed between the herniated uncus and the free margin of the tentorium.
3. Any of the nerves may be involved by a process of basal meningitis (tubercular, syphylitic or carcinomatous) or by allergic process like in Guillain-Barre syndrome.
4. *The third nerve is commonly compressed by an aneurysm of the posterior communicating artery.*
5. Localised meningitic process (secondary to mastoiditis) may involve the fifth, sixth and seventh cranial nerve *(Gradinego's syndrome)*.

6. Any pathology in the region of the cavernous sinus or superior orbital fissure would involve all the oculomotor nerves along with the ophthalmic division of the fifth cranial nerve. Such lesions include *cavernous sinus thrombosis, carotico-carvernous fistula, intracavernous aneurysm of internal carotid artery or a tumour* (pituitary adenoma or a meningioma) invading the cavernous sinus. Not an uncommon condition in our country is the syndrome of painful ophthalmoplegia (Tolosa-Hunt syndrome) which mimicks any cavernous sinus lesion.

The cause is perhaps an inflammatory process involving the periosteum of the superior orbital fissure or the sheath of the intracavernous carotid artery. There is intense pain in the distribution of the ophthalmic branch of Trigeminal along with rapid development of oculomotor palsies. The condition responds dramatically to corticosteroids.

Systemic medical disorders like diabetes and atherosclerosis at times causes isolated oculomotor lesion perhaps by causing small infarcts of the nerve trunks.

Diseases of the ocular muscles will closely mimick oculomotor nerve involvement. The common conditions are Thyrotoxicosis, Myesthenia Gravis and progressive ocular myopathy. In any case of isolated oculomotor palsy, it is important to think above and rule out Myesthenia by an Edrophonium Test.

## The Pupils

### Anatomical considerations

Pupillary size is determined by the balance of action between a ring of constrictor fibres innervated by the parasympathetic and radially arranged dilator fibres innervated by the sympathetic. Parasympathetic overactivity thus causes pupillary constriction and paralyses pupillary dilatation. The reverse is the case with the sympathetic.

### Parasympathetic pathways and the pupillary reflexes

When a beam of light is focussed on one eyeball, the pupil of the same side as well as of the opposite side constrict (light reflex). The light stimulus is carried from the ipsilateral retina by the optic nerve, the chiasma and the optic tract to the lateral geniculate body; wherefrom it is relayed to Edinger-Westphal nuclei of both sides lying in the midbrain. This nucleus is in fact a part of the third nerve nucleus and gives rise to the pre-ganglionic parasympathetic fibres. These traverse with the third nerve and on entering the orbit terminate in the ciliary ganglion. The post-ganglionic fibres originate from this ganglion and pass as the short ciliary nerves which innervate sphincter pupillae muscle in the iris.

The parasympathetic fibres are also concerned with the accommodation reflex necessary for near vision where in addition to pupillary constriction, medial conjugate deviation of the eyes occurs to bring a near object to focus. The impluses originated from the visual cortex and then pass to the frontal lobe by way of occipito-frontal fibres. From here, descending fibres terminate in the midbrain around Edinger-Westphal nuclei as well as the third nerve nuclei which is necessary for causing pupillary constriction and medial convergence by contraction of both medial recti muscle. The final common pathway, is of course, the third cranial nerve itself.

### Sympathetic pathway

The central sympathetic pathway, of course, starts in the hypothalamus and descends down in the cervical spinal cord to terminate around cells of the intermedio-lateral horn of the spinal grey column. Preganglionic fibres start from here and pass out via the $T_1$ ventral nerve root and enter the cervical part of the sympathetic chain wherein they ascend up to the superior cervical ganglion. Post-ganglionic fibres start from here and pass along the sheath of the internal carotid artery to enter the cranial cavity and orbit. In the eye they supply not only the dilator pupillae muscle but also the unstriped muscle of the eyelid (Mueller's muscle) which elevates the eyelid passively.

## LESIONS OF THE PARASYMPATHETIC PATHWAY

The end result is a dilated fixed pupil without any light reflex.

1. Optic atrophy always causes a fixed dilated pupil on the side of the lesion *(amblyopic pupil)*.
2. Partial lesions of the optic nerve, (**usually** due to a demyelinating disease) cause afferent pathway lesion with a *Muscus Gunn Pupil.* The normal eye shows a brisk pupillary reaction to bright light. But in the abnormal eye, the reaction is slow and incomplete. It may be so brief that it may start to dilate immediately.
3. In a lesion of the optic tract with hemianopia, light focussed on the affected half field of vision will not elicit a light reflex *(hemianopic Wernicke's pupil).* This test differentiates an optic tract from a radiation lesion but in practice is usually very difficult to elicit due to dispersion of light in the eye.
4. Upper midbrain compressive or destructive lesions will also cause pupillary abnormalities e.g. in case of pinealoma. In this condition paralysis of upward gaze also occurs **(Perinaud's syndrome).**
5. Lesions anywhere in the course of the third nerve may interrupt pupillary parasympathetic fibres. This, however, is not universally true as partial lesions are common where the pupil escapes. Compressive lesions are usually complete. Irregularity of pupillary size is the earliest sign of uncal herniation (causing ipsilateral third nerve compression) in a case of cerebral SOL.
6. **Argyll-Robertson Pupil (ARP)** : This is the hallmark of neurosyphilis but similar pupil may rarely be found in diabetes, peroneal muscular atrophy and facial hemiatrophy. The characteristic features of ARP include :-
   (a) Small irregular pupils
   (b) Loss of light reflex
   (c) Preservation of accommodation reflex
   (d) Absence of response to mydriatics
   (e) Patchy depigmentation of the iris.

The site of the lesion responsible is debatable. Although originally thought to be in the periaqueductal grey matter in the midbrain, a more plausible site is perhaps in the region of the ciliary ganglion or in the substance of the iris itself:

7. **Holmes-Adie (or Tonic) pupil :**

The tonic pupil is a widely dilated circular pupil which is usually unilateral and which reacts very slowly to light but smartly to accommodation. This is usually associated with the absence of knee and ankle jerks but the etiology is unknown. In most cases this is a chance finding but may be baffling to the clinician if this condition is not thought of.

8. Isolated loss of accommodation reflex only is a rarity. This classically occurs in diphtheria and is fully recoverable.

## LESIONS OF THE SYMPATHETIC PATHWAY :

Lesions anywhere in the course of the sympathetic pathway to the eye causes a Horner's syndrome. The features of the fully developed syndrome include :

1. The affected pupil is smaller (miosis) due to reduced pupillo-dilator activity. This asymmetry is more obvious in darkness. The light and accomodation reflexes are present but reduced.
2. Mild to moderate ptosis of the eyelid — due to paralysis of the sympathetically innervated Mueller's muscle.

3. Impairment of sweating (anhydrosis) of the affected half of the face. This results if the lesion is proximal to the superior cervical ganglion.
4. Enophthalmos (i.e. sunken eye due to dryness of the intraorbital structures) although described in literature, is rarely seen.
5. Loss of **cilio-spinal** reflex : this is a sympathetically mediated reflex **wherein** pinching the skin of the neck produces ipsilateral pupillary dilatation.

As *Horner's syndrome* may result from either a pre-ganglionic (proximal to superior cervical ganglion) or a post-ganglionic lesion, it becomes at times important to differentiate between the two. This is usually done by using Adrenaline (1 : 1000) eye drops. This produces no effect on a pre-ganglionic Horner pupil but causes marked dilatation in case of a post-ganglionic lesion due to phenomenon of denervation supersensitivity.

**Common causes of Horner's syndrome :**

A. **Central lesions :** (Pre-ganglionic)

**Brain stem :** Vascular lesions (classically posterior inferior cerebeller artery occlusion causing Lateral Medullary Syndrome), demyelination and tumours.

**Cervical cord lesions :** Syringomyelia and intramedullary tumours like gliomas and ependymomas.

B. **Peripheral lesions :**

**D1 root lesions** (pre-ganglionic) : The commonest cause is compression by an apical bronchogenic neoplasm (Pancoast Tumour). All cases of Horner's syndrome must always have a chest X-ray for this reason.

**Cervical sympathetic chain** (Pre- and post-ganglionic) : Common causes of damage include neoplastic infiltration, surgical exploration, and trauma to the neck.

**Intracranial sympathetic fibres : (Post-ganglionic) :**

Theoretically, the internal carotid nerve plexus may be damaged by lesions in the cavernous sinus causing Horner's syndrome. But this is rarely seen in clinical practice as parasympathetic damage due to involvement of the third nerve usually determines the pupillary response. A transient form of Horner's syndrome due to involvement of ocular sympathetic fibres occurs during attacks of cluster headaches (a variant of migraine).

**Pupillary abnormalities in an unconscious subject :**

Normally reacting equal pupils indicate a functioning brain stem and is a reassuring sign.

As described earlier, the earliest sign of progressive cerebral (uncal) herniation is an ipsilateral pupillary dilatation. Jonathan Hutchinson described sequential pupillary changes following rapidly rising intracranial pressure usually due to extradural haematoma following head injury. The pupil on the side of lesion is first constricted and then dilates; the same sequence of events then follows on the other side.

Bilateral fixed dilated pupils usually denote *irreversible brain stem damage.* The only toxic causes of such changes are glutethamide, atropine and amphetamine poisoning.

Bilateral pin-point pupil is also a ominous neurological sign usually occurring in pontine or intraventricular haemorrhage along with hyperpyrexia. Opiates, of course, produce similar pupillary abnormality.

## THE FIFTH CRANIAL (TRIGEMINAL) NERVE

**Anatomical considerations :**

Motor and sensory fibres of the fifth nerve emerge by two separate roots from the lateral surface of the pons, lying close to the origins of the seventh and eighth cranial nerves at the cerebello-pontine angle. The two roots pass up to the petrous tip where the sensory root expands to form the gasserian ganglion and the motor root passes below the ganglion. The ganglion gives rise to the three principal divisions of the fifth nerve — namely ophthalmic (first division), maxillary (second division) and mandibular (third division). The first two are purely sensory while the third division is joined by the motor roots of the fifth nerve. The first division supplies the skin of the forehead, upper eyelid, side of the nose and the scalp up to the vertex. It also carries general sensations from the cornea and conjunctiva. The second division supplies the skin over the cheek, the zygomatic region and the temple. The third division has its sensory supply in the skin overlying the lower jaw (excluding the angle which is supplied by C2 root) and upper part of the pinna. The motor root, through the mandibular division, supplies all the muscles of mastication and the tensor palati.

The fibres of the sensory root on entering the pons divide. Those concerned with touch terminate in the principal sensory nucleus situated in the pons.

Those carrying pain and temperature pass downwards as the spinal tract of the trigeminal which terminate in its nucleus/which extends down as far as the upper part of the cervical spinal cord. The fibres from the ophthalmic division occupy the lower most part of the tract and those from the mandibular division the highest part. Second neuron pathway fibres from this nucleus form the spinal lemniscus which cross the midline and ultimately join the spino-thalamic tract to end in the thalamus.

**Assessment of fifth nerve function :**

This is assessed by the following —

1. Sensory : Testing sensations like touch, pain and temperature in the two halves of the face in the distribution of the three divisions of the nerve. Trigeminal sensory loss should never extend below the lower border of the mandible.

2. Motor : Motor power and wasting, if any, are noticed in the muscles of mastication which include the masseter, temporalis and the pterygoids. Weakness of the last group of muscles, causes, jaw deviation to the side of the lesion on opening the mouth.

3. Reflex : Two reflexes are mediated by the nerve — one superficial (corneal reflex) and one deep (jaw jerk).

The fifth nerve constitutes the afferent limb of the corneal reflex and the facial nerve the efferent. Hence a lesion of either nerve will abolish the corneal reflex. In order to differentiate between the two the consensual reaction is looked for.

The jaw reflex is sometimes inelicitable in normal people. It attends clinical significance only when it is very brisk and this usually signifies a bilateral pyramidal lesion above the level of the pons.

**Lesions of the trigeminal nerve**

A. In the brain stem such lesions usually involve the spinothalamic tract, hence cause loss of pain and temperature sensation with preservation of light touch (dissociated sensory loss). Important causes include a vascular lesion like thrombosis of the posterior inferior cerebellar artery and syringobulbia. In the former condition a crossed hemianalgesia results due to involvement of the ipsilateral spinal tract and the spinothalamic tract carrying sensation from the opposite half of the body. In syringobulbia the expanding syrinx first involves those fibres which represent the most caudal parts of the distribution of all three divisions causing sensory loss first in the periphery of the face which gradually converge upon the nose and the lip as the compression increases.

B. **Outside the brain stem :**

1. The nerve may be involved at its point of attachment to pons by an expanding tumour

specially an acoustic neuroma. Trigeminal sensory loss will be associated with ipsilateral nerve deafness and facial paralysis.

2. A neuroma may also arise from the trunk of the nerve itself or the gasserian ganglion.
3. The first division of the nerve is usually involved in lesions in the cavernous sinus (described earlier).
4. The first division is also involved in Herpes Zoster.
5. Isolated trigeminal motor or sensory neuropathy has also been described.

## TRIGEMINAL NEURALIGA

Trigeminal neuralgia (T.N.) is a paroxysmal disorder characterised by brief attacks of severe pain within the territory of one or more divisions of the fifth nerve. It is also known as tic doulourcux because of the facial muscle spasm which occurs as a response to sudden intense pain. Females are affected more often than males and it is rare before middle life. In most occasions the disease is of unknown aetiology (idiopathic form). Rarely when it occurs in the young, it may be manifestation of multiple sclerosis or even a tumour involving the nerve.

In the idiopathic form, abnormalities have been described in the biopsy of the nerve root. Many cases have aberrant arteries impinging upon the root or there may be pressure for small tumours. Degenerative changes have also been described in the trigeminal ganglion itself which are thought to be the result of arteriosclerosis involving the small blood vessels in the ganglion. In the elderly, demineralisation of the base of the skull with upward tilting of the petrous pyramid may cause angulation and irritation of the nerve root. Mechanical stretching of the root may also occur in the elderly as a result of downward descent of the contents of the posterior fossa.

Whatever might be the underline pathology, the end result is a generation of repetitive stimuli at the site of damage and then spreading through the nerve to give rise to the paroxysms of pain.

**Clinical features :**

The pain is sudden, sharp, electric shock like in quality lasting for a few seconds to a minute. Very often it comes in bouts of repetitive attacks. It strikes with dramatic suddenness and may cause an involuntary exclamation, cessation of speech, contraction of the face on the affected side and watering of the eye.

The pain is usually limited to one division of the nerve usually the second or the third division and only occasionally in both. Isolated supraorbital neuralgia is rare. The pain will never extend beyond the territory of the fifth nerve and this differentiates T.N. from atypical facial pain which is of psychogenic origin.

The pain may be precipitated by acts of chewing, talking, smiling, shaving, cold air, eating icecream or drinking hot beverages. There is usually a "trigger spot" touching which can immediately bring on pain. In severe cases patients suffer from extreme depression and anxiety and may forego eating or drinking. Many patients may have tooth extraction under the false belief that the pain is originating in a bad tooth.

In idiopathic cases neurological examination is usually normal. Finding physical signs like loss of sensation or depressed corneal reflex should suggest a secondary cause for neuralgia.

Such cases should be investigated with skill. X-rays particularly basal view to look for the exit foramina (which may be eroded by tumours) and C.T. scanning. If demyelination is suspected C.S.F. study for immunoglobulin and evoked potentials should be performed.

**Treatment :**

A. **Medical therapy :** Most cases in the earlier stages respond well to medical treatment. Carbamazepine is the drug of choice and can be used in dosage varying from 300 to 1200 mg. per day. Side-effects include aplastic anaemia, agranulocytosis and thrombocytopenia. Hence periodic blood counts will be necessary. Once control is achieved, the dose may be reduced to a maintenance level that is sufficient to keep the patient pain-free. Treatment needs to be continued from months to years as recurrence is common.

Phenytoin can be used singly or in combination with Carbamazepine and gives comparable results. The dosage requirement varies from 200 to 600 mg per day and is adjusted to achieve a serum level of 15 to 20 mcg per ml. Side-effects include gum hyperplasia and ataxia.

Other drugs which have been tried include Clonazepam and Sodium Valporate.

B. **Surgical therapy** : Surgical therapy is indicated only when medical treatment has proven ineffective.

When the pain is limited to one division of the nerve a mandibular, infraorbital or supraorbital neurectomy or local injection of alcohol may suffice. However, regeneration of the nerve occurs with recurrence of pain.

When 2nd and 3rd divisions are involved ganglion may be injected with alcohol. This often leaves permanent anaesthesia and occasionally causes loss of corneal sensation and subsequent ocular damage. On occasions, the pain recurs on an anaesthetic face. For these reasons, alcohol injection of ganglion is not preferred now-a-days.

The most commonly used surgical procedures are gangliolysis, suboccipital craniectomy with decompression of the trigeminal nerve and trigeminal tractotomy.

Percutaneous radio frequency trigeminal gangliolysis is performed under local anaesthesia with radiographic control to guide the probe in the foramen ovale. The technique gives very good results in expert hands and is particularly suitable for elderly patients.

Suboccipital craniectomy with decompression of the trigeminal nerve is a more radical approach with the unique advantage that it produces pain relief without any sensory loss. The sensory root is visualised using an operating microscope and the source of compression is identified, which is usually an aberrent artery. A small non-absorbable sponge is placed between the nerve and the object.

Trigeminal tractotomy i.e. division of the spinal tract of the trigeminal, is needed for cases who are resistant to gangliolysis and decompression and is rarely performed nowadays.

## THE SEVENTH OR FACIAL NERVE

**Anatomical considerations** :

The facial nerve contains four different components which include —

(a) Motor efferent fibres supplying the muscles of facial expression and the platysma of the neck.

(b) Secretomotor efferent fibres to the lacrimal and salivary glands.

(c) Sensory afferent fibres conveying taste from the anterior two-thirds of the tongue via the chorda tympani nerve.

(d) Sensory afferent fibres from the external auditory meatus.

The motor nucleus of the facial nerve is in the lower pons and the fibres emerging from it loop round the nucleus of the sixth cranial nerve before coming out of the brain at the cerebello-pontine angle along with nervus intermedius and the eighth cranial nerve. It immediately enters the internal auditory meatus along with the eighth nerve and runs a tortuous course through the temporal bone in the facial canal before coming out through the stylomastoid foramen. It then passes forwards into the parotid gland where it divides to form the parotid plexus from which branches supply the facial musculature. Within the facial canal lies the geniculate ganglion and two branches of the nerve, namely, the nerve to the stapedius and chorda tympani nerve.

The superior salivary nucleus is the secretomotor nucleus for the submandibular and lacrimal glands. The preganglionic parasympathetic fibres are carried in the nervus intermedius and pass through the geniculate ganglion, some fibres then travelling in the greater superficial petrosal nerve to the sphenopalatine ganglion. Postganglionic fibres then pass to lacrimal glands and the glands of nose and palate.

The secretomotor fibres for the submandibular gland pass through the chorda tympani nerve to relay in the submandibular ganglion, postganglionic fibres from which supply the submandibular and sublingual glands.

The chorda tympani nerve arises from the facial nerve in the facial canal 6 mm proximal to stylomastoid foramen and leaves the tympanic cavity to join the lingual nerve through which its fibres are distributed to the anterior two-thirds of the tongue for carrying taste sensation. The taste fibres in the chorda tympani relay in the geniculate ganglion and central fibres pass to the nucleus of the tractus solitarius.

**Facial paralysis**

Facial paralysis may be due to —

1. A supranuclear or upper motor neuron (UMN) lesion involving the pyramidal fibres destined for the facial nucleus.
2. A supra nuclear lesion involving those fibres only which are concerned with emotional facial movements leading to mimic facial palsy.
3. Lesions involving the facial nucleus or the nerve itself.
4. Disorders of the facial muscles (e.g. facio-scapulo-humoral muscular dystrophy, dystrophia myotonica and myesthenia gravis).

A UMN facial palsy is distinguished by the fact that the upper facial muscles are relatively spared. This is due to bilateral pyramidal innervation of those parts of the facial nucleus controlling movements of the upper face. In a lower motor neuron lesion, however, upper and lower facial muscles are affected equally.

Emotional movements of the face are controlled by a separate group of upper motor neurons and hence these are spared in case of a hemiplegia. Isolated involvement of this pathway, characterised by appearance of facial asymmetry only during emotional expressions, indicates a lesion of the opposite frontal lobe and is called mimic facial palsy.

## NUCLEAR AND INFRANUCLEAR LESIONS OF THE FACIAL NERVE

**Central (Pontine) lesions :**

1. Cerebrovascular disease
2. Demyelinating disease
3. Pontine tumour
4. Syringobulbia
5. Poliomyelitis

**Peripheral lesions :**

A. Temporal bone :

1. **Infections**
   Bacterial : otitis media, syphilis, leprosy.
   Viral : varicella, mumps, herpes zoster, infectious mononucleosis

2. Tumours : Facial neuroma, acoustic neuroma, leukaemia
3. Granuloma : Sarcoidosis (causes recurrent and/or bilateral facial palsy)
4. Autoimmune : Guillain-Barre syndrome (bilateral facial palsy)
5. Metabolic : Diabetes, uraemia
6. Vasculitis : Polyarteritis
7. Trauma : Surgical operations in mastoids, temporal bone fracture
8. Idiopathic : Bell's palsy

B. **Parotid Gland**

1. Trauma
2. Sarcoidosis
3. Parotid tumour

A lesion within the temporal bone is associated with loss of taste in the anterior two-thirds of the tongue if it involves the nerve proximal to the origin of the chorda tympani. Herpes zoster of the geniculate ganglion deserves special mention which is known as the syndrome of Ramsay Hunt. One or more of the following symptoms may occur — pain in the ear and palatoglossal arch, vesicles with a similar distribution, loss of taste of the anterior two-thirds of the tongue, facial paralysis and deafness.

## BELL'S FACIAL PARALYSIS

Sir Charles Bell described the structure and function of the facial nerve in 1829 following which all diseases affecting the facial nerve were called Bell's palsy. With recognition of some causes of facial palsy like herpetic infection, the term Bell's palsy is now restricted only to the idiopathic form of peripheral facial nerve paralysis. The exact aetiology is unknown and a vascular ischaemic lesion of the nerve probably occurs in the region of the stylomastoid foramen. Other aetiological factors which have been suggested include a viral infection and an immunological damage of the nerve.

### Clinical features

Bell's palsy is almost always unilateral. The onset is sudden and often follows exposure to a draught. Frequently there is pain at the onset in the mastoid region. Paralysis of facial muscles cause the mouth to be drawn on the healthy side and the eye on the affected side fails to close. Due to absence of blinking, there is impairment of absorption of tears which tend to overflow the lower lid. On attempting to close the eyes, on the affected side the globe remains visible in an upturned position *(Bell's Phenomenon).* The nasolabial furrow is flattened on the affected side and the patient is unable to blow his cheeks or to whistle. Food tends to collect in the vestibule of the mouth and there is difficulty in gargling.

Many patients complain of a transient numbness on the affected side of the face although there is no actual fifth nerve involvement as evidenced by an intact crossed corneal reflex. The corneal reflex on the affected side will be absent due to damage to the efferent limb, i.e. the facial nerve.

When the chorda tympani nerve is involved there is loss of taste in anterior two-thirds of the tongue and involvement of the nerve to stapedius causes hyperacusis.

In long-standing cases due to failure of eye closure exposure keratitis and conjunctivitis may result.

### Treatment

It is important to understand the natural history of the disease in order to rationalise treatment. The facial nerve is acutely inflammed and oedematous within the facial canal. Treatment must, therefore, be directed at mitigating the effects of the inflammation.

The function of the nerve is interrupted in most cases by a reversible conduction block. In the first group full recovery usually takes place but not in the latter as repair can only be by regeneration of axons, some of which, either by misdirection or by branching will innervate muscles other than those it originally supplied. The aim of treatment is, therefore, to prevent axonal degeneration or denervation of the facial muscles.

When there is no denervation, recovery soon begins within a few days and completes within a few weeks. All those who recover completely show some return of movement within first four weeks. When any denervation has occurred there will be some degree of permanent weakness combined with associated movement (synkinesis) due to misdirection of axons. For example, the eye may close on pursing the lips or the angle of mouth may move up when the eyebrow is raised. An interesting form of late sequelae of facial palsy is the syndrome of crocodile tears in which tears pour from the affected eye during eating. This is due to faulty reinnervation when the salivary autonomic fibres in the facial nerve are misdirected to the eye.

Denervation occurs early within the first four days of onset. Treatment to prevent denervation must therefore also be early. It is difficult, however, to detect such cases so early even by electromyography and electrical stimulation tests. Hence, if effective treatment exists it should be given to all complete palsies seen within a week of onset. Incomplete palsy is a good prognostic sign and the decision to treat such cases must depend on the relative risk of the treatment employed. Bad prognostic signs in complete palsy include pain, advanced age, loss of taste sensation and hyperacusis. Electrogustatometry is currently being evaluated to pick out cases with early denervation.

A short rapidly tapered course of high dose prednisolone given soon after the onset has been claimed to be effective in reducing the incidence and severity of denervation and is widely practised. Although all cases might not respond satisfactorily, if there is no contraindication like diabetes or peptic ulcerations, cases seen within a week of the onset should be treated with an initial prednisolone dose of about 60 mg. per day reducing to zero over 10 to 15 days. It is useless to carry on treatment with steroids for weeks if recovery does not take place. In a large series including both complete and incomplete palsies, 88% of treated patients made complete recovery and a further 11% had only minor sequelae.

Combined with this medical treatment active and passive facial muscle exercises should be encouraged to prevent development of contractures. Galvanic stimulation of the facial muscles, although widely practised, is of debatable value.

Surgical treatment has been based on the rational purpose of decompressing the facial nerve in the canal to prevent denervation. Unfortunately this approach is ineffective. Residual weakness when gross can, of course, be helped by plastic surgery.

## THE EIGHTH CRANIAL (VESTIBULO-COCHLEAR) NERVE

**Anatomical considerations :** The eighth nerve carries impulse from the highly specialised organs, the organ of corti and the vestibular apparatus situated in the depth of the internal ears. The cochlear nerve carries sound vibrations from the hair cells of the organ of corti through the spiral ganglion in the cochlea, to the cochlear nuclei in the brain stem. Majority of the fibres cross and run in the lateral fillet to terminate in the medial geniculate body and are then relayed to superior temporal gyrus, where sound is finally interpreted.

Impulses carried in the vestibular nerves arise in the labyrinth, induced by movement of endolymph, which affect the hair cells in the ampullae of the semi-circular canals and the otolith organs in the utricle and saccule. The semi-circular canals are three in number on each side. Activity in the canals is transmitted through the vestibular nerve and ganglion to the vestibular nucleus in the brain stem. These nuclei have connections with the cerebellum, the oculomotor nuclei, nuclei of the upper cervical nerves and the temporal lobes. These interconnections are necessary for maintenance of posture and balance during head, neck and eye movements.

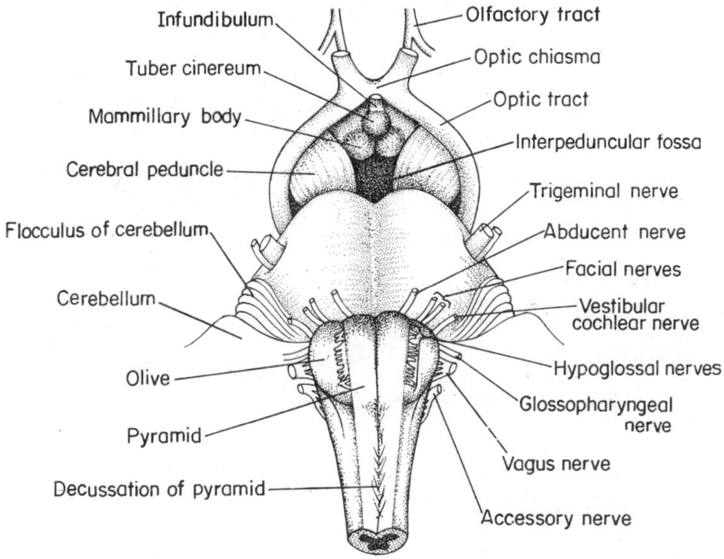


**Fig.12.7 : Medulla oblongata, pons and Cranial nerves emerging at different levels.**

## Test of auditory function

Simple bedside tests of auditory function include testing with a wrist watch as well as by whispered voice. The tuning fork tests help to distinguish between hearing loss due to middle ear disease (conductive deafness) and that due to eighth nerve damage (perceptive deafness). Two tests are commonly employed.

**Rinne's test :** Here a 512 Hz tuning fork is held on the mastoid until it is no longer audible. It is then moved in front of the external ear and normally it should still be audible (i.e. air conduction is more than bone conduction : AC$>$BC). This situation also persists in case of perceptive deafness but is reversed (i.e. BC $>$ AC) in conductive deafness. Further differentiation rests on Weber's test.

**Weber's Test :** In this test the vibrating tuning fork is held on the centre of the forehead and normally it should be heard equally in both ears. In perceptive deafness, Weber is lateralised to the healthy ear but in conductive deafness it is lateralised on the affected side.

**Audiometry :** This gives a quantitative measurement of hearing. Pure sounds of known frequency and intensity are presented to the patient via earphones. For each frequency the intensity at which the sound is perceived is plotted on a standard graph, from the shape of which it is possible to differentiate perceptive from conductive deafness. Classically high frequency loss is characteristic of nerve deafness and low frequency loss occurs in middle ear disease.

In loudness recruitment test, sound stimuli of the same frequency but of different intensities are presented to either ear and the patient is asked to state at which intensity the sound is heard with the deaf ear as loud as that heard in the normal ear. In conductive deafness, the ratio between the intensities required to produce equal loudness in the two ears remains the same for all intensities. In nerve deafness due to lesion in sensory end organ in the cochlea (e.g. Meniere's disease) the difference between the two ears diminishes or may disappear as the intensity rises.

This phenomenon however does not occur in lesions of the nerve trunk itself (e.g. acoustic neuroma).

## BRAIN STEM AUDITORY EVOKED RESPONSE (BAER)

This is a recently developed highly sophisticated electrophysiological test by which not only hearing can be tested but also neural activity in the cochlear, auditory nerve and brain stem pathways can be studied.

The test can also be done in the newborn, infants and in unconscious patients to test the integrity of the brain stem. A series of clicks are presented to the ears through the earphones and evoked potentials are recorded with the help of the scalp and mastoid electrodes. Five potentials are usually recorded, each of which denotes activity of one part of the auditory pathway. From the amplitude and latency of such potentials, localisation of lesions is possible.

**Causes of conductive deafness :**

These include all diseases of the external ear, middle ear and eustachian tube.

**Causes of perceptive deafness :**

1. **Cochlear lesions :** Meniere's disease, advanced to sclerosis, drug toxicity and vascular lesions.
2. **Lesions of nerve trunk :** Post-inflammatory lesions, toxic nerve damage, cerebellopontine-angle tumours like acoustic neuroma and traumatic injuries.
3. **Central lesions :** Pontine vascular lesions and rarely brain stem demyelination.

**Vestibular Function Tests :**

1. **Gait and Stance :** Unilateral disorders of vestibular function causes the patient to veer or fall to the side of the lesion. This is also true for cerebellar hemispheric lesions as well.
2. **Nystagmus :** Careful examination of spontaneous eye movements are very important (vide *infra).*
3. **The Caloric Test :**

   This test is based on the fact that the hair cells can be stimulated by convection currents set up in the semi-circular canals if they are heated or cooled. The lateral canal is most suitable to study. The patient's head is held back at 60° to bring these in vertical position, at which stage it is easier to produce convection current.

Water at 30°C and at 44°C is irrigated into each ear in turn and this produces easily observed nystagmus as the canals are stimulated or inhibited. The duration of nystagmus is measured which normally lasts for about two minutes.

If the semi-circular canals or the eighth nerve are damaged, absence or defective response to both hot and cold water in the affected ear will be found. This is called canal paresis. Classically it occurs in Meniere's diseases, acoustic neuroma and vestibular neuronitis.

The central connections of the vestibular nerve are such that cold water in one ear has the same effect as hot water in the other. If nystagmus cannot be induced in one side (e.g. cold water failing to induce nystagmus in the left ear and warm water in the right) it indicates that the vestibular nucleus of the appropriate side (in the example cited in the right side) is defective. This is called directional preponderance and indicates a central brain stem lesion.

## NYSTAGMUS

Nystagmus may be defined as a failure of maintenance of ocular posture causing rhythmical oscillations of the eyeballs. The amplitude of movement may be equal in two phases *(pendular nystagmus due to poor vision)* or may be jerky with a slow and quick phase alternating *(Jerk nystagmus due to labyrinthine or brain stem dysfunction).* The direction of jerk nystagmus is named after the direction of the fast phase. The amplitude of the movement is greatest on looking to the side, towards which the quick phase occurs.

When nystagmus of this sort is elicited only on deviation of the eyes to the side of the fast phase it is said to be of first degree. If the nystagmus, in addition to above, is also present on looking straight ahead, it is called second degree nystagmus.

Third degree nystagmus is even present when looking to the opposite direction to that in which the fast phase is beating.

Normal subjects may show jerk-nystagmus if lateral gaze is maintained at extreme range outside the limits of binocular vision for a long period. An exaggeration of this phenomenon may also occur in myasthenia gravis. To be clinically significant and pathological in nature, nystagmus must occur within thirty degrees of the midline (i.e. well within the binocular field of vision) and must be sustained.

## TYPES OF NYSTAGMUS AND THEIR LOCALISATION

(1) **Vestibular nystagmus :** Acute vestibular disturbance due either to viral infection (vestibular neuronitis), vascular lesions, trauma or due to an attack of Meniere's disease shows horizontal jerk nystagmus with or without a rotatory component. The direction of the quick phase is usually away from the side of lesion. Gaze in the direction of quick phase increases the frequency and amplitude of the nystagmus (Alexander's law). Vertigo accompanies the nystagmus and subsides with its disappearance. Diagnosis of vestibular cause is suggested by the presence of tinnitus and/or hearing loss.

(2) **Positional nystagmus :** This is elicitable in patients who give history of positional vertigo (i.e. vertigo on lying down, sitting up or turning over in bed). Nystagmus may be provoked by the patient being rapidly laid down supine on a couch with his head over the end of it and turns to one side. With a peripheral lesion (e.g. in the labyrinth as in benign positional vertigo) nystagmus appears after an interval of few seconds and may be rotatory in nature. This usually occurs when the affected ear is downmost. It is often associated with severe vertigo but the nystagmus fatigues away quickly and is difficult to reproduce in the subsequent minutes.

In contrast, in case of a central lesion causing positional nystagmus, nystagmus appears immediately on head turning, is not associated with vertigo and is often reproducible.

(3) **Brain stem nystagmus :** Multidirectional nystagmus is classical of brain stem lesion. Vertical nystagmus (nystagmus beating in vertical direction and not nystagmus elicited on vertical gaze) is always due to a central lesion and is never labyrinthine in origin. Common causes include Wernicke's encephalopathy, multiple sclerosis, brain stem vascular episodes, brain stem gliomas and drug toxicity. The classical example of the latter is phenytoin toxicity seen in epileptics but may also occur with benzodiazepines and barbiturates. Drugs causing vestibular damage like streptomycin and gentamycin usually do not cause spontaneous nystagmus.

(4) **Ataxic nystagmus :** This results from damage to the medial longitudinal bundle which interconnects the nuclei of the 3rd, and 6th cranial nerves and is necessary for conjugate eye movements. An internuclear ophthalmoplegia results with paralysis of horizontal lateral gaze. Jerk nystagmus is exaggerated in the abducting eye. This condition is almost pathognomonic of brain stem demyelination.

(5) **Cerebellar lesions :** Lesions of cerebellar hemispheres produce jerk nystagmus with the fast phase towards the side of the lesion. Lesions of the vermis usually cause truncal ataxia but no nystagmus. Degenerative cerebellar diseases also do not usually cause nystagmus.

(6) **Congenital nystagmus :** This is usually of the pendular type and may be present even on looking straight ahead. Usually this is due to poor visual acuity acquired early in childhood due to congenital optic atrophy, macular degenerations, high myopia, toxoplasmosis, albinism etc. It may also be familial when vision may be normal.

A variant of this may develop later in life in people working in dark environment for a long time (Miner's nystagmus).

(7) **Optokinetic nystagmus :** In normal subjects viewing passing objects from a moving train alternating slow and fast eye movement are seen. Pursuit movement track the retreating target and when it reaches the limit of the lateral gaze a quick movement takes the eyes back to fix on the next forward target. This response depends on the integrity of the frontal and occipital connections. In clinical practice optokinetic response is tested by moving a striped drum in front of the eyes in various directions. Unilateral hemispheric lesions e.g. a right parietal lesion, will cause loss of optokinetic nystagmus when the drum rotates such that the stripes run from left to right. Loss of quick phase is also seen in supranuclear ophthalmoplegias. (e,g. in progressive supranuclear palsy). Testing for optokinetic response is a very useful way to differentiate between hysterical blindness and organic blindness of cortical origin where the pupillary reflexes and the fundal appearance remain normal.

(8) **See-saw nystagmus :** In this type as one eye raises it rolls in towards the medial angle and the other falls rolling outwards. This form of nystagmus is generally due to a large parasellar tumour.

(9) **Convergence-retraction nystagmus :** In this type as the eyes look upward a jerk nystagmus is seen in which the fast phase brings the eyes towards each other in a convergence movement. Viewed from the side it appears as though the eyeballs are being pulled back into the head. This rare phenomenon occurs with lesions in the pineal region.

(10) **Downbeat nystagmus :** On lateral gaze specially below the horizontal meridian downbeating (fast phase downwards) jerk nystagmus developed. This is pathognomonic of a lesion in the region of the cervicomedullary junction at the foramen magnum like-platybasia or Arnold-chiari malformation (herniation of cerebellar tonsils).

(11) **Periodic alternating nystagmus :** In this type horizontal nystagmus occurs alternating in direction every minute or two. Hurried examination may miss the alternating sequence. Likely pathology includes vascular or degenerative lesions involving the brain stem at the level of the vestibular nucleus.

(12) **Spasmus nutans :** This rare self-limiting disease of infants consists of head nodding, torticollis and nystagmus of pendular or jerk type in horizontal, oblique or vertical plane.

## NINTH, TENTH AND ELEVENTH CRANIAL NERVES

**Anatomical considerations** (Fig.12.8) : These three nerves emerge together from the lower part of the brain stem. The ninth or glossopharyngeal nerve carries general sensation from the pharynx and also carries taste sensation from the posterior one-third of the tongue. The tenth or vagus nerve supplies motor fibres to the muscles of the palate, pharynx and larynx. The accessory nerve has two components. The cranial part joins the vagus to supply the laryngeal muscles and the spinal part supplies the sternomastoid and the trapezius muscles. These three nerves emerge together from the skull through the jugular foramen and in this situation come in close proximity to the hypoglossal nerve and the cervical sympathetic.

**Clinical aspects :** The glossopharyngeal nerve constitute the afferent limb of the gag reflex, the efferent limb of which is constituted by the vagus nerve. Paralysis of the vagus causes dysphagia, nasal regurgitation of food, nasal intonation or hoarseness of voice.

Lesions of the spinal accessory cause weakness of the trapezius causing drooping of the shoulder and of the sternomastoid causing difficulty in turning the neck to the opposite side.

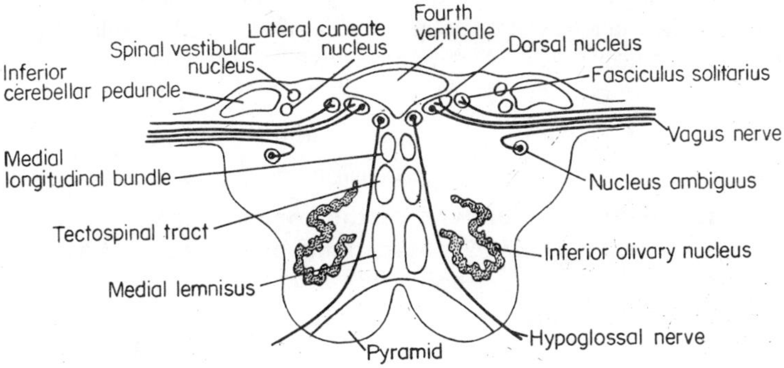


Fig.12.8 : Section through fourth, ventricle showing vagal nerve nuclei and hypoglossal nerve.

**Jugular foramen syndrome :** Lesions in the region of the jugular foramen involve the ninth, tenth and eleventh cranial nerves and may also involve the hypoglossal and cervical sympathetic causing Horner's syndrome. Such lesions include intracranial tumours like neurinomas arising from the nerves, meningioma and epidermoid tumours. Extracranial lesions which may involve the same area include an infiltrating nasopharyngeal carcinoma or a glomus jugulare tumour.

Other lesions affecting the muscles of deglutition and laryngeal muscles include infective polyneuritis affecting the cranial nerves, poliomyelitis, motor **neuron disease**, polymyositis and certain forms of muscular dystrophy (**Fig.12.8**).

**Glossopharyngeal neuralgia :** Attacks of severe pain occur in the throat when fluid or food is swallowed. The condition is similar to trigeminal neuralgia. This may be of idiopathic type or may be symptomatic when the nerve may be compressed by aberrant vessels or adjacent tumours. All such cases need full investigations to exclude the latter possibility. The idiopathic form responds to carbamazepine and **phenytoin** but resistant cases would need section of the nerve with posterior **cranial fossa exploration**.

## TWELFTH OR HYPOGLOSSAL NERVE

**Anatomical considerations :** Hypoglossal is the motor nerve of the tongue. The nucleus of the nerve is situated in the medulla and the nerve originates by four rootlets which correspond to the four cervical myotomes which migrated to form the muscles of the tongue. The nerve leaves the cranial cavity through the hypoglossal canal of the occipital bone in close proximity to the nerves which traverse the jugular foramen. In the neck the nerve passes downwards and forwards to reach the tongue.

**Clinical aspects :** Unilateral lower motor **neuron** lesion of the hypoglossal causes paralysis of the muscles of the corresponding half of the tongue. The paralysed half-atrophied tongue causes the overlying mucosa to be thrown into folds and the tongue deviates to the side of the lesion on protrusion. Such a lesion may result from an infarct in the anterior part of the medulla causing **ipsi lateral** hypoglossal paralysis and contralateral hemiparesis, due to damage to the pyramidal tract before decussation. The facial muscles are spared. This is called medial medullary syndrome.

Isolated lesion of the hypoglossal nerve during its passage through the hypoglossal canal can occur but is uncommon.

The nerve may also be involved in lesions in the region of the jugular foramen as described in the previous section.

Bilateral lower motor neuron lesion of the hypoglossal causes atrophy of the whole tongue with difficulty in protrusion and difficulty in articulation of the linguals (e.g. t and d) Fibrillations commonly occur. Common causes of bilateral lower motor hypoglossal lesion include motor neuron disease and syringobulbia.

In unilateral upper motor neuron lesion (for example cortical or capsular lesion) the tongue deviates away from the side of lesion on protrusion and usually there is no wasting.

Bilateral upper motor neuron paralysis of the tongue occurs, as a result of the lesions involving both corticospinal tracts above the medulla (pseudobulbar palsy). In such cases though true wasting does not occur, the tongue appears smaller than normal owing to spastic contraction of the muscles. There is difficulty in protruding the tongue associated with slurring of speech (spastic dysarthria).

## CEREBROSPINAL FLULD AND HYDROCEPHALUS

*G.C. MOOKERJEE*
*M.K. MUKHERJEE*

---

**Introduction :**

The term "Hydrocephalus" is derived from the two words "Hydro" and "Encephalon", which means accumulation of excess water (fluid) inside the cranial vault. The "water" inside the cranial vault represents the **cerebrospinal fluid** (CSF). Increase in the total quantity of the intracranial fluid in the brain substance causes raised intracranial tension but not hydrocephalus as in pseudomotor cerebri or cerebral oedema.

Normally the entire cavity enclosing the brain and the spinal cord has a volume of about 1950 ml, and only about 150 ml of this volume is occupied by the CSF. Actually this 150 ml of fluid is contained in the ventricles of the brain in the cisterns around the brain and in the subarachnoid space around both the cerebral hemispheres and the spinal cord. All these chambers or spaces are interconnected with one another.

The major function of the CSF is to cushion the brain tissue within the solid and bony vault and project it from sudden physical trauma. The brain tissue and the CSF both have almost the same specific gravity and as such the brain floats in the fluid.

**Formation of the (CSF) :**

It is formed from three different sources –

(1) the choroid plexuses inside the ventricles of the brain, mainly the lateral ventricles – the bulk portion of the fluid is formed here.

(2) the blood vessels of the meningeal and ependymal linings of the chambers containing the CSF.

(3) The blood vessel of the brain and the spinal cord.

The **choroid plexus** is a cauliflower-like tuft of blood vessels covered by a thin layer of cuboidal epithelial cells which contain plenty of mitochondria and vacuoles and it projects into the temporal horns of the lateral ventricles, the posterior portions of the third ventricle and the roof of the fourth ventricle.

The CSF is being formed continually and also being reabsorbed continually into the blood through the veins via the arachnoidal villi and through the "perivascular spaces" of the brain.

**CSF Pressure :**

CSF pressure varies normally between 80 and 150 mm. water with an average of 130 mm. water (equivalent to 10 mm Hg). In spite of the fact that there is a continuous secretion and absorption of the CSF the pressure of the fluid is regulated at a constant level by : (1) the rate of fluid formation and (2) the resistance to circulation and hence absorption through the arachnoidal villi. The CSF pressure rises or decreases with the rise or fall of either of these two factors.

**Composition of CSF :**

It is a clear, colourless, transparent fluid which does not coagulate on standing. Its reaction is alkaline and contains about 0 to 5 lymphocytes per cubic mm. Its specific gravity is between 1.004 and 1.006.

Chemically it represents colloid-free plasma with some variations in its crystalloid composition. Of the important constituents its protein content and sugar content are respectively much less and slightly less than those in plasma whereas the chloride content is much above than that in plasma.

With all these physiological backgrounds, the pathological basis in the development of hydrocephalus can be discussed subsequently as follows.

## AETIOPATHOLOGY OF HYDROCEPHALUS

This can be discussed under two headings :

1. Congenital
2. Acquired

1. **Congenital causes :**

(a) **Arnold-Chiari Malformation :** It is a congenital defect in the posterior fossa where a tongue-like projection of the cerebellum and the choroid plexus extend with an enlarged fourth ventricle into the spinal canal through the foramen magnum thereby stretching and kinking backward the upper cervical spinal cord. This condition is frequently associated with spina bifida and meningomyelocoele and may lead to hydrocephalus.

(b) **Dandy-Walker Malformation** (also known as atresia of the foramina of Magendie and Luschka) — here some congenital septa or membranes block the outlet of the fourth ventricle and as such the fourth ventricle is ballooned out into a large cavity above which lies the cerebellar vermis.

(c) **Congenital atresia or forking of the aqueduct of Sylvius :** Here in this condition the upper portion of the aqueduct is grossly narrowed which again may be forked or obstructed by a transverse septum. This leads to the hydrocephalus of the lateral and the third ventricles.

(d) **Agenesis of corpus callosum :** Partial or complete — this condition is often associated with lipomas and meningiomas at the site of the developmental defect. Pneumoencephalogram is diagnostic.

2. **Acquired causes :**

(a) **Trauma :** e.g. birth injuries, head injuries, intracranial haemorrhages especially intraventricular haemorrhage leading to secondary stenosis of the aqueduct of Sylvius are the common causes.

(b) **Inflammation :** Especially of the meninges and the brain (meningitis, encephalitis and meningo-encephalitis) or inflammatory reaction to subarachnoid bleeding at birth or later in life, may lead to gliosis of the aqueduct or obliteration of the subarachnoid space.

(c) **Neoplasms and space occupying lesions :** Like tuberculomas, gliomas, organised subdural haematomas or abscesses — all may produce obstructive hydrocephalus. Again a tumour of the choroid plexus (particularly choroid plexus papilloma which usually occurs in children below 2 years or age) may rarely cause hydrocephalus due to over-production of the CSF.

Other neoplastic conditions which might cause hydrocephalus in the paediatric age group include — colloid cysts attached to the choroid plexus of the third ventricle, chordoma, pituitary adenomas and pinealoma.

(d) **Miscellaneous :** Apart from the above conditions there are some conditions commonly grouped under a single heading of "Pseudotumor Cerebri" (also known as benign intracranial hypertension) which embraces different clinical entities all of which cause over-production of the CSF with mild to moderate gradation of hydrocephalus especially among the paediatric age group. It has been found in association with various infections especially otitis media hyper- and hypo-vitaminosis A, tetracycline - toxicity, sudden withdrawal of steroids, hypothyroidism, hypoparathyroidism and Addison's disease. It is a self-limiting condition and prognosis is usually good.

### Classification

From treatment point of view hydrocephalus can be classified with two types: 1) Communicating type and (2) non-communicating type of hydrocephalus whereas from anatomical point of view it can also be classified under two types — (a) Internal and (b) External type of hydrocephalus.

(a) **Communicating type :** In this type of hydrocephalus, as the name signifies there is free communication between the cerebral ventricles and the subarachnoid space. It usually is due to abnormally over-production of the fluid by the choroid plexuses of the ventricles in the newborn infants. This type leads to a huge accumulation of the fluid due to excessive production the amount of which progressively becomes more and more than the amount which can re-enter the venous system through the arachnoidal villi, leading to huge collection of the fluid both inside ventricles and in the subarachnoid space outside the brain.

(b) **Non-communicating type :** In this type as the name signifies, there is no free communication between the cerebral ventricles and the subarachnoid space, and instead there is a block or obstruction (and hence also called obstructive type) to such a free flow of liquid.

Actually speaking, the terms 'communicating' and 'non-communicating' are misleading as has been emphasised by some authors as both the types, strictly from pathological point of view, are due to some form of anatomical or physiological obstruction between the points of formation and absorption of the fluid.

### Internal & External types of hydrocephalus :

These two anatomical types are differentiated depending upon the anatomical site of greatest enlargement of the CSF spaces, whether ventricular or extra-ventricular.

### Clinical Features :—

**Onset :** In case of congenital hydrocephalus it is present at birth or becomes manifested and apparent within a short time after birth, usually within a few months of life and progresses quite rapidly producing wide range of symptoms and sequelae.

In case of acquired hydrocephalus, it usually develops later in life, in association with or as sequelae to the conditions predisposing to it and the progress is not as rapid as in the case of congenital type.

**Progress :** The progress of the process and the symptoms arising out of it vary widely — may be rapid or slow and steadily progressing, intermittent or even remittent, depending upon the cause, especially in case of obstructive type where the obstruction may be complete or partial or intermittent.

In either type the *classical picture, especially among the infants is dominated by enlarged or an enlarging head due to enlargement of the skull in all diameters with bulging and tense fontanels, wide gaping at cranial suture lines, prominent and dilated scalp veins on shiny scalp protruding forehead with bulging eyebrows. The eye sign is known as the "Sun-set sign"* characteristically by a visible sclera above the iris due more to the retraction of the upper eyelid than to the pressure on the orbit. Other eye signs are failure to gaze and strabismus and papilloedema ultimately leading to optic atrophy. The "papilloedema" which means "the swelling of the optic disc which can be seen with the help of an ophthalmoscope" is due to high pressure in the optic sheath (the dura mater in the orbital region of the frontal lobe of the brain extending as a sheath into the orbit around the optic nerve and this is pierced by the retinal artery and the vein a few millimetres behind the eyeball on their way to and from the eye along with the optic nerve) due to raised cerebrospinal fluid-tension which impedes the flow of blood in the retinal veins thereby also raising the retinal capillary pressure, ultimately resulting in retinal oedema. As the tissues of the optic disc are much more distensible than those of the remainder of the retina, the optic disc becomes more and more odematous than the remainder of the retina and swells into the cavity of the eye. Other manifestations in infants specially include mild to moderate diplegia, hyperactive reflexes with irritability, a high-pitched cry, fretfulness, ear pulling, head rolling convulsive seizures, vomiting and failure to thrive and gradually leading to a lethargic baby with drowsiness.

**Investigations :**

Investigations form a very important step in the correct diagnosis of the cause of the condition and of the site of obstruction if there be any so that early and definite approach for the treatment can be instituted.

The important investigations are :

(1) Straight X-ray of the skull — PA, AP, basal and lateral views or any other special view in some cases requiring them.

(2) Tomograms in different planes to localise any tumour or growth.

(3) Electro-encephalogram (EEG) — if necessary serial.

(4) Brain scanning (with the isotope RISHA — Radioactive Ionised Human Serum Albumin).

(5) Carotid angiogram

(6) Pneumo-encephalogram (wherein air or helium or oxygen is introduced into the subarachnoid space, usually in the lumbar region, sometimes by cisternal puncture under general anaesthesia) but cisternal puncture should be avoided in patients suspected to be suffering from Arnold-Chiari malformation).

(7) Ventriculogram (wherein gas is put directly into the ventricular system through a patent fontanel of an infant or through a trephine-hole in older children as adults in whom the fontanel is not patent).

(8) Echoencephalogram and especially CT-scan in localising a tumour.

## DIAGNOSTIC CRITERIA

**In infants and very young children :-**

Symptoms of irritability, restlessness, vomiting, failure to thrive along with an enlarged or enlarging head is noted by serial measurements plotted on a head chart.

Bulging fontanels and separation at cranial suture lines will be evident.

Positive transillumination test and "Setting-sun" eye-sign associated with features of rise of intracranial tension are noted in established cases. There may be associated congenital malformation.

**In Older Children and Adults :**

History of onset and progress along with the history of past illness suggesting inflammation of the brain and/or the meninges symptoms of headache, vomiting and dimness of vision may draw attention.

"Crack-pot" sign on percussion of the skull, presence of papilloedema on ophthalmoscopy along with features of raised intracranial tension are strongly suggestive.

**Differential Diagnosis**

This should be made in (1) infants and young children with the possible causes of enlargement of head and in (2) older children and young adults with all possible causes of increased intracranial tension with or without enlargement of head.

**In Infants and Young Children with possibilities of enlarged head :**

**Normal variations of skull**

It should be borne in mind that slight and simple enlarged appearance of the head is somewhat within normal variations from infant to infant and as such an enlarged or enlarging head should be confirmed only after serial measurement of the head and plotted against a head chart and compared with percentile variations.

**Prematurity :**

In premature babies also the head apparently looks enlarged in comparison to other body measurements and this is normal. Here also the gestational history and the features of prematurity along with serial measurements of the head will not call for detailed investigations.

**Familial :**

In certain families the head at birth and even after birth appears to be somewhat bigger than the average as a "family trend" and as such this possibility should be borne in mind before the diagnosis is inferred.

**Large Baby :**

Especially the babies of diabetic mothers are as a whole large in comparison to average and serial head measurements and absence of other features of raised intracranial tension will clinch the clue.

**Subdural Effusion and/or haematoma :**

A localised swelling usually conforming to the shape of the underlying cranial bone along with or without the presence of the ecchymosis under the scalp with a history of birth trauma or any other trauma helps to exclude the possibility of hydrocephalus. X-ray of the skull is diagnostic and in doubtful cases subdural tap should be undertaken both for the sake of diagnosis and to release the effect of compression on the underlying brain tissue.

**Rickets :**

This condition also leads to separation (rather delayed union) of sutures with an enlarged head but should never be mistaken for hydrocephalus. The following points in favour of rickets will help to recognise ricket :

(1) It is usually common between 4 months and 2 years of age.

(2) There is diffuse round prominence of the parietal regions as well as of the frontal regions (this is also true of congenital syphilis) and as such there are four prominent bony bulges with an anteroposterior and a transverse groove between them thus forming the "hot cross bun" shape. Frontal bossing is also prominent.

(3) Craniotabes is the earliest sign of rickets which may appear as early as 3 months of age and is a softening and thinning of an area of the skull — commonly in the occipitoparietal region of the skull, which indents on pressure and rebound often with a crackle. (This may also be found normally in prematures.)

(4) Presence of funnel-shaped or pigeon-shaped chest.

(5) Presence of Harrison's groove corresponding to the costal insertions of the diaphragm.

(6) Rachitic rosary — enlarged costochondral junctions.

(7) Presence of kyphosis or lordosis of the spine with prominent and protuberant abdomen.

(8) Presence of enlargement of the elbows, knee, ankles and bow legs in older children.

(9) Raised alkaline phosphate concentration in blood with usually a low blood phosphorus level and rarely with a low blood calcium level (causing infantile tetany).

(10) Presence of characteristic X-ray findings most prominent at the lower ends of the Ulna and Radius — showing typical cupping, spreading, fraying, stippling of the ends of the shafts, spurring and decreased density of the shaft with unusually prominent trabeculae.

**Congenital Syphilis —**

This condition also leads to hydrocephalus and some enlargement of the head because of the so-called "hot-cross bun" appearance as in rickets, but the usual features of congenital syphilis make this condition unmistakably distinct from all other alike conditions. The diagnostic features are :

(1) Presence of a family history along with —

(2) "snuffles" with a mucopurulent discharge occasionally bloody with upper-lip excoriation;

(3) Characteristic lesions of skin and mucous membrane including "rhagades" (radiating fissured scars) around the angles of the mouth and "condylomalata" (flat raised plaques in the anogenital area);

(4) Parrot's paralysis (Pseudoparalysis);

(5) Characteristic X-ray findings — multifocal osteochondritis at the metaphyses of the elbows, wrists, knees and ankles, symmetrical periostitis and osteomyelitis of the long bones, Wimberger's sign — bilateral moth-eaten appearance of the medial aspect of the proximal tibia.;

(6) Hepatosplenomegaly, lymphadenopathy — particularly epitrochlear, choreoretinitis;

(7) Characteristic CSF changes and finally positive anti-treponema antibodies test (TPI test and FTA-ABS test) and other serological tests for syphilis in blood.

**Mega encephaly :**

This is a rare condition in which a child has an unusually large brain (and as such has large head) of poor quality without hydrocephalus. Diagnosis is easily made by pneumoencephalogram.

**Hydranencephaly :**

This is another rare condition in which the head of the infant is full of CSF, with little brain tissue. The diagnosis is easily established by transillumination in a dark room and also by air studies.

**Gargoylism :**

In this condition, apart from hydrocephalus there is a peculiar facies, hepatosplenomegaly, congenital corneal opacities (along with a peculiar sabot-shaped deformity of the second and third lumbar vertebrae with kyphosis, mental retardation, enlargement of the pituitary fossa when the child becomes a little older than the infant stage).

Neoplastic conditions involving the skull and the brain which produce asymmetric enlargement of the head with or without hydrocephalus. All these conditions are diagnosed by clinical examinations and investigations.

**Causes of enlarged head**

**In Older Children :**

The causes mentioned earlier have all to be considered along with the following additional possibilities :

Normal variation among middle-aged males an increasing prominence of the forehead, mostly over the frontal areas due to slow enlargement of air cells of the frontal air sinuses and is not pathological. This prominence of the forehead makes the eyebrows appear overhanging the eye.

**Acromegaly :** This condition also leads to some enlargement of the head but the involvement of the skull bones is much less than the involvement of the lower jaw and the phalanges of the hand and the feet, giving the face a characteristic appearance and the whole skeleton an overall enhanced growth pattern. Besides, this condition often leads to bilateral temporal hemianopia. X-ray of the skull (lateral view) often exposes an enlarged sella turcica due to hypertrophy of the pituitary body to which the disease is due.

**Primary and Secondary neoplastic conditions involving skull bones :** these mainly lead to asymmetric enlargement of the head and a close clinical examination and the history of the case will clinch the diagnosis and differentiate them from hydrocephalus.

**Treatment**

It is to be borne in mind that, among infants, about 40 per cent of all cases do undergo spontaneous arrest. Surgical interventions, as such, should be reserved to cases in which serial measurements of head circumference show progressive and rapid enlargement of the head and clinical effects raise intracranial tension. Among older children and adults, about 100 per cent of them need surgical treatment.

Before any surgical measure is undertaken, all attempts should be made to confirm the cause of hydrocephalus, its nature and whether communicating or non-communicating type and the exact site of obstruction.

**General Measures :** Maintenance of nutrition and electrolyte balance of the body fluids either by oral or by intravenous feeding.

**Surgical Measures :** Once the patient is being prepared well to bear the stress and strain of surgical intervention, the plan for surgical treatment should be sorted out. The same should be undertaken by an efficient neurosurgeon in a well-equipped neurosurgical unit.

Two types of surgical approaches have been tried.

(1) Reduction in the production of excess CSF by — fluid restriction, blood-letting, choroid plexectomy — all these measures and procedures are not much beneficial and backdated and have been abandoned in favour of the second type of procedure.

(2) Bypass operations comprising of bypassing the point of obstruction by diverting and shunting the CSF to normal or artificial sites for absorption or excretion.

In pure aqueductal obstruction with adequate subarachnoid system, Torkildsen's operation draining CSF . from the lateral ventricle to cisterna magna by using a plastic tube.

Other bypass operations are :

(1) Between the ventricular system and lesser peritoneal sac or the pleural spaces.

(2) Between the ventricular system and the superior venacava or the atrium using the Spitz-Holter or the Pudenz-Heyer valves to prevent reflux of blood—this is the most popular and widely practised procedure at present.

(3) Between the lateral ventricle or in cases of communicating hydrocephalus, between spinal theca and the ureter after nephrectomy. (This operation leads to a negative electrolyte balance because of huge loss of C.S.F. via urine and as such supplementary sodium or ammonium chloride has to be given by mouth daily).

The risks of such bypass operations include —

(1) Obstruction to the passage of CSF because of blockage inside the tubes which sometimes call for a revisional surgery.

(2) Septicaemia and bacteriaemia due to colonization of organisms of the artificial valves.

(3) Multiple pulmonary thrombosis with pulmonary hypertension and heart failure.

The result of surgery is very difficult to assess. Without surgery, the mortality rate is very high, as high as 75 per cent. But with surgery the survival rate is about 75 to 80 per cent and among survivors the I.Q. is more or less retained within normal limits.

**Prognosis**

Prognosis should be guarded in hydrocephalic patients. The prognosis with and without surgical interventions has been discussed earlier. Many patients, even after successful surgery, suffer from emotional complexes.

Paraparesis, ataxia, urinary incontinence (if hydrocephalus is associated with meningomyelocele) and defective vision. The chance of a revisional surgery is also pretty high in cases of bypass operations.

## CEREBROVASCULAR STROKES

### (Syndromes of cerebral strokes : Cerebro-vascular accidents)

*G.C. MOOKERJEE*

---

**Introduction**

Blockage of one or more cerebral vessels due to atheroma, thrombosis, occlusion, or rupture of a blood vessel may lead to sudden or rapid loss of brain function which is clinically described as "stroke". A large number of clinical patterns may occur depending on the extent of pathological alternations produced by the lesion which may be due to the following conditions :

(1) Cerebral thrombosis in atherosclerotic vessels;

(2) Cerebral emboli — source usually cardiac;

(3) Cerebral haemorrhage — due to sudden rupture of atherosclerotic or aneurysmal blood vessels;

(4) Subarachnoid haemorrhage is also due to vascular leaking usually at the circle of Willis;

(5) Middle meningeal artery may break due to trauma also causing a stroke;

(6) Vascular malformations often remain symptomless but suddenly may leak causing intra-cerebral haemorrhage. These congenital vascular abnormalities may be :

(i) Looping, kinking or tortuosity of cerebral vessels;

(ii) Aneurysmal dilatation;

(iii) Arteriovenous malformation;

(iv) Fibromuscular dysplasia;

(v) Dissection of internal carotid artery.

These congenital abnormalities are often causes of stroke in younger age group. A stroke may be easily precipitated when hypertension is associated, in these cases. Hypertensive crises may also lead to hypertensive encephalopathy or even stroke.

**Pathogenesis**

The initial process which leads to a stroke syndrome consists of ischaemia of a part of the brain due to blockage of a large or small vessel by clot or atheroma. Arteritis is rare but rupture of a vessel causing cerebral or subarachnoid haemorrhage is not so uncommon in the elderly. In the young it may occur in presence of congenital vascular abnormalities mentioned above especially in presence of hypertension. Hypertensive encepalopathy, cerebral oedema and migraine may be mistaken for a stroke.

The net result of the vascular occlusion is anoxia of a part of the brain, which, if not reversed soon by collateral circulation, will lead to local infarction with or without haemorrhage.

Brain cells are highly susceptible to anoxia as well as hypoglycaemia. Brain receives 20% of its blood supply of the total cardiac output. Hence severe fall in B.P. and cardiac arrest may cause loss of consciousness. Lack of oxygen supply to brain cells may lead to neuronal necrosis within 5 to 7 minutes.

Infarction of the brain may occur at any site but usually certain parts are more vulnerable where end-arterial supply is not supported by adequate collaterals.

Middle cerebral artery which supplies the most important functional part of the brain is highly susceptible due to presence of end-arteries supplying the areas adjoining internal capsule putamen and globus pallidus.

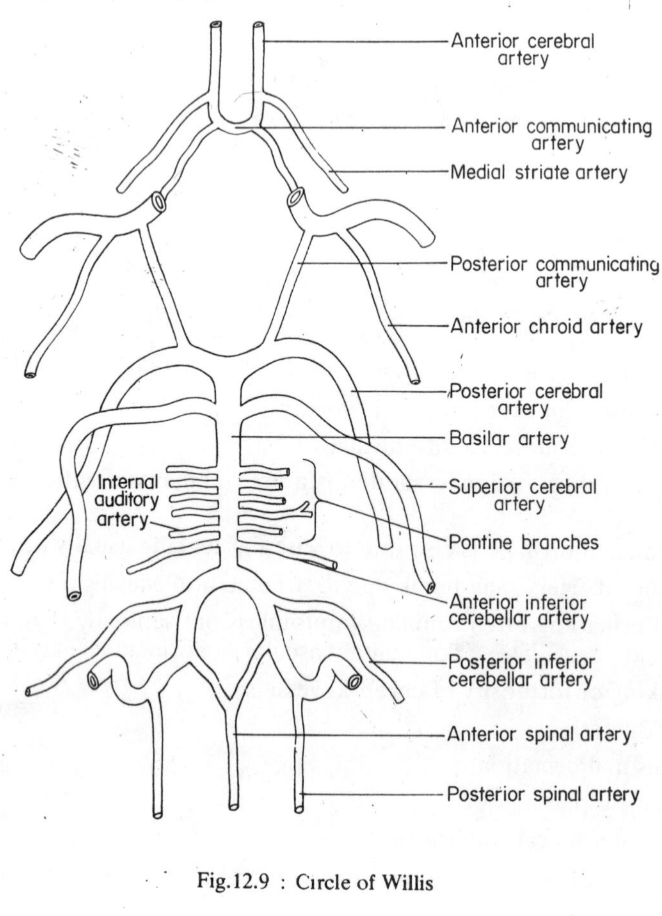


Fig.12.9 : Circle of Willis

Internal cerebral haemorrhage may occur anywhere if there are aneurysms, hypertension being the precipitating factor. A common site is circle of Willis (Fig.12.9). Head injury however is an entirely different problem. The only important point to remember is that even a trivial head injury in elderly, often forgotten, may lead to an intracranial haematoma and lead to hemiparesis after a few weeks.

Various clinical patterns of stroke-syndrome will occur depending of the vascular territories affected, size and extent of damage produced.

The following vessels may be involved :

(1) Internal carotid artery
(2) Middle cerebral artery
(3) Anterior cerebral artery
(4) Anterior choroidal artery
(5) Vertebro-basilar artery
(posterior cerebral and vertebral vessels).

Each of these syndromes can be usually recognised on careful clinical examination. C-T Scan is however very helpful.

**Lacunar infarcts :**

Besides the above vessels, occlusion of small perforating branches of the circle of Willis, anterior, middle or posterior cerebral vessels (end arteries) can produce infarcts in deeper regions of the brain. These are called **Lacunar infarcts** causing syndromes of acute stroke.

Pure motor hemiplegia may be a presenting feature when a lacunar infarct involves the posterior part of the internal capsule. The infarcted area later forms a cyst-like space, hence called lacuna.

The other syndromes due to lacunar infarcts involving branches of lenticulo-striate artery may also occur.

Dysarthria-clumsy-hand syndrome with severe speech defect, facial palsy and paretic tongue may occur due to lacunar infarct in the genu and anterior limb of internal capsule.

Hemi-chorea, hemi-ballismus and pseudobulbar syndromes may also occur. Atypical lacunar stroke may cause severe dysarthria, dysphagia, spasticity of all limbs. There may be paroxysms of laugh and cry.

Hemi-sensory syndrome, a pure sensory syndrome may occur due to involvement of thalamic vessels. The patient may experience loss of sensation on one side of the body or have abnormal sensation of burning and heaviness of one side.

Some of these cases were earlier considered as hysteria, when these basic pathologic changes were not well understood. Lacunar infarcts can be diagnosed in most cases if CT scan is done within 7-10 days of the attack but very small infarcts can still be missed. However, prognosis is usually good as these cases recover quite well within a few weeks.

The classical clinical presentation of a cerebral stroke is hemiplegia with or without loss of consciousness.

**Causes of Hemiplegia**

(A) **Acute or dramatic onset**

(1) Cerebral haemorrhage including middle cerebral artery haemorrhage (Fig.12.10).
(2) Subarachnoid haemorrhage
(3) Cerebral embolism causing cerebral infarction
(4) Hypertensive encephalopathy
(5) Recurrent cerebral ischaemia.

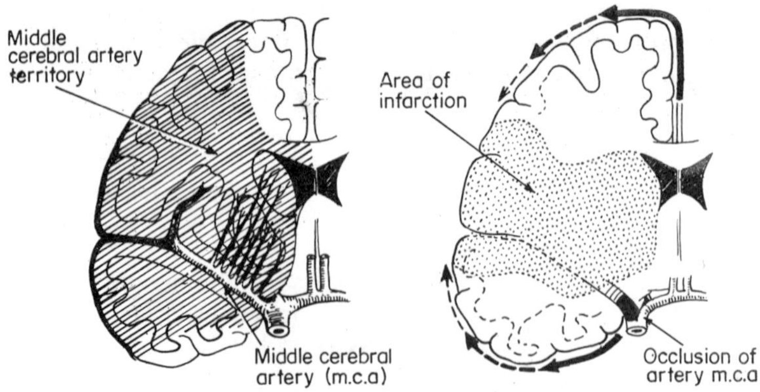


Fig.12.10 : Occlusion of Middle Cerebral Artery

(B) **Gradual onset**

(1) Cerebral thrombosis and cerebral infarction

(2) Cerebral abscess

(3) Chronic subdural haematoma

(4) Cerebral tumours

**Intra-cerebral haemorrhage :**

Non-traumatic spontaneous intracerebral haemorrhage occurs usually in the elderly, rarely in the young, due to rupture of atherosclerotic vessel or due to rupture of an aneurysm in the circle of Willis, causing subarachnoid haemorrhage (Fig.12.9). Sometimes subarachnoid haemorrhage is also associated with intracerebral bleeding due to pre-existing adhesion of the aneurysmal vessels with the brain tissue adjoining above the circle of Willis. Intracerebral haemorrhage may also be sometimes associated with leak of blood into the sub-arachnoid space.

Clinically, however, attempts are usually made to distinguish these conditions, although in some cases it may be difficult due to overlapping of the pathological processes.

**Role of Hypertension**

It should be clearly understood that systemic hypertension often plays a very important role in the aetiology of cerebrovascular accidents (CVA), though it can occur in the old people due to atherosclerosis even without much hypertension.

Presence of microaneurysms or berry aneurysms are sometimes found in the cerebral vessels especially at the circle of Willis. The most common site of rupture is internal capsule though it may occur anywhere, e.g. external capsule, parietal white matter, base of the brain (aneurysmal), cerebellum and brain stem.

Sometimes a cerebral aneurysm may rupture into brain stem and form an intracerebral haematoma, without any blood in CSF.

**Clinical Features**

In majority of the cases it is possible to make a clinical diagnosis about the nature of pathology whether the patient has cerebral haemorrhage, thrombosis, embolism, spontaneous subarachnoid haemorrhage or TIA.

In some instances special investigations may be necessary. Sometimes encephalitis may also cause hemiplegia, cerebral tumours also may cause spontaneous haemorrhage into the tumour, presenting an acute stroke. T.I.A. has been described in a separate chapter.

In general, onset and type of hemiplegia depends on the underlying lesion, the size of the infarct and extent of damage. The typical triad is :

(1) Hemiplegia

(2) Loss of consciousness, stupor or semicoma

(3) Neck stiffness, if there is subarachnoid haemorrhage.

Hemiplegia is initially flaccid in type. Head is turned on one side. Eye signs consist of unequal pupils which later may be dilated and fixed. But in case of brain-stem haemorrhage the following eye signs are present :

(1) Pinpoint pupils

(2) Skew-deviation of eyes

(3) Intermittent downward movements of the eyeballs

(4) Absence of acute vestibular reflex i.e. absence of eye movements, if the internal ear is perfused with ice-cold water.

General examination of stroke patients will reveal stuporose, semi-comatose or comatose patients, except in cases when thrombosis has very slowly developed or in some cases of lacunar infarction. These patients of lacunar infarction present with aphasia, monophagia or hemiparesis without loss of consciousness. These patients may also improve quickly in many cases.

Associated hypertension, L.V. hypertrophy, I.H.D., mitral valve disease, diabetes mellitus or syphilis may be present.

The classical CNS findings are as follows :

(1) Pupils — as described above

(2) There is facial asymmetry (note naso-labial fold which is flattened) and stertorous breathing or cheyne-stoke breathing; rate is usually slow in cerebral haemorrhage. The cheek on affected sides blows in and out.

(3) Flaccid paralysis of limbs on one side.

(4) Deep reflexes are absent in the beginning, later gradually spasticity develops on the affected side. Earlier the spasticity develops, better is the prognosis.

(5) Plantar reflexes may be absent or extensor in both sides in comatose cases but later on remains extensor on the paralysed side.

(6) Abdominal and cremasteric reflexes are also lost.

(7) Incontinence of bladder and bowel initially but later on there may be retention of urine.

(8) Spontaneous limb movements and rarely convulsion may occur in some cases.

**Course and prognosis**

The final outcome of acute stroke depends chiefly on the nature and extent of brain damage. About 75 to 80% cases are due to infarction while 20 to 25% are due to haemorrhage. Prognosis is worse in cerebral haemorrhage. Brain-stem infarction has relatively lower mortality but haemorrhage in this region is always serious. Various associated factors which influence the prognosis are :

(1) Extent of cerebral damage. Larger the area involved worse is the prognosis, C-T scan is helpful for assessment. Infarcts also are less dangerous than haemorrhage.

(2) Rapid development of haemorrhage or infarction.

(3) Age of the patient is important. Higher the age, greater is the possible mortality.

(4) Associated I.H.D. hypertension, diabetes mellitus or severe chest infection makes the prognosis worse.

Clinical forecast is difficult, so prognosis should be guarded.

Deep coma remaining unchanged for over 48-72 hours or semicoma proceeding to coma for over first 24-48 hours, indicates bad prognosis.

In my own experience, however, a few cases have survived who remained in deep coma for 5 to 9 days with good recovery. In one case a patient who was in coma for 15 days survived, under care of an experienced medical officer who remained at patient's residence day and night. These are exceptional cases but support the dictum, never give up hope, while express your guarded prognosis.

Early return of spasticity is a good sign. If spasticity does not develop within four to six weeks the chance of useful recovery is remote.

**Investigations**

**Blood Examination :**

It is essential to check blood for malaria parasite in the tropics while routine blood tests e.g. TC, DC, Hb, ESR, sugar and urea are usually done as a routine. Additional tests e.g. liver function tests, uric acid, creatinine etc. may be considered, if required.

**ECG** is useful while chest skiagram may sometimes be required.

**Urine** should be examined daily for 2 to 3 days and later on culture may also be done to assess presence of urinary tract infection, especially if catheter is used.

**Radiology**

X-ray of the skull may be helpful in some cases as some cerebral tumours show calcification. Presence of fracture skull or evidence of haematoma may also be noted.

X-ray chest may also be useful in showing cardiac enlargement, presence of aortic aneurysm or a malignant new growth.

**CSF** — L.P. may be done carefully to exclude haemorrhage from infarction but if C.T. scan can be done L.P. is not routinely necessary unless **SAH** is suspected. In developing countries, however, CSF still remains a useful tool of investigation.

Examination of CSF is done carefully to measure CSF pressure and to detect blood in CSF. Routine biochemistry and cytology should also be checked.

Fundoscopy should be done in all cases as far as possible before lumbar puncture. Careless drainage of large amount of CSF in patients with high CSF pressure may result in conning of the brain stem.

Brain-scan may not show a positive picture in all cases in the first few days but positive scan is usually obtained by the first weekend. Technetium 99m pertechnate is injected for the scan and a Gamma-camera is used. Positive scan areas appear yellow to red, called "hot-areas", while normal areas are blue.

**Angiography**

Angiography is not routinely done but is a very useful investigation in expert hands. Mortality of 1-2% may occur. Its usefulness has been reduced where C.T. scan is available but still it is useful in diagnosing the vessels involved and especially when carotid endarterectomy is proposed. Aneurysms are clearly detectable.

**EEG**

EEG has relatively no importance except where epileptic fits are present. It can detect difference in the electrical activities of each cerebral hemisphere and locate a disturbed focus. It has no place as a routine test.

**C.T. Scan**

C.T. scan is a great advance in the investigation of cerebrovascular accidents.

More recent non-invasive technique consists of ultrasound and Doppler technique. Possibly nuclear magnetic resonance (NMR) technique will become more perfected in the near future.

Carotid phono-angiography and oculoplethysmography are also used to study vascular tree for detecting arterial disease.

Another new development in this direction is positron-emission tomography. In this new technique positrons are used instead of electrons.

Finally, however, it should be realised that clinical approach with simpler tests is adequate in most cases, while special sophisticated investigations are necessary for special situations.

**Management**

The most important aspect of the treatment is careful nursing care and supportive therapy to maintain vital processes. The management can be divided into the following steps :

(1) Emergency care and transfer of the case to a hospital

(2) Case of acute stroke during the first week

(3) Convalescing stroke-patient

(4) Long-term management and rehabilitation.

First decision is to decide whether to transfer the patient to a hospital or treat the patient at home. This will depend on socio-economic status, attitude of the relatives, complications present and availability of qualified nurses and doctors. In developing countries conditions vary a great deal. Transportation is not only difficult in rural setting, sometimes impossible. Expert neurological advice and facilities as well, are hardly available in large number of cases occurring in out-of-town areas. Hence the general practitioner is the best man to manage the case within limited resources.

It is, however, interesting that unexpected recoveries may occur if the patient is cared for by good nursing and simple supportive care.

Up to date there is no specific drug therapy which substantially may help to a significant degree.

The following points are to be considered in acute stages :

(1) Inhalation of oxygen may be helpful in acute stages

(2) Prevent choking, falling back of tongue, vomitus or during attempts to feed when patient is in coma

(3) Airway tube should be used in cases of coma

(4) Attention to bladder is important. An indwelling Foley's catheter should be used when there is retention of urine and every possible care to control urinary tract infection is important.

(5) I.V. fluid during first 24-48 hours to maintain fluid electrolyte balance in mandatory. Additional calories can be provided by 25% glucose 25 to 50 ml at 3 to 4 hour intervals by I.V. shots slowly given via venous line.

(6) Once the patient is stable I.V. fluid may be discontinued and Ryle's tube feeding should be started till patient is able to take his feeds. Both I.V. fluid and Ryle's tube feeding can be done where considered necessary.

**Special Therapeutic Regimes**

**Cerebral oedema** — Many methods are in vogue for reduction of cerebral oedema. These are as follows :

(1) **Steroid hormones** — are very commonly used in mild to heroic doses. Presence of high BP or diabetes mellitus are contraindications.

**Dexamethasone** — 5 to 20 mg is recommended as starting dose followed by 4-8 mg × 4-6 hourly for 5-7 days by I.M. or I.V. route.

(2) **Frusemide** may be used in doses of 40 to 80 mg I.V. to be repeated 8-12 hourly for 2-3 days, taking care about electrolyte imbalance.

(3) **Mannitol** 20% has been used in doses of 300 ml given daily for 2 or 3 days. Low molecular weight dextran (Lomodex) is also used.

Some reports suggest that dexamethasone or I.V. mannitol is disappointing, while others continue to use it.

(4) **Anticoagulants** — The only indications is in case of T.I.A. and vertebro-basilar insufficiency or rarely in cases of 'stroke-in-evolution'. It is risky in old atherosclerotics and therefore its use is very limited. CSF must be free from blood if anticoagulants are prescribed and all other contraindications are excluded. The method is the same as in cases of myocardial infarction.

(5) **Antiplatelet agents :**

(a) Aspirin in dosage of 300 mg is prescribed three times daily after feeding. It is cheap and useful but not without risk of gastric bleeding.

(b) Dipyridamole 100 mg may also be given three times daily with or without aspirin. It is claimed that the combination is more effective, especially in cases of T.I.A. or stroke-in-evolution.

(6) **Sulphinpyrazone** — has been recently recommended as another useful drug. Dose 200 mg four times daily.

All these three drugs are anti-platelet adhesion reducing agents and hence should be useful in preventing vascular thrombus formation.

(7) **Glycerol** — Oral glycerol 1.5g per kg. of body weight in four divided doses may be helpful in reducing cerebral oedema.

(8) **Low molecular dextran** (e.g. Lomodex) may be helpful as anti-sludging agent — especially in thrombotic or embolic infarcts.

(9) **Antibiotics** should be given as indicated.

(10) **Vasodilators** — Cerebral vasodilators once in vogue are not any more recommended. In fact they may be more harmful in diverting more blood to healthy areas while infarcted area may be depleted (so-called steal-phenomenon).

(11) **Pyritinol (Encephabol)** is another drug which is worth consideration. In the author's experience it appears to be a useful agent to be used in acute stroke.

Dose — 200 mg amp to be given slowly I.V. × 12 hourly for 2 to 4 days, later on oral therapy may be instituted.

(12) Codergocrine mesylate Inj. 0.3 mg/ml (Hydergine) is also being used in acute strokes.

**Stage of convalescence :**

Patient gradually recovers with some degree of neurological deficit which should be periodically reviewed.

Physiotherapy is started in bed by regular changes of posture several times daily even in acute stage. As soon as patient is conscious, active physiotherapy should be started daily. Some patients remain flaccid for a few weeks, hence they cannot actively participate, but all possible movements must be continued.

Other patients will improve rapidly, but some of them become spastic limiting their ability to participate in active physiotherapy so successfully. Associated disorders, e.g. hypertension and diabetes should be vigorously treated, but attempt to reduce high B.P. in acute stage is not recommended.

Attention to diet depending on lipid profile, obesity, diabetes and renal insufficiency, if any, is very important.

**Surgical treatment :**

Scope of surgery is limited, especially in developing countries. It may be considered by experts in the following situations :

(1) S.A.H. or T.I.A ;
(2) Carotid artery stenosis or insufficiency ;
(3) Extraction of clots during acute stage, very rarely successful ;
(4) Microvascular or intracranial bypass surgery. Only a very few patients may be benefited in special centres, scope being limited in this part of the globe at present.

No treatment however can be considered as specific. Opinions vary and statistics remain unconfirmed. Even heroic surgical methods e.g. evacuation of clots were practised but controlled trials were not impressive. Restoration of blood supply by endarterectomy or anastomotic surgery by joining superior temporal artery to a suitable intracerebral vessel (EC-IC bypass) are being attempted.

With the help of C.T. Scan follow-up, it may be possible in future to evaluate these techniques. Readers may refer to a book discussing critical approach to stroke problems by D.T.Wade et at ("STROKE" published by Chapman and Hall Medical (1985) Cambridge).

**Rehabilitation :**

The basis of long-term management is gradual rehabilitation. Some people are fortunate to recover extremely well to go back to their original work with minimal disability. But 75% of victims will have varying degree of disablement limiting their future performance. Most unfortunate patients will remain bed-ridden with spastic limbs on the right side as well as aphasic, while they may be mentally able to realise their disablement. Each patient will have his own problem, regarding social, economic and domestic affairs.

Most of our hospitals are not able to cope with these problems and there are very few centres for management of these cases for proper rehabilitation programme. Long-term physiotherapy, occupational therapy and psychotherapy are the three triads of rehabilitation. Speech therapy should be started where trained speech therapy is available, otherwise attending physician should guide.

Depression (melancholia) in these patients is a great problem. Antidepressant drugs and psychotherapy are most important.

Some patients with left hemispheric lesions may require speech therapy. Many patients will do well with special shoes and various gadgets for their daily self-help regime.

## CEREBRAL VEINS AND VENOUS THROMBOSIS

Intracranial veins and venous sinuses may be affected by infection or thrombotic process. This process may lead to serious intracranial infections e.g. leptomeningitis, suppurative encephalitis or brain abscess.

The infection usually reaches into the intracranial veins or venous sinuses from face, scalp, dental infections, air sinuses or middle ear. Aseptic venous thrombosis may also occur due to infections of mouth, air sinuses or middle ear. Aseptic venous thrombosis may also occur due to oral contraceptives, marasmic states, severe dehydration or polycythaemia.

**Clinical features**

The following clinical syndromes are usually encountered :

**Cavernous sinus thrombosis**

This usually follows pyoderma in face e.g. boils around lips in particular. The onset is acute with high fever, toxaemia, severe headache and ocular signs, consisting of chemosis, oedema of eyelids, and proptosis.

The 3rd, 4th and 6th cranial nerves are paralysed with pain in the eyes. Papilloedema may follow. All these are due to thrombosis of the cavernous sinus. Usually the condition is unilateral but the other eye may also be involved.

**Transverse sinus thrombosis**

Acute febrile illness with toxaemia, headache and vomiting heralds the onset. Focal signs develop due to extension of thrombotic process to other sinuses.

Superior sagittal sinus involvement causes paraparesis while extension to other venous sinuses leads to various focal neurological presentations e.g. hemiparesis, faciobrachial paresis or paralysis of cranial nerves.

**Superior sagittal sinus thrombosis**

The onset in acute as in above conditions associated with paraparesis or rarely hemiparesis, aphasia, even epileptiform seizures.

**Thrombosis of cortical veins**

In addition to febrile episode, focal symptoms and signs will depend on the area of the brain involved by thrombosis. Accordingly monoparesis, hemiparesis, epileptic seizures may occur.

**Treatment**

The condition needs intensive treatment with antibiotics and supportive therapy. Rarely surgical interference may be required.

## CEREBRAL TRANSIENT ISCHAEMIC ATTACKS

*N.N. SARANGI*

Transient ischaemic attacks (TIA) are episodes of temporary and focal cerebral dysfunction of vascular origin, which are thought to result from ischaemia too brief to cause infarction. The main clinical importance of TIA is its recognition as a precursor of major thromboembolic stroke. Basic background patho-physiological factors behind TIAs and major strokes are the same. TIAs may be regarded as brief temporary strokes where focal neurological signs resulting from brief ischaemia completely reverse themselves.

To define an episode as TIA, a time-limit of 24 hours has been traditionally accepted as the upper limit of duration of each episode. When these are of longer duration, but still reversible, a terminology of RIND (Reversible ischaemic neurological deficit) is used to define them.

Thus TIA is defined as "an acute disturbance of focal neurological function with symptoms lasting less than 24 hours and assumed to be due to a vascular disease of an arterial embolic or thrombotic kind, neurological signs of no functional significance are usually found subsequently"

**Clinical Picture**

Clinical picture depends on the arterial territory involved. In each individual case, recurrent episodes tend to be identical.

Attacks may be :-

Carotid territory TIAs, or vertebrobasilar territory TIAs. Carotid territory TIAs may be :-

(1) Transient hemisphere attacks, or

(2) Transient mono-ocular blindness (Amaurosis Fugax).

Transient hemisphere attacks show different forms of contralateral focal, neuro-deficit-like transient hemiparesis or partial involvements like facial weakness, upper or lower limb weakness, or weakness of hands and feet, different form of dysphasias, temporary visual field defects, or temporary parietal lobe dysfunctions.

Transient monoocular blindness presents as ipsilateral monoocular visual loss which clears gradually. Vertebrobasilar TIA's show various presentations like dizziness, diplopia, dysarthria, complete or partial weakness of one or both sides, gaze paralysis, dysphagia, ataxia, impaired hearing, vomiting or hiccough.

**Differential Diagnosis**

TIAs are to be differentiated from the following conditions, among others, which are associated with transient episodes of possible neurological system involvement.

Epilepsies — Unconciousness, frank convulsions, bladder or bowel incontinence, or tongue biting are usual in TIA, and EEG is almost always normal in TIA. Stokes Adams attacks — Focal neurologic manifestations are rare in SA attacks and convulsion or unconsciousness are rare in TIA.

Peripheral labyrinthine disorders including Meniere's syndrome and positional vertigo are not associated with symptoms or signs of brain stem involvement whereas ischaemic attacks involving brain stem are likely to be associated with diplopia, vertical nystagmus, numbness, weakness, dysphagia etc.

Migraine accompaniments of visual, motor and sensory symptoms may be confused with TIAs A careful history of periodic hemicrania and vomiting is helpful. One may rely also on family history, age and sex of the patient.

Diabetic patients particularly on drugs may have focal symptoms like TIA during hypoglycaemia and one should assess the diabetic status of these patients.

**Mechanism of TIA :**

Most important mechanism in operation, at least in most case of carotid territory TIAs is embolism of atheromatous or thrombotic materials from a proximal source to distal parts, where these produce brief periods of ischaemia, before being promptly fragmented re-establishing circulation in the affected region. Arterial sources of embolism with radiologically identifiable lesions of carotid stenosis or occlusion are recognised in many of these cases. Cardiac source is the second important source of emboli.

In severe stenoses, distal insufficiency caused as a result of transient complete occulsion of the stenosed part by platelet fibrin materials has been proposed to be another contributing factor where embolism may be an epiphenomenon but not directly responsible for TIA episodes. Mechanical or haemodynamic factors with kinking of arteries of fall of B.P. may be important in vertebrobasilar TIAs.

There is some correlation between the duration of the attacks and expectation of major artery stenosis or occlusion, and intracranial branch artery involvement. In patients where episodes are brief lasting less than an hour, averaging around 10 minutes some chances of major arterial obstruction are more likely to be associated with intracranial branch artery involvement.

**Management :**

Though the major importance of TIAs are their recognition as precursors of major thromboembolic strokes, associated vascular pathological changes in coronary circulation, make them vulnerable to risks of death due to myocardial infarction.

Thus the aim of treatment is prevention of recurrence of TIAs, prevention of stroke, and prevention of death due to stroke and non-stroke causes.

Choice of treatment :

A. Medical treatment with —
   (a) Anticoagulants
   (b) Anti-platelet agents
   (c) Supportive measures like antihypertensive therapy in hypertension.

B. Surgical treatment of appropriate surgically remediable vascular lesion with —
   (a) Carotid endarterectomy
   (b) Extracranial intracranial bypass surgery.

Following plan may be useful for assessment of TIA patients for management.

Cases are evaluated clinically to exclude conditions like :

(1) Systemic blood diseases like polycythaemia or severe anaemia;
(2) Cardiovascular diseases;
(3) Haemodynamic factors like postural hypotension, neck artery narrowing (important in vertebrobasilar TIAs) etc.

Rest may be presumed to have a cerebral vascular pathology.

If facilities are available, these cases are assessed for their fitness for vascular surgery.

A. If they are unfit for surgery, proper treatment of hypertension — anti-antiplatelet agents are tried.

   In normotensive patients — anticoagulants or antiplatelet agents are given.

B. If they are fit for surgery — angiography is done in normotensive patients with or without clinical evidence of extracranial carotid artery disease.

Surgical treatment is undertaken if an accessible surgically remediable lesion is found.

Otherwise :

1. In normotensives — anticoagulant or antiplatelet agents are given.
2. In hypertensives — antihypertensive with or without antiplatelet treatment is given.

**Anticoagulants :**

Heparin and coumarin agents like bishydroxycoumarin or warfarin are most commonly used.

Anticoagulants may be continued for three months to one year and if recurrence follows reduction or discontinuation, treatment may be reinstituted to be continued indefinitely.

Therapy may cause many problems, particularly dangerous haemorrhagic complications and must be given only in cooperative patients without any history of bleeding disorder and with facilities for good laboratory control under the supervision of an experienced physician.

Heparin is used in a dosage of 5000 to 10000 units I.V. initially and continued every 6 to 8 hours. Oral anticoagulants may be started simultaneously and heparin may be discontinued often for 2 to 3 days. Average maintenance dose of bishydroxycoumarin is 5 to 75 mg. and that of warfarin 2 to 15 mg. daily.

Antiplatelet agents are less likely to cause haemorrhagic complications and are preferred.

**Antiplatelet agents :**

Platelet behaviour plays an important role in the pathogenesis of T.I.A. During the phase of platelet activation with platelet aggregation, arachidonic acid derived from platelet phospholipids are converted to prostaglandins $PGG_2$ and then to $PGH_2$ by cyclooxygenase. $PGH_2$ is converted to thromboxane $A_2$ by thromboxane synthetase in platelets which is a powerful vasoconstrictor and platelet aggregator $PGH_2$ is also converted to prostacyclin $PGI_2$ in the vascular endothelium, which is a powerful natural vasodilator and platelet antiaggregator. Thromboxane $A_2$ inhibits and prostacyclin $PGI_2$ stimulates adenyl cyclase and thereby respectively decrease and increase cyclic AMP. A rise of ADP acts as a promoter and that of AMP as an inhibitor of platelet aggregation. Cyclic AMP is degraded by phosphodiesterases.

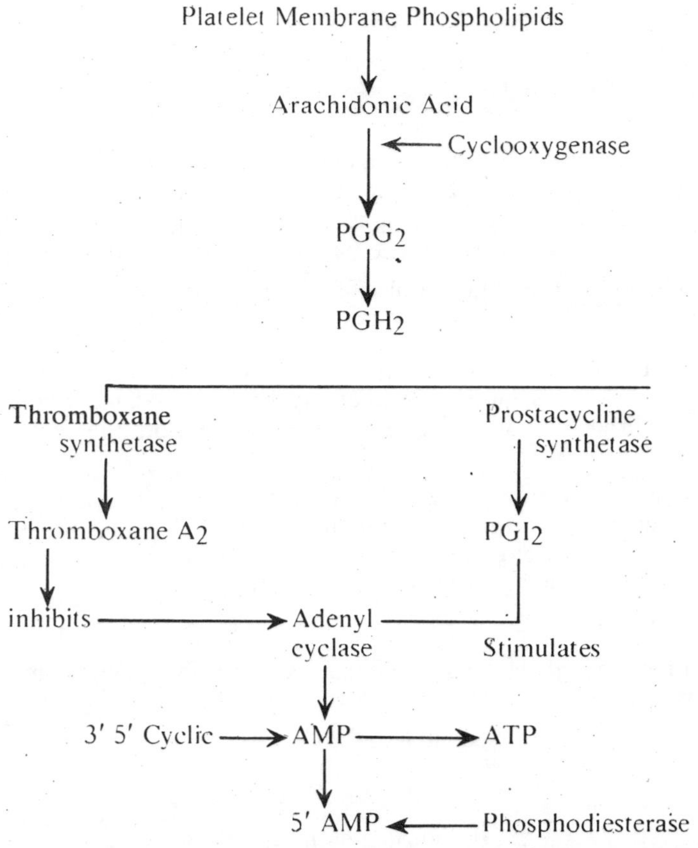


Drugs which alter platelet behaviour and interfere with platelet aggregation are used in treatment of TIAs. Clinically useful agents are aspirin, dipyridamole and sulfinpyrazone. Aspirin intraactivates platelet cyclooxygenase and inhibits synthesis of pro-aggregatory thromboxane $A_2$. Aspirin however, inhibits cyclooxygenase system in vascular endothelium as well where it inhibits synthesis of prostacyclin, a potent endogenous inhibitor of platelet aggregation. A low dose aspirin therapy within 300 to 325 mg. daily is used now, which will be sufficient to inhibit thromboxane $A_2$ synthesis, but will not inhibit prostacyclin synthesis.

Sulphinpyrazone is also an inactivator of cyclooxygenase, but whereas aspirin induced inactivation is irreversible, sulphinpyrazone induced inactivation is temporary and reversible. It is used in a dosage of 200 mg. thrice a day.

Dipyridamole inhibits phosphodiesterase and increases cyclic AMP level in platelets. Platelet antiaggregatory behaviour is associated with a rise in platelet cyclic AMP level. Dose is 50 to 100 mg thrice a day.

**Surgical management :**

This can only be done in specialised neurosurgical units. Arteriography may be done only if the patient is a potential surgical candidate and facilities for surgery exist. Patients with **stenosis of** one carotid artery in its extracranial part are most ideal candidates for surgery.

# INTRACRANIAL NEOPLASMS

*D. ROYCHOUDHARY*

**Definition**

True intracranial neoplasms are tumours arising from cerebral tissues, meninges, nerves, nerve sheaths and intracranial blood vessels. Besides these, there are a number of pathological lesions which behave like intracranial tumours, i.e. space occupying lesions (S.O.L.) e.g. cysts, aneurysms, tuberculomas, chronic abscess, subdural haematoma and now-a-days rarely seen gummata.

In the present chapter intracranial neoplasms will be discussed.

**Pathology**

Intracranial tumours may occur at any age and suprisingly it is one of the common causes of childhood malignancy. Tumours arising from embryonic nest, malignant tumours of cerebellum and brain-stem are fairly common in the first decade of life. Both the sexes are almost equally affected.

The rapidity of onset of symptoms is chiefly dependent upon distortion of the CSF circulation rather than on the actual size and growth of the tumour. A small benign tumour in the posterior aspect of the third ventricle or close to the aqueduct will produce symptoms more quickly than a malignant tumour in the frontal pole or posterior parietal region.

**CLASSIFICATION :**

This classification, though lacking in details, is clinically oriented and is useful for the practitioners of medicine :-

A. Primary — 80%   B. Secondary — 20%

**Primary**

(1) Glioma — 42%
(2) Meningioma — 18%
(3) Pituitary — 10%
(4) Neurilemmoma — 8%
(5) Others — 2%

**Gliomas :**

Tumours from glial cells are the commonest type of brain tumours. Previously gliomas were thought to arise from primitive cell rests, but present concept is that the de-differentiation of adult glial cells gives rise to various types of tumour.

Gliomas are subgrouped as follows :

(2) Astrocytoma – grade I to IV
(2) Ependymoma – grade I to IV
(3) Oligodendroglioma
(4) Neuroastrocytoma
(5) Medulloblastoma.

**Astrocytoma :**

Commonest variety of gliomas. Adults are commonly affected though involvement of cerebellum and brain stem is observed in younger are group. Cystic changes in the tumour are quite common which often may be solitary and of considerable size. Highly malignant astrocytoma is called glioblastoma.

**Ependymoma :**

Whitish firm tumour arises from ependyma. The fourth ventricle is the commonest site. Choroid plexus papilloma, a tumour of early age, once considered as tumour of separate category, is now considered as a low grade papillary ependymoma and lateral ventricle is the common site. Oligo-dendro-glioma is a slow growing tumour of fourth and fifth decade and calcification is more common than other varieties of gliomas. Despite controversy, neuroastrocytoma is preferred to be grouped under gliomas and the incidence is very low. Medulloblastoma is predominant in cerebellar midline structures in children. It is locally invasive and through the C.S.F. may metastatise in the spinal canal.

**Meningioma :** It arises from the cells of the arachnoid membrane and is slightly more common in females. Highest age incidence is between 40 and 50 years. The common sites are in areas where arachnoid villi are normally present along the superior sagittal sinus, the convexity of the hemispheres, olfactory groove and the sphenoid ridge. Less common sites are suprasellar region posterior fossa and lateral ventricles. Meningiomas usually compress the brain but sometimes may be locally invasive. Malignant change is uncommon. The overlying bone may show osteolytic or osteoblastic changes with actual invasion of bone but maintaining its benign nature.

**Pituitary Tumours :** Most of the tumours of this group arise from the cells of anterior lobe and adenoma of chromophobe-cell is the commonest variety. This develops in adult life and expands the sella initially. As it grows, it extends upwards and compresses the optic chiasma and adjoining structures.

Signs of hypopituitarism do not develop till at least 70 per cent of the pituitary tissue has been affected. Tumour of acidophil cells is less common than chromophobe adenoma and either acromegaly or gigantism develops depending on the onset of tumour. In majority of these cases biopsy material from operation reveal in the stain with eosin-haematoxylin, preponderance of chromophobe cells which outnumber acidophilic cells. Thus it is difficult to correlate the clinical features and number of acidophil cells.

The small sized tumour of the basophil cell is rare and is usually found at autopsy. Excessive secretion of ACTH from the basophil cells induces hyperplasia of adrenal cortex and hypersecretion of cortisol results producing Cushing's syndrome. However, in most of the cases of Cushing's syndrome, adrenal cortical hyperactivity is independent of basophil adenoma.

Craniopharyngiomas originate in the embryonic rest of epithelial cells, possibly the remnant of Rathke's pouch in the suprasellar region. Though the lesion is congenital, symptoms usually develop after the age of 10 years. The tumour is mostly cystic and contains yellow or brownish oily fluid with high cholesterol content.

**Neurilemmoma :** It is derived from the Schwann cells of nerve sheath and majority are found to arise from the eighth cranial nerve. Involvement of fifth and second cranial nerves is also seen. It is common in third and fourth decades. The tumour usually develops in the internal auditory meatus and grows slowly eroding the bone and protrudes in the intracranial cavity. When it reaches the subarachnoid space, the protein secretion from the tumour causes rise in the CSF protein. Eventually it reaches the cerebellopontine angle producing classical clinical features.

**Other tumours :** A variety of tumours which constitute only 2% of the intracranial tumours in this group —

(1) Skull tumours (osteoma and osteochondroma).

(2) Tumours of developmental origin (colloid cyst of the third ventricle chordoma, dermoid cyst, epidermoid cyst).

(3) Pinealoma

(4) Blood vessel tumour

(5) Sarcomas including tumours of reticuloendothelial system (Hodgkin's disease, Leukaemia) are included in this category.

Skull tumours can be diagnosed from straight X-rays but for the diagnosis of other varieties of this group, investigations including C.T. Scan are necessary and at times diagnosis can only be made at operation or after biopsy.

**Secondary Tumours :**

The incidence of metastatic tumours has gone up in recent years due to better diagnostic facility with CT scan. Bronchus, breast, kidney, thyroid, G.I. Tract, uterus and prostate are the sites of primary growth in majority cases. These are blood borne metastases and are located frequently in the territory of middle cerebral artery posterior to Sylvian fissure. Ventricular metastasis and carcinomatosis of meninges are uncommon. Direct extension of nasopharyngeal carcinoma into the intracranial cavity by eroding the bone of the base of the skull occurs in rare cases.

The metastasis of cerebral malignant tumours outside the central nervous system was once considered to be unknown. But in recent years occasional reports of such metastasis are coming up in the literature.

**Clinical Features**

As intracranial tumours are mostly malignant irrespective of age, early diagnosis is imperative for better prognosis. This is possible only when the clinician is conversant with the diverse clinical presentation of intracranial tumours.

**Raised intracranial tension :**

Factors which contribute to the rise in intracranial pressure are :

1. Mass of the tumour
2. Surrounding oedema around the tumour
3. Venous engorgement
4. Obstruction of CSF circulation.

The last factor determines the rapidity of development of clinical features of raised intracranial tension. It develops very late in sellar tumours and acoustic neurinoma which are benign and circulation of CSF is not affected till late stage.

**Clinical Diagnosis :** The following points are important :

**Headache :** It is mostly due to stretching of cerebral blood vessels and partly due to stretching of dura. Early morning headache is common. It may be dull but at times intense and may be even intermittent indicating fluctuation of intracranial pressure. Both generalised and localised headache are seen. Occipital headache is common in posterior fossa tumor.

**Vomiting :** It is more common in early morning with headache but is rarely "projectile". Persistent vomiting in infants and children without apparent gastrointestinal trouble should arouse suspicion of raised intracranial tension. Nausea is usually absent.

**Visual disturbance :** Diplopia due to third or sixth cranial nerve palsy sometimes develops early in the disease. In posterior fossa neoplasm, papilloedema develops earlier than supratentorial tumors.

In frontal, temporal occipital lobe tumors papilloedema may not develop for some time as ventricular distortion and CSF obstruction are minimal. Prognosis is better if diagnosis can be made before the onset of papilloedema.

Vision is maintained in spite of papilloedema for a considerable time. Failing vision signifies gross papilloedema or postpapilloedic optic atrophy and visual recovery in such cases is uncertain even after effective treatment. Unilateral primary optic atrophy develops in sphenoid ridge and olfactory groove meningioma by its proximity to the optic nerve and subsequently papilloedema develops on the opposite side (Foster Kennedy syndrome).

**Convulsive seizure :** Raised intracranial tension produces generalised convulsion in about 10 per cent cases. Tumours located close to cerebral cortex give rise to convulsion more frequently and may even preceed other clinical manifestations.

**Vertigo :** Though dizziness and unsteady gait may be features of raised intracranial tension, yet true vertigo is a rare symptom.

**Alteration of vital functions :** Raised intracranial tension for considerable period produces hypoxia of the vasomotor centres resulting in bradycardia and elevated blood pressure. Respiration is also involved when conscious level deteriorates.

**Alteration of mental state and conscious level :** Confusion and disorientation in space develop when tumour produces raised intracranial tension. Impairment of memory, irritability and lack of concentration are early features. Dementia and incontinence of urine, though may result from raised tension, are more common in frontal lobe tumours.

**False Localising Signs :**

These may be confusing :

(1) Cranial nerve palsy — Unilateral or bilateral third or sixth nerve palsy result from the distortion of the brain stem due to rise in intracranial pressure.

(2) Bilateral extensor plantar responses

(3) Bilateral grasp reflexes

(4) Endocrine disorders caused by enlarged third ventricle.

(5) Signs of vascular occlusion — rapidly expanding tumour may compress cerebral vessels and produce acute features like hemiplegia and aphasia and may be mistaken for stroke.

**Enlargement of head :** It is observed when tumour develops in infancy and early childhood and may be mistaken for primary hydrocephalus.

**Localisation of Tumours**

**Frontal lobe :**

Alteration of mental state like lack of alertness, confusion, disorientation even dementia with urinary incontinence is observed.

Grasp reflex should be examined both in the upper and lower limbs and when present is of great diagnostic value.

Long tract signs on the opposite side develop when cortico-spinal fibres are involved.

Anosmia of the side of lesion, expressive aphasia. Jacksonian fits on the opposite side are other important localising signs.

As mentioned eariler, papilloedema develops in late stage only.

**Parietal Lobe :**

Tumours in this region produce cortical sensory disturbance which is very difficult to elicit, particularly when alteration of mentation supervenes.

Due to proximity to the motor area of frontal lobe, pyramidal signs on the opposite side develop subsequently. Agraphia if elicitable is of great localising value.

In deep-seated parietal lobe tumours — opposite lower quadrantic homonymous visual field defects develop and perimetry and scotometry should be done in all cases of suspected intracranial tumours.

**Temporal Lobe :**

Anteriorly placed tumour produce uncinate fits (hallucination of smell and taste, smacking of lips and tongue); medially placed tumour may, particularly outburst of rage may be seen.

Disturbance of memory (de javu phenomenon) and crossed upper quadrantic homonymous visual field defect are characteristic features. In left sides tumour aphasia may develop.

Tinnitus and auditory hallucination are useful localising features suggesting tumour near auditory cortex.

## OCCIPITAL LOBE :

The characteristic focal sign of occipital lobe neoplasm is visual field defect in the form of crossed homonymous hemianopia but in early stage quadrantic field loss may be evident in perimetry. Macula is spared. Visual object agnosia and generalised convulsion preceded by usual aura may be present.

### Cerebellum :

This is a common site for childhood brain tumour. Medulloblastoma in first decade and astrocytoma in second decade should be suspected in cerebellar neoplasma.

In midline cerebellar tumour, features of raised intracranial tension including papilloedema become evident early.

Truncal ataxia may be missed if gait is not examined. Tonic fits develop when mid-brain is compressed from midline when tumour extends laterally ipsilateral limb ataxia and nystagmus can be elicited.

Nystagmus is more evident on lateral gaze to the side of lesion.

Hypotonia, positive finger-nose-test, disorder of speech (slurring and jerky articulation) and adiadochokinesis will be evident as the tumour expands into the cerebellar hemisphere.

### Cerebello Pontine Angle Tumour :

Acoustic neurinoma is the commonest tumour in this site and meningioma is next common. Tinitus is an early symptom: vertigo and nystagmus develop subsequently.

Corneal reflex is diminished quite early on the side of lesion.

Ipsilateral cerebellar signs indicate that the tumour is of considerable size.

Dysphagia and dysarthria are late manifestations due to involvement of ninth and tenth cranial nerves.

### Brain Stem Tumour :

Glioma is common and is seen in younger age group. Papilloedema develops late.

Multiple cranial nerve palsies (third to seventh) with long tract signs on one or both sides are suggestive of brain stem neoplasm.

Weber's syndrome, Benedikt's syndrome, Perinaud's syndrome develop depending on the site of involvement of the brain stem by the tumour.

In late stage decerebrate rigidity develops. Appearance of nystagmus and ataxia indicates involvement of cerebellar connections.

Sensory changes are the result of destruction of ascending sensory pathways.

### Pituitary Tumour :

Chromophobe adenoma — the commonest type of benign tumour and for a considerable time the growth is at the expense of sellar enlargement without producing symptoms.

When the dura of the diaphragmatic sella is stretched by the tumour, dull frontal headache may develop which is usually ignored by the patient.

The presenting feature is usually visual disturbance,the patient hits against wall or persons while walking due to constriction of field of vision and driving of car becomes difficult.

Perimetry reveals quadrantic field defect in the early stage and classical bitemporal hemianopia subsequently.

Hypopituitarism, as mentioned earlier, does not develop till 70% of the functioning tissues are involved. Oligo-menorrhoea followed by amenorrhoea in female and impotency in male develops.

Other features are — weakness, scanty hair, low metabolic rate and obesity.

**Eosinophilic Tumour :**

Gigantism develops in adolescence and acromegaly in adults. Due to fibrous hyperplasia, of skin and subcutaneous tissue become thick, especially of fingers and lips; tongue becomes bigger in size and may be protruding.

Over-growth of the bone is most evident in skull, face, mandible, hands and feet. The movement becomes slow and kyphosis is common.

Hyperglycaemia and glycosuria may develop.

Impairment of sexual functions is seen both in male and female. Lactation in nulliparous women is sometimes seen both in clinically diagnosed chromophobe adenoma and eosinophil tumour due to overproduction of prolactin.

**Basophil Tumour :**

It is a rare clinical entity which affects females more than males and is manifested by progressive adiposity, masculine hair distribution, amenorrhoea and hyperglycaemia. Classically it cannot be distinguished from Cushing's syndrome resulting from the adrenal hyperplasia.

**Craniopharyngioma**

The features are typical :

Raised intracranial tension;

Retarded growth and delayed puberty;

Visual disturbances consist of dimness of vision and ophthalmoscopic finding of primary optic atrophy;

Diabetes insipidus may develop when supra-opticoneurohypophyseal pathway is involved.

**Intraventricular Tumours :**

In third ventricular colloid cyst intermittent intense headache without localising sign may be the only feature.

In tumour of the lateral ventricle and fourth ventricle, features of progressive raised intracranial tension are seen. Diagnosis is often missed till ventriculography or CT scan is done.

**Investigations :**

**Radiological examination :**

(a) X-ray chest — plain X-ray of chest — PA view should be done as a routine in all patients. Presence of tuberculous lesion may be an indication of tuberculoma of brain, when raised intracranial tension of focal seizure is presenting feature. Evidence of pulmonary metastasis may be a pointer that the intracranial lesion is a secondary neoplasm.

(b) X-ray Skull — PA, AP and lateral views of X-ray skull are taken in all cases. Though in about 40% patients kull X-ray be normal, yet one of the following abnormalities will be of great value :

(i) Evidence of raised intracranial tension is — sutural diastasis, silver beaten appearance, erosion of posterior clinoid process.

(ii) Lateralising sign — Shift of pineal calcification from midline.

(iii) Localising signs — abnormal calcification is seen in oligodendroglioma, astrocytoma and meningioma. Erosion of bone or new bone formation is seen in meningioma.

Enlargement of sella is seen in pituitary adenoma and tumours which produce enlargement of third ventricle.

(c) **Electroencephalography (E.E.G.)** — Positive findings are present in 80% patients when the tumour is of long duration. Focal abnormalities in the form of theta and delta waves are of great importance. Other positive findings are : loss of background activity, reduction of amplitude of alpha wave, spike and sharp wave surrounding the tumour mass. In deep-seated tumour or small tumour and posterior fossa tumour, EEG findings are normal.

(d) **Echoencephalography** — Shift of midline echo is evident with A-scan echography and with B-scan echography tumour area may be outlined. The use of ultra sound (1500 metres per second) is one of the important non-invasive investigations for localisation of tumour.

(e) **Angiography** — This is the most commonly used neuro-radiological investigation in the management of intracranial tumours. Even when localisation of tumour has been done by non-invasive methods like B-scan echography and CT scan or isotope-scan (vide infra) — angiography is imperative to assess the vascularity of tumour. By percutaneous puncture water soluble iodine containing dye such as meglumine iothalamate (Conray 280) is injected into the neck either in the carotid or vertebral artery and serial films are taken of the skull to visualise the vascular pattern of the brain. Tumour is diagnosed from the shift of normal vessels and from the presence of new abnormal vascularity.

(f) **Isotope Encephalography** — After injecting radio-active isotope (99m TC — Technetium) into the Vein,Brain Scanner is used to demonstrate differential absorption of isotope in normal and diseased brain. But this investigation may not be able to differentiate tumour from blood clot or infarct for which other investigations like angiography or CT scan will be necessary.

(g) **Computed Tomography (CT scan)** also known as Computerised Axial Tomography (CAT-scan) is of immense value in localisation of early lesion and has revolutionised the system of neuroradiological investigations. As this is non-invasive and is more informative, this CT scan is done preliminary to angiography or isotope-scanning. Ventriculography (vide infra) is now seldom required for the diagnosis of intracranial tumours, in centres, where facility for CT scan exists.

Angiography is now employed only to assess the vascular pattern of tumours prior to surgery.

(h) **Ventriculography** — This investigation helps to localise intraventricular tumour as well as posteriorly placed tumour which cannot be diagnosed by angiography. As mentioned earlier, the CT scan has greatly replaced this investigation. Through a burr hole-water soluble iodine containing contrast like 'Conray 280' is introduced in the right lateral ventricle and X-rays are taken which show ventricular outlines. By ventricular displacements distortion or filling defect space occupying lesion can be diagnosed. As it is an operative investigation, some additional risk is involved in ventriculography and great discretion is exercised to proceed with this investigation.

(i) **Pneumoencephalography** was a very useful investigation in pre-CT scan era for diagnosis of small tumours without evidence of raised intracranial tension. To ascertain the superior extension of sellar tumour, this has a useful place in investigation. With the advent of CT scan, it is now less commonly used. In sitting position air is introduced through lumbar puncture 20-30 cc in fractional doses and by manipulation of head, entry of air in the cisterns and ventricles is achieved, X-ray films are then taken in different positions of visualise the ventricular systems and cisterns.

(j) **C.S. fluid study** — In presence of evidence of raised intracranial tension lumbar puncture is risky and is not done. But for early diagnosis of brain tumour, C.S. fluid study may be helpful. Rise in CSF protein and in some cases detection of malignant cells may contribute substantially. Its greatest utility is in the differentiation of brain abscess and tuberculous meningitis from brain tumour as in all these conditions papilloedema and other evidences of rise in intracranial presence are present in later cases. It is important to remember that brain abscess and tuberculous meningitis may be afebrile and infective nature is not suspected till CSF findings are known. But before doing lumbar puncture angiography or CT scan should be done in patients with papilloedema to assess the probable complications that may follow L.P. In acoustic neurinoma high protein is found is CSF.

**Diagnosis** — Clinical suspicion of intracranial tumour is of prime importance for early diagnosis. Investigations in well-equipped neurology centres will clinch the diagnosis. CT scan will help in early detection. In some cases differentiation of tumour from other causes of space occupying lesions (e.g. tuberculous, cyst, abscess, granuloma) is difficult. When pituitary tumour is suspected, pituitary function test is desirable. In eighth cranial nerve tumour, audiometry, vestibular tests and CSF study are useful adjuncts. In haemangioblastoma, erythrocytosis with elevated haemoglobin is observed.

**Prognosis** — Amongst primary tumours, as majority are malignant, long-term prognosis is not bright. But with the advances of surgical technique, anaesthesiology, radiotherapy and chemotherapy the result of treatment is the same as that of other malignancies of the body.

In benign tumour some may be in the vicinity of vital structures e.g. acoustic neurinoma, sphenoid ridge-meningioma — when complete removal is not possible and some morbidity is unavoidable. In most of the centres operative mortality is less than 10%. Morbidity in the form of visual defect, motor paresis, speech defect and pituitary dysfunction are present in some cases depending on the sites of tumour. Early diagnosis will minimise neurological deficits. Post-operative convulsive seizure can be tackled with anticonvulsive drugs.

**Treatment** — Most of the tumours are now accessible and surgical removal is undertaken for primary tumours. Use of operating microscope has facilitated near complete removal of meningioma and acoustic neurinoma with gratifying results.

For solitary metastasis — surgical excisions is undertaken. For multiple metastasis, chemotherapeutic agents like cyclophosphamide, azathioprine, vincristine and other allied groups of drugs are available.

In primary malignant tumours surgical removal followed by post-operative radiation or chemotherapy is used.

In tumours of postcranial fossa, there is considerable rise in intracranial pressure due to obstruotion of CSF circulation. In the first stage ventriculoatrial shunt is done to reduce the intracranial pressure and in the second stage posterior fossa is explored for removal of tumour. This two-stage operation has considerably brought down the mortality of posterior fossa neoplasma.

In late stages, when the patient is brought in a drowsy state, quick reduction of intracranial pressure is indicated. 20% Mannitol by I.V. drip or 10% glycerol intravenously is effective to bring down intracranial pressure. Furosemide by intravenous route is also effective. These agents should not be use for a long time because they induce rebound cerebral oedema of varying grade, though with glycerol rebound oedema is minimal.

**Steroid in Brain tumour**

In all tumours, praticularly of malignant tumours there are considerable peritumoral cerebral oedema. This oedema regresses effectively with dexamethasone. Initial high dose up to 20-40 mgm may be given but usually 10 mgm is adequate in majority cases. For 4-7 days dexamethasone is continued in the dosage of 4-8 mgm 4 hourly and then the operation is planned. This preoperative steroid therapy has considerably changed the prognosis and post-operative complications. Once this is given pre-operatively it has to be continued during as well as after operation for few days. Though steroid in large dosage can produce gastric haemorrhage, the overall beneficial effect of steroid in the treatment of tumour outweighs its complications.

During chemotherapy and radiotherapy, dexamethasone is a useful adjunct to combat cerebral oedema. Following operation for pituitary tumour, steroid may have to be given for prolonged period.

Steroid should be started only after completing all investigations. Early institution of steroid particularly before doing isotope scan may result in a normal scan even when there is a tumour. Previously some of the brain tumours were misdiagnosed as benign intracranial hypertension as there used to be clinical improvement and also brain scan used to be negative due to reduction of oedema with steroid.

Judicious use of steroid, ventriculoatrial shunt before definitive surgery followed by radiotherapy and/or chemotherapy have considerably improved the outlook of brain tumour treatment. Physiotherapy and psychotherapy are also invaluable in the management of brain tumour. Anti-convulsive drugs may have to be used in selected cases to prevent and control convulsive seizures.

## NEUROSYPHILIS

*G.C. MOOKERJEE*
*K.A. KABIR*

### INTRODUCTION

Neurosyphilis or syphilitic affection of the nervous system has become a rare disease compared to what it was in the early part of this century. Nervous system is affected in secondary and tertiary stage of syphilis. In secondary neurosyphilis, symptoms are mainly headache and malaise but sometimes mild form of meningitis may also occur. If CSF is examined this stage, pleocytosis is detected.

In tertiary stage of syphilitic affection of the nervous system, two types of lesion are found e.g. :

(1) Meningovascular type — where meningeal vessels are obliterated, resulting in neuronal destruction.

(2) Parenchymatoms type — where neuronal parenchyma is directly affected resulting in cerebral dysfunction.

In meningovascular syphilis there is either involvement of blood vessels of meninges of brain or spinal cord. There may be cranial or spinal pachymeningitis involving the dura. Leptomeningitis of basal meninges is common and may lead to adhesive arachnoiditis involving the cranial nerves. The third nerve is most commonly involved. Hydrocephalus may also occur due to blockage in C.S.F. pathway. The principal lesions in tertiary neurosyphilis is endarteritis obliterans leading to thrombosis of vessels and necrosis of the part supplied by that vessel resulting in "gumma" formation.

Neurosyphilitic disease may be classified as follows :

(A) **Parenchymatous syphilis**

(1) General paralysis of Insane (G.P.I.)

(2) Tabes dorsalis

(3) Tabo-paresis

(B) **Meningo-vascular syphilis**

(1) Syphilitic meningitis

(2) Cerebral pachymeningitis or leptomeningitis

(3) Cerebral gummatous lesions

(4) Cervical pachymeningitis
(5) Syphilitic amyotrophy
(6) Erb's syphilitic spinal paralysis
(7) Chronic meningomyelitis
(8) Syphilitic radiculitis
(9) Acute transverse myelitis

## GENERAL PARALYSIS OF INSANE OR GENERAL PARESIS (G.P.I)

General paresis was first described by Bayle in 1822. Out of 12 neurosyphilis cases, there were five cases of general paresis, four meningovascular syphilis and three tabes dorsalis.

This condition occurs usually 10 to 15 years after the primary syphilis. Males are more often affected.

In G.P.I. the principal feature which initially attracts attention of relatives is dementia. It is due to cerebral cortical atrophy, specially affecting anterior part of cerebral hemisphere. The meningeal layers become thickened and there is infiltration of lymphocytes.

The patient who was previously alert and active gradually becomes slow and manifests intellectual deterioration.

There is often change in habits and general interests. He may develop grandiose ideas and boasts of knowledge, wealth and status. He becomes careless about his dress, forgets easily and confabulates to compensate for his inability to remember things.

Gradually tremors may develop in tongue, lips and fingers. These are fine tremors and the tongue tremors are characteristic forward and backward movements, known as "trombone tremors . Articulation is also affected and gradually slurring speech may develop.

There may be involvement of pyramidal tracts and the plantar reflexes become extensor. Incontinence of urine and stool also occurs. Epileptiform fits are frequent and in the terminal stage the patient becomes bed-ridden, dirty and incontinent. Argyll-Robertson pupils are characteristic of neurosyphilis. The pupils are small, irregular and unequal. The pupils do not react to light but accommodation reflex is preserved, as a result they respond to convergence.

When G.P.I. is associated with tabes dorsalis, the plantar response is lost and the syndrome is called taboparesis.

## TABES DORSALIS

As the name implies, in tabes dorsalis there is degeneration of posterior root and posterior columns of spinal cord, especially in the thoracic and lumbosacral regions. Males are the common victims.

The onset is usually insidious. The patient suffers from paroxysmal attack of "lightening pain" usually localised. Each attack lasts for a few seconds, may be in the same place or may shift from place to place. It is exacerbated by intercurrent illness. Paraesthesia is common in the lower limb. The patient may complain as if he is walking on cotton wool. The skin is hypersensitive to touch. Pain and paraesthesia are due to irritation of degenerating sensory fibres. The patient rapidly develops ataxia partly due to loss of position sense and impairment of co-ordinating fibres. Romberg's test is positive. Patient walks with a broad base and may like to use a stick. He goes forward with high stepping gait. Ataxia is aggravated in the dark.

There is loss of sphincter control, usually resulting in retention of urine. Sometimes the patient may present with painless perforating ulcer of the foot. Swollen and unstable joint is known as Charcoat's joint. Physical signs include hypertoxicity, loss of ankle and knee jerks, absence of position, joint and vibration sense; bilateral ptosis with some compensatory wrinkling of forehead constitutes a typical tabetic facies. Argyll-Robertson pupils are also present.

The A.R. pupil is due to involvement of colliculonuclear and sympathetic fibres in periaqueductal grey matter.

Ataxia is due to posterior column lesion and affection of posterior roots. The patient tries to compensate by visual aid. If his eyes are closed, he becomes ataxic as noted while washing face in wash basin. This is the basis of Romberg's sign.

In course of time peripheral vision is reduced but central vision remains normal. Optic atrophy may develop in some cases. Visceral crisis may occur in form of epigastric pain associated with vomiting (gastric crisis), rectal pain (rectal crisis), laryngeal stridor (laryngeal crisis). Sometimes acute bladder pain with stranguiry may occur.

**Investigations**

In neurosyphilis there is lymphocytosis in C.S.F. and its protein content is elevated (40-100 mg) :

Serologic test – Serologic test includes the following :

(1) Non-treponemal and (2) treponemal.

Non-treponemal tests include VDRL and RPR (Rapid plasma reagin).

The specific treponemal serologic tests include TPI (treponemal) immobilisation test and FTA-ABS (flourescent treponemal antibody – observed) test. In practice the non-treponemal tests are used for screening and specific treponemal tests for confirmation of diagnosis.

**Treatment**

There is no single established schedule for treatment of neurosyphilis. Penicillin is the antibiotic of choice. Aqueous procaine penicillin-G is given by I.M. injection in dosage of 600,000 units daily for 15 days or benzathene penicillin 2.4 million units I.M. weekly for 3 weeks.

Treatment-resistant cases are treated with short acting penicillin in very large doses e.g. 20 million units I.V. for 10 to 14 days.

In late stages the patient has to be hospitalised. Aqueous crystalline penicillin 2-4 million units I.V. may be given four hourly for ten days.

In cases of penicillin allergy, tetracycline or erythromycin 500 mg is given four times a day for 30 days.

All patients require follow-up three monthy, for the first year and six monthly for the second year. Clinical and CSF studies must be made. Sometimes second course of treatment may be required.

**Meningovascular syphilis**

This form is due to affection of meningeal or vascular structures or both tissues. It may present as mild meningitis causing headache, irritability, low grade fever and general ill-health. Basal meningitis may cause cranial nerve palsies including A.R. pupil. If large cerebral vessels are involved, cerebrovascular accidents may occur.

CSF changes consist of raised protein, increased cells with lymphocytic predominance and positive serology for syphilis.

Sometimes the symptoms may be so mild that CNS signs and symptoms are absent but changes in CSF may be characteristic. These cases are often missed. Therefore in all cases of syphilis follow-up for involvement of CNS is recommended. Periodic CSF studies are mandatory for final test of cure after primary or secondary stage therapy is duly completed. Only serological tests are not enough to declare a full cure. If CSF changes are suggestive, full treatment for neurosyphilis should be given.

In G.P.I. or advanced cases of neurosyphilis there is risk of Herxheimer reaction. This can be prevented by giving steroid therapy. Usually prednisolone 40 mg daily may given for first 3 to 4 days to be gradually tailed off. Procaine penicillin may be started on fourth day in usual dosage, and continued for 15 to 21 days.

If erythromycin or tetracycline is given in cases of penicillin allergy, the dose should be 500 mg six hourly for 15 to 20 days. The old method of fever-therapy or malaria induction therapy is no longer practised.

### Spinal forms of neurosyphilis

Spinal endarteritis may involve anterior or posterior spinal artery leading to thrombotic occlusions of the vessel concerned. The affected grey matter suffers infarction. This results in acute transverse myelitis. Anterior spinal artery occlusion results in damage to anterior horn cells and spinothalamic tract. So there will be LMN lesion at the level of lesion and loss of crude touch, pain and temperature sensation below the segment of lesion.

If posterior spinal artery is affected, postero-lateral white matter and posterior horn cells (Gall & Burdach's tract) will be affected. There will be loss of all sensation below the level of lesion with pyramidal (UMN) type of lesion below the segment affected.

The other spinal forms of neuro-syphilis are :

**Erb's syphilitic spinal paralysis** — A rare disorder causing spastic paraplegia without sensory loss; sphincter control also is lost.

**Syphilitic amyotrophy** — is due to damage of anterior horn cells in the cervical region. Therefore the lesion results in muscular wasting in upper limbs especially in shoulder girdles, upper limbs and hands. Lower limbs may remain normal or may develop spastic paralysis; sphincter disturbances are also rare.

**Chronic meningomyelitis** — It usually occurs in the thoracic region of the spinal cord. Pain is common and features of chronic transverse myelitis will be present.

Treatment of all these forms of syphilis is the same as described above.

# EPILEPSY

*G.C. MOOKERJEE*
*K.A. KABIR*

## INTRODUCTION

The term 'epilepsy' is a Greek word 'epilepsia' meaning a seizing. 'Epilepsy' is a syndrome rather than a disease, characterized by chronic, recurrent, paroxysmal changes in neurological functions of the brain, clinically manifested by musculo-skeletal convulsions with or without loss of consciousness. Each episode of neurological function is termed a 'seizure'. The convulsive disorders of brain may be motor, sensory, cognitive or emotional events. Actually the pattern of fits will depend on the area of the brain from where abnormal discharge is occurring. However, sometimes there are no convulsions at all but only brief spells of 'absence attacks'. Absence attacks or sometimes temporal lobe attacks may not be diagnosed and children are often stamped as inattentive, lazy or stupid. Sometimes they are referred to psychiatrists. An EEG in these cases may be used, which may show paroxysmal discharge of petitmal pattern.

## PATHOPHYSIOLOGY OF EPILEPSY :

The incidence of epilepsy appears to be about 0.5 to 2 per cent in the general population, females being affected more than males. In developing countries it appears to be 20 to 25 per thousand population (WHO report). Experimentally it has been found that certain special parts of brain are susceptible to electrical and chemical stimuli resulting in seizure. These are motor cortex, temporal lobe, amygdala and hippocampus.

The repetitive and stereotype nature of epileptic seizure suggests that these areas become unstable due to some ill-understood mechanism, influenced by yet unknown metabolic or vascular abnormalities.

A single attack without recurrence may be due to syncope while repeated episodes would suggest it to be idiopathic epilepsy or hysteria or some intracranial or metabolic complications. Stoke Adam's syndrome points to a cardiac cause and therefore both cardiac and cerebral lesions should be taken into account during evaluation of convulsive episode.

Electroencephalography (EEG) recordings or normal brain reveals alpha rhythm of 8-13 cycles per sec (c.p.s.) while during sleep the waves are slower.

In grand mal epilepsy, there is high voltage paroxysmal discharge of electrical activities which may be focal or generalised. In focal lesion the EEG discharges are due to local brain damage. Many metabolic disturbances may also be associated with epileptic seizures.

## BIOCHEMISTRY OF SIEZURES

There is an alteration in the membrane permeability with increase in extracellular potassium concentration and decrease in extracellular calcium concentration which affects the function of cerebral tissues. Both have profound influence on neuronal excitability, neurotransmitter release and neuronal metabolism. There may be increased amount of released neurotransmitter and neuropeptides. During seizure there is increased blood flow, glucose utilization, alteration in oxidative metabolism and local pH. All these may be responsible for attacks as in case of "Todd's paralysis'.

There are two kinds of neurotransmitters, inhibitory and excitatory. The inhibitory one is gamma-amino-butyric acid (GABA) and the excitatory is acetylcholine. Experimentally seizures can be produced by blocking inhibitory mechanisms i.e. by agents which antagonise GABA. There may be some abnormality in the GABA inhibitory system. The anti-epileptic drugs such as phenobarbital, benzodia-zepines and valproic acid act by enhancing GABA media inhibiting in the brain.

Even repetitive subthreshold electrical stimulus can evoke a seizure discharge. Thus spontaneous seizures may occur without any further electrical stimulation. This is the so-called 'kindling' phenomenon.

## AETIOLOGY :

Heredity, age and sex are the important factors in the aetiology of epilepsy. Epilepsy can be broadly classified into two types :

(1) Acquired type where the specific cause can be determined by investigation.

(2) Idiopathic type – where no specific cause can be found out. This constitutes about 75% of all cases.

### Acquired epilepsy

Amongst the acquired causes, congenital malformations, birth trauma, asphyxia and hyperpyrexia are important factors, in all age groups. Brain tumour and cerebral atherosclerosis are the most important causative factors after the age of 30 years. It constitutes about 30 per cent of patients with new focal seizures. Therefore if a patient has developed epileptic fit for the first time after the age of 30 years, very detailed investigations are necessary.

### Classical causes of epileptic seizure

| | |
|---|---|
| Infant<br>(0-2 yrs.) | Congenital malformation,<br>Genetic disorders.<br>Intracranial birth injury<br>Acute infection<br>Metabolic disturbances (hypoglycaemia hypocalcaemia, hypomagnesemia, pyridoxine deficiency) |

| | |
|---|---|
| Child<br>(2-12 yrs.) | Idiopathic<br>Acute infection<br>Trauma<br>Febrile convulsion |
| Adolescent<br>(12-18 yrs.) | Idiopathic<br>Trauma<br>Drug and alcohol withdrawal<br>Arterio-venous malformation |
| Young<br>(18-35 yrs.) | Trauma<br>Alcoholism<br>Brain tumour |
| Older adult | Brain tumour<br>Cerebrovascular disease<br>Alcoholism<br>Metabolic disorders (uremia) hepatic failure, electrolyte abnormality, hypoglycaemia. |

## MAJOR EPILEPSY

(Grand mal or generalized seizure) : It can occur in any age group and may be due to many pathological processes. It consists of (1) preconvulsive or prodromal symptoms of the aura followed by (2) tonic-clonic convulsions. There may be precipitating factors such as mental excitement, fatigue or alcoholic drinks. In the prodromal phase usually there is an emotional upset either in the form of excitement or depression which usually lasts for minutes or even hours. Sense of impending attack or the "aura" is the most important component of grand mal epilepsy. Aura is a subjective sensation produced at the beginning of the epileptic discharge and perceived by the patient before the loss of consciousness. The nature of aura may be helpful in locating the site of epileptic focus in the brain. Aura may be of various kinds, e.g. sense of fear or unreality (jamais Vu) or familiarity (deja Vu), a peculiar epigastric sensation (butterflies in the stomach), unpleasant odour (olfactory hallucination), different types of visual or auditory hallucinations (simple flashes of light or balls of fire or simple hearing of words or phrases). Sometimes these attacks, preceded by visual or auditory aura are considered as supernatural heavenly phenomena and attacks are given religious hue. Vertigo or subjective giddiness is a common aura. There may be sensory auras, such as tingling, numbness or 'electric shocks or motor' auras of chewing or 'smacking' of lips. Sometimes the convulsion may begin with turning of head to one side (the adversive attack) or flexion of the upper limb.

The convulsions usually begin with an 'epileptic cry' that is a harsh scream due to expiration of air through the partly closed vocal cords, immediately followed by loss of consciousness. The patient hurts himself and the marks of injury are usually present in an epileptic patient. The convulsion proper is a phase of tonic spasm of muscles, symmetrical on both sides of the body, head and eyes are related on one side while the mouth is drawn to one side due to facial spasm (Fig.12.11). The upper limbs are adducted at shoulders and flexed at the elbow and wrists. The fingers are flexed at the metacarpophalangeal and extended at the interphalangeal joints, with adducted thumb. The lower extremities are extended with inverted feet. The respiratory muscles are in spasm and the respiration stops, hence the patient becomes cyanosed. This stage lasts for a few seconds.

This is followed by clonic phase which consists of short, interrupted jerks. Froth cames out of the mouth and the tongue may be bitten. Incontinence of urine may occur. The tendon reflexes may be absent, the plantar may be extensor.

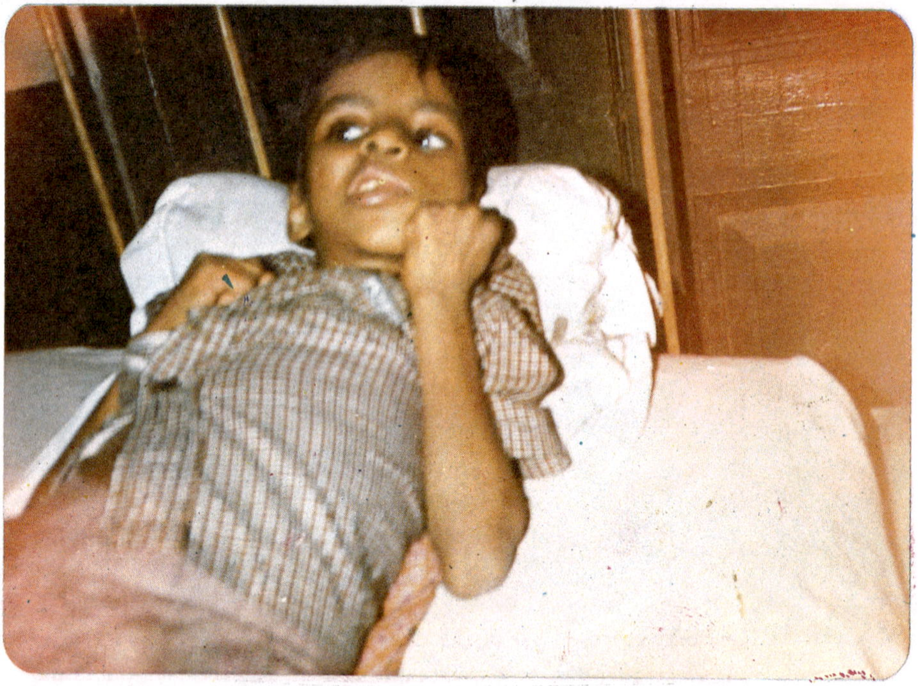

Fig.12.11 : A typical Jacksonian fit (*Patient of Islamia Hospital*)

After the clonic phase, the patient regains consciousness and usually complains headache. In some patients there may be post-epileptic automatism. There may be residual evidence of neurological signs such as hemiparesis or monoparesis, sensory disturbances and dysphagia. The positional paralysis is called "Todd's paralysis" which may last for minutes or even hours.

In 20% cases the grand mal seizure may be nocturnal, otherwise it occurs annually or several times a year. In females, menstrual period or pregnancy may be precipitating factors.

**Other Varieties of Epilepsy**

In mild epilepsy attack there may be transient loss of consciousness which is called petit mal epilepsy, sensory epilepsy, myoclonic epilepsy and infantile spasms are various other types which must be recognised.

**Petit mal or Focal Epilepsy :**

Petit malepilepsy is not associated with convulsions. The attacks always begin in young children (6-14 years of age), rarely appear first time in adult. The child stares blankly, their eyes roll up beneath the upper eyelids. The child stops talking and will cease to do any work which he was doing. The attack lasts for a second or two only, after which the patient becomes normal again. He does not recollect the incidence. Occasionally there may be a myoclonic jerk or twitching of the upper extremity. The attack may occur many times a day.

## TEMPORAL LOBE EPILEPSY :

(Psychomotor epilepsy)

This condition is now renamed as complex partial seizures, this old name was expressive of the disorder. It is due to epileptiform activities in the temporal lobe areas including hippocampus, amygdala or limbic system.

The patients usually experience a peculiar aura of smell, emotional, visual or sensory experience. He may have hallucinations during which he may see large figures of animals or humans (Macropsia) or minute objects (micropsia) before the attack. He may suddenly feel that he has gone to a place, where he has been before or feel an emotional experience of remote day, or recall events of previous birth (De la vu phenomena). Any of these varied experiences may be followed by a phase of automatism during which she may do some activity as well as even break things, play musical tune, walk about aimlessly and may get injured or injure others. This phase of highly skilled activity is not remembered at all when he comes round.

He may become comatose after the phase of automatism and remember nothing of these actions after this attack is over. EEG shows unilateral or bilateral spikes or slow waves in the temporal and adjoining areas.

## JACKSONIAN EPILEPSY

The site of lesion is the precentral gyrus. The seizure begins either in thumb, index finger, the angle of the mouth or great toe. The convulsion then usually spreads centrifugally and becomes bilateral when consciousness is lost. Jacksonian epilepsy is always organic in nature.

### Sensory epilepsy :

This sensory equivalent of motor, Jacksonian epilepsy consists of paraesthesia usually involving a part or the whole of one side of the body. The lesion is usually at the parietal lobe but the consciousness is retained.

### Myoclonic epilepsy :

Sudden brief repetitive or single muscle contractions of one part or whole of the body. The site of lesion is usually the reticular formation of brain stem.

### Akinetic epilepsy :

There is sudden loss of muscle tone resulting in fall without any warning. Seizures are of short duration, consciousness is also lost but he soon regains consciousness. In catalepsy, the attack is similar but consciousness is not lost. The patient suddenly falls without warning and remains helpless where he falls while he is fully conscious.

### Infantile spasms

This occurs in infants characterized by sudden shock-like flexion of the arms and often flexion of the head, neck and trunk with drawing up of knees (salam attacks). There are abnormalities of dendritic developments in pyramidal neurons of frontal cortex.

### Status epilepticus

Status epilepticus is a medical emergency in which patient gets recurrent episodic epileptiform convulsions without relief. The patient becomes unconscious and develops tonic and clonic convulsions, cyanosis and high fever. Blood pressure may be raised. Sudden withdrawal of anti-epileptic drugs or too rapid change of medication is frequently followed by status epilepticus.

### Diagnosis :

Meticulous history taking is important for the provisional diagnosis of epilepsy as physical and neurological examinations cannot be properly done during fits. Epileptic attacks must be differentiated from paroxysmal fits due to organic brain disorders,e.g. hypertensive encephalopathy and organic brain diseases including brain tumours.

## LABORATORY INVESTIGATIONS :

In view of convulsive episode it may be necessary to do this following tests depending on this clinical background :

(1) Complete haemogram and malarial parasites

(2) Blood urea, creatinine and glucose

(3) Serum electrolytes

(4) Liver function tests

(5) CSF study

The above tests may be necessary as a known epileptic may develop severe infection, malaria, renal or liver failure and electrolyte imbalance. Each test is certainly not required in all cases.

X-ray skull, EEG, ECG even CT scan may be required. Brain tumours may sometimes present with recurrent convulsions. Epileptiform fits occurring for the first time in adult age should be further investigated.

**CSF Studies :**

After severe seizure there may be slight increase in CSF pressure and protein and cell count.

X-ray skull should be done to detect asymmetry of skull caused by birth trauma, maldevelopment, abnormal calcifications, shift of calcified pineal body or signs of increased intracranial pressure. A chest radiograph may detect presence of any pulmonary infection, tumour or cardiac enlargement.

**EEG**

EEG is helpful in diagnosis but a normal ECG does not exclude epilepsy. On the other hand, 10 to 15% of normal subjects may reveal EEG abnormalities, who have no fits. Hence clinical background is very important.

However, certain patterns are useful in the diagnosis.

**Computerized axial tomography (CT Scanning)** is particularly helpful in detection of any abnormality suspected in adults with seizure of recent onset. Cerebral angiography is useful to detect any vascular abnormalities of the brain.

Radioactive isotopic gamma camera brain scanning has been also used for the diagnosis.

## PROGNOSIS

Prognosis of epileptic attack is not bad provided thorough medical treatment can be instituted.

After the first attack he should be treated and followed up for a sufficiently long time for at least three years after the cessation of last attack or even indefinitely in some cases. Death may occur in status epilepticus, during a nocturnal attack due to asphyxia and face being buried in a pillow. Fracture of rib, dislocation of shoulder have been reported due to violent convulsions. Some children with 'petit mal' may develop grand mal attack at adolescence.

## TREATMENT

Treatment of the patient with seizure consists of :

(1) Suppression of seizure
(2) Elimination of causes of seizure, if possible
(3) Exclusion of organic causes
(4) Treatment of psychosomatic disorder which is always associated with this type of patient
(5) Rehabilitation.

Suppression of seizure can be achieved by avoiding precipitation factors, e.g. alcohol, physical and emotional stress and by presenting anti-epileptic drugs. The ideal anti-epileptic drug should inhibit the discharge without side-effects but no such drugs are available, hence side-effects. Should be carefully watched especially because the drugs are to be given on long-term basis.

It is also wise to start treatment with a single drug at the onset and try to control with one drug only, if possible. If this does not succeed a second drug may be tried or combination may be used.

The choice depends chiefly on the diagnosis of the type of epilepsy. The idiopathic or primary type, i.e. generalised form due to genetic defect of the neurons dependent on the neurochemical transmitters. The partial epilepsies are often due to local malformation or injuries in the part of cerebral cortex.

It is most important therefore to diagnose the type of seizures before correct drug therapy can be given.

It is also important that hysteria is not mistaken for epilepsy. The most useful drugs used nowadays are phenobarbitone, phenytoin, diazepam, carbamazepine, ethosuximide and the latest being valproic acid. It is again stressed that before drugs are started, be sure that it is epilepsy and try to classify it correctly. Patients suffering from non-neurological cases of blackout, e.g. hysteria, Stoke Adam's syndrome, cardiac arrhythmias and simple faints should not be mistaken for epilepsy. It is better to wait and watch, while carrying out appropriate biochemical, cardiological and radiological investigations including angiography. CT scan or gamma camera scan, if indicated. It is better to be sure in the beginning than to start long-term life-long treatment. *The duration of treatment may be at least three to five years while some patients will require life-long treatment.* Phenobarbitone and phenytoin are good combination in the treatment of epilepsy. It is better to use one of them initially. Even phenobarbitone may alone be adequate in cases. Unfortunately all the anti-epileptic drugs have a tendency to produce drowsiness, dysarthria, ataxia, often blurred vision and diplopia. These are more common with primidone and hydantoinates. Reduction of dose may reduce or ameliorate the symptoms. Macrocytic anaemia is common with prolonged use of many drugs, e.g. phenytoin. Sometimes it can be prevented with the administration of folic acid in dosage of 5 mg daily. Paradoxically it may sometimes induce more seizures. Phenytoin may induce involuntary movement, blood dyscrasia. Frequent blood count, urine analysis and liver function tests are advocated while treating the patient to evaluate the function of respective organs. Generalised grand mal and focal motor seizures are usually treated with a combination of phenobarbital and hydantoin.

In some cases phenobarbital can be substituted by primidone (Mysoline). This powerful drug is given in a dosage of 250 mg thrice or four times daily (125 mg thrice daily for young children).

The combination of primidone and phenobarbital is contraindicated because of their combined sedative effect. Clonazepam in dosage of 1.0 mg daily and sodium valproate (200 mg thrice daily up to 600 mg daily) can be given both in grand mal and petit mal epilepsy. In some resistant cases chlordiazepoxide 5-10 mg thrice daily, diazepam 2-5 thrice daily, beclamide 500 mg thrice or four times daily are administered along with usual regime.

In petit mal, ethosuximide, in a dosage of 250 mg, two, three or four times daily is now the drug of choice. In resistant case trimethadione and paramethadione in dosage of 300 mg thrice daily may have to be added along with ethosuximide. However, their possible toxic effects must be watched for. For partial and generalised tonic-clonic seizure phenobarbitone, phenytoin, carbamazepine and valproic acid are all used. Valproic acid, however, is very useful in all kinds of primary generalised epilepsy.

**Status epilepticus**

It is a medical emergency and needs immediate treatment to eliminate the risk of brain damage. Adequate airway and oxygenation must be established, if necessary, by endotracheal intubation. Anticonvulsants such as diazepam 10 mg can given intravenously which may be repeated once or twice within 15 to 20 minutes interval.

Vital function must be maintained. See that the patient does not injure himself. A padded tongue depressor or a plastic airway tube should be introduced to prevent choking. Patency of airway should be taken care of.

Be careful not to inject cerebral depressants if the cause is suspected to be alcohol or CVA. Known epileptics may develop diabetic coma or hypoglycaemia, if he is a diabetic.

Phenytoin may also be used but it is not available freely. In our experience diazepam is good enough to control fits.

Loading dose of phenytoin is quite high (750 to 1500 mg) and is not well tolerated. It is better to use diazepam initially followed by oral phenytoin. Recommended dose is 2 to 5 mg/kg of body weight. Most patients are already on this drug, hence maintenance dose may be continued or may have to be increased, if necessary. Sometimes newer drugs, e.g. valproates may be introduced.

Paraldehyde may be useful when all drugs fail. Dose of first drug to be injected is 4 to 5 ml. in each buttock, i.e. total 8 to 10 ml.

Rarely sodium thiopentone may have to be given 0.5 to 1.0g I.V:

In mild cases the patient may be controlled by intramuscular injection of 125-250 mg of phenobarbitone sodium followed by 120 mg every hour for several hours. The patient should be nursed flat and preferably in the semiprone position. If unconsciousness is prolonged, nasal feeding should be started.

ACTH and adrenocortical steroid are now used in the treatment infantile spasms.

Epilepsy is not regarded as primarily a psychological disorder. However, depression, anxiety, hysterical manifestations may occur in epileptic patients and sometimes these may be precipitating factors for seizure.

**Antidepressant and/or Tranquilizers**

Antidepressant and/or tranquilizings drugs are helpful. Some patients may be hospitalised for such problems. Certain antidepressant drugs (e.g. imipramine) may potentiate the epileptic discharge, whereas chlordiazepoxide and diazepam have an anti-convulsant effect.

It is desirable that an epileptic patient should as far as possible live a normal life. Children should attend schools, but teachers must be sympathetic and helpful. They should be allowed to take part in sports under careful supervision. Certain risks of everyday life must be explained to the patient, his parents and friends. The patient should not swim in deep water unaccompanied. Adults should carry out a sedentary occupation. Occupation involving working at heights, near fire or working with heavy machinery or driving vehicles is obviously not advisable.

There is no bar for the patient to get married, but certain possible risks regarding pregnancy and hereditary transmission of disease to children should be explained by counselling. Good hygiene in epileptic patient should be maintained. Moderate exercise is desirable. Alcohol is best avoided.

**SURGERY :**

Surgical treatment may be very helpful in selected cases when medical treatment has failed.

However, selection should be made after thorough and detailed neurological investigations.

Small post-traumatic hematomas, glial scars or nodules or localised cysts may cause focal seizures and these may be surgically removed, if located by EEG brain scan or CT scan. In some cases neurosurgery have been preferred to do lobotomy under sterotactic control. Hippocampus, temporal lobe isthmus or tracts from uncas has been removed. Corpus callosum section or massive hemispherectomy also has been done for intractable epilepsy with behaviour disorder and deteriorating intellectual function.

## MIGRAINE

*G.C. MOOKERJEE*
*B. KHAN*

### INTRODUCTION

Migraine is a common disorder characterised by recurrent attacks of headache usually unilateral associated with nausea, vomiting, disturbance of vision and sometimes giddiness. It commonly occurs when the person gets up early in the morning. It may be also bifrontal, occipital or generalised headache. Females are more commonly affected. Attacks are first noticed in adolesence or adults but rarely it may start in the childhood.

**Aetiology :**

Familial incidence is well-known. It is transmitted by dominant inheritance and many members in a family may be affected. Intelligent, over-conscientious, ambitious and energetic people suffer more than other people.

Many factors are known to precipitate the attack of migraine. Anxiety, emotional disturbances, flashing light, excessive noise, uncorrected refractive errors and premenstrual phase may precipitate migrainous attacks. Tyramine containg food, cheese, chocholate, onion, fried food, sherry and red wines may precipitate the headache. Pregnancy causes remission of attacks in majority of cases.

**Pathogenesis**

The pain of migraine is due to constriction and later dilatation of arteries of the scalp, orbit and external carotid as well as basilar artery. This has been confirmed experimentally by inhalation studies of radioisotope Xenon$^{133}$ during the aura. Dilatation of vessels leads to oedema of musculature of vessel wall, oedema of surrounding structures and vascular spasm causing the headache.

Various vasoactive humoral substances seem to act on the hypothalamus causing the vessel wall changes but the exact nature of bio-chemical reaction and mechanisms is not fully understood. Noradrenaline, 5-hydroxytryptamine (5 H.T.), tyramine, histamine, reserpine, serotonin and bradykinins are correlated in the pathogenesis of migraine.

**Clinical features :**

The migrainous attacks usually begin at puberty but the onset can also occur rarely in the middle age. Headache comes in recurrent spasms and pain stays from hours to few days. Paroxysmal nature of attack may recur after few days to several months. Before the headache, subjects may experience prodromal sensory symptoms. They occur during the vasoconstriction phase and usually may last for 10 to 30 minutes. Prodromal symptoms are visual changes in the from of white or coloured visons, zigzag lines in vision blurred, patchy or distorted images or temporary hemianopia. Paraesthesia in the form of numbness or muscular weakness may be felt in the upper limbs which gradually spreads to other hand and around mouth and tongue. In some patients with left-sided headache, transient aphasia may be noticed before pain.

Actual headache comes after the sensory aura and it usually begins in the supra-orbital area or temple of one side of the cranium. Later it may be localised or spread to other parts of the head. The side of headache may or may not concide with the side of sensory changes. The side of head affected may be the same or different in different attacks. In classical attacks of migraine, pain is severe and throbbing in nature, associated with nausea or vomiting, photophobia, and sweating. During the attacks the person does not like to take part in conversation nor does he like to eat, smoke or even drink fluids. He prefers to remain in dark room because of photophobia. A good sleep during might may relieve his pain.

Some fortunate persons get mild form of headache with or without prodromal symptoms. Hemiplegic migraine is characterised by unilateral paraesthesia or temporary paralysis. In ophthalmoplegic migraine, there are signs of temporary oculomotor nerve palsy and diplopia.

**Differential Diagnosis**

(1) Brain tumour or intracranial aneurysm also presents with headache in spasms with prodromal symptoms. Presence of papilloedema and specific neurological changes and sometimes CSF changes are helpful in diagnosis.

(2) Intermittent headache with tingling sensation in limbs may occur in pheochromocytoma and hypertension.

(3) Frontal headache, unilateral in distribution is a feature of chronic sinusitis. It starts in the morning and increases gradually during the day. There may be signs of upper resipratory tract infection or tonsillitis.

(4) Subdural haematoma presents features of headache with or without neurological deficit. History of trauma, lateralising signs, and CSF examination will help in diagnosis. C.T. scan is confirmatory.

(5) Post-head-injury headache may also cause headache of recurrent type. History of injury and absence of any physical signs are helpful.

(6) Cerebro-vascular accident and cerebral haemorrhage may lead to episodic headache during convalescence but this is not difficult to diagnose.

(7) Dental neuralgia can easily be recognised as local signs will be present.

(8) Headache of neurosis may sometimes be difficult to differentiate from migraine, because the personality type is also similar in both cases. Headache of neurosis may also come in paroxysms. It lasts longer in duration and interval between two attacks is usually shorter.

(9) Vomiting and diarrhoea of migraine may be have to be differentiated from abdominal causes.

**Investigations :**

Usually the diagnosis of migraine is made by taking good history, clinical examination and its follow-up. But in atypical cases the following investigations may be necessary :

(1) X-ray skull PA, lateral and Towne's view

(2) Ophthalmoscopy

(3) Lumbar puncture to study C.S.F. pressure, cytology and biochemistry

(4) Electro-encephalogram (E.E.G.)

**Special Investigations :**

(1) Carotid and basilar angiography

(2) Pneumo-encephalography

(3) Brain scanning and ultrasonic studies

(4) C.T. scan when necessary.

**Treatment :**

There is no specific cure for migraine, hence various measures are to be adopted to combat the problem. It is good to explain the nature of the disease to the patient, so that he can take some preventive measures, which may reduce the number of attacks.

Avoidance of situations which precipitates the attack is important. Late nights, TV shows, movies, alcohol, smoking, flashing lights and some dietary articles may be known factors causing attacks. These can be eliminated as far as possible.

Tranquilizers e.g. diazepam or phenobarbitone can be regularly taken in small doses when attacks are frequent. Tricyclic antidepressants and MAO inhibitors are sometimes useful; when using these drugs take care regarding adverse drug combination.

**Acute attacks** should be treated with aspirin or paracetamol and codiene wherever possible. These may relieve minor or moderate attacks, often with additional diazepam. For severe attacks ergometrine tartarate may have to be used. Oral preparations containing ergometrine tartarate 1.0 mg plus 100 mg of codeine are available in the market. One tablet followed by second one after half an hour may be required. Sometimes oral ergometrine causes nausea and vomiting, so 1.0 mg of the drug may be given sublingually or as aerosal. Many patients prefer rectal suppository or even by I.M. injection in dosage of 0.5 mg. In severe attacks oxygen inhalation may also help.

Massage of head with menthol eucalyptus containing ointments may also be helpful. For prevention of repeated and frequent attacks methysergide (a serotonin antagonist) may be useful (1.0 to 3.0 mg T.D.S.) but its rare adverse effect is retro-peritoneal fibrosis.

Other drugs like prochlorperazine, clonidine, chlordiazepoxide, diazepam and barbiturates may be used in different times in judicious manner than rather to use any one drug for many years continuously. There is some evidence that migraine is less common among diabetics. In two diabetic clinics in Calcutta under our care, there was not a single migrainous subject among 1500 diabetics. Possibly attention to avoid hypoglycaemia and prevention of prolonged fasting may be helpful.

The disease usually has tendency to get spontaneous remission by the fourth decade, so the patient has to live with it for many years.

## DEMYELINATING DISEASES

*G. C. MOOKERJEE*
*K. A. KABIR*

The demyelinating diseases are an important group of nervous system disorders because of its frequency and the disability they produce. The demyelinating process is however patchy destruction of myelin sheath. Surprisingly, in this group of diseases myelin sheath of central nervous system is involved, peripheral nerves are spared possibly because of difference of their chemical composition. Usually the axons are spared. The patchy destruction is usually accompanied by acute inflammatory process.

The aetiology of the demyelinating diseases is obscure. Acute forms are sometimes familial and may also occur after acute infection often due to viral infection. It has been recorded even after vaccination. There is an apparent inter-relationship between genetic, infective, immunological and biochemical mechanism. The aetiological and clinical classifications are difficult. The present classification is based on clinical and pathological findings.

(1) Multiple sclerosis.
(2) Acute disseminated encephalomyelitis.
(3) Acute haemorrhagic leucoencephalomyelitis.
(4) Neuromyelitis optica of Devic's syndrome.
(5) Diffuse sclerosis or Schilder's disease.

Demyelination can be produced experimentally in animals and man by drugs or toxins such as cyanide intoxication, arsphenamine treatment of syphilis or diphtheria-toxin, vit $B_{12}$ deficiency. But in all the above conditions patchy destruction is limited to peripheral nerves.

## MULTIPLE SCLEROSIS

Multiple sclerosis is the modern name of disseminated sclerosis. From autopsy studies it is revealed that there are scattered areas of glial scarring or sclerosis in central nervous system, but the peripheral nerves and axons are usually spared. In acute lesions, there is oedema with spreading edge and lymphocytic reaction. Oligodendrocytes which are supposed to be responsible for myelin formation are either absent or abnormal.

Gliosis gradually develops in the plaques but the lesions are not systematically distributed. Therefore symmetrical clinical features are absent in multiple sclerosis.

**Aetiology :** The exact aetiology of multiple sclerosis is unknown.

However, emotional stress, trauma infection, surgery and pregnancy are often precipitating factors. It usually affects young adults around 20 to 30 years, with female predilection. The female and male ratio is 3 : 2. It is almost absent in Equator but the disease process proceeds away from the Equator with a peak of 150 per 10,000 people in northern latitude. Multiple sclerosis is more common in higher socio-economic groups. There is usually positive family history. Various infections, injury or emotional upsets and even pregnancy may precipitate a first attack of multiple sclerosis.

There is strong evidence that multiple sclerosis is an autoimmune disease. The lesions of multiple sclerosis and those of experimental allergic encephalomyelitis (EAE) are auto-immune diseases induced by immunization with myelin in animals and are identical.

There is fall of T-lymphocytes and the rise when the disease is in remission stage. There is increased IgG production in CSF which may be due to hyperactivity of B-cells in brain. Viral theory cannot be also excluded as 'virus-like' particles have been observed from either autopsy or biopsy material from MS patients of which the most important are tubular structures resembling myxovirus nucleocapsids. Morphological study of "virus like" structures and serological resemblance of patients of MS and measles, suggest close relationship of measles with MS.

**Clinical features :**

The disease is characterized by exacerbations and remissions. The clinical picture is determined by the location of foci of demyelination.

Weakness and ataxia are often the precipitating features, which brings the patient for medical attention. The chief symptoms are weakness of limbs, ataxia, tremor, sensory symptoms, e.g. tingling and numbness of limbs, ophthalmic symptoms, e.g. ocular pain, dimness of vision and diplopia (double vision). Nystagmus can be demonstrated. Ophthalmoscopy may reveal swelling optic disc and temporal pallor.

Sensory symptoms are sometimes very annoying, producing so-called 'useless hand syndrome'. Lhermitte's sign may be suggestive of the diagnosis. The test consists of flexion of the neck which results in electric shock like sensation in the back and limbs.

Muscular wasting is very rare. Incoordination usually in upper limbs, in the form of "intention tremor" is a frequent symptom in MS. In finger-nose test, the tremor increases in amplitude as the finger approaches the nose. Tremor of the head is due to cerebellar involvement. Acute retrobulbar neuritis is present in about 85 per cent cases of MS. There is pain in eye with ocular movement and blurred vision. Eyes are tender on pressure and central scotoma may be present larger for red and green than for white; usually optic disc is normal during the acute stage. Ocular symptoms deteriorate within a few days but vision improves in a few weeks. In chronic cases there is temporal pallor of the optic discs. In 70 per cent cases nystagmus may be present. It is usually absent on central fixation and appears in conjugate deviation bilaterally.

Articulation may be slurred in early stage due to either spastic weakness or to ataxia of muscles of articulation or both. The 'syllabicor' 'scanning' speech is typical in late cases where cerebellum is involved.

Impairment of position and joint sense may be present due to affection of posterior columns of the spinal cord. Acute paraplegia with complete loss of motor and sensory function below mid-dorsal level may be the presenting features of MS in some cases.

Exaggerated tendon reflexes associated with the clonus as well as flexor or extensor spasms may occur in late stages. Extensor plantar response may occur due to affection of corticospinal tract.

Sphincter control is disturbed. In the early stages hesitancy or precipitancy of micturition is common. Retention or reflex evacuation of both urine and stool may occur in late stages. Impotence is common, sweating is impaired. Some emotional control is disturbed leading to involuntary laughter or tears especially in late stage. Dementia also may occur in some cases. Deafness is rare, but vertigo is common.

The common clinical features in young adults are weakness and spasticity of lower limbs, ataxia, intention tremor, defective sphincter control, nystagmus and temporal pallor of optic disc. The classical triad of Charcot, nystagmus, intention tremor and scanning speech is present only in 10 per cent of cases.

**Laboratory tests :**

Though diagnosis of multiple sclerosis mainly depends on clinical findings, laboratory tests are helpful in confirmation in some cases. Cell counts are predominantly lymphocytes usually slightly increased in CSF but more than 50 cells is rare. IgG level which is usually less than 12% CSF may be increased but the total protein level is rarely elevated.

Myelin debris and even myelin basic protein determined by radio immuno-assay appears during the attacks of the disease. It appears that IgG is formed within the nervous system in this disease. Oligoclonal bands may be seen in electrophoresis.

Presence of complement factor Cg in CSF is low. Slowing of conduction tested by visual evoked potential (VEP) is revealed in 80 per cent cases. VEP test is helpful detection of addition sites in suspected cases. Low-density lesions within white matter usually in a paravertical or subcortical distribution detected by CT scan are an adjunct to diagnosis of MS. Nuclear magnetic radiation (NMR) gives useful information about pathology.

**Diagnosis**

Multiple sclerosis should be suspected when symptoms and signs cannot be explained by a single pathology. MS usually presents symptoms in one leg and signs in both legs. Waxing and waning is an important pointer. Weakness, ataxia, intention tremor, nystagmus and ocular signs are the sine qua non of the diagnosis. In differential diagnosis many conditions, e.g. spinal tumour, Friedreich's ataxia, cervical spondylosis, subacute combined degeneration, retrobulbar neuritis and transverse myelitis should be considered. Neuromyelitis optica may closely simulate MS. In Friedreich's ataxia, there is diminution of ankle jerks, later on knee jerks, scoliosis and pes cavus, and extensor response. Unlike MS the disease takes a slow progressive course.

Lost tendon reflexes, gastric achylia, megaloblastic anaemia and low serum $B_{12}$ are the characteristic findings of subacute combined degeneration. X-ray cervical region, spine myelography, CT body scan are helpful in the diagnosis of cervical spondylosis and spinal tumour.

**Prognosis**

Generally patients reach the terminal stage within 5-25 years.

Disease has a variable course. Sometimes acute cases may be fatal within a few months. In a few fortunate cases there may not be a second attack after the first remission. The terminal stage may be distressing when the patient becomes invalid with ataxia, weakness and spasticity.

**Treatment**

The treatment of multiple sclerosis is unsatisfactory.

The aim of the treatment should be :

(1) To treat the acute attack

(2) Relief of symptoms e.g. tremor, spasticity, urinary problems and visual failure.

(3) Prevention of relapse.

Though the disease has natural tendency to have remission and relapse spontaneously, the glucocorticoid administration speeds up the recovery, ACTH or prednisolone are used but ACTH is preferable in a dosage of 80 units intravenously for 3 to 7 days followed by intramuscular injections over the next 2 to 3 weeks. Prednisolone is given orally in a dosage of 60 mg daily in divided doses for 3 to 7 days gradually tapering over next 2 to 3 weeks. Long-term steroid therapy is not advocated. These drugs act via mechanism other than immune response probably by reducing oedema and inflammation and thereby increasing the conduction of demyelinated nerve.

Immuno-suppressive agents such as azathioprine (immuran), cyclophosphamide may be tried to reduce the number of relapses.

Spasticity is best controlled by Baclofen in dosage of 30 to 100 mg per day. Baclofen is a gamma-aminobutyric acid compound and it has a few side-effects. Tremors are difficult to relieve, however trial of propranolol 40 to 320 day may be done. Occasionally tremor of the arm may well respond to contralateral cryothalamotomy.

For urinary problems, intermittent catheterisation is better than continuous in-dwelling of catheter. Women can be trained in self-catheterisation.

Any infection may cause deterioration, hence appropriate antibiotics should be used whenever indicated.

Physiotherapy must be done regularly and prevention of nutritional deficiency is essential.

Occupational therapy, counselling and judicious planning are essential for chronic and debilitated cases. Pregnancy is better avoided within two years of acute attack because of associated fatigue and weakness.

Glutenfree diet and sunflower-oil polyunsaturated fatty acids may be useful to prevent relapses.

## ACUTE DISSEMINATED ENCEPHALOMYELITIS

**Acute perivascular myelinoclasis**

### INTRODUCTION

Acute disseminated encephalomyelitis (ADE) is a rare neurological complication following vaccinations, e.g. smallpox or rabies vaccine or some viral infections such as chickenpox, measles, mumps, as well as non-specific respiratory infections. Incidence is about 1 in every 30,000 vaccinations. It affects either brain or spinal cord or both. Nerve roots are usually involved. There is an acute perivascular distribution.

### PATHOLOGY

Macroscopically there is congestion and oedema of the nervous system. Microscopically there is marked perivascular infiltration of lymphocytes and plasma cells. Zonal demyelination occurs in white matter especially around veins. Oligodendrocytes are either absent or pyknotic. Fat-laden macrophages are found around the demyelinated areas. Changes are found mostly in cerebral white matter, pons, middorsal, lumbar and sacral region.

It is due to hypersensitivity of the nervous system to viral multiplication with products of viral injury.

### CLINICAL FEATURES

Children and adolescents are more vulnerable. The onset is abrupt with headache, fever, delirium with frequent convulsion leading to stupor and even coma may occur.

There are signs of meningeal irritation, monoparesis or hemiparesis. When brain stem is involved, nystagmus, ocular palsies and pupillary changes may be found. Some cases may be present as spinal cord syndrome.

Cerebellar signs are often present. CSF is always abnormal in protein content (50-100 mg%) and lymphocyte count (10 to a few hundreds). The mortality may be around 20 per cent, whole 80% cases recover within a period of weeks or months.

### TREATMENT

ADE responds dramatically to high doses of glucocorticoids given for four to six weeks and carefuly nursing as well as supportive therapy.

## ACUTE NECTROTIZING HAEMORRHAGIC ENCEPHALOMYELITIS

Acute necrotising haemorrhagic encephalomyelitis (ANHE) is an acute fulminating disease of central nervous system occurring within a few days following an upper respiratory infection. Autopsy shows marked destruction, even liquefaction of white matter of one or both hemispheres. Areas of small haemorrhagic spots are found in the brain. Histological findings are identical with those of acute disseminated encephalomyelitis with perivascular foci of demyelination.

The clinical course resembles that of acute disseminated encephalomyelitis, rapidly deteriorating to fatality within two or three days. Neurological signs are frequently unilateral or bilateral CSF findings show polymorphonuclear pleocytosis up to 2000 cells and considerable increase in protein content. The exact aetiology is not yet established.

## NEUROMYELITIS OPTICA OR DEVIC'S DISEASE

To disease is characterized by massive demyelination of optic nerves and tracts of the spinal cord.

### Pathogenesis

The exact aetiology is not known. It usually follows an acute attack of transverse myelitis. Extensive loss of myelin sheath is observed in both optic nerves, chiasma and tracts of the spinal cord.

Mononuclear lymphocytic infiltrations are also observed both in demyelinating areas as well as throughout the spinal cord.

### Clinical features

The disease usually begins with febrile sore throat along with headache. Bilateral optic neuritis or a retrobulbar neuritis usually follows an attack of spinal lesion. Papilloedema and bilateral central scotoma are also present.

Paraplegia with retrobulbar neuritis may be presented with sensory impairment and sphincter disturbances. Quadriplegia may also occur. The optic nerve lesion may precede, follow or may simultaneously occur along with spinal lesion. There may be complete recovery in lucky few while relapse and remission may occur as in M.S.

This may be a variant of M.S. or a separate clinical syndrome cause of which is not known.

Management — symptomatic and supportive.

## DIFFUSE CEREBRAL SCLEROSIS OR SCHILDER'S DISEASE

### Encephalitis periaxialis diffuse

This is a progressive neurologic disorder characterized by progressive mental and visual deterioration. There are two forms of this disorder, associated with spastic paralysis, originally described by Schilder in 1912.

(1) Genetically determined and associated with adrenocortical atrophy.

(2) Sporadic massive, well-defined usually symmetrical demyelination in white matter of cerebral hemispheres, occurring without any obvious cause.

In Schilder's cases diffuse sclerosis, translucent, greyish gelatinous areas were observed in the posterior parts of both cerebral hemispheres, axons being spared.

### Clinical features

Healthy children may be the victims. Onset may be rapid or insidious. Headache, giddiness, intellectual impairment are the first symptoms. Fever is exceptional. It may be followed by epileptiform attacks, aphasia, weakness and incoordination of limbs. Visual disturbances are due to destruction of optic radiations. When one occipital lobe is involved, contralateral homonymous hemianopia is present. Nystagmus is common. In acute cases there is cerebral oedema raised intracranial pressure and papilloedema.

Progressive spastic weakness gradually develops. It may become fatal within 2 to 3 years with quadriplegic decerebrate rigidity and dementia.

**Treatment**

Treatment is unsatisfactory. ACTH and steroids are ineffective. Management is entirely supportive.

## DISORDER OF EXTRAPYRAMIDAL SYSTEM

*P.K. SETHI*

Disorder of extrapyramidal system manifests, as or by combination of abnormal involuntary movements (dyskinesias), and change in muscle tone disturbance in bodily posture. Functionally extrapyramidal system includes not only basal ganglion nuclei, but also related structures in the brain stem as well as extensive neural network of connections with other parts of nervous system. Caudate nucleus and putamen are collectively called striatum, which has to & fro extensive connection with pallidum. Thalamus is another important integrative station. These along with subthalamic nucleus, red nucleus and substantia nigra and its multifarious connection with brainstem constitute the system. Thus these nuclear masses along with their connections with each other and with certain parts of reticular system cerebellum and cerebrum make up an anatomic-physiologic unit that is called "as the extrapyramidal system".

What is the function of this system ? In lower animals it is highly developed and is not dominated by the cerebral cortex. In men, where cerebral cortex is highly developed, its role is presumed to be secondary to pyramidal system. According to one of the latest views this system cannot initiate movements but is capable of exerting, modulating and reinforcing influence on movements of cortical origin. Thus movements have their origin in cerebral cortex and are mediated through pyramidal tract but are modified/influenced appropriately reflexly through extrapyramidal system. Hence, it is best to view both the systems i.e. pyramidal and extrapyramidal acting in unison and balance. Disorder of extrapyramidal system may give rise to one or all of the followings :-

(i) Abnormal involuntary movements i.e. tremor, chorea, athetosis, dystonia, ballism.

(ii) Changes in muscle tone.

(iii) Disturbances in bodily posture.

In spite of several detailed clinical and experimental studies it is not always possible to associate a particular deficit or involuntary movements with specific anatomical site of lesion in basal ganglion. This is so as the basal ganglion, as stated above, has extensive connections and in the disease process lesions are seen in more than one place.

During the past decade, great strides have occurred in neuro-chemistry suggesting that the disease of this region should not be considered in terms of specific anatomic-physiologic disturbance of extrapyramidal system only but in terms of neurotransmitter balance imbalance. Basal ganglions are rich in neurotransmitter agents, notably acetyl choline (ACH), dopamine (DA) and gamma-aminobutyric acid (GABA). There is a complex system of enzymes and substrates available in these regions responsible for storage, release and degradation of these neurotransmitters. Neurophysiologically one may visualize that there is a balance between the inhibitory transmitter, e.g. DA and GABA on one side and the excitatory neurotransmitter, viz. ACH on the other side. When there is depletion of the former, i.e. dopamine deficiency resulting in relative cholinergic hyperactivity it may lead parkinsonism. On the other hand dopamine hyperactivity and/or chlolingeric hypoactivity results in hyper kinetic phenomenon as seen in Huntington's Chorea.

However, this is a relative simple explanation and many more questions remain to be answered. These hopefully will be answered as our knowledge about neurotransmitter increases.

## THE PARKINSONIAN SYNDROME (PARKINSONISM)

In 1817, James Parkinson first described the major manifestations of this syndrome. The clinical description as provided by him has not been excelled as yet. The disease is characterized by tremors, muscular rigidity and abnormality of postural reflexes. It is one of the most frequently encountered diseases of basal ganglion and prominent cause of disability. It may occur in isolation or with other neurological disabilities, hence it is best to regard it as a syndrome.

It can be classified as primary or secondary (symptomatic) where cause of parkinsonism is known. Primary parkinsonism or Paralysis Agitans is the one described by Parkinson and called as Parkinson's disease.

## PRIMARY PARKINSONISM or PARKINSON'S DISEASE

(Paralysis Agitans)

Most of the cases of Parkinsonism fall under this category. The disease frequently begins after the age of 50 years, although rarely juvenile parkinsonism is also known.

Exact aetiology of the disease is not known. Neuropathologically the most striking finding is loss of pigmented neurons in substantia nigra, locus ceruleus, and pigmented brain stem nuclei. Neurochemically there is deficiency of striatal dopamine, thus leading to imbalance between dopamine and cholinergic influences resulting in parkinsonism. But question which remains the unanswered is what leads to the loss of these pigmented neurons containing dopamine in this area.

The disease begins insidiously, the early symptoms may be difficult to perceive and may be overlooked as part of aging. Slight tremors or stiffness and slow gait may be easily ignored by the relatives or even by the patient himself. As the disease develops the major neurological findings are as follows :

(i) Paucity of facial expression

Emotional expressions are difficult to come by, with face becoming mask-like with infrequent blinking. There may be blepharospasm. The skin takes on oily quality.

(ii) Tremor

Tremors take several forms. "Pill rolling" tremor of thumb and finger is most common. Tremors are typically present at rest, but diminish or disappear on action. It differs from that of anxiety, thyrotoxicosis and due to intoxication by being slower, of greater amplitude and more rhythmic. The rhythmic beat coincides with alternating burst of activity in agonist and antagonist muscles in EMG. Arm, jaw, tongue, eyelids and foot may also be involved.

(iii) Rigidity

Muscular rigidity may slowly creep in. This is readily evident on passive movements of limbs when cogwheeling is noticed rather than smooth flowing easy motion.

(iv) Akinesia

Patient may have marked difficulty in initiation of movements, he may be very slow in voluntary movements with unexpected arrests. Originally it was thought that the rigidity interfers with facility of movement but now it is believed that it is akinesia which leads to poverty of movements. There may be absence of arm swing in walking, sudden turning or getting up from chair. Infrequency of swallowing and slowness of chewing may develop. As disorder of movement worsens, handwritting becomes small (micrography) and cramped. Walking becomes slow and shuffling, frequently individual losing his balance. Individual may have difficulty in initiating gait but once having started seems to be chasing his centre of gravity (festinating gait). The speech may become slow and monotonous.

(v) Postural abnormality

The attitude may be stooping with tendency to let his head fall forward. Later there may be deformities of trunk, hands and feet.

**Management**

Most patients will require life-long therapy. In addition to specific drug therapy, supportive therapy in form of encouragement and physical therapy to avoid deformities are to be emphasized.

**Drug therapy**

Drug therapy is based on consideration of the dopaminergic/cholinergic balance. The object is either is (1) to increase available dopamine or dopamine agonist at the cholinergic site in the neostriatum or (2) to reduce cholinergic activity with anticholinergic agents.

a. **Anticholinergics**

These are time honoured useful drugs either used alone or in conjuction with L-Dopa, with which they have synergistic effect. In a mild case, especially when the tremor is most prominent problem these alone suffice. Commonly used drugs are :

(i) Trihexyphenidyl Hcl (Pacitane, Artane) 2 mg tab

(ii) Procyclidine Hcl (Kemadrin) 2.5 mg, 5 mg tab

(iii) Benzotropine (Cogentin) 1 mg, 2 mg tab.

Treatment should be initiated with small doses such as Trihexylphenidyl, 2 mgm three times a day, and then gradually increased until further increases yield no additional benefit or gives side effect which are not acceptable. Commonly well-tolerated side-effects of anticholinergic drugs include dry mouth, blurred vision and dizziness. Other, often serious, side-effects are toxic psychosis, constipation, urinary retention and precipitation of glaucoma.

A number of other agents, with mild central anticholinergic properties have been found useful, e.g. diphenhydramine (Benadryl), orphenadrine (Dispal) etc. Benadryl in particular in divided dosages up to 50 mrm a day is useful as adjunct to L-Dopa.

b. **Levodopa**

Levodopa has been the greatest breakthrough in treatment of parkinsonism especially for akinesia. The initial oral dose is 500 mg/day in divided doses after food, increasing by increments of 250 mg/day every third day, until the maximum tolerated dose (usually in range 3 to 6 g. total/daily) is reached. If the dose is increased too rapidly nausea will be the limiting factor, it may be helped by cyclizine 50 mgm 30 minutes before food. Other adverse reactions include postural hypotension, psychiatric disturbance, rarely cardiac dysrhythmias. Long-term effects are still being evaluated. Sooner or later patient may develop dyskinesia : choreiform movements of hand and feet, grimacing and mouthing movement. These may respond to stoppage of drugs or decrease of dosages, thus calling for constant supervision. Another interesting phenomenon associated with long-term L-Dopa therapy is "on-off" phenomenon, where patient who was responding fairly well to therapy may not only stop responding but develop severe akinesia, hypotonia, and apprehension. This may last for a few hours to a few days. Period of drug holidays is recommended. Sadly L/Dopa therapy benefit may decline after about 2-3 years.

**Levodopa – DOPA – decarboxylase inhibitor combination.**

The concurrent use of a peripheral decarboxylase inhibitor, carbidopa, has allowed reduction of L-Dopa does so as to avoid peripheral side-effects. In combination one begins the use of L-Dopa 100 mgm together with carbidopa 10 mg (sinemet 100/10) three times a day.

c. **Amantadine hydrochloride** (symmetrel) 100 mgm daily, increasing to 100 mg twice a day has also been found helpful in the treatment of Parkinson's disease. The benefit is occasionally short-lived. Intermittent use has been advocated. The drug may act by increasing dopamine release at the synapse in the neostriatum.

d. **Other drugs**

Other new dopamine receptor agonists are currently under investigation. Bromocriptine (an ergot alkaloid) may help by reducing the need for high dose of L/dopa and has been found useful.

The antidepressants imipramine (Tofranil) and amitriptyline are minimal effective when used alone, but in combination with anticholinergic agents or levodopa they may be of great help in relieving the depressive symptoms which many patients may have.

## SECONDARY OR SYMPTOMATIC PARKINSONISM

Poisoning with carbon monoxide, manganese and other heavy metals, infectious process such as encephalitis, cerebral trauma and rarely brain tumour in region of basal ganglion may give rise to Parkinson-like symptoms. Diffuse cerebral arteriosclerosis may give neurological signs superficially resembling Parkinsonism called pseudoparkinsonism.

Drug induced Parkinsonism has assumed great importance in recent years. The use of neuroleptics as psychotherapeutic or antiemetic agents has resulted in a number of extrapyramidal syndrome. In some cases the symptoms may be dose related, in others there may be individual hypersensitivity. Abnormal movements involving face, tongue and head may predominate. Grimacing, mouthing movements, dystonia or akathisia (restless fidgety state) have to be recognised. The symptoms usually disappear within a few days of stopping of the drug but sometimes these may persist for a long time or may be permanent. Anticholinergic drugs such as trihexyphenidyl etc. help to control Parkinsonism. Recently it has been shown that the abnormal movements may be controlled by the administration of choline chloride.

### Essential Tremors (Familial Tremors)

Familial tremor is usually seen in one or both hands, it is increased by voluntary movement and there is family history of the condition. Usual age of onset is before age of 25 years. Tremor improves with alcohol intake. There is no associated rigidity with tremors as compared to Parkinson's disease. Some of these patients respond very well to $\beta$-blockers propranolol in dosage of 120 to 180 mgm a day in divided doses.

### Senile Tremors

Senile tremor usually appears first in the head and is often limited to it; when it spreads to limbs, it is increased by volitional movements. Rigidity is absent.

### Choreas

Chorea refers to brief, rapid, semipurposive, non-repetitive, explosive movements. They involve upper and lower limbs, face, trunk and head. They may occur so rapidly that the individual may appear in constant motion. They differ from tics in being unpatterned and non-reproducible. Exact anatomical site giving rise to chorea is controversial, however pathological lesions are commonly found in striatum. Choreiform movements may occur in number of disease entities. Two important conditions are :

## ACUTE CHOREA

(Sydenham's or infectious chorea, St vitus dance)

This disease in encountered primarily during childhood between ages of 5 and 25 years. Females manifest these symptoms at least twice as often as males. Acute chorea may occur in association with a variety of conditions viz. encephalitis/encephalopathies, occurring with exanthema, with pertussis and diphtheria, vascular disease, tumours and degenerative processes of the basal ganglion. However, commonest association is with rheumatic fever. Other manifestations of rheumatic fever, i.e. carditis. arthritis or valvular disease may precede, coincide or follow acute chorea. The movements may occur at rest, get accentuated by movements and disappear in sleep. Facial grimacing, difficulty in speech, chewing and swallowing may be present.

Acute chorea is self-limited disease. Recovery occurring in two to six months. Bed rest and sedatives are of help. As there is high incidence of rheumatic valvular heart disease complicating acute chorea, prophylaxis as for rheumatic fever is recommended.

## HUNTINGTON'S DISEASE – HEREDITARY CHOREA

This is a good example of human disease inherited as Mendelian dominant of autosomal type with full penetrance. Hence 50 per cent of children of epileptics will invariably be affected the disease is relatively rare. Sporadic cases may occur.

Pathologically, widespread degenerative changes with cell loss and reactive gliosis are found, primarily in the cerebral cortex and caudate nucleus. Recently it has been found that glutamic acid, decarboxylase and choline acetylase activity are reduced in the basal ganglion.

The first signs usually appear between the ages of 30 and 45. These are usually choreiform movements which are faster, more jerky and bizarre than Sydenham's chorea. Subsequently dementia slowly develops, which progressively increases requiring admission to a mental hospital in 10 to 15 years. Occasionally dementia may precede involuntary movements. The EEG shows a low voltage, featureless record. Computerized axial tomography or pneumoencephalography demonstrates selective atrophy of caudate nucleus.

There is no specific treatment which alters the course of underlying disease or fatal outcome. Symptomatic control of choreiform movements may be accomplished by the use of neuroleptic agents such as haloperidol, chlorpromazine to tetrabenazine or recently by choline chloride.

## ATHETOSIS

Athetosis is characterised by slow, sinuous writhing movements (mobile spasm). These occur when pathological conditions involve the basal ganglion, particularily putamen, in addition to corticospinal tract. Most cases are congenital, being due to a primary disorder of myelination of striatal neurons, with glial formation, developing in intrauterine life. Other cases are due to cerebral anoxia at birth, by Kernicterus, Wilson's disease, damage to basal ganglion during the exanthematous disease or in the elderly from cerebrovascular disease.

The movements may affect distal part of the limbs as well as proximal. Facial grimacing may be present. Movements are more slow than chorea, but occasional gestures of both conditions are to be observed, hence the term choreo-athetosis. Similar but slower movements of the proximal parts of the limbs and of the trunk are termed as torsion dystonia.

There is no specific treatment but pallidotomy and thalamotomy may be of value, particularly for dystonia. Physiotherapy may help in promoting muscular relaxation.

## HEMIBALLISM

Hemiballism is characterised by violent, flinging movements. The lesion is invariably in contralateral subthalamic nucleus, the Corpus Luysii. A variety of pathological processes, viz. tumour or infectious diseases involving this area may give rise to hemiballism, but most cases are as a result of cerebrovascular accident either haemorrhagic or occlusive. Initially the movements may be so violent that they may exhaust the individual. However, in most instances, the initial intensity decreases gradually and in six to eight weeks the movements may stop spontaneously.

## TIC (HABIT SPASM)

A tic is a sudden, abrupt, rapid, purposeless, involuntary contraction of a muscle or a group of functionally related muscles occurring at irregular intervals. This may be eye blinking, shrugging of the shoulder, head shaking, gesture of the limbs or face, etc. A tic often develops as a neurotic manifestation.

No effective treatment is available.

An unusual form of generalised tic (Gilles de la Tourette's disease) encountered in childhood, has facial twitching, continuous gestures associated with echolalia, foul language or obsessional ideas. The disease is progressive unlike simple tics.

Haloperidol in divided dosage of 6 to 20 mgm may be effective in controlling the movements and verbal outbursts.

## SPASMODIC TORTICOLLIS

This condition is characterised by involuntary movements affecting many cervical muscles on both sides of the neck. It may occur as a sole manifestation of extrapyramidal disease or may be associated with other neurological signs. It may also be manifestation of hysteria. The movements consist of spasmodic rotation, flexion and extension of the cervical spine in the anterio-posterior and lateral planes.

It has to be differentiated from congenital torticollis due to fibrosis following haematoma of sternomastoid muscle which is present from birth. Local disease of the cervical spine, muscle or lymph node may also cause torticollis.

It is an intractable disease. Sedation and physiotherapy are employed with varying results. Surgical division of the spinal accessory nerves or of the cervical nerves should be tried only if the disability is intolerable.

## DISEASES OF THE PERIPHERAL NERVES

*P.K. SETHI*

Although structure and function of the peripheral nervous system (PNS) are relatively simple, the disease affecting this system stands out as a difficult subject in neurology. Faced with the problems affecting the PNS, the physician has to ascertain two things. First, that the peripheral nerves are being affected and, secondly, to find out the exact aetiology. It is the latter one which is not always easy to establish. In recent years, with the advent of electrophysiological studies in human beings (nerve conduction velocities and electromyographic studies) and better histo-pathological studies of nerve and muscles, more insight has been gained into this aspect.

A rational approach to the disease/disorder of the peripheral nerves should be based on their fundamental structures. The cells of the origin lie in the motorneurons of the spinal cord. The motor roots are composed of the emerging axons of the anterior and lateral horn cells; they terminate on muscle fibres, or sympathetic or parasympathetic ganglion. The peripheral axons of the dosal root ganglion cells constitute the sensory nerve fibres.

The axons thus formed are enveloped by a series of Schwann cells forming the fatty myelin sheath. There is intimate symbiotic relation between the axon and its myelin, although morphologically they are independent. Thus a disease process may involve one without much involving the other.

The motor and sensory fibres are large protoplasmic extension of their respective parent cells in the spinal cord. The long axon depends upon the intact healthy metabolism of the parent cell for its nutrition. A disorder of function of nerves thus may occur if some insult occurs at the level of parent cell, or dysfunction in metabolism of ensheathing myelin nor if something goes wrong with rich vascular supply by the nutrient arteries to nerve or combination of these factors. Further these nerves pass through narrow foramens (intervertebral and cranial) and some of these may pass through tight compartments peripherally (e.g. median nerve between carpal ligaments). This explains the susceptibility of some nerves to compression and entrapment.

### General Clinical Features

There are certain general clinical features which may characterize the disease of peripheral nerves. These may be motor, sensory, trophic or autonomic dysfunction.

Motor weakness may be prominent symptom. In generalised polyneuropathies muscles of lower limbs are affected first and more severely than those of hand or forearm. The trunk and respiratory muscle may also get affected. In mononeuropathy corresponding muscles supplied by the nerve affected show weakness. Weakness of muscle may be slowly followed by atrophy. The rule is that tendon reflexes are markedly diminished or completely lost.

Sensory loss occurs when sensory fibres are involved like motor function, sensation tends to be more affected in the distal segments of the limbs. As the disease worsens, the sensory loss may spread to more proximal part and may involve ,all the modalities of sensation. Vibration sense is more often affected than the touch and position sense. The paraesthesia like numbness and tingling sensation may dominate in symptomatology.

**Autonomic Dysfunction**

In diabetes and certain other polyneuropathies, when autonomic nervous system is involved there may be symptom/signs of autonomic dysfunction. This may be in the form of diarrhoea, weak bladder and bowel sphincters and overflow incontinence, sexual impotence, small or medium size unreactive pupils and anhydrosis, etc. In long-standing slowly progressive polyneuropathies, the feet, hands and spine may become deformed.

**Work-up of a case of polyneuropathy**

Once the diagnosis of peripheral neuropathy has been thought of on above referred clinical features, attempt has to be made for establishing the possible aetiology. A detailed history of onset, whether acute, subacute or chronic, any preceding history of fever, infectious conjunctivitis, innoculations, vaccinations, any history of antecedental trauma; history suggestive of metabolic disorder, viz. diabetes or porphyria, history of chronic alcoholism or possible toxin or drugs, signs suggestive of malnutrition may help to suggest the diagnosis in a particular case. Time spent on such a pursuit may be richly awarded. In laboratory work-up appropriate biochemical tests may be done to rule in or out a particular entity suspected. Measurement of nerve conduction velocities and electromyographic studies may shed further light. CSF studies may help and nerve biopsy may further confirm diagnosis in certain setting.

**Classification**

Several ways of classification are possible.

* Depending upon course of illness
  acute, subacute, chronic.
* Depending upon anatomical distribution
  Mononeuropathy, mononeuritis multiplex, localized radiculopathy, generalised polyneuropathy.
* Depending upon type of function affected
  sensory, motor, mixed.
* Depending upon pathology
  axonopathy (Predominant axon involvement), Schawanopathy (Predominant myelin involvement)
* Depending upon aetiology

**Generalised Polyneuropathies**

In this group, there is a generalised affliction of all nerves. The most common clinical picture is symmetrical involvement of motor and sensory nerves, first manifest at the distal part of limbs as already described. The course of the disease may be acute, subacute or chronic.

Aetiology : List of causes is really a long one.

Some of the important ones are as follows :

Heredo-familial diseases : -- Peroneal-muscular atrophy, Charcot-Marie-Tooth type of neuropathy, hypertrophic interstitial neuropathy (Dejerine-sottas disease), hereditary sensory radiculoneuropathy, Refsum's disease.

Infections : Leprosy, herpes zoster, brucellosis, infectious - hepatitis, infectious mononucleosis, typhoid fever, mumps, diphtheria.

Allergic neuropathies : Guillian-Barre's syndrome (Acute infective Polyneuritis), neuralgic amyotrophy, serum neuropathy.

Metabolic : Diabetes mellitus, uraemia, porphyria, amyloidosis.

Nutritional deficiency : Vitamin $B_{12}$ deficiency, neuropathy alcoholism, beriberi, pellagra, pyridoxin deficiency and malabsorption syndrome.

Toxic : Lead, arsenic, mercury, gold triorthocresylphosphate, carbon disulphide, benzene derivatives.

Several drugs : Dilantin, furadantin, isoniazide, metronidazole, clinoquinol, sulphonamides, stilbamidine, perhexiline, vincristine, Doriden etc.

Collagen disease & Vascular disorder : Polyarteritis nodosa and other vasculitis may cause mononeuritis multiplex.

Neoplasm : Carcinoma of the bronchus and other neoplastic tumours.

*Note* : Polyneuropathy may be the first manifestation of malignancy. There are many other rare causes for which larger neurological texts should be referred to.

**Pathology**

The polyneuropathies show segmental demyelination and axonal degeneration in various combinations. The former, a patchy affair involving the myelin appears as primary event in diabetes, diphtheria, Guillian-Barre's syndrome, carcinomatous neuropathy and lead neuropathy, whereas in neuropathy due to alcohol, porphyria and isoniazide axonal degeneration seems to be primary. This distinction has practical importance as the motor conduction velocities are far more depressed in former where myelin is involved.

Certain features peculiar to common forms of polyneuropathy are discussed below.

**Acute 'Infective Polyneuritis' (Guillian-Barre's Syndrome)**

This disease is characterized by the acute and usually febrile onset of rapidly spreading polyneuritis, with or without implication of cranial nerves, there is usually a considerable increase in the protein content of the cerebrospinal fluid without much of pleocytosis.

The disease is encountered in all parts of the world and in all seasons. A mild respiratory or gastrointestinal infection may precede the neuritic symptoms by 1 to 3 weeks. Other preceding events may include viral exanthema and fevers, vaccinations or surgical procedure. The exact cause is not known but allergic pathology is suspected.

After the above antecedent event, weakness occurs, progressing to paralysis, starting in the periphery and sweeping rapidly up to the legs, arms and trunk. Paraesthesias in the form numbness and tingling is quite common, although there may not be an actual sensory loss.

Bilateral facial weakness is quite common, other cranial nerves may also get involved. The paralysis is flaccid, deep tendon reflexes are lost and the plantar responses are usually flexor. Death may occur because of respiratory or bulbar paralysis, unless prompt action is taken for respiratory support. There may be accompanying changes in autonomic parameters.

**Diagnosis :** The protein content of the spinal fluid is often normal for the first few days, then starts rising (100 - 1000 mg per 100 ml), cell count may be normal or slightly raised (albumino-cytological dissociation).

The presence of paraesthesias and sensory changes helps to exclude poliomyelitis. The neuritis of acute porphyria is distinguished by abdominal pain, a rise of blood pressure, mental symptoms, convulsions, and the presence of porphyrinuria. Diphtheritic polyneuritis is usually preceded by evidence of the local lesions in the nose, throat or skin and before the onset of polyneuropathy there is usually blurring of vision due to weakness of accommodation. Other causes of rapidly ascending paralysis are rabies, antirabies-inoculation reaction and potassium intoxication.

**Treatment :**

The key to therapy is respiratory assistance at the earliest sign of respiratory embarrassment and careful nursing. The disease may remit naturally in the majority of cases. The possibility of an autoimmune mechanism provides a rationale for use of corticosteroids. However, there is no convincing evidence about its beneficial effect. According to some, it may retard recovery (Oxford Text Book of Medicine, 1985 ELBS 21.41). Physiotherapy and proper positioning of limbs should begin once the condition of the patient is stabilized.

**Polyneuritis due to leprosy**

This is probably the most common disease of peripheral nerves in the world today. Disease is particularly frequent in India and Central Africa.

It is an infectious neuritis, being due to direct invasion of nerves by acid-fast myobacterium leprae. Details of the disease have been discussed under the chapter on leprosy. It is to be emphasized that the nerves are thickened and in distinction to other polyneuropathies tendon reflexes are usually preserved in leprosy, despite widespread sensory loss. High index of suspicion is required and disease should not be missed, as it is a treatable condition.

## NEURALGIC AMYOTROPHY

*(Paralytic Brachial Neuritis)*

Neuralgic amyotrophy is characterized by pain in the region of one or both shoulders, lower motor neuron paralysis of some of shoulder girdle muscles and minimal sensory loss. Disease affects young adults. There may be antecedental history of upper respiratory infection, or vaccination/innoculation. As the paralysis sets in, there is marked restriction in the movement of shoulder girdle muscles especially abduction. Gradually wasting sets in. With physiotherapy, analgesics and supportive care recovery occurs gradually with return of good motor power, although wasting of muscles may persist.

**Alcoholic Polyneuropathy**

Pain is usually severe. Other evidence of alcoholism such as tremors, hepatopathy or cardiomyopathy may be present.

**Lead Neuropathy**

Lead poisoning causes pure motor neuropathy, usually within distribution of the radial or lateral popliteal nerves. Wrist drop may be common presentation. Other clinical features of chronic lead poisoning are anaemia with punctate basophilia of red cells, blue line on gums. There may be colicky pain in abdomen, and in children there may be mental changes and seizures due to lead encephalopathy.

**Diabetic Polyneuropathy :** This is discussed under diabetes.

**Mononeuritis multiplex :** This is a condition in which several nerves are involved concurrently or serially. Clinical signs are limited to discrete neural territories. Examples are leprosy, polyarteritis, vasculitis, diabetes and sarcoidosis.

**Mononeuropathy :** This term denotes affection of single nerve. Trauma, sustained pressure and entrapment are the common causes. Ulnar nerve at the elbow, radial nerve in middle of upper arm, and common peroneal nerve at the head of fibula are frequently involved. The signs are those of lower motor neuron paresis and sensory loss in the distribution of respective nerves. Generally complete recovery occurs in four to six weeks.

As emphasized in the beginning nerves may get compressed whenever they pass through rigid anatomical structures giving rise to entrapment neuropathy. Compression of the median nerve in carpal tunnel is the commonest entrapment syndrome. It occurs most frequently in middle age. It may be seen in myxoedema, pregnancy, rheumatoid arthritis. The patient complains of pain, tingling or electric-shock-like sensation in thumb and index finger supplied by affected median nerve. Pain may be severe at night. The condition may be disabling. The pain can be reproduced by light percussion of affected median nerve near wrist — 'Tineal sign'. Management consists of treatment of cause, local hydrocortisone injection or surgical decompression.

The lateral cutaneous nerve of thigh may be frequently entrapped at the inguinal ligament giving rise to paraesthesia and pain over the anterolateral aspect of thigh referred to as meralgia paraesthetica.

**Nutritional neuropathy**

Deficiences due to members of the B-complex group may cause neurological disturbances as follows :

(1) Aneurine or thiamine (vitamin $B_1$) deficiency causes beriberi neuropathy. Wernicke's encephalopathy is a special syndrome which may occur due to $B_1$ deficiency especially among alcoholics.

(2) Pyridoxine vitamin ($B_6$) may cause infantile convulsions as well as polyneuropathy. The latter may especially occur during prolonged I.N.H. therapy.

(3) Nicotinic acid or niacin (vitamin $B_7$) deficiency may cause dementia, dermatitis (pellegra), ataxia and polyneuropathy.

(4) Pentothenic acid deficiency as typically causes burning feet syndrome, described by Gopalan.

(5) Cyanocobalamin or vitamin $B_{12}$ deficiency may cause subacute degeneration of spinal cord with achylia gastrica. Many of these deficiencies occur in combination in famine-stricken areas or among prisoners of war (captivity cord syndrome). Details of various vitamin disorders are discussed in a separate chapter.

**Polyneuritis of unknown cause**

In spite of extensive investigation, in a large number of cases of polyneuritis the exact cause may not be found out, sometimes even at autopsy. If the disease is relapsing and remitting, hypertrophy of nerve may be present. Some of these patients may respond to steroid, usually given in desperation while others may not respond to steroid or relapse when steroid is stopped.

## RADIAL NERVE PALSY

**Causes**

Prolonged external pressure on the radial nerve, e.g. use of crutch, pressure on inside the upper arm due to alcoholic slumber with arm hanging down the edge of the bed or chair (Drunkard's or Saturday night palsy). It can also be due to trauma or fracture of the upper end of humerus.

When the lesion is high up in the axilla all the muscles supplied by $C_{3-8}$ are affected leading to paresis or paralysis of all the muscles supplied by it. Extension at elbow is not possible due to paralysis of triceps and extension of wrist and fingers is also not possible resulting in wrist drop. Sensory loss is usually not much evident or variable.

If the injury is in the lower part of humerus, triceps, bracho-radialis and extensor carpi radialis longus escape paralysis.

**Treatment**

If there is no lack of continuity of the nerve i.e. when it is due to pressure effect, recovery occurs in due course. Splinting is necessary and orthopaedic supervision is recommended.

## MEDIAN NERVE PALSY

**Causes** — Trauma, injury to shoulder or shoulder dislocation and carpal tunnel syndrome.

There is inability to pronate the forearm. Flexion of terminal phalanges and abduction of thumb at right angle to the palm is not possible. Ulnar deviation at the wrist is noted. Wasting of thenar muscles will occur in due course. Sensory loss may be noted in the terminal phalanges of index and middle fingers.

**Treatment**

Splinting is necessary with orthopaedic supervision. Rarely surgical suturing may be necessary if nerves are divided due to trauma.

## ULNAR NERVE PALSY

**Cause** — Local trauma at the elbow joint or pressure while sleeping or during anaesthesia.

Leprosy is an important cause.

There will be numbness of the little finger and hypothenar area of the palm. Clawhand will result. Sensory loss is limited to little finger and inner half of the ring finger. Wasting of hypothenar and interosseous muscles will occur. Ulnar side of forearm also will show muscular wasting.

**Treatment**

Leprosy — Treatment required with appropriate drugs discussed elsewhere in this book.

Traumatic causes require surgical care.

## POLIOMYELITIS

(Infantile paralysis, Heine medin disease)

*G.C. MOOKERJEE*
*K.A.KABIR*

**Introduction**

Poliomyelitis is an infectious diseases caused by coxsackie-like viruses which have predilection for anterior horn cells and brain stem motor nuclei causing lower motor neuron type of paralysis of the affected muscles.

There are three distinct immunologically different types of polioviruses e.g. Type 1 (Brunhilde), Type 2 (Lansing) and Type 3 (Leon). These is no cross-immunity between them. Polioviruses are spherical particles measuring 30$\mu$ diameter and can be found in throat, respiratory passage or faeces of the patients. It can also be isolated from C.S.F. in acute stage. Usual route of infection is through ingestion from alimentary tract. Respiratory tract may also be an alternate route. Viruses travel via autonomic nerves to the spinal cord. Haematogenous and lymphatic spread is also possible. Raw tonsillar bed after tonsillectomy and even injection sites are common route of entry of polioviruses and that is why prophylactic inoculation and tonsillectomy should be abandoned during epidemic.

Incubation period is 7-14 days but may vary from 3 to 35 days. Macroscopically the spinal cord is congested, oedematous soft and minute haemorrhagic spots are detected. Histologically, grey matter of spinal cord and brainstem are also affected. Signs of degeneration are found in anterior horn cells. There is perivascular cuffing mainly with lymphocytes. After acute stage there is regeneration of nerve cells which have not been severely damaged.

Nerve cells which are severely damaged completely disappear and the corresponding anterior roots and peripheral nerves show degeneration. The affected muscles are atrophied with a relative increase of fat and connective tissue.

## CLINICAL FEATURES :

In the developing countries children in the age group of two and five years are the common victims. The disease is rare below one year and above 25 years. The incidence of poliomyelitis is going down with the increasing use of poliovaccine. Clinical features :

(1) Subclinical type : In this type there are no clinical signs and symptoms but there is development of immunity.

(2) Abortive type : Exposure to virus leads to general constitutional symptoms such as fever, headache, malaria, facial congestion, diarrhoea or vomiting without any involvement of nervous system.

(3) Pre-paralytic stage : Along with the constitutional symptoms there are signs of meningism without any paralysis. Marked pleocytosis is present in the C.S.F.

(4) Paralytic : In very small number of cases typical paralysis supervenes commonly involving lower limbs with or without cranial nerve involvement.

The paralytic stage representts two forms :

(1) Spinal form and (2) Brain stem form.

### Spinal Form :

The paralysis is preceeded by fasciculation, pain in the muscles and tenderness. The paralysis may be localised or widespread. Usually distal muscles below knee are affected but thigh muscles may also be involved. In severe cases trunk muscles as well as all four limbs and neck muscles may be involved. Patient may not be able to lift his head from bed due to neck muscle paralysis. When it is less extensive the paralysis is asymmetrical and patchy involving lower limbs only. Usually the process of paralysis occur overnight and within 24 hours.

Paralysis leads to wasting of muscles. Depending on the extent of muscles affected there may be sublaxation of joints or contracture of muscles.

### BRAIN-STEM FORM

(Polioencephalitis)

In this type motor nuclei of the brainstem are affected leading to paralysis of facial, pharyngeal, lingual and rarely ocular paralysis. Cardiac and respiratory centres may also be affected rarely.

## DIAGNOSIS :

In the pre-paralytic stage the disease is differentiated from other causes of meningism. In poliomyelitis, CSF shows pleocytosis, with predominant lymphocytes high protein content with normal sugar level. Cell count is usually within 500 per UL.

In adult poliomyelitis it should be distinguished from acute transverse myelitis and Guillain-Barre syndrome. In acute transverse myelitis, there is flaccid paralysis with extensor plantar response, loss of sphincter control and sensory loss. In Guillain-Barre syndrome, paralysis is proximal and CSF does not show pleocytosis.

When the patient is seen after many years of acute attack, it should be distinguished from motor neuron disease and syringomyelia. In the former, fasciculation is present while dissociated sensory loss is present in the later.

## TREATMENT :

Chiefly the treatment is supportive. The important points are :

(1) Maintain airway where there is respiratory complication and watch should be carefully made for cranial nerve and respiratory muscle involvement.

(2) Polio-bed, if available, is very useful, otherwise maintain comfortable position in firm mattress, with sponge pads, sand-bags and footboard etc. for optimum limb position.

(3) Change of position and give warm compress by wet packs in the initial stages.

(4) **Judicious use of analgesic and antispastic drugs are useful. Aspirin, propoxyphene and** diazepam the chief drugs to be used.

(5) Maintain nutrition by proper feeding specially if chewing is difficult and where swallowing is a problem. Tubal feeding may be necessary.

(6) Retention of urine and faecal impaction may become problems and require special nursing care.

(7) Hypertension, hypotension or tachyarrhythmia should be watched and treated accordingly.

(8) When there is respiratory paralysis, intubation and ventilatory support is necessary.

(9) When acute stage subsides i.e. temperature becomes normal and limbs are not tender and painful, careful physiotherapy should be started. Overzealous physiotherapy may end in more deformities.

(10) Properly fitting braces and splints may be necessary in many cases.

## COMPRESSION OF THE SPINAL CORD

*G.C. MOOKERJEE*

### INTRODUCTION

Compression of the spinal cord may be due to causes in vertebral column, meninges and in the spinal cord itself.

Important causes of compression of the spinal cord are —

(1) **In the vertebral column :**

(a) Trauma causing vertebral fracture, vascular damage or whiplash injury due to acute stretch-damage of the spinal cord.

(b) Protruded I.V. disc.

(c) Metastatic new growth— commonly prostatic, bronchus and breast carcinomas.

(2) **In the meninges :**

Meningioma, neuro-fibroma, lymphomas, leukaemias,epidural abscess, tuberculosis or syphilitic meningitis.

(3) **In the spinal cord :**

Gliomas, ependymoma or malignant metastasis.

The effects on the spinal cord (Fig.12.12) may be due to direct pressure effect or by causing local oedema due to venous obstruction. Ischaemia may occur due to occluded blood supply.

If the compression is relieved early, recovery is possible, but if the nerves or nerve-cells are damaged due to prolonged pressure or ischaemic changes chance of recovery is remote.

### CLINICAL FEATURES

In acute traumatic injury paralysis occurs rapidly, otherwise in most cases cord compression produces gradual and progressive appearance of signs and symptoms.

In cases of injury or metastasis the onset is acute, especially if the blood supply is occluded. Local new growths are usually slow growing. These may be extramedullary (i.e. growing from structures outside spinal cord) or *intramedullary* (i.e. growing from structures within the spinal cord). Disc protrusion is a common cause of cord compression. New growths or disc prolapse may either cause pressure on nerve roots or on the spinal cord directly or may cause occlusion of arterial blood supply, resulting in loss of function of structures involved. If the cause can be removed before permanent neuronal damage has occurred, considerable functional recovery may be possible. *Hence early diagnosis is most important.*

Suspicious symptoms are local pain, aggravated by coughing, sneezing or movement of the spine.

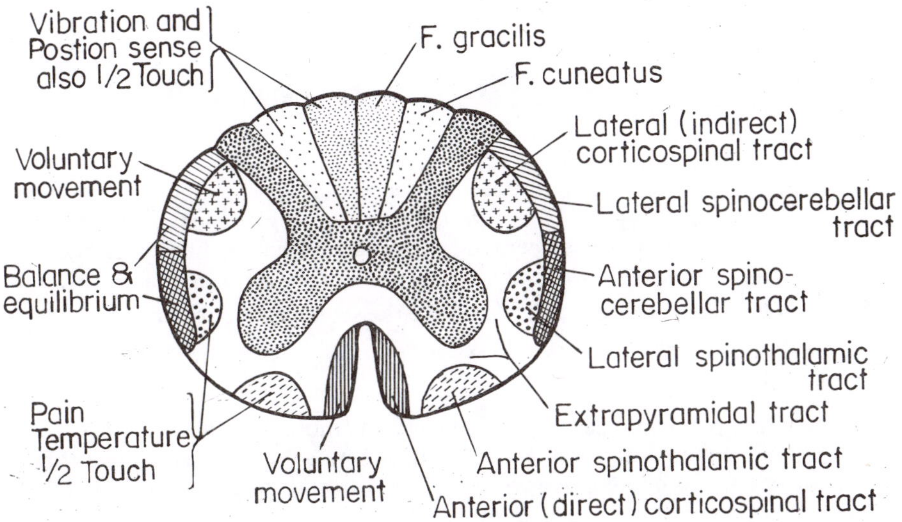


Fig.12.12 : Cross section of a normal spinal cord.

There may be root pains and local discomfort over the spine. The clinical features will depend on the level of lesion. Numbness, paraesthesia, cold or hot sensations may be felt. Motor paralysis may gradually be noticed. Segmental localisation is most important to find out the level of lesion.

Involvement of posterior root gives sensory deficits in the particular segment. If motor root is involved, LMN lesion of the same segmental distribution will occur. Affection of one half of the spinal cord will result in Brown-Sequard syndrome. If descending motor fibres are affected, there is UMN paralysis below the segment of the lesion. Bladder and bowel control may be affected.

Therefore, segmental landmarks should be carefully learnt and remembered. *Quadriparesis or quadriplegia* may occur when the lesion is above fifth cervical segment. Lesion at this level causes UMN type of paresis of all four limbs.

If the lesion is situated between fifth cervical and first thoracic segment of the spinal cord, there will be segmental sensory deficit of upper limb with LMN type of lesion, while the lower limb will have spasticity due to UMN lesion.

If the lesion is situated above twelve thoracic segment, there will be spastic paraplegia associated with sensory level in appropriate level. However, it should be remembered that a tumour or haematoma in the region of falx cerebri (e.g. meningioma) may also cause spastic paraplegia.

As the spinal cord ends at the level of first lumbar vertebra, lesions below this level cannot compress the cord but may only affect the spinal roots resulting in root lesion. If the tumour is large enough, it may damage the cauda equina as a whole resulting in so-called "cauda equina" syndrome.

Hence it can be seen that anatomical relations of the spinal segments and vertebral column is important (Table 12.1).

Table : 12.1 — Anatomical relations of cord segments

| Spinal cord segment | Vertebral body |
|---|---|
| $C_8$ | Lower $C_6$ and upper $C_7$ |
| $T_6$ | Lower $T_3$ and upper $T_3$ |
| $T_{12}$ | $T_9$ |
| $L_5$ | $T_{11}$ |
| Sacral | $T_{12}$ and $L_1$ |

From Table 12.1, it is possible to correlate the segmental levels of cord, roots and vertebra. Seventh cervical spine is also a good landmark as from this level spines of each vertebra can be located. It is also to be noted that seven cervical vertebrae contain eight segments and eight pairs of cervical roots emerge almost horizontally. $C_1$ has no sensory root. In infancy, lower tip of cord ends at the level of $L_4$, while in adults it is $L_1$. Lower the segment of cord, longer the root and exit is also obliquely and downwardly oriented.

**Sensory localisation**

Each segment of the spinal cord has a pair of sensory and motor-root which joins on either side to form the nerves which emerge out of intervertebral foramina on either side of vertebral column. Each nerve root has a cutaneous territory of supply through posterior root which is called a *"dermatome"*. Thirty-one pairs of spinal nerves have overlapping areas of sensory supply. Section of one particular sensory root does not produce much recognisable sensory impairment. However, pressure on a particular sensory root causes typical pain sensation i.e. "root pain". When two or three segments of cord are affected, definite bands or areas of sensory impairment will be manifested. Localisation of sensory disturbances of any segment can be diagnosed at which the highest level of sensation is impaired if there is a band of hypo- or hyper-aesthesia. This can be learnt from sensory localisation charts (Table 12.2).

If two sides are not equally involved loss of sensory level is asymmetrical. When spinothalamic tract is affected, loss of pain and temperature sensation occurs at specific level. As pain fibres cross at a lower level than heat and touch fibres, the loss of these modalities will vary with same lesion. The "pointer sensory" levels are to be noted for rapid bed-side diagnosis.

Sacral neoplasms may be difficult to detect. There is no root pain but vague sacral discomfort may be present. Coxalgia is often a pointer. These patients come late to the neurologist and too late to the neurosurgeon.

Table : 12.2 — Important segmental sensory areas

| | | |
|---|---|---|
| $C_3$ | — | Sides of the neck,<br>Posterior part of mandible and ear. |
| $C_6$ | — | Outer areas of arm, forearm, areas of hand including thumb, index finger and thenar part of palm. |
| $C_8$ | — | Inner part of forearm and hand, including 3rd to 5th digit. |
| $T_1$ | — | Area covering ulnar border of forearm up to wrist. |
| $T_3$ | — | Area covering upper precordium and axilla |
| $T_5$ | — | Band encircling the trunk at nipple level |
| $T_8$ | — | Band-like area encircling lower costal margin |

*Table Contd.....*

*Table contd.....*

| | | |
|---|---|---|
| $T_{10}$ | — | Mid-abdomen at the umbilical level |
| $L_1$ | — | Inguinal region and lower abdomen |
| $L_2$ | — | Lower lumbar area and front of the thigh. |
| $L_4$ | — | Antero-medial aspects of the leg to medial aspect of dorsum of the foot up to hallux. |
| $L_5$ | — | Outer area of the leg and dorsum of the foot including 1st to 3rd toes. |
| $S_1$ | | Sole of feet except great toe and lower half of posterior surface of leg. |
| $S_2$ | — | Posterior aspect of the thigh, leg, sole and plantar aspect of toes. |
| $S_4$ and $S_5$ | — | External genitalia including perineum. |

The crux of the diagnosis lies in the fact that lesion of plexus or peripheral nerve causes different kinds of sensory impairment than produced by lesions of the segments or roots.

## MOTOR LOCALISATION

The skeletal-muscles are also supplied in segmental fashion through motor roots and each segmental unit is called a "myotome".

Similar to *myotomes* and *dermatomes;* segmental supply of all internal organs are also supplied by the spinal segments. These are called *"enterotomes"* but this is not clinically so easy to localise.

## MOTOR SEGMENTAL DIAGNOSIS

Each segment of the cord has lower motor neuron cells clustered in the anterior horns. Skeletal muscles receive their nerve supply from anterior-horn cells on segmental basis while most skeletal muscles receive their supply through two or three motor roots, depending on the size of the muscles. Segmental supply of motor nerves shown in Table 12.3 : ...

Table : 12.3 — Segmental motor supply to skeletal muscles

| | | |
|---|---|---|
| $C_4$ | — | Supraspinatus and infraspinatus |
| $C_5$ | — | Biceps, deltoid, brachialis,<br>Supinator longus |
| $C_6$ | — | Pronators of forearm |
| $C_7$ | — | Triceps, extensors of wrist and fingers |
| $C_8$ | — | Flexors of wrist and fingers |
| $D_1$ | — | Small muscles of the hand |
| $D_2$ to $D_{10}$ | — | Intercostal muscles |
| $D_7$ to $D_{12}$ | — | Muscles of the abdominal wall |
| $L_2$ to $L_3$ | — | Abductors of thigh |
| $L_2$ to $L_4$ | — | Extensors of knee |
| $L_4$ to $S_1$ | — | Abductors of thigh |
| $L_4$ to $L_5$ | — | Anterior tibial muscles |
| $L_5$ to $S_1$ | — | Peroneal group of muscles<br>Small muscles of foot and calf-muscles |
| $L_5$ to $S_2$ | — | Hamstrings |
| $L_4$ to $S_2$ | — | Gluteal muscles. |

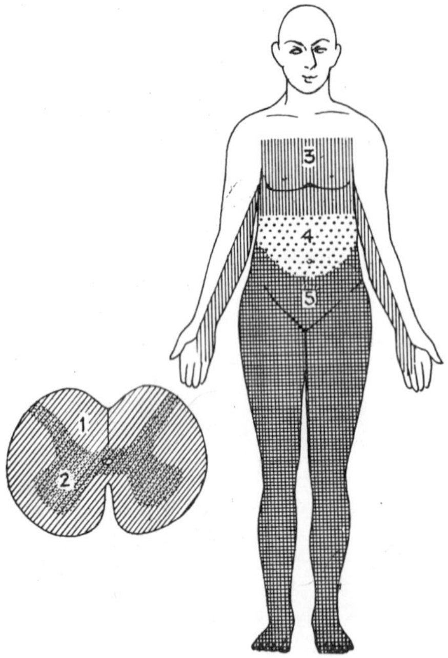


Fig.12.13(a) : Complete transection of the cord.

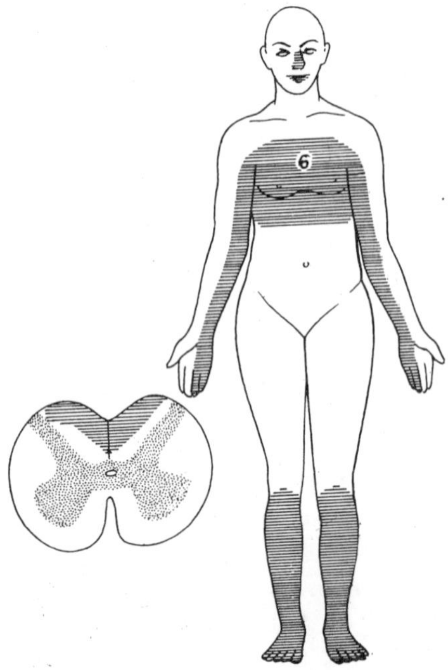


Fig.12.13(b) : Posterior Column lesion in tabes dorsalis showing areas of cutaneous analgesia. Lesion in the lower cervical and upper thoracic

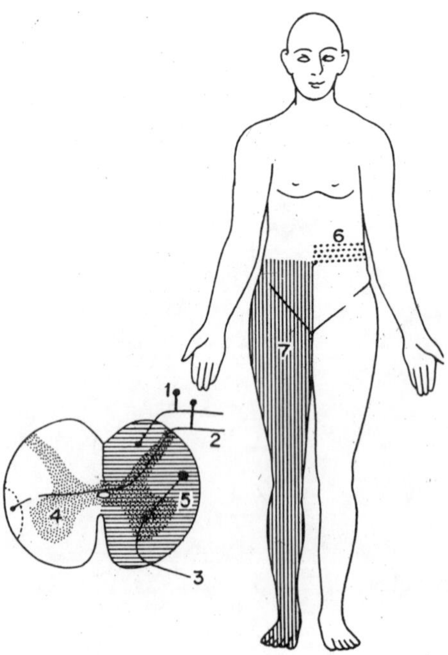


Fig.12.13(c) : Unilateral loss of temperature and pain sensation in hemi section or the cord. (at T12) 1 & 2. Posterior roof; 4-normal side of cord; 3 & 5 affected sidé; 6 band of analgesia on the affected side; 7 loss of pain and temperature sense on the opposite side.

In complete transverse lesion of the cord all voluntary movements of skeletal muscles at end below the lesion are lost. At the segmental level, LMN lesion will cause loss of tone and reflexes as well as wasting of segmental muscles. Below the level it shows UMN type of paralysis. However, if the lesion is acute there will be flaccid paralysis during the stage of spinal shock and spasticity may occur later, when some recovery is taking place. Assessment of the wasting of skeletal muscle should be carefully made. Wasting is often overlooked as there may be hypertrophy of the neighbouring muscles. Deep reflexes and plantar response should be tested to localise the level of damage. Above the level of lesion the reflexes are normal, while at the level of damage reflexes are reduced or lost. Below the level of lesion reflexes are exaggerated unless there is spinal shock. Plantar response will be extensor in case of UMN lesion.

Table 12.4 shows the segmental level of important deep reflexes.

Table : 12.4 — Important reflexes showing localisation of segments

| | | |
|---|---|---|
| $C_5$ | — | Biceps and supinator jerks |
| $C_6$ | — | Pronator jerks |
| $C_7$ | — | T.iceps jerks |
| $D_7$ - 12 | — | Abdominal reflexes |
| $L_2$ | — | Cremaster reflexes |
| $L_3$ - 4 | — | Knee jerks |
| $S_1$ | — | Ankle jerks |
| $S_1$ | — | Plantar reflexes |

Fig.15.16(a), (b), (c) and (d) illustrate some typical cord lesions

## BROWN-SEQUARD SYNDROME

Any lesion affecting one half of the spinal cord may damage pyramidal tract, spino-thalamic tract as well as posterior column of the cord of the involved side. This is known as Brown-Sequard syndrome. Pyramidal lesion on the side of lesion causes weakness with spasticity on the side of lesion but pain and temperature sensation is lost on the opposite side. The upper level of the loss of pain and temperature sensation on the opposite side will be a few segments below the level of lesion, as fibres which are involved at the site of entry into the cord causes a band of analgesia and thermo-anaesthesia on the same side just below the lesion.

Involvement of the posterior column is not always present, but when it is affected, loss of position and vibration sense occurs on the same side of the lesion.

## AETIOLOGIC DIAGNOSIS OF CORD COMPRESSION

Only about 10% of spinal tumours are intramedually consisting of ependymoma and gliomas. The remaining extramedullary tumours may be intradural or extradural. Secondaries are also usually extradural.

When pain is the chief presenting feature, it may be diagnosed as rheumatism, colitis, G.B. disease, hepatitis or renal pain. A good neurological examination, assessment of muscular wasting and determination of any sensory loss only reveal the diagnosis.

## HINTS ON LOCALISATION

1) History should be taken carefully especially regarding injury, fall and any symptoms of bladder dysfunction as well as sexual incapacity.
2) Note if the patient has real root pains, girdle pain, hyperalgesia, hyperaesthesia or sensory loss at any level.
3) Tenderness over the spines is also suspicious.

4) Wasting of muscles and its segmental distribution, if any, is noteworthy.
5) Determine the deep reflexes carefully. The jerks are lost at the level of lesions and may be exaggerated below the level of lesion, unless there is spinal shock.
6) Plantar response, abdominal reflexes and cremasteric reflexes should always be tested.

**DIFFERENTIAL DIAGNOSIS**

1) Motor neuron disease — Wasting of muscles, fasciculation, absence of sensory loss and no sphincter disturbances are characteristic.
2) Subacute combined degeneration — There are lesions of pyramidal tract and posterior column of cord, associated with macrocytic anaemia, achylia gastrica, megaloblastic bone marrow.
3) Syringomyelia — The deep jerks may be lost associated with dissociated sensory loss, tropic skin changes and congential defects, e.g. pes cavus etc.
4) Multiple sclerosis — Remission and relapse of symptoms, nystagmus, intention tremor, ataxia and temporal pallor of optic disc are characteristic.
5) Syphilitic meningomyelitis — A.R. pupil, VDRL test and CSF findings are helpful.
6) Parasagittal intracranial tumour — may cause spastic paraplegia.

**INVESTIGATION**

1) CSF — studies may be helpful. High protein content with normal glucose and cell count are strongly suggestive features. CSF may be xanthochromic. Queckenstedt's test may be positive.
2) X-ray of the spine should always be taken, the part to be studied depends on clinical data. It may show evidence of caries spine, possible disc lesion or metastatic deposits.

   A very significant finding is flattening of pedicles and increased interpedencular distances, due to expanding lesions in the spinal canal. Tumours of nerve roots cause erosion and widening of I.V. foramina.

**TREATMENT**

1) Surgical treatment may be considered where possible. Intramedullary tumours are difficult to excise, hence only irradiation therapy may have to be done. Decompression provides temporary relief from pain and possibly some functional improvement.
2) Decompression of spinal cord surgically followed by irradiation may be done in cases of epidural spinal metastasis.
3) Steroids may also be used in high doses in short courses to relieve pain.
4) Certain tumours, e.g. meningioma can be removed successfully with considerable functional recovery. Similarly, disc problems can be surgically well managed.
5) Symptomatic treatment to relieve pain, reduce spasticity and control of bladder infection is important.

## DISC PROLAPSE SYNDROME

*G.C. MOOKERJEE*

### CERVICAL SPONDYLOSIS

This is due to degenerative changes in the intervertebral discs of cervical vertebrae causing prolapse of nucleus pulposus which causes pressure effects on the cervical nerve roots. Pressure on nerve roots will result in root pains in areas of the nerve supply. Thus pain may be felt in shoulder, arm, forearm and fingers.

Commonest site is disc between sixth and seventh cervical vertebrae but sometimes more than one disc may be affected and several roots may be involved unilaterally or even bilaterally. The pain is aggravated by movement of the neck, jerking, sneezing and coughing.

The syndrome may come in acute form or as a chronic condition. The effects of compression are further aggravated due to presence of osteophytic outgrowths.

The pressure may be on the spinal cord or on the roots. Acute syndrome usually presents with root pains while chronic pressure effects may cause spinal cord compression and paraparesis, due to midline herniation.

The roots usually affected are as follows :-

$C_5$ — Reduced biceps jerk and sensory loss occur in the lateral side of arm. Muscles chiefly affected are biceps, deltoid and brachioradialis.

$C_6$ — Supinator jerk is diminished due to affected brachioradialis muscle. Sensory loss occurs in the lateral side of forearm and thumb.

$C_7$ — Triceps jerk is affected and triceps muscle is wasted; sensory loss is not so marked but may be present in middle finger.

$T_1$ — Finger flexors are weak and intrinsic muscles of hand and finger flexor are affected. Sensory loss may be present in the medial side of the arm and forearm up to little finger. Vertigo may be associated symptom. Rarely dysphagia may occur.

Cord compression may cause symptoms of paraparesis with increased KJ, AJ and extensor plantar response.

## DIAGNOSIS

Clinical signs along with X-ray picture of cervical spine suggest the diagnosis. AP, lateral and oblique views may be taken. Radiology will show diminished I.V. disc spaces and presence of osteophytes with loss of normal cervical curvature. The cervical spine looks straight in the lateral view.

Myelography or discography may be done when surgery is contemplated.

## TREATMENT

Rest in bed with neck support may be sometimes necessary. Some cases will require plastic collar for the neck properly fitted to provide support to the neck. It should be used during the day but removed during sleep. A roll of soft towel should support the neck during sleep or a soft pillow may also be used for this purpose. Neck support with collar may be required for one to three months.

Intermittent traction may be arranged if no relief is obtained with above methods. Keep close watch for any pressure effect on the spinal cord and if this is present, surgical decompression may be considered in expert hands.

# LUMBAGO

*(Lumbar disc syndrome)*

Degeneration and herniation of lumbar discs causes lumbago syndrome. In most cases (about 60%, the discs between $L_5$ and $S_1$ are involved while in 30% cases discs between $L_3$ and $L_4$ are involved. Both also may be involved in about 10 to 20% cases.

The patient gets pain along the distribution of sciatic nerve along with tingling sensation. Sensory loss may also develop. The pain is aggravated by movements, jolting, jerking, sneezing and coughing. The neurological findings may be detected as follows :

1) Patient is unable to lift up the leg due to pain. Extension of the leg at the knee joint with flexed thigh will also cause pain (Lasegue's sign).

2) There may be scoliosis due to spasm of sacrospinalis muscle. The segmental signs and symptoms will be present.
3) When $L_4$ is affected, K.J. is depressed, sensory loss may be present in the medial side of the calf muscle, weakness develops in quadriceps, ilio-psoas and adductors of the thigh.
4) When $L_5$ is affected, extensors of toe and ankles are affected. Sensory changes and pain being limited to lateral side of calf and dorsomedial foot.
5) When $S_1$ is affected, A.J. is depressed, extensors of toes are weak. Posterior aspect of the calf is usually affected causing pain and sensory loss.

X-ray picture of lumbar spine may show reduced disc-space and osteophytic changes. Myelography and CSF studies may be required when compression on cauda equina is suspected. CSF protein may be raised.

Differential diagnosis should be made from other causes of cord compression syndrome already discussed under spastic paraplegia.

**TREATMENT**

Rest and non-steroidal analgesics are given as for cervical spondylosis, but when pain is severe, epidural injection of procaine may be necessary. Suitable local support by lumbar jacket or belt may also be required in some cases.

Surgical decompression may also be necessary if the above measures fail to relieve.

## CONGENITAL AND DEGENERATIVE DISORDERS

*G.C. MUKHERJEE*
*K.A. KABIR*

### MOTOR NEURON DISEASE

It is a degenerative disease affecting anterior horn cells of the spinal cord, motor nuclei of medulla and corticospinal tract. The disease usually affects adults in age group of 30 to 60 years, usually sporadic in nature but familial incidence is often noted. Rarely it affects infants and children, e.g. Werdnig-Hoffman disease and Kukelberg Walender syndrome. As a result, different syndromes are presented depending on which system of tracts are predominantly affected. When corticospinal tracts are predominantly affected it is called amyotrophic lateral sclerosis and when the brunt falls on medullary nuclei it is called progressive bulbar palsy. Trigeminal motor nuclei, nucleus ambiguus, dorsal nucleus of vagus and hypoglossal nucleus are commonly affected. The 3rd and 4th nerve nuclei almost invariably escape.

**Pathology :**

Macroscopically nothing conspicuous is visible in the spinal cord; anterior horns or cerebral cortex appears smaller than normal. Microscopically there is degeneration of affected cells. There may be axonal degeneration of ventral roots and peripheral nerves.

As the disease process affects both lower and upper motor neurons, there is combination of symptom complex, e.g. wasting of small muscles of hands, forearm, arm or shoulder muscles, weakness, clumsiness along with fasciculation. Dysarthria may be the presenting symptom when medullary nuclei are first affected, causing atrophy of tongue. In amyotrophic lateral sclerosis lower limbs show the typical presentation of upper motor neuron paralysis. Disproportionate weakness is noted in the upper limb due to both lower motor and upper motor neuron paralysis.

Sphincters are usually spared, but there may be precipitancy or difficulty in micturition in late stages.

## CLINICAL TYPES

**Five types are recognised :**

1) **Progressive bulbar palsy** — In this type bulbar nuclei are primarily affected, hence there are symptoms and signs of cranial nerve involvement. Presenting features will be difficulty in chewing, swallowing, coughing, speech and even breathing. Tongue becomes atrophied, palatal weakness is evident with depressed gag reflex and pooling of saliva. Pursing and whistling become impossible.

2) **Pseudobular palsy** — In this type cortico-bulbar fibres of both sides are degenerated, hence there is UMN type of involvement of the cranial nerves. The typical findings are contracted but spastic tongue, which does not easily move.

   Limb involvement is often affected, consisting of weakness, spasticity, wasting and fasciculations. This is due to upper and lower motor neuron involvement. Sphincters are usually spared.

   Patients with bulbar or pseudobulbar involvement have poor prognosis and usually die of pulmonary infection within three to five years.

3) **Progressive spinal muscular atrophy** — Degeneration of anterior horn cells in the spinal cord leads to progressive weakness and LMN-type of paralysis in all four limbs. Weakness, muscular fasciculation and wasting are the typical features.

4) **Primary lateral sclerosis** — This is typical upper motor neuron involvement affecting all four limbs.

5) **Amyotrophic lateral sclerosis** — Both upper and lower motor neurons are affected, producing weakness, spasticity, wasting in all four limbs. None of the above syndromes have any sensory deficit.

## INVESTIGATIONS

CSF findings are normal. Serum creatine phosphokinase is somewhat elevated but not as high as in muscular dystrophies. Biopsy of wasted muscles shows histological features of denervation.

EMG shows effects of chronic partial denervation, with abnormal spontaneous activity in resting muscles. A reduction in number of motor units during movement may be recorded. Motor conduction velocity may be impaired slightly but sensory side is normal.

Recently hexosaminidase deficiency has been reported in juvenile spinal muscular atrophy. In this variety low levels of hexosaminidase-A have been reported in blood. Rectal biopsy also presents abnormal findings.

## TREATMENT

There is no curative treatment. Hence the management consists of symptomatic and supportive measures.

Anti-cholinergic drugs, e.g. amitriptyline, atropin and trihexyphenidyl may be helpful if drooling is present. Propanthelene 15 mg twice daily also may help. Spasticity becomes a real problem, which may be eased with diazepam or baclofen.

Surgical measures, e.g. tracheostomy, gastrostomy or cricopharyngo-myotomy, may be the end-stage supportive care in bulbar palsy cases.

Physiotherapy is necessary throughout the life-time of these patients. Nutrition has to be provided at all costs; when normal feeding is difficult in bulbar palsy, tubal feeding and parenteral nutrition may be required.

# HEREDITARY ATAXIAS

There is a group of hereditary or familial disorders due to degenerative changes in spinocerebellar, corticospinal tracts and bulbo-cerebellar fibres. Optic nerve may also be affected. These disorders occur in families with typical features of ataxia associated with dysarthria, intention tremor, nystagmus and congenital deformities, e.g. pes cavus, spina bifida or scoliosis. Even congenital heart disease may be associated.

The clinical types occurring in different members of the families appear to be similar repetitions.

Several types occur depending on the combination of involvement of cerebellar, cortical and spinal connections. The typical syndromes are :

1) Friedrich's ataxia
2) Marie's ataxia
3) Olivo-ponto cerebellar degeneration
4) Roussey-Levy syndrome
5) Bassen-Kornzweig syndrome
6) Refsum's syndrome

**Friedrich's ataxia**

The most common age of onset is 10 to 30 years. Ataxic gait and reeling tendency along with speech defect are typical features. Ataxia is first noted in lower limbs, then spreads up. "Staccato" or scanning speech is classical and diagnostic muscular hypotonia, intention tremor and nystagmus are detected on clinical examination. Deep jerks are lost with extensor plantar response. Vibration sense, joint sense and sense of position are affected due to affection of posterior column.

Optic atrophy and even dementia may also occur. Associated congenital skeletal deformities e.g. pes cavus, scoliosis or spina bifida may be presented. ECG changes showing conduction defects e.g. heart block may be noted.

**Marie's ataxia**

It is a progressive disorder of middle age or early adult life due to cerebellar degeneration associated with pyramidal tract involvement.

**Olivo-ponto-cerebellar degeneration**

Usually presents in later age group in adults. Ataxia and dysarthria along with intellectual deficiency are notable features. Optic atrophy also is associated.

**Roussey-Levy syndrome**

It is different from Friedrich's ataxia in the following respects :

a) Plantar response is flexor;
b) Posterior column is spared so there is no loss of vibration and position sense;
c) There is no dysarthria or nystagmus.

**Bassen-Kornzweig syndrome**

It has similar features like Friedrich's ataxia but has additional features, e.g. steatorrhoea and acanthocytosis. Lipoprotein abnormalities have been reported (absence of $\beta$-lipo proteins).

**Lefsum's syndrome**

Features of Friedrich's ataxia are associated with retinitis pigmentosa and deafness.

## SYRINGOMYELIA

*G.C. MOOKERJEE*
*K. KABIR*

### INTRODUCTION

Syringomyelia is considered as a degenerative disorder of the spinal cord where the defect consists of enlarged central canal resulting in so-called "Syrinx formation" most commonly in the upper part of spinal cord. These cavities are possibly due to imperfect fusion of the neural tube, but exact cause is not really clear. Syringomyelia may be "communicating" extending upward up to medulla (syringobulbia) or "non-communicating". The "non-communicating" variety is usually associated with spinal injury or trauma and confined to lumbar or lower dorsal cord region. Syringomyelia is often associated with other congenital anomalies e.g. Chiari type-1 (congenital extension of cerebellar tonsil below foramen magnum) or spina bifida or large naevi over spinal skin.

These cavities are central and therefore when these cysts enlarge, the immediate brunt falls on the spinothalamic tract which crosses anterior to the central canal, while posterior column is spared. Hence there is loss of pain and temperature sensation on both sides of the segments involved, while light touch and proprioceptive sensation remain unaffected (sensory dissociation) Fig.12.14. Later, it affects the anterior horn cells causing lower motor neuron type of weakness in affected segments and spasticity in lower limbs due to pressure on pyramidal tracts. Plantar response becomes extensor.

Tropic changes are very common and include ulcers, with delayed healing, cyanosis, hyperkeratosis and thickening of fingers. Charcot's joints are common in the shoulder and elbow. Atrophy, demineralisation with destruction of joint surfaces are the common radiographic findings.

The salient features are :

1) Segmental atrophy
2) Areflexia
3) Sensory dissociation (see Fig.12.14)
4) Loss of pain and temperature sensation.
5) Pyramidal involvement (in late stages in lower limbs)
6) Syringobulbia — there is involvement of lower cranial nerves (bulbar palsy), motor and sensory loss over both sides of face.

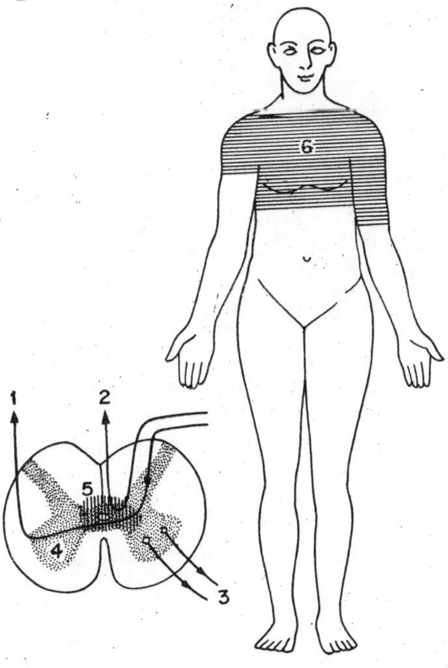


Fig.12.14 : Dissociated sensation in syringomyelia

It should be noted that though there is dissociated sensation over a few segments, there is normal sensation above as well as below the affected area. This is due to involvement of central region damaging the crossing spinothalamic fibres.

## INVESTIGATIONS

Investigation includes X-ray spine and myelography where there is doubt. CSF is only helpful when there is a block showing raised protein content. In some cases air encephalography or ventriculography may be needed.

In these patients who have Arnold Chiari malformation, radiological abnormalities are noted in plain X-ray of skull and cervical spine.

C.T. scan reveals caudal displacement of fourth ventricle.

## TREATMENT

Arnold Chiari malformation associated with syringomyelia may be surgically treated. Post-traumatic syringomyelia may require expert surgical handling.

Syringomyelia or syringobulbia otherwise should be treated symptomatically. Physiotherapy which delays contractures and reduces spasticity is very useful, as there is no curative treatment. Aim is to apply physical therapy to reduce spasticity. Diazepam also may help due to its action on spinal inter-neurons, influencing supra spinal centres.

Dentrolene has been used in some cases of spasticity with some success.

Syringomyelia is progressive, but there may be spontaneous arrest of the disease in some cases. Sudden aggravation of symptoms occurs with minor injury.

## NEURO FIBROMATOSIS

*(Von Recklinghausen's disease)*

This condition consists of multiple tumour and formation presenting as fibromatous growth in the skin or within the body. It may be a single tumour or multiple nodular growths arising out of neurilemma sheath, hence can occur anywhere in the body, where nerve trunks or nerve roots are presented (Fig.12.15).

It is an autosomal dominant disorder resulting in these fibromatous tumours anywhere in the body. Gliomas, meningiomas and pheochromocytomas (chromaffin origin) may be associated with neuro-fibromatosis.

Multiple discrete movable lumps of various sizes may occur all over the body or only in one or two sites of varying sizes. It may present as solitary neurofibroma in the cranial nerves (especially VIII nerve) or in the spinal nerve roots.

The nerve trunks can also be thickened and sometimes there may be a diffuse plexiform growth.

Cutaneous growths are of varying sizes and usually do not cause much difficulty except the ugly appearance. Cafe-au-lait patches of pigmentation are presented in the skin in many cases. Deep neurofibromatosis may cause local pressure effects. These may undergo cystic changes. Rarely there may be malignant changes.

In intraspinal or intracranial types, the protein level is CSF is raised.

X-ray studies may reveal that internal auditory meatus or intravertebral foramen is enlarged due to local expanding neurofibroma.

### Treatment

In case of spinal or cerebral compression effects or malignancy, surgical removal may be necessary.

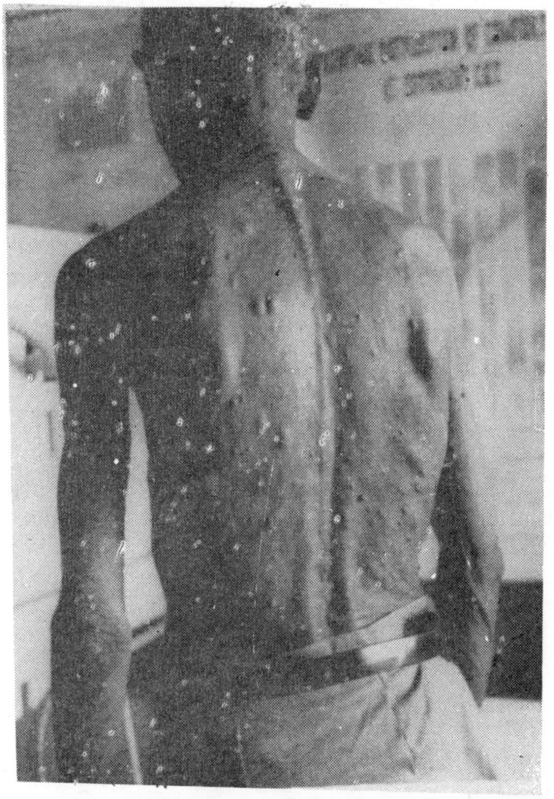

Fig.12.15 : Neuro-fibromatosis/Von-Reckling hausens disease *(Editor's case)*

## DISORDER OF MUSCLES

*SHYAMAL SEN*

### INTRODUCTION

The derivative meaning of the word 'muscle' is amusing; the Latin word 'musculus' means a mouse, the usual fusiform shape tapered at both ends gives a distance resemblance to the mouse, hence the name. Volume-wise muscle is the largest single organ of the body of which it forms about one-fifth by weight. There are more than 600 muscles in the body.

A voluntary muscle is composed of muscle fibres, each of which is multinucleated cell consisting of many fibrils, sarcoplasm and number of discrete organelles including mitochondria, ribosomes, Golgi apparatus, glycogen granules and lipid droplet. Each fibre which varies in length from a few millimetres to many centimetres and the thickness from 10-100 micron is enclosed in a sacrcolemmal sheath, deep to which the muscle nuclei are situated. Each has a motor end-plate in which the nerve fibres terminate and make contact with it. Muscle fibre contains fine fibrillar structure called filaments which are made of actin and myosin. The highly organised arrangement is responsible for the function of contractile system of the muscle. The sarcoplasmic reticulum and the 'T' system are tubular network (transverse system of fibres) which play an important role in contraction and relaxation of the muscle fibre (Fig.12.16).

A motor unit is a group of muscle fibres supplied by an anterior horn cell. The larger cell bodies of anterior horn cell give rise to alpha motor-neurons which supply the extrafusal muscle fibres; smaller cell bodies give origin to the gamma neurons which supply the intrafusal fibres of muscle spindles.

Contraction of the muscle fibres which make up a motor unit is preceded by electrical excitation of the fibre membranes. Ultra structure of skeletal muscle has demonstrated that the unit structure of individual myofibril is the sarcomeres extending for one Z-line (situated in the midst of 'I' band) to the next. True muscle disorders are distinct from neuromuscular disorders in that the diseases affect the muscle primarily and not secondary to disorder of the nerves. The term 'myopathy' has been defined as any disease or syndrome in which there are pathological, biochemical or electrophysiological changes in the muscle tissue of the voluntary musculature in absence of any involvement of central or peripheral nervous system. The term 'muscular dystrophy' has been reserved for genetically determined myopathies.

**Primary myopathy or muscular dystrophies**

The disease is heredo-familial, but the forms of late onset tend to be sporadic. The familial form affects males more commonly than females.

**Classification**

There are various forms of muscular dystrophies, classified by earlier authors on the basis of distribution of the muscles affected. Later on,it was observed that genetic distribution of these disorders follows a definite pattern and as such a clinico-genetic classification has been accepted. A number of varieties of these disorders have been described. Only the important are included here :

**A : X-linked**

1. Sex-linked recessive type severe — (Duchenne)
2. Sex-linked recessive (mild) — (Beker)
3. Benign with early contracture — (Dreefuss)

**B : Autosomal dominant**

1. Facio-scapulo-humeral (Landouzy & Dejerine)
2. Scapulo-peronial muscular dystrophies
3. Distal type of muscular dystrophy-infantile and adult onset
4. Ocular myopathy
5. Oculo-pharyngeal

**C : Autosomal recessive**

1. Limb-girdle type (Scapulo-peronial)
2. Childhood muscular-dystrophy (excepting Duchenne)
3. Congenital muscular dystrophies

## AETIOLOGY

Aetiology is not yet understood but as has been already stated a genetic factor is very much suspected and in many cases it has been demonstrated in animal models. The familial forms affect males more than females.

**PATHOGENESIS :** The pathogenesis of the muscular dystrophy remains elusive, but there are currently three hypotheses under active consideration at this time.

1. **Vascular theory :** Possibilities are inadequate blood supply leading to degenerative changes in dystrophic vessels. An abnormal amount of catecholamine in intrafibrillar substance of muscle in muscular dystrophy (MD) leads to vasoconstriction of capillaries are called sick motor neuron hypothesis.
2. **Neurogenic theory. :** Decrease in motor units implying decrease in anterior horn cell, so called sick motor neuron hypothesis.

3. **Membrane theory :** There is a genetically determined abnormality in surface membrane of the muscle fibre in MD. The theory is supported by the leakage of muscle enzymes from sarcoplasm, through muscular membrane into the serum in MD. The membrane abnormality is present in known carrier and has also been demonstrated in erythrocytes in patients with MD. The various factors, apart from genetic, in causation of sarcolemmal defect leading ultimately to cell necrosis are depicted in the following diagram :

GENETIC ABNORMALITY IN A VARIETY OF MD

---

Deficiency of vit E
Selenium
Biotin

Lack of energy due to ischaemic
hypoxia mitochondrial defect
Excessive muscular work

Trophic

Infective agents
Agents

Immunological

Sarcolemmal Defect

Increased net influx of $Ca^{++}$

Excess uptake of $Ca^{++}$ by Mitochondria

Functional and later structural damage of Mitochondria

Lack of energy

Elevated cytoplasmic $Ca^{++}$ level

Hypercontraction of muscle fibres

Dissolution of Z-bands by CA proteases

Cell necrosis

**(After Arongemann & Pemma (Lancet – 1,692– 674, 1976)**

## PATHOLOGY

The histological appearances are essentially the same in all forms of MD varying according to the rapidity of the disease process in the individual case. In MD, the muscle fibres show a patternless variation in size, some being larger and some smaller than normal.

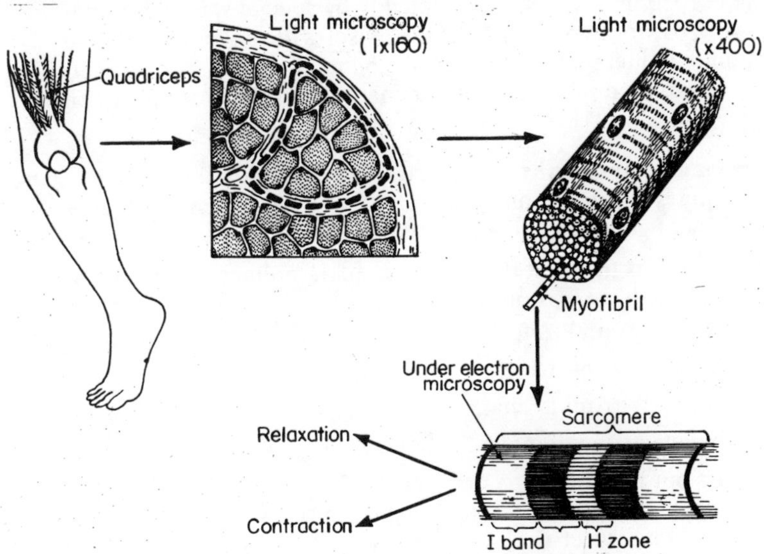


Fig.12.16 : Normal Pattern of Skeletal muscle *(Diagramatic)*

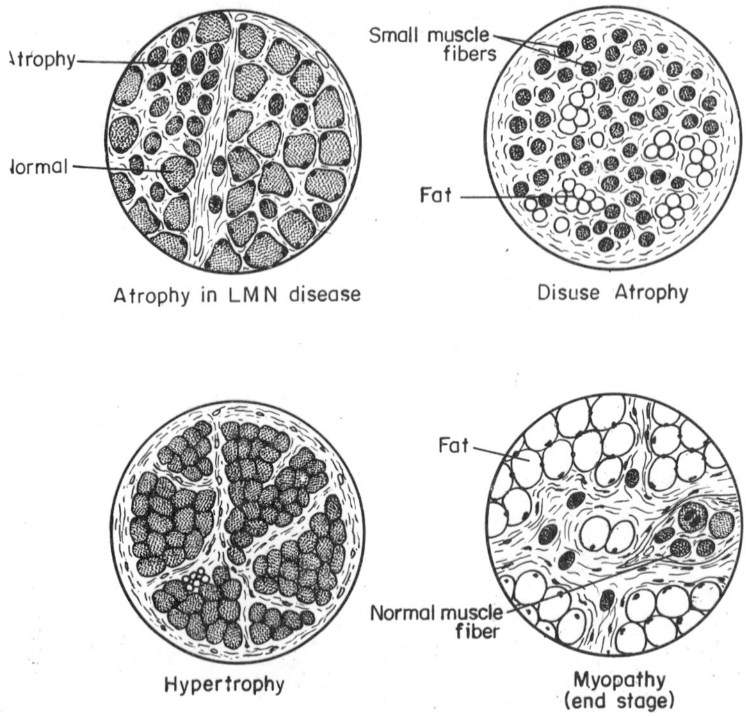


Fig.12.17 : Various histological types of lesions in disease of muscles.

Sarcolemmal nuclei are generally more prominent that usual and some are found deep within the fibre (migration of sarcolemmal nuclei). There are various degrees of degeneration and phagocytosis of muscle fibres. There is no perivascular cellular infiltration when the disease process is slow but fatty replacement of muscle fibres are seen. Myelinated nerve fibres are seen intact and sometime curbed up (seen microscopically by special staining) due to loss of muscle bundles. In patients with pseudohypertrophy of the muscles the enlargement is due to an increase in the amount of fat and an increase in the bulk of the muscle fibres. In patients with myotonic dystrophy long rows of sarcolemmal nuclei are a characteristic abnormality (Fig: 12.17).

## CLINICAL FEATURES

**Duchenne type muscular dystrophy :** By usage and definition this is the more frequent and dreaded type of dystrophies in infancy and early childhood described by Duchenne. In our MD series it forms about 75% of genetically determined myopathies.

**Genetics :** Female carriers transmit the disease to male siblings but themselves do not suffer from the disease; thus family history is obtained from maternal side. The carrier female may be identified with about 80% accuracy) as follows :

(a) Creatine kinase test of serum (which is highly elevated)

(b) Muscle biopsy (slight dystrophic changes)

(c) Slightly myopathic electromyogram

Age of onset is 3-5 years but may occur as early as the first year of life,seldom after tenth year. Frequent fall or tendency to fall after the child has learnt to walk with fair stability draws the attention to the parents. The onset is insidious and sometimes it is difficult to pinpoint the beginning of the disease. Subsequently difficulties in rising from floor or climbing stairs awkward peculiar gait and inability to run properly may be noticed. These relate to the early involvement of pelvifemoral muscles. Later shoulder girdle muscles are affected and there is progressive disability of getting up from the floor or from bed and inability to perform daily activities of life; finally the child is confined to bed or chair before the age of twelve years. Total disablement is frequent during second decade of life aggravated by obesity, kypho-scoliosis and cardio-respiratory embarrassment.

Clinical signs include weakness and wasting of the pelvifemoral and shoulder girdle muscles with unusually large calves, quadriceps and the deltoid muscles with so-called pseudohypertrophy as they are weak on muscle testing. Hypertrophy of calves is seen almost in all cases and of the tongue in about 25% of the cases. The weakness is clinically evident by a waddling gait and the peculiar way the child resorts to when he is asked to get up from a supine position. He first turns on his face and then uses the hand to sit up; then again uses his hands to lift his trunk and finally assumes a posture "Climbing up his own legs" Fig.12.18 (a) and (b). This latter part of the manoeuvre is sometimes termed as Gower's sign. When he is observed from front while he is standing he has a wide base, as obvious pordotic stance with protruberant abdomen; when observed from the back apparent winging of scapula is noted. The muscles affected in the upper limbs include serrati, pectoralis, latissimi, biceps and brachioradialis while in the lower limbs they are iliopsoas, quadriceps, glutei and anterior tibial muscles. The forearm and hand muscles, gastrocnemius and foot muscles retain average power until late in the illness. The deep reflexes are maintained till late and the ankle jerk is last to go. Apart from muscle involvement, there is no other neurologic deficit.

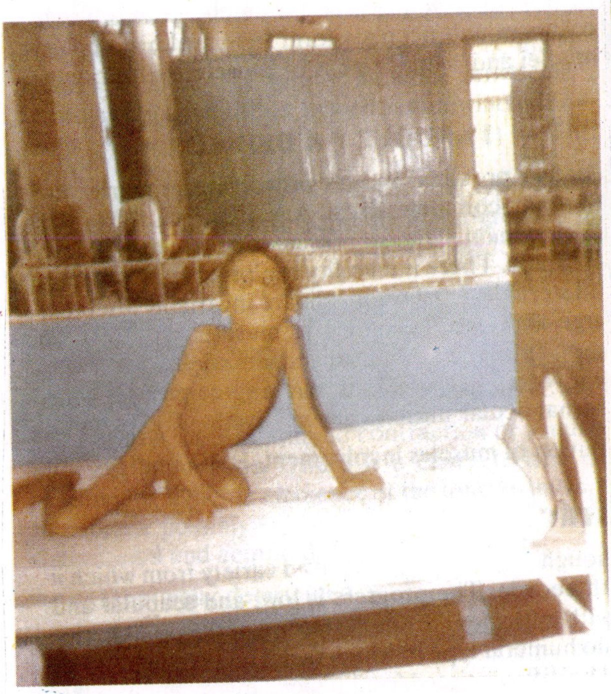

Fig.12.18 (a)

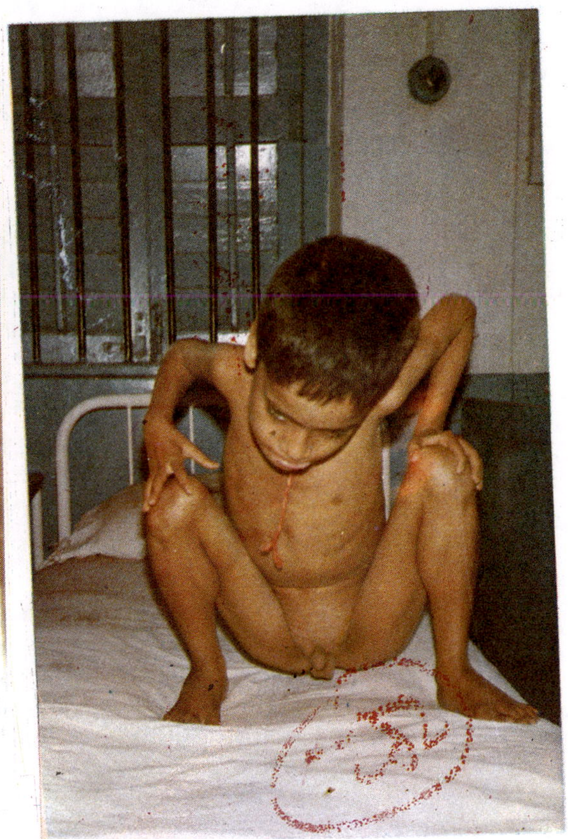

Fig.12.18 (b)

Pseudo-hypertrophy muscular distrophy
*(Photo : Dr.K. Kabir — Islamia Hospital)*

Other systemic involvement includes the heart, the respiratory systems, the bones and mental functions.

Cardiac involvement is in late stage and manifests in tachycardia and congestive failure. ECG changes are seen early e.g. slurring of QRS or deep Q and prominent R in right chest lead is a common feature; bundle branch block, elevation or depression of S-T segments are sometimes seen. ECG changes are seen in about 50% of cases. Respiratory involvement is mainly due to lack of mobility of respiratory muscles and skeletal changes of thorax due to lack of muscular support. The respiratory functions are greatly affected and proneness to infection is a difficult clinical problem in the last stage. The shaft of long bones is thin due to disuse atrophy and shows gross osteoporosis in X-ray pictures.

The child is mildly or moderately retarded and I.Q. is around 60-70. Some diffuse non-specific EEG changes have been noted.

**Diagnosis :** This is suggested by early onset of the disease in a child with history of recurrent falls and defective gait. The family history on the maternal side is present in about 40% of cases. Gower's sign, the bulky calf and deltoid, the stance and the gait are characteristic. Testing for muscles shows characteristic distribution of muscle involvement.

**Laboratory tests :** The serum enzyme CPK, CPK-MB, SGPT, LDH are all elevated. The CPK should be routinely done and may be elevated to 10,000-20,000 units in early stage and falling with progress of the diseases.

**EMG :** Shows short duration, low amplitude polyphasic motor unit potentials and a near normal interference pattern.

**Muscle biopsy :** Biopsy should be done in appropriate muscle and must be sectioned in both transverse and longitudinal section special histochemical staining is not of much use in routine diagnosis. As already indicated affected muscles will show loss of fascicular pattern with variation in fibre size. Hyalinisation, flocculo-granular changes and necrosis form the usual histological feature. There is migration of sarcolemmal nuclei and replacement of muscle by fibro-fatty tissue.

## FACIO-SCAPULO-HUMERAL TYPE OF MD – (LANDOUZY & DEJERINE)

This is a slowly progressive dystrophy affecting proximal muscles involving primarily the muscle of shoulder and face, with long remissions and complete arrest. Age of onset is 6-20 years and is usually autosomal occurring in either sex dominant. Clinical presentation is with difficulty in raising arm above shoulder, with winging of scapula. There is inability in closing eyes, pressing lips or whistling. The lower part of trapezius and sternal part of pectoralis are invariably affected, while the deltoids may seem inordinately large and strong. The other muscles involved are sternomastoids. Serratus magnus, rhomboid, supraspinatus, latissimus and later deltoids. Biceps working is less than triceps. Pelvic muscles are involved later and to a mild degree giving rise to lordosis and pelvic instability, occasionally external ocular muscles are involved.

Diagnosis is clinched by age of onset, distribution of muscles involvement. EMG findings and muscle biceps. SCPK is seldom very high.

## SCAPULOPERONEAL MUSCULAR DYSTROPHY

Again an autosomal dominant type of MD though there is a rare X-linked variety from which it differs is having a later onset in second to fifth decade. The progress is low, and scapular and peroneal group of muscles are affected often with initial foot drops. Some are of the opinion that it is incomplete or abortive form of facioscapulo humeral type in which facial involvement is late and mild feature. Scapuloperoneal MD should be differentiated for neurogenic scapuloperoneal syndrome (a form of spinal muscular atrophy of varying genetic transmission).

## DISTAL TYPE (OF GOWER)

This is a rare form and its existence is debated by many. The process usually begins in small muscles of the hands and slowly spreads prominently. In the thigh,anterior tibial and calf muscles are affected first. The condition is benign and proximal muscles weakness occurs in few more severe cases. The juvenile form described by Beimoral was subsequently found to be neurogenic.

## OCULAR MYOPATHY (PROGRESSIVE EXTERNAL OPHTHALMOPLEGIA)

The symptoms may begin at any age i.e. early childhood to old age. They usually start with ptosis; involvement of facial muscles or some proximal muscle is not uncommon. There is progressive limitation of ocular movements without significant diplopia. Absent of fatiguability and diurnal varieties differentiate it from ocular myasthenia, but a similar progressive external ophthalmoplegia associated with clinical features of central nervous system involvement and retinal degeneration complicate the diagnosis, but this usually occurs in children.

There is, however, a distinct group of external ocular muscle involvement with dysphagia, to which the name 'oculopharyngeal myopathy' has been given.

## LIMB GIRDLE MYOPATHIES OF LATE ONSET AND DOMINANT INHERITANCE

The onset is in late teens and slowly progresses to seventh decade in some cases. It is usually autosomal recessive in their gentle transmission, may well be heterogenous and autosomal dominant in the inheritance. Proximal lower-limb weakness predominates but affection of quadriceps effect may be mild. Serum enzyme activity may be normal.

## CHILDHOOD MUSCULAR DYSTROPHY

Usually autosomal recessive in inheritances and many MD in childhood in girls are of this type. Some, however, would belong to neurogenic type (spinal muscular atrophy). They are usually pelvifemoral in onset and onset may be as early as in Duchenne but progress is comparatively slow and patients become unstable to walk in their early twenties. The distribution of affected muscles resembles those of Duchenne type.

## CONGENITAL MUSCULAR DYSTROPHY

These have been described in two forms, the benign non-progressive variety and the rapidly progressive one. The former includes genetically autosomal recessive variety with or without årthrogryphosis multiple, as well as many include a variety of non-genetic myopathies acquired *in utero.*

A few cases of rapidly progressive type have been described. They present with severe hypotonia at birth with subsequent progressive muscular wasting and weakness. Serum CPK level is often normal or only a little raised.

# MYOTONIC DISORDERS

Myotonia is the continued contraction of a muscle which persists after cessation of voluntary effort of stimulation. There is a characteristic dimple induced in the affected muscle after percussion (in thenar eminence or the tongue) and appears to be due to dysfunction of sarcolemmal membrane possibly related to chloride conduction. Broadly there are two types — Genetically determined and acquired drug induced

Genetically determined :

Myotonia congenita (autosomal dominant & autosomal recessive type)

Paramyotonia congenita

Dystrophia myotonica

Chondrodystrophic myotonia.

[ *Photographs and figures are included by the editor.* ]

# MYASTHENIA GRAVIS

*G.C. MOOKERJEE*

## INTRODUCTION

Myasthenia gravis (M.G.) is a disorder of transmission of nerve impulse through myoneural junction, resulting in muscular weakness and fatigue of some groups of skeletal muscles. Bulbar, proximal limb muscles and respiratory muscles are commonly involved. There is defective conduction of nerve impulse at the myoneural junction due to shortage of functioning acetylcholine receptors. The defect can be alleviated by administration of anti-choline esterase drug, e.g. edrophonium or neostigmine.

## AETIOLOGY

It is now established that in M.G. there are circulating antibodies to acetyl choline receptor (Ach R). The T–lymphocytes (thymic) as well as B-lymphocytes also are involved in this process. These circulating antibodies to Ac HR get fixed in the receptor sites, resulting in depletion of functioning receptor units on the post-synaptic membrane. Hence myoneural transmission is affected. Thus M.G. may be considered as auto-immune disease and truely it is sometimes associated with thyrotoxicosis, diabetes mellitus, collagen diseases, e.g. rheumatoid arthritis and SLE.

## PATHOLOGY

Histological changes consist of atrophy of skeletal muscles, abnormalities in nerve-endings and motor end-plates. There are infiltrations of lymphocytes (lymphorrhages). Focal necrosis may also be present.

## CLINICAL FEATURES

The disease occurs in all age groups and affects both sexes; but females usually predominate. Commonest presentation is fatigue and muscular weakness involving bulbar muscles, usually noticed at the end of the day. Proximal limb muscles may also be affected so that climbing up stairs may be difficult or tiring. The following symptoms may occur due to affection of bulbar muscles : (Fig.12.19) ptosis (drooping eyelids) diplopia, difficulty of chewing meat or swallowing food and slurred speech. Nasal regurgitation or choking due to aspiration of fluid into respiratory passage may occur. Ptosis of one or both eyes is often the first symptom. The patient may feel well after a night's rest but worse at the end of the day. She is a tired person in the late evenings and has difficulty of speech and eating problem at dinner. External ocular muscles are incordinated resulting in double vision. Complete ophthalmoplegia may occur but pupils are normal. Weakness of the orbicularis oris presents with myasthenic smile (myasthenic snarl). Gradually weakness of jaw, palatal palsy and facial muscular weakness may develop (causing expressionless face). Whistling is not possible. Later swallowing problems are troublesome. Even head is bent down the chest and becomes difficult to lift it up due to weakness of neck muscles.

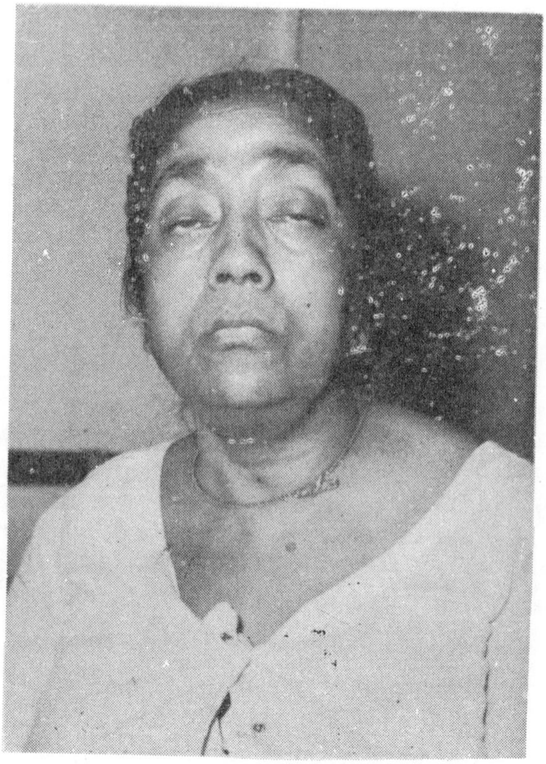

Fig.12.19 : Myasthenia Gravis *(Editor's case)*

There may be proximal muscular weakness but the sensory function and deep reflexes are preserved. Muscular wasting can only occur at late stages.

## DIAGNOSIS

The best way to establish the diagnosis by giving I.V. injection of edrophonium hydrochloride (Tensilon), which immediately relieves the symptoms for some time. The symptoms come back as soon as drug action is over, which is usually about three minutes.

The initial dose is 2.0 mg of the drug to check the sensitivity, followed by 8 mg I.V. EMG and electrical testing may also be done before and after the therapeutic test. Intramuscular injection of neostigmine (1.25 mg) with 0.6 mg of atropine may also settle the diagnosis as the improvement lasts half an hour to one or two hours. Provocative tests are sometimes done by using curare or quinine but are dangerous and may be left for the neurologists.

Differential diagnosis is to be made from other causes of bilateral ptosis and myopathies but the therapeutic test is always convincing.

## TREATMENT

Initially the treatment is started with neostigmine tablet 15 mg four to six times daily. Abdominal colic and diarrhoea may also occur. Most cases can be maintained by pyridostigmine 60 mg tablet given at six hourly or eight hourly intervals. Dose has to be adjusted and larger or more frequent administration is required towards the evening, before eating or delivering lectures. Too much dose also causes trouble (cholinergic crisis), i.e. exaggeration of symptoms. Its muscarinic side effects can be controlled by propantheline hydrochloride 15 mg twice daily or Inj. atropin 0.6 mg subcutaneously. These, however, can be combated by oral propantheline or Inj. atropine.

Intractable cases may require administration of corticosteroids, which should be started in small dosages, e.g. 5 mg of prednisolone three times daily up to 30 mg per day. Larger doses may cause trouble. Close observation is preferable in a hospital.

Azathioprine is occasionally used and may be combined with steroids. In some cases intensive medical care is required. Anti-cholinesterase drugs, ephidine, aldosterone inhibitors, steroids and azathioprines may also fail, when plasmapheresis to remove the circulating antibodies may be useful. Where this is not possible thymectomy may be carefully considered.

However, some cases go downhill within two to three years in spite of treatment, on the other hand spontaneous remission is also well-known, which may or may not relapse again.

### Surgical treatment

In some cases when thymoma is present, thymectomy is helpful but radiotherapy is sometimes recommended before surgery. The place of thymectomy in routine treatment of MG cases is controversial.

# CHAPTER – 13
# RHEUMATOLOGY

*SANAT KUMAR SARCAR*

## INTRODUCTION

The Greek word "Rheumatism" means catarrhal changes of the mucus. In large number of joint disorders, there is actual alteration of the joint mucin, the polysaccharide hyaluronic acid. Some like to term this group of diseases as arthritis, i.e. lesions in the articular and periarticular structures. Though difficult, a working definition is suggested.

## DEFINITION

Rheumatology is the science of rheumatic diseases, affecting articulo-periarticulo-muscular structures (loco-motor system) and other connective tissues of the human body (systemic diseases), characterised by pain, swelling, stiffness and limitation in the joints, with other systemic symptoms and signs.

## CLASSIFICATION

There are a large number of rheumatic diseases or arthritis, little over 100 in number, known from ancient times all over the world. In India 'Ayurvedic system', all kinds of chronic joint disorders with pain are termed 'BAT'. The "International League against Rheumatism" and "American Rheumatism Association", both had presented two different big lists or classification charts. For practical purposes, we may simplify them into seven major groups :-

I. **Inflammatory group of Rheumatic disease of known infectious agents :-**

(a) **Bacterial** Brucella. Gonococcus. Mycobacterium tuberculosis. Pneumococcus. Staphylococcus. Salmonella. Streptobacillus Moniliformis (Haverhill fever). Treponema pallidum (Syphilis). Treponema pertenme (Yaws) etc.

(b) Rickettsial

(c) Viral

(d) Fungal

(e) Parasitic etc.

II. **Inflammatory Polyarthritis of Unknown Aetiology :-**

(a) Rheumatoid arthritis. Still's disease. Psoriatic arthritis. Reiter's Syndrome

(b) Ankylosing Spondylitis

(c) Rheumatic Fever

(d) Group of "Intermittent Periodic Arthritis Syndromes"

(e) Enteropathic Arthritis.

III. **Degenerative Joint Diseases :-**

(A) Axial or Spinal involvement, e.g. Spondylosis

(B) Peripheral (Proximal/Distal), e.g. Osteoarthrosis (Osteoarthritis)

They may be (a) primary, or (b) secondary.

IIV. **Traumatic and/or Neurogenic disorders :-**

(a) Traumatic arthropathy, — due to direct trauma resulting in haemorrhage, exudation, and injury to different musculo-skeletal structures (articular & periarticular)

(b) Postural and occupational group — due to indirect trauma, stress or strain, etc.
(c) Neurogenic arthropathy, — charcot's joint, shoulder-hand syndrome. Syringomyelia, diabetic neuropathy.

V. **Arthritis related to known Metabolic, Biochemical or Endocrinal disorders of bones and joints :-**

(a) Gout, pseudogout, articular chondro-calcinosis
(b) Onchronosis, hematochromatosis & Wilson's disease
(c) Rheumatic disorders in endocrinopathies — in hyperparathyroidism, acromegaly,
(d) Haemoglobinopathies (e.g. Sickle cell disease)
(e) Haemophilia
(f) Gaucher's disease
(g) Scurvy (hypo-vitaminosis C).

VI. **'Connective tissue' disorders, including "Diffuse Collagen diseases" :-**

(a) Systemic lupus erythematosus. (S. L. E.)
(b) Polyarteritis nodosa
(c) Scleroderma (Progressive systemic sclerosis)
(d) Polymyositis and dermatomyositis
(e) Mixed connective tissue diseases (M.C.T.D.).

VII. **Non-articular rheumatism or "Painful syndromes" :-**

(a) Intervertebral disc lesions, and low back syndromes
(b) Tendinitis, peri-tendinitis, bursitis etc.
(c) Fibrositis, myositis and myalgia, fascitis
(d) Tenosynovitis
(e) Carpal tunnel syndrome
(f) Shoulder-hand syndrome, etc.

Besides, the above seven classical groups, "**Tumour and Tumour like conditions**", e.g. multiple myeloma, synovioma, giant cell tumour of tendon sheaths, metastatic lesions in bones & joints, benign tumours of articular tissues present painful joints with rheumatic disorders.

## CLINICAL PRESENTATIONS IN RHEUMATOLOGY

(i) **History taking in Rheumatology :-**

It is needless to emphasize the importance of skillful history taking in rheumatology, as in all other types of diseases. Some special questions are to be answered, regarding the joints :-

(a) How it started ? Sequence of involvement of joints
(b) Number of joints involved, with locations-axial or peripheral, proximal or distal.
(c) Pattern of joint involvement-symmetrical or asymmetrical; migratory, or shifting; or multiple joints involved at a time.
(d) Time-intensity — Acute or chronic; periodical or constant; self-limiting or progressive.
(e) History of trauma is to be noted :- direct or indirect; chronic stress & strain; occupational stress or trauma; posture in lying, sitting, standing & working.

(ii) **Subjective Symptoms Local & General :-**

(a) **Pain** — is the chief symptom of the rheumatic disorders, which causes immense suffering, and results in physical and mental disability. This unpleasant sensory manifestation must be thoroughly understood. Its **site** (from superficial or deep structures), **time-intensity, nature** (acute, chronic, sharp, dull etc.), **character** (depending on structures involved), **distribution** (localised, diffuse, referred etc.) **time period** (continuous, intermittent etc.) are to be noted and analysed. Similarly, the **results of pain,** e.g. muscular rigidity, tenderness, mental reaction, and other reflex clinical phenomenons are to be correlated. So proper analysis of pain help in the diagnosis and management.

(b) **Stiffness/rigidity** — may be to articular swelling, or of periarticular origin. Morning stiffness, stiffness after rest, tansitory, periarticular swelling of O.A. etc. Muscle guard or spasm resulting from pain, may give rise to stiffness. So magnitude, particular time, duration and accompanying features with stiffness are to be recorded.

(c) **Limitation of movements** — in the joints — may be due to pain, internal joint structure involvement, or ankylosis. Periarticular structures and muscle spasm or contractures may cause limitation. The amount in degrees and range of limitation, i.e. inner, middle or outer range should be mentioned.

(d) **Swellings** — are of different natures — fluctuating or tense swelling may be due to effusion or exudation inside the joints; hard swelling due to bony overgrowths; firm periarticular soft tissue swelling etc.

(e) There may be other **systemic symptoms,** e.g. atrophy, fatigue, emotional disturbances, etc.

(iii) **Objective signs and methods of examination**

e.g. swelling, tenderness, local sign of inflammation etc, are to be detected by clinical examination as stated below :-

A. **Local Examinations** are made, and a joint chart is maintained.

I. **Inspection** (Look & Compare).

(a) **Skin** — Colour changes, shiny or tense, abnormal creases, any break etc.

(b) **Contour or shape** of joints and limbs, swelling, wasting, shortening etc.

(c) **Position and alignment** — of joints and limbs.

(d) Any **deformity** or not.

II. **Palpation** (Feel & Compare) : -

(a) **Skin** — It is moist or dry, rough or smooth, warm or cold, skin sensations — are charted graphically.

(b) **Soft Tissues & Joints :**

1. Swelling as discussed.
2. **Tenderness** — localised, or "all over"; **gradation of tenderness :-**

Grade I. — Patient complains of tenderness on deep pressure.

Grade II. — Patient whines on deep pressure.

Grade III. — Patient 'withdraws the part' on localised pressure.

Grade IV. — Patient withdraws before the part is touched — 'touch me not' attitude, tenderness all over due to inflammation, e.g. gout, and acute inflammatory flares.

3. Thickened synovium, or other structures, can be felt.

4. In case of any soft tissue swelling — its shape, size, surface, consistency, edge and attachments should be determined.
5. Fluid accumulation in the joints should be determined by 'fluctuation test', 'tap method' and 'bulge test', by demonstrating the displacements of fluid.
6. Joint stiffness, or laxity (subluxation and dislocation) are recorded.
7. Crepitations — are different natures, — e.g. coarse bony grating, coarse cartilagenous crepitations, medium cartilagenous crepitations and rubbing, fine soft tissue crepitation and rubbing.
8. Signs of inflammations : Heat, erythema, etc.

(c) Bones — are to be palpated for tenderness, localised thickening, shortening, any irregularity of surfaces, any bony growth, or spurs, or nodes, or lumps. The size (progressively increasing or not ?), shape, site, edge, consistency and tenderness of any abnormal bony lump should be determined. Any bending of the bones is to be noted.

III. **Movements in Joints** (Move and Compare) :-

(a) **Active movements** through full range, and any limitations and pain in particular ranges are noted.

(b) **Passive movements** through permitted full range are performed to find out any limitation and pain in any range; any increased or abnormal movements.

B. General examination of the different systems of the body.

**DIAGNOSTIC AIDS :** Skiagram and laboratory tests are definitely of much help, which will be also discussed with individual diseases.

**X-ray Examination of Bones and Joints**

| General | Bones | | Joints & Periarticular Structures |
|---|---|---|---|
| | Bone as a whole : | Components : | |
| 1. Site | 1. Shapc & Outline | 1. Cortex | 1. Joint space — intact or not, diminished or increased |
| 2. Contour or shape of the limb or spine as a whole | 2. Density & mineralisation | 2. Medulla | 2. Joint line |
| 3. Maturity, age & ossification | 3. Architecture & intactness | 3. Periosteum | 3. Periarticular swelling |
| 4. Alignments of all the bones and joints of the part examined | 4. Position & allign-ment with neighbouring structures | 4. Any abnormal outgrowth or swelling | 4. Soft tissue shadows (e.g. Psoas shadow) |
| 5. Any abnormal radio-opaque shadows | | | 5. Any other abnormal shadows, and radio opacity (e.g. myositis) ossificaces). |

N.B : The part examined should be always compared with normal side of the body or normal specimen.

IV. **Joint Deformity** — Whether postural or structural (fixed), congenital or acquired is to be determined.

V. **Muscle Power** is tested and noted numerically – 0,1,2,3,4 & 5; and a progress chart is maintained. Any wasting deficiencies is noted.

VI. **Functional testing** should be done at intervals and 'Activities of Daily Living (A.D.L.) chart and 'Work Chart' are to be maintained.

VII. Some special clinical tests for different regions (Specific Rheumatological Examinations) are done to help in the diagnosis of different diseases, which will be discussed with different diseases.

**Special X-ray Examinations :**

Arthroscopy
Arthrography

**Laboratory tests :**

1. Joint structures examinations :-

**Synovial fluid analysis** — may be done after it is aspirated aseptically, in the following ways :-

A. **General Examination** —

1. Volume — normal, increased, or diminished.
2. Colour — clear to pale yellow (normal), white, purulent, or xanthochromic (yellow) Blood fluid is due to trauma.
3. Clarity — transparent (normal), opaque, or translucent.
4. Viscosity — normally very high; may be low or very low (watery).
5. Mucin clot — good (normal); fair, or poor.
6. Spontaneous Clot — Normal synovial fluid does not clot, as it lacks in fibrinogen, prothrombin, factors V and VII etc. But pathologic fluids do clot; rapidity and size vary with the underlying lesion.

B. **Microscopic Cytology** —

1. Total W.B.C. count per c.m.m.

**Normal** = less than 150. Increased in pathological conditions. In degenerative lesions up to 3,000 and in inflammatory conditions 3,000 and much above.

2. Differential leucocytic count —

Normal — polymorphonuclear cells are less than 25%. In inflammatory lesions — much above 25%, up to 90% even.

3. Wet smear inspection by polarised and phase contrast microscopy —

(a) "Inclusion body cells" or "ragocytes" (rasin cells), originally called "RA Cells". It is not disease specific, may be found in joint fluids of inflammatory disorders. They are polymorphonuclear leucocytes with ingested or phagocytosed material, including immunoglobulin G and M.Rh factors, fibrin, antinuclear factors, immune complexes and DNA particulars.

(b) Classic "L.E. Cells" are seen in Write's stained smears. It consists of a W.B.C. with a large purple-red homogeneous globulin inclusion body, which compresses the nucleus against the cell membrane.

It must be differentiated from "tart" cells, polymorphonuclear W.B.C. that have phagocytosed nuclear debris.

(c) "Reiter's Cells" are not again disease specific (an inconstant feature of Reiter's syndrome) has been found in many inflammatory joint fluids. The cells are macrophages with ingested polymorphs (dead and degranulated).

(d) In rheumatoid arthritis, the synovial fluid is found to contain a large number of lymphoblasts, over half of all large mononuclear cells.

**Crystals in synovial fluid :-**

| CRYSTALS | DISEASES |
|---|---|
| (i) Monosodium urate monohydrate (M S U ) | Gout |
| (ii) Calcium pyrophosphate dihydrate (C P P D) | Pseudo-gout |
| (iii) Dicalcium phosphate<br>(iv) Apatite | In calcifications and Degenerative lesions. |
| (v) Adrenal corticosteroid esters | Iatrogenic post-infection flare. |

**BLOOD EXAMINATIONS**

| | | | |
|---|---|---|---|
| Cellular Component : | Haemoglobin & type of anaemia | Total W.B.C. Platelet count | Differential Count |
| | Inclusion bodies and abnormal cells. | | |
| Plasma Component : | E.S.R | Serological reactions (e.g. for Rh factor etc). | |
| | Immunoglobulins antibodies — IgG, IgA, IgM, IgD, IgE. | Serum Proteins — Albumin, Globulin, Fibrinogen — C.R.P. | |
| | Auto-antibodies — e.g ANA, anti-DNA etc. | 'Complement' plasma Proteins, e.g. C3, C4 etc. | |

C. **Microbiologic tests :-**

(a) Culture for bacteria, fungi, viruses, or tubercular bacilli.

(b) Smear & culture of joint fluid for microbes, for detection of their antigens by counter-current immuno-electrophoresis.

D. **Serologic tests**

(a) Total protein content — Normal — 1.8g/dl.

(b) Total Haemolytic Complement (C H50) — titration : It measures the functional activity of all complement component proteins in synovial fluid — Normal — very low level of C' H50.

E. **Chemical tests for :**

(a) Glucose.
(b) Protein.
(c) Enzymes.

II. Synovial membrane — Biopsy & histology
III. Subchondral Bone
IV. Articular Cartilage

**Extra articular biopsy :**

(i) Subcutaneous Nodules and other depositions.
(ii) Muscle Biopsy.

To determine the type of anaemia, Mean Corpuscular Volume (MCV) and Mean Corpuscular Haemoglobin (MCH), should be determined :-

— Macrocytic, Normocytic, or Microcytic
— Hyperchromic, Normochromic or Hypochromic.
} Type of anaemia.

The study of lymphocytes and lymphoblasts are important. Inclusion bodies and abnormal cells were discussed under Synovial fluid examination.

**Erythrocyte Sedimentation Rate (ESR)**

It is the "single important laboratory test" which indicates and is proportionate to the inflammatory activity in the connective tissue diseases. It is the property of the plasma component, and is influenced by the fibrinogen, and alpha-and gamma-globulins content in plasma.

It is not a specific or diagnostic test, ESR is normal in degenerative conditions and fibrositis. In congestive heart failure, especially in young patients with rheumatic carditis, the E.S.R. is lowered. According to some rheumatologists, the C-reactive protein (CRP) and hepatoglobin are more accurate than the ESR for serial evaluation of rheumatoid activity and are not depressed by hormone therapy.

The invading agents (e.g. bacteria, rickettsia, virus etc.) and foreign antigens trigger on the defensive mechanism (immunocomplex response) of the body to produce antibodies (which are of different types and natures) and 'antigen-antibody complexes'.

Immunoglobulins (Ig) are antibodies and are heterogenous proteins, synthesised primarily in plasma cells, and is formed in serum and extra-cellularfluids. Five major classes of immunoglobulins (Ig) are —

IgG, IgA, IgM, IgD, and IgE..

They are studied by electrophoretic and immuno electrophoretic analysis of serum and urine.

'Antigen - antibody complexes' again activates the compliment system consisting of 18 plasma proteins, which helps the defensive mechanism of the host to recognise the foreign antigen and to generate the mediators. They are responsible for haemolysis of antibody sensitised B.B.C.

Sometimes, the defensive reactions become "out of bounds" and produce antibodies against host's own structures, without recognising them. They are called 'auto-antibodies', e.g. antinuclear antibodies (ANA), anti-DNAantibodies etc. They are useful in diagnosis and prognosis of the cases.

## EPIDEMIOLOGY OF RHEUMATIC DISORDERS :-

A disease should be understood and studied from all aspects, so that it can be efficiently diagnosed, treated and controlled. Epidemiology means the effect of the disease on population at large. ('Epi' means upon; 'demos' means people; 'logy' means science). This broad methodology is related to —

| Clinical Medicine — to determine specific treatment (Curative), and 'Diagnostic Criteria'. | Laboratory Diagnosis (Diagnostic) | Public Health — Control of the disease (Preventive) |
|---|---|---|

The methodology includes the study of prevalance, distribution, and all the associated factors releated to the disease, by population survey. The following aspects of the disease are recorded and studied :-

1. Prevalance (P), incidence or rate of occurrence (I), average duration of the diseases (D), in a given population, of a demarcated area. $P = I \times D$. are determined.
2. The following factors which influences the disease incidence (I) and prognosis are :- 'Onset-age', Sex, Races and Socio-economic condition, etc.
3. The disease is studied and 'classified'; and also specified with 'Diagnostic Criteria' determined
4. Sensitivity and specificity of the disease in a given population.
5. Where the disease is infectious or communicable or not.
6. The methods of control of the disease.
7. The 'causation' of the disease, and the associated factors, i.e. the complete aetiology is thoroughly studied.

In rheumatology, most of the disease have multifactorial aetiology; interactions of those factors with the body's defensive mechanism produces a complicated immuno-complex pathogenesis. These interactions of multiple factors are related to the 'Host', 'Causative agents' and 'Environmental conditions'. Primary cause of aetiology is thus obscured, and the triggering factors come to the limelight, which are either exogenous precipitating factors, or endogenous predisposing factors in the host. Epidemiological studies show a large number of factors influencing the disease, but the original definite cause or infection is still not known. The initial primary infection of short duration starts an immuno-complex mechanism in the body, which again sets up secondary infection or infection-like mechanism affecting some selected structures (e.g. joints) along with systemic manifestations giving rise to the characteristic picture of the disease.

The 'Host factors' influencing the disease are Age, Sex, Race, Hereditary factors, different susceptible systems or organs of the body, etc. The causative agents may be bacteria, virus, mycoplasma, or rickettsia with their antigenic structures. The environmental conditions influencing the disease are toxic materials, climatic conditions, geographical distributions etc.

The aim of this chapter is to impress the importance of studying the rheumatological disorder from different scientific angles to diagnose them specifically, and to treat and rehabilitate the chronically ill patients in the society as tolerant, productive and happy individuals. The incidences of these diseases are no more thought to be rare in this country as in the past. With the increased expectation of life, increased stress and strain of modern life, and better diagnostic methodology are bringing more rheumatological cases to the limelight, not only in this country but all over the world. The medical students and the clinicians are expected to get more benefit from reading this chapter, once before and re-reading it again after they have studied the individual diseases, discussed in the following chapters.

To conclude, a simple survey-chart of some of the rheumatological disorders or syndromes are presented to have a glimpse of the diseases to be studied. Table 13.1 presents important features of these disorders. Fig.13.1 presents bird's eye view.

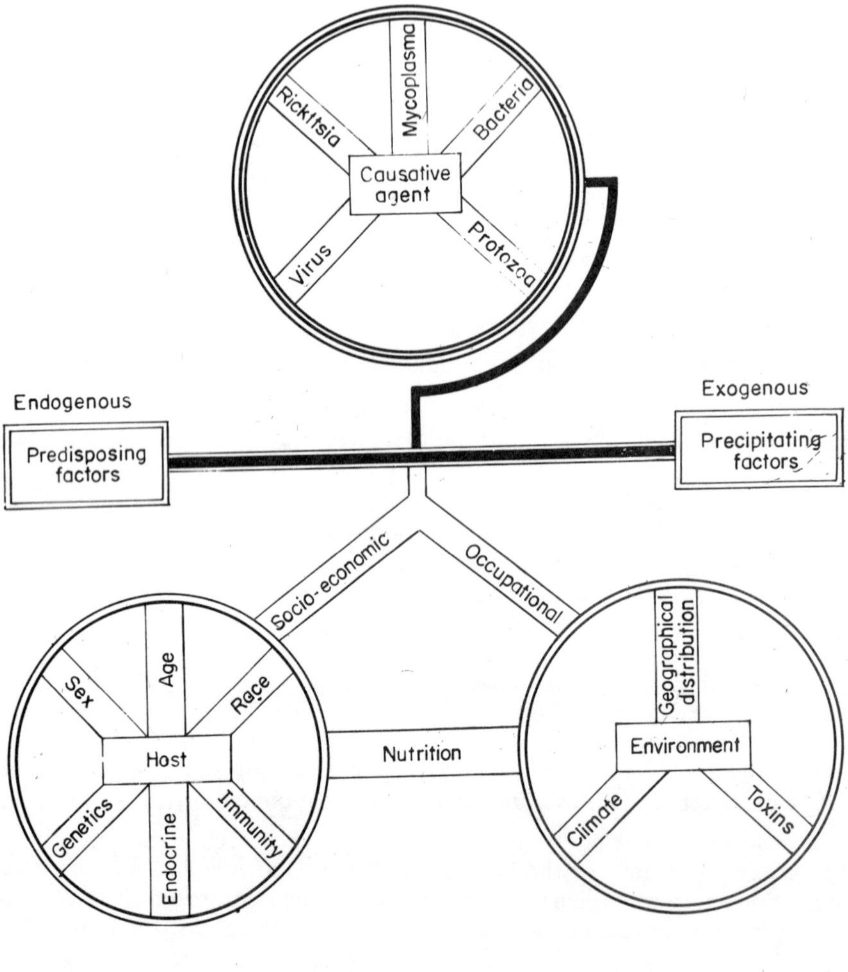


Fig.13.1 : Multifactorial contributions to etiology :
(Tricycle : 'Host' – 'Causative agent' – 'Environment')

**Table 13.1 : Rheumatoid Disorders and Syndromes**

| RHEUMATOLOGICAL DISEASES/SYNDROMES | AGE (IN YEARS) | SEX RATIO (M = MALE) (F = FEMALE) | RACIAL SUSCEPTIBILITY B = Black W = White | GENETIC PREDISPOSITION | CARDINAL FEATURES | GEOGRAPHICAL DISTRIBUTION & CLIMATIC VARIATION : |
|---|---|---|---|---|---|---|
| 1. **Spondylo-arthritic** Syndromes :- 1. Rheumatoid Arthritis | All ages Increases with age | F : M = 3 : 1 | All races | Polygenic pattern of **inheritance associated** with histocompatible antigen – HLA – $DW_4$ | **"Morning stiffness" Progressive symmetrical polyarthritis, with remissions and exacerbations & Systemic S/S. Normocytic hypochromic anemia. X-Ray – Erosive arthritis. Rh factor – 60% (+) ve, or 40% negative.** | Sporadic/Endemic, – all over the world. |
| 2. Ankylosing Spondylitis | 15 to 35. **– Young adults** | M : F = 4 : 1 | All races | Histocompatible cell surface antigen HLA – B 27 positive in (63 to 96% cases) | Progressive Arthritis and ankylosis of S.I. joints and spine, with acute pain & stiffness. Associated features – Iritis, Prostatitis, non-specific Urethritis, and Ulcerative colitis. | Sporadic/Endemic – all over the world. |
| 3. Reiter's Syndrome | 20 to 40 – young adults | M > F Common in young males | All races | Histocompatible lymphocyte surface antigen H L A – $B_{27}$, positive in 70 to 96% cases. | 'H' of (i) sexual intercourse transmission, (ii) Epidemic **dysentery.** ***Clinical 'triad'*** :- Polyarthritis, – Urethritis, – Conjunctivitis. + Muco-cutaneous lesion, diarr-**hoea/dysentery & fever. Sero-negative for Rh factor.** | Sporadic/Endemic + occasional Epidemic with epidemic dysentery. |
| 4. Psoriatic Arthritis | 15 to 55. – common in young adults (30 to 35) | F : M = 1.04 : 1 | All races | Multifactorial pattern of inheritance – Histo-compatible typing – H L A – BW 17, H L A – B 13, H L A – B12, H L A – B 27 positive in 70% cases. | – Skin lesions of psoriasis. – **Asymmetric poly-arthritis** of hands and feet, S.I. jts. and spine. – **X-ray shows errosive and** atrophic arthritis. –Sero-negative for Rh factor | Sporadic/Endemic – all over the world. |
| 5. Enteropathic Arthritis | 25 to 45 | Peripheral (a) Arthritic Group (M : F = 1:1) **(b) Spondylitis Group.** (M : F = 2.4 : 1) | All races | H L A – B 27 – antigen positive in 70% cases. | – Peripheral Arthritis and/ or Spondylitis. – Erythema nodosum and stomatitis. – Colitis, Proctitis, – **Uveitis** (Eye). – **Seronegative (Rh factor).** – **X-ray shows erosive** arthritis, Periarteritis & **marked periarticular soft** tissue swelling. | Sporadic/Endemic + occasional Epidemic on tropical country – Worse in summer. |

| | | | | | | |
|---|---|---|---|---|---|---|
| II. **Degenerative Group** Osteoarthrosis (osteoarthritis)<br>A) Primary —<br>B) Secondary — | After 40. | F > M | All races except Eskimos get less | **Unknown inherited pre-disposition** | — Painful swelling and stiffness of weight bearing joints mainly, with other **peripheral joints**<br>**Heberden's Nodes —**<br>— Instability and deformity of joints. X-ray : Degenerative changes, with — lipping, osteophytes, and cysts. Seronegative for Rh factor. | Sporadic and Endemic, in aged persons all over the world. |
| III. **Metabolic disorder :-** Gout | Over 30 | M > F | In all races; more in intellectual people. | **Inherited inborn error of metabolism; Genetically determined or acquired.** | **Acute onset** — Extremely painful, tender, monoarticular (90%) arthritis, with little constitutional symptoms, beginning at night usually 1st M.T. of **great toe.**<br>**Chronic** Poly-articular arthritis, — recurrent attacks with intervals of complete freedom. **Serum uric acid** — 6.8 mg/dt. or more (Normal) 3.5 mg/dt.) —<br>**X-ray** — Erosive punched out changes and over-hanging margins. | All over the world. |
| IV **Collagen Diseases :**<br>1. "Systemic Lupus Erythromatosus (SLE) | Any age. (Peak age = 15 to 25) | F : M = 9 : 1 i.e. 90% patients are female | All races. B : W = 4 : 1 | — Immune deficiency, particularly $I_gA$ & $C_2$ Histocompatible antigens H L A — A10 & H L A — B18 present | Chronic inflammatory disease with remissions and **exacerbations affecting multiple systems due to vasculitis :-**<br>(i) Skin rash (e.g. butterfly rash). (ii) Arthritis without deformity/Arthralgia.<br>(iii) Nephritis. (iv) Serosites — **(pleural effusion, pericarditis)** (v) Nervous system-(psychosis, convulsion etc.) | All over the world<br>All climate (worse in cold) |

| | | | | | | |
|---|---|---|---|---|---|---|
| 2. Polymyositis and<br><br>Dermatomyositis : (Classified into five clinical types) | All ages.<br><br>— Bimodal peak :<br>— 10 to 14<br>— 45 to 64 | F : M<br><br>= 2 : 1 | All races,<br><br>B : W<br>= 4 : 1 | Positive mediated through hyper-sensitivity. | Inflammatory and degenerative lesions of striated muscles, resulting in spontaneous remissions and exacerbations of (i) symmetric myalgia (weakness and atrophy). (ii) Skin lesions on face, neck, arm etc.<br>(iii) Arthritis without deformity/Arthralgia. (iv) Raynaud's phenomenon.<br>(v) Dysphagia etc. | All over the world.<br>All climate — worse in cold. |
| 3. Progressive Systemic Sclerosis (P.S.S.) or Scleroderma. | 30 to 50 | F : M<br>= 4 : 1 | All races,<br>B : W<br>= 4 : 1 | Immunologically determined; genetic predisposition present. | Generalised progressive, with characteristic 'CREST' syndrome :-<br>C = Calcinosis.<br>R = Raynaud's — Phenomenon<br>E = Esophageal dysfunction<br>S = Sclerodactyly.<br>T = Telangiectasis. | All over the world.<br>Worse in cold climate. |
| 4. Polymyalgia rheumatica | Over 50 | F M | Usually Caucasian Race | Genetic predisposition present | Sudden onset of —<br>(i) Severe pain in neck, back, shoulders, upper arms & thighs.<br>(ii) **Morning stiffness and swelling — + +**<br>(iii) Non-specific systemic features :-<br>fever, anorexia, weight loss, lassitude, apathy and depression.<br>(iv) Often associated with Carpal-tunnel syndrome.<br>(v) High E.S.R., high fibrinogen and anaemia.<br>(vi) Dramatically relieved with steroids. | |

# RHEUMATOID ARTHRITIS

*G.C. MOOKERJEE*

## INTRODUCTION

Although the precise cause of rheumatoid arthritis (R.A.) is not yet established, it is possibly true that in genetically predisposed persons, continuous antigenic stimulation (be it viral or bacterial) may lead to a chronic synovial injury and gradual destruction of joints if the process is not arrested by treatment. The histocompatibility antigen HLA-DRw4 is found in 70% or patients with R.A. (Harrison, 1983) and in most patients the serum and joint fluid may contain heterogeneous antibodies called rheumatoid factors. These are IgA/IgG and IgM antiglobulins as well as antinuclear and anticollagen antibodies. Much evidence has collected to show that autoimmune phenomena and excessive immune complex activity are present in this disease. It is also evident however, that the rheumatoid factors by themselves are not solely responsible for the pathogenesis of R.A. since they are found in many other chronic infections.

The presence of immune complexes, complement components, together with lymphocytes and plasma cells on particular cartilage synovium and in the phagocytic cells of the joint are also suggestive of the immunological mechanism in the causation of R.A. Immune complexes in R.A. do not require an exogenous antigen but are formed by the IgG, Rh factors when these IgG molecules possess both the antibody specifically and the antigenic determinant. The activation of complement components leads to influx of neutrophils into the joint and therefore the synovial fluid contains complement components, total haemolytic complement and their breakdown products.

The causes of tissue injuty in R.A. are :-

(a) Phagocytosis of immune complexes by polymorph leucocytes liberate lysosomal enzymes and the superoxide ion which damages cell membranes, kills cells and depolymerized hyaluronic acid.

(b) Macrophages release enzymes that degrade joint structures.

(c) Collagenase cleaves collagen, making it susceptible to other proteases, depolymerized protoglycans.

(d) Prostaglandins (produced by synovial cells) stimulate osteoclasts and cause bone resorption while osteoclast activating factor from mononuclear leucocytes also enhances the process.

(e) Plenty of T cells in the synovium release lymphokins leading to inflammation of joints.

All these factors lead to destruction of articular cartilage and subchondral bone which are the features of R.A.

The extraarticular features of R.A. probably are due to humoral immune mechanisms involving immune complexes having IgM or IgG Rh factors and patients with acute vasculitic lesions have minimally depressed serum complement levels.

## EPIDEMIOLOGY

R.A. may occur in all age groups but is commonly seen in the 3rd and 4th decades. Women to men ratio is about 3 : 1. Cold climates may aggravate symptoms, but do not alter the course of the disease. Poor living conditions in developing countries also aggravate it.

## PATHOLOGY

Initially there is infiltration of the synovial membrane and overlying connective tissue with lymphocytes, plasma cells and macrophages which leads to swelling and congestion along with an increase in effusion of synovial fluid into the joint spine during the active phase leading to hypertrophy of the synovial membrane and ultimately granulation tissue (pannus) is formed under the articular cartilage, which is progressively destroyed. Finally fibrous adhesions form between the layers of the pannus across the joint space leading to fibrous or bony ankylosis, while adjacent muscles atrophy. All these factors cause subluxation of the joint. Subcutaneous nodules (caused by small vessel vasculitis) have central areas of fibrinoid material (swollen and fragmented collagen fibres), fibrinous exudate and cellular debris. These zonal areas are surrounded by a pallisade of radically arranged proliferating mononucleal cells. The nodule is encapsulated by loose fibrous tissue. These granulomatous lesions may occur in pleura, lung, pericardium, sclera and over pressure points (e.g. elbows, sacrum). Lymph nodes may be hyperplastic showing numerous lymphoid follicles with large germinal centres, plasma cells are numerous in the sinuses and medullary cords of the lymph nodes. Histologically the nodes may sometimes resemble giant follicular lymphoma.

**Predisposing causes**

(1) Heredity and familial tendency are both important factors.

(2) Septic focus is often blamed but not definitely proved. But better not to have them.

(3) Environment — Damp climate is often blamed. It is common in India also.

(4) Infection, trauma, nutritional deficiency may have some role to play.

(5) Psychological trauma often precipitating and aggravating factor.

## CLINICAL FEATURES

The disease usually comes into the scene in most unsuspected manner. At the beginning there is mild ache and stiffness of small units of the hands, wrist and feet, especially in the morning called morning stiffness. Even these symptoms may be preceded by muscular aches and they symptoms may gradually start in one or two joints often symmetrically. Unlike migrating arthritis or rheumatic fever, arthralgia or arthritis and periarthritis lingers on and gradually other joints are affected over months or years.

Proximal interphalyngeal joints (P.I.P.) and later metacarpophalyngeal joints (M.C.P.) are commonly involved in early stages, joints gradually become swollen, tender, warm with tense dusky skin surface. Movements become very painful, small joints bear the main brunt but wrists, ankle and elbow joints may be later on affected but shoulder, hip and spinal joints are usually spread.

Rarely R.A. starts as an acute disease with high lever, polyarthritis, vasculitis and rheumatoid pneumonia.

Raynaud's phenomenon is often present. Tenderness, warmth and swelling (the synovium becoming palpable as boggy tissue around the joints) and a bluish discolouration in fair skinned persons is characteristic. The severity of the disease is reflected in the atrophy of surrounding muscles, while a limited range of movement leads to "swan-neck, cock-up-toes and boutonniere" deformities. Volar subluxation and ulnar deviation of the metacarpo-phalyngeal joints along with tender nodules and tenosynovitis may cause the "trigger finger", (or carpal tunnel syndrome, if median nerve is pressed while flexion contractures of knees and hips greatly hinder ambulation. Subluxation of the atlanto-axial joint may cause cord compression leading to bladder dysfunction. Sphincter disturbances and even sudden death. Temporomandibular joint involvement makes chewing difficult and hoarseness of voice may result due to affection of crico-arytenoid joints; even severe upper airway obstruction is possible.

A popliteal cyst may develop with synovitis of the knee joint due to herniation or rupture of synovium posteriorly, which may rupture stimulating thrombophlebitis and may be confirmed by arthrography. Rheumatoid vasculitis produces nail fold thrombi, small infarcts on the volar surface of hand digital gangrene and ulcer of the calf and ankle, while motor-sensory symptoms result from vasculitis of the vasa nervorum and the cranial, mesenteric and even coronary vessels may become involved. Keratoconjunctivitis sicca (Sjogren's syndrome), uveitis, episcleritis may occur and a nodule may perforate the sclera (scleromalacia perforans). Dysphagia and dysparunia may also occur. Involvement of the lungs consists of development of single or multiple nodules, diffuse interstitial fibrosis, pleural effusion and rheumatoid pneumonitis.

The pleural fluid may show low glucose/high LDH level. In patients with pneumoconiosis, multiple pulmonary nodules along with rheumatoid arthritis is called "Caplans syndrome". Pericarditis with cardiac tamponade is rarely seen. Aortic regurgitiation, conduction abnormalities and myocardial infarction (involvement of coronary vessels) may also occur. Rheumatoid arthritis may also affect initial valves leading to rheumatoid mitral stenosis (known as Jaccuad type of mitral stenosis). Splenomegaly, lymphadenopathy (generalised) and amyloidosis (causing renal failure) may occur rarely.

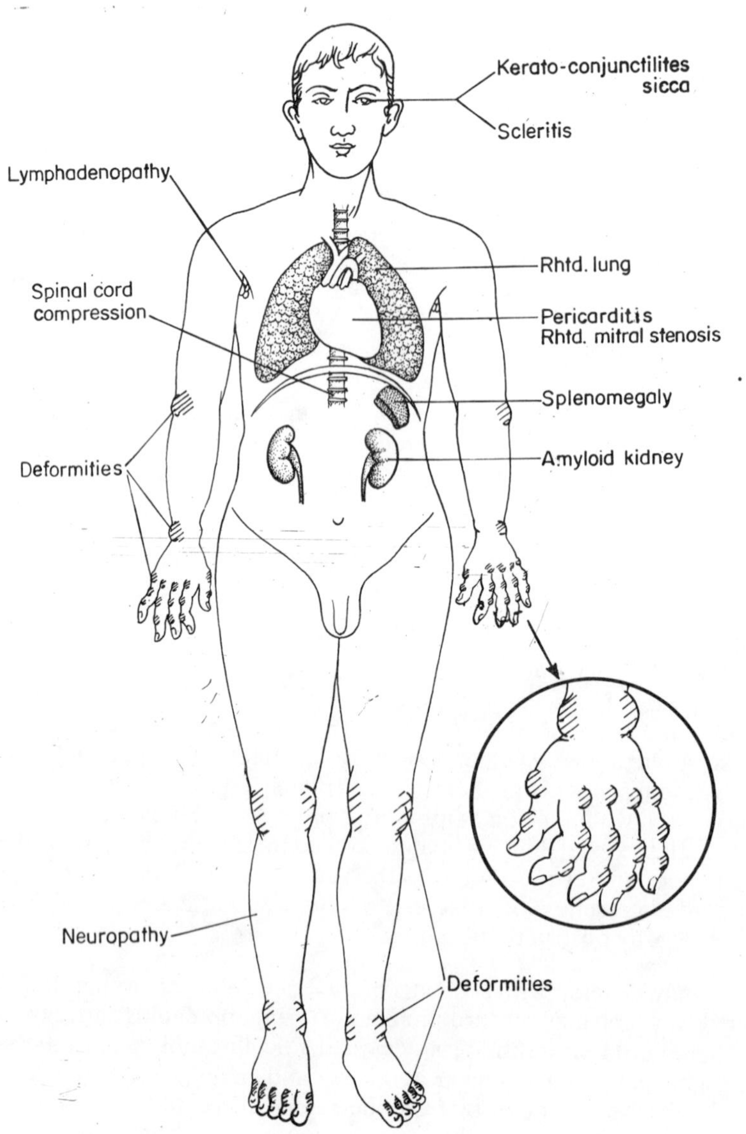


Fig.13.2 : Manifestations of rheumatoid arthritis

**Felty's syndrome** is R.A. splenomegaly and neutropenia.

**Still's disease** is Juvenile R.A. characterised by high spiking fever, polyarthralgias, myalgias, maculopapular rashes, pericarditis, sore throat, pneumonitis, lymphadenopathy, splenomegaly and pain abdomen.

## COURSE

It is highly variable but a high titre of Rh. factor, multiple nodules and vasculitis, proclaims a poor prognosis. Usually it is a chronic disease.

## LABORATORY FINDINGS

Normocytic, normochromic (or hypochromic) anaemia with a low serum iron and total iron binding capacity is found, together with mild leukocytosis, eosinophilia, thrombocytopenia and high ESR level (sometimes neutropenia may be present). Raised ESR usually indicates activity of disease, but this is not always so and Coomb's test may be positive. Haemolytic anaemia is sometimes seen. Elevated gamma globulin and $alpha_2$ globulin with low albumin is seen on protein electrophoresis. The Rose Waller test (Sheep cell agglutination test or SCAT) may be positive in 70% of cases. Human erythrocyte agglutination test (HEAT) or the differential agglutination test (DAT) is used to detect IgM Rh. factor. The SCAT is sensitive but it is not specific but the HEAT and DAT tests are specific but not so sensitive.

Significant titres are SCAT 1 : 32, DAT 1 : 16 and Latex fixation test 1 : 20. The Rose Waller test may be positive in SLE, scleroderma and Sjogren's syndrome as well as many other diseases like sarcoidosis, chronic liver disease etc. Antinuclear factor is present in 30% of R.A. patients.

## RADIOLOGY

Initially only soft tissue swelling of joints may be seen, but with progressive periarticular osteoporosis, narrowing of joint spaces with marginal erosions and ultimately "cup & pencil" deformities and massive bone resorption (arthritis multilans) develop. Marginal sclerosis and osteophyte formation indicate secondary osteoarthritis.

## DIAGNOSIS

Clinical picture, elevated ESR, positive Rh. factor, and radiological findings usually clinch the diagnosis.

Low total haemolytic complement (CH 50) in synovial fluid is common; rarely arthroscopy and synovial biopsy is required to exclude tuberculosis, pigmented villonodular synovitis and synovial tumours. Gram's stain excludes any infective aetiology.

### General measures

This consists of rest to mind and body. Attend to joint pain, optimum position of limbs and support. Splinting may be initially required in acute stage and physiotherapy is absolutely essential.

Analgesics, sedatives, good diet, iron and additional vitamins may be prescribed, where indicated.

Expert physiotherapy, hydrotherapy, warm bath, paraffin bath help in relief of pain and allow movements.

### Drug therapy

The drugs used in RA belong to three groups; anti-inflammatory agents, remission inducing agents and immune suppressive (cytotoxic) agents.

However, in all cases it is better to give a trial to aspirin group, as they are cheap and effective. But aspirin may also cause gastro-intestinal bleeding rarely.

**Anti-inflammatory agents** — At first the non-steroidal anti-inflammatory drugs (NSAID) are to be used; these are aspirin, phenyl-butazone, oxyphenbutazone, indomethacin, propionic acid derivatives (e.g. ibuprofen, ketoprofen, naproxen), 2nd generation propionic and acetic acid derivatives (e.g. flurbiprofen), salindac, alcofenac, fendofenae, and tolmetin), 3rd generation propionic acid derivatives (e.g. piroxicam, feribufen) feriamates (e.g. mafenomic acid, flufenamic acid). Enotic acid derivation (e.g. azarpropzone, feprazone).

Among the new ones declofenac sodium (Diclomax, voveran) appears to be promising.

**Gluco-corticoids** are considered anti-inflammatory drugs. Since they do not alter the cause of the diseases, in spite of possible remission, their long term use even in low dosage, is not recommended in view of side-effects. Sometimes intraarticular steroid (hydrocortisone) injections may tide over acute problems. However, judicious steroid therapy may sometimes be essential.

**Remission Inducing Agents** — These drugs may modify the course of the disease and they may be used simultaneously with the NSAID. These include penicillamine and gold salts (gold sodium thiomalate called Myocrisin) gold thioglucose (Solganol) and suranofin (an oral form). The gold salts are slow-acting suppressive anti-R.A. drugs, which have been proved to reduce disease activity, as well as to decrease erosive charges. Due to their toxicity (dermatitis, stomatitis, pruritus, membranous glomerulonephritis) they are to be used only in patients with active progressive disease with erosive/deformative changes, with nodules and/or high titer of Rh. factor, or patients requiring high doses of steroids and not responsive to antimalarials.

**Antimalarials** — In many patients chloroquine phosphate (250 mg daily) or hydroxy-chloroquine sulphate (200 mg b.d.) have shown clinical benefit. Long-term use may cause nausea, diarrhoea, rash, haemolytic anaemia, ototoxicity and neuromyopathy. Deposits on the cornea and even retinopathy may occur causing permanent visual damage. Clinical improvement usually occurs after 8 to 12 weeks and prolonged treatment for over six months may be required. Some authorities recommend that it should not be given more than ten months, and it longer treatment is required, it should be used only ten months in a year. Even daily dose of 250 mg may be toxic if used without break; weekly dose should be kept below 1750 mg. It is better to give it six days in a week. So they should be used very carefully and ophthalmological assessment every three months is advisable. These drugs however do not retard progression of radiological changes.

**Immuno-Suppressive agents** — These drugs are used only life-threatening extra-articular manifestations not responding to the previously mentioned agents and in steroid dependent patients.

**Azathioprine** (1.25 mg/kg to 2-5 mg/kg of body weight) is effective, but dosage must be reduced in patient receiving allopurinol. The side-effects are nausea, vomiting, stomatitis, diarrhea, hepatitis and bone marrow suppression. Fortnightly blood counts are essential for monitoring.

**Cyclophosphamide** — This alkylating agent is effective in dosage of 1-2 mg/kg while side effects include alopecia, bladder toxicity, azoospermia and anovulation, as well as G.I. tract disturbance, bone marrow suppression and teratogenesis. Urinalysis and blood counts should be checked fortnightly, 6-mercaptopurine, chlorambucil and methotrexate are also rarely used.

**Levamisole** — This anthelmintic is an immuno-modulator, which augments T-lymphocyte response, polymorph and macrophage chemotaxis and phagocytosis and may be effective in R.A. in dosage of 150 mg weekly.

There is however a great risk of agranulocytosis even with two weekly blood counts. The drug needs further evaluation.

**Surgical treatment** — Surgical decompression and synovectomy of wrist joint and tendon sheaths, are often needed when other measures fail.

Reconstructive tendon surgery, osteotomy, arthrodesis, and arthoplasties with or without prosthesis may be essential for rehabilitation. Total hip replacement has been performed with remarkable success in recent years.

**Supportive therapy** — Attention to general health, eradication of septic foci especially dental care and psychotherapy are all very important. Anxiolytic drugs and tranquilizers also may be required. In acute stage rest is essential for two to four weeks. Splints may be needed for short periods with active exercise of muscles. Anaemia should be treated with iron therapy. Warm baths, wax-baths and warm swimming pool exercises are often rewarding.

## GOUT

*G.C.MOOKERJEE*

### Definition

It is a group of disorders associated with hyperuricaemia giving rise to deposits of monosodium urate, monohydrate crystals on various body tissues like joints, tendons and the kidney causing inflammatory arthritis, tenosynovitis, cellulitis, bursitis, urolithiasis or urate nephropathy and tophaceous deposits. Although all cases of gout must necessarily have hyperuricaemia, all cases of hyperuricaemia does not lead to gout and asymptomatic hyperuricaemia is commoner than gout.

**Epidemology** — Post-pubertal males are most commonly affected, and hyperuricaemia correlates positively with obesity, haemoglobin, high social class, high alcohol habit, high protein intake and urban habitant. Thus gouty arthritis is a disease of the affluent sedentary classes.

The normal plasma uric acid level varies between 0.12 and 0.42 mmol (2 and 7 mg/100 ml.) and hyperuricaemia exists when levels above 0.42 mml/litre in adult males and above 0.36 mmol/1 in adult females is found.

**Aetiology of Hyperuricaemia and Gout** — An increase in the production of uric acid or a decrease in the excretion or a combination of the two mechanisms may cause hyperuricaemia and these mechanisms are determined by many genetic and environmental factors.

(a) Increasedproduction occurs in about a quarter of all gout patients and they are hyperexcreters of uric acid (as long as the kidney functions normally). Myeloproliferative disorders, psoriasis, HGPRT deficiency, $G_6$ PD deficiency.

(b) Decreased excretion occurs in three quarters of gouty patients. Some genetic defect in the fractional urate excretion is said to be present (e.g. lactic acidaemia in alcoholism, exercise, starvation, vomiting, toxaemia of pregnancy or renal failure in diabetics, pyrazinamide, low dose aspirin, hypertension, hyperparathyroidism, myxoedema and Down's syndrome.

(c) Certain specific enzyme defects may lead to hyperuricaemia, and these should be suspected when gout occurs at an early age, where there is a family history of gout or when tricacid lithiasis is the presenting feature. (e.g. deficiency of GHPRT (Lesch-Nyham syndrome) PRPP (phosphoribosyl, pyrophosphate synthetase, overacting, hypoxanthene-gunanine-phosphoribasyl transferase $G_6$ PD deficiency glucose 6 phosphatase deficiency).

(d) Idiopathic, when no other cause can be detected.

## ACUTE GOUT

### CLINICAL FEATURES

The metatarsophalangeal joint of the great toe is the commonest site of the initial attack, in 70% cases, after which the ankle, knee, small joints of hands, feet, and elbow following that order of frequency. The onset may be severe, during sleep or may also be insidious. The joint is red, hot, swollen with shinny overlying skin. Pain and tenderness is present. Fever with leucocytosis and high ESR may be present, but prodromal symptoms like anorexia, nausea, or mood changes may be seen in the insidious type. Untreated may have spontaneous remissions in a few days or weeks, followed by desquamation and pruritis. Acute attacks may occur after unusual physical exercise, surgery, systemic illness, trauma, allopurinol therapy, uricosuric drugs, severe dietary restriction, diuretic drugs or alcohol excess. After the first attack, there are usually repeated attacks until it becomes a continuous state of acute or subacute gout.

**Chronic gout** — Tophaceous deposits characterize chronic gout, and they can cause cartilage and bone erosion, severe functional impairment and gross joint deformities. They are to be found in the pinna, bursae and tendon sheaths, or in the carpal tunnel, if the median nerve is compressed. Rarely paraplegia or heart block may occur depending on the site of deposition.

When glomerulosclerosis, renal tubular obstruction, tophi formation lead to hypertension, it invites secondary pyelonephritis and chronic urate nephropathy may result. Sometimes this may occur without any inborn error of metabolism on autosomal dominant inherited disease.

Ischaemic heart disease, diabetes mellitus, obesity, type-IV hyperlipoproteinemia and hypertension may all be associated with gout and hyperuricaemia.

## INVESTIGATIONS

(1) Blood uric acid level (not conclusive)

(2) Synovial fluid aspiration and examination under polarised light may be done. In acute cases the serum uric acid level may be normal, especially in joints treated with allopurinol or NSAID. X-ray pictures are not useful because by the time characteristic changes appear (punched but erosions soft tissue swelling of tophic) the diagnosis has been already established.

## TREATMENT

Acute attacks of gout need urgent relief as the condition is very painful. The drug of choice is colchicine to be started without delay, i.e. as soon as signs of exacerbation takes place. To start with, dosage should be 1.0 mg every 2 hours till the pain stops or toxic symptoms appear. In 80% of cases acute attacks are relieved by colchicine. Total dose varies from 4 to 6 mg on the first day. Diarrhoea and abdominal pain can be relieved by belladonna or atropine preparation along with diphenoxylate (Lomotil).

**Colchicine** is, however, contraindicated if there is suspicion of peptic ulcer or hepatorenal disease. Usually most patients learn to use the drug in future attacks. Once the acute pain relieved, the dosage of the drug is reduced till the joint swelling subsides and is then gradually tailed off.

**Indomethacin, phenylbutazone and oxyphenbutazone** are also very effective drugs and can be used as alternative drugs. Though these drugs do not cause abdominal cramp, vomiting and diarrhoea, yet these are not tolerated in peptic ulcer cases. Toxic effects may rarely occur even in short-term courses.

**Steroids and ACTH** are also remarkably effective but these are never routinely used, unless patients are not relieved with the above drugs or there are contraindications. Moreover, once steroids and ACTH are discontinued, there is always a chance of relapse.

**Uricosuric drugs** — These drugs reduce the production of uric acid and help excretion of urates in urine. These are indicated when repeated attacks are occurring and they produce very good results when used concurrently with small doses of colchicine (0.5 mg two or three times daily).

**Probenacid (or Benemid)** — It is given in dosage of 0.5 to 2.0 g daily combined with or without colchicine and can be very useful in reducing uric acid. Rarely causes nephrotic syndrome.

**Sulphinpyrazone (Anturan)** is given in dosage of 100 mg twice or thrice daily up to 400 mg per day.

Side-effects should be watched. Rarely causes bone marrow depression.

**Allopurinol (Zyloric)** — It is a drug which acts as xanthine oxidase inhibitor and so it reduces plasma urate, as also help in mobilizing tophaceous deposits. Dose 100 mg twice or thrice daily. Toxic effects should be watched, for it can produce renal damage and even epidermal necrolysis.

Symptomatic and supportive treatment should also be done, e.g. use of sedatives, analgesics and antibiotics in presence of associated infection, diabetes mellitus. I.H.D. and hypertension are often associated and require careful management.

## PROPHYLACTIC TREATMENT

In having gouty nephropathy, or recurrent attacks, chronic gouty arthritis or markedly raised urate levels, prophylactic treatment is advised.

Side-effects should be carefully watched. Rarely it produces leucopenia, hepatic damage and occasionally haemosiderosis.

## PROPHYLACTIC TREATMENT

In having gouty nephropathy, or recurrent attacks, chronic gouty arthritis or markedly raised urate levels, prophylactic treatment is advised.

Allopurinol inhibits conversion of xanthine to hypoxanthine and uric acid. It is started with 300 mg daily along with colchicine 0.5 mg BD, many weeks after the acute attack and the dose may be gradually raised up to 900 mg daily.

Probenacid (0.5 g to 1 gm BD) or sulphinpyrazone (100 mg TDS) together with colchicine acts as uricosuric agent and are very effective, but they should not be used in gout with over-production of uric acid and gross uricosuria, in renal failure and in renal stones.

The patient is advised to eat less proteins, avoid alcohol, and reduce weight for obesity.

Surgery may be required to remove tophi sometimes.

# SPONDYLOARTHRITIS

*G.C. MOOKERJEE*

## INTRODUCTION

People who are seronegative for IgM rheumatoid factor and who suffer from a variety of common articular, extra-articular and genetic ailments, belong to a group of disorders known as the "seronegative spondyloarthritides".

The group includes ankylosing spondylitis, psoriatic arthritis, Reiter's syndrome and reactive arthritis, enteropathic arthritis associated with Crohn's disease, ulcerative colitis, Behcet's syndrome, Whipple's disease and juvenile chronic arthritis.

Clinicopathological features common to this group of disorders are : (a) an asymmetrical seronegative inflammatory oligoarthritis, (b) sacroilitis and/or in some cases spondylitis (c) arthropathy which has a tendency to develop inflammatory lesion of tendinous attachments to bone, (d) arthritis associated with anterior uveitis, (e) high prevalence of HLA-B27 histo-compatibility antigen, (g) familial tendency.

## AETIOLOGY

An abnormal response to an infective mechanism coupled with genetic predisposition is nowadays thought to be the cause of the seronegative spondyloarthritides. "Yersinia Enterocolitica" has been identified as the infecting organism causing the reactive arthritis that follows dysentery. Reiter's syndrome follows bacterial dysentery, but in most of the other disorders among the group the infective organism is yet unknown. Also the role of the presence of HLA-B27 is still not clear since this is only a marker for immune response genes, autoimmune reaction initiated by the modification of HLA-B27 positive cellular receptors due to the inciting organism, (which may also render the cells nerve susceptible to cytotoxin lymphocytes) is another possibility regarding the causative mechanism. Thus a person possessing the HLA-B27 gene is not necessarily predisposed towards this disease.

## ANKYLOSING SPONDYLITIS (A.S)

### DEFINITION

Progressive stiffening and finally fusion of the axial skeleton brought about by a chronic inflammatory arthritis usually of the sacroiliac joints and spine.

Young men between 20 and 30 years are most commonly affected and the m-f ratio is 9 : 1, although incomplete variants of the classical disease may equalise the ratio . Certain ethnic groups show prevalence (e.g. Haida Indians), and so does first degree relatives of patients with psoriatic arthritis, inflammatory bowel disease, Reiter's syndrome and of course ankylosing spondylitis itself. 90% of patients are HLA-B27 positive, and faecal carriage of Klebsiella species (especially during exacerbations)may be aetiologically significant. Associated prostatitis, may not however show any infective organism in the prostatic fluid.

### CLINICOPATHOLOGICAL FEATURES

The pathological hallmark of the disease is the presence of "syndesmophytes" which is new bone formation at the function of vertebral bodies and annulus fibrosus of intervertebral discs. due to the heading of enthesopathic foci, leading to bony ankylosis of the spine (bamboo spine of X-ray). The enthenopathy comprises multiple foci of inflammation containing lymphocytes and plasma cells at ligamentous attachments to bone causing bony erosion.

Low back pain and stiffness of insidious onset and chronic nature with exacerbations and remissions, occasional radiation of pain to thigh or buttock, and early morning stiffness are characteristic of A.S., although some may present with acute symptoms resembling lumbar disc prolapse. There is pain on sacroiliac compression, all movements of the lumbar spine are restricted. While symptoms or signs of nerve root compression is significantly absent, cases presenting with symptoms referable to thoracic or cervical spine usually display evidence of previous involvement of the costovertebral may cause chest pain aggravated by breathing. Tenderness over prominences such as iliac crest, ischial tuberosity and greater trochanter, Achilles tendinitis and plantar fascitis are characteristic features.

**INVESTIGATIONS :** Rheumatoid factors — negative
Antinuclear factors — negative

Synovial fluid complement levels — not reduced. Routine blood examination usually displays raised ESR.

### RADIOLOGY

Although early X-rays may be normal, eventually irregularity and marginal sclerosis progressing to fusion is seen, especially in lower parts of joints. Syndesmophyte formation, ossification of anterior longitudinal ligament leading to "squaring" of vertebrae, erosion and sclerosis and anterior corners of vertebrae and factal joint changes are all common and typically, progressive ossifications lead to the "Bamboo spine", with erosive changes in symphysis pubis, ischial tuberosities and peripheral joints. Osteoporosis and atlanto axial dislocation may occur.

Negative X-rays may prompt a radionuclide bone scan but this is a non-specific test showing blood flow and turnover of bone.

D/D — Prolapsed lumbar vertebral disc, trauma causing low back pain and other spondyloarthrities are to be considered in differential diagnosis. Degenerative joint diseases display no systemic manifestations and occur in elderly. Benign senile hyperostic spondylosis may resemble, but here the osteophites extend horizontally (not vertically from the edges of the vertebral bodies and while the sacroiliac joints is intact the disc spaces are often narrowed. Peripheral joint involvement, such as the M.T.P. and great toe may be confused with gout pseudogout, infective arthritis or any other seronegative inflammatory arthritis.

# MISCELLANEOUS JOINT DISORDERS

## REITER'S SYNDROME

### INTRODUCTION

Reiter's syndrome is suspected if there is a tetrad of arthritis, non-specific urethritis, mucocutaneous lesions and conjunctivitis, especially if it occurs after attack of enteric infection with samlonella chlamydia, shigella or yersine organisms. Sometimes it is called "Reactive arthritis".

Patients coming to the venereal disease clinic suffering from arthritis are sometimes diagnosed as Reiter's syndrome but these may be cases of gonococcal arthritis and not Reiter's syndrome. Male to female ratio is 50 : 1, but the male preponderance may be due to the fact that women often ignore the symptoms of urethritis and the disease is overlooked. Subjects with HLA-B27 positive histocompatibility antigen, have greater susceptibility in contracting this disease.

### CLINICAL FEATURES

An acute onset with oral lesions, urethritis, conjunctivitis, and arthritis appear simultaneously about one to three weeks after dysentery or sexual exposure. Systemic symptoms like fever, weight loss and vasomotor changes in the feet are often present, chiefly knee and ankles are involved.

Arthritis may subside spontaneously but in about 15% cases there is recurrence without any relapse of dysentery. Sometimes low back pain and stiffness due to sacro-ileitis may occur.

Serum rheumatoid factor and antinuclear factors are negative but in 75% of cases, HLA, B-27 may be detected.

Mucocutaneous lesions consist of stomatitis, and keratoderma blenorrhagica.

Sometimes carditis may occur leading to aortic incompetence. However, spontaneous remission may occur though tendency to relapse is well known.

### RADIOLOGY

Reduction of joint space, erosive changes, and periarticular osteoporosis are noted especially when the disease is protracted or there is recurrence.

Periostitis is present specially in metacarpal bones and in phalanges. Characteristic "fluffy" calcaneal spurs may be seen. The sacroileitis may be present as in spondylitis but isolated bony spurs and paravertebral ossification is present in the spine unlike ankylosing spondylitis.

### TREATMENT

Mainly symptomatic and supportive. In acute stage rest and use of nonsteroidal anti-rheumatic drug is resorted to, as in rheumatoid arthritis. Aspiration of joints having effusion and injections of steroids may also be required. Systemic steroids are very occasionally necessary. Anterior uveitis may be a medical emergency and it should be treated by topical sub-conjunctival or systemic corticosteroids. Rarely severe arthritis and intractable keratoderma blenorrhagica justify the use of cytotoxic drugs. Tetracycline is the drug of choice for the non-specific urethritis but the drug does not affect other symptoms nor does it alter the course of the disease.

## BEHCET'S SYNDROME

### DEFINITION

This syndrome was described by the Turkish dermatologist Dr. Behcet. Recurrent oral and genital ulceration associated with uveitis, sero-negative recurrent arthritis are the characteristics of this disease. The major criteria include inflammatory arthritis of large joints, epididymitis, intestinal ulceration, thrombophlebitis and neuropsychiatric symptoms. If all major criteria are present, it is said to be "complete" syndrome, while if only three major criteria are present it is incomplete. The knees, ankles, wrists and elbows are most frequently involved in arthritis.

Sometimes eyes are badly involved leading to blindness. Uveitis, keratitis, hypopyon and even optic neuritis may occur, CNS involvement consists of encephalitis, cranial nerve palsies and spinal cord lesions.

There may be leucocytosis and high ESR.

### TREATMENT

When arthritis is the dominant presentation treatment is similar as in the case of rheumatoid arthritis. But antibiotics may be necessary for infected ulcerations. Corticosteroids and immunosuppressive therapy are used in severe and serious cases. Follow-up is essential as there is tendency to relapse and remission.

## WHIPPLE'S DISEASE

The disease is manifested by diarrhoea, pain in the abdomen, arthritis and malabsorption in the gut. Anaemia, gastrointestinal bleeding, lymphadenopathy and fever may occur. Usually there is non-erosive and asymmetrical oligoarthritis, but occasionally some patients develop spondylitis..

Very rarely extraarticular features like meningo-encephalitis, peripheral neuropathy, pericarditis or pleurisy may develop.

### INVESTIGATIONS

ESR is raised, often very high, during the acute phase may persist at high level long after symptoms have subsided.

### DIAGNOSIS

PAS positive macrophages in small intestinal biopsy confirms the diagnosis of Whipple's disease. Certain rod-shaped organisms which are as yet not identified have been detected by electron microscopy in the lamina propria and synovial membrane of affected persons.

### TREATMENT

Treatment consists of supportive measures and use of tetracycline 1.0 to 2.0g per day, which may have to be given for a few months.

Anaemia and hypoproteinemia will need appropriate therapy including blood transfusion.

### ENTEROPATHIC ARTHRITIS

Ulcerative colitis and Crohn's disease display two different types of sero-negative inflammatory arthritis.

Sacroileitis is seen in patients with ulcerative colitis of Crohn's disease along with ankylosing spondylitis, but they are not affected by the intestinal disease process and pursue an independent course. High incidence of HLA-B27 positive cases is seen.

### ENTROPATHIC SYNOVITIS

This is a non-erosive oligo-arthritis, acute and migratory in nature usually affecting the weight bearing joints; sometimes wrists and small joints of the fingers and toes may be involved. Arthritis is primarily dependent on bowel disease, e.g. ulcerative colitis and Crohn's disease. Arthritis often occurs in association with aphthous mouth ulcers and erythematous rashes which disappear following total remission of ulcerative colitis. There is no specific treatment for arthritis, as arthritis settles down bowel disease is controlled.

## JUVENILE CHRONIC ARTHRITIS

*(Juvenile Chronic Arthritis or Still's Disease)*

Juvenile chronic arthritis may start with severe lymphadenopathy, hepatosplenomegaly, pleurisy, pericarditis and high intermittent fever along with systemic disturbances. There may be a striking degree of retardation of growth, along with weight loss and often transient erythematous rash appearing with rise of temperature.

Leucocytosis, anaemia and raised ESR are noted. Rheumatoid and antinuclear factors are negative. Usually most children improve after a few months but some cases have recurrent attacks which may progress to a severe chronic polyarthritis.

## SEROPOSITIVE POLYARTICULAR DISEASE

It occurs in about ten per cent of children with juvenile chronic arthritis and girls are more commonly affected than boys, usually after eight years of age. It is very similar to adult onset, rheumatoid arthritis and erosive changes are commonly seen. Nodules and vasculitis along with low grade fever and anaemia are all present.

Rheumatoid factor and antinuclear factors are positive in 75% cases.

## IMPORTANT GUIDELINES ABOUT USE OF NSAID IN RHEMATOID DISORDERS

(1) Many new drugs have appeared in the market in recent years and it is becoming difficult to choose a safe drug as almost of all of them are capable of producing gastrointestinal complications, liver damage, blood dyscrasias, renal failure, toxic epidermal neurolysis and Stevens - Johnson syndrome (Brit. Med. Jour. Vol.292, 1986 CMS update pages 1190-1191 gives an excellent details of drug reaction due to NSAID).

(2) It is advisable not to prescribe these drugs wherever possible and avoid it in cases of peptic ulcers or of there is history of P.V. disease.

(3) Always it should be given after meals and antacids.

(4) Start with minimum dose and in Editor's view salicylates, aspirin (being cheapest and effective) and Ibuprofen are best drugs to start initially.

(5) Avoid use of indomethacin indiscriminately specially slow-release indomethacin preparations are dangerous.

(6) Sale of these drugs over the counter without prescription should be stopped.

(7) Combination of NSAID with oral steroids may also be done after very careful consideration.

(8) Watch for adverse drug reactions.

(9) Assess hepatorenal health while prescribing these drugs.

(10) Regular follow-up is essential.

# CHAPTER – 14
# MANAGEMENT OF FLUID AND ELECTROLYTE IMBALANCE

*N.C. DAS*

To arrive at a plan of treatment, one has to consider :

(1) What *imbalance* is present now and what is their magnitude ?

(2) What *additional loss* can be expected during treatment ?

(3) What are *daily requirements* for fluids & electrolyte ?

For each one of these, the need for –

(a) Water
(b) Sodium
(c) Potassium
(d) Other electrolytes
(e) Acid-base adjustment

should be assessed separately and added together for replacement.

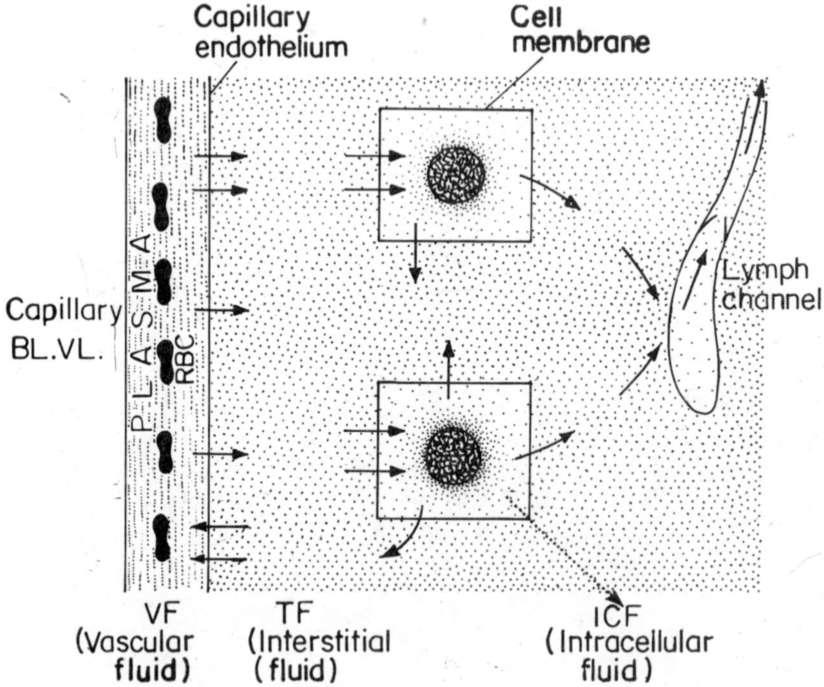


Fig.14.1 : Distribution of body water in different compartments. Movements of water shown by arrows.

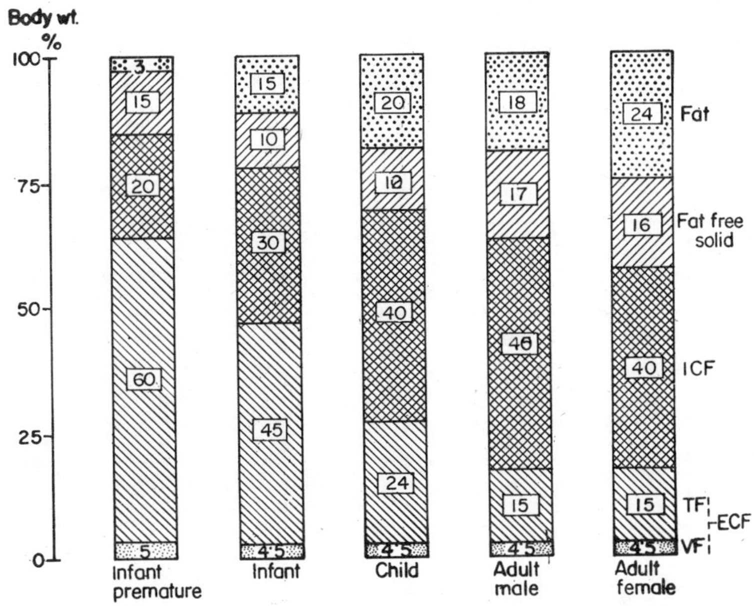


Fig.14.2 : Percentage of body of fat and fluid content by age.

**Points to remember**

(1) Adequate renal function simplifies fluid therapy. Renal function is adequate if the **first** urine void in the morning is protein-free, glucose free and has sp.gr. of 1016 or higher **and** pH of 5.8 or lower.

(2) **Normal electrolyte concentration in serum**

| | | |
|---|---|---|
| $Na^+$ | = | 135 – 145 mEq/L |
| $K^+$ | = | 3.5 – 5.5 ,, |
| $Cl^-$ | = | 82 – 115 ,, |
| $HCO_3^-$ | = | 22 – 29 ,, |
| Ca | = | 4.0 – 5.5 ,, |
| Mg | = | 1.5 – 2.5 ,, |

(3) **Urine electrolyte concentration mEq per litre (random specimen)**

| **Tubular activity** | **Sodium** | **Potassium** |
|---|---|---|
| Normal | more than 40 | more than 40 |
| Conserving (early) | 10-30 | 20-30 |
| Maximal retention | less than 5 | 15-25 |

**Essential Investigation**

If the patient is thirsty and dry, fluid deficit or imbalance exists. Following investigations must be done :

(1) Blood haematocrit (HCT) value (42 to 52% Normal)
(2) Serum sodium, potassium and chloride
(3) Serum protein (total)

(4) Urine volume, in past 24 hours
(5) Urinary sodium and potassium
(6) Urine specific gravity and reaction
(7) Blood pH – if potassium deficit is indicated.

## CHART - I

To find out the *type of imbalance* follow this chart :

| IMBALANCE | SERUM | | | | | URINE | | TYPE OF FLUID REQUIRED |
|---|---|---|---|---|---|---|---|---|
| TYPE | Hae-mato-crit (Hct.) | $Na^+$ | Cl | $K^+$ | Protein | Volume | $Na^+$ | for replacement |
| 1) Hypertonic dehydration | ↑ | ↑ | ↑ | – | – | ↓ | + ve or low | Electrolyte free water (5% glucose) |
| 2) Hypotonic dehydration | | | | | | | | |
| (a) True $Na^+$ depleletion | ↑ | ↓ | ↓ | – | – | ↑ | –ve absent | Sodium containing fluid |
| (b) Water intoxication | ↓ | ↓ | ↓ | – | – | ↑ | +ve | Restrict IV fluid |
| (c) Chronic over expansion of ECF (sick cell syndrome) | ↓ | ↓ | ↓ | ↓ | ↓ | ↑ | –ve | Restrict water & sodium. Give fresh blood, plasma, glucose, potassium, insulin |
| 3) Inadequate ADH seretion | – | ↓ | ↓ | – | ↓ | Normal | +ve | Treat cause |

Compare with investigation results, and finally decide about the type of fluid required for replacement.

## CHART - II

To find out the magnitude of **water deficit,** follow this chart.

The chief symptoms and signs of water deficit are thirst, oliguria and hypernatremia. Each three mEq of serum sodium concentration rise above normal (of 145 mEq) indicates a deficit of at least one litre of water.

**Clinical signs of water depletion**

| *Clinical feature* | *Magnitude of fluid deficit* |
|---|---|
| Thirst only | 1.5 litres or less |

| | |
|---|---|
| Marked thirst<br>Dry mouth, groin or axilla<br>Serum sodium increased<br>Urine sp. gr. increased<br>Hct, skin turgor, BP normal | 1.5 - 4 litres |
| Intolerable thirst<br>Marked hypernatremia<br>Oliguria ++<br>Body wt. decrease<br>Hct. increased slightly<br>Apathy, stupor | 4 litres or more |

If not corrected, hyperosmolar coma and death.

## CHART - III

To find out the magnitude of **sodium deficit,** follow this chart

Serum sodium concentration alone is not a reliable guide to sodium need. A low serum sodium more often indicates water-excess than sodium deficit.

**Clinical signs of acute sodium depletion**

| *Signs and symptoms* | *Magnitude of deficit* |
|---|---|
| Furrowed tongue<br>Neck veins collapsed<br>Hct elevated, serum sodium normal<br>Urine sodium less than 40 mEq/L<br>Tachycardia<br>Anorexia<br>Little or no thirst<br>No craving for salt | Up to 450 mEq of Na+<br>(3 litres of ECF loss) |
| Hct rise ++<br>Oliguria<br>Hypotension<br>Apathy, nausea<br>Serum sodium low | More than 600 mEq of Na+<br>(more than 4 litres of ECF loss) |

Hypovolemic shock and death.

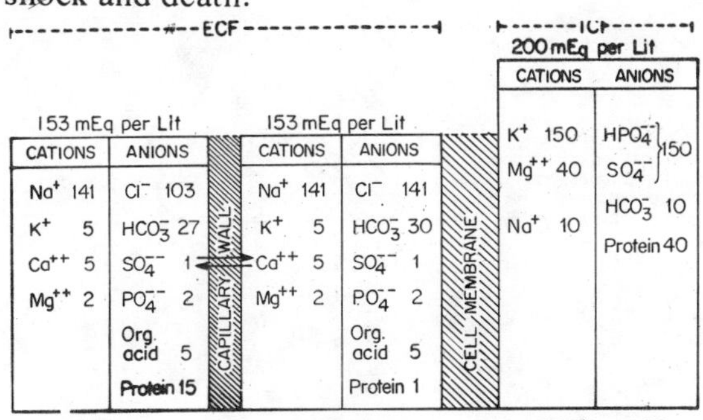


**Fig.14.3 : Norheal concentration of electrolytes in mEq/Ltr. in different compartments of the body.**

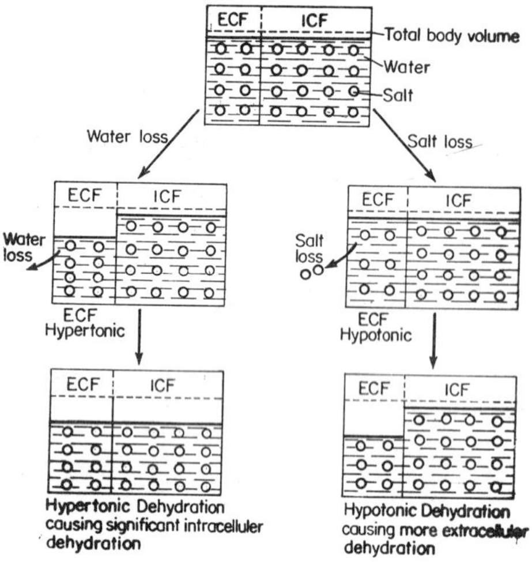


Fig.14.4 : Shows ECG & ICE Volume changes in hypertonic and hypotonic type of dehydration.

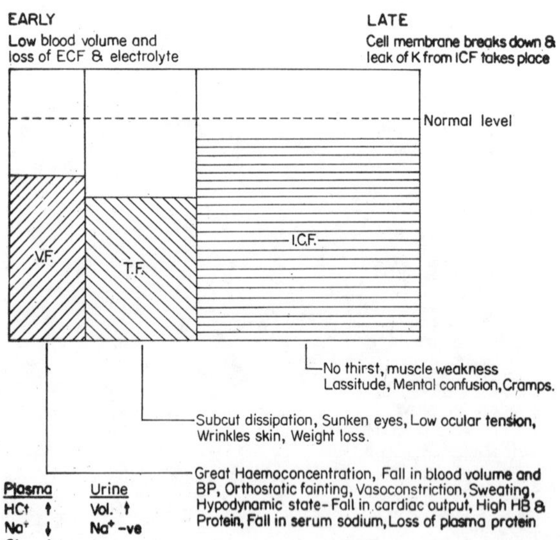


Fig.14.6 : Effects of True sodium depletion.

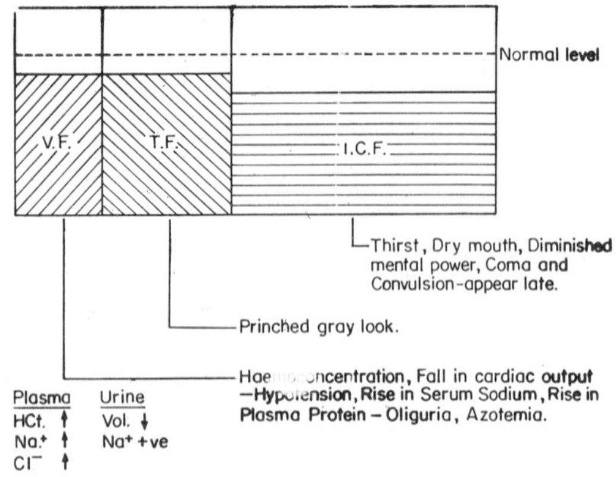


Fig.14.5 : Hypertonic dehydration effects of water loss

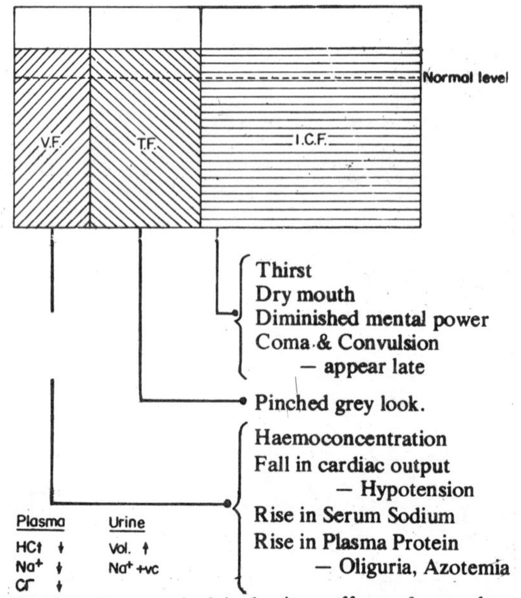


Fig.14.7 : Hypertonic dehydration : effects of water loss.

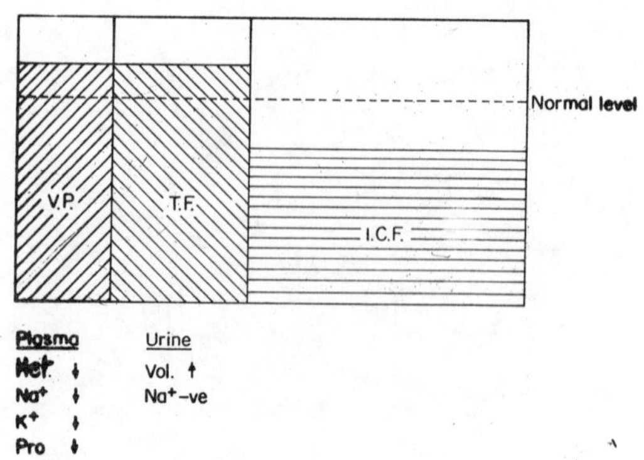


Fig.14.8 : Effects of chronic expansion of E.C.F. (chronic wasting disease).

## CHART - IV

**To find out the magnitude of potassium imbalance follow this chart :**

Early signs of potassium depletion are vague.

(a) Malaise, weakness, paralytic ileus and distension are noticed in hypokalemia in early stage.

(b) Muscular paresis, ectopics, sagging S-T or low voltage inverted-T are signs of severe hypokalaemia.

Only one percent of the total body potassium is in serum, therefore serum potassium value does not reflect the amount of potassium deficit in the body.

Total Body potassium (mEq per Kg)

| *Clinical State* | *Male* | *Female* |
|---|---|---|
| Normal | 45 | 35 |
| Moderate wasting | 32 | 25 |
| Severe wasting | 23 | 20 |

To find out the exact amount of body potassium deficit check :

(1) pH of the blood
(2) Serum potassium value
(3) Weight of the patient
(4) Degree of wasting, if any, of the patient.

Then using the Nomogram estimate the exact amount of potassium deficit, the patient is suffering and replace at a rate of only 20 mEq per hour (even in severe hypokalaemia).

BODY $K^+$ CAPACITY (mEq per Kg)

| Normal | Male | Female |
|---|---|---|
| Normal | 45 | 35 |
| Moderate wasting | 32 | 25 |
| Severe wasting | 23 | 20 |

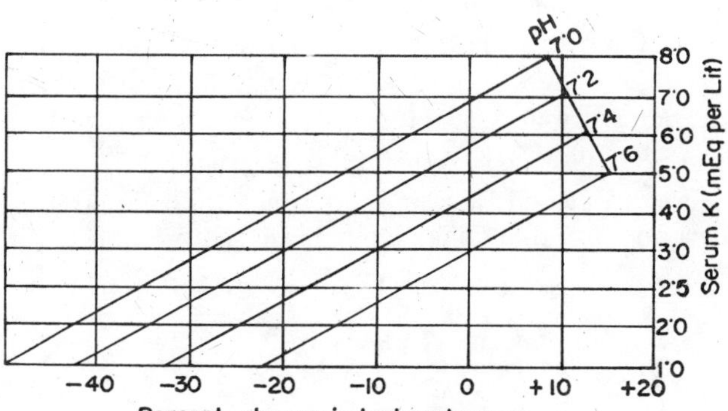


NOMOGRAM : for calculation of depletion or excess of total body Potassium.

Step 1 – using serum K and pH, determine percentage change in body $K^+$

Step 2 – using body wt and clinical state, determine total body $K^+$ capacity

Step 3 – Multiply total body capacity by percentage change of $K^+$ to obtain an estimate of $K^+$ deficit or excess.

Fig.14.9 : Nomogram for calculation of potassium **deficit**.

**Example**

Patient is female with moderate wasting; body weight 50 kg.
pH = 7.4, serum $K^+$ 3 mEq/L.
Therefore, her total body potassium should be 25 × 50 = 1250 mEq
From Nomogram we find she is having — 10% deficit of potassium.
Thus her total potassium deficit = 10% of 1250 mEq = 125 mEq.
For treatment 125 mEq of $K^+$ will have to be given at the rate of 20 mEq of $K^+$ per hour.

## CHART - V

**Additional losses during treatment**

The additional losses may be due to :

(1) G.I. secretion loss e.g. vomiting, gastric suction, fistula etc. Gastric suction losses amount to usually 500 to 1000 ml.
(Chloride and water loss is predominent)

(2) Increased insensible loss resulting from fever, hyperventilation, high environmental temperature.

| Addl. allowance to be made | Fever (F°) | Environmental temperature (F°) | Resp. rate |
|---|---|---|---|
| None | 101° — or less | 85°7 or less | 35 or less |
| 500 ml | 101° — 103° | 85° — 95° | over 35 |
| 1000 ml | 103° or more | 95° or more | |

(3) Increased water and salt loss from sweating.

| **Degree of sweating** | **Addl allowance for 24 hours** | |
|---|---|---|
| | **Water (ml)** | **Sodium (mEq)** |
| Moderate intermittent | 500 | 25 |
| Moderate continuous | 1000 | 50 |
| Profuse continuous | 2000 or more | 75 or more |

(4) Increased renal loss of water and salt following enforced osmotic diuresis e.g. Mannitol, urea, Dextran 40.
Mannitol 12.5 Cm each will enforce excretion of —
water = 125 ml; $Na^+$ = 10 mEq/L; K = 2 mEq/L.

(5) Third space loss — sequestrated ECF in tissue space following trauma or post-operative cases. (Exposed peritoneum 1 mm thickness increase ≡ 1000 ml N. sodium chloride sol loss)

(6) Plasma loss from burns, granulating wound, via drainage tubes.

## CHART - VI

**Maintenance requirement**

Water and electrolytes required daily for maintenance in adult above 40 kg.

| **Requirement** | **Per day** | **Per hour** |
|---|---|---|
| Volume (water) | 35-40 ml per Kg. | 100 ml per hour (fixed) |
| Sodium | 40-100 mEq | 3 mEq ,, |
| Potassium | 40-80 mEq | 2 mEq ,, |

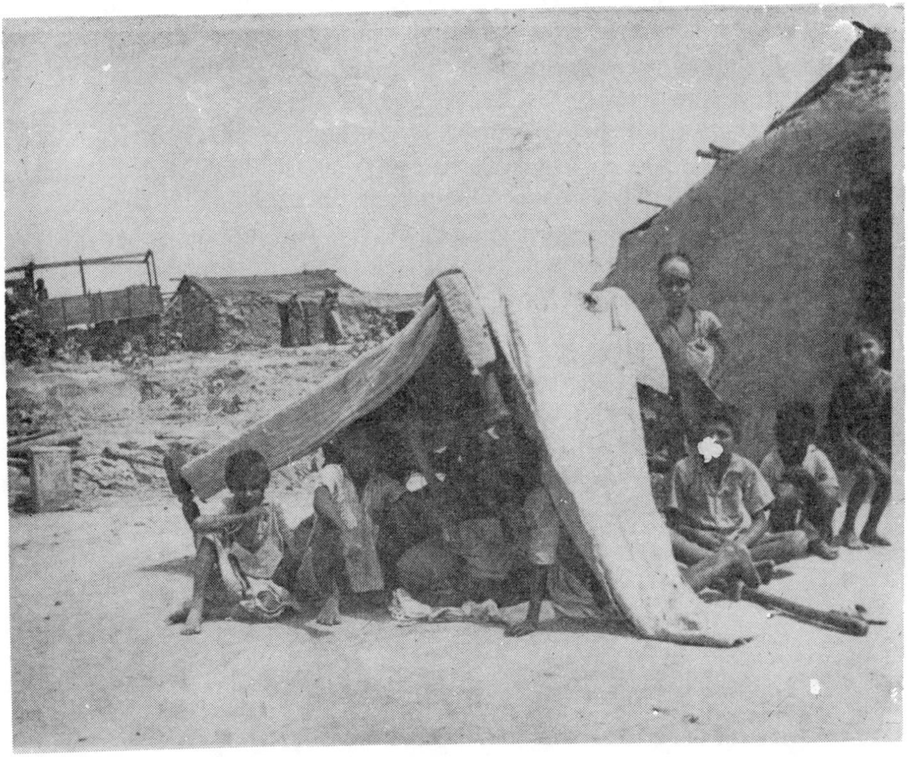

Fig.14.10 : A typical poorman's resting place in summer cause of rapid dehydration of sick people is obvious *(Photo — Editor's)*

**Note :**

(a) The maintenance volume of water allows for both normal sensible and insensible losses per day. Daily urine loss is included in this figure. The smaller figure is used when stress-induced antidiuresis is present; the larger figure is used for routine situations.

(b) Sodium excretion in urine is usually 40-200 mEq per day in adults. Basal losses via other routes are not important.

(c) Potassium excretions in urine is usually 40-100 mEq per day and this obligatory loss of $K^+$ continues even in presence of potassium depletion.

(d) Calcium and magnesium loss via urine and faeces is extremely small and usually do not require replacement.

## CALCULATION OF IMBALANCE

(a) From chart I to IV, *present imbalance* for water, sodium and potassium can be determined.

(b) From chart V, *additional losses* during treatment can be determined.

(c) From chart VI, *maintenance requirement* can be determined.

Adding a, b and c, total imbalance can be estimated.

**Formation of fluid and electrolyte order**

(1) Period of evaluation should usually be every 24 hours; but for very ill patients it may even two hours.

(2) **Calculated total requirement** for **water, sodium** and **potassium** separately for the treatment period, by adding the following :

(a) **Half** of the estimated magnitude of present imbalance ('A' above);

(b) Loss anticipated during treatment period ('B' above);

(c) Maintenance requirements for the number of hours in the treatment period ('C') above;

(3) (a) Fluid order should be to administer the total calculated requirement within the treatment period, (i.e. generally 24 hours; for very sick cases 2 hours);

(b) Fluid and electrolyte requirements should be converted into standard IV, solutions in bottles, with concentration amount of various electrolytes;

(c) Infusion rate of I.V. fluids should be as required.

| **Infusion Drops per min.** | **Approx. ml per hour** | **Approx. litres per day** |
|---|---|---|
| 5 | 20 | 0.5 |
| 15 | 60 | 1.4 |
| 30 | 120 | 2.9 |
| 50* | 200 | 4.8 |
| 75 | 300 | 7,2 |
| 100 | 400 | 9.6 |
| 120 | 480 | 11.5 |
| 150** | 600 | 14.4 |
| 200 | 800 | 19.2 |

* Maximum rate for hypertonic solution via peripheral veins

** Maximum rate for isotonic solution, without monitoring.

Use the formula, or for drop rates

Number of litres in 24 hours × 11 = No. of drops per min.

(4) (i) Predict the outcome of treatment.

(ii) Check during treatment period and make adjustments.

(iii) Re-evaluate after the proposed period of treatment and fresh assessment of fluid and electrolyte requirement for next period of treatment should be done.

**Note :**

(1) A balanced electrolyte solution (Ringer Lactate sol) is preferable as the medium for supplying $Na^+$ need and water. If the patient is acidotic, use 0.6 m sodium lactate solution, if patient is alkalotic, Normal saline solution is indicated.

(2) Ordinarily –

(a) Limit infusion rate to 500 ml per hour i.e. 120 drops per min.

(b) Limit $K^+$ infusion rate to 20 mEq per hour.

(c) Lower leg veins should not be used for I.V. infusion.

(d) C.V.P. monitoring essential for rapid infusion or in heart failure cases.

(e) Add Ascorbic acid 300 mgm and vitamin B Complex to one bottle daily.

(f) Intake-output chart must be maintained.
Do not try to replace urine loss. It is accounted in daily maintenance requirement.

**Example**

History – 55 year old man, 70 kg. history of duodenal ulcer, vomiting severely and complaints of epigastric pain. Extremely thirsty.

Physical — T = 102° F°. BP = 100/70 (no postural hypotension) P = 100/min, skin, axilla and groin dry, Tongue furrowed, skin-turgor fair. Urine passed about 30 ml in last 12 hours.

Lab reports — Serum : Na+ = 154 mEq, K+ = 2.2 mEq, HCt = 38%, pH = 7.52
Urine : sp. gr. = 1032, Na+ = 22, K+ = 3; pH = 6.0

**Interpretation**

(1) **Severe water deficit :** (3000 ml + approximate) Reasons — Vomiting, Thirst ++, Dry axilla and groin; urine less, urinary sp. gr. high; Hct normal; Hypernatraemia Serum Na+ rise = 9 mEq above normal of 145 mEq = three litres of ECF loss.

(2) **Moderate Na+ deficit :** (250 mEq approximate) Reasons — Vomiting; Furrowed tongue, poor turgor, tachycardia. Urinary Na+ low; ECF loss nearly 3 litres.

(3) **Severe Hypokalemia :** (350 mEq approximate) Reasons — Irregular pulse, serum K+ low, Urinary K+ moderately low, (conserving) paradoxical aciduria (serum pH alkaline 7.5 and urine acidic).

Using Nomogram changes of body K+ = −11%
Total body K+ being 45 × 70 kg = 3150 mEq.
Deficit of K+ amounts to 11% of 3150 mEq = 350 mEq.

**Thus, fluid requirements for 12 hours**

| | | Water | Na+ | K+ |
|---|---|---|---|---|
| (a) Half of deficit (existing) | | 1500 ml | 100 mEq | 175 mEq |
| (b) Maintenance requirement for 12 hrs. | | 1250 | 50 | 40 |
| (c) Likely losses | (i) G.I. | 1000 | | |
| (in 12 hours) | (ii) Temp | 500 | 60 | 10 |
| ∴ In 12 hours, we will give | | 4250 ml | 210 mEq | 225 mEq |

**Fluid orders for 12 hours**

**Note :** Total K+ deficit cannot be made up within 12 hours treatment since rate of administration should not be more than 20 mEq/hour.

(a) First 2 bottles = 1000 ml, 5% dextrose with 0.45% saline at 200 drops per min watch urinary output. — 1½ hrs.

(b) 3rd & 4th bottle = 1000 ml. — same solution at 120 drops per min (Add 40 mEq of Kcl in the bottle) — 2 hrs.

(c) 5th & 6th bottle = 1000 ml same solution 60 drops per min (Add 60 mEq. of Kcl in bottles) — 4 hrs.

(d) 7th & 8th bottle = 1000 ml. 5% Dextrose only at 60 drops per min — 4 hrs.

Add : 60 mEq of Kcl in the bottles
+ Ascorbic acid = 150 mgm } in one of the bottles
+ B Complex

11½ hrs. to 12 hrs.

**5% Dextrose with 0.45% saline**

| | Na+ | K+ | Calories |
|---|---|---|---|
| per litre | 77 mEq | 74 mEq | 200 |

**given in 12 hours.**

water = 4000 ml
Na+ = 231 mEq
K+ = 60 mEq
Cl = 222 mEq

# CHAPTER 15
# GASTROENTEROLOGY

## MODERN INVESTIGATIVE PROCEDURES

*G.C. MOOKERJEE*
*M.L. SAPRA*

### Introduction

Until recently the diagnostic methods in gastroenterology including liver diseases were limited to radiological contrast studies e.g. barium meal, barium enema, oral and intravenous cholecystography, repeated stool examinations, sigmoidoscopy or proctoscopy, gastric acid accretion studies, pancreatic function tests and biochemical liver function tests. Invasive tests like liver biopsy and splenoportography are also done but may be accompanied with complications.

There has been a revolution in investigative procedure during recent years with the availability of ultrasound imaging, computed tomography, radioisotope scanning, percutaneous transhepatic cholangiography (PTC), upper gastrointestinal endoscopy using flexible fiberoptic endoscopes, colonoscopy and retrograde endoscopic pancreaticocholangiography (ERPC).

Majority of these procedures are atraumatic. Most of them are, however, expensive and demand sophisticated technology and are not freely available. These tests can only be carried out at specialized centres. In a developing country like India, it will probably take a long time for these tests to be freely available but it is considered important that all medical students and practitioners should know about them and their value in diagnosing difficult cases.

### Ultrasound Imaging or Scanning USS :

Once the equipment is available, it is one of the most painless, relatively inexpensive and atraumatic investigations. It can be done as an out-patient and takes a very short time. The results depend, of course, on the quality of the machine and expertise of the person using it. It is easy to make wrong interpretation due to inexperience. The procedure has got no contraindications, although excessive gas in the abdomen may not allow proper imaging. It is especially in the diagnosis of gastrointestinal diseases related to liver, gall bladder and pancreas. Some of the indications for ultrasonography have been summarized as below :

(1) Delineation of abdominal masses and their relationship to different abdominal viscera. It also helps to detect cystic or solid S.O.L.

(2) Confirmation of hepatomegaly and splenomegaly;

(3) Demonstration of space occupying lesions in the liver and their nature whether solid or cystic. It is particularly useful in diagnosing metastases in the liver, liver abscesses and hepatic cysts.

(4) Aspiration of liver abscesses and liver biopsy from a particular site under ultrasonographic guidance.

(5) Study the effects of treatment by watching the size of the lesion and its regression during frequent follow-up examinations.

(6) Guided aspiration biopsy from different abdominal organs or masses.

(7) Diagnosis of portal hypertension and confirmation of patency of portal vein. One can also confirm whether a porto-systemic shunt is patent or not.

(8) Demonstrate even small cysts, SOL'S and abscesses.

(9) Supports the presence of congestive heart failure by demonstrating dilated hepatic veins and inferior vena cava.

(10) Demonstration of gall bladder and biliary duct diseases. The availability of latest real-time gray-scale ultrasonographic equipment has made ultrasonography as the primary investigation for demonstration of gallstones. It is as accurate as oral cholecystography, can be performed rapidly and is cost-effective.

It can be used in acutely ill and jaundiced patients and the patient is not exposed to ionic radiations. Accuracy of this procedure in demonstrating gallstones is 95-99 per cent.

(11) It is a very safe and most direct method to detect biliary tract obstruction and differentiates extra hepatic from intra hepatic jaundice. It may also indicate the site of obstruction and helps in aetiological diagnosis. However, it is not always possible to diagnose the precise aetiology by ultrasonography.

(12) Study of pancreatic disorders — Ultrasonographic examination of the pancreas is performed to help in diagnosis of pancreatitis and its complications like pseudo-pancreatic cyst and detection of pancreatic carcinoma. It is not, however, always possible to examine pancreas ultrasonographically and computed tomography and ERCP should be done in such doubtful cases.

(13) Study of alimentary tract — Ultrasound has still not been found to be of much use in study of alimentary tract because luminal gas is a physical barrier. Contrast barium studies will continue to be the main diagnostic tool in these cases. However, modern flexible endoscope is an additional and very effective tool.

**Computed Tomographic (CT) Scanning :**

Availability of whole body computed tomography (CT Scan) has generated an interest in investigation of gastrointestinal diseases. Its main advantages are superb density and spatial resolution of images. It is non-invasive, exposes the body to less radiation than a barium enema and is fairly rapid.

The major limitation, however, is the cost and its limited availability.

The major uses of CT scan in gastrointestinal diseases are in :

(i) Diagnosis of liver, pancreatic, splenic and gastrointestinal diseases

(ii) Staging of malignant disorders

(iii) Planning of treatment

(iv) Assessing response to therapy

(v) Guiding biopsies and drainage.

The greatest advantage of CT Scan is that it can image the entire abdomen at one sitting and hence too many investigations for different organs are not required.

**Radionuclide Imaging or Scanning :**

Large variety of radiopharmaceuticals are used. There has been tremendous improvement in radioisotopic imaging technology in recent years, particularly in the field of gastroenterology. These studies are very safe, non-invasive and exposure to radiation is more or less the same as in case of any standard radiological examination. The radionuclide is given in a tracer dose orally or intravenously and quantitation is done by external monitoring with a scintillation camera. Availability of computer system to help in analysis of results has further simplified and improved the technique.

The different radiopharmaceuticals used are : I-131 rose bengal, Au 198 gold colloid, Tc99m sulphur colloid (most commonly used at present technetium 99m and Gallium 677). The main clinical conditions where radionuclide scanning may be of help are :

(a) Evaluation of liver-splenic size, contour, location, uniformity of colloid distribution and presence of 'Cold' lesions.

(b) Evaluation of hepato-cellular disease :

(i) Nonhomogeneous colloid distribution

(ii) Hepatomegaly

(iii) Splenomegaly

(iv) Increased uptake of colloid by spleen and bone marrow

(c) Evaluation of space occupying lesions in the liver —

(i) Hepatic metastases

(ii) Hepatic cysts (ultrasonography is adequate)

(iii) Liver abscesses (ultrasonography is adequate)

(iv) Primary hepatocellular carcinoma

(d) Hepatobiliary imaging :

It is particularly useful in diagnosis of acute cholecystitis, evaluation of cholestasis and biliary tract abnormalities.

(e) Detection and localization of site of bleeding in gastrointestinal tract.

(f) Evaluation of gastrooesophageal reflux.

**Upper Gastrointestinal Fiberoptic Endoscopy**

Fiberoptic endoscopes are made up of two types of fibre bundles — one carries light down to illuminate the visual field and the other carries the undistorted image back to the examiner's eye. The shaft also contains wire control for multidirectional movement of the tip. One or more separate channels are available for suction and biopsy. This gives an excellent view of all mucosal surfaces of the oesophagus, stomach and duodenum. Observations can be made regarding presence of focal benign or malignant lesions diffuse mucosal changes, motility, intraluminal obstruction, or extrinsic compression. Along with providing direct visual impression of the pathology, there is provision for taking directed biopsy for histopathology from suspicious lesions. Material for cytological examination can also obtained. In addition to being used in diagnosis, recently fiberoptic endoscopes are being used more frequently for therapeutic procedures such as dilatation of benign oesophageal strictures, removal of foreign bodies and treatment of upper gastrointestinal bleeding. The greatest advantages over rigid endoscopy are case of introduction without anaesthesia, greater and hence better diagnostic efficacy and minimal complication rate. Main complications include rarely perforation, bleeding and medication reactions, cardiopulmonary failure and very rarely. As compared to radiology of upper 'GT tract', this technique is more sensitive and specific for diagnosis of upper GI lesions. With single contrast barium studies done in good centres the correct diagnosis is obtained in 60-70% of upper GI lesions as compared to 98-100% with fiberoptic endoscopy. With double contrast and combination of double contrast mucosal relief views followed by single contrast Ba-examination the success rate in diagnosis goes up to 85-90%. But this technique takes longer time, requires special expertise and there is more radiation danger.

**Fiberoptic Colonoscopy**

This is an important diagnostic and therapeutic adjunct for the management of colonic diseases. Diagnostic colonoscopy is useful in diagnosis of abnormal or equivocal barium enema findings, unexplained rectal bleeding, to evaluate the complications of inflammatory bowel disease, surveillance for development of carcinoma in inflammatory bowel disease. A direct biposy of the lesion as well as cytology-material by brush can be obtained. The most useful therapeutic technique is colonoscopic polypectomy. In some instances haemorrhage from vascular lesions can be controlled by colonoscopic electro or photo-coagulation. A thorough cleaning of the large gut is required prior to performing colonoscopy. In hands of expert, caecum can be reached in 85-95% of cases.

### Endoscopic Retrograde Cholangiopancreatography (ERCP)

This employs fiberoptic endoscopy and techniques of radiography in the study of biliary and pancreatic diseases. Side-viewing endoscope is used. After entering the second part of the duodenum, ampulla of Vater is located and cannulated and desired duct system, either pancreatic or bile ducts can be outlined by injecting contrast media through the endoscopic catheter. It requires both endoscopic and radiographic skills. It is a fairly safe procedure in expert hands with a success rate of 82 to 93 per cent. But it is a costly procedure and requires plenty of technical expertise. It has made the diagnosis of pancreatic and biliary diseases easier. Evaluation of biliary tree is mostly required in cases of obstructive jaundice whereas evaluation of pancreatic duct is indicated in cases of chronic pancreatitis and carcinoma of pancreas.

Therapeutically ERCP is used for performing sphincterotomy and removal of retained stones from common bile duct. It can also be used for introducing an endoprosthesis across malignant bile duct strictures. Complication rate is about 3%. In addition to medication reaction, complications of endoscopic procedure these include development of acute pancreatitis and cholangitis.

### Percutaneous Transhepatic Cholangiography (PTC)

This is another important diagnostic aid in visualizing biliary tree in addition to ERCP. In fact details of biliary tree are better delineated with this method. With the advent of Chibas needle which is fine and flexible, the procedure has become very safe. The needle is introduced percutaneously through the intercostal space into the liver. The stylet is withdrawn, contrast material is injected slowly as the needle is withdrawn until the ductal system is entered. This whole procedure is done under fluroscopic control. After proper positioning of the patient and manipulating in different positions, radiographs of the whole ductal system are taken to delineate the site of obstruction. In obstructed biliary system the success rate is 90 to 100%. In non--obstructed biliary tracts the success rate has been in the range of 75 to 80%. Complications of the procedure include bile peritonitis, haemorrhage and septicaemia, Coagulation parameters must be normal before performing PTC as is the case with all invasive, investigations on liver. In suspected biliary obstruction,antibiotics should be started one day prior to procedure. PTC can also be used for external or internal drainage of bile in obstructed biliary duct prior to life in malignant structures.

## DISEASES OF THE DIGESTIVE SYSTEM

*G.C. MOOKERJEE*

### Introduction to Gastroenterology

The function of the digestive system is to receive food in the mouth, chew it and mix it well with saliva, pass it down through oesophagus into stomach for further digestion, by the action of acid gastric juice. Some nutrients are absorbed but most of the food material requiring further processing are sent downwards to be digested by the action of bile, pancreatic juice and succus entericus. Absorption of digested food takes place in the small intestines and the remaining material passes into large gut where water is particularly absorbed. The remaining mass which is almost solid is excreted as stool. Thus the functions of digestive system are as follows :

(1) Reception of food
(2) Digestion of food
(3) Process of onward and one way transmission
(4) Absorption of nutritional substances
(5) Excretions of waste product i.e. evacuation of stool.

The object or the whole process is to procure nutrition for tissue metabolism required for survival. In case of unicellular protoplasmic amoeba the process is simplest but in humans it involves multiple organs, e.g. mouth, tongue, teeth, coordinated action or oropharyngeal, oesophageal and gastrointestinal (G.I.) muscles. The integrity G.I. tract alone is not enough. Thoracic cage, abdominal cavity and its contents may affect G.I. function. Disorder of neurological origin or vascular insufficiency may cause derangement of G.I. tract. Many systemic diseases may produce G.I. disorders while symptoms of diseases of spine, meninges, heart and pleura may be mistaken for G.I, disorders.

Besides, the function of reception, digestion, and absorption of food as well as excretion of water the G.I. tract also has a special role in defence mechanism. It also secretes many hormones to control the secretion of various digestive juices. It protects its own mucosa by secretion of mucus and a rapid turn over of epithelial cells. Special immunological mechanism is also involved in this defence mechanism.

**Symptoms of G.I. Tract Disorders :**

The major symptoms of deranged G.I. tract will depend on the site of pathology and its anatomical relations. As digestive tract traverses an extensive course from head to perineum, its symptomatology is often varied and confusing.

The symptoms of G.I. tract include anorexia, nausea, vomiting, abdominal pain, distension, gaseous eructation, passage of too much flatus, dysphagia, diarrhoea and dysentery. Heart burn and lower chest pain are very important symptoms which may be due to gastric, biliary or even ischaemic heart disease. Acid reflux, sudden regurgitation of food occurs in gastro-oesophageal disorders.

The analysis of each symptom should be made in relation to history. Analysis of pain is most important. Its site, type, time, duration, recurrence, radiation, relief and relation of food must be evaluated. These details will be dealt in the discussion on various G.I. disorders.

The most important object is to come to a diagnosis, which in case of G.I. disorders is sometime extremely difficult even after stool tests, gastric analysis and time-honoured radiological investigation as well as intestinal biopsy. However, modern radioisotopic scanning and ultrasonography have made tremendous advance in the diagnosis of G.I. disorders.

Hence clinical evaluation of digestive system disorders begins at the mouth and ends in the anus. It includes proper examination of lips, tongue, teeth, gums and oropharyngeal areas. It then involves proper examination of chest as well as abdomen and finally it may require an internal examination in many cases.

**Oral Cavity**

Patients may complain of dry mouth, painful areas, sore tongue, difficulty of chewing or swallowing, lack of taste, burning tongue, toothache or oral ulcers. All these may affect his nourishment due to inability to eat properly. However, in some instances patients have no oral symptoms and yet may have important clues in the oral cavity. Hence careful and proper examination of oral cavity, tongue,. tonsils, teeth, and gums is essential.

Some important points as follows :

Lips may be cracked in winter or due to lip-biting (a neurotic habit) but vitamin B complex deficiency diseases may cause cheilitis. Lips are pale in anaemia and swollen in angioneurotic oedema or inflammation. Stellate cicatrices around the lips proclaim congenital syphilis (ragadies). Chancres, epitheliomas, fungal fissures (perleche) also occur in lips.

Treatment will depend on the aetiology.

**Teeth & Gums**

Neglect of evaluating early diseases of teeth and gums may result in a lot of problems. Pyorrhoea alveolaris and dental caries may not only cause faulty digestion or loss of teeth in early life but it may be responsible for continued oral sepsis which may lead to rheumatic disorders and even nephritis.

Gums may reveal many important clues to important disorders. Gums may be inflammed due to local infection or appear swollen and congested in leukaemias, agranulocytosis, scurvy, pupura and Vincent's angina. Actinomycosis causes greenish yellow discharge which microscopically will show sulphur granules. Pigmentation of gum may occur in some tropical people as well as in Addison's disease. Blue lines in the free margin of gums may be seen in lead and bismuth poisoning.

Oral mucosa may be affected due to leucoplakia which are specially noted among smokers and tobacco chewers. It may be seen in tongue and oral mucosa; whitish patches are seen, which later on hardens and fissured and even may become malignant. Oral ulcers known as stomatitis are most troublesome. Syphilitic ulcers may occur in various stages of syphilis including gummata of tertiary stage.

**The Tongue**

Proper examination of tongue is most rewarding. Abnormality of tongue may be due to diseases of tongue itself or due to effects of diseases elsewhere, causing alterations in size shape of tongue and its mucosal appearance. During examination of tongue, note its surface, mucosa shape, its movements as well as its size or bulk.

Commonly tongue may be coated with whitish patches which is not abnormal unless it is thickly coated with curdlike areas with areola. On scraping the surface bright red or even bleeding surface is noted. This is due to thrush, i.e. fungal affection by candida albicans.

It usually occurs in bottle-fed children or under poor hygienic condition or in marasmic children.

Leucoplakia may be seen as flat whitish patches on the surface of tongue. Look into the buccal mucosa and gums for similar lesion. These are due to hypertrophy of the papillae which later on gets atrophied in patchy areas. Causes are too much smoking, tobacco chewing, syphilis while some are pre-malignant conditions. Hence, whenever there is suspicion biopsy must be ordered.

Colour of tongue normally is greyish white. It is pale in anaemia, bright red or scarlet red (so called fiery tongue) due to niacin deficiency. It is dark red beefy tongue in riboflavin deficiency. Polycythaemia vera causes bluish red tongue. Pellagrous tongue is usually of magenta colour. Patchy pigmentation may be seen in Addison's disease. But melanin pigments may sometimes be seen as black patches.

Coated furred tongue is often noted in mouth breathers, heavy smokers, alcoholics as well as in people with chronic colonic or hepatic disorders.

Dry coated tongue is noted in high fever, dehydration and ketosis. Raspberry tongue has scattered red dots, seen in scarlet fever not common in this country; strawberry tongue is due to progression of glossitis causing epithelial excoriation, giving a strawberry appearance. Ulcers may form on the tongue due to ulcerative stomatitis, vincent's angina, pemphigus, syphilis, herpes, malignancy, dental injury. Whenever there is doubt, biopsy should never be delayed.

Syphilitic lesions occur in form of primary chancre, Hutchison's Wart, mucous patches, snailtrack ulcers, leucoplakia or even gummata, depending on the stage of syphilis. Malignancy usually occurs in the margins, usually single indurated ulcer. Regional lymphnode is enlarged.

In severe dehydration tongue may appear dry and small in size, Atrophy may be noted also in pseudobulbar palsy (small pointed conical tongue). Hemiatrophy of tongue is seen in unilateral hypoglossal nerve involvement. Deviation may also occur in hypoglossal nerve involvement.

Spasm of tongue may occur in hysteria, chorea or disseminated sclerosis (D.S.). Immobile tongue occurs in bulbar palsy, advanced amyotrophic lateral sclerosis, syringomyelia, tabes dorsalis or advanced malignancy.

Tremor of tongue may be seen in bulbar palsy, encephalitis, chronic alcoholism, delirium tremens, GPI, parkinsonism, D.S., toxic fevers, especially severe typhoid fever, etc.

**Geographical Tongue**

Map-like areas develop due to desquamation of mucosa in patches. These patchy areas are surrounded by proliferating whitish margins consisting of heaped epithelium.

Improvement of nutrition, oral hygiene and general health are the basis of treatment.

**Enlarged Tongue :**

Angio neurotic oedema may cause painless enlargement but may extend downwards causing laryngeal oedema, a serious medical emergency. Even tracheostomy may be required. Acute glossitis may cause acutely painful enlargement of tongue due to streptococcal infection, which should be treated with penicillin group of drugs or erythromycin and supportive therapy. Macroglossia or large tongue may occur as a congenital defect or in acromegaly, cretins, myxoedema, amyloidosis or due to abscess or new growth, e.g. haemangioma, lipoma, lymphangioma and malignancy.

## METHODS OF INVESTIGATION OF G.I. TRACT DISORDERS

Investigation will depend on the finding of clinical history, physical examination, i.e. examination of abdomen by inspection, palpation, percussion and auscultation. Tests for presence of fluid must be carefully done whenever abdomen is distended and there is suspicion of ascitis. Digital examination and proctoscopy may be required whenever there is a history of difficulty or pain during evacuation or history of blood P.R. or continued dysentery.

Sigmoidoscopy is considered if there is chronic dysentery or history of rectal bleeding.

Most cases will not require modern and sophisticated methods of investigation. It is preferable that expensive investigations are ordered after a specialist consultation when dealing with poor people. Careful clinical assessment by an experienced consultant, will be much less expensive than a C.T. Scan.

**Stool :** Inspection of stool is most important. However, this is often neglected and small samples are sent to the laboratory. If these are examined several hours after passing stool it has very little value.

Stool must be inspected as fresh as possible or in office practice, try to get a proper description of stool from the patient himself, explaining to him what you want to know.

Stool may be brownish watery in simple diarrhoea, mixed with blood and mucus with faeces in amoebic dysentery, tar coloured in upper G.I. bleeding.

Giardial infection may produce simple diarrhoea but the patient has a feeling or urgency to evacuate, associated with noisy expulsion of foul-smelling faecos with gas. In cholera stool is rice-water in colour and passage of stool is painless and frequent. When solid normal-looking stool contains streaks or drops of fresh blood, it is usually due to haemorrhoids. Stool of ulcerative colitis is mixed with fresh or altered blood. Frank blood may also be passed. In all these cases, P.R. and procto sigmoidoscopy should be considered. Where the whole faecal matter is black like coal tar, it is called malaena. It is due to bleeding from upper gastrointestinal tract. Malabsorption syndrome causes bulky frothy stool. Routine examination of stool must be done to find out presence of pus cells, RBC's macrophages, undigested materials, intestinal parasites, parasitic ova and cysts, segments of worms etc. Organisms can be cultured if necessary, but fresh stool should be used. Hanging drop preparation is done for diagnosis of cholera. Microscopic G.I. bleeding may occur due to peptic ulcers, ankylostomiasis, frequent asprin intake and mucosal erosions. This is detected by occult blood test. However, bacteriology of small intestinal flora can be checked by collecting sterile sample by sterile Ryle's tube passed into the upper intestines or still better by endoscopes.

**Radiology**

Plain radiograph of abdomen may be very helpful in determining shape and size of enlarged, organs, presence of gas causing distension of gut, gas under diaphragm, etc. giving important information. A chest radiograph simultaneously taken gives additional information regarding the roof of abdomen.

Barium meal X-ray studies show the movement of opaque barium along the gut and thus motility and movements of oesphagus, stomach and intestines can be observed directly during screening as well as series of pictures can be taken and mucosal pattern, ulcers, new growth can be diagnosed in most cases. The barium follow-through will show the appearance and movements of the whole of the G.I. tract down to rectum. Barium containing enema and radiological study are particularly done for visualizing of the shape, size, mucosa, constrictions, diverticula, new growths and ulcerative lesions of large gut. It is, however, somewhat uncomfortable for the patient especially in aged or cardiac patients.

X-ray exposure to female abdomen may be injurious to foetus in early months of pregnancy. Enquiry should be made regarding the last menstrual period (LMP) and X-ray exposure to women at risk should be avoided. It is considered first 10 days (10-days rule) from onset of LMP is safe for radiological examination of females of child-bearing age.

**Ultrasonography**

This method of investigating the abdomen by ultrasound waves and recording photographs has become extremely useful in detecting stones in gall bladder, renal calculi, cysts and abscesses. Foetal body can be seen and its development as well as deformities can be made out.

**Radioisotope scanning**

This is also a very valuable method especially in hepatic and splenic disorders. Radioisotopic uptake reveals the health of tissue cells and may detect cold areas due to cysts, abscesses, new growth or metastasis.

**C.T. Scans**

This is another excellent method of investigation which reveals sliced view of abdominal organs at various levels. Due to large installation cost its availability is limited to affluent countries though several units are now available is India.

**Secretory Studies**

**Pentagastrin test**

By the method "basal acid output" and "maximum acid output" are estimated. A synthetic polypeptide (pentagastrin) is used to stimulate gastric juice secretion.

The patient fasts overnight and if he is on cimetidine, drug is discontinued for 48 hours prior to the test. In the fasting state in the morning gastric juice is aspirated and all secretions are collected for one hour. Then Inj. pentagastrin is injected S.C. and samples of juice are collected for further one hour.

**Usefulness of the test**

(1) Large volume of basal collection suggests pyloric spasm or obstruction.

(2) Absence of acid suggests possibility of gastric carcinoma.

(3) High basal acid suggests Zollinger Ellison syndrome.

**Pancreatic function tests**

Pancreatic juice is collected by duodenal incubation under X-ray control. At first gastric juice is aspirated as much as possible. Then tube is pushed into the duodenum and injections of secretin and pancreozymin are given I.V. and the juices are collected for one hour for estimation of bicarbonate, amylase and trypsin. The juice is also microscopically examined for RBC, cytology and malignant cells.

In malabsorption state with steatorrhoea, if the G.T.T. cruve is diabetic in type, it is suggestive of advanced pancreatic disease or pancreatic carcinoma. In pancreatic insufficiency the volume of juice, bicarbonate level and enzyme contents are all diminished. The modern method, however, is to carry out endoscopy, collect the juices directly as well as visualise the local pathology. Biopsy can also be taken simultaneously.

**Endoscopy**

Rigid metallic instruments, e.g. oesophagoscopes and sigmoidoscopes were in vogue to carry out endoscopy in the past. Later on around 1940, the semiflexible gastroscopes were introduced. Very few experts were using this method till Japanese introduced gastro-camera. This is a tiny camera which is introduced into the stomach and multiple pictures are taken blindly.

However, gastrointestinal investigation was completely revolutionised since the principle of fiberoptic light transmission originally patented in Britain (Baird 1928; Hopkins & Kapany 1954) was utilised by the technical expertise of American and Japanese collaboration.

During present decade oesophago-gastro-duodenoscopy and colonoscopy are being used more and more. This is now available in India also in many special centres. Modern endoscopy instruments are flexible tubes containing a series of glass bundles instead of lenses used in the past. These bundles are 2-4 mm in diameter and there are many thousands of fine glass fibres which transmit light by internal fibre to fibre reflections.

With these modern endoscopic instruments, biopsy can be easily made from the suspected areas and juices can be aspirated, even gall stones can be removed in some cases. Polyps and F.B.'s. can also be removed and strictures can be overcome. In acute bleeding, haemorrhage can be controlled successfully.

However, it must be realised that proper training and experience of the doctor behind the instrument is most important. The problem today however is acutely felt in developing countries where funds, instruments and experts in this field are lacking.

However, it must also be realised that even if these instruments and experts are available, value of barium meal X-ray studies will still remain as primary diagnostic stool. Endoscopy is an additional method of diagnosis and specially valuable in barium negative dyspepsias. The additional value of endoscopy is where other methods fail to elucidate the pathology and still clinical grounds exist for further investigation.

## DISEASES OF THE MOUTH

*G.C. MOOKERJEE*

**Introduction**

Mouth receives food, masticates, mixes the food with alkaline saliva containing the enzyme ptyalin and then pushes the bolus into oesophagus for onward passage to stomach. Ptyalin breaks polysaccharides into disaccharides.

Defects of teeth, painful gum, oral ulcers or neuromuscular incordination will affect the digestion of food.

A good set of teeth and proper chewing habit is extremely important for good health. Rapid eating habit, i.e. swallowing food bolus without proper chewing is a common cause of indigestion. Oral hygiene is essential for the health of teeth and gum. Timely warning to children will save lot of trouble in later years both from the points of good health and economy. Sweet-eating in schools is a bad western habit which has now become widespread in this country also, leading to increased incidence of caries of teeth among school children. Periodic dental inspection should be made a compulsory routine from school-going age.

## PYORRHOEA ALVEOLARIS

It is the commonest oral sepsis due to lack of oral hygiene. Gingivitis is the starting-point. Inflammation involves papillary or marginal gingiva, due to bacterial infection plus calcareous and mucin deposits in the free gum margin. Inadequate oral hygiene leads to collection of food debris which liberates acid substances causing periodontitis. If periodontitis is not treated it causes bone resorption, separation of gingiva and teeth and progressive local infection (pyorrhoea alveolaris). This kind of oral sepsis is not only a local disease but it may be responsible for many crippling disorders from rheumatism to nephritis.

**Treatment**

Expert dental care must be rendered to save the teeth. Even aspiration of pus from gum abscess may cause pulmonary complications, e.g. pneumonitis and lung abscess. Antibiotics will help a lot but extraction of tooth may be necessary. It is most important that doctors should routinely inspect oral cavity and prevent dental decay and lot of old-age problems.

The habit of eating chocolates and lozenges will as 'pan' (betel leaf) and tobacco or cigarette smoking are the major causes of dental problems.

## STOMATITIS

Stomatitis is an inflammatory disease of oral mucous membrane, with or without ulceration, caused by multiple factors e.g. :

(1) **Bacterial**

e.g. Vincent's organism, fusiform bacillus, H. streptococci, C. diphtheriae, M. tuberculosis, T. pallidum.

(2) **Viral :**

e.g. Measles, chicken-pox, herpes virus and no more existent smallpox.

(3) **Fungal :**

e.g. Candida albicans and moniliasis.

(4) **Nutritional :**

Deficiency of B-complex vitamins e.g. Riboflavin, niacin, cyanocobalamin and folic acid. Deficiency of vitamin C causes scurvy, heralded by bleeding gums.

(5) **Mechanical :**

Smoking of tobacco, 'pan-chewing' (due to lime and catechu), neat alcohol drinking, toothpastes (not properly washed out) and too hot food.

(6) **Immunological** — IgA immunoglobulin deficiences, especially occurring in infants and children.

Many underlying diseases, e.g. diabetes mellitus, leukaemia and malignancies are often in the background.

**Catarrhal stomatitis :**

Usually occurs due to causes described under mechanical causes of stomatitis. Bad oral hygiene may be a singular cause.

**Treatment**

Removal of precipitating agents, alkaline mouth wash and bland diet.

## APHTHOUS STOMATITIS

In this condition tiny ulcers appear, which often enlarge and coalesce. Yellowish sloughs may appear.

They come and go in crops and cause painful mouth with excessive salivation leading to difficulty in mastication. Even speech is affected due to local pain.

**Treatment**

It is very intractable to treatment; spontaneous remission may occur but recurrence is also fairly frequent. Meticulous oral hygiene is essential.

Bland diet, liquid or semi-liquid at the beginning, is essential to maintain nourishment. Oral toilet, hydrogen peroxide or alkaline mouth wash or short course of tetracycline mouth wash (0.5%) may be tried. Hydrocortisone succrets are often quite useful. Give attention to vitamin B complex intake. High doses of vitamin C (1000 mg per day) may be tried with glucose.

## VINCENT'S ANGINA

(Ulcero-membranous stomatitis)

It is an acute ulcerative condition affecting oropharyngeal muscosa and gum-tissue, causing a lot of discomfort, salivation and difficult mastication. Greyish-white sloughs are seen with superficial membrane formation, which can be easily removed. Regional lymph nodes are enlarged, causative organisms are fusiform bacillus and borelia Vincenti.

The most important differential diagnosis is from diphtheria. In diphtheria, membranes are commonly seen in tonsillar and peritonsillar area or pharyngeal mucosa and not usually in inner cheek and gums. The chief differentiating feature being that the diphtheretic membrane is tough and cannot be easily removed by a swab. It can be removed by a pair of forceps, resulting in raw bleeding surface. Bacteriology confirms the diagnosis.

**Treatment**

Inj. procaine penicillin 5,00,000 units given I.M. twice or thrice a day for 5 to 7 days is sufficient but mild cases can be treated with oral antiseptic lozenges, sucked every two or three hours. Oral hygiene, vitamins and supportive therapy should be given as usual.

## MONILIASIS

(Thrush)

It is due to candida albicans commonly seen in malnutrition states and in debilitating diseases, children often are victims. The lesions appear as small pin-head painful white spots, which coalesce and become extensive patches (pseudomembrane).

Diagnosis is made by inspection and confirmed by microscopy.

**Treatment**

1% Gentian violet or still better nystantin paint and local toilet is usually adequate. Attention to general health, nutrition and underlying diseases must be given.

## GANGRENOUS STOMATITIS

(Cancrum oris)

It used to be common when Kala-azar was endemic and inadequately treated. It may also occur due to vincent's organisms. H. streptococci, when there is gross malnutrition or advanced malignancy elsewhere.

**Treatment**

Attention to underlying disease, oral hygiene, appropriate antibiotics and later reconstructive surgery. If there is active leishmaniasis. it should be treated properlv.

## DISEASES OF OESOPHAGUS

**Introduction**

Oesophagus or gullet is a fibro-muscular tube through which food materials are transmn from oropharynx into the stomach. The oesophageal mucosa is lined by cuboidal cells and the tube has sphincter-like mechanism both at upper and lower ends so that swallowed food does not regurgitate. The upper oesophageal sphincter (UOS) is at the level of cricoid cartilage, i.e. junctions of crico-pharynx and oesophagus and lower oesophageal sphincter (LOS) is at the oesophago-gastric junction.

The sphincters automatically open when the food is being passed and transmitted downwardly by peristaltic waves of the oesophagus, otherwise these sphincters remain closed.

The cardinal symptoms of disorder of oesophagus are dysphagia and pain.

Whenever a patient complains of one or both of these symptoms, it is essential to urgently investigate to exclude cancer and achalasia.

## DYSPHAGIA

**Oesophageal causes**

Common causes are :

1. Cancer of the oesophagus
2. Cardiovascular diseases with enlarged heart especially left auricle, pressing on the gullet
3. Intrathoracic tumour pressing on the oesophagus
4. Acute oesophagitis leading to stricture : swallowing of strong alcohol, corrosive agents or acid injury, oesophageal reflux as in hiatus hernia
5. Accidental instrumentation injury causing stricture
6. Achalasia cardia.

**Rare causes are :**

1. Collagen disease, e.g. scleroderma and dermatomyositis
2. Plummer Vinson syndrome
3. Diverticula or pharyngeal pouch
4. Congenitally short oesophagus
5. Chaga's disease
6. Diffuse idiopathic oesophageal spasm.

Pharyngeal disorders may also simulate dysphagia

1. Painful conditions of oro-pharynx — Acute tonsillitis, stomatitis, retropharyngeal abscess and dental pain
2. Bulbar or pseudobulbar palsy.

## ACHALASIA CARDIA

(Cardiospasm)

Achalasia means "unable to relax". Cardiospasm is a misnomer. Chaga's disease due to trypanosomiasis also causes achalasia.

**Aetiopathology**

The disease involves whole of this oesophagus causing ineffective contraction of smooth muscles and incordination of peristalsis. The lower oesophagus does not relax, while upper two-thirds of oesophagus do not have adequate propelling peristalsis. The lower oesophageal muscles become thicker while upper two-thirds go on dilating. The basic defect is lack of adequate neuronal supply in Auerbach's plexus. In Chaga's disease, the Auerbach's plexus is destroyed not only in oesophagus but also in whole or GI tract, so that achalasia, megaduodenum, megacolon, even megaureter can occur. Aetiology of achalasia cardia, however, is unknown.

**Clinical Features**

The cardinal symptoms are dysphagia and regurgitation of food taken many hours before.

Dysphagia occurs both for solids and liquids and is more marked when attempt is made to eat in a hurry. Regurgitation of food into respiratory passages during sleep may cause aspiration pneumonitis. Another important feature of regurgitation is absence of acid taste. Initially dysphagia is intermittent, later it becomes permanent causing huge dilatation of oesophagus. Gradually there is progressive loss of weight.

### Diagnosis

A chest radiograph usually suggests the diagnosis. Enlarged oesophageal outline with a fluid level is noted behind the cardiac silhoutte. Barium swallow picture clearly shows the oesophageal pathology but does not exclude carcinoma at the lower end of oesophagus. Therefore, oesophagoscopy should be done to exclude carcinoma.

### Treatment

All cases should be referred to a thoracic surgeon as there is no medical treatment. Isosorbide dinitrate or **nifedipine** may be helpful in mild cases. The surgical management consists of :

1. Hydrostatic dilatation of the narrow segment by bougies, hydrostatic or pneumatic balloon through oesophagoscope.
3. Heller's operation, i.e. cardiomyotomy.
3. Endoscopic myotomy.

It is however essential that presence of carcinoma to be excluded.

## ACUTE OESOPHAGITIS

### Causes

1. Corrosive agents swallowed accidentally or for suicidal attempts
2. Gastric juice reflux
3. Monilial infection in seriously ill chronic invalids.

### Treatment

Depends on underlying aetiology. Antacids, demulcents and bland diet to reduce acidity. **Ranitidine orally or parenterally may be useful. Prevent reflux of acid juice from stomach by** avoiding prolonged gastric intubation. Antiemetics may be used to control vomiting. Acute oesophagitis due to acid and corrosive damage has been discussed in the chapter on poisoning.

## CHRONIC OESOPHAGITIS & OESOPHAGEAL HIATAL HERNIA

Chronic oesophagitis is due to mucosal damage of lower end of the oesophagus due to reflux of acid gastric juice into oesophagus. This may occur due to incompetence of oesophago-gastric junction. Normally lower oesophageal sphincter and the diaphragmatic sphincter chiefly prevent reflux of acid juice into oesophagus. Even mucosal ulcerātion and bleeding may occur. If the condition is allowed to persist the lumen may become narrowed due to fibrosis.

### Oesophageal Hiatal Hernia

The oesophageal hiatus in the dome of diaphragm is formed by a splitting of the fibres of the right crus and this forms a pinch cock action, preventing regurgitation of gastric juice. Weakness of this area or raised intraabdominal pressure (e.g. pregnancy, ascitis, intraabdominal tumours etc.), old age, obesity, emaciation etc. are possible factors.

Three types of hiatal hernia are possible e.g. :

1. Sliding variety (oesophago-gastric)
2. Rolling (para oesophageal)
3. Mixed type, i.e. both sliding and rolling.

**Clinical features**

The chief symptom is heartburn and dysphagia. Heartburn is aggravated especially on lying down or bending and after a large meal. It is more common in elderly and obese people. Females suffer more than males. Water brush due to regurgitation and salivation can be quite troublesome. Regurgitation of gastric juice may cause severe aspiration pneumonitis. Haematemesis can be severe. Anaemia is often prominent.

**Diagnosis**

History and symptomatology suggest the diagnosis. It is confirmed by barium meal study confirming presence of hiatus hernia.

Sometimes symptoms are present but barium study fails to demonstrate it. In severe cases oesophagoscopy and biopsy may be done only if malignancy is suspected. Modern fiberoptic flexible oesophago-gastroscopes are excellent for diagnosis.

**Treatment**

Patient should be advised to take small meals three hourly and avoid spicy diet, alcohol, betel chewing, tobacco chewing and smoking. They should not go to bed immediately after meals. Frequent administration of antacids may be required i.e. after each meal or whenever symptoms occur. Xylocaine viscous is often useful before meals.

Oral metoclopramide 10 mg. three times a day half an hour before meals may help. If still there is acid reflux especially in co-existing peptic ulcer, can be given parenterally if symptoms are severe and especially if there is haematemesis. Postural precaution is important. Bending should be avoided.

Diet regime initially should be in the line of peptic ulcer. Most cases will improve and can be controlled by medical treatment. Surgery is required only in a few cases if medical treatment fails.

## PARAOESOPHAGEAL HERNIA

In this rare condition a small part of oesophagus rolls alongside into chest but the lower oesophageal sphincter is normal. If the herniation is small, it hardly causes any symptom, but if large portion of stomach becomes intrathoracic breathlessness and cardiac embarrassment may occur.

Auscultation of the chest may reveal stomach movements due to peristalsis in left lower chest unless the hernia is very small.

Barium-radiography settles the diagnosis.

## OESOPHAGEAL SPASM

Diffuse oesophageal spasm may be due to lack of neuronal defect as in case of achalasia but whole of the oesophagus is affected due to incoordinated peristalsis.

**Clinical features**

Symptoms usually occur during swallowing or even due to emotional stress.

Discomfort in chest, retrosternal pain may mimic cardiac angina. Dysphagia is not a so prominent symptom.

**Diagnosis**

Barium radiograph demonstrates wavy oesophageal outline, known as 'corkscrew oesophagitis'.

**Treatment**

Most cases require assurance tranquilizers and slow eating habit. Proper mastication and slow deglutition should be encouraged. Glyceryl trinintrini or pentaerythrol tetranitrate as used for ischaemic heart disease may also help. In very rare instances cardiomytomy may be considered.

## DIAPHRAGMATIC HERNIA

It is due to incompetence of the left cupola of diaphragm which is usually a congenital defect or may be acquired in old age

In a newborn it can cause acute respiratory difficulty but diagnosis can be easily made by auscultation, as tinkling intestinal sounds can be heard in the left side of the chest. Plain X-ray of the chest settles the diagnosis.

**Treatment**

Surgical treatment should be done except in old people whose postural care may only be necessary.

## CARCINOMA

Carcinoma oesophagus is common in India and it constitutes about one third of all G.I. cancers.

Habit of drinking too hot food, tobacco chewing, strong neat alcoholic drinks are possible causes. For details of aetiopathology reference should be made to surgical text book but it is necessary to stress that any dysphagia with or without thoracic pain or discomfort during swallowing should be urgently investigated by barium meal X-ray examination of the oesophagus. A 'rat-tail' type of radiological picture suggests the diagnosis. As early lesions are likely to be missed in X-ray study,fiberoptic oesophago-gastroscopy should be carried out so that even small lesions can be detected. Sometimes these cases are mistaken for I.H.D.

**Treatment**

The case should be handed over to a cancer centre so that both surgical and oncological review is possible. The possible methods of treatment available today are :

(a) Surgical operation using prosthesis.

(b) Chemotherapy using mitomycin-C, bleomycin, methotrexate, cyclophosphamide and suitable drug combinations.

(c) Radiotherapy with or without surgery, depending on the stage.

## BENIGN TUMOURS

Adenomas and liomyomas may occur in oesophagus. When growth enlarges it may cause bleeding or produce dysphagia.

**Treatment** – Surgical.

# ACUTE GASTRITIS

*G.C. MOOKERJEE*

Acute gastritis is a definite clinical entity, which occurs due to a variety of clinical conditions e.g. emotional stress, shock or toxic materials damaging the mucosa. If gastric mucosal barrier is damaged acid-peptic digestion of mucosa may occur.

**Causes :**

Irritant food
Alcohol
Salicylates
Aminophylline
Cortico-steroids
Phenylbutazone
Indomethacin.

Idiosyncracy to some drugs e.g. sulpha drugs, iodides, tetracyclines.

Staphylococcal food poisoning.

In addition acute corrosive poisoning is a very well — known cause

**Clinical features :**

In mild form there is epigastric discomfort and often local tenderness. Nausea and loss of appetite may occur.

In severe cases acute epigastric pain, vomiting or even upper gastro-intestinal bleeding may occur causing haematemesis followed by malaena.

Early gastroscopy settles the diagnosis.

**Treatment :**

Early cases will improve with antacids, and bland diet, causative factor being removed e.g. withdrawal of drugs or alcohol.

Acute corrosive gastritis needs intensive care as follows :

1. Cold water lavage
2. Liquid antacids 2-3 hourly
3. Cold milk by Ryle's tube
4. Use of demulcents
5. Intravenous fluids or blood transfusion
6. Attention to coagulation defects if any

(Refer to the section on poisoning for further details).

## "ACUTE DILATATION OF STOMACH"

It is usually a post-operative complication after major abdominal surgery or trauma but sometimes it occurs due to toxaemia of an acute infective process.

Its pathogenesis is not clearly understood. The stomach becomes hugely dilated with mucosal congestion and contains large quantity of gas, mucus, and gastric juice but containing little acid.

**Clinical feature :**

The onset is characterised by rapid abdominal distention and repeated vomiting; loss of fluids and electrolyte leads to hypovolaemic shock. In surgical cases it usually occurs after 48 hours and the patient rapidly deteriorates very promptly. Distension of abdomen and shock are prominent features. There may be abdominal discomfort due to distension but no severe pain.

**Treatment :**

1. Omit oral feeds
2. Gastric suction to aspirate gastric contents
3. Correction of fluid electrolyte loss
4. Judicious use of anti-biotics.

## "SUPERIOR MESENTERIC ARTERY SYNDROME"

This is also known as duodenal ileus and it is due to compression of 3rd part of duodenum by the superior mesenteric artery which crosses the 3rd part of duodenum.

Symptoms usually occur in some thin persons when they walk about after heavy meal. Vomiting may occur. Relief occurs on lying in bed in prone posture, when compression is relieved due to prone position. A barium meal X-ray taken in erect posture shows dilatation of duodenal loop, proximally.

## VOLVULOUS OF STOMACH :

A very rare conditon, which occurs due to twisting of stomach along its long axis, fixed between oesophagogastric junction and duodenum. Sometimes there may be a gastric neoplasm or chronic gastric ulcer.

**Clinical features**

In acute volvulous there is acute abdominal pain with nausea which heralds the onset. A palpable mass is felt in the epigastric region.

Volvulous if chronic, there is epigastric discomfort, gargling after meal and palpable mass felt in the epigastrium.

**Treatment :** Surgical.

## PEPTIC ULCER SYNDROME

*G.C. MOOKERJEE*
*A.K. SEN SHARMA*

**Aetiology**

Peptic ulcer is caused by the digestive action of hydrochloric acid and pepsin on the mucous membrane of the upper gastrointestinal tracts when mucosal resistance is poor. It occurs mainly in the stomach, first part of duodenum, less commonly in post-bulbar duodenum, distal duodenum and jejunum especially in case of Zollinger Ellison (Z.E.) syndrome. Due to presence of peptic mucosa, it can occur in Meckel's diverticula. As a matter of fact any part of gastrointestinal tract which has contact with hydrochloric acid and pepsin may develop an ulcer.

Duodenal ulcer is commonest peptic ulcers and may occur in teenage, young and old people and all over the world. In India it is commonest among rice-eating south Indians (especially Tamil Nadu and Kerala) and Bengalis while less common among those in northern India, who are wheat-eaters. Males are more affected than women.

Various factors like tobacco-smoking or tobacco chewing, spicy food, hot food, improper chewing habit (lack of proper salivary digestion), mental stress, too much tea or coffee drinking are all blamed. However, familial and genetic susceptibility appears to be more significant. People with blood group 'O' appear to be non susceptible.

However, the real cause of peptic ulcer formation is still not clear.

Steroids, aspirin, aminophylline, non-steroidal anti-inflammatory and analgesic drugs definitely play an important role. Strong alcoholic drinks especially gulped without food also play a significant role. Diluted alcohol taken with snacks are not harmful. Many disorders are known to be associated with peptic ulcer, e.g., infectious hepatitis, cirrhosis of liver, chronic pancreatitis, primary hyperparathyroidism, polyendocrine disorders, thermal burns, severe trauma and brain tumours. Chronic bronchitic may develop gastritis or even gastric ulcer due to too such oral aminophylline group of drugs.

**Patho-Physiology**

There have been considerable advances in the understanding of aetiology, pathophysiology, biochemistry as well as in its medical treatment. Lower part of the oesophagus lined by columnar epithelial cells is vulnerable to acid gastric juice. In presence of hiatus hernia, reflux oesophagitis with ulceration may be caused by constant or repeated contact with gastric juice.

Stomach consists of fundus, body, antrum and pylorus. It is highly vascular organ supplied by three sets of vessels (e.g. left gastric, right gastric and short gastric vessels). In the lesser curvature branches of left gastric artery anastomoses with the branches of right gastric artery. The greater curvature of the stomach is supplied by left gastro-epiploic artery. In fundus, branches of short gastric arteries spread with multiple branches.

The mucosa of the stomach consists of surface of epithelium and multiple glandular cells. Parietal cells secrete hydrochloric acid and chief cells liberate pepsin; G-cells located in the antrum and duodenum are responsible for gastrin secretion. G-cells have endocrine function which secrete "gastrin" hormone. Besides these, there are plenty of mucus glands.

*Control of gastric secretion is a complex phenomena :*

(1) Nervous control — Two sets of vagus nerves (para sympathetic) control the acid secretion directly acting with acetylcholine of the parietal cells. Vagus nerves are also responsible for gastric secretion by G-cell in the antrum.

(2) Gastrin is gastrointestinal hormone, responsible for humoral control of acid secretion. Circulating gastrin molecules are of different molecular sizes. Larger molecules of gastrin remain in the circulation for longer time. Smaller molecules though more active, disappear quickly Gastrin is secreted by G-cells in the stomach and to some extent in duodenum. The secretion of gastrin is influenced by many factors e.g. distension or stomach, alkalisation of antrum, calcium, and also magnesium levels, as well as by glucagon, VIP, GIP, and increased activity of vagus nerves. Secretion is inhibited by hyperacidity and produces feedback mechanism.

(3) Mast-cell lying in the gastric mucosa secretes histamine which also stimulates acid secretion. There are receptors for histamine to act on the parietal cells which secrete hydrochloric acid by a complex mechanism.

**Pathogenesis**

Normal cell population of parietal cells in normal individuals is about a billion but higher (2-3 billions) in case of subjects with duodenal ulcer.

Maximum acid secretion is about 40 mEq per hour in patients of duodenal ulcer (normal being 18-20 mEq per hour) although in many patients it may be normal. Thus it appears that it is difficult to correlate these two factors in some cases.

Pentagastrin and histamine provocation test increases the acid secretion during intraprandial period. Increased acid secretion indicates higher population of parietal cells or its increased sensitivity to various responsible agents mentioned earlier.

**Defence mechanism**

A complex mechanism plays a great role for protection of gastric and duodenal mucosa from the various aggressive agents e.g. acid pepsin, bile, pancreatic enzymes and other exogenous agents. Physiologically continuous regeneration of the epithelium, covering of mucus coat, protection of $HCO_3$, and prostaglandins are also protective factors.

*Zollinger Ellison syndrome* — In this condition there is formation of giant or multiple and recurrent ulcers mainly in the duodenum. This is due to a non-beta islet cell tumour of the pancreas, which secretes gastrin. Rarely it occurs in oesophagus. There is high blood gastrin level leading to excessive secretion of acid, associated with fulminant recurrent and multiple ulceration. It can be diagnosed by presence of high acid secretion (80–100 mEq per hour) and immunoassay of high level of plasma gastrin. The condition is to be treated by total gastrectomy. Other factors of high blood gastrin level may be due to hyperplasia of G-cell mass in the antrum and failure of inactivation by kidneys.

*Gastric Mucosal Barrier* — Gastric surface epithelium is impermeable to certain ions and restrict the back flow of H-ions from the lumen to blood and movement sodium in the opposite direction. This phenomena known as "gastric mucosal barrier". Impairment of this mechanism appears to be the cause of gastric ulcer.

*Effect of bile and pancreatic enzymes* — The bile and pancreatic enzymes produce damage of stomach mucosa. Reflux of bile and pancreatic enzymes in excess, in the stomach due to incompetent pylorus may produce gastric ulcer.

*Gastric blood flow* — Gastric arteries enter the stomach from submucosal plexus in the submucosal layer. From this plexus, submucosal arteries branch off and supply the rich subepithelial network of capillaries. This gives adequate protection by continuous cell regeneration. But in old age this rich blood flow may be restricted due to atherosclerosis and break the protective mechanism leading to gastric ulcer formation.

**Clinical features**

Symptoms will depend on the location and stage of the ulcer. In tropics many tropical bowel disorders may present symptoms of upper abdominal dyspepsia, which may be confused with peptic ulcer. Flatulence, epigastric discomfort, heart-burn, acid eructations are often confusing symptoms which may not only occur due to peptic ulcer but also may occur in chronic amoebiasis, chronic pancreatitis, colonic disorders as well as due to helminthiasis.

Indiscriminate orders for routine barium meal X-ray study may be reported as "presence of Ascaris-check stool" However, ulcer and ascaris both may persist. However, careful stool examination may be helpful. It is better to put the patient on vegetarian diet for three days and check stool for occult blood as well as for ova, parasites and cysts.

It is also stressed that gastric ulcer may not have ,classical or diagnostic symptoms or signs, hence whenever in doubt, refer the patient for endosocopy. It may discover presence of gastric ulcer missed in barium meal studies and may reveal early malignancy.

*Pain*

Epigastric or vague abdominal pain is a characteristic and predominant presenting symptom. Careful analysis of symptoms may help in distinguishing between chronic duodenal and uncomplicated peptic ulcer and between peptic ulcer and other disorders that mimic peptic ulcer.

(1) *Location of pain*

(a) Duodenal ulcer — well localised in epigastric or subxiphoid area.

(b) Gastric ulcer — epigastric area, often not well localised, even vague discomfort only.

(c) Oesophageal ulcer — Substernal or subxiphoid area.

(d) Postbulbar ulcer — low epigastric or hypogastric region.

*Note* : Dogmatic pronouncements about site and nature of lesion should never be made on the basis of pain location. Even cardiac and gall-bladder pain may be mistaken for chronic peptic ulcer, or oesophagitis.

(2) *Character of pain*

In duodenal ulcer pain is steady in empty stomach. Patients usually learn to relieve themselves by taking cold milk, biscuits or even plain water. It is variously described as "gnawing", "burning", "aching", "hunger pains", "dull", "sense of fullness" or "gas pain", etc.

(3) *Intensity of pain*

It is directly proportional to site, type and chronicity of ulcer. The pain located around left of mid-epigastric region being lowest in duodenal, intermediate in gastric and highest in post-bulbar or stomal ulcers.

Size of ulcer and the patient's sensitivity to pain are important. Serosal involvement, as in penetrating ulcer may cause radiation of pain to spine. Rhythmicity is important. Spontaneous remission and relapses may occur giving false-positive results of therapeutic trials. In duodenal ulcer, onset of pain is about one and a half to two hours after meals. It often comes at night (between midnight and early morning. There is a cycle food → comfort →(2 hrs) → pain.

In gastric ulcer, pain appears soon after meals; pain is seldom present at night and on awakening. Sometimes it is only vague discomfort.

Pain may radiate to the spine. Duration of pain is usually 30—90 minutes.

Both duodenal and gastric ulcers show periodicity i.e., pain occurs for days and months, subsides for many months and then recurs to repeat the cycle.

(4) *Relieving factors*

In duodenal ulcer food (especially milk) and antacids usually bring immediate relief.

In gastric ulcer food brings little or no relief, but may cause aggravation of pain. Pain is however relieved by antacids.

(5) *Nutrition*

In duodenal ulcer patient eats bland high calorie diet quite well, specially milk and gains weight.

In gastric ulcer, patient is afraid to eat and loses weight progressively.

Loss of weight and unexplained anaemia are often pointers.

Gastric cancers are often diagnosed ,too late so be careful and suspicious.

*Stool Examination* for occult blood — if properly done may be a pointer — though it is a non-specific test.

*Radiology* remains the major diagnostic tool in our country because facilities for endoscopy are not yet widely available. Barium meal study be done by a competent radiologist himself who can employ special techniques and manoeuvres to demonstrate small lesions so that more than 80% cases of peptic ulcer can be demonstrated.

**Limitations of Radiology**

(a) About 15—20% lesions cannot demonstrated.

(b) Benign nature cannot be ascertained in certain cases and so gastroscopy and exfoliative cytology are indicated.

(c) Superficial ulcers may not retain barium and are missed.

(d) Distal duodenal, oesophageal and stomal ulcers are difficult to demonstrate; Endoscopy is indicated.

**Endoscopy** — Fiberoptic flexible gastroscopy will detect over 90% lesions including ulcers of distal duodenum, oesophagus, stomal ulcers, superficial ulcers and those near the angulus along the lesser curvature. Ulcers can be directly visualised, photographed and contents scraped for cytological studies with the modern fiberoptic endoscopes fitted with camera. Unfortunately the scope of this valuable diagnostic tool is limited in our country. False positives may be diagnosed in the hands of not-so-experienced.

Limitations — Lesions situated higher up in the lesser curvature, posterior wall and parts of cardiac end and fundus cannot be visualised. These cases are often mistaken for anginal pain and wrongly treated till too late.

**Gastric Juice Analysis** — It is usually unnecessary and troublesome to the patient. One hour basal acid output coupled with maximal histamine (also Betazole or Pentagastrin) stimulation provides useful information. Traditional troublesome methods used in olden times are now not necessary.

*Indications :*

(a) To exclude malignancy.

(b) When Zollinger-Ellison syndrome (Z.E.) is suspected.

*Value of Gastric juice study :*

(a) True achlorhydria (defined as a condition where the gastric acid pH does not fall below 3.5 under maximal stimulation) excludes benign peptic ulcer. It is common in gastric carcinoma and invariably present in pernicious anaemia.

(b) Hyperchlorhydria or hypersecretion is normally seen in duodenal ulcer.

(c) Hypochlorhydia or normal secretion is seen in gastric ulcer.

(d) High basal secretory activity of 10-30 mEq and a ratio of basal to maximal stimulation secretion of 0.6 or more is characteristic Z-E syndrome.

Serum gastrin level should be estimated if features of Z-E syndrome are present. It is ten times more than the normal value.

*Provocation tests* — There are two main provocative tests where stimulants are used for maximal secretion of acid by parietal.

(a) Basal acid out put (BAO); The test is done in fasting state in the morning.

A Ryle's tube is introduced into the stomach and gastric juice is aspirated by low pressure suction pump. The volume is measured and acid level is determined. Then four samples are taken at 15 minutes interval for one hour and acid concentration is measured. This is called BAO.

Maximum concentration of acid after stimulation either by injecting pentagastrin histamine or is estimated. The acid secretion after stimulation is known as peak acid output (PAO).

If the peak acid output is abnormally high (80 to 100 mEq) it is an indication to assay blood gastrin level for the diagnosis of Z-E syndrome.

***Serum gastrin levels***

Estimation of gastrin level is indicated in the following conditions :

(1) Giant ulcer not healed by adequate treatment.

(2) Multiple ulcers.

(3) Recurrent ulcerations.

(4) Multi-glandular disease with peptic ulcer.

(5) Massive haematemesis or perforation of peptic ulcer inspite of good medical treatment.

These are suggestive of the diagnosis of Z-E syndrome, if proved early treatment can be carried out either by intensive medical therapy or surgical resection of the stomach (total gastrectomy).

Other indications of radio-immunoassay of gastrin are the study of gastrin level after stimulation in or achlorhydric conditions e.g. gastric carcinoma, pernicious anaemia and total vagotomy. In none of these conditions there will be rise in gastrin level.

**Treatment**

The methods of the treatment :

(1) Reduce the acid content of the stomach (HCL)

(2) Promote healing of ulcer.

(3) Prevent complications.

(4) Maintain nutrition of the patient.

(5) Prevent invalidism.

*Reduction of acid content of stomach*

*Antacids* : Antacids act either by chemical neutralisation (sodium bicarbonate, calcium carbonate or magnesium hydroxide) or by absorption (aluminium hydroxide).

Antacids were used in the past as a regular programme for treatment of ulcer. There was inadequate information about the efficiency and their complications. Sodium bicarbonate preparations are not used now due to short-term action and rebound effect of acid secretion respectively. Most potent antacids are aluminium hydroxide and magnesium hydroxide in the treatment of peptic ulcer. The liquid form of these products are most useful to be taken at three or four hourly intervals.

*$H_2$-receptor antagonists*

$H_2$-receptor antagonists inhibit acid secretion of the parietal cells.

The first drug introduced was cimetidine ($H_2$-receptor antagonist). It reduces fasting and food-stimulated acid secretion by 95 to 70% respectively. It is beneficial in the treatment of duodenal ulcer as well as gastric ulcer. The ulcer heals up within six to 20 weeks. Then requires maintenance dose for a few weeks. Side-effects e.g. mental confusion, impotency, gynaecomastia may occur rarely but specially in those requiring parenteral injections. Dose — 200 mg tablet three times daily before meals and 400 mg at bed time. Treatment should continue for three to four months at least.

(ii) Ranitidine is better $H_2$-receptor antagonist then cimetidine and has less side effects. Mode of action is more elaborate than cimetidine. Treatment should continue for about two to three months.

Both drugs are expensive for our poorer patients, who often discontinue treatment once relief starts. This leads to relapse. In my opinion (G.C.M) proper dieting, antacids and anti-cholinergic drugs may still be useful in treatment of early duodenal ulcers. Autopsy studies of medico-legal cases also reveal evidence of healed ulcers, although there were no symptoms of peptic ulcer in lifetime of these cases.

**Pharmacological action**

*$H_2$-receptor antagonists :*

(a) Reduce the acid secretion by parietal cells.

(b) Increase gastric mucosal regeneration.

(c) Increase synthesis of prostaglandins (endogenous).

(d) Increase gastric mucosal blood flow.

(e) Increase gastric mucosal bicarbonate secretion.

(f) Increase transmucosal potential difference.

*Carbanoloxone sodium*

It is disodium salt of glycyrrhizinic acid obtained from liquorice. It possibly causes increase of gastric mucus more helpful in gastric ulcer than duodenal ulcers.

Due to its aldosterone-like effect retention of sodium and water and excess potassium loss may occur. Prolonged use may cause hypertension, hypokalaemia and even CCF. Diuretics and potassium supplements may help but spironolactone should not be used as it will reduce its therapeutic efficiency.

Deglycyrrhizinized liquorice is practically devoid of the side-effects and it appears to be helpful in both gastric and duodenal ulcers.

Dose — Two tablets six times daily for 6 to 8 weeks usually.

*Sucralfate* — It increases the mucosal resistance. It is sucrose octa — sulphate basic aluminium salt, which has protective action against pepsin action. In the stomach when pH is below 4, profuse polymerisation and cross linking of the product results in formation of sticky gel. The gel adheres to the base of the ulcer and give protective action. It also prevents exudation from the base of the ulcer and also absorb pepsin, trypsin and bile salt. It is non-systemic alternative to $H_2$-receptor antagonist without much side-effects or potential for systemic drug interactions. It should not be used in patients with impaired renal function and patients under 18 years. It can be used during lactation especially nursing mother so that there is no harmful effect on the new born.

Dose — One tablet 1.0 g one hour before meals and at bed time.

Antacid should not be taken with or within one hour of its administration because due to alteration of pH polymersation may be effected. Tetracyclines and $H_2$-receptor blockers should be kept in mind. These are constipation, diarrhoea, dry mouth, back pain, headache and drowsiness.

*Emotional factors*

Psychological factors should be taken into account. All stressful factors aggravate the disease. In case of necessity hospitalisation of the patient requires consideration for complete physical and mental rest. Stressful environment can then be eliminated.

*Exogenous factors*

(a) Patient should be advised to stop smoking.

(b) Alcohol should be avoided or be reduced to minimum in addicts and not be taken in empty stomach. Addicts otherwise may violently react to sudden discontinuance of alcohol. However, most patients become teetotaller when properly advised.

(c) Drugs like aminophylline, aspirin, non-steroid anti-inflammatory drugs are to be avoided.

**Diet**

In the past various special diets were in vogue but it has now been established by many controlled trials that bland diets or milk diets are not particularly helpful. Diet should be planned according to patient's previous food habit and subjective reactions. However, some items are not tolerated well. The principles are :

(a) Diet should have adequate calories and generally non-spicy.

(b) Oriental cooking with lot of spices and too much fatty fried food is usually not tolerated.

(c) Food cooked in water vehicle with small amounts of cooking oil, smashed potato and soft vegetables are usually tolerated.

(d) Milk based puddings and sweets made of clotted milk are good.

(e) Milk has stimulating secretagogue effect, hence do not actually depress acid secretion but milk-made sweets e.g. Sandesh or Bengal-rasogollas are usually well tolerated. Similarly, boiling milk clotted by fresh lime (chhana) is very good.

(f) Meals should be regularly taken while tea and coffee be avoided.

(g) Patients will however give an idea of items of food not tolerated.

(h) In acute phase liquid and semi-liquid diet is necessary when cold sweet milk with antacids has to be given. Some patients do better with artificial preparations of milk e.g. Horlicks and Complan type of milk food.

**Duodenal ulcer**

Adequately treated with the above regime duodenal ulcers should heal within 8-10 weeks. Patient should be treated with a single drug either cimetidine or ranitidine and maintenance therapy will reduce recurrences. In poorer population, it may be economically impossible to provide these drugs for two to three months but even three to four week's course followed by cheaper drugs e.g. belladonna preparations and antacids may be successful. No useful purpose will be served if drugs like ranitidine are taken for a few days or in as-you-like-it bases. Colloidal-bismuth is also a cheaper substitute. If the subjective symptoms persist or relapse after the maintenance therapy, patient should be given another course of drug or combination of drugs with careful supervision. If the symptoms still persist it should be presumed that the case may require surgical treatment. Blood gastrin level should be checked and if hypergastrinaemia is present, diagnosis of Z-E syndrome is considered and proper surgical treatment should be arranged.

**Gastric ulcer**

If the ulcer is not very large it should be healed within 8-12 weeks. If it does not, endoscopic evaluation should be done. Repeat-biopsies to be taken even if earlier biopsy did not reveal malignancy. If proved to be benign another course of treatment may be continued, with bed rest. If the ulcer is not healed with proper medical treatment the case should be subjected to surgery. Whenever possible, endoscopy should be the guiding factor. Radiology is only an alternative.

**Complications**

Following complications are encountered.

(a) Bleeding peptic ulcer is one of the most important causes of upper gastrointestinal haemorrhage. It can occur in adults as well as in old people, the latter being more susceptible. Most commonly the posterior duodenal ulcer bleeds though ulcer in other sites may also bleed.

Clinical manifestations e.g. haematemesis and malena or both depends upon the severity and site of bleeding. In duodenal ulcer there may not be any haematemesis but severe malena may be present. Unless patient is a known case of peptic ulcer, diagnostic problems may arise. The other conditions of upper GTT bleeding are portal hypertension, acute gastric erosions (after taking drugs like aspirin, steroid and non-steroid-anti-inflammatory drugs), Mallory Weiss syndrome, acute gastritis and gastric carcinoma.

In case of bleeding peptic ulcer, the general health is good and there may be history of pain and other vague dyspeptic symptoms. In portal hypertension patient may have hepatic facies, spider navi, enlarged spleen. In Mallory-Weiss syndrome sudden bout of vomiting, epigastric or retrosternal pain is followed by blood vomit. Acute gastric erosions will give history of taking drugs but it does not mean that there may not be an existing ulcer also. Interpretation is most valuable. Enlarged left supraclavicular lymph nodes etc. are signs of advanced gastric carcinoma.

Patients with moderate to severe bleeding will present signs of shock e.g. low B.P., rapid pulse, cold limbs and sweating. If the BP is rapidly falling with rising pulse rate, the rate of bleeding is severe and urgent replacement of blood or even emergency surgery may be necessary. Immediate management should depend upon the clinical evaluation of internal haemorrhage when active bleeding has stopped. CVP measurement (where feasible) will help in assessing the amount of replacement therapy.

During active bleeding oral feeding is not allowed but cold water or even small feeds of iced milk be given. Till blood is procured, intravenous 5% glucose-saline should be continued. I.V. ranitidine 2 ml. four to six hourly should be given. Once the patient is stable, start cold milk with antacids as well as oral ranitidine, the treatment of choice. Soft diet is gradually introduced. Food is also a good antacid and promotes confidence to the patient as well as nutrition.

If bleeding continues or recurs, endoscopy is procedure of choice. In well-equipped centres manned by experts, selective angiography may be done. Continuous bleeding or recurrence may be an urgent indication of emergency surgery specially in elderly people, instead of delaying tactics.

It must also be remembered that operative risk is more if the operation is carried out during the bleeding but pros and cons have to be carefully assessed between the physician and surgeon.

## SURGICAL TREATMENT OF PEPTIC ULCER

*A.K. SEN SARMA*

**Introduction**

Various types surgical treatment of peptic ulcer have been evolved during the third and fourth decade of this century. The aim of all these operative measures is to minimise the acid secretion either by ablating the neurogenic influence or by reduction of parietal cell and G-cell mass. The results of these operations are still being reviewed from time to time in various surgical units of the world.

Latest development of the knowledge of pathophysiology of peptic ulcer is the discovery of H-receptor antagonist. This has revolutionised the medical treatment of uncomplicated peptic ulcer. Thus the indications of surgical treatment is now restricted. The gastroenterologist is not that enthusiastic as before, for taking up cases for surgery without fair trial with modern medical treatment. However, the treatment of gastric ulcer is still handicapped due to possible presence of ulcer-cancer.

**Indications of surgery**

(1) Uncomplicated duodenal ulcer — failure of medical treatment means non-healing of ulcer even after repeated courses of treatment with modern medical therapy and recurrence of ulcer inspite of continued maintenance dose. Endoscopy is helpful in confirming presence of ulcer.

(2) Gastric ulcer should heal within 10 to 12 weeks of medical treatment. If it does not heal endoscopic biopsy must be done before the starting a second course of drug therapy. The surgical treatment in case of gastric ulcer should be liberal than that of duodenal ulcer.

(3) Complicated peptic ulcer

Definite indications for surgery are —

(a) Perforated peptic ulcer

(b) Pyloric stenosis

(c) Hour glass deformity of stomach

(d) Repeated bleeding ulcer or continued bleeding

(e) Malignancy proved by endoscopic biopsy.

As already discussed in the management of bleeding peptic ulcer, the indications of operative treatment of bleeding ulcer are :

(1) Elderly patients with heavy and continued bleeding

(2) If the bleeding is heavy and continuous inspite of continuous blood transfusion along with parenteral cimetidine or ranitidine and other supportive therapy.

However, it must also be remembered that operative mortality and morbidity increases when surgery is undertaken during active bleeding. Therefore if possible if better to take the decision after due consideration of the background factors.

**Different types of operations**

Neurogenic disruption :

(1) Truncal vagotomy ⎤
(2) Selective vagotomy ⎦ with drainage

Ablation or reduction of parietal cell mass and 'G'-cell mass.

(1) Subtotal gastrectomy in duodenal ulcer

(2) Total gastrectomy in Zollinger Ellison syndrome

(3) Partial gastrectomy in gastric ulcer.

Combination of both vagotomy and anterectomy may also be done in some cases.

**Truncal Vagotomy**

This is original vagal-interruption surgery initially coupled with gastro-jejunostomy, subsequently with pyeloroplasty. This is being practised for a long time. Main trunks of left and right vagus are cut in between ligature at the lower part of the oesophagus. The lower part of the oesophagus is exposed classically by retracting the left triangular ligament otherwise also, subhepatic exposure of the oesophagus is practised. Main aspect of this operation is to cut the vagal trunk before any gastric branch comes out. Sometimes few branches of Vagi, come out from higher situation and if this is not appreciated during operation some degree of operative failure of vagotomy with recurrence of ulcer may be caused. Thus sufficient experience is required for this operation. In an inexperienced hand failure rate of vagotomy increases.

**Drainage Operation**

(a) Gastro-jejunostomy is anastomosis of the stomach with proximal jejunum well away from the pylorus. It is a retro-colic anastomosis.

(b) Pyloroplasty — The principle of this operation is to enlarge the outlet of the stomach by cutting pyloric sphincter longitudinally and closed transversely by a single layer stitches with dexon or silk.

(2) Selected vagotomy — It is a vagal interception leaving the branches supplying pancreas and biliary tree. This is also combined with drainage operations. This technique was practised to reduce diarrhoea as complication of truncal vagotomy.

(3) Highly selective vagotomy — Aim of this operation is to disrupt all the branches of vagus supplying the stomach except antrum.

**Ablation of parietal cell and 'G' cell mass**

(1) Subtotal gastrectomy was widely practised in the middle of the century but the operation is not so popular now, due to increase in mortality and morbidity in comparison to other operations. The operation consists of ablation of two-thirds of the stomach so that it removes large segment of parietal cells and G-cell mass. After resection, anastomosis is done with proximal jejunum. It is a retrocolic anastomosis.

(2) Total Gastrectomy — It is a desperate operation to remove the whole stomach and carry out oesophago-enterostomy. Duodenum is completely diverted so that food goes straight down into the jejunum. This operation is done in Zollinger Ellison syndrome.

(3) Partial Gastrectomy — This is the operation of choice in gastric ulcer, common site of the ulcer being in the lesser curvature of the stomach. After resection, remaining stomach is anastomosed with the duodenum (Billroth — I) or with the proximal jejunum (Billroth — II).

*Combination of both* — Truncal vagotomy with anterectomy will depress the neurogenic acid secretion by parietal cells and excision of antrum will decrease the humoral factor by reducing gastrin by 'G'-cells in the antrum.

**Discussion**

Diagnosis of peptic ulcer should be established not only by clinical features but should be confirmed routine Ba-meal and or endoscopy.

Indiscriminate medical therapy without correct diagnosis leads to waste of both time and money. Timely investigation is worth while because many upper abdominal disorders may mimic peptic ulcer syndrome.

Therefore once the diagnosis is certain and other associated ailments are excluded proper regime of medical treatment should be started and the case is closely followed. Most cases of the duodenal ulcer respond to medical treatment but in case of gastric ulcer close follow up is necessary for the fear of malignancy. However, it is essential that all suspected gastric ulcer cases should have endoscopic evaluation whenever possible, specially if symptoms continue inspite of good medical treatment.

All complicated peptic ulcers should be treated by surgery. Associated ailments e.g. Diabetes, hypertension and ischaemic heart disease should be stabilised before the operation.

In all obstructive complications, water and electrolyte imbalance should be corrected. Negative nitrogen balance should also be combated.

In bleeding duodenal ulcer, it is always better to give a complete curative surgery i.e. partial gastrectomy and ligation of bleeding ulcer with vagotomy.

Perforated duodenal ulcer should be treated with suturing of the perforation with peritoneal toilet. These cases should be followed up and in some cases a definite surgery is required at a later date.

Partial gastrectomy, subtotal gastrectomy, vagotomy with drainage operations etc. are the choices of operations. Decision also depends upon the experience of the surgeon. With vagotomy and drainage operation mortality is minimum but the recurrence rate of ulcer is higher.

Partial gastrectomy or subtotal gastrectomy — recurrence rate is less but the mortality and morbidity is higher. Morbidity of these operations is due to smallness of stomach and gastro-intestinal hurry. This is known as post-gastrectomy syndrome e.g. dumping syndrome, anaemia, bilious vomiting, diarrhoea and hypoglycemia.

## "PYLORIC OBSTRUCTION"

### (Gastric outlet obstruction)

*G.C. MOOKERJEE*

The term pyloric obstruction as commonly used in surgical text books should better be changed to "obstruction of the gastroduodenal pathway" or "pyloroduodenal" or "gastric outlet obstruction". Obstruction in any luminal path may be due to muscular spasm, or to a growth in the lumen or a mass pressing on the lumen of the gut from out side.

**Causes :**

(1) **Chronic duodenal ulcer or pre-pyloric gastric ulcer :** (or channel ulcer). Causing obstruction due to pylorospasm, fibrosis, or oedema.

(2) Pyloric carcinoma

(3) Congenital hypertrophic pyloric stenosis (or adult type).

**Clinical features :**

Abdominal discomfort, feeling of fullness in the epigastrium and vomiting are early manifestations. These are usually preceded by a long history of duodenal or gastric ulcer, which if absent, leads to the suspicion of pyloric carcinoma.

The symptoms of the underlying pathology should draw attention to its possibility. Physical examination may show signs of anaemia and dehydration even tetany, though some may remain reasonably well, being feed with large amounts of milk.

Vomiting brings much relief but the patient may eat just after vomiting. In the begining vomiting is sudden and recently eaten food is brought out. Later when the stomach starts to dilate and becomes atonic, large vomits will occur containing food ingested many hours earlier. The vomited food is then foul smelling due to putrefaction of food ingested even a day or two before. There is usually no bile (because of the obstruction).

Progressive anaemia, and weight loss will occur due to malnutrition and signs of avitaminosis will occur in late stages. Loss of electrolytes and $H^+$-ions, will result in alkalosis.

**Diagnosis :**

Pyloric obstruction should be suspected if an excess of 100 ml. of gastric content after fasting overnight is present or if it contains foul smelling food residue. History is important.

Inspection may show gastric peristalsis from left hypochondrium to the right hypochondriac region. Two or three waves may occur following each.

Palpation stimulates these peristalsis waves. A large lump, hemispherical or like a golf ball, may be felt.

On auscultation, a splashing noise can be heard or "the succussion splash" is demonstrable by gently shaking the patient from side to side.

**Investigations :**

(1) **Gastric juice** — can be aspirated which is foul smelling and putrid in late cases. There is no bile.

(2) **Blood picture** shows anaemia. In late cases there is low plasma electrolytes and evidence of alkalosis.

(3) **Blood Urea** may be raised due to dehydration.

X-ray pictures with barium meal shows hugely dilated stomach and the meal remains there even after 8 to 12 hours.

**Management :**

Surgical consultation should be made as early as possible.

(1) In pyloric obstruction, due to spasm or oedema, symptoms will improve by medical treatment.

(2) Anti-cholinergic drugs should be discontinued if it is being used.

(3) Daily gastric washing should be done carefully once or even twice even four hourly for three to four days.

(4) Antacids specially in liquid form should be given 3 or 4 hourly with semiliquid meals or soft non-irritating semisolid diet. Milk, vegetable soup, dal, egg, molten rice, pressed rice (chira) boiled in milk, biscuits, butter, jelly, pudding, etc. should be given. If daily aspiration indicates no reduction of residual juice and food residue indicates stagnation in stomach, surgical intervention, is essential.

(5) Dehydration and electrolyte disturbance must be properly corrected by intravenous fluids. Three to four litres of fluid may be required in 24 hours.

Medical treatment will be no use in cases where obstruction is due to scar tissue or hypertrophic pyloric stenosis or malignancy. However, in modern times, gastroscopy and biopsy may be helpful, otherwise aetiological diagnosis is made in the operation theatre.

## CARCINOMA STOMACH

*G.C. MOOKERJEE*

Cause of carcinoma stomach is unknown, but may be related to presence of N-nitroso compound in the diet. Genetic element is important incidence, being higher among people with blood group-A. Other predisposing factors are pernicious anaemia and achlorhydria.

Gastric carcinoma is not so common in India, yet it requires to be considered in the differential diagnosis of all cases of upper abdominal symptoms specially in middle age and elderly people. Only five per cent patients of gastric carcinoma are below 40 years of age. It is more common in Japan, Chile and the Scandinavian countries. Its incidence appears to be falling in U.S.A. and U.K. Mean age group is 55 yrs, and men are affected twice as other as women.

Data from Tata Memorial Hospital, Bombay, suggests gastric cancer is about 1.5% of all malignant neoplasma. Average age of onset is 56 years and is very rare before 30 years. Men suffer 3 times more than females; possibly many Indian females from rural areas die undiagnosed.

Gastric cancers are discussed in detail in surgical text books but it is a very important to stress to the students and general practitioners that gastric carcinoma may be surprisingly silent hence when upper abdominal symptoms are persisting inspite of treatment in patients of elderly age group, investigations to exclude carcinoma are mandatory. So called clinical diagnosis of gastritis, peptic ulcer, amoebiasis, colitis are often responsible for missed diagnosis of gastric malignancy. Emaciation, palpable mass in the abdomen, jaundice and coffee ground haematemesis are late signs, when nothing can be done surgically.

Presence of Virchow's gland in the neck, hard fixed enlarged lymph glands (at the root of left side of neck called Troiser's sign) or axillary or umbilical lymph glands proclaim distant metastasis. It is only the family doctor who can make an early diagnosis, so that surgical treatment can be considered.

If proper treatment does not improve symptoms of peptic ulcer or if upper abdominal discomfort e.g. anorexia, nausea or epigastric discomfort does not improve with medical treatment, if there is anaemia or loss of weight in an elderly patient with vague dyspepsia, the patient must be investigated to exclude carcinoma. Alteration of bowel habits, nausea & vomiting (pyloric tumour), dysphagia (tumour at cardiac end) are other presenting symptoms.

Three pre cancerous conditions must be remembered :

1. Chronic gastric ulcer
2. Pernicious anaemia with achlorhydria & gastritis
3. Polyposis of stomach (single or multiple).

**Types of gastric carcinoma**

*Chatterjee BP*

1. Antral 60%
2. Pyloric 15%
3. Fundus and cardia 6%
4. Greater curvature 4%

*Macroscopic types*

1. Ulcerative 33%
2. Proliferative 27% (cauliflower type)
3. Infiltrating or scirrhous 15%
4. Colloid 5%
6. Combined type 20%

*Histological types*

1. Adenocarcinoma
2. Squamous-cell carcinoma.

**Investigations :**

(1) The simplest of all tests is to examine the gastric juice. Presence of blood, achlorhydria or hypochorhydria and gastric pH above 6.0 specially after pentagastrin test in strongly suggestive of gastric carcinoma. Exfoliative cytology may show malignant cell in gastric juice.

Occult blood in stool will be strongly positive. Advanced cases will cause progressive anaemia, gross emaciation,coffee ground vomiting, black stool, pain in abdomen, tenderness over epigastrium with palpable lump, metastatic enlargement of lymph gland, jaundice, ascitis, and oedema. Left supraclavicular gland is felt (Virchow's gland).

Rectal examination may show presence of enlarged lymph glands in the rectovesical pouch, such diagnosis is of no value.

Loss of weight, anaemia and raised ESR are often pointers. A well done barium meal will be positive in 80% of cases.

In modern times, gastroscopy with biopsy and brush cytology has been extremely useful for early diagnosis and should be done more frequently specially in barium negative but suspicious cases. It is worth stressing that early diagnosis of gastric carcinoma depends on the doctor's ability to suspect it, because many early cases may have very insignificant symptoms.

In 25% cases symptoms suggest peptic ulcer. It may however, be noted that chronic gastric ulcer rarely causes malignancy. In view of the late diagnosis, early cases do not reach the surgeons and at the present time 5 years survival after surgery is hardly above 10%. Over 50% cases are commonly diagnosed too late for surgery.

**Treatment :**

In early case here the growth has no apparent metastasis, gastrectomy is done but where metastases has occurred, partial gastrectomy, or gastrojejunostomy may be done to relieve symptoms. Chemotherapy with Adriamycin and 5-fluro-uracil (5 F.U) quite useful palliative measure. Radiation therapy also may be necessary along with 5 F.U. Small nutritional feeds and drugs like metoclopramide, phenothiazones, pentazocaine, pethidine or morphine may be required for relief in advanced cases.

**Prognosis** is generally bad as usually diagnosis made late but with modern endoscopy early diagnosis should be possible and 5 years survival rate should improve.

## ABDOMINAL TUBERCULOSIS

*G.C. MOOKERJEE*

Abdominal tuberculosis may mimic many abdominal disorders hence may be missed in early stages.

**Pathology**

The basic pathology is the same as tuberculosis anywhere else. Abdominal tuberculosis may be due to :

(1) Direct intestinal invasion from contaminated utensils, infected milk (raw or unboiled). Cheap hotels and wayside eating cabins in tropics are major sources. This group is called 'Primary'.

(2) Swallowing of heavily contaminated sputum from pulmonary lesion may cause abdominal tuberculosis (secondary).

Tubercle bacilli enter the mucosa and are engulfed by macrophages and invade lymphoid follicles and cause typical transverse ulcers in the intestinal wall. The peyer's patches are typically affected. The organisms may go into mesenteric lymph glands causing 'tabes mesenterica' or affect peritoneum resulting in plastic peritonitis or tuberculous ascitis. It may also spread causing genitourinary tuberculosis.

Depending on the structures involved abdominal tuberculosis may present, in the following ways :

(1) *Small intestinal tuberculosis* — Small intestinal mucosal lesions lead to formation of submucosal lesions breaking down into typical deep transversely placed ulcer. The initial lesions are in the Peyer's patches. The lesions are often localised in small segments or may be extensive.

(2) *Iliocaecal tuberculosis* is localised in ileocaecal region and presents as hypertrophic or hyperplastic lesion. This may be felt as localised lump in the R.I.F and is therefore, to be differentiated from amoeboma, carcinoma, Crohn's diseases, appendicular mass or lymph gland enlargement.

(3) Glandular tuberculosis may also occur in the abdomen. It is often insidious in occurance and may heal with calcification or may end in "tabes mesenterica".

(4) Peritoneal tuberculosis may be due to primary lesion in lungs or abdomen and may cause ascitis or chronic plastic peritonitis.

**Clinical features**

As already mentioned, abdominal tuberculosis may mimic many acute, subacute and chronic intraabdominal conditions. The typical features will depend on the type of pathological lesions present as follows :

(1) *Tuberculous peritonitis* This is often seen in developing countries but rare in advanced countries. The patient will present with abdominal discomfort, poor appetite, indigestion and fever of varying grades. In the early stage, ascitis is small and may be missed if careful examination is not made. It has to be differentiated from malignancy and ascitis due to other causes. I have come across many cases of cirrhosis of liver with tuberculous ascitis, where cirrhosis was due alcohol or malnutrition. Treatment of tuberculosis, correction or malnutrition and stopping alcohol in future may lead to many years of active life.

(2) *Ilio-caecal tuberculosis.* — The usual presenting features are, intermittent colicky abdominal pain in the right iliac fossa and around umbilicus. Patients often say there is some distension within the abdomen associated with recurrent colicky pain. Fever of varying grades, gargling and borborygmi may be present. Constipation may be a feature. Pain is aggravated with purgatives. Signs of intestinal obstruction may gradually develop. On palpation a lump may be felt which is often diffuse and tender. This has to be differentiated from amoeboma, carcinoma, Crohn's disease etc. Hence P.V. or P.R. examination must be done.

(3) *Luminal or intestinal tuberculosis* manifests with cramp, colic and colitic symptoms. Diarrhoea, colicky or vague abdominal pain, flatulence, anorexia, nausea and even vomiting may occur. Loss of weight, varying grades of fever with vague abdominal symptoms are often the only features. Neglected cases may end in haemorrhage, perforation of bowel or fistula formation which are rare now-a-days. Abdominal palpation reveals doughy and tender abdomen.

**Prognosis**

Prognosis is good provided diagnosis is not too late. Once surgical complications have occured, troublesome problems are to be tackled.

**Treatment**

The chemotherapeutic treatment of abdominal tuberculosis is not different from pulmonary tuberculosis. With modern drugs, nine months treatment on the average is usually adequate. (Refer to the chapter on tuberculosis). It is better to start treatment with rifamycin 450 to 600 mg daily plus INAH 300 mg and pyrazinamide 1.0 to 1.5 g daily, depending on body weight. After two months pyrazinamide is discontinued and ethambutol is given (15 mg/kg of B.W.).

When there is hepatic insufficiency. I have omitted rifamycin and used streptomycin 0.75 to 0g daily. Old patients rarely suffer from abdominal tuberculosis. However, in old patients streptomycin can cause trouble but cautious use of streptomycin (where rifamycin can not be used), 0.75 g twice or thrice a week can be trouble free.

In tuberculous ascitis, perfect cure can be achieved but sometimes addition of oral prednisolone 30—40 mg daily with antacids after meals may be necessary for about three weeks, to be tailed off within six weeks. Usual precautions should be taken.

For tense ascitis paracentesis may have to be done a few times but should done only if it is necessary to relieve the patient's symptoms. Prednisolone in these cases quickly improves the condition.

Surgical interference is rarely necessary now a days, for intestinal obstruction, fistula formation or perforation etc.

# MALABSORPTION SYNDROME

G.C. MOOKERJEE

Malabsorption of essential food factors e.g. carbohydrates, proteins, fats, minerals and vitamins may gradually lead to malnutrition and loss of weight. Deficiency symptoms will develop associated with clinical features consisting of diarrhoea, abdominal discomfort, flatulence, anaemia and weight loss. In early stages these cases are often mistaken for chronic colitis and are wrongly treated by repeated course of antibiotics and anti-amoebic drugs. The initial clinical picture of vague ill health and indefinite bowel disorders with diarrhoea causes confusion in diagnosis and treatment.

Careful history taking and inspection of stool, may be more rewarding than sending a lump of stool to the laboratory for routine testing.

## Causes of Malabsorption syndrome

Any reason which upsets normal digestive process may result in malabsorption.

Broadly the defects are of two types :

(1) Disturbed digestive process due to lack of enzymes or bile or intestinal hurry due to surgical operations e.g. gastroenterostomy or partial gastrectomy (Polya type of surgery). Digestion may also be affected due to shortage of bile or pancreatic diseases (e.g. chronic pancreatitis, carcinoma or cystic fibrosis. Colonisation of bacteria in upper small intestine may also be responsible by interfering with bile-acid-micelle formation. Tropical sprue is a syndrome of unknown aetiology also causes malabsorption syndrome (vide infra).

(2) Mucosal disorders e.g. tuberculosis, tropical sprue. Crohn's disease, giardiasis, Whipple's disease and lymphangiectasia etc. are also causes of malabsorption.

(3) Vitamin $B_{12}$ deficiency also may be responsible by causing lack of intrinsic factor.

## Clinical features

Diarrhoea (steatorrhoea), anaemia, loss of weight and abdominal distension are the common features. Inspection of stool is a must and offensive smelling loose, pale, bulky stool floating in water is very suggestive.

Hypocalcaemic tetany, haemorrhagic manifestation (vitamin K — deficiency) and evidence of multiple vitamin deficiency may be noted. Even rickets in children and osteomalacia in adults may occur. Oedema occurs due to hypoalbuminaemia.

## Diagnosis

Inspection of stool helps in diagnosis. Absorption tests are often done to find out defective absorption of nutrients e.g. glucose, fat, vitamin $B_{12}$ etc. Xylose absorption test is also done. Biopsy of jejunum settles the diagnosis. Exclusion of pancreatic or hepatic disorders may be necessary.

Barium meal X ray of G.I. tract reveals dilated loops, appearance of segmentation of small gut with flocculation or barium meal.

*Topical sprue* is of unknown aetiology which may occur among foreign visitors or even in local people of tropics. Deficiency of fat and d-xylose absorption vitamin $B_{12}$ or folic deficiency are noted. Besides demonstration of absorption defects, jejunal biopsy is helpful in diagnosis.

*Lactose intolerence* also presents as malabsorption syndrome, specially common in West. This may follow in a bowel infection. Hydrogen-breath-test is helpful in diagnosis of lactose intolerance.

## Coeliac disease

In this type of malabsorption there is abnormally reactive mucosa due to ingestion of wheat, oats, barley or rye starches. Immunological mechanism may be responsible. The mucosal villi shows subtotal atrophy. The disease occurs in early childhood but rarely noted in early adult life.

Sometime the disease predisposes to lymphoma of small gut. Hence this should be kept in mind when relapse of symptoms occurs after some years.

**Treatment**

Replacement therapy and attention to nutrition are most important. Gluten-free diet is necessary for coeliac disease. Lactose is to be avoided for lactose intolerance i.e. milk or milk products should be withdrawn. Special artificial formula-foods are available but some are to be imported hence quite expensive (See Appendix). Parenteral vitamin $B_{12}$, folates and iron therapy will usually be required. Parenteral calcium injections once to thrice a week and monthly vitamin D injections may be necessary. Low fat, high protein diet along with vitamin B complex injections to be given if signs of deficiency are present.

Pancreatic enzymes are given in pancreatic insufficiency.

Bile acids do not help if there is bile acid deficiency, as they pass to the large gut causing interference of water and salt absorption. Judicious use of cholestyramine in doses of 6 to 12 g daily may help.

Blood transfusion may often be helpful.

## IRRITABLE BOWEL SYNDROME

*G.C. MOOKERJEE*

**Introduction**

It is a syndrome suggestive of colonic dysfunction in which patient suffers life-long disability consisting of vague abdominal discomfort or pain, irregular bowel movements resulting in constipation or diarrhoea, sometimes associated with depressed appetite, belching, nausea and even vomiting.

The aetiology is unknown but recently it is suspected that dysfunction of smooth muscles of G.I. Tract may be responsible possibly caused by dietary factors, stress, drugs, gastrointestinal hormones or smooth muscle incordination.

According to symptomatology two clinical types are recognised

(1) Spastic colon type

(2) Painless diarrhoea type

The former group is more common.

**Aetiology**

Though aetiology is unclear, the following possible mechanisms may be responsible.

(1) Abnormal gut-motility : Normally two types of smooth muscle contractions are seen in G.I. tract :

(a) Segmental movements which reduces the diameter of the lumen and slows the stream of faeces. This is called "a" – type contractions.

(b) Propulsive mass peristaltic movements which occur periodically and propel large quantities of faeces from one region to another. This is called "b" type contractions.

Predominent 'a' type contractions (segmental) cause constipation while 'b' type contractions cause diarrhoea.

In recent studies by several gastroenterologists (Thompson D.C., Corbett C.L. and Whorwell P.T.) it was shown that patients of IBS display increased colonic motility when disturbed by hormones, drugs or emotional stimulation, although under resting conditions they are the same as normals.

The pain is due to distension of some segments of both the large as well as the small bowel. Irregular contractions often lead to prolonged episodes of pain. Even the oesophageal sphincter may show dysfunction.

(2) *Myoelectric activity*

The intrinsic myoelectric activity of the colon plays an important role in the control and coordination of colonic musculature.

(3) ***Hormones*** : Cholecystokinin, increases colonic contractions and may reproduce postprandial pain.

(4) *Psychological factors* : Emotional stress is believed to play an important part. Patients of IBS are irritable, anxious, and suffer from depression, hostility and various anxiety symptoms.

(5) ***Diet*** : Food intolerance is believed to be an important agent in some cases.

(6) *Neurological factors* : It seems excitability of neuronal plexus of the gut may play an important but possibly secondary role in IBS patients.

(7) ***Drugs*** : Antacids, antibiotics, beta-blockers, dopamine-blockers and narcotics may induce IBS is many patients.

(8) *Postinfective* : Gastroenteritis is often the starting point of some patients of IBS.

**Clinical features**

*Pain* : The pain in IBS may be chronic, intermittent or arching. Although 90% patients may have pain, the type of pain may vary in the same patient in different times. It may occur in hypogastrium, right iliac fossa, right upper quadrant of abdomen or epigastrium. Referred pain may occur in shoulder, lumbar or sacroiliac joints, Proctalgia fugax may also occur in IBS.

The pain is relieved by defecation or passage of flatus.

**Disturbed Bowel Habit :** There may be diarrhoea or constipation or both. The faeces may be pellet like, and the patient feels the evacuation is incomplete. There may be excess of mucus in stool. In the painless diarrhoea type, urgent diarrhoea occurs, in the morning or during or after a meal. Distension, nausea, flatulence, and borborygmi may occurs. Nonspecific systemic symptoms like headache, lassitude, depression and anxiety may occur. The chief symptoms in IBS are :-

(1) Distension of abdomen
(2) Relief of pain with bowel movement
(3) Loose bowel movement with abdominal discomfort or pain
(4) Frequent bowel movement without pain
(5) Too much mucus in stool
(6) Feeling of incomplete evacuation may be present.
(7) Constipation with intermittent passage of pellets of stool or constipation followed by diarrhoea.

**Diagnosis :** The diagnosis is usually suspected when patient in apparently good health has the symptoms described above.

The usual signs of any chronic illness are not found in IBS, thus malnutrition, anaemia and fever are usually absent. However, when symptoms continue for months or years patient develop food-fads or may not eat well and may develop anaemia and loss of weight.

The distal colon may be tender, rectal examination may be painful and reveals hard faeces in the rectum.

The caecum is filled with gas.

Sigmoidoscopy reveals absence of any other disease, and rapidly contracting sigmoid suggest the spastic type. However, in elderly and old patients, malignancy must be excluded. Endoscopy and radiological studies should be done.

**Management**

The relative importance of constitutional psychological and dietary factors should be considered.

The patient must be reassured, since many patients believe they have cancer, so his confidence must be restored after proper investigations. Anxiety or depression must be treated with tranquilizers or antidepressant drugs. Adjustment of diet is sometimes useful.

**Anticholinergic drus**

The anticholinergic drugs reduce muscle tone and peristalsis along the entire G.I. Tract. Since also effect, other smooth muscles of the body, there are side effects such as blurred vision, drying of salivary secretions, tachycardia and palpitation.

In patients with narrow angle glaucoma, raised intraocular pressure may cause complications. Urinary retention may also take place specially in elderly.

**Musculotropic agents :**

Some drugs affecting gut motility e.g. metoclopramide and more recently mebeverine have been used to modify abnormal smooth muscles of G.I. Tract. These drugs reduce intracellular calcium level of smooth muscles and reestablish their normal function and appear to be useful agents in IBS, specially mebeverine. Most of these patients however go from doctor to doctor and from clinics to hospitals and are in the risk of being treated repeatedly with various antibiotics and antiamoebic drugs and may finally become a neurotic individual with feeling of "no chances of recovery". Proper indoctrination will save many cases of permanent invalidism.

## ULCERATIVE COLITIS

*G.C. MOOKERJEE*

**Introduction**

Ulcerative colitis is a chronic inflammatory disease of colon which may have an acute or insidious onset. Clinically it is difficult to differentiate it from amoebic or bacillary dysentry and most often the disease is diagnosed by exclusion. The disease is rare in tropics, where amoebiasis, giardiasis and bacillary colitis are more common, hence most cases are initially treated with antiamoebic drugs or antibacterial agents.

The aetiology is still not established and therefore the following probable aetiological factors are blamed :

(1) Bacteria — are sometimes associated but these are secondary invaders.

(2) Auto-immunity — a possibility but not proved. Immunological factors are suspected as serum antibodies e.g. IgA level is often raised.

(3) Food allergy — some cases do well after withdrawal of milk & milk products, crabs, prawns or eggs. The disease however is more common in the west than in tropics.

**Pathology**

The disease may affect whole of the colon starting usually from recto-sigmoid zone. Sometimes it presents as ulcerative proctitis which may remain localised for sometime. It may get cured or may extend upwardly to sigmoid and finally may involve the whole of large intestine. Small intestine is generally spared, but rarely extension may occur into terminal ileum. Sigmoidoscopic appearance is so typical that diagnosis can be made by looking into the reddish, velvetty, angry mucosa of rectosigmoid. But in acute stage it is almost impossible to introduce the instrument. The mucosa is often severely inflammed and ulcerated, may extend into the depth gut-wall causing perforation. Repeated relapses may result in fibrosis and narrowing of lumen with development of features of obstruction. Microscopically mucosal capillaries are engorged with infiltration of inflammatory cells specially in lymphoid tissues and ultimately may result in necrosis with poor healing tendency.

Inflammatory cells are lymphocytes and plasma cells. Bleeding from congested mucosa may be small, recurrent or severe haemorrhage per rectum. In **Crohn's disease** the inflammation may extend deep into muscular coat and serosal layer, which is not usual in ulcerative colitis.

### Clinical features

Ulcerative colitis usually affects people during **peak** period of life i.e. after twenties and becomes rare after 40 years of age. Stress and strain as well as psychological factors are often associated. It often starts as acute diarrhoea or dysentry and lingers into chronic stage. Blood and mucus containing stool suggests and attack of dysentry. Sometime it has an insidous onset with diarrhoea having a few loose stools with a little blood and mucus.

Some cases of ulcerative colitis are limited to rectum only. In this type there may be no diarrhoea and stool may be semiformed or even nearly — solid in appearance, but is coated with plenty of mucus or muco-purulent exudate and blood.

On examination patient may not be looking sick in early stage but later on, he will become anaemic and undernourished due to chronic blood loss and diarrhoea causing poor absorption. There may be febrile episodes, abdominal colic, nutritional deficiency and electrolyte imbalance.

Most cases may have and many courses of antiamoebic and antidiarrhoeal drug therapy.

### Investigations

Stool examination reports are variable. Sometimes there will be plenty or RBC's and pus cells in stool. Some other times there will be scanty RBCs or pus cells or even indefinite findings.

Blood picture will reveal iron deficiency or even macrocytic anaemia with occasional leucocytosis.

### Diagnosis

Sigmoidoscopy and preferrably **fiberoptic** endoscopy settle the diagnosis. The **naked** eye appearance of mucosa in usually diagnostic. However, biopsy is desirable.

**Sometimes sigmoidoscopy and endoscopy is not possible due to lack of experts or acute painful** state. Barium enema X-ray study of large gut is useful.

### Complications

(1) Haemorrhage
(2) Stricture or obstruction
(3) Rectal prolapse
(4) Perforation of gut
(5) Carcinoma which may be multicentric
(6) Toxic megacolon

Toxic megacolon is a serious disorder where there is colonic obstruction with colonic distension, fever and toxaemia.

### Treatment

Rest is very important as well as maintainence of nutrition by special dieting. Avoid items of diet which aggravates diarrhoea. The aim is to give complete nutritional support by low residue **diet, artificial milk preparations or by avoiding milk, eggs, crabs or prawn where indicated. Fluid and electrolyte balance must be corrected.**

### Corticosteroids

Oral corticosteroids may have to be given in acute cases, usually prednisolone 10 mg three or four times daily may be adequate to be given initially for two to three weeks. Gradually it should be tailed off in three to six weeks.

Sometimes it may be necessary to give Inj. ACTH if oral prednisolone is not tolerated or contraindicated. Inj. ACTH acthergel 40 units once or twice daily should be adequate and may be withdrawn gradually.

Side effects of steroid therapy should be watched carefully.

In some cases retention enema of hydrocortisone (100 mg) or betamethasone 8 mg per day may be used. In ulcerative proctitis suppositories of corticosteroids are also used.

**Salazopyrine**

It is a recognised drug which is often successful in ulcerative colitis. It is better to give a trial of this drug before steroids are used.

**Dose :** 3 to 8 g. daily in 3 to 4 divided doses. Toxic effects are rare but if side effects are noted the drug should be discontinued. When drug is tolerated it should be continued till remission occurs. It should be continued if possible in lower dose e.g. 1.0 g T.D.S. or Q.D.S. for a few weeks in cases where relapses have occured in the past.

Azathioprine or 6-mercaptopurine have been occasionally used in resistant cases but effects are not very encouraging. Moreover side effects are often severe in these anaemic and under nourished patients.

**Surgery**

Ileostomy with colectomy and excision of rectum may be done where medical treatment has failed. Expert surgical expertise is required.

## CROHN'S DISEASE

*G.C. MOOKERJEE*

**Introduction**

In modern times Crohn's disease and ulcerative colitis are classified in the group of Inflammatory Bowel Diseases (IBS), as both are basically chronic Inflammatory disorders of unknown aetiology involving the G.I. Tract. Crohn's disease is characterized by localised areas of non-specific granulomatous inflammation of the bowel, while in ulcerative colitis, the pathological changes are not segmental as in Crohn's disease.

*In ulcerative colitis* inflammatory features are well marked in large gut, bleeding per rectum is common and rectum is almost always involved. The sigmoidoscopic picture of red, angry and congested mucosa is diagnostic.

Crohn's disease was originally called *regional ileits* or enteritis, because of its tendency to involve the terminal ileum. It is now well known that it can occur anywhere in the G.I. Tract including the buccal mucosa, oesophagus and duodenum, ileum & jejunum and even large intestine. When Crohn's disease affects small intestine segmentally it is called regional ileitis. Ulcerative colitis may coexist with Crohn's disease.

In tropical countries both diseases are not so common, while many tropical bowel diseases and tuberculosis of the bowel may produce many features mimicing chronic inflammatory bowel diseases (I.B.D.). Patients presenting with recurrent diarrhoea or chronic recurrent dysentery are plenty in tropical practice. Most of them are due to chronic amoebiasis while giardiasis, schistosomiasis, bilharziasis are found in certain areas only. A clinician in the tropics must recognise these disorders from so called chronic inflammatory bowel disease (I.B.D.).

**Aetiology** — The cause of Crohn's disease is unknown but it has been suggested that the following factors may be involved :

(1) Genetic predisposition : It occurs in families, more common in white Jews.

(2) Infective cause : Pseudomonas infection-yet to be proved.

(3) Immune mechanism : It is a possible basis, IBD also occurs in gamma-globulinaemia.

(4) Psychological — Emotional stress exacerbates IBD, but emotional stress may also be caused by the disease. This may result in a vicious circle.

**Pathology**

*Macroscopic :* The intestine is oedematous so that the lumen is markedly reduced, almost closed. The oedematous mucosa displays a "cobble stone" pattern, which may have linear ulcerations and fissuring. The lesions are interspaced by normal mucosa (unlike ulcerative colitis), thus producing "skip lesions". Enlargement of mesenteric lymph nodes and thickening of mesentry occurs.

*Microscopic :* All the coats of the intestinal wall are affected, showing varying grades of inflammation. Hyperplasia of lymphoid follicles, granulomas, deep crepts or fissures may occur. The clefts may cause fistula formation, resulting in fistula between bowel and bladder or bowel and uterus or vagina, or adjacent loops of intestines.

**Clinical features :** Any age, any sex may be affected, but most common ground 40 years of age.

Depending on the part of the gut affected, the clinical features vary and may mimic many diseases including appendicitis when the onset is acute.

In chronic cases, abdominal pain is usually common specially in the lower right quadrant. Palpation reveals local tenderness and muscle guarding, P.R. examination may demonstrate palpable mass which may also be felt per abdomen. Such ileocaecal mass may have to be differentiated from ileocaecal tuberculosis, appendicular mass or new growth. In children lymphadenitis specially should be considered.

If there is vigorous borborygmi, along with nausea and vomiting with colic abdominal pain, intestinal obstruction may be suspected. There are usually many acute attacks of colicky pain in the course of the chronic disease, due to subacute obstruction.

Reduced surface area for absorption and disturbance of the biliary enterohepatic circulation due to involvement of ileum, protein losing enteropathy (due to inflammed mucosa) and bacterial colonisation in fistulae may occur. This leads to the malabsorption syndrome. Diarrhoea occurs without frank blood, mucus or pus, unless colon is involved, while involvement of the anal canal presents skin tags, perianal abscesses and fistula.

Generalised features like weight loss, low grade fever, moderate anaemia and clubbing may occur. Erythema nodosum, ankylosing spondylitis, iritis, enteropathic arthritis, and aphthous stomatitis may occur in some cases. There may be hydronephrosis due to involvement of right ureter entangled in abdominal mass of intestines.

**Investigations**

(1) Sigmoidoscopy is very helpful in diagnosis while modern method of colonoscopy is more useful in diagnosis.

(2) Alteration of mucosal pattern, ulcers and the marked narrowing of the lumen of a segment causing the "String Sign" is pathognomonic of the disease, and is evident in barium pictures of G.I.T.

(3) Barium enema may demonstrate involvement of the large gut which if involved in its entire length, may be difficult to distinguish from ulcerative colitis.

(4) Stool for occult blood may be positive, and microscopic examination shows RBC and or pus cells.

(5) Blood examination shows anaemia and hypoproteinaemia. Schilling Test may be abnormal.

(6) Diagnosis may be established by rectal biopsy or perianal skin tag biopsy in some but not all cases. Now-a-days most cases will be diagnosed by fiberoptic colonoscopy by which visual appearance can be recognised and also biopsy can be taken.

**Differential diagnosis**

In Tropics, chronic amoebiasis, giardiasis and tuberculosis must be excluded.

Pseudomembranous colitis due to prolonged antibiotics may cause acute diarrhoea sometimes dysentery.

Shigella, salmonella, yersina, campylobactor infection, etc. are not so difficult to differentiate as they produce acute enteritis. When prolonged it may be mistaken with acute ulcerative colitis.

Beechet's syndrome is characterised by ocular involvement (conjunctivitis & uveitis), oral ulcers, urethritis and in females vulvo-vaginitis.

**Treatment**

The medical treatment consists of supportive treatment as recommended in cases of chronic bowel diseases.

*Supportive therapy* consists of providing adequate nutrition by easily digestible, low residue diet. Raw vegetables and fibrous fruits are not tolerated. Prepared milk-products, may be added with vitamin supplements, and iron salts may be required.

*Antibiotics*

These are not routinely necessary unless evidence of bacterial infecton is present. Sulphasalazine (salazopyrine) as well as appropriate antibiotics may have to be used as in case of ulcerative colitis. Metronidazole is useful in enterocutaneous fistula.

*Steroids*

A report from National cooperative Crohn's disease study (Gastroenterology : 1979, 74, 825) reveals that prednisolone and sulphasalazine are useful in acute stage of Crohn's disease while azathiaprine is not useful.

Steroid therapy should be considered in presence of diffuse disease and in acute forms.

Oral prednisolone (or equivalent drug) in dosage of 30 to 40 mg daily should be started initially for two to three weeks and then may be reduced and tailed off. In some cases small doses may have to be continued for weeks but avoid prolonged therapy whereever possible.

Another method is to give 15 to 40 mg on alternate days till symptoms subside to gradually fail off.

*Salazopyrine* is given 2 to 3 g daily, in divided doses as in ulcerative colitis. It appears to be more effective in colonic rather than ileal disease. Dose should be gradually reduced to 1 to 2 g daily for maintenance for several weeks. Prednisolone plus salazopyrine do not appear to have additional advantage.

*Azathioprine of 6-mercaptopurine* has been tried in Crohn's disease but its value appears to be uncertain hence not to be routinely used.

Recently metronidazole has been advocated in perianal Crohn's disease (Gastroenterology 79; 357, 1980) but prolonged use of this drug is also likely to produce complications. Further reports are awaited.

**Surgery**

Surgery is indcated in complicated cases due to fistula, bleeding and obstruction failure of medical therapy is also a relative indication.

# CONSTIPATION

*G.C. MOOKERJEE*

## Introduction

Incomplete and infrequent evacuation of dried, hard faeces is known as constipation. Although there may be wide variation in the amount and frequency of passage of stool, usually most individuals have one evacuation in 24 hrs, and this by habit, is usually in the morning hours.

## Causes

Constipation may be a functional disorder or due to wrong diet, organic local lesion or a generalised systemic disease. The pernicious habit of neglecting the nature's call to defecate, weak abdominal wall, sedation, or post operative complications are common causes of constipation. Since defecation is a reflex process, the suppression of the urge to defecate may cause the reflex to be dulled.

A low residue diet may produce too little roughage, or sometimes autonomic dysfunction may lead to spastic colon causing constipation.

Certain gastrointestinal diseases e.g. pyloric stenosis,intestinal obstruction, carcinoma colon or diverticulitis may cause constipation. Local painful conditions e.g. and fissures, thrombosed piles or ischiorectal abscess are also responsible.

Pressure on the colon as in pregnancy, uterine fibroids or pelvic malignancy may also lead to constipation. Drugs like opiates, codeine, $CaCO_3$, anticholinergic drugs and ganglion blockers cause constipation.

## Clinical features :

Many people have a fixed idea regarding the frequency of bowel movement, and they may develop a neurosis becoming bowel conscious. They develop functional symptoms and go on taking purgatives and enemas off and on. This may become a vicious circle.

**Faecal stasis :** However, constipation may be associated with the many symptom complexes, producing nausea, anorexia, flatulence and is caused by distension of the bowel. Tongue may be coated. A few days of constipation is followed by large foul smelling stool.

**Drastic purgatives :** are often used which may cause loss of electrolytes are dehydration. Repeated soap-water enema (if not evacuated) may get absorbed to produce the water-intoxication syndrome causing weakness and drowsiness, convulsions or even coma. Saline enemas may produce over-hydration causing oedema and pulmonary congestion. Old people sometimes suffer a lot due to chronic constipation.Features of abdominal discomfort, colicky pain, efforts to pass stool often causes fainting. Even features of intestinal obstruction may occur.

These cases are to be carefully handled and conservatively treated lest they may go to operation table in the hands of inexperienced. Two illustrations are cited :

**Case I —** A patient aged 82 years in a nursing home was recommended surgery for subacute intestinal obstruction by a senior surgeon and a Gastroenterologist but the patient left the nursing home against medical advice and conservative treatment relieved all symptoms. The patient has remained well since this episode three years ago.

**Case 2 —** An elderly lady used to get repeated attacks of abdominal colic lasting for 18 to 24 hours due to severe constipation. She was usually relieved by an ounce of liquid paraffin two or three times in course of 24 to 48 hours. Her constipation was usually aggravated by too many sleeping pills for chronic insomnia. There was no organic disease.

**Colonic neurosis —** This may develop from young age, and is often due to bad bowel training by the parents of the child. Often the urge to defecate is suppressed because of cold weather, laziness or anxiety (as before going to school). Sometimes over-anxious parents may inadvertently give purgatives unnecessarily.

**Spurious Diarrhoea** — This may occur in old age, due to impaction of hard faeces in the rectum causing constipation while purgatives produce the passage of liquid stool by the side of the impacted mass. Rectal examination confirms the diagnosis.

**Investigations** should be undertaken for piles, prolapse, and fistula in all constipated patients as well as a thorough clinical examination of the patient should be done. Enquire regarding fluid intake, roughage in diet, previous bowel habit, drug intake and any evidence of systemic disease. Change of life's routine may cause constipation. A young man on completion of university education gets a job in an industry where his duty hours are in shifts e.g. from 6 A.M. to 2 P.M. or 2 P.M. to 9 P.M. and night duty of 9 P.M. to 6 P.M. Consider he has to leave his house at 4 to 5 A.M. to reach in time. This kind of change of normal life may cause serious problems in bowel habit.

A newly married girl in a middle-class family with one toilet to share with many, is also a likely candidate.

So before special investigations are ordered these personal problems should be enquired into.

**Treatment**

In general, constipation occurring in the younger age group is not serious, and should be managed by counselling and alteration of food habits rather then by purgatives or laxatives. Fluids should be given adequately. High roughage diet plenty of green vegetables should be added to the diet.

Regular physical exercises or certain special 'Yogic asanas' may be helpful. Abdominal exercises and self massage of abdomen before toilet may be tried.

*Indigenous drugs*

*Hydrophilic colloids* swell up in presence of water, and thus increase the bulk helping bowel movement. 'Isabgool' is such a drug which is cheap and is often very useful. Its husk or seed both are used but seeds appear to be more helpful. Powdered dry "Bael" fruit or a few senna-pods soaked in warm water in form of 'senna' tea often helps.

**Enemas**

These should be avoided routinely but low enemas, or suppositories may be necessary in bedridden or comatose patients.

*Liquid paraffin* may be used but it soils clothes and prevents absorption of fat soluble vitamins.

*Milk of magnesia* is a mild laxative and may be used when required but castor oil is best avoided.

In very old people hard scybella may cause symptoms of subacute intestinal obstruction. Semiliquid diet, liquid paraffin or milk of magnesia, etc. should be judiciously used. In stubborn cases, digital clearance of rectum after an over-night retention enema of olive oil (150 — 200 ml) may be required. Constipation is best treated by liquid paraffin, olive oil, soap water enemas or suppositories in these cases.

Toilet training and prompt response to natural urge of defecation is important. Neglect to attend nature's call is often an initiating factor.

Psychotherapy and repeated reassurance may be required in stubborn cases.

## DIARRHOEAL DISORDERS IN CHILDHOOD

*C.M. BANERJEE*

According to WHO report, infant mortality due to diarrhoea is around 40%. In India, it is the leading cause of death in children below three years. Roughly, every pre-school child suffers two or four attacks of diarrhoea in a year with a mortality of 1 to 4%. Mortality is higher among low-income group families.

**Definition**

Diarrhoea is a symptom characterised by frequent passage of loose and abnormal stools. If blood and mucus are present, it is dysentery. Diarrhoea may be acute, recurrent and chronic. It may be mild, self-limited or severe with high fever, dehydration and collapse.

**Aetiology**

Over 80% of acute diarrhoea occurs in infants and children below three years. The incidence declines in the older age group.

The predisposing factors are flies, open-air disposal of faeces, malnutrition, poverty, poor hygiene, lack of safe drinking water, ignorance and superstition. In India, religious congregations, "melas", open-air wayside eating restaurants, are responsible for epidemics. In malnourished infants, immunological incompetence is another important factor causing high mortality and frequent attacks. Infective diarrhoea is rare in breast-fed infants as mother's milk contains anti-infective antibodies like Ig A and Ig D. Infective diarrhoea is common among bottle-fed infants. Hence greater emphasis should be placed on breast-feeding. Rather feed the mother as well as possible. Diarrhoeas may occur due to anteral infection as well as parenteral causes.

**Enteral infection**

(1) *E. coli* is the commonest bacteria in all age groups. E.coli of different sero-type cause epidemics in nurseries, hospitals, schools and residential hostels. This type of E.coli is invasive as in case of shigella, producing inflammation of intestines and stools contain blood and mucus. Another type of E.coli releases entero-toxic agent like V. cholera. It is not invasive.

(2) *Shigella group* e.g. Shigella Flexner, Sh. Boyd, Sh. Shigella, Sh. sonna.

(3) *Salmonella group* is responsible for seasonal diarrhoea and carrier state. e.g. S.Typhi, S.Para-typhi, S.typhimurium, S. enteridis, S. Hidelberg and S. Newport.

(4) *Staphylococcal infection* occurs in bigger children due to food poisoning and through carriers, prolonged administration of antibiotics is another cause encouraging super infection.

(5) *V.Cholera and El tor Vibrio* cause epidemics of cholera. Occasionally, Klebsiella proteus, pseudomonas, pyocyaneous etc. may cause diarrhoea. In cold countries campylobactor which is a vibrio causes abdominal pain and diarrhoea due to consumption of infected chicken flesh.

(6) *Viral :* Influenza, poliomyelitis, measles, adeno-viruses, rota-virus and coxsackie virus may cause diarrhoea.

(7) *Parasitic :* E. histolytica, giardia lambia, round worms, tapeworm, threadworm, hookworm also strongloides stercoralis and trichuris trichura cause acute recurrent and chronic diarrhoea in children, especially in school-going age group. Malaria may produce acute diarrhoea with blood and mucus in stool.

(8) *Fungal :* Candida albicans causes thrush and diarrhoea among neonates especially among bottle-fed.

**Parenteral infection**

Pneumonia, meningitis, urinary tract infection, mastoiditis, and septicaemia may cause acute diarrhoea. Septicaemia is a cause of diarrhoea, especially in low-birth-weight babies.

*Dietetic :* When colostrum changes to normal mother's milk and when meconium changes to stools, there may be frequent stools in the neonates. This is physiological diarrhoea and needs no treatment.

In the underfed babies there may be hunger diarrhoea. The stools are frequent, small, greenish and sticking to the diapers.

In over-fed babies there may be frequent large stools, while excessive sugars, fats and fatty acids, spicy foods may cause diarrhoea. Recurrent diarrhoea may be due to food intolerance or food allergy; milk, wheat-gluten, fish, egg and groundnut may cause allergic diarrhoea in some children.

The incidence of acute diarrhoea increases during weaning period (weaning diarrhoea).

*Endocrine disturbances :* Like hyperthyroidism, hypoparathyroidism, and adrenal tumour may cause acute diarrhoea in older children.

*Iatrogenic :* Broad spectrum antibiotics and many other drugs cause changes in bacterial flora producing diarrhoea (due to staphylococci and candida).

Rarely, pseudomonas entero-colitis may occur, diarrhoea being severe and prolonged.

*Emotional :* In older children nervous tension, anxiety, depression and fear cause diarrhoea. Often there is family history. Post-prandial diarrhoea belongs to this group.

*Miscellaneous :* Hirschprung's diseases may cause diarrhoea in neonates and necrotising enterocolitis is also a rare cause.

**Causes of neonatal diarrhoea**

(1) Physiological diarrhoea
(2) Parenteral infection and deep sepsis
(3) E.Coli infection
(4) Lactose intolerance
(5) Unconjugated bile-acid diarrhoea
(6) Thrush
(7) Milk allergy
(8) Congenital chloridorrhoea
(9) Necrotising enterocolitis
(10) Hirschprung's disease

**Causes of chronic diarrhoea**

Common causes are :

(1) Amoebic dysentry
(2) Malnutrition
(3) Disaccharidase deficiency
(4) All causes of recurrent diarrhoea

**Causes of recurrent diarrhoea**

(1) Amoebiasis and giardiasis
(2) Malabsorption syndrome e.g. coeliac diseases and fibrocystic disease of the pancreas, protein-losing enteropathy
(3) Abdominal tuberculosis
(4) Ulcerative colitis
(5) Crohn's disease
(6) Cirrhosis of liver
(7) Immunological deficiency with malnutrition.

**Clinical features of acute diarrhoea**

The biochemical changes are always more important. The fundamental disturbance lies in loss of water and electrolytes, causing dehydration, which may be isotonic, hypotonic, and hypertonic depending on the proportion of water and salts loss. In isotonic dehydration the ratio of electrolytes to water is undisturbed though their sum total in body fluids is reduced. When more water than electrolytes is lost hypernatraemia or hypertonic dehydration occurs. While if more salt then water is lost then hypotonic especially among malnourished children and 15% are hypertonic.

Dehydration may be mild, moderate and severe.

*In mild cases :* The child loses 5% body weight, may pass 5-6 stools, is pale irritable, with slightly sunken eyes and fontanelle (if not closed). Tongue is still moist, acidosis is not noticeable, stool may be green or yellow.

*Moderate cases :* (Loss of weight — 5% to 10%). Stools may be 10 or more, child is ill, irritable or drowsy, with sunken eyes and fontanelle with dry mucous membrane and inelastic skin. If the skin on the abdomen is pinched it very slowly retracts to the surface. Acidosis is usually present, though not marked.

*Severe cases :* (Loss of body weight is more than 10%). There are too many loose motions with marked constitutional symptoms like shock and peripheral failure. The pulse is thready and rapid with low blood pressure. There is oliguria or anuria. Eyes are sunken, marked depression of fontanelle. The abdominal skin is inelastic.

Breathing is deep and rapid due to acidosis. There may be convulsion. If the loss of body weight is more than 15% the condition becomes irreversible with all the previous symptoms being more marked. The child is in coma with anoxia; abdomen is sunken or in case of hypokalaemia there may be distension and tympanitis resulting in paralytic ileus. Plasma sodium level is less than 130 m Eq/L.

The extracellular fluid is hypotonic. To maintain electrolyte balance there is shift of water to intracellular compartment resulting in oedema of brain and liver tissue and there is more loss of potassium, and bicarbonate by the kidneys. The child is first drowsy, then comatose with convulsion. Thirst is absent. Tongue may be moist.

**Hypernatraemia :** Plasma sodium exceeds 150 m. Eq/L E.C.F. fluid is hypertonic; to maintain electrolyte balance water shifts from cells into extracellular compartment resulting in shrinkage of brain cells. Hence subdural and intracerebral haemorrhage may occur.

The child in hyperirritable and has profound thrist. All the signs of dehydration are exaggerated and there may be hyperpyrexia.

**Hypokalaemia :** In acute diarrhoea this is quite common due to loss of potassium with stools and due to vomiting, acidosis and toxaemia. The child is lethargic and flabby with hypotonia of muscles, loss of deep reflexes, distension of abdomen with marked tympanitis resulting in paralytic ileus; there is tachycardia with characteristic ECG charges.

*Acidosis :* Here the $CO_2$ combining power is lower than 20 m. Eq. per litre. In severe acidosis, the child is drowsy and respiration is deep and may be 80-100 per minute, urine may contain ketone bodies.

The sequelae of recurrent and chronic diarrhoea are :

a. Growth failure
b. Malnutrition
c. Immunological deficiencies
d. Prolapse of rectum
e. Psychological changes in the child.

**Diagnosis**

Routine examination of stools, macroscopic and microscopic examination is sufficient for starting treatment. For etiological diagnosis well-equipped laboratory is required for stool culture with sensitivity tests, estimation of Na, K, $CO_2$ combining power and other electrolytes Hb concentration, blood urea and creatinine etc.

**Management**

**Remember five "D"s :**

(1) Diagnosis (aetiological) as far as possible
(2) Dehydration should be assessed
(3) Drugs
(4) Diets
(5) Disaccharidases deficiency must be watched.

Nowadays the emphasis is on domiciliary treatment rather than hospitalisation, mild and moderate cases can be treated at home; present experiences show that oral hydration if started with the onset of any diarrhoea may prevent the child from getting into severe stage. What is required is the health education emphasising oral hydration in rural areas and urban slums in our country. Hospitalisation is required for severe cases with shock and peripheral failure, and marked acidosis. If parenteral therapy is required for moderate cases this can be done at home with scalp vein canula, which is now available.

The WHO formulation oral hydration is :

Sodium chloride 3.5 gm
Sodium bicarbonate 2.5 gm
Pot. Chloride 1.5 gm
Glucose 25 gm

To be dissolved in 1 litre of boiled water. Many preparations conforming to the formula are now available in the market. According to WHO, children rehydrated with oral solution have their appetite restored quickly and improve their nutritional state. In rural areas mothers may be instructed to dissolve in one litre of boiled water one level teaspoon (about seven pinches) of dry common salt and enough sugar to sweeten and use this fluid.

Oral fluids 10-20 cc/kg/hour may be given for 48 hours by which time dehydration is virtually controlled. Even where parenteral therapy is given, the maintenance therapy can be continued with oral hydration. Once the child can take fluid by oral route 30 cc to 60 cc oral fluid is given after every stool is passed.

Where parenteral fluid is to be given isotonic saline with 5% glucose M/6 lactate solution or Ringer lactate or Hartman's solution are given as indicated.

**Fluid requirement of acutely dehydrated children**

Commonly 5% glucose in half normal saline is used to combat acute dehydration.

Usual method is to give 120 to 200 ml/kg in 24 hours intravenously but in severe cases 45 to 60 ml/kg is given in first four hours of treatment.

However, in the new-born it may be safer to use a quarter strength saline after initial treatment with half-normal glucose for 12 to 24 hours.

When severe metabolic acidosis is present 1/6 molar lactate should be given to start with 30 ml/kg body weight, which may be repeated after a few hours if acidosis persists (assessment is by Astrup micromethod). Each ml. of 8.4% sodium bicarbonate is 1 mEq. The bicarbonate requirement may be roughly calculated as follows :

Body weight in kg $\times$ 0.35 $\times$ base deficit in m. Eq/hour (considering that 35% of B.W. is extracellular fluid).

Potassium deficiency is correctable by oral K-salt but in severe cases specially where vomiting continue, intravenous potassium chloride may be necessary. Hypertonic dehydration and water intoxication are sometimes real problems and these have been discussed in detail in this chapter on water and electrolyte balance.

If vomiting does not stop or if there is abdominal distension and intestinal hurry, parenteral therapy has to be continued till the child can take fluid orally. When isotonic solution is used for initial therapy intravenously, potassium should be given orally 1-3 gm daily. In severe hypopotassaemia, potassium has to be given by I.V. drip in 1-3 mEq/kg dose. In hyperpotassaemia digoxin, insulin and calcium are of value. For hyponatraemia with 3% NaCl in 5% glucose may be followed by isotonic saline while monitoring of electrolytes should be done. Frequent electrolyte studies are essential to properly tract these cases.

**Specific drugs**

Choice of drugs depends on aetiology. When the diarrhoea is due to too much food, wrong food or under-cooked or irritable food, no specific drug therapy is required.

Indications of specific drug therapy are as follows :

*Sulpha drugs* : Can be used in mild cases. They are economical. Sulphadimidine which is absorbable can be used in 100 — 150 mg/kg/day done in 4 doses. Sulphaguanidine and Thalazole are also good for dysentery.

*Sulphamethoxazole :* Trimethoprim, Co-trimoxazole, may be employed in some cases. Trimethoprim should not be used in infants below 6 months. Resistance of E.coli and shigella to sulpha drugs has been reported.

*Chloramphenicol :* Avoid use of this drug and it should not be given to prematures, newborns, anaemic and malnourished children. It produces grey baby syndrome and depression of bone marrow. Routine use of this drug is forbidden.

*Ampicillin* 100—200 mgm/kg orally or parenterally 5—7 days. Drug rash and pseudomembranous enterocolitis should be watched for.

*Nalidixic acid* has also been used in some epidemics due to shigella in adults as well as children, where resistance was noted to commonly used drugs.

*Streptomycin :* It is given orally in 100 mgm.kg/day dosage in four divided doses singly or in combination with chloramphenicol. It is effective even in gram negative infections. Better avoid this.

*Furazolidine :* Besides E.Coli and salmonella, giardia and E.histolytica respond to it. But haemolytic anaemia due to glucose 6 phosphate dehydrogenase deficiency may occur; carcinogenic effects have also been reported. Dose 6 mg/kg for 5 days.

*Kanamycin*

In septicaemia and staphylococcal infection in newborn, I.M. kanamycin 10—15 mg/kg/day may be given for 3 to 5 days. Note nephrotoxicity and 8th Nerve damage may sometime occur.

*Gentamycin* may be required in pyocyaneous and pseudomonas infection. Dose 3—5 mg/kg a day I.M. in divided doses. It is also nephrotoxic antibiotic and should not be used in viral, diarrhoea or unless specially indicated. Diarrhoea due to milk allergy, lactose intolerance and pseudomembranous (enterocolitis) and non-specific diarrhoea.

For giardiasis and amoebiasis, metronidazole or tinidazole or furazolidine are used.

*Tetracycline* oral or I.M. should not be given to infants and children below 8 years as they cause staining of teeth and deposition in growing bones and occasionally produce pseudomotor cerebri syndrome.

Bismuth, pectin and kaolin may be given in mild cases but opium preparations should be avoided. Lomotil, though it is very effective in adults it may cause adverse symptoms in infants and children below 3 years and may cause paralytic ileus. Therefore it should not be used in infants and children Inj. chlorpromazine given I.M. 5 mg is effective for vomiting. In persistent vomiting stomach wash with water is sometimes beneficial, for abdominal distension oral potassium chloride 0.5 to 1 gm thrice a day may be used.

*Diet :* The present concept is not to starve the child. If there is nausea and vomiting, if the child cannot retain anything stop feeds for 8-12 hours; otherwise continue breast feed or give ½ to 1/3rd diluted artificial milk available locally. Half-cream milk, lactic-acid milk or even sweetened condensed milk in 1 to 8 dilution can be given. Full strength formula should be reached gradually especially if there is distension and intestinal hurry. For bigger children bland diet with cereals may be started avoiding high protein and high fat diet. Banana, curd, apple pudding, pulp of "Bael" fruit may be given as tolerated.

Early feeding management prevents marasmas which is common after acute diarrhoea.

**Disaccharidase deficiency**

In some normal babies and in some diarrhoea cases deficiency of enzymes for lactose and rarely sucrose may be seen. Lactose deficiency may be primary or seconday. Primary deficiency is uncommon, usually seen in premature babies, because lactose is developed just before gestation. It is formed in brush border of epithelial cells of villi of small intestine. In the absence of lactase, lactose is not hydrolysed into galactose and glucose to be absorbed. Hence there is increase of osmotic load of intestinal contents causing diarrhoea.

Besides diarrhoea there may be abdominal distension and colic. Lactose is converted into lactic acid, hence the stool is highly acidic causing redness of periantal skin.

Secondary lactose deficiency occurs in infantile diarrhoea, especially viral diarrhoea. Other infections, milk allergy, prolonged use of antibiotics like neomycin, colimycin and kanamycin also cause secondary lactose deficiency.

**Diagnosis** is by detecting acidity, presence of reducing substance in the watery stool by Benedict's solution and identifying lactose by paper sugar paper chromatography. In primary cases intestinal mucous membrane biposy which is rather difficult may be done.

**Treatment :**

(1) Stop all lactose preparations including milk.

(2) *Feeds :* Small babies may be given soyabean milk, milk protein, butter and arrowroot. Butter milk of over-ripe curds, washed several times, contains no lactose. Hence it can be given. Secondary lactose intolerance disappears after a few months. No antibiotics should be given.

**Milk allergy**

A small percentage of infants and children develop allergy to milk protein, especially lactoglobulin of cow's and buffalo's milk. The symptoms start when breast milk is changed to bovine milk. In addition to diarrhoea there is vomiting, abdominal colic and distension. There may also be wheezing and cough. If this condition is suspected,milk should be totally stopped. The symptoms will disappear only to appear in 48 hours if milk is started again.

**Treatment**

(1) Stop all milk;

(2) Correct dehydration and feedings;

(3) Soyabean milk and arrowroot for infants. For older children egg, jelly animal proteins, cereals and fruits like banana should be given;

(4) To desensitize the child milk should be gradually introduced starting with drops. It may take many months before the child can tolerate milk;

(5) Wheezing and cough cannot be treated by any medicine if milk is not stopped.

### Necrotising Enterocolitis :

Occurs in low birth weight infants, in infants having multiple transfusions with repeated umbilical catheterisation and in infants with Hirschprung's disease. Bowel stasis and intestinal wall ischaemia multiple ulcers, sloughing of the epithelium with haemorrhages are the pathological changes. X-ray shows dilated intestines with air bubbles in the walls. Peritonitis and perforation are common. From 3rd or 4th day after birth the baby passes frequent water stools containing blood and mucus vomiting, abdominal distension and paralytic ileus, rectal prolapse may occur.

Prognosis — grave

Treatment — symptomatic with antibiotics

### Pseudomembranous Enterocolitis

It may occur during or soon after antibiotic therapy, characterised by frequent stools with blood and mucus, colics, nausea, vomiting, abdominal distension sigmoidoscopic appearance is generalised inflammation of mucosa of colon with raised thick yellowish white pseudomomembrane. This condition is rare in children but seen in adults. Treatment is symptomatic. All oral fluids stopped, nasogastric suction began, appropriate intravenous fluids and nutrients given.

## ACUTE APPENDICITIS

*A.K. SEN SARMA*

Acute appendicitis is a common cause of acute abdomen which requires urgent operative treatment. Incidence seems to be increasing especially in the western world due to dietary habit. Mortality is very much reduced due to discovery of various antibiotics, early diagnosis and early surgery. Appendix is an elongated cul-de-sac projecting from the caecum near the ileocaecal junction. It can attain various positions e.g. ileal, pelvic, paracaecal and retro-colic.

It can be affected in two ways :

(1) Blood borne infection causing enlargement of lymphoid tissue in the wall, producing obstruction of the lumen further aggravates the situation.

(2) Primary obstruction by impaction of faecolith, small stones or seeds ingested with food.

Inflammation of the wall and obstruction of the lumen is produced by stasis and oedema. This is in addition to thrombosis of the vessels jeopardising blood supply leading to gangrene, perforation and peritonitis. Simultaneous protective mechanism, however, comes to localise the inflammation. The greater omentum (policeman of the abdomen) tries to localise the process and forms an inflammatory appendicular lump or appendicular abscess. Failure to localise results in general peritonitis, severe toxaemia and even death, if not promptly treated.

### Clinical features

The following are the cardinal symptoms at the onset of the disease.

(i) Pain is the most prominent feature, it starts around the umbilicus or epigastrium and quickly settles down in right iliac fossa.

(ii) Fever is usually not high in majority of cases, but usually the temperature is slightly elevated.

(iii) Nausea and later vomiting appear. Patient looks toxic with coated tongue, malaise, fever and elevation of pulse rate. Tenderness over the McBurney's point with muscle-guard i.e., localised rigidity, hyperaesthesia, Rovsing's sign are all the features of acute appendicitis.

Tenderness can be elicited during rectal examination. If the treatment is delayed, there may be general peritonitis associated with high fever, tachycardia, tenderness and rigidity all over the abdomen, impairment of intestinal movement, weakening of bowel sounds and distention of abdomen. These features are due to gangrene and perforation of inflammed appendix.

### Differential diagnosis

There is no difficulty in diagnosis if the classical features are available. Some cases especially with highly placed appendix it may be mistaken for acute cholecystitis, perforated peptic ulcer. Due to retrocaecal position it can produce frequency of micturition and loin pain simulating ureteric calculi. Some gynaecological diseases may mimic acute appendicitis. Regional ileitis may also be confused with acute appendicitis. Viral lymphadenitis of right external iliac group of glands in children may be confused and may be mis-diagnosed as acute appendicitis. Chronic appendicitis, recurrent appendicitis should be diagnosed with great reservation. Chronic amoebiasis which is very common in tropical countries should be kept in mind while diagnosing chronic appendicitis.

### Treatment

As already stated acute appendicitis should be treated by surgery. Once clinical diagnosis is made, blood examination usually shows high leukocyte count with increased polymorph but it may also be normal. Nothing should be given by mouth. Intravenous fluids should be started and plan for operation should be organised. Broad spectrum antibiotic should be started from the beginning. Apendicular abscess should be drained extra-peritoneally. Internal appendicectomy to be carried out later. In more complicated cases where general peritonitis has developed, aggressive management with laparatomy will save the life of the patient along with supportive therapy.

### Treatment

Conservative treatment with rest, I.V. fluids and antibiotics is allowed only in special circumstances e.g. if there is a well organised lump and where there is no immediate surgical arrangement available in remote places and in mid-sea. However, patient can be transported quickly. Nowadays in all large ships facilities for operative treatment are available.

## CARCINOMA OF COLON AND RECTUM

*A.K. SEN SARMA*

Carcinoma of colon is usually an adeno-carcinoma. The incidence is more common in the western world in comparison to this country, Africa and South-East Asia. This is probably due to dietary habits with low-roughage and high-protein type diet.

### Pathogenesis

It is more common in the left, colon and rectum, which constitutes 75% of the total cases. The right colon and the transverse colon have almost equal incidence.

Carcinoma primarily 'de novo' is more common than the secondary carcinomatous change which occurs in ulcerative colitis and multiple adenomatous polyph. The actual aetiological factors of carcinoma colon are not well established. However, habitual constipation due to intake of low residue diet, prolonged contact of carcinogens in contact with the colonic mucosa may be one of the important causes in the western world.

It can be polypoidal, ulcerative and constricting type producing intestinal obstruction. In anaplastic or undifferentiated types, there is rapid growth of tumour with the necrosis, perforation and paracolic abscess.

### Spread

1) *By lymphatics*

   It goes through epicolic lymphatic channels and drains into the lymphatics along with superior and inferior mesenteric vessels. Some cases of carcinoma of lower part of rectum extent up to anal-canal and may spread to the inguinal lymph nodes to the external iliac group.

2) *Blood borne*

   It spreads along the portal radical to the liver.

3) *Intraluminal spread*

It is not very uncommon and multiple carcinoma can be seen.

4) **Local spread**

These are usually multiple in cases of ulcerative colitis and multiple adenomatous polyp. Severity of the disease will depend on histological grading.

**Diagnosis**

(i) Alteration of bowel habits is one of the cardinal symptoms of carcinoma colon. This includes alternating constipation and diarrhoea associated with borborygmi, excessive mucus and passage of blood per rectum. This symptom should create suspicion and calls for detailed examination and investigation. Blood and slime is more common in carcinoma rectum. Progressive constipation with sub-acute large bowel obstruction are the features of stenosing type of carcinoma of left colon whereas diarrhoea is the feature of caecal carcinoma.

(ii) Anaemia is very common in carcinoma of colon. Unexplained anaemia and loss of weight in elderly males should raise suspicion.

(iii) Abdominal lump can be felt in the flank of the abdomen with or without features of intestinal obstruction. In late cases where the tumour is metastasised ascitis, nodular liver, and malignant cachexia are present. This is too late for any treatment.

**Investigation**

The patient should be investigated for the assessment of the general condition including anaemia, cardio-respiratory diseases and diabetes by detailed examination of the patient as a whole. Blood examination, post-glucose meal test for sugar, X-ray of the chest and E.C.G. etc. should also be done.

**Special investigations**

1) *Rectal examination :*

By finger and proctoscope. Usually most of the carcinoma rectum can be felt by the finger during rectal examination and seen during proctoscopy.

2) *Sigmoidoscopy*

By this investigation tumours of the rectum and sigmoid colon are visualised.

3) *Colonoscopy :*

It is a mandatory instrumentation to see the whole colon for single or multiple tumour. Visualisation of the whole colon is required specially in cases of multiple adenomatus polyph. Punched biopsy should be taken for histological confirmation. Unfortunately it is not available in developing countries except in large city hospitals.

4) *Ultra-sound scan and C-T scanning :*

Sonograms or C-T scan will help in detecting hepatic secondaries.

5) *X-ray studies :*

In our part of the world, barium-meal enema is still very much practised especially as facilities of endoscopy are limited.

**Management**

The treatment of carcinoma colon and rectum is basically operative. Carcinoma colon can be present with acute on chronic obstruction. In such cases two stage operations are required. Firstly, relief of obstruction by proximal defunctioning colostomy followed by second stage which consists of recession of the affected portion of the bowel.

If there is no obstruction the management will be as follows :

1) General assessment of the patient correction of cardiovascular disease, respiratory disease, diabetes, anaemia and any other co-existing disability.

2) Bowel sterilisation : Light diet and then liquid diet, repeated bowel-wash will clear the faecal mass from the bowel. Simultaneously oral antibiotic should be given for five days prior to operation.

3) Electrolyte estimation and correction of electrolyte imbalance, if any.

The following operations are usually required for the tumour of various regions :

1) Right hemi-colectomy in case of caecal growth. Extended hemi-colectomy in case of growth in the ascending colon.

2) The removal of transverse colon with distal one-third of ascending colon and proximal part of descending colon.

3) Left hemi-coloctomy in case of sigmoid colon cancer.

4) Abdomino-perineal recession with proximal and colostomy in case of carcinoma rectum.

5) Anterior recession with colorectal anastomosis in case of high rectal cancer.

## DIVERTICULITIS

*A.K. SEN SARMA*

In this condition there are multiple acquired diverticuli in the large gut especially in sigmoid colon. It occurs in the age group of 40-60 years. It is commonly seen in the western world due to wrong dietary habits discussed before. In this country and other parts of Asia and Africa this disease is not so very common. This epidemiological difference is due to intake of high-fibre-containing bulky food taken in this part of the world. Whereas in the western world food is low residual and there is less bulk of faecal mass.

### Pathology

The sigmoid colon is commonly involved. These are acquired pulsion diverticuli, due to increased intraluminal pressure primarily caused by spasm of pelvi-rectal junction. In order to propulse the faecal content, the muscle coat hypertrophies and during this process pulsion-diverticulum projects through the muscle fibre. Diverticuli are actually mucosal projections of the bowel and retain its original blood supply. Diverticuli are usually silent, diagnosed accidently during radiological examination : Sometimes it can develop infection (diverticulitis) giving rise to vague lower bowel dyspeptic symptoms. It can perforate and present features of acute abdomen; slow leak may form a para-colic abscess, which may burst or may produce fistula. Internal fistula is sometimes seen as cysto-colic or, colo-colic fistula. Due to hypertrophy of the muscle, the lumen of the gut may be reduced giving rise to colonic obstruction.

### Diagnosis

Most uncomplicated diverticular disease usually does not give rise to any symptoms. As the disease progresses patient may complain of vague lower bowel dyspeptic symptoms, e.g. alteration of bowel habit, alternate constipation,diarrhoea and borborygmi. This can be present as painful and tender lump in the left iliac fossa when complicated with infection or paracolic abscess.

As already mentioned patient can present with all the features of acute abdomen and requires careful laboratory investigation urgently. Rarely it can give rise to excessive mucus per rectum. In case of repeated attacks of infection there is deterioration of health characterised by malaise, loss of appetite, loss of body weight and bleeding P.R.

### Investigation

In all cases of lower bowel dyspeptic symptoms radiological study with barium enema should be done. Diverticulosis can be easily diagnosed by barium meal appearance characterised by multiple diverticular sacs seen as projections close to the bowel wall. After evacuation of the barium with air insufflation technique, the diverticuli are better visualised as residual barium remains in the diverticulum. Associated findings of narrowing of the bowel, thickening of the bowel wall and lack of haustration may be present.

**Endoscopy :** Sigmoidoscopy and colonoscopy are mandatory instrumentations to exclude concomitant malignancy. In such cases multiple punch biopsy may be taken for histological study.

**Blood examination :** Haemogram and ESR are done for general assessment. Blood sugar, E.C.G. and X-ray chest are required to exclude associated diseases, if any.

**Cystoscopy :** It will be required if there is evidence of cystocolic fistula characteristic by the evidence of cystitis and passage of air while micturating.

**Treatment**

Once the diverticular disease is diagnosed patient should be kept in observation. He is advised to take bulky and high residual food, bulk producing laxative containing cellulose, *isobgul & bael* fruits etc.

**Treatment of complicated cases**

1) Inflammation : Acute inflammatory stage should be treated as acute abdomen conservatively.
2) In chronic form where there is chronic obstruction surgical resection of the affected portion of the gut should be considered.
3) In case of perforation : Acute abdomen should be treated urgently. Peritoneal toileting and de-functioning colostomy to save the life of the patient. Subsequently surgical resection to be considered in later days.
4) Paracolic abscess : It should be drained extra-peritoneally, if required proximal colostomy should be simultaneously performed.
5) In cases of internal fistula resection of the affected portion of the bowel should be carried out.

## HIRSCHSPRUNG'S DISEASE

*G.C. MOOKERJEE*

Hirschsprung's disease or megacolon is caused due to congenital absence of myenteric nerve plexus in the upper rectum and pelvic colon. It may sometimes extend more proximally in the ascending colon. In Chaga's disease also similar condition may occur due to destruction of nerve plexus by trypanosomiasis. Mega-colon may rarely be acquired due to obstinate constipation, which however does not produce so much dilatation of sigmoid colon as in Hirschsprung's disease.

The presenting feature is severe constipation in the newborn, associated with progressive abdominal distension and then vomiting. Abdominal examination does not help the diagnosis but P.R. examination reveals empty rectum.

Radiological examination with barium settles the diagnosis. Treatment is surgical removal of the affected segment of large gut. In acquired megacolon, treatment is usually conservative. Cretinism should be excluded. Diet adjustment, laxatives and enemas usually helpful; very rarely surgical help may be required.

# ABDOMINAL ULTRASOUND IMAGING

*S.K. SHARMA*

**Introduction**

Diagnostic imaging includes the various scanning techniques in current use. These include ultrasound, C.T. scanning, radio-nuclide imaging and the latest modality is MRI i.e. Magnetic Resonance Imaging. The term "Scan", therefore, when unspecified, becomes confusing as it includes all these different modalities.

It is important to appreciate the application and limitations of these modalities under different clinical settings. They are all complementary to each other as they do not always provide the same information in a particular clinical condition. Each has its own advantages and limitations, knowledge of which will ensure that the most suitable procedure is carried out during the investigation of a diseased condition. This will result in saving both time and money and also quicker initiation of proper therapy.

**Ultrasound**

Ultrasound is high frequency sound-waves (1-10 MHZ) inaudible to the human ear, which are produced in a transducer. As these sound-waves pass into the body it is reflected back towards the transducer from various tissue inter-faces and organs. Analysis of the reflected sound-waves takes place within the machine and a composite picture of a section of the body is produced in the T.V. screen. As the transducer scans the body, numerous such sections are produced in transverse, longitudinal and oblique planes. These sections can also be photographed after freezing them on the T.V. screen.

**Grey-scale ultrasound**

This involves selective amplification of low-level echoes and permits visualisation of fine internal structures of organs. Strong echoes appear white and the weaker ones in varying shades of grey, depending on the strength of that echo.

**Real time ultrasound**

Here slices of the portion being scanned are produced at a rapid rate of 15 - 200 frames per second on the T.V. screen. This sequential presentation of images enables visualisation of moving structures e.g. heart and blood vessels.

**Doppler effect**

When an ultrasound beam reflects off a stationary surface the frequency of the reflected beam is the same as that of the generated beam. If the surface from which the ultrasound is being reflected is in motion, the reflected ultrasound will be at a different frequency from that of the generated ultrasound. The latter is the Doppler effect and can be used to measure the flow profile across a blood vessel and hence to calculate the blood flow volume.

**Advantages of ultrasound**

1) It is non-invasive and requires no special patient preparation.
2) It provides information on structural boundaries and demonstrates anatomy well.
3) The depth of anatomical structures or pathological masses from the skin surface can be measured by ultrasound.
4) Ultrasound can differentiate between solid masses (tumours) and fluid containing masses (cysts)
5) As it is harmless to the patient, foetus and staff, examinations can be repeated and the method can be safely used in pregnancy.
6) Moving structures e.g. heart can be studied by ultrasound.

## Clinical application

*Limitations of ultrasound*

1) As ultrasound is reflected off air-containing organs, it is unsuitable for examination of lungs and intestines.
2) Bones cannot be examined by ultrasound as it cannot pass through them.

*Preparation of the patient for ultrasonography*

| | | |
|---|---|---|
| 1. Liver | : | No special preparation. If patient has been bed-ridden, laxatives may be required. |
| 2. Gall Bladder | : | Nothing by mouth except water 12 hours before examination. |
| 3. Pancreas | : | Laxatives, if patient is constipated. Light bland meal should be given prior to examination. |
| 4. Obstetrics, Gynaecology, Prostate and urinary bladder. | : | Patient must attend with full bladder. |

5. No special preparation required for kidneys, spleen, thyroid, breast, heart and aorta.

## Hepatic disorders

*Normal sonographic appearance*

The liver parenchyma appears homogenously grey with branches of the portal veins and hepatic veins within it, which appear as tubular structures. Walls of portal vein branches which contain fibrous tissue appear echogenic and can be traced towards the porta. Hepatic vein tributaries can be traced towards the inferior vena-cava and their walls do not appear echogenic. **Normal biliary radicles and hepatic artery branches are not visualised within the liver parenchyma**

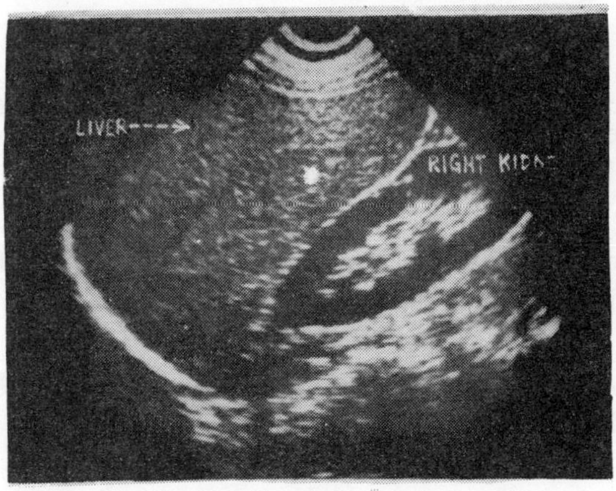


**Fig.15.1 : Normal liver and right kidney**

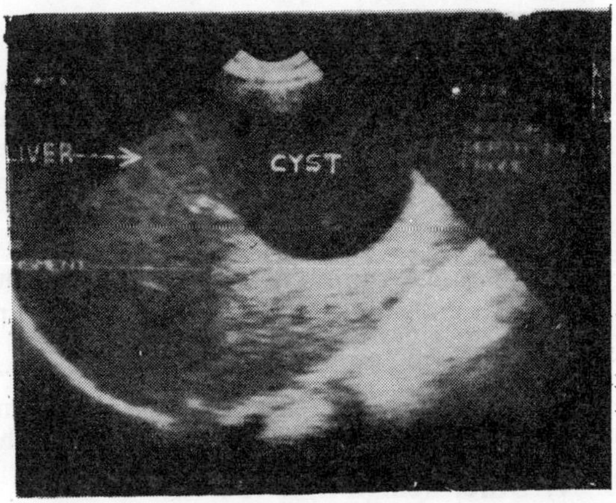


**Fig.15.2 : Liver cyst seen as a well-defined round mass with posterior enhancement of echoes**

**Focal liver disease**

The varied appearance on ultrasound of the different focal liver diseases permits a more accurate differential diagnosis than is possible with techniques like isotope scanning and CT.

1) **Simple liver cysts**

They are common incidental findings and appear as rounded echo-free areas with smooth walls and posterior enhancement.

2) **Poly-cystic liver disease**

Multiple echo-free cysts are seen in the liver which is enlarged. It may be associated with poly-cystic kidneys. Some of the liver cysts may show internal echoes due to haemorrhage.

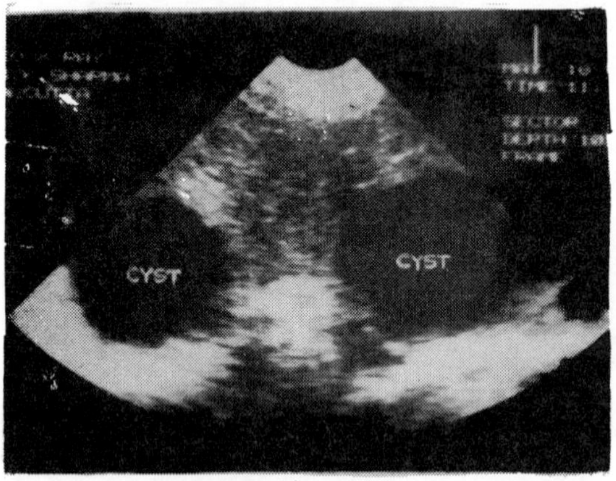


**Fig.15.3 :** Multiple simple cysts in the liver

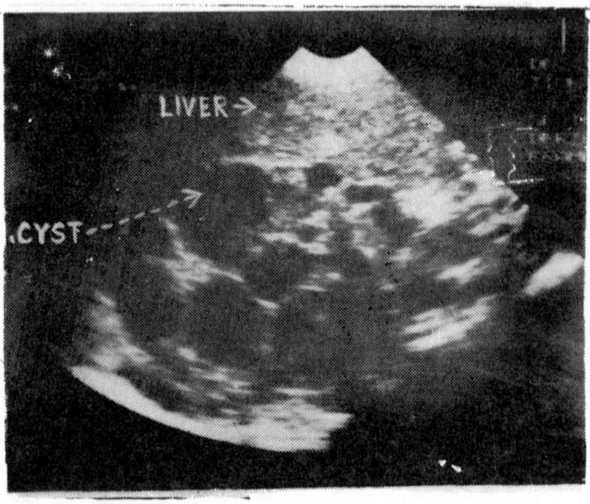


**Fig.15.4 :** Hydatid cysts of the liver seen as multiple echofree areas in the right lobe

3) **Hydatid disease**

It may appear as a cystic lesion quite indistinguishable from a simple cyst. When daughter-cysts form, multiple septa which represent walls of compressed daughter-cyst are seen.

4) **Liver abscess**

These appear as hypoechoic lesions mainly in the right lobe of the liver. Its margins may be well defined or sometimes even poorly defined. Necrotic tissue and debris within the abscess can be recognised. Ultrasound is useful in not only detecting abscesses but in guiding needle aspirations of contents for bacteriological study and therapeutic drainage.

5) **Liver trauma**

Haematomas can be recognised by ultrasound and their appearance varies with the state of organisation, being echo-free at first and later showing internal echoes.

6) **Haemangioma**

These are the commonest benign liver tumours. The capillary type appears echogenic while the cavernous type is relatively echo-free. They tend to be situated near the liver surface.

7) **Other benign liver tumours**

These are rare lesions and include adenoma and focal nodular hyperplasia. Adenomas are associated usually with oestrogen intake and appear as an hyperechoic ill-defined heterogenous mass.

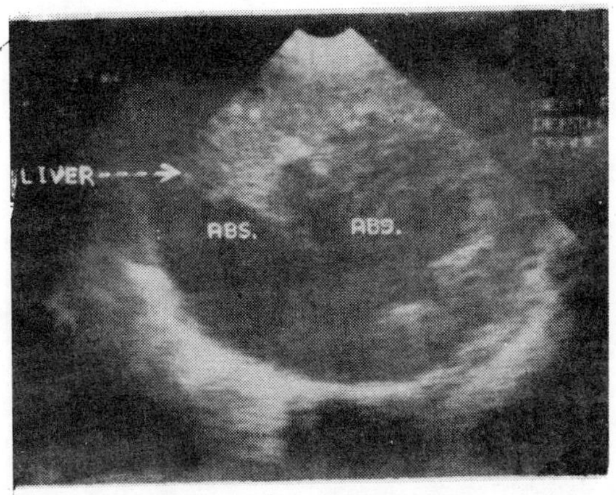


Fig.15.5 : Large hypoechoic lesion in Right lobe of liver extending upto subphrenic region. Liver abscess

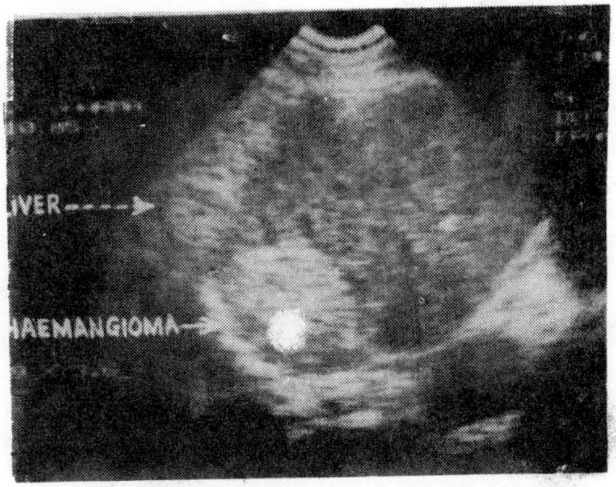


Fig.15.6 : Liver haemangioma seen as an echogenic mass in the posterior aspect of the right lobe

8) **Primary Hepatoma**

Three main microscopic patterns exist – nodular form, massive form and diffuse type. The last type is very difficult to diagnose by ultrasound. The nodular and massive types are recognised as masses of high, low and mixed echoes in the liver.

9) **Focal liver metastasis**

Focal liver deposits are usually multiple and may appear echogenic, echopoor, cystic or necrotic. Calcified deposits can also occur. Depending on the type, the origin of the primary tumour can be sometimes predicted.

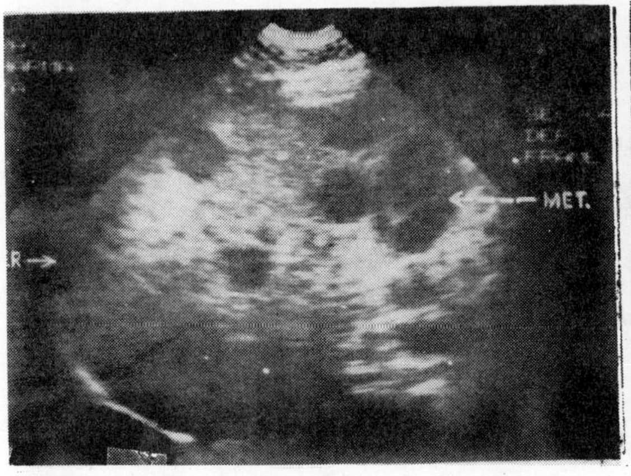


Fig.15.7 : Hypoechoic metastasis in liver. Multiple rounded masses seen in the right lobe of liver

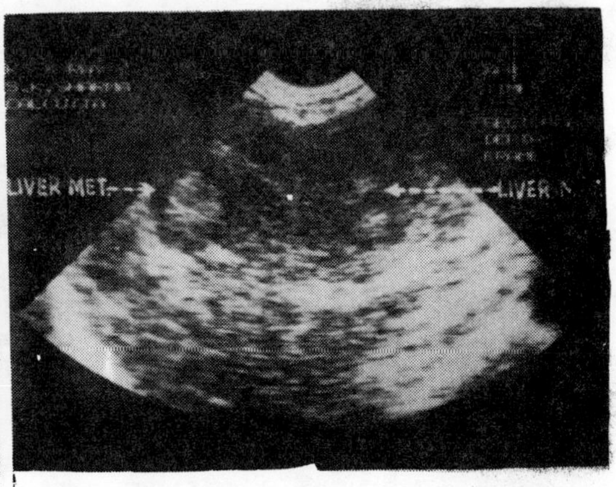


**Fig.15.8 : Two well-defined rounded masses with hypoechoic rim in right lobe of liver Metastatic deposits**

**Diffuse liver disorders**

Detection and differentiation of diffuse liver disorders by ultrasound is difficult unless the changes are gross.

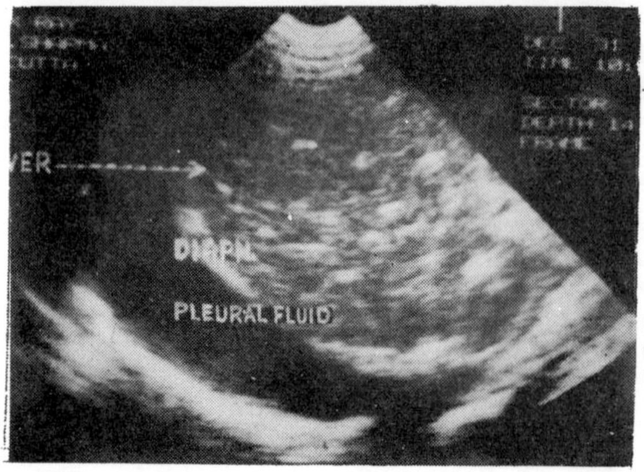


Fig.15.9 : Hepatitis. Liver parenchymal echoes are diffusely heterogenous and portal vein walls show increased echogenicity.

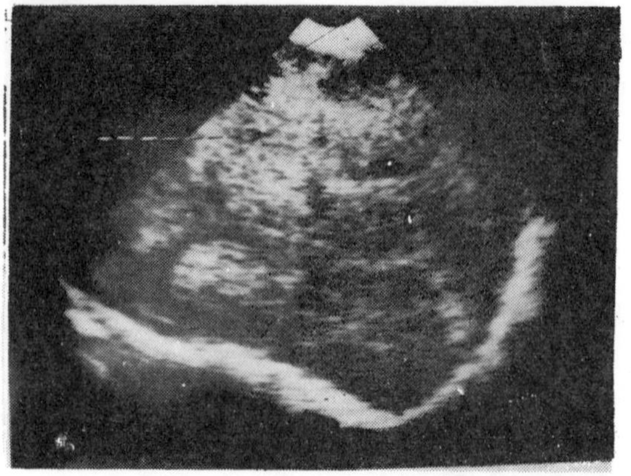

Fig.15.10 : Diffuse liver metastasis liver; parenchymal echoes are grossly hetrogeneous.

The following pathological changes can be detected by ultrasound :

1) Fatty change
2) Cirrhosis
3) Hepatitis
4) Miliary malignancy

*Fatty liver*

Here the enlarged liver shows an echotexture which is uniform but finer than normal with some increase in attenuation leading to difficulty in imaging the posterior part of the liver The liver also appears much brighter than normal.

*Cirrhosis*

On ultrasound examination appearances of cirrhosis may be divided into those of liver itself and the associated findings.

Liver findings may be variable and non-specific. The liver may show high level echoes and portal vein walls are not seen distinctly. In addition,the liver parenchyma may show a fine texture with attenuation of echoes posteriorly. Surface nodularity due to regenerating nodules can also be recognised.

Associated findings include presence of ascites and evidence suggestive of portal hypertension. A portal vein diameter of more than 1.5 cm and presence of varices near the splenic hilum and sometimes recanalization of the umbilical vein can be found with portal hypertension.

*Hepatitis*

Ultrasonically their detection and differentiation is difficult. In acute hepatitis the liver appears hypoechoic throughout — 'dark liver' whereas in chronic hepatitis, liver pattern is bright. Hepatitis associated with patchy necrosis produces a 'moth-eaten' pattern.

**Diffuse malignancy**

Three types are recognised by ultrasound — 'moth-eaten', 'miliary' and 'dark' or 'hypoechoic' type.

The first type is due to widespread focal diseases where the normal liver tissue is almost replaced by the tumour. Ill-defined confluent regions of altered reflectivity is seen throughout the liver.

The miliary type shows a fine texture throughout the liver. These changes are very subtle and may be difficult to recognise.

Low level echoes or hypoechoic liver is encountered in some forms of malignancy, mainly lymphoma.

**Biliary system**

*Normal sonographic appearance*

The normal gall bladder in the fasting state appears as a pear-shaped organ with smooth walls. Bile within it is echo-free. The cystic duct can sometimes be traced from its neck, but the level where it joins with the common hepatic duct cannot usually be identified.

The common bile duct which is formed by the union of the right and left hepatic duct is seen as a tubular structure anterior to the portal vein with the hepatic artery lateral to it. The normal bile duct at the level of the porta measures less than 6 mm. in diameter. Unless dilated, the duct cannot usually be traced beyond the porta.

*Preparation for biliary scanning*

The patient should be fasting for 8 hours prior to the examination so that the gall bladder is well distended with bile. Visualisation of the extrahepatic biliary tree may become difficult due to intestinal gas and a loaded colon. A mild laxative and an anti-flatulent the night prior to the examination may be necessary.

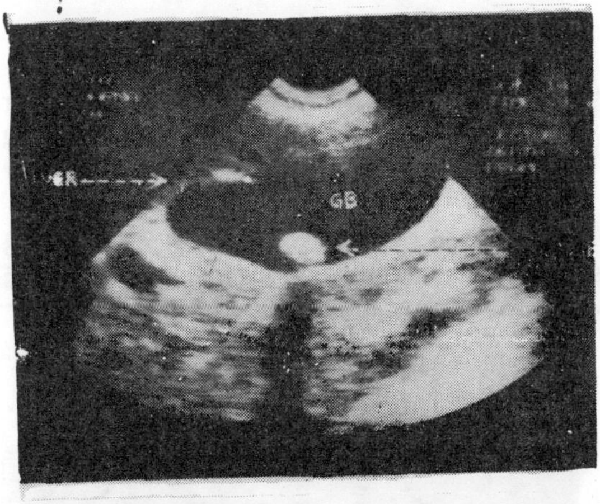


Fig.15.11 : Gall bladder showing a single stone with dense posterior shadowing

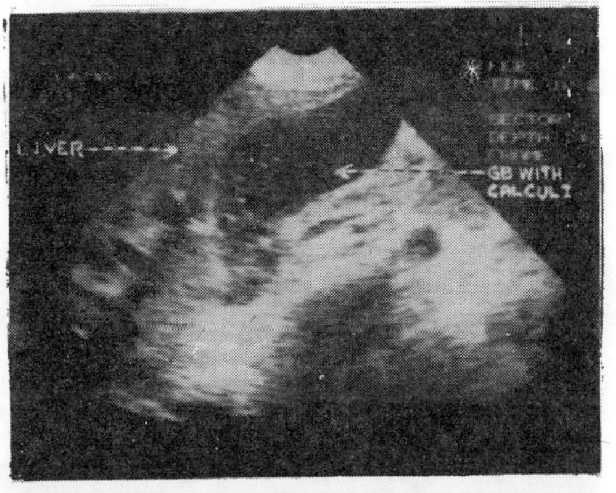


Fig.15.12 : Gall bladder showing multiple small non-shadowing stones

## Gall Bladder Disease

*Gall stones*

These appear as echogenic intraluminal shadows and produce prominent posterior shadowing which shift when the patient's position is changed. Cholesterol polyps and calcifications in the wall can also give this appearance but they do not shift with change of the patient's position.

*Sludge*

Faint diffuse echoes in the dependent portion of the gall bladder with no evidence of posterior shadowing is characteristic of biliary sludge or "echogenic bile"

*Carcinoma*

It appears as a fixed intraluminal mass which may invades and destroys the gall bladder wall. It is

**almost always associated with gall stones. Invasion of the liver by the tumor can be recognised in later stages.**

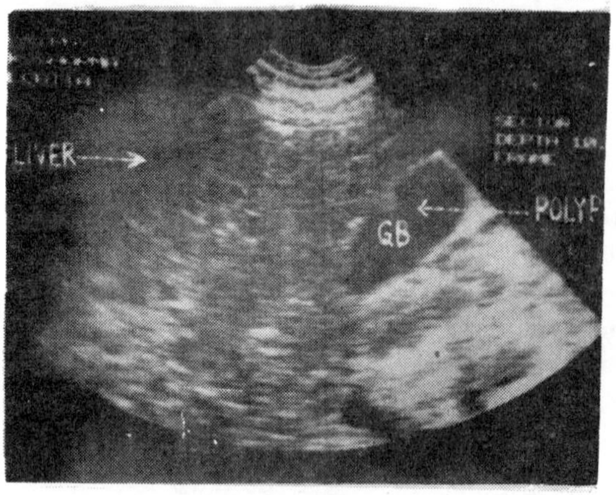


Fig.15.13 : Polyp of Gall bladder. A small hypoechoic mass seen in relation to anterior wall. It is non-shadowing and not mobile

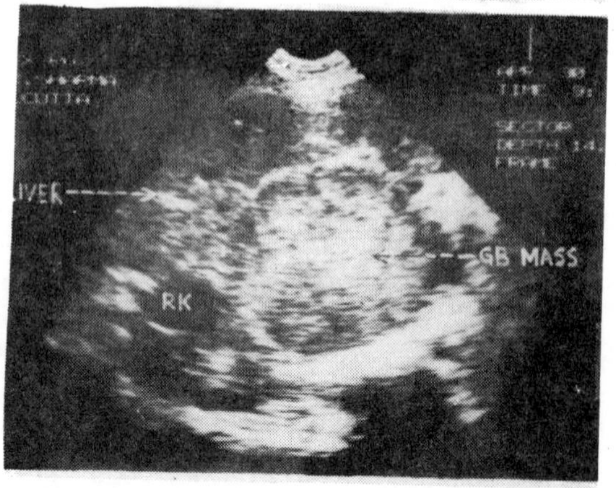


Fig.15.14 : Mass containing mixed echoes arising from Gall Bladder. Liver adjacent to mass shows metastatic deposits. A case of Gall Bladder neoplasm

*Non-visualised gall bladder*

Ultrasound is an excellent modality to further investigate cases of non-visualised gall bladder on cholecystograms. In most cases ultrasound will show a contracted gall bladder containing stones and at times a normal sized gall bladder showing no stones but having thick walls – "acalculous cholecystitis"

In many instances, the gall bladder may not be visualised by ultrasonography. This occurs when the gall bladder is completely packed with stones so that no bile remains in it. These ,stones appear as echogenic foci with posterior shadowing and the walls of the gall bladder are not seen.

**Obstructive Jaundice**

**Differentiating obstructive from non-obstructive jaundice is very reliable by ultrasound.**

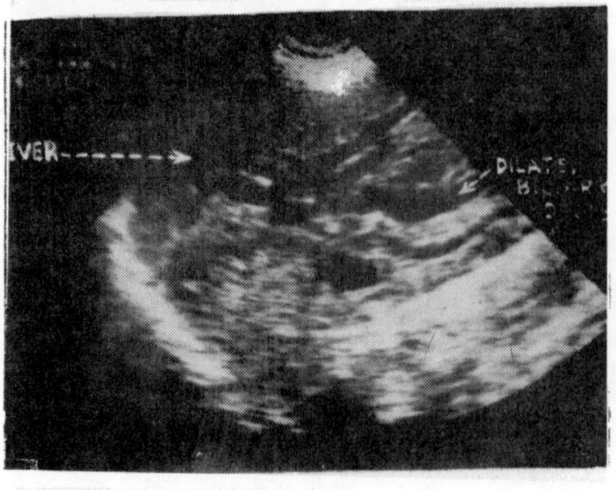

Fig.15.15 : Dilated intrahepatic biliary radicles in obstructive jaundice

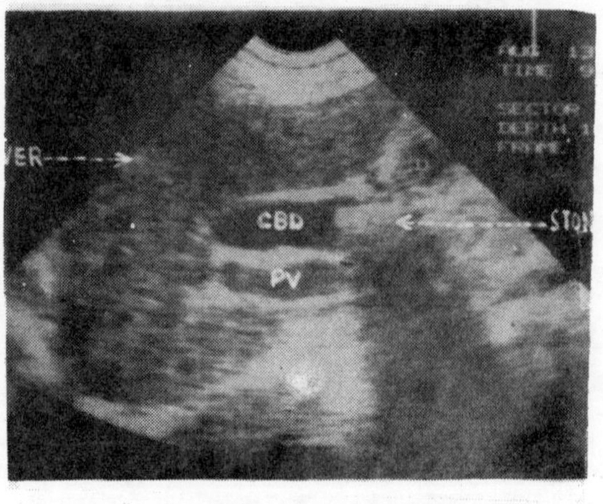


Fig.15.16 : Dilated CBD showing a fairly large calculus in its proximal part with dense posterior shadowing in a case of obstructive jaundice.

Dilated intrahepatic biliary radicles and dilated CBD are very easily identified by ultrasonography. When dilated, the CBD measures 6 mm or more at the porta hepatis. In post cholecystectomised patients, however, the CBD may measure upto 10 mm in diameter without evidence of obstruction. Apart from differentiating obstructive from non-obstructive jaundice, sonography can also reveal the cause and level of obstruction in most instances. When CBD obstruction is proximal, the cause e.g. stones, growth, etc. can be identified in most cases. With distal obstruction, however, the cause is always not apparent due to gas in the duodenum which obscures this portion of the duct. With pancreatic head neoplasms or peri-ampullary pathology, the CBD can usually be seen upto its terminal portion. In the former case, the neoplasms may be evident and a dilated pancreatic duct can also be seen. Masses, e.g. enlarged lymphnodes, gall bladder neoplasms etc., which can give rise to obstructive jaundice due to extrinsic pressure on the CBD at the porta level can also be recognised by ultrasound.

## PANCREAS

Pseudocysts which are fairly common and usually present with abdominal lump can be recognised by ultrasound. Chronic pancreatitis and pancreatic abscesses can also be diagnosed. Pancreatic head tumours which usually cause obstructive jaundice can also be evaluated.

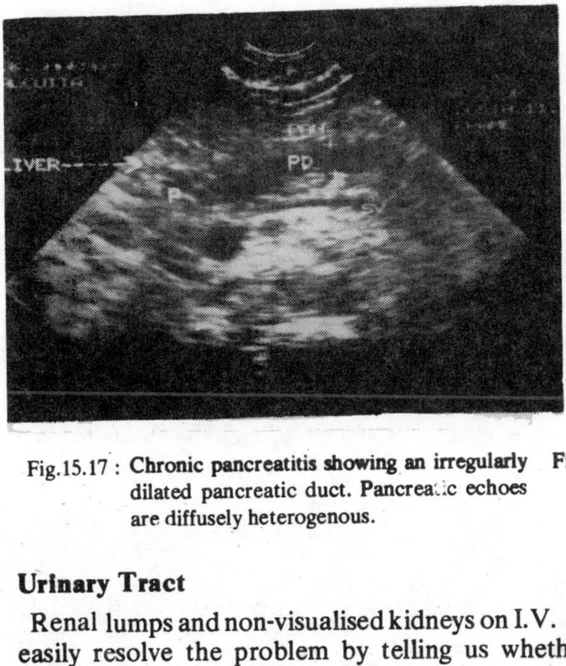


Fig.15.17 : **Chronic pancreatitis showing an irregularly dilated pancreatic duct. Pancreatic echoes are diffusely heterogenous.**

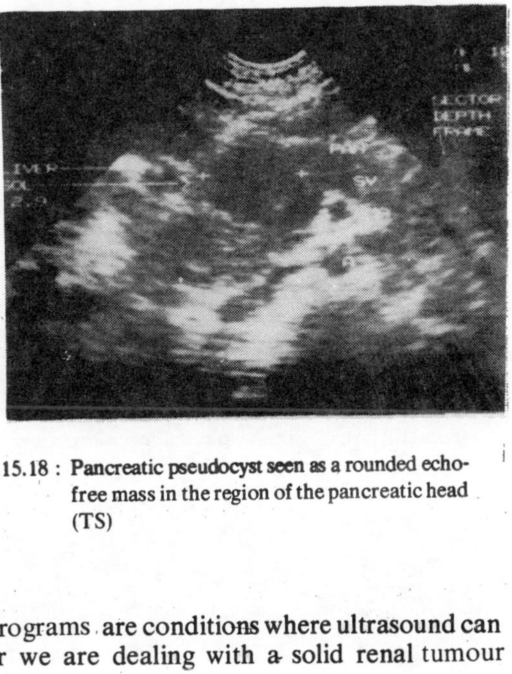

Fig.15.18 : **Pancreatic pseudocyst seen as a rounded echo-free mass in the region of the pancreatic head (TS)**

## Urinary Tract

Renal lumps and non-visualised kidneys on I.V. urograms are conditions where ultrasound can easily resolve the problem by telling us whether we are dealing with a solid renal tumour (malignant), cyst or hydronephrosis.

Renal parenchymal disease can be evaluated though it is not always possible to be specific. Though large renal stones are easily detected, very tiny stones are difficult to diagnose. Pyonephrosis and perinephrosis abscesses can also be assessed.

Ultrasound is very helpful in the follow-up of renal transplants as it can detect both acute and chronic rejections. Urinoma and lymphocele which may form after transplant operations can also be detected.

Various congenital anomalies of the kidney e.g. fusions, malrotations, agenesis, hypoplasia etc. can be detected.

Normal ureters cannot be visualised by ultrasound. However, dilated ureters can be detected.

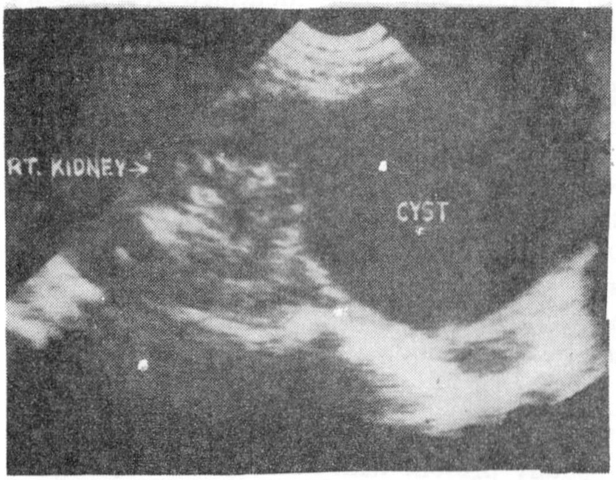


Fig.15.19 : Echofree mass in lower pole of right kidney represents a simple renal cyst

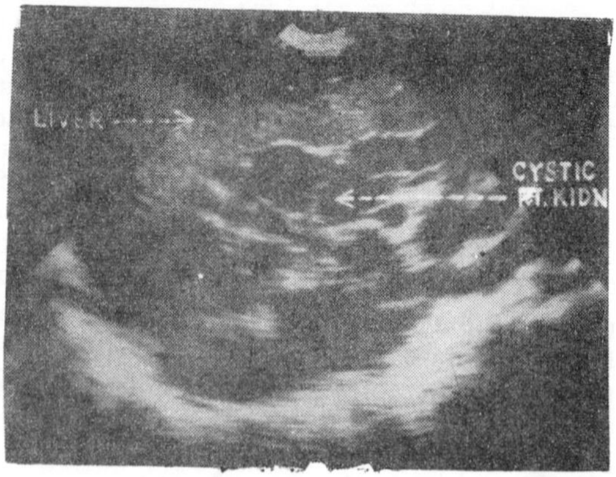


Fig.15.20 : Polycystic kidney; Multiple cystic area seen involving the entire right kidney. Normal liver tissue seen anteriorly

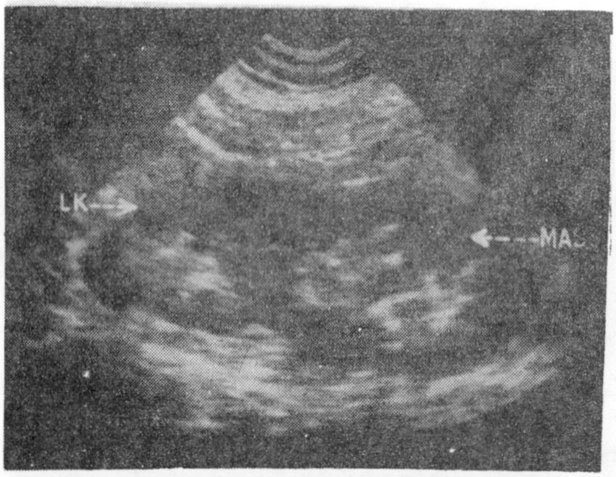


Fig.15.21 : Renal cell carcinoma. A hypoechoic mass in lower pole of left kidney with distortion of central echocomplex

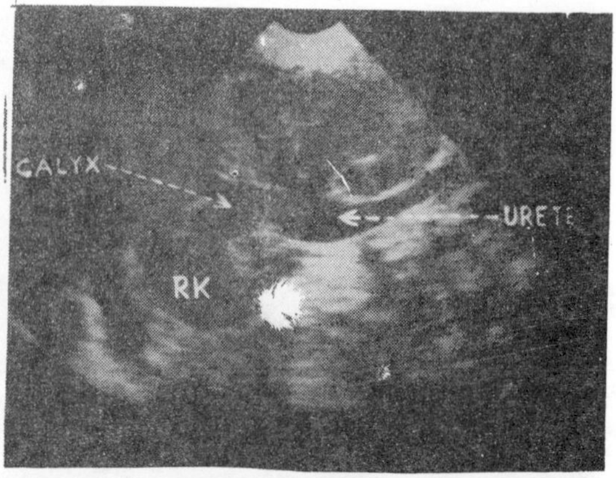


Fig.15.22 : Left kidney showing early hydronephrotic changes. Dilated proximal ureter is also seen.

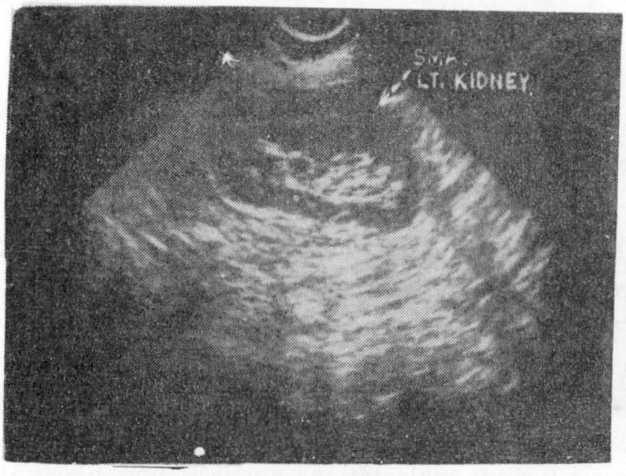


Fig.15.23 : Chronic inflammatory disease of the kidney. Small-sized kidney showing increased echogenicity of cortex

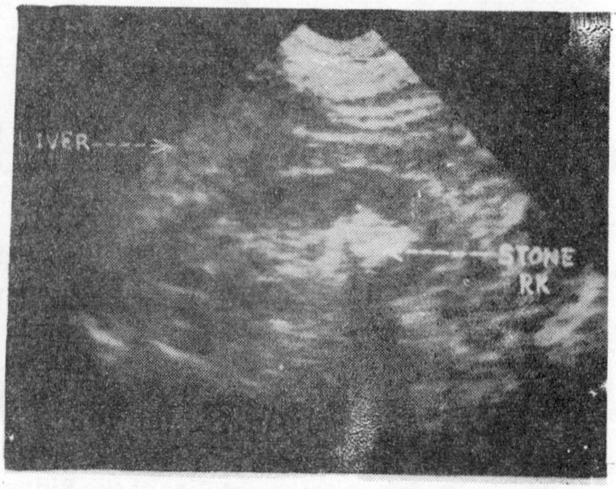


Fig.15.24 : Echogenic focus in lower calyx of right kidney with posterior shadowing from a stone

Urinary bladder when distended with urine is well visualised and stones and tumours can be detected. Ultrasound can also help in the staging of the bladder tumours. Enlarged prostate due to benign hypertrophy or carcinoma can be distinguished.

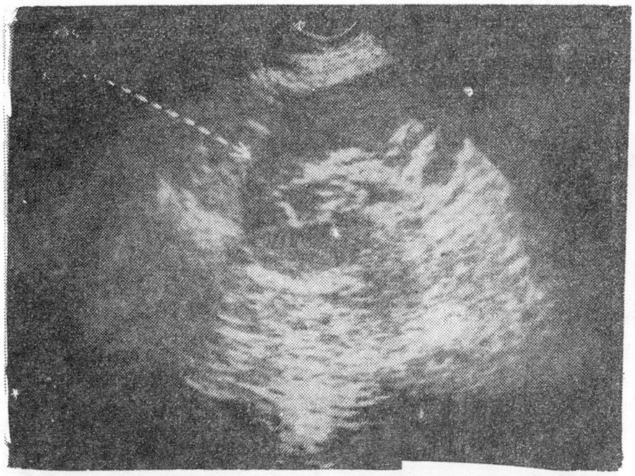

**Fig.15.25 : Transplanted right kidney in iliac fossa showing mild calyectosis**

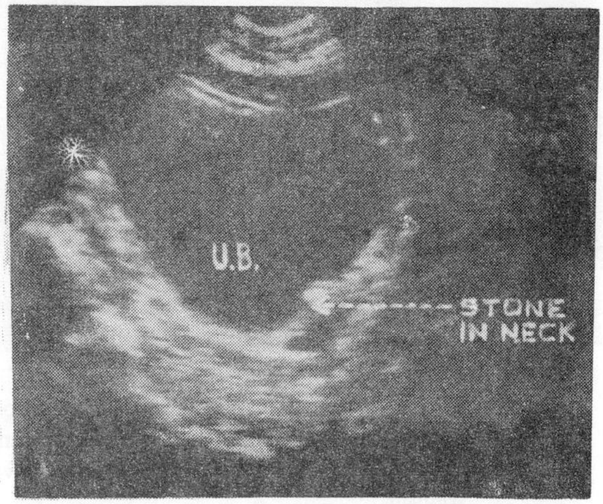


**Fig.15.26 : Distended urinary bladder showing a small calculus near the neck**

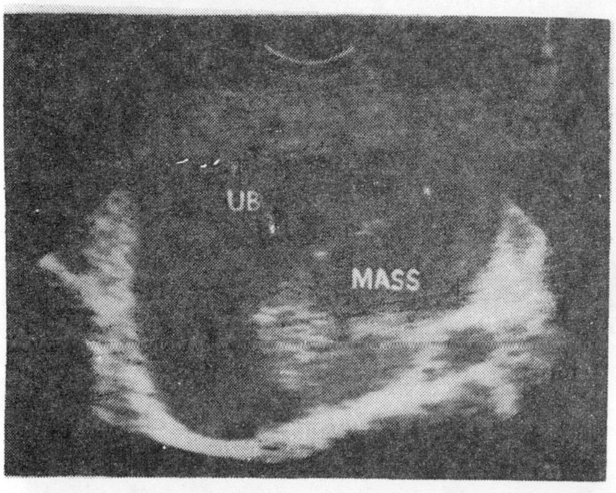


Fig.15.27 : Distended urinary bladder showing a large hypoechoic mass with a broad base which represents a papilloma. L.S.

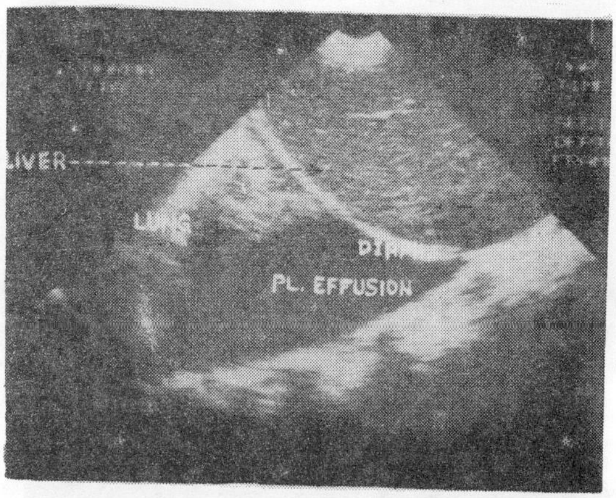


**Fig.15.28 : Right-sided pleural effusion seen as an echo-free area above the right dome of diaphragm.**

### Retroperitoneum

Ultrasound can detect enlarged lymph nodes in the retroperitoneum due to lymphoma, metastasis, tuberculosis etc. Soft tissue tumours e.g. sarcoma and fluid collections e.g. haematoma, abscesses etc. can be detected.

### Aorta

Size and site of aortic anomalies can be evaluated and thrombosis within it can also be identified. Post-operative assessment of aortic graft is possible by ultrasound.

### Spleen

Splenic cyst, abscess and metastasis can also be recognised by ultrasound.

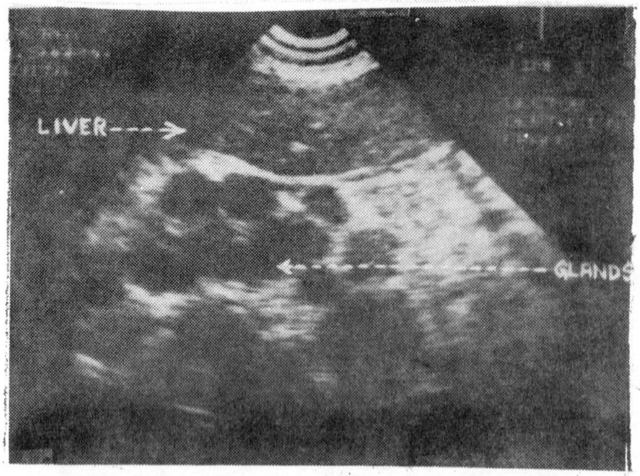


Fig.15.29 : Retroperitoneal lymphadenopathy. Hypoechoic lobulated masses are seen in pre and para-aortic regions and also pre and paracaval regions

## Abdominal Lump

Ultrasound can evaluate the precise nature and relationship of abdominal masses. Intestinal origin of a mass can also at times be predicted by ultrasound.

## Ascites

Very small amount of free peritoneal fluid can be detected by ultrasound.

Similarly small amounts of pericardial or pleural effusions may be detected.

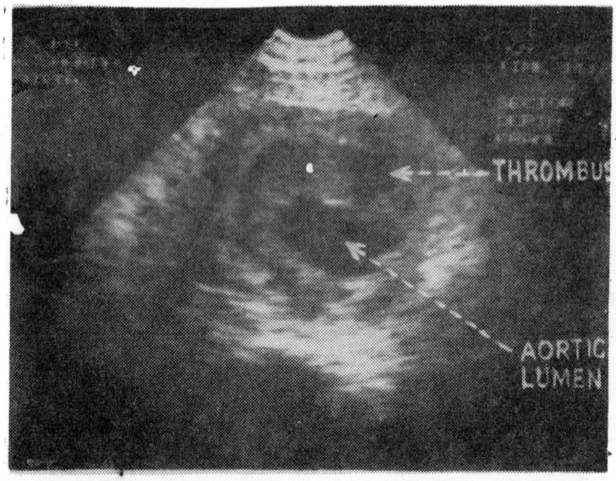


Fig.15.30 : Aortic aneurysm with intramural thrombus. T.S.

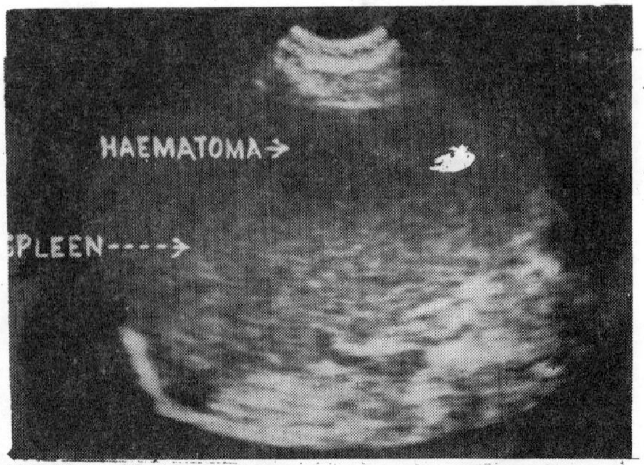


Fig.15.31 : Splenic hematoma seen as an oval hypoechoic area with low level internal echos in anterior aspect of spleen

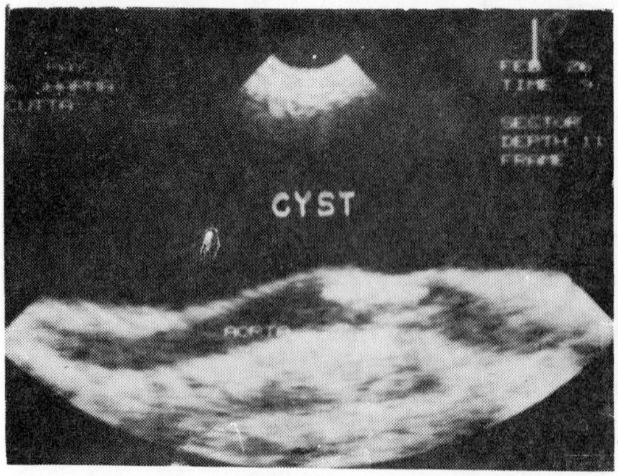


Fig.15.32 : Huge mesenteric cyst appearing as echofree mass in the abdomen

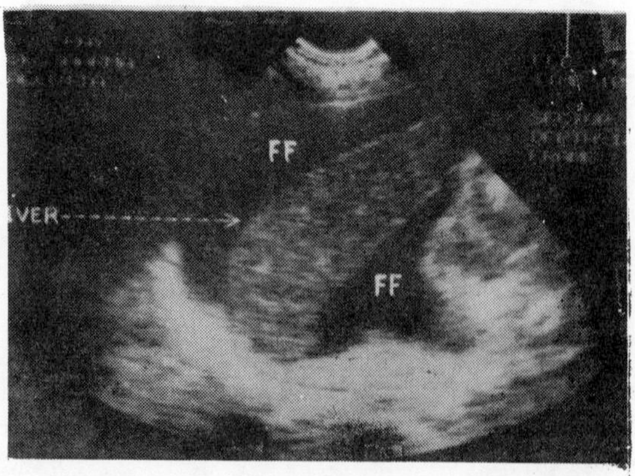


Fig.15.33 : Ascites in cirrhosis. Free peritoneal fluid (FF) is seen occupying the supra and sub-hepatic spaces

# CHAPTER 16
# DISEASES OF LIVER, GALL BLADDER AND PANCREAS

## LIVER FUNCTION TESTS

*G.C. MOOKERJEE*

There are wide varieties of laboratory tests to assess liver function but no single test is universally helpful. The clinician should select those tests that are most appropriate to the particular clinical situation. For instance, in an uncomplicated case of viral hepatitis, only serial urine examination may be quite adequate. Unless there is some special clinical indication expensive tests are not required. Interpretation of the results may also depend upon values of tests done serially, so as to assess the evolution or the course of disease. The important and most useful liver function tests are presented.

(1) *SERUM BILIRUBIN* : The spectrophotometric method is ideal for determining serum bilirubin, which measures the two pigment fractions conjugated and unconjugated bilirubin.

(a) Conjugated bilirubin, i.e. water soluble bilirubin diglucuronide gives a direct reaction with the diazo reagent, (sulphanilic acid), the normal level being less than 0.25 mg/100 ml. It is raised in predominant hepatocellular disease. Since it is normally absent in the urine, bilirubinuria in a jaundiced patient always suggests conjugated hyperbilirubinaemia, most probably due to hepatobiliary disease.

(b) Unconjugated or lipid soluble bilirubin gives an indirect reaction with the diazo reagent, the normal level being 0.3 to 1.0 mg/100 ml.

Unconjugated bilirubin is raised in haemolytic states (due to over-production of bilirubin) and in Gilbert's syndrome (due to inability to transport bilirubin across the liver).

Total serum bilirubin should be less than 1.0 mg in normal individuals.

(2) *URINARY BILIRUBIN* : Bilirubinuria is measured by the foam test, Harrison's spot test or the Ictotest tablet or strip-dip method, and it may be detected even before clinical jaundice sets in. In the presence of jaundice, bilirubinuria suggests conjugated-hyperbilirubinaemia while its absence points to haemolytic diseases or Gilbert's syndrome (which is a congenital unconjugated hyperbilirubinaemia).

(3) *URINARY UROBILINOGEN* : It can be measured only in fresh urine samples by the Watson method (normal 0.2 to 1.2 units) and while its usefulness is limited. Its complete absence for over a week indicates complete biliary obstruction (i.e. no bile is entering the intestines).

(4) *SERUM ENZYME ASSAY* : In the absence of bone disease or pregnancy, a markedly elevated serum alkaline phosphate indicates impaired hepatic excretory function, because increased enzyme synthesis occurs as a sequelae to extra or intra-hepatic cholestasis. It may be measured in Bodansky units (normal 1.5 to 4.5 units) or in King-Armstrong units (normal 4 to 13).

In parenchymal liver disorders, there is only a small rise (6 to 10 Bodansky) while in metastatic liver disease, it may be the only abnormality of routine liver function rests. In obstructive jaundice (due to cholestasis, stone or new growth, blocking common bile duct it may be increased to 3 to 10 times of normal value. It may also be raised in bone disease in certain physiological states like late pregnancy and in growing children.

(5) *NUCLEOTIDASE* : This enzyme level is raised in liver disease, but not in bone disease so that concurrent measurements of both alkaline phosphatase and 5-nucleotidase may help differentiate the two conditions.

*TRANSAMINASES*

The two enzymes known to be of value are :

(1) Serum asparate aminotransferase (AST) previously known as SGOT
(2) Serum alkaline aminotransferase (ALT) previously known as SGPT

AST (SGOT) is found in many tissues, especially in heart, liver and skeletal muscles. ALT (SGPT) is chiefly found in liver but in smaller quantities in kidneys and skeletal muscles. These enzymes are raised due to any parenchymal damage to liver. Therefore, these are elevated quite early and are early indications of liver cell damage. Raised AST (SGOT) usually indicates acute myocardial damage, while raised ALT (SGPT) alone may be useful in detecting hepatic cellular damage. The normal values are within 40 karman units for each. (In I.U, ALT-SGOT is 5 to 15 U and AST-SGPT is 5 to 30U).

In viral hepatitis,there may be a rise of ALT even in the prodromal phase, while during the jaundiced phase, it may be 500 to 1000 karman units which later on falls rapidly as the condition improves. In acute hepatic necrosis ALT (SGPT) may be even 2000 to 3000 karman units. High rise may be seen also in drug induced hepatitis, acute exacerbations of chronic active hepatitis and in hepatic congestion due to heart failure, while in infectious mononucleosis, up to twice the normal-value may be reached. In obstructive jaundice the rise is small. Of the two, ALT (SGPT) is more specific for liver disease and serial measurements may be useful to follow the course of liver disease. 5-Nucleotidase — is an enzyme which specifically indicates liver disease but difficult to measure in routine practice.

*LACTIC DEHYDROGENASE (LDH)*

This is not routinely useful as estimation of total LDH does not give us much clue to the site of tissue damage, as the enzyme is widely distributed in almost all organs. However, by fractionisation method, five tissue specific isoenzymes may be determined to locate the organ damage. High serum level particularly suggests metastatic carcinoma of liver. Moderate rise occurs in acute viral hepatitis.

*GAMMA (γ) GLUTAMYL TRANSPEPTIDASE (GGT)*

The most sensitive indicator of hepatocellular damage is glutamyl transpeptidase (GGT), which may rise even after heavy drinking before other abnormalities are appreciable. So it is a very useful test for alcoholic liver disease and early hepatic injury. (Normal : 7 to 30 I.U.).

*SERUM PROTEINS :* Protein synthesis, especially albumin production falls whenever there is chronic severe liver damage. In acute liver disease, there is not much change in plasma albumin as the half life is about three weeks.

Albumin (normal 3,5 to 5 g/100 ml) may be decreased in subacute and massive hepatic necrosis, chronic active hepatitis, and all other extensive parenchymal liver disease, while globulin (normal 2 to 3.5/100 ml) may be raised in chronic inflammatory disorders.

Neoplastic and inflammatory liver diseases produce high levels of $alpha_2$ globulins, while some patients with bile duct obstruction may have also high globulin levels.

Electrophoresis is the best method to estimate the concentrations of $alpha_1$, $alpha_2$, beta and gamma globulin.

Serum electrophoresis produces typical densitometric scans, which gives characteristic graphic patterns in certain diseases of the liver as well as in other pathological stages e.g. nephrotic syndrome, collagen diseases, myelomatosis etc.

*CLOTTING FACTORS :* Many clotting factors are produced in the liver, and the one stage prothrombin time (reflecting activities of prothrombin) fibrinogen level and factors V, VII and X may indicate health of the liver.

These are not routinely measured but may have to be assessed in patients before any surgical procedure (including biopsy) is undertaken.

*SERUM AMMONIA* : In severe hepatocellular necrosis, the liver is unable to convert ammonia to urea, resulting in markedly raised serum ammonia level. It is elevated in hepatic encephalopathy but the level of ammonia does not always correlate with degrees of encephalopathy. It may be due to the fact that other metabolites also contribute to the pathogenesis. The normal level of serum ammonia is 0.8 to 1 µg/ml of blood. The test should be performed immediately.

*BLOOD LIPIDS* : Total cholesterol (normal 130 to 230 mg/100 ml) and cholesterol esters (normal 50 to 70% total cholesterol) may be decreased in acute or chronic liver diseases while in cholestasis a moderate to extreme rise of total cholesterol occurs but with reduced level of esterified fraction. Serum triglycerides are also raised in hepatic cholestasis a moderate to extreme rise of total cholesterol occurs but with reduced level of esterified fraction. Serum triglycerides are also raised in hepatic cholestasis.

*IMMUNOLOGIC TESTS* : Antimitochondrial antibodies are found in primary biliary cirrhosis (and also in some cases of drug hepatitis) while in chronic active hepatitis there may be antinuclear antibodies and anti-smooth muscle antibodies. In long incubation viral hepatitis (hepatitis B virus), the detection of hepatitis B-surface antigen ($HB_S$ Ag) is confirmatory evidence. Alpha feto-protein is a valuable test in the diagnosis of hepatoma.

*BROMSULPHALEIN EXCRETION TEST (BSP)* : An intravenous injection of 5 mg/Kg body weight is given, followed by sampling of venous blood, from a different site after 45 minutes. Normally less than 5% of the injected dye remains in plasma, because most of the dye is taken up by the hepatocytes and excreted into the bile, and is thus an indication of the secretory capacity of the liver. It is not used widely, because it is of non-specific value and may also be raised in heart failure, shock, ascites or fever. Rarely the dye may cause anaphylactic reactions.

It should be realised that all these tests are not required in all cases of liver disease. Clinician should order a few tests depending on the clinical setting and facilities available.

Most cases of viral hepatitis can be treated on clinical grounds and urine tests, while other tests are required in special situations discussed in relevant chapters of this volume.

Many other special investigations may have to be done to investigate liver disease, especially of chronic varieties as mentioned below :

*RADIOLOGIC PROCEDURES* : Plain X-ray of the abdomen : Only gross hepatomegaly or hepatic masses that distort the diaphragm may be detected. Enlarged spleen which is not palpable may be detected also. Calcified stones of gall bladder, biliary tree, pancreas, echinococcal cysts and haemangiomas may be detected.

Metastatic tumour mass may be found in lungs in a skiagram of the chest.

*BA MEAL X-RAY OF G.I. TRACT* : In portal hypertension, oesophageal varices may be visualised in barium swallow, while an enlarged left lobe of liver may displace the stomach laterally and anteriorly. Enlarged head of pancreas may produce irregularities of 2nd part of duodenum.

*CHOLECYSTOGRAPHY & CHOLANGIOGRAPHY* : Oral or I.V. cholecystography are done to detect gall bladder disease but cannot be performed in presence of jaundice.

An experienced radiologist using a fine needle, may be able to cannulate and visualize a major dilated duct to detect an obstructive lesion in 90% cases, although the normal or small ducts associated with intrahepatic cholestasis are more difficult to cannulate.

*Endoscopic retrograde cholangiopancreatography (ERCP)*

Using the fiberoptic duodenoscope, the ampulla of Vater can be cannulated under direct vision and contrast material injected into the biliary and pancreatic ducts thus enabling the bile ducts to be visualised radiographically in jaundiced patients. It is specially useful in suspected carcinoma of head of pancreas or ampulla of Vater, because in addition to contrast studies biopsies brushings for cytological study can be obtained. There is no risk of bile peritonitis but acute pancreatitis may be a complication in rare instances.

*ANGIOGRAPHY* : Selective angiography of superior mesenteric and hepatic arteries has replaced splenoportography because it enables clinicians to visualize both arterial (hepatic) and venous (hepatic & portal) systems. It is helpful in diagnosis of cirrhosis of liver, primary and secondary S.O.L. as well as to visualize collateral circulation in portal hypertension.

*RADIOISOTOPIC SCANS OF LIVER (SCINTISCAN)*

Three types of scans are used :

(1) The colloidal scan which depends on uptake of labelled colloid by Kupffer cells.

(2) The Rose-Bengal scan in which this dye is taken up and excreted by hepatocytes.

(3) The gallium (Ga) scan in which radionuclide 67-Ga is concentrated in neoplastic and inflammatory tissues more than in normal hepatocytes. Hepatomas will therefore produce an area of reduced uptake or bare areas by the colloid scan or Rose-Bengal scan, but an area of increased uptake 'hot spot' will appear while using the 67-Ga scan. The colloid scan 3 cm in diameter, the Rose-Bengal scan is used to differentiate intra from extra hepatic cholestasis, while the 67 Ga scan is used for diagnosis neoplastic infiltration in a cirrhotic patient.

*ULTRA – SONOGRAPHY*

Ultrasound is useful in detecting mass lesions (tumours, cysts or liver abscess) as well as gall-stones. It is more useful and safe as it is independent of liver function.

Small lesions up to 1 to 2 cm. can be accurately visualized and upper abdominal ultrasound scan can help in deciding possible causes of extrahepatic biliary obstruction. It is preferable to C.T. scanning because is it less expensive but quite useful.

*COMPUTERIZED TOMOGRAPHY (CT SCAN)*

It is a non-invasive but accurate and reliable method for diagnosing mass lesions in liver or pancreas. It is specially useful in differentiating between intra-hepatic fluid collections (e.g. S.O.L. cysts, abscess, haematomas) as well as in dilatation of gall bladder, extra-hepatic ducts or portal vein.

*Other Diagnostic Procedures* : Percutaneous needle biopsy is safe, simple and very valuable diagnostic tool in diffuse parenchymal disorders, as also in disseminated focal diseases (granulomas) Major indications of liver biopsy include :

(1) Unexplained hepatosplenomegaly

(2) Cholestasis of uncertain cause

(3) Persistently abnormal liver function tests

(4) Suspected systemic or infiltrative disease (Sarcoidosis or miliary tuberculosis)

(5) Suspected primary or metastatic tumour

*It is contraindicated in :*

(1) Impaired haemostasis

(2) Infection of right pleural space or septic cholangitis

(3) Severe anaemia or ascites

(4) Non-co-operative patient and

(5) Non-availability of compatible blood

*Peritoneoscopy or Laparoscopy*

The abdominal serosal lining, liver, gall bladder, spleen and other abdominal organ scan all be visualized with this technique with minimum discomfort and hazard. In suspected intra abdominal malignancy it may obviate the need for exploratory laparotomy. Diagnosis is made by inspection or directed needle biopsy.

# VIRAL HEPATITIS

*M.L. SAPRA*

## INTRODUCTION

Viral hepatitis may be defined as a systemic viral infection in which hepatic cell necrosis and hepatic inflammation are responsible for characteristic clinical, biochemical, immunoserological and morphological features. It is caused by at least three (may be more) viral agents each of which has distinct immunoserologic characters and epidemiologic features. These viral agents are known as Virus A.B and non-A, non-B.

In addition to these three viruses primarily causing hepatitis, several other viruses may cause hepatitis e.g. cytomegalovirus, Epstein-Barr virus, herpes simplex, Lassa fever virus and Marburg virus. Yellow fever virus causes epidemic in South America and Africa.

### History

Episodes of jaundice have been described as early as the fifth century B.C. in Babylonia. The term 'epidemic jaundice' appeared in the writings of Hippocrates in Greece. Since then many outbreaks of jaundice have been described particularly amongst military population. Initially jaundice was thought to be due to obstruction of bile passages. Role of hepatic necrosis and inflammation as cause of jaundice was recognised only after development of percutaneous needle biopsy of the liver in 1930 in Denmark. Infectious aetiology was suggested by Pickles in 1930s. In 1947 Maccallum suggested that virus of infectious hepatitis should be called virus A. Hepatitis A virus was discovered in 1973 by Feinstone and colleagues by immune electron microscope. The existence of a form of viral hepatitis that was transmitted by direct inoculation of human blood or its derivatives was recognised in 1883 — mostly spread by small-pox vaccination. Other epidemics have been described after percutaneous form of therapy for syphilis. Artificially transmitted malaria for the treatment of neurosyphilis, was also accompanied by jaundice in some cases. Convalescent serum for prevention of infectious diseases caused epidemics of jaundice in 1930s to early 1940s. During World War II, pooled plasma used for treatment of battle casualties caused post-transfusion jaundice.

In 1947 MacCallum suggested the name Hepatitis B virus as cause of serum hepatitis.

Discovery of Australia antigen in 1963 by Blumberg and colleagues started a new era in the history of viral hepatitis. The antigen now designated as HBSAg was shown subsequently to be the surface material of the hepatitis B virus.

### Hepatic Pathology

The essential lesion is an acute inflammation of the entire liver. Along with liver cell necrosis there is leucocytic and histiocytic infiltration. The necrosis is most marked in centre of lobules and the cellular infiltration is greatest in portal tracts. The sinusoids show hyperplasia of Kupffer cells. Fatty change is absent. Acidophil bodies as well as ballooning of cells may be seen. There may be centrizonal cholestasis. In some cases focal spotty necrosis is seen. Bile duct proliferation is common. Reticulin network is usually well preserved and helps in regeneration of liver in proper form. Occasionally the necrosis may be confluent,so-called submassive necrosis. In massive fulminant necrosis the whole lobule is involved.

The basic pathology of virus A.B and non-A non-B hepatitis is almost identical. Histological changes are found even before the development of jaundice. A new virus known as Delta virus is discovered which is associated with superinfection with Hepatitis-B Virus.

**Clinical features :**

Viral hepatitis when symptomatic may be anicteric or icteric. The symptoms of anicteric hepatitis are essentially the same as those of icteric disease but there is no apparent jaundice. The clinical course of the disease is almost similar to icteric type but the duration of illness is less. Most patients with icteric hepatitis are symptomatic although occasional jaundiced patient may be asymptomatic.

Febrile symptoms predominate in early phase of acute illness. Fever or feverish feeling and anorexia are the most predominant symptoms. The fever is usually between 99°F and 101°F but occasionally reaches 102°F to 104°F. Anorexia is severe, merely smell of food often induces nausea. Aversion to smoking in smokers, is one of the earliest symptoms. Nasal discharge and sore throat also occur during prodromata in 10-20% of cases.

In viral hepatitis,vomiting is generally not severe but nausea is annoying. When vomiting becomes more severe it may indicate severe liver damage. Abdominal discomfort or pain particularly in right hypochondrium is common due to stretching of liver capsule as it enlarges, 94% of patients note change in colour of urine to dark brownish. This occurs before jaundice becomes obvious. Onset of jaundice is usually associated with disappearance of distressing symptoms. Itching is not always present but may occur in severe cases due to too much bile salt in circulation.

Stool colour is pale or muddy in early stage due to inflammatory obstruction in bile passages. Other less well-known symptoms are skin rashes, lymphadenopathy, arthralgia, myalgia, irritability and insomnia, Frank arthritis is sometimes observed in cases of virus B hepatitis. In almost all patients there is tenderness over the liver varying from mild tenderness to very severe degree.

Hepatomegaly is common, but rarely massive. Massive necrosis leads to a small and soft liver. The spleen is palpable in 5-15% of the patients and posterior cervical lymph nodes may be enlarged. Spider angiomata, palmar erythema and transient gynaecomastia, have been described without underlying chronic liver disease.

Atypical cases present with cholestasis, features being predominant and resemble mechanical obstruction to bile ducts.

**Laboratory tests**

Total white cell count within normal limits is the usual finding in viral hepatitis although leucopenia has been described in a few cases. Rarely agranulocytosis, thrombocytopenia or pancytopenia develop during viral hepatitis. Examination of urine occasionally shows proteinuria but bilirubinuria is usually present during preicteric stage. The serum bilirubin determination is one of the most frequently utilized laboratory tests. With onset of the icteric phase, the serum concentration usually rises for 10-14 days in the average adult direct reacting fraction being predominant.

In most patients maximum concentration is less than 10 mg/100 ml although up to 20 mg/100 ml. may be observed in a few patients. The rate of decline from the peak levels is more gradual.

Assays of aminotransferase activities are most popular, laboratory test to detect parenchymal injury. They are sufficiently sensitive and specific tests. Aminotransferases may start rising 7-10 days before the onset of symptoms of hepatitis. The peak level is usually reached in the first week after symptoms begin. The levels vary between 500 to 5000 iu/ml. The level of alanine aminotransferase (SGPT or ALT) is usually higher than that of aspartate aminotransferase (SGOT or AST). Once acute illness subsides, fall to normal levels is quite rapid.

In a typical case of viral hepatitis, serum alkaline phosphatase activity may be normal. Marked elevations occurs in association with intrahepatic cholestasis.

The prothrombin time is usually within five seconds of the control values in a typical case of viral hepatitis.

**Diagnosis**

Presence of viral hepatitis may be suspected on epidemiological grounds if the patient's illness resembles and is related to viral hepatitis in his or her associates. In the sporadic case, epidemiological features are less helpful. The diagnosis of typical viral hepatitis is usually established by recognition of characteristic clinical features, laboratory tests and course of illness during the period of observation. In patients with *atypical forms* of viral hepatitis diagnosis is more difficult and may require liver biopsy and histological examination. *Drug induced hepatitis* may closely resemble viral hepatitis. A complete drug history is essential. *Alcoholic hepatitis* has also to be considered in differential diagnosis. History of prolonged and excessive alcoholism, moderate elevation of aminotransferases, and mild jaundice with hepatomegaly favours alcohol induced disease. Gamma-glutaryl-transferase (G.G.T.) is also high in alcoholic liver damage. Estimation of G.G.T. is specially useful in alcoholic hepatitis. Jaundice in alcoholic liver is a serious sign. Sometimes *cholestatic form* of viral hepatitis is confused with extra hepatic biliary tract obstruction.

## VIRUS A HEPATITIS

This disease is caused by a small RNA enterovirus of picorna group. The virus can be identified in the stools of the patients from about two weeks before until one week after the onset of jaundice. It can also be identified in human liver biopsies during acute stage by immuno-fluorescence. Chronic carriers are not known. The virus can be transmitted to marmosets and chimpanzees. These two animals form the animal model for study of virus A hepatitis. The virus can also be grown in tissue cultures. A serum antibody (Anti-HAV) appears as the stool becomes negative for virus. These anti-HAV are of two types :

1) IgM anti-HAV implies a recent infection. This antibody appears within a few days and persists only for two to six months. This is more helpful in diagnosis.
2) IgG anti-HAV remains elevated for years after acute infection and is the antibody responsible for life long immunity to further infections with hepatitis A.

**Epidemiology**

Incubation period is 15-50 days. Age group 5-14 years is the group most affected. With improving hygiene the prevalence is decreasing world-wide.

Disease occurs in two forms : sporadic and epidemic. Mode of spread is chiefly by faecal-oral route. There is no spread by semen, urine or nasopharyngeal secretions. Homosexuals also acquire this infection by way of oral sex. Most sporadic cases follow close person to person contact. Explosive water-borne and food-borne epidemics have been described. Intensity of faecal exposure as well as number of susceptible as in a given population determines the attack rate of hepatitis A. In underdeveloped countries where poor hygiene and sanitation exists, there is evidence of continuing hyperendemicity and extremely high inapparent infection rates in early childhood resulting in long-term immunity. Attack rate in adult population is very low. Similar pattern exists, in closed institutions for mentally retarded in developed countries. Because neither persistent viraemia nor persistent faecal excretion of HAV has been established, it is believed that HAV is maintained in the populations by serial transmission from acutely infected patients to susceptibles. No reservior of infection has been demonstrated in human beings.

Use of human-sewage for soil fertilization can result in frozen-fruit-related epidemics. Ingestion or raw prawn and oysters from polluted water is known to have caused some epidemics.

Contamination during preparation has resulted in transmission with other foods. Water borne epidemics are due to contamination of usual water supply or due to ingestion of contaminated water not meant for consumption. Contact with non-human primates like newly imported chimpanzees, monkeys, gorillas etc. is another method for spread of virus A hepatitis.

Veterinarians, zoo workers, research scientists and other handlers exposed to these animals are at risk. Transmission of hepatitis A from man to primate and then back to man by faecal-oral route seems likely. Role of flies and cockroaches in spread of virus A hepatitis has not been proved convincingly.

## VIRUS B HEPATITIS

This disease is caused by hepatitis B virus which is a DNA virus. This type of hepatitis was firmly recognized in 1965 with the discovery of Australia antigen by Blumberg and colleagues in Philadelphia. Australia antigen is now known to be surface of the hepatitis B virus and is termed as hepatitis B surface antigen (HBSAg). The disease can be transmitted to chimpanzees. Virus has not been grown in tissue cultures.

### Serological markers of HAV hepatitis

1) *Hepatitis B surface antigen (HBSAg) :*

The antigen appears in blood after about six weeks of infection and usually disappears in three months. Persistence for more than six months is indicative of a carrier state. Of the various methods for its detection, radioimmunoassay (RIA) and enzyme linked in immunosorbent assay (ELISA) are the best so far as sensitivity and specificity is concerned. HBSAg may be detected in hepatocytes of carriers and chronic hepatitis cases.

2) *Antibody to hepatitis B surface antigen (anti HBS)*

The antibody appears late, some three months after the onset of illness and persists. The levels are rarely high. 10-15% of patients with acute type B hepatitis never develop antibody. Anti-HBS appears to confer immunity.

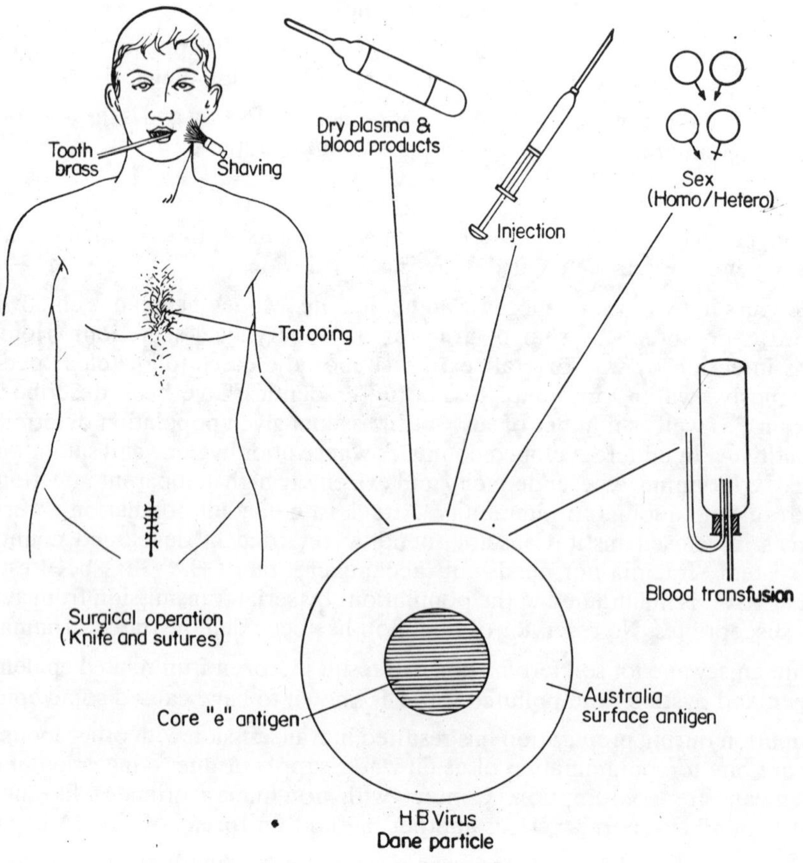


Fig.16.1 : Mode of spread of hepatitis—B-virus

3) *Antigen associated with hepatitis B (HBsAg)*

The antigen appears about one week of illness and usually disappears in two weeks. Persistence of HBsAG implies carrier state and prolongation of disease.

4) *Hepatitis B core antigen (HBcAg) and its antibody (anti-HBc) :*

HBCAg is rarely detected in serum. It is mostly detected in liver biopsy specimen by immunoflourescence whereas anti-HBC is present in serum. It may be useful in diagnosing acute hepatitis B where tested for HBSAg are negative.

These markers are of some importance in diagnosing chronicity and identifying infectivity. HBeAg, DNA polymerase IgG anti HBc imply ongoing infectivity.

**Epidemiology**

Type B hepatitis is spread largely by whole blood and its products (Fig.16.1).

*Classification of human blood and blood products according to risk of transmitting viral hepatitis is as follows :*

*'Average-risk' materials*

Whole blood
Packed, washed or frozen RBCS
Fresh frozen plasma
Single donor platelet concentrates
Single donor granulocyte concentrates

*'Safe' materials*

Albumin
Plasma protein fraction
Immune serum globulin
Hyperimmune globulin

Semen and saliva are also possibly infectious. Other body fluids may contain HBsAg but not virus particles and hence are non-infectious. The disease is also transmitted by intimate, often sexual contact.

*Groups in which acute and chronic type B Hepatitis should be suspected are :*

- Immigrants from the Mediterranean countries, Africa or the Far East.
- Drug abusers
- Homosexuals
- Neonates of HBsAg, HBeAg-positive mothers
- Hospital staff particularly of renal oncology units.
- Patients with renal failure, reticuloses, cancer, organ transplants
- Staff and patients of hospitals for mentally retarded
- Post transfusion (paid donors)
- Surgeons and dentists.

Vertical transmission that is infection passing from a mother to foetus or neonate is particularly important.

Other opportunities for parenteral infection include the use of unsterile instruments for dental treatment, ear piercing and manicures, prophylactic inoculations, subcutaneous injections, acupuncture and tattooing.

Blood sucking arthropods e.g. bed bugs and mosquito, may be important vectors, in tropics.

**Non-A Non-B Hepatitis**

The common types of virus hepatitis can now be identified. Virus A hepatitis is diagnosed by the serum IgM antibody which is detected in the acute attack and for a next few weeks afterwards. Hepatitis due to virus B is diagnosed by the hepatitis B surface antigen (HBs Ag) – Hepatitis due to Epstein barr virus and cytomegalovirus infection is excluded by relevant physical finding and laboratory investigations.

There remains a large number of patients with virus hepatitis where the cause is unknown. These cases have been designated as due to non-A non-B virus. The agent/agents concerned have not been identified. Following observations favour the existence of more than one NANB hepatitis viruses :-

(i) Multiple episodes of virus hepatitis in same individual that could not be attributed either to HAV HBV or other viruses.

(ii) Different incubation periods – Long Incubation and Short Incubation

(iii) Different modes of spread-parenteral as well as faecal, as in Indian epidemics.

(iv) Sequelae of chronic hepatitis very common in parenteral transmission whereas no chronic hepatitis in water borne epidemics of India.

(v) Electron microscopic study of liver biopsy specimen revealing two different type of changes in different NANB hepatitis.

NANB hepatitis agents have been successfully transmitted to chimpânzees and also from one chimpanzee to other chimpanzees.

No serological markers have been identified so far.

**Epidemiology**

NANB hepatitis is particularly associated with transfusion of blood and blood products. It may account for 80-90% of post-transfusion hepatitis where routine screening of donors has virtually eliminated hepatitis B. This type of spread is more akin to HBV hepatitis. In addition to this type or spread NANB hepatitis may be responsible for up to 25% of sporadic cases of viral hepatitis.

Particularly affecting population of lower socio-economic status thereby raising the possibility of close person to person contact. In India most of the epidemics of NANB hepatitis have been water borne resembling spread skin to HAV hepatitis. Vertical transmission from mother to foetus has been studies in detail.

**Type A, Type B and Non-A, Non-B Hepatitis Contrasted**

| | A | B | NANB |
|---|---|---|---|
| Virus | RNA | DNA | DNA |
| Experimental animal | Marmoset | Chimpanzees | Chimpanzees |
| Tissue culture | Yes | No | No |
| Incubation period (days) | 15-20 | 50-60 | 7-50 |
| Spread | | | |
| Blood | No | Yes | Yes |
| Faeces | Yes | No | No |
| Saliva | Yes | Yes | No |
| Vertical | No | Yes | Yes |
| Intrafamily | Yes | Yes | Yes |
| Acute attack | Mild | Severe | Mild |
| Onset | Acute | Insidious | Insidious |

| | | | |
|---|---|---|---|
| Serum sickness | No | Yes | No |
| Mortality | 0.5% | 1-5% | 1-3% |
| Chronicity | No | Yes (10%) | Yes |
| Liver cancer | No | Yes | ? |

**Treatment of acute attack :**

Treatment has little effect in changing the course of the disease. Limited bed rest in acute stage is important. They can be allowed up when they feel better irrespective of depth of jaundice. They should rest after meals. Convalescence is allowed when the patient is asymptomatic, liver is no longer tender and serum bilirubin is less than 1.4 mg/ml. The period of convalescence should be twice the period spent in bed. No benefit occurs from the low fat diet except that it is not palatable, hence patient may not able to eat well. Usual diet in hepatitis is composed of the food most appetizing to the patient. Supplements of vitamins, aminoacids, etc. are not essential. Corticosteroids do not accelerate the rate of healing, do not alter the degree of liver necrosis and also do not assist in immunity. In virus hepatitis use of corticosteroids as a routine is not justified. On the other hand, use in acute hepatitis may favour relapses and chronicity.

**Follow-up**

The patient should be seen four weeks after discharge and if necessary at monthly intervals for the next three months. Special attention should be paid towards recurrence of jaundice and size of liver and spleen. Serum bilirubin, albumin and transaminase levels should be checked. If initially positive for HBsAg, serum should be checked for this. Exercise should be undertaken within limits of fatigue. Alcohol should be denied for 6-12 months. Diet should be unrestricted.

**Chronic sequelae**

Hepatitis A infection never becomes chronic so is the waterborne type of NANB hepatitis.

**Benign sequelae**

1) *Prolonged viral hepatitis (1-4%) also known as chronic lobular hepatitis.* Four months is the time-limit beyond which adults would be considered to have a prolonged course.

   Symptoms, physical findings and laboratory abnormalities continue to persist. Cirrhosis does not develop in affected patients.

2) *Relapsing hepatitis (15 to 18%)* — This refers to an illness in which the patient who has apparently had complete recovery following an acute episode of viral hepatitis manifests a recurrence of the original symptoms and findings on one or more occasions usually within six months of the original illness. Recurrences are milder. Most common causes thought of are early and excessive physical activity, consumption of alcohol and use of corticosteroids during acute episode of hepatitis. This type of hepatitis may be difficult to differentiate from a second attack due to another hepatitis virus.

3) *Chronic persistent hepatitis* manifests by persistence of laboratory abnormalities for long period of time without progression to more severe hepatic dysfunction in an asymptomatic on mildly symptomatic individual with historical evidence of preceding bout of hepatitis. This diagnosis is confirmed by follow up examinations that show no evidence of disease progression and liver biopsy revealing typical histological changes. It does not progress to cirrhosis.

**Serious sequelae** : These are —

1) Chronic active hepatitis
2) Cirrhosis
3) Primary hepato-cellular carcinoma
4) Aplastic anaemia
5) Glomerulonephritis
6) Necrotizing vasculitis

**Carrier state following viral hepatitis**

There is no evidence that hepatitis A leads to development of a prolonged carrier state. Neither viraemic nor faecal carriers of HAV have been recognized.

In HBV hepatitis in approximately 5-10% of patients, serum will remain HBsAg, positive for more than three months indicating the development of a carrier state. There are no clinical or laboratory features of acute infection in such cases. The carrier state may not be life-long because carraige rate of HBsAg appears to decline with increasing age. Prevalence ot carrier state varies from 0.1 to 0.5% of the general population in USA while it approacnes 20% in the Far East.

A viraemic carrier state in NANB viral hepatitis has been established by transmission experiments or man and chimpanzees. Exact prevalence rates are not known but may be as high as for HBV.

**Immunoprophylaxis of viral hepatitis**

Viral hepatitis is endemic in tropical countries. Prophylactic immunization therefore has gained a lot of importance, these days with recent advances in knowledge.

Immunoglobin preparations available for prophylaxis are of two types :

(a) Immune serum globin (ISG)

(b) Hepatitis B immune globin (HBIG).

Prophylaxis for viral hepatitis type A : For intimate household and institutional contacts, a dosage of 0.02 ml/Kg is recommended. It may either abort infection or modify it to make it mild anicteric disease.

A dosage of 0.05 ml/Kg is recommended for travellers from developed countries visiting endemic areas for more than 4 months. This dose may have to be repeated every 4-6 months. No suitable vaccine has been made so far.

**Prophylaxis for type-B Hepatitis :** So far HBIG (Hepatitis B Immuno globin) was being used for post exposure cases in two doses of 0.05 to 0.07 ml/Kg within 7 days and 30 days of exposure and ISG (Immune serum globin) in a dosage of 0.05 ml to 0.07 ml at every 4 months interval for preexposure prophylaxis.

However, with the emergence of a safe vaccine for active immunization againt HBV now, the above indications are being re-evaluated.

No suitable preparation has developed so far for immunoprophylaxis against Non-A Non-B type of hepatitis.

**Prevention**

Notification of disease is important because it leads to early detection and hence identification of method of spread.

Virus — A : Prevention lies in perfect sanitation. The virus is excreted in faeces, hence proper disposal of faeces for as long as two weeks before the occurrence of jaundice, isolation and quarantine of patients and contacts can not be expected to significantly influence the spread of hepatitis. Ordinary methods of sterilization of water including chlorination are in effective. Boiling for 10 minutes is a safe guard. Linen and other clothing soiled by patients should be autoclaved or boiled. Contamination of food, water and milk directly or indirectly by contacts or patients or by sewage should be prevented. Boiled water should be used during epidemics.

Virus — B : This is controlled by avoiding the use of blood products unless really indicated. All prospective blood donors should be screened for HBsAG by radio-immunoassay. Blood donor should be rejected if they have been in contact with hepatitis cases or have suffered from hepatitis during previous six months or if their blood is suspected to have been responsible for a case of post transfusion hepatitis. Exclusion of commercial donors and HBsAg positive donors reduces considerably the frequency of post-transfusion hepatitis.

As far as possible, sterile disposable equipment should be used for medical, dental and public health procedures.

## FULMINANT HEPATIC FAILURE

*(Acute massive hepatic necrosis)*

*G.C. MOOKERJEE*
*M.L. SAPRA*

**Definition :**

It is a clinical syndrome which results from sudden or severe deterioration of hepatocellular function. It is characterised by mental changes, confusion, stupor and coma as a result of hepatic encephalopathy. The condition should not be confused with liver failure due to pre-existing chronic liver diseases. Usually it occurs within eight weeks of onset of acute liver disease.

**Aetiology :**

The commonest cause is viral hepatitis. The infection may be due to hepatitis virus A, virus B, or non-A non-B viruses. The relative incidence of these viruses as the responsible factors has yet to be established but it appears that virus B and non-A non-B infections are more often complicated by fulminant hepatic failure than virus A infections.

Next to viral hepatitis, other important aetiological factor is drug toxicity. There are a large number of hepatotoxic drugs which may cause toxic liver damage but those commonly blamed for fulminant hepatic failure are paracetamol over-dosage, halothane when given repeatedly, antitubercular drugs particularly INH, tetracyclines given intravenously, mono-amino-oxidase inhibitors (phenelzine, iproniazid) and aldomet.

Fatty liver of pregnancy is another condition which is associated with fulminant hepatic failure. Acute alcoholic hepatitis may also lead to fulminant hepatic failure. Surgical shock and gram-negative septicaemia are other uncommon aetiological causes. Carbon tetrachloride poisoning which was frequently mentioned as cause of acute liver cell failure is hardly ever used these days. It may be emphasised that viral hepatitis is the most common cause of fulminant hepatic failure.

**Clinical picture**

The clinical picture is dominated by features of hepatic encephalopathy. The neuro-psychiatric features are :-

(a) Clouding of consciousness and fetor hepaticus
(b) Personality changes and antisocial behaviour
(c) Nightmares, headache and dizziness
(d) Delirium, mania and fits
(e) Violent behaviour
(f) Flapping tremors.

Decerebrate rigidity dominates the clinical picture later on. The plantar reflexes which remain flexor till late in the disease become extensor. The ocular reflexes usually remain brisk.

Depression of brain-stem function is reflected by respiratory and circulatory failure, cardiac arrhythmias and hypertension.

Depth of jaundice has no correlation with neuropsychiatric changes which may even develop before jaundice appears in early stages of illness. Later on however, the jaundice becomes deep and the liver shrinks in size.

Coma is divided into four stages, stage — I being the prodromal and stage 4 being deep coma.

The clinical picture later on may be dominated by features of any one of the following complications :-

(a) Haemorrhage
(b) Respiratory failure
(c) Hypoglycaemia
(d) Renal failure
(e) Infection
(f) Hypertension
(g) Cerebral oedema
(h) Biochemical and electrolyte disturbances.

## INVESTIGATIONS

Serum bilirubin is usually raised and so are the amino-transaminase levels SGPT (ALT), SGOT (AST) levels however have no relation to the ultimate prognosis. The levels usually fall during the terminal stages.

Serum albumin levels may fall in later stages and this indicates a poor prognosis.

Prothrombin time is increased and a coagulogram may show deficiency of other coagulation factors. Platelet count may be low. Hb levels and leucocytic count are generally normal unless active bleeding is taking place.

Cerebrospinal fluid is normal and lumbar puncture is not indicated unless the diagnosis is in doubt. Electroencephalogram (EEG) usually shows typical features in the form of waves of increasing amplitude and decreasing frequency. EEG should be done daily if possible because it has also got a prognostic significance. Blood ammonia levels may be raised.

Hypoglycaemia may be encountered in a good number of cases. Blood gas analysis and X-ray chest may help in assessing the respiratory functions while electrocardiogram may show evidence of cardiac arrhythmias.

Urine analysis, blood urea and serum creatinine will help in diagnosing renal damage.

Serum electrolytes, calcium bicarbonate and magnesium levels should be estimated in each case to find out any electrolyte and acid base disturbance which needs correction.

### Prognosis

It is still very poor in spite of so many advances in methods of treatment and understanding of the condition. Mortality varies between 60 to 90%. Those cases who recover however recover fully without leaving behind any evidence of chronic liver disease.

Bad prognostic signs are :-

(a) Depth of coma-majority of cases in grade 4 coma usually end in fatality.
(b) Long duration of coma
(c) Persistence of overt bleeding
(d) Development of renal failure and respiratory failure
(e) Advanced age of the patient
(f) Marked laboratory evidence of hepato-cellular damage particularly increased prothrombin time.

Etiology of fulminant hepatic failure generally has no bearing on the prognosis.

### Management

The patient should be admitted to an intensive care unit and constantly be watched for complications e.g. cardiac arrhythmias, respiratory failure, renal failure, massive gastrointestinal haemorrhage and septicaemia.

Monitoring of vital parameters, level of consciousness, liver functions, blood sugar, calcium phosphate and electrolyte levels is essential and should be done regularly. Size of the liver should be marked daily.

The patient should be managed on the lines of any other case of coma and care of respiratory passages, skin, bladder and bowel taken properly.

It is essential to supply calories in the form of glucose which should be given as a 10% infusion continuously. Supplements of 50 ml. of 50% glucose should be given whenever blood glucose level falls below 100 mg%. Adequate supplements of potassium chloride should be added. 10 ml. of 10% calcium gluconate may be required in some cases. Magnesium supplements may also be needed occasionally. Ascorbic acid in a dosage of 500 mg. daily may be added to the infusion. Frequent check up of electrolytes in plasma is very helpful. Although portosystemic encephalopathy is a minor problem in such cases, the following measures are taken to avoid it :-

(a) Restrict protein intake completely

(b) Bowel wash daily

(c) Neomycin 1.0g. six hourly orally daily is usually recommended. However, in Editor's opinion amoxycillin or ampicillin is preferrable, because small amounts of neomycin may be absorbed to produce toxic effects. Reasonable sterilization of gut can be achieved by ampicillin or amoxycillin).

(d) Sedation to be avoided. If considered absolutely essential, then 25 mg phenargan or 30 mg phenobarbitone parenterally may be used.

(e) Lactulose 15 to 60 ml. orally every six hours may be given to reduce absorption of ammonia from the intestines by producing increased frequency of stools, lowering pH of stools and altering the gut flora.

Parenteral Vit K supplements have no role to play correcting the bleeding diathesis. Heparin to treat disseminated intravenous coagulation has also not proved to be of any real value and in fact may precipitate massive gastroduodenal haemorrhage.

Cimetidine or Ranitidine I.V. is now used routinely as a prophylactic to prevent upper gastro-intestinal haemorrhage in cases of fulminant hepatitis. Dose-2 ml ampoule 6 hourly.

Use of L-dopa helps to awaken some patients but the drug has not been found to be helpful in changing the prognosis. Respiratory failure and renal failure are serious complications in these cases and should be treated as and when they develop.

Corticosteroids have no role to play in the management of fulminant hepatic failure and should be avoided. In fact, their use may lead to serious complications like gastric erosions, infection and acute pancreatitis.

Liver has got tremendous power of regeneration although factors controlling this are not known. Many measures of temporary hepatic support before the regeneration taken place have been tried but have so far not been of much use in actually changing the prognosis.

(a) Exchange transfusion

(b) Plasmapheresis

(c) Haemodialysis

(d) Extracorporeal liver perfusion

(e) Charcoal haemoperfusion.

The aim of all these procedures is to remove the toxic metabolites till the patient's liver recovers or a liver transplant can be given. Liver transplantation is, however, still in the realm of experimental surgery.

## LIVER TRANSPLANTATION

First liver transplantation was successfully performed by C.S. Welch in 1955. Starzel and his unit, performed first heroic operation of hepatic transplantation. Since then over 500 reported cases have come to light with varying survival rates. One year survival is now about 60% which is very encouraging. One case has survived 19 years (Sheila Sherlock 1986). The most important problem is to get a donor, who should be an irreversibly brain-damaged subject and is free from liver disease. Further ABO blood and tissue compatibility must be satisfied.

At present this operation therefore is only available in a few centres expertising in transplant surgery.

# JAUNDICE

*G.C. MOOKERJEE*
*M.L. SAPRA*

Jaundice or icterus is due to an increase in the serum bilirubin in blood resulting in yellowish colouration of skin, sclera, mucus membrane or urine. Normal serum bilirubin is mostly unconjugated and its normal range is between 0.5 and 1.0 mg/100 ml. Clinical jaundice appears when the serum bilirubin level rises above 2 mg/1U/ml. Type of bilirubin depends on the aetiology of jaundice.

**Bilirubin Metabolism**

The major amounts of serum bilirubin is derived from red blood cells when they are broken down after about 120 days of their normal life span. The globin from haemoglobin of red blood cells is separated and 'Haem' molecule is coverted in the reticuloendothelial cells to biliverdin and finally bilirubin (Table :16.1).

The effete red blood cells, however, contribute only 80-85 per cent of serum bilirubin. The remainder is derived from :

1) 'Haem' formed during haemoglobin synthesis
2) Red cell precursors in the marrow
   "infective erythropoiesis"
3) By-product of porphyrin metabolism in the liver involving cytochrome, myoglobin, catalase and other heme-containing enzymes.

The bilirubin thus liberated is unconjugated and is insoluble in water. It is however bound by serum albumin and due to its protein-bound state and insolubility in water, it cannot be excreted by the kidneys. This albumin-bound-bilirubin enters the liver cells from the plasma, the exact mechanism of this transport is not clear. In the microsomes of the liver cells, it is conjugated with glucuronic acid. The immediate glucuronyl-donor is uridine diphospho-glucuronic acid and the enzyme concerned is glucuronyl transferase. This process of conjugation makes the bilirubin water soluble. From the microsomes the conjugated bilirubin is excreted into the biliary canaliculi.

The biliary canaliculi join together to form large bile ducts which ultimately discharge the bilirubin into the duodenum along with the other constituents of bile. Major portion of this conjugated bilirubin is not reabsorbed by the intestinal mucosa and is excreted in the stools partly as bilirubin-glucuronide or in altered states. The intestinal bacteria alter bilirubin-glucuronide into urobilinogen and related compounds through a series of enzymatic reactions. These are also called sterco-bilins which render normal colour of stool. This urobilinogen is by the cells into the the bile. An "enterohepatic" circulation for urobilinogen thus exists. A small amount of this urobilinogen (less than 4 mg daily) however escapes into the blood and is excreted in the urine.

Table 16.1 : Formation of Bilirubin and Urobilinogen

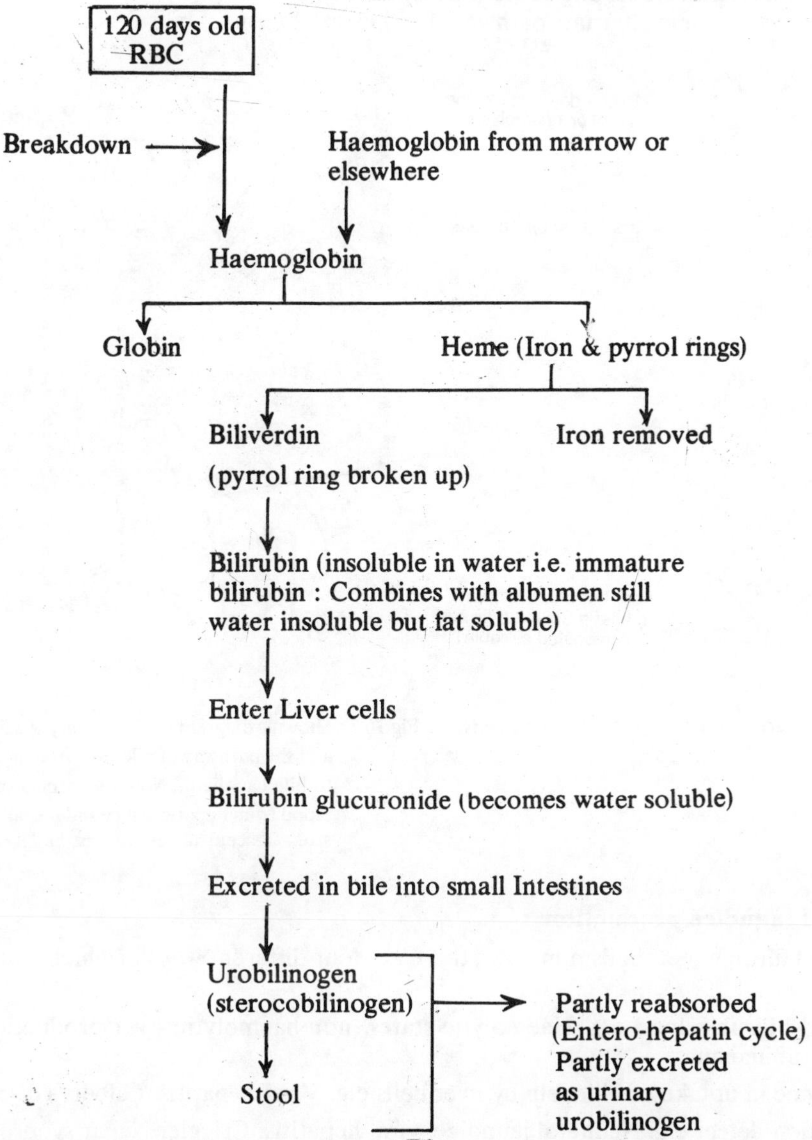


This quantity in the urine is usually not sufficient to give a positive qualitative Ehrlich's test Daily faecal urobilinogen output ranges between 50 and 300 mgm. In cholestatic jaundice this is greatly reduced while in haemolytic jaundice this will be very much increased. The average life of RCBs being 120 days, in an adult about 6.3 G of haemoglobin is broken down every day :

| | | |
|---|---|---|
| Average blood volume | — | 5 liters |
| Average haemoglobin | — | 15 g/100 ml. |
| Total circulating haemoglobin | — | $15 \times 10 \times 5 = 750$ g |
| Haemoglobin catabolised daily | — | $750/120 = 6.3$ g |

This gives rise to about 250 mg bilirubin daily. In addition to this about 30 mg bilirubin is derived daily from sources other than effete red blood cells as discussed already. This daily output of urobilinogen in stools and urine is however considerably less- about 100-200 mg. It is obvious therefore that some alternate pathways for the metabolism of bilirubin must be available.

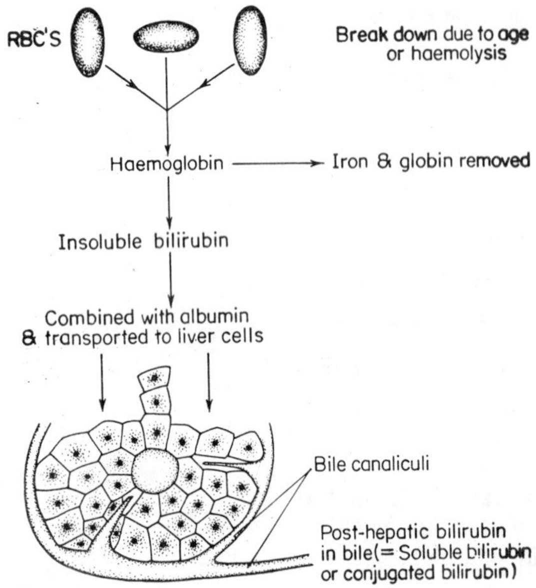


Fig.16.2 : Biliburin formation from red blood cells.

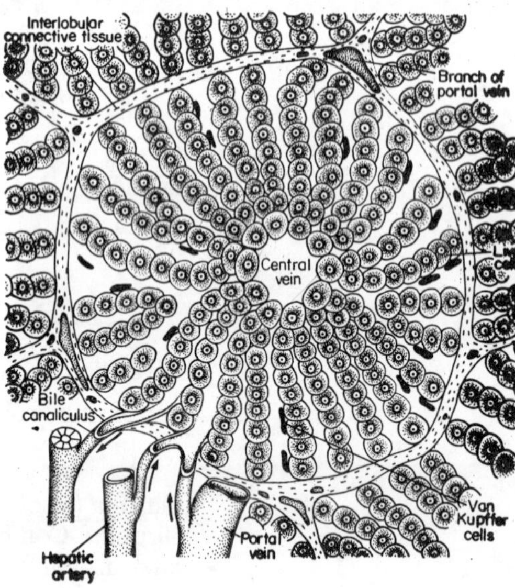


Fig.16.3 : Showing diagrammatic anatomy of a liver lobule and the pathway of bile-flow from hepatic cells to bile canaliculi. Note the circulatory path of blood from hepatic artery and portal vein in the sisusoids central vein drains the blood out.

**Mechanism of Jaundice production :**

Keeping the bilirubin metabolism in view, there are four different ways in which jaundice can develop :

1) Increased bilirubin load e.g. Haemolytic states, non-haemolytic over production, shunt hyperbilirubinaemia.
2) Disturbance in uptake of bilirubin by liver cells e.g. Viral hepatitis, Gilbert's disease
3) Conjugation defect e.g. Neonatal jaundice, viral hepatitis, Criggler-Najjar syndrome
4) Bilirubin excretion defect :
   (i) Intrahepatic e.g.
   Drug Jaundice, Viral hepatitis
   Rotor syndrome, Dubin Johnson syndrome
   (ii) Extrahepatic obstructioh of common bile duct e.g. stone or stricture in bile duct or carcinoma head of pancreas or ampulla of Vater.

It is important to remember, however, that more than one mechanism may be responsible in an individual case e.g. viral hepatitis.

**Classification of jaundice :**

There are different ways in which jaundice can be classified. A simple method would be to classify it on the basis of type of serum bilirubin encountered i.e.

1) Jaundice due predominantly to unconjugated bilirubin
2) Jaundice due predominantly to conjugated bilirubin.

Another useful classification is based on the pathological mechanisms giving rise to jaundice i.e :

1) Haemolytic jaundice (prehepatic)
2) Hepatocellular jaundice (hepatic)
3) Cholestatic jaundice
   (a) Intrahepatic cholestasis (intra hepatic bile duct)
   (b) Extrahepatic cholestasis (post hepatic)

A classification based on the fundamental derangement in the bilirubin metabolism has already been discussed under the heading of mechanism of jaundice production.

It must be emphasized, however, that in an individual case, more than one "type" of jaundice may be present. It is felt that consideration of various types of jaundice under the following headings is more useful and practical :

1) Haemolytic jaundice
2) Hepatocellular jaundice
3) Cholestatic jaundice
4) Drug jaundice
5) Congenital hyperbilirubinaemias.

**Haemolytic Jaundice :** There is increased bilirubin formation due to excessive destruction of red blood cells. Jaundice due to unconjugated hyper-bilirubinaemia develops when the liver cannot cope with the excessive load.

The following clinical features are usually observed :

1) The jaundice is usually mild. Serum bilirubin levels normally do not rise above 4 mg/100 ml. Most of the serum bilirubin is of unconjugated type.
2) The spleen is generally enlarged due to excessive haemolysis by reticuloendothelial system.
3) A certain amount of anaemia (haemolytic anaemia) is usually present.
4) There may be history of remissions and relapses. Fever, abdominal pain and arthralgia may be present during relapses. Pruritis is absent.
5) Stools contain large amounts of stercobilinogen and are highly coloured. Increased amounts of urobilinogen are present in the urine. There is no bilirubin, however, in the urine. It is therefore also called achlouric jaundice.
6) Reticulocytosis is invariably present.
7) Liver function tests including serum aminotransferases and BSP retention are wichin normal limits.

The common conditions which may give rise to haemolytic jaundice are :

1) Congenitial defects in the red blood cells e.g. Congenital spherocytosis, sickle cell anaemia, thalassaemia.
2) Extracorpuscular factors acting on red blood cells e.g. Infections, auto-immune acquired haemolytic anaemias, incompatible blood transfusions, tissue infarcts (pulmonary), Rh-factor in compatibility.
3) Drugs.

**Hepato-cellular Jaundice :**

The jaundice in these cases is due to damage to the liver cells. The mechanisms responsible for production of jaundice are :

1) Defective uptake of unconjugated bilirubin by the damaged liver cells.
2) Defective conjugation in the microsomes.
3) Cholestasis due to canalicular obstruction by the swollen inflammed hepatocytes.
4) Regurgitation of bile from damaged cells into hepatic circulation. The classical example of hepatocellular jaundice is viral hepatitis. Other conditions which may produce hepatocellular jaundice are :
   (a) Infections like leptospirosis, yellow fever and septicaemias.
   (b) Drugs like iproniazid, isoniazid, halothane, heavy doses of tetracyclines and paracetamol, carbon tetrachloride (also vide infra)

Both conjugated and non-conjugated types of serum bilirubin are raised in hepatocellular jaundice. There is marked rise in serum amino-transferases (more than 100 I.U. per litre) and only moderate rise in alkaline phosphatase. Hepatocellular jaundice must be differentiated from extrahepatic cholestasis because unjudicious surgical intervention in these cases may lead to fulminant hepatic failure. Detailed features of hepatocellular jaundice have been discussed under viral hepatitis.

## DRUG JAUNDICE

This subject has assumed great importance during the last few years or so. Large number of drugs are metabolized by the liver, chiefly by the enzymes in the hepatic microsomes. The biochemical processes involved are mainly oxidation, reduction, hydrolysis, conjugation or acetylation. During this process some of the drugs of their metabolic products may produce liver damage and jaundice. More than 100 drugs are recognised today, as potentially hepatotoxic. Many new ones are being added to the list with rapid introduction of powerful chemotherapeutic agents. It is therefore very important to consider chemical compounds as potentially hepatotoxic and therefore history of drugs intake by the patient should form an essential part of investigation of all cases of jaundice.

Metabolism of the drugs by the liver may result in the following effects :

1) It may become more potent e.g. phenylbutazone
2) It may becomes less potent e.g. pethidine
3) It may become clinically effective e.g. cyclophosphamide (not effective otherwise).

It is also important to remember that some drugs may induce enzyme induction in the liver cells. Their continued use makes them less effective because they are metabolized at a faster rate because of enzyme induction. Inactivation of another drug may also be accelerated in this way and untoward reactions may occur e.g. the effect of phenindione is decreased when phenobarbitone is being given simultaneously. Bleeding may be precipitated in a well controlled case if the latter is suddenly stopped. This property of enzyme induction due to drugs is being utilized therapeutically in certain clinical situations e.g. phenobarbitone reduces the level of serum bilirubin in neonatal jaundice.

The different mechanisms which may be responsible for drug jaundice are :

1) Haemolytic reaction
2) Hepatitic reaction
3) Cholestasis :
   (a) Sensitivity type
   (b) Non-sensitivity type
4) Direct hepatotoxicity

It is not possible however, to always define the mechanism responsible in an individual case. There is considerable overlap and more than one mechanisms may be responsible in a particular case. The problem is complicated further by the fact that more than one drug may have been administered simultaneously. The methods in use to predict possible hepatotoxicity of a drug are :

a) *Animal experiments* : It has not been useful to predict hypersensitivity type of reaction. The response in humans may otherwise also be different.

b) *Clinical experiments* : The parameters used to assess liver damage are serum aminotransferase levels and BSP retention. Small deviations from normal may however disappear with continued administration of the drug and it is difficult to say therefore whether these abnormalities were due to hepatotoxicity or normal variations.

c) *Needle biopsy of the liver* : It is not possible to do it in every case. Drug hepatitis may however be difficult to differentiate from viral hepatitis even by electron microscopy.

d) *Challenge experiments* : Some of the drug reactions may proceed to a stage of fulminant hepatic failure. It is not always considered ethical therefore to challenge the individual with the same drug again if it is likely to be hepatotoxic.

**Haemolytic reactions :** Haemolytic drug reactions are however common in individuals with glucose 6-phosphate dehydrogenase deficiency. The important drugs which may precipitate haemolysis and jaundice in these cases, are antimalarials particularly phenacetin 8-aminoquinolines, sulphonamides, PAS and chloramphenicol etc.

**Hepatitis like reactions :** The drugs commonly in use and incriminated are indomethacin, monoamino-oxidase inhibitors like iproniazid, halothane and except for the fact that the onset is usually afebrile and serum aminotransferase levels are not very high. Since there is no diagnostic laboratory test for the latter it is difficult to differentiate them. The possibility of a coincident viral infection is however always there.

Hepatitis like reactions are not related to the dose or duration of the drug therapy. They may develop even weeks after stopping the drug therapy. The incidence is not high but what is significant is very high mortality rate (20-30 per cent). The condition should always be kept in mind whenever a patient develops hepatitis while on any of the above mentioned drugs. The treatment is the same as for viral hepatitis.

**Direct Hepatocellular Necrosis :** These drugs are known as hepatotoxic agents and produce cellular necrosis. The degree of liver damage is dose-dependent. Other organs particularly the kidneys, gastro-intestinal tract and the brain are also damaged. The common drugs leading to this type of reaction are carbon tetrachloride, heavy doses of intravenous tetracyclines, paracetamol taken in suicidal doses, over dose of ferrous sulphate and cytotoxic drugs like 6-mercaptopurine and metho-trexate. Irradiation to the liver can also produce similar results.

Symptoms appear shortly after exposure to the drug. Abdominal pain, nausea, vomiting and diarrhoea reflect gastro-intestinal involvement, renal failure appears due to kidney damage and confusion with coma are manifestations of central nervous system involvement. Jaundice usually appears in 24-48 hours. The offending agent should be removed and the patient treated for renal and acute liver failure on conventional lines.

**"Hypersensitivity" type cholestasis :** The commonest drug giving rise to this type of reaction is chlorpromazine. Other phenothiazines may also produce a similar reaction. The reaction is not dose dependent and may occur several days after the drug is stopped. The incidence is quite high about one per cent of all cases taking chlorpromazine for a week or more develop this type of jaundice.

The onset is usually insidious but may be associated with prodromal features suggestive of viral hepatitis. Sensitivity rashes, eosinophilia and recurrence on re-exhibition of the drug are important features suggestive of a hypersensitivity reaction. Pre-existing liver disease does not increase the risk to this type of jaundice and phenothiazines are therefore not contraindicated in liver damage. The jaundice is usually mild and disappears after 3-4 weeks. But it may persist for months and even years in some patients and may be confused with surgical jaundice. It is important to avoid surgery in these cases which may precipitate hepatic failure. Deaths due to fulminant hepatic failure have been however recorded in a few cases.

Other drugs which may produce hypersensitivity type of cholestasis are oral hypoglycaemic agents, antithyroid drugs, nitrofurantoin and thiazide group of diuretics.

**Non-hypersensitivity type of Cholestasis :** This reaction is dose dependent and jaundice will develop in anybody who takes the drug for a sufficient period. Features of hypersensitivity are absent. Cholestasis is absent. It is usually encountered after methyl-testosterone and anabolic steroids. Jaundice generally subside after the offending drug is stopped. The importance of avoiding surgery in these cases has been already stressed.

In addition to the types of drug reaction described above, it must be emphasized that some drugs are capable of producing both hepatitic as well as cholestatic features and features of both may be present in jaundice due to these drugs. These drugs are PAS and other antitubercular drugs, oral hypoglycaemic agents, sulphonamides, methyl-dopa, erythromycin estolate and oleandomycin.

Jaundice may also develop as a part of hypersensitivity reaction to drugs like penicillin, sulphonamides and phenindione.

Cholecystographic media may produce jaundice by competition with excretion of bilirubin. Drugs like sulphonamides and salicylates may compete with serum albumin for binding sites and produce jaundice. Jaundice may also develop following consumption of food contaminated with insecticides and fungi.

## CHOLESTATIC JAUNDICE

The word 'chole' means yellow in Greek and is used in medicine for bile and 'stasis' is "arrest". Any jaundice which is due to failure of 'mature bile' to reach the duodenum, after conjugation in the hepatic microsomes should be considered under cholestatic jaundice. The obstruction to the flow of bile may be inside the liver i.e. "intra-hepatic cholestasis" or outside the liver in larger biliary passages — 'extra hepatic cholestasis'. The terms cholestatic jaundice and obstructive should be considered inter-changeable although some people use cholestasis for only intrahepatic obstruction. It should be appreciated that the clinical and biochemical features of intra and extra-hepatic cholestasis are more or less similar and it may be sometimes difficult to differentiate between the two. The importance of this differentiation however cannot be over emphasized. Surgical treatment which is essential in most cases of extra-hepatic cholestasis may prove fatal in a case of intrahepatic cholestasis by precipitating fulminant hepatic failure.

The factors which are responsible for clinical manifestation of cholestasis are :

1) Failure of the bile to reach the intestines.
2) Accumulation of bile in the blood stream
3) The effect of bile components on the liver cells.

They produce following features common to all forms of cholestasis :

1) Light coloured stools.
2) Reduction of faecal urobilinogen
3) Absence of urinary urobilinogen
4) Hypoprothrombinaemia.
5) Malabsorption of fats and fat soluble vitamins.
6) Jaundice due to conjugated bilirubin
7) Itching

8) Hypercholesterolaemia
9) Elevation of serum alkaline phosphatase
10) Mild increase in serum transaminase levels
11) Failure to excrete BSP and cholecystographic dyes.

*Intrahepatic Cholestasis* : The various mechanisms which may produce intrahepatic cholestasis are :

1) Swollen liver cells may press upon their surrounding biliary canaliculi.
2) There may be some genetic defects in the handling of conjugated bilirubin.

The important etiological causes of intrahepatic cholestasis are :

1) Viral hepatitis
2) Drugs — e.g. phenothiazines, Methyl testosterone, Nitro-furadantin, Chlorpropamide, Nor-ethynodrel and Sulphadiazine.
3) Alcoholic hepatitis
4) Primary biliary cirrhosis
5) Septicaemic conditions
6) Pregnancy — rarely
7) Dubin Johnson and Rotor syndromes — very rare.

The clinical features common to cholestasis of both types are present and have been already discussed. Pruritis is very marked. The jaundice is usually insidious in onset and not preceded by any prodromal illness except in cases of cholestasis due to viral hepatitis. Hypersensitivity type of drug jaundice may be associated with skin rashes and eosinophilia. The general health of the patient is usually good. The liver may be enlarged but can be non-tender. The stools may be acholic and urobilinogen absent in the urine if the obstruction is complete. Investigations reveal increased conjugated serum bilirubin, alkaline phosphatase and cholesterol levels. Electrophoresis of serum proteins shows rise in $\alpha$—2 and $\beta$-globulins. The serum amino-transferases are only moderately increased. Liver biopsy reveals excessive bile in biliary canaliculi, Kupffer cells and liver cells. The changes are more marked centrilobularly. Degenerative changes may be seen in some of the hepatocytes. Changes due to the underlying disease producing cholestasis are present.

Intrahepatic cholestasis is usually self-limited and the prognosis is excellent in most of the cases. The jaundice and cholestasis may however persist for a long time in some cases.

*Extra-hepatic Cholestasis* : The common causes of extrahepatic obstructions are :

1) Gall stones
2) Stricture of the bile duct
3) Carcinoma head of pancreas
4) Chronic pancreatitis
5) Carcinoma of bile ducts
6) Pressure on the bile duct at the porta hepatitis due to metastatic lymph nodes, amoebic liver abscess or hydatid cyst.

General features of cholestasis are similar to intrahepatic cholestasis. Pruritis is however not so severe as in intrahepatic cholestasis. Pruritus is however not so severe as in intrahepatic type. Fever with rigors, appreciable abdominal pain, leukocytosis and occult blood in the stools are however important features which suggest extra-hepatic cholestasis. Liver is enlarged but not tender. Absence of hepatomegaly is strongly against a diagnosis of extrahepatic obstruction. Positive blood cultures signify cholangitis and are strongly in favour of extrahepatic obstruction. The jaundice and colour of stools may vary if the obstruction is intermittent as is likely in a bile duct stone. There is progressive increase in jaundice however in cases of carcinoma head of the pancreas.

Liver function tests reveal findings similar to those seen in intrahepatic cholestasis.

**How to manage a case of cholestasis :** All attempts should be made to differentiate intra-hepatic cholestasis from extra-hepatic cholestasis. A detailed history, physical examination and routine investigations like urinary urobilinogen, colour of stools and occult blood in stools, leucocytic count, liver function tests including serum bilirubin and its type, alkaline phosphatase, aminotransferase levels, prothrombin time and electrophoresis of serum proteins, plain X-ray films of the abdomen and barium meal studies of stomach and duodenum should be carried out in each case.

If a diagnosis of extrahepatic cholestasis can be established, then elective surgery should be carried out to relieve the obstruction.

In cases where there is some doubt of intra-hepatic cholestasis, the patient must be observed for a period of at least 4 weeks before surgery is thought of. It is unlikely that a period of wait in a case of extrahepatic obstruction is likely to harm the patient very much. In intra-hepatic cholestasis, surgery may be dangerous. During the period of observation, clinical examination and investigations outlined above should be periodically repeated. Following additional investigations may be of help to differentiate between intra-hepatic and extra-hepatic cholestasis :

1) "Steroid Wash" — Administration of 40 mg prednisolone daily in divided doses for 5 days brings down the serum bilirubin level by more than 40 per cent in a case of hepatocellular jaundice. The fall in cases of extra-hepatic jaundice is much less and only transient. The mechanism of action of steroids is not exactly known. It is likely that the metabolism of bilirubin by some alternate pathways is enhanced.
2) Liver Biopsy — Jaundice per se is not a contraindication to liver biopsy. There is however increased risk of bleeding. Biliary peritonitis may develop as a complication in cases with extrahepatic obstruction. Biopsy findings may be helpful to differentiate between intra-hepatic and extra-hepatic cholestasis. The value is however rather limited. Therefore it is usually avoided in jaundiced patients.
3) Percutaneous transhepatic cholangiography — Aspiration of bile through a needle introduced into the liver through the abdominal wall indicates biliary tract obstruction. A contrast medium can be injected through the needle to visualise the dilated ducts as well as the site of obstruction. If an obstruction is demonstrated, a laparotomy should be performed on the same day to avoid biliary peritonitis. This procedure is being increasingly used these days and appears to be one of the best means available at present to differentiate between extra-hepatic and intra-hepatic cholestasis.

In difficult and undiagnosed cases a laparotomy should be performed if the jaundice shows no signs of regression after a period of six weeks. An operative cholangiogram and liver biopsy must be performed in cases where no extra-hepatic obstruction is found. Laparotomy however is no substitute for thorough observation and detailed investigations which must be carried out in such cases. The physician and the surgeon should have a close liasion and co-operation in all difficult cases of cholestasis during the entire period of observation. Sonogram and C.T. scan may be very helpful.

## CONGENITAL HYPERBILIRUBINAEMIAS

Familial or congenital disorders of bilirubin metabolism may give rise to jaundice which may be due to :

a) Rise in unconjugated serum bilirubin
b) Rise in conjugated serum bilirubin

These are rare conditions but the importance of recognising these conditions lies in the fact that they are mostly benign conditions and may be confused with other causes of jaundice. These patients are often submitted to repeated investigations and may even be submitted to a laparotomy. They should therefore be considered in the differential diagnosis of jaundice when other common conditions have been excluded.

**Conditions associated with unconjugated hyperbilirubinaemia :**

*Gilbert's Disease or Syndrome :*

It is commonest type of congenital hyperbilirubinaemia, inherited as an autosomal dominant gene. The disease is usually detected after an attack of viral hepatitis when mild icterus persists after recovery or it may be discovered accidentally while the patient is being investigated for some other illness. The serum bilirubin is generally below 3.Omg/100 ml but the levels fluctuate. Infections and fatigue may produce vague abdominal discomfort, nausea and vomiting, increase in jaundice and serum bilirubin leavels. Other liver function tests including BSP retention are within normal limits. The liver histology is normal. The condition is probably due to defective uptake of bilirubin by the liver cells. The prognosis is excellent and it must be differentiated from viral hepatitis and haemolytic jaundice.

*Criggler-Najjar Syndrome :*

It is a very rare condition. The importance of recognising it however lies in the fact that this is one form of congenital hyperbilirubinaemia which may produce kernicterus and be fatal if not treated in time. The defect lies in the conjugation of bilirubin by liver cells. Severe and persistent jaundice appears on the first or second day after birth and kernicterus may develop. The main danger is during first few weeks of life because alternate pathways for metabolism of serum bilirubin develop subsequently. Other liver function tests and liver histology are normal. Treatment consists of cholestyramine therapy and exchange blood transfusions.

*Primary 'Shunt' hyperbilirubinaemia :*

Bilirubin is formed in excess from sources other than effete red blood cells. The possible sources are erythroid precursors in the bone marrow and directly from haem. The mode of inheritance is unknown. The condition is rare.

*Familial neonatal hyperbilirubinaemia or Lucey-Driscoll hyper-bilirubinaemia :*

The hyperbilirubinaemia is seen only in neonatal period. It may be due to presence of some unidentified inhibitor in the serum. The condition should be differentiated form physiological jaundice of the newborn.

**Conditions associated with conjugated hyperbilirubinaemia :**

*Dubin-Johnson Syndrome :*

The diagnostic feature in this condition is presence of masses of brown pigment granules in liver cells. Fresh liver biopsy specimen locks chocolate brown in colour. The pigment is probably related to melanin. The jaundice in these cases shows marked fluctuations. It deepens with intercurrent illnesses and constitutional symptoms and malaise may appear during these exacerbations. Bilirubin is present in the urine because the hyperbilirubinaemia is conjugated. Serum bilirubin is usually less than 6 mg/100ml. BSP excretion test shows higher retention at 90 and 120 minutes than at 45 minutes. The other liver function tests are within normal limits. The liver may be enlarged and tender in some cases. The defect in these cases lies in the transport of conjugated bilirubin from liver microsomes to the biliary canaliculi. The condition carries an excellent prognosis.

*Rotor Syndrome :*

It is more less similar to Dubin-Johnson Syndrome except for the fact that the liver cells do not show pigment deposits. The prognosis is excellent. Diagnosis is by liver biopsy.

[This chapter has been updated from the book on "Diseases of the Liver" by the authors, originally published by Current Tech. Lit Pvt. Ltd., Bombay, 1973].

# CIRRHOSIS OF LIVER

*D.N. GUHA MAZUMDAR*

## Introduction

It is a condition of diffuse fibrosis of liver disorganising the lobular architecture with connective tissue bands uniting centrilobular zones with portal tracts and nodular parenchymal regeneration. Hepatocellular necrosis is always the initiator of this disease involving all parts of the liver without necessarily affecting each lobule.

## Pathogenesis

Necrosis of liver cells may occur as a result of nultiple aetiologies, collapse of reticulin framework as a result of hepatocellular necrosis is followed by formation of new fibroblasts which leads to collagenesis. Factors responsible for this stimulation to collagen formation is not known. Its cells, the perisinusoidal fat storage cells are strong suspects as being transformed into fibroblast and may be responsible for intralobular collagen formation. Collagenesis progresses from a reversible to an irreversible state. The distribution of initial fibrotic process varies e.g. in alcoholism and congestive cardiac failure it is centrizonal whereas in viral hepatitis or haemochromatosis it is periportal. Fibronectin, a glycoprotein present on the liver cells surface probably binds the collagen and organizes hepatocytes growth during healing response. The regenerating nodules and adjacent fibrosis disturb the hepatic vascular tree. Portal hypertension develops as a result of impediment of blood flow and development of internal fistula. Oesophageal and gastric varices develop and splenomegaly occurs as a result of portal hypertension.

Ascites develops as a result of multiple factors in cirrhosis. These are : (1) decrease of colloid osmotic pressure due to decreased albumin synthesis by liver, (2) portal hypertension, and (3) increase of hepatic lymph production because of hepatic venous outflow obstruction. More fluid enters the peritoneal cavity than leaves it and ascites develops. Reduction of effective intravascular volume takes place and this in turn leads to secondary hyperaldosteronism resulting in retention of sodium and water from distal renal tuble. A viscious cycle develops and further ascites is produced.

Cirrhosis has to be differentiated from nodule formation within the liver as in Felty's syndrome of partial nodular transformation. Similarly, this is not the same as hepatic fibrosis. One of the important cause of portal hypertension in India is non-cirrhotic portal fibrosis in which fibrous septa spread out of the portal tract in a linear or trabecular fashion, the aetiology of this condition is not known. Fibrosis in the portal region also occurs in congenital fibrosis. Interlobular fibrosis of the liver occurs in granulomatous liver disease. Depending on the preponderance of the size of the nodules, the cirrhosis may be micronodular (frequently in alcoholics) macronodular (frequently following viral hepatitis) or mixed.

## Aetiology of cirrhosis :

(1) Viral hepatitis : Type B, Non-A Non-B.
(2) Cryptogenic
(3) Alcoholic
(4) Toxins and drugs
Amanita phalloides toxin
Methotrexate
Methyldopa
(5) prolonged cholestasis — intra or extrahepatic
(6) Immunological — Lupoid hepatitis
(7) India childhood cirrhosis

(8) Metabolic
e.g. Haemochromatosis, Wilson's disease
— anti-trypsin deficiency
Type IV — glycogenesis, Galactosaemia
Congenital tyrosinosis.

(9) Hepatic venous outflow obstruction
e.g. Veno-occlusive disease, Budd Chiari syndrome, constrictive pericarditis.

**Clinical Features**

About one-third of patients suffering from cirrhosis may be asymptomatic being diagnosed at autopsy. A history of past jaundice or pain abdomen or prolonged alcohol intake may be available in some cases, but most of the cases of cirrhosis in our country are cryptogenic.

Patients may complain of considerable weight loss, weakness, anorexia, flatulence, nausea and vomiting. He may present with haematemesis or melena due to gastrooesophageal variceal bleeding. After a few months patient notices abdominal fullness due to ascites and at this stage he may present himself to the physician. Various complications of advanced cirrhosis of liver is shown in Fig. 16.4 There may be symptoms of bleeding tendency e.g. epistaxis, purpura or menorrhagia due to defect in the synthesis of coagulation factors (Prothrombin, Factors VII, IX) with or without thrombocytopaenia due to hypersplenism.

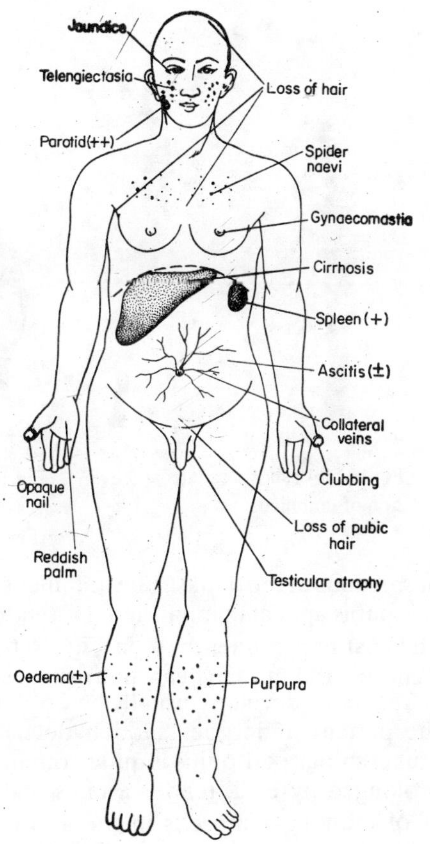


Fig.16.4 : Important complications of cirrhosis of liver.

Signs of hepatocellular failure are frequently apparent. There may be low grade fever. Jaundice is seldom conspicuous, except in cases associated with chronic hepatitis or cholestasis. The skin is dry and inelastic and the body hair may be scanty. There may be prominent venules over the face and vascular spiders scattered over the head and upper body. In males gynaecomastia and testicular atrophy may be present. All these cases are believed to be due to an excess of circulating oesterogen being not inactivated by the damaged liver. Anaemia, hypochromic and microcytic, are common and due to blood loss. Occasionally macrocytic anaemia does occur. Oedema of feet occasionally develops because of hypoalbuminaemia. Finger clubbing, cyanosis, and hyperdynamic circulatory state may be seen in a few patients and are probably due to venoarterial shunting of blood in multiple pleural and intrapulmonary telengiectasis. Increased melanin deposition in the skin may lead to generalised pigmentation. The patient may complain of hypersomnia or inversion of sleep rhythm.

On examination patient's mental state will depend upon presence or absence of neuropsychiatric manifestations. Ascites is common, though not invariably present. It may appear suddenly or develop insidiously over the course of months.

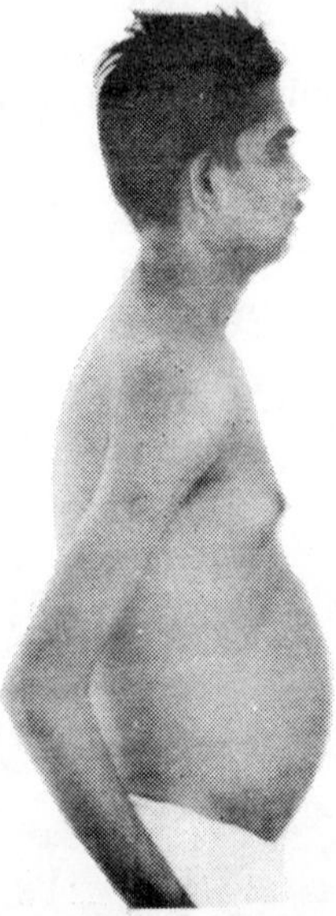

Fig.16.5(a) : shows gynaecomastia and action in cirrhosis of liver *(Editor's case)*

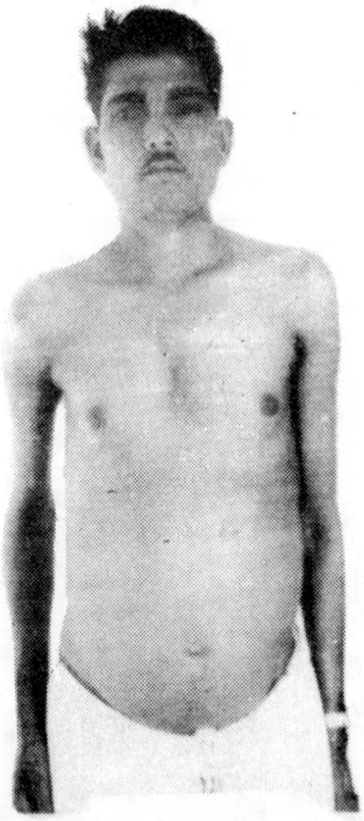

Fig.16.5(b) : shows asicitis and eversion of umbilicus.

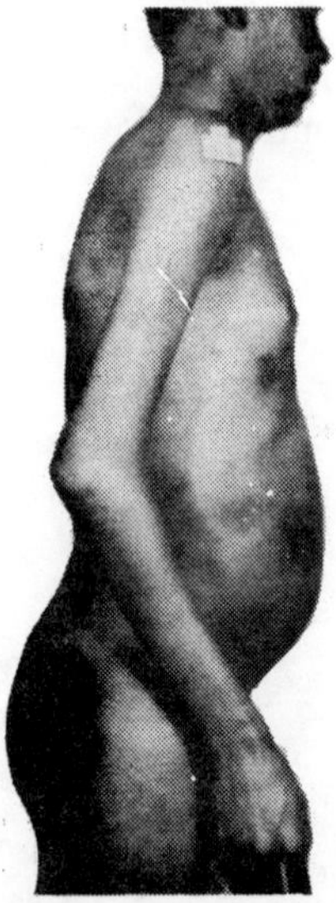

Fig.16.5(c) : The same patient after a year showing patchy skin pigmentation.

The fullness is particularly conspicuous in the flanks. The umbilicus is everted and the distance between umbilicus and symphysis pubis appears diminished. Distended veins radiating from the umbilicus (flow away from umbilicus) are frequently seen Fig. 16.6. Protein concentration of ascitic fluid rarely exceeds 1-2 gm per 100 ml. Higher values suggest infection or malignancy, spontaneous bilateral peritonitis frequently develops, usually by Coliform bacilli and Streptococci and should be suspected if the patient undergoes sudden deterioration, particularly with encephalopathy. Complicating tuberculous peritonitis is quite common in our country. It should be suspected in presence of prolonged pyrexia, tender ascites and presence of high protein content and increased number of mononuclear cells in the ascites fluid. Splenomegaly and abdominal wall venous collaterals indicate portal hypertension. The spleen is usually hard and is usually moderately enlarged. Communication between portal and systemic veins frequently lead to collateral circulation. The sites are at the lower end of the oesophagus and upper end of the stomach (their rupture produces haematemesis and melena), the anus and lower rectum (their rupture leads to bleeding piles), at the umbilicus through the paraumbilical veins running along falciform ligament (caput medusae) and between retroperitoneal and diaphragmatic veins, and omentum, colon and spleen. Oesophageal varices could be demonstrated by barium swallow examination of lower end of oesophagus and endoscopy. Transcutaneous splenoportography or venous phase of coeliac axis angiography will demonstrate the collaterals arising out of the splenoportal system and gross distortion of intrahepatic pattern of the branches of portal vein.

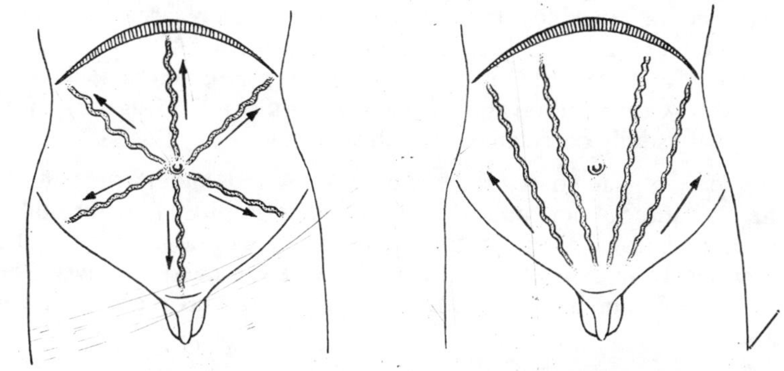


Fig.16.6 : Direction of vensus blood flow suggesting site of obstruction

## Investigations

Biochemical tests may be quite normal in cirrhosis. But the concentration of plasma albumin is usually reduced and the globulin level is elevated. The reduction of albumin is due its diminished synthesis by the liver while increased globulin due to increased serum antibodies to gastrointestinal tract antigens, particularly E.coli which bypass Kupffer cells in the liver and produces antigenic stimulus to other organs, particularly the spleen. There may be slight increase in serum transaminase or gamma glutamyl transpeptidase, and a constant excess of urinary urobilinogen level. The prothrombin time may be prolonged and non-responsive to vitamin K injection. Serum alkaline phosphatase concentration is usually normal. Forty-five minutes Bromsulphalein retention is

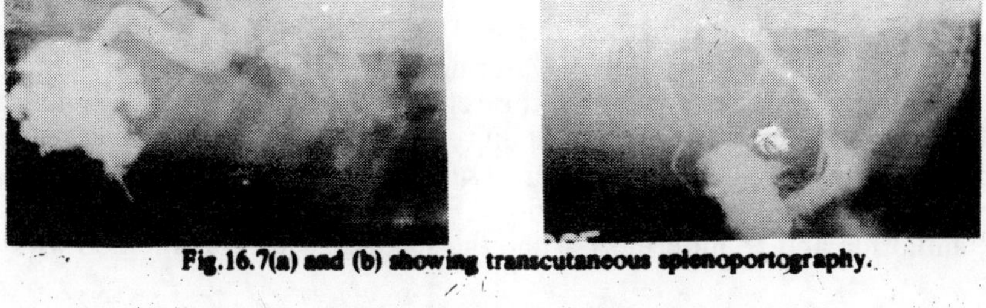

**Fig.16.7(a) and (b) showing transcutaneous splenoportography.**

more than 5 per cent even in cases where other tests of liver functions are found to be normal. The two-hour post-prandial plasma total bile acid level is usually increased. Liver biopsy is not only helpful to confirm the diagnosis but also helps in knowing the aetiology or cirrhosis and degree of activity present in the liver.

**Course and Prognosis**

Patient suffering from cirrhosis may progress to chronic or intermittent episodes of neuropsychiatric manifestations. Features of neuropsychiatric manifestations are alterations of sleep rhythm, personality changes, intellectual deterioration, flapping tremor, confusion, stuporosity of coma. Encephalopathy may follow intake of sedative drugs, intake of high protein diet, use of excessive diuretic leading to hypokalaemia, or taking out of much fluid from the peritoneal cavity, infection or gastrointestinal bleeding E.E.G. changes (usually large bilaterally synchronous slow wave) are characteristic and depends upon the degree of severity of encephalopathy. It is due to cerebral intoxication (probably nitrogenous) by intestinal contents which have not been metabolised by the liver. Arterial blood ammonia level (normal is 0.8-1 $\mu$g/ml) is usually found to be elevated and its level usually correlate well with severity.

Death sometimes occurs due to severe haematemesis and melena in spite of good liver function. Spontaneous bacterial peritonitis, tuberculous peritonitis, hepatorenal syndrome are some of the other complications. There is increased incidence of hepatoma in patients suffering from cirrhosis. Cirrhosis, though usually a progressive disease, need not always be so. In some cases, e.g. in Wilson's disease and haemochromatosis the fibrosis may regress following treatment.

**Prognosis**

Prognosis depends on many factors. The prognosis is not good if ascites is present and is worse if large doses of diuretics are needed to control it. Jaundice is a serious sign.

Neuropsychiatric complications, developing in the couse of progressive hepato-cellular failure indicate bad prognosis, where as those developing chronically and associated with large portal systemic collateral circulation respond well to restriction of protein intake. Gross hypoprothrombinaemia (serum albumin $<$ 2.5 gm%), persistent hypoprothrombinaemia, uncorrected by Ir Vitamin K. persistent hyponatraemia (serum sodium $<$ 120 mEq/L) not related to diu therapy, persistent hypotension are of grave prognostic sign. Prognosis is better if decompens has followed gastrooesophageal haemorrhage, in alcoholic cirrhotics if they abstain, if the liver is big and if there is no ascites.

**Treatment**

Though medical treatment does not influence the course of established portal hypertension, an adequate medical measure can influence the prognosis of cirrhosis by favouring regeneration of parenchymal cells, prevention of progression of fibrosis and reduce the development of fluid retention and encephalopathy. Adequate mixed diet and avoidance of alcohol intake are helpful in some cases where nutritional deficiency and chronic alcoholism are thought to be responsible for progression of the disease. A diet of 1 gm of protein per Kg. body weight with a calorie intake of 2000-3000/ day is adequate unless malnutrition is obvious. If oedema or ascites is present salt free protein addition may be helpful. Other dietary supplements, e.g. yeast, thiamine, riboflavin, niacin, choline and methianine are supposed to be of value in these cases. Protein restriction is to be made to patients showing evidences of encephalopathy.

Ascites and oedema may diminish by bed rest and salt restriction having a diet containing sodium chloride 0.5 gm per day. Restriction of water intake to the volume equal to the previous day's fluid loss may be made. If the response to this regime is not satisfactory (weight loss is less than 1 gm in 4 days) diuretics may be used. Potent diuretics are thiazide, frusemide, bumetamide, pyretamide and ethacrynic acid. These are powerful saluretic and kaluretic agents and need oral potassium supplementation (by potassium chloride). Poorly saluretic conserving potassium are spironolactone, amiloride and triamterine. When the second group is combined with the first group, potassium chloride supplements are reduced or may be unnecessary. Complications like encephalopathy or hepatorenal failure may be avoided by treating the ascites slowly. In resistant cases paracentesis of small quantity of fluid may have to be done followed by infusion of dextran, salt poor albumin etc. Refractory ascites may be tackled by porto-caval anastomosis (though it increases the incidence of èncephalopathy) or peritoneal venous shunt (Le Veen Shunt) connecting peritoneal cavity with superior vena cava.

If the patient develops haematemesis or melena the patient should be hospitalized. Blood transfusion has to be given. Stress induced mucosal ulcers are frequent and Cimetidine I.V. or Ranitin is given. If bleeding continues, Vasopressin 20 units in 100 ml of 5% dextrose may be given over 10 minutes period and repeated every 2-4 hours. It reduces portal venous pressure as a result of mesenteric vasoconstriction. Colicky abdominal pain and coronary vasoconstriction are its side-effects. If G.I. bleeding still persists then it can be controlled by using a Sengstaken – Blackemore tube. The tube possesses two balloons which when inflated exert pressures on varices in the fundus of stomach and lower part of oesophagus. If bleeding still persists emergency meso-caval shunt surgery may be done. Alternative procedure is transhepatic variceal sclerosis by injection human thrombin and gel foam through a catheter introduced into the variceal supply vein (left gastric and short gastric) through portal vein. Patients who survive acute haemorrhage or who have recurrent variceal bleeding, portal systemic shunt surgery or injection sclerotherapy may be instituted Classical porta caval shunt is easier to perform but has the disadvantage of completely stopping hepatic blood flow through portal system and hence runs the risk of high incidence of encephalopathy. Distal splenorenal shunt obviates this problem partly but is more difficult to perform. Recently a new technique of graft interposition splenocaval shunt has been developed in Calcutta and it is easier to perform without much reduction of hepatic blood flow. Alternately, sclerosing agents like ethanolamine oleate or sodium morrhuate may be injected into the oesophageal varices through a needle passed through fiberoptic endoscope. Veins are injected sequentially every one to four weeks. The procedure is not easy to perform and complications include perforation of oesophagus, mediastinitis, aspiration pneumonia, abnormal motility of the oesophagus etc. However endoscopic sclero therapy can not be done when patient is actively bleeding.

Hepatic encephalopathy, though usually terminal, may sometimes be reversible.* Dietary proteins are to be stopped and the bowel is to be emptied of nitrogen containing material by bowel wash. Neomycin 1 gm 4 times a day may be given for one week. All diuretics are to be stopped, fluid and electrolyte balance to be maintained. Lactulose 10-30 ml orally three times a day may be given. Its mechanism of action is not known, but it may facilitate ammonia utilization by gut bacteria by providing a carbohydrate source. Potassium deficiency may be treated by oral use of potassium chloride or administration of fruit juice. Levodopa, a precursor of dopamine can pass blood brain barrier and may be used to increase the cerebral dopaminelevel as there is some suggestion that encephalopathy occurs due to defect, in dopaminergic neurotransmission. However, few patients are benefited with this agent. Bromocriptine, a specific dopamine receptor agonist with a prolonged action is also currently being tried for its treatment.

Specific therapy for cirrhosis is unsatisfactory. Colchicine inhibits assembly of collagen and increase collagenase production. Beneficial results are reported following its use but this is a toxic drug. Corticosteroid therapy in chronic active hepatitis (autoimmune type) is helpful in reducing active hepatic inflammation and collagenesis. Cirrhosis associated with certain diseases are as follows :

### Haemochromatosis

The condition develops following increased iron absorption over many years and is likely to be due to autosomal recessive inheritance. Fibrosis occurs as a result of increased iron deposition in the liver.

* One patient (see fig.16.5) survived five episodes of coma and died during 6th attack due to C.V.A. *(Editor's case)*

Similar changes are also seen in the pancreas, heart and endocrine glands. The patients are usually middle-aged men with pigmentation, hepatomegaly, diminished sexual activities, diabetes. The slaty-gray pigmentation is due to increased melanin in the basal layer or the epidermis. Ascites is usually uncommon and the liver appears enlarged. Though the spleen is palpable but features of portal hypertension are not common. The serum iron is raised (normal 125 mg/dl) and the serum transferrin is about 96% saturated (normally 30%).

Diagnosis can be confirmed by needle biopsy of liver. The iron content of liver is found to be much elevated and hepatocytes will be seen loaded with iron by special staining for iron. Repeated blood letting by venesection (500ml per week) helps in taking out iron from iron storage sites. Oral chelating agent e.g. desferrioxamine may also be used for this condition.

**Wilson's Disease**

Wilson's disease, inherited as autosomal recessive genetic trait may also present as cirrhosis. It is associated with increased deposition of copper in the liver and basal ganglia. Ceruloplasmin, an $\alpha$ 2 globulin responsible for transport of copper in plasma is reduced and the serum copper level is also reduced. Cirrhosis develops insidiously and may or may not be associated with neurological manifestations of basal ganglia lesion. The patients are usually young, and clinically present with vascular spiders, splenomegaly, ascites and portal hypertension. The copper content of liver biopsy material is much elevated (normally $< 55 \mu g/g$ dry weight of liver tissue). Penicillamine which chelates copper and increases it urinary excretion is used for its treatment 1-2 gm of D-penicillamine hydrochloride orally in four divided doses, may be used for a prolonged period. The drug may produce toxic reactions, e.g. rashes, aplastic anaemia, leucopenia, proteinuria and S.L.E. like syndrome. The drug need to be continued throughout life and doses should be adjusted depending upon the response.

**Biliary Cirrhosis**

Biliary cirrhosis is a condition which develops following chronic inflammatory lesions of the interlobular bile ducts, bile ductules and periportal liver cells. True cirrhosis develops late and usually takes a micronodular feature. It could be primary in which chronic granulomatous inflammation and damage of the interlobular bile ductules are followed by ductular proliferation, scarring and cirrhosis. The aetiology of the condition is unknown, but immunological mechanisms are related to initiation of the bile duct injury. It can be secondary to obstruction of the common bile duct for a prolonged period. The clinical features of impaired bile excretion (cholestasis) include progressive and prolonged jaundice, protracted itching, development of xanthelasma, steatorrhoea, hepatomegaly and marked elevation of serum cholesterol and alkaline phosphatase. a patient suffering from primary biliary cirrhosis is usually a female between ages of 40 and 59 frequently presenting with pruritus without jaundice. Jaundice may never develop but usually appears within 6 months to two years. In some cases jaundice and pruritus develop simultaneously. Liver is usually enlarged and spleen palpable. In contrast to many other forms of cirrhosis, there are few other signs of liver cell failure except biliary excretion. Steatorrhoea and associated malabsorption of fat soluble vitamins may lead to diarrhoea, purpura and osteomalacia. Associated other diseases include rheumatoid arthritis, dermato-myositis, sjogren's syndrome, autoimmune thyroiditis and finger clubbing.

Life expectancy is 6-7 years after the condition is diagnosed. Serum IgM level is very high and mitochondrial antibodies are detected in the serum. Treatment is mainly symptomatic and supported by use of intramuscular injection of fat soluble vitamins and calcium supplement. Pruritus is treated by use of cholestyramine. Corticosteroids are contraindicated because of their effect on bone in producing further demineralization. D. Penicillamine is used to reduce liver copper level (as it is elevated in primary biliary cirrhosis) and its affection on the immune system. Portal systemic shunts may be carried out to those who present with bleeding from oesophageal varices as the operation is usually well tolerated by the patients.

### Cardiac Cirrhosis

Long-standing right-sided cardiac failure in patients suffering from valvular heart diseases, constrictive pericarditis or cor pulmonale may lead to cirrhosis. The pathologic features are characterised by fibrosis around central vein extending outwards as linear scars ultimately producing nodular regeneration and cirrhosis. The liver is found to be enlarged firm and irregular. The clinical condition is associated with ascites and peripheral oedema. Mild abnormalities of liver function tests may be observed. Bleeding from oesophageal varices is rarely seen. Proper diagnosis and treatment of underlying cardiovascular disease would prevent the occurrence of cardiac cirrhosis.

### Indian Childhood Cirrhosis

This type of cirrhosis occurs between the ages of 1 to 5 years and is encountered in the Indian subcontinent. There is a tendency for affection of more than one child in the same or closely related families. The aetiology of the condition is not known. On histology, the liver cells appear swollen with disintegration of cytoplasm which appears as dense eosinophilic mass with fuzy outlines.

Mallory's hyaline is common and occasionally abundant. Lymphocytes, neutrophils and histiocytes pervades through the entire lobule. Diffuse fibrosis involving most of the lobules throughout the liver may lead to splenomegaly and portal hypertension. The cirrhosis is typically of micronodular type. Abundant ductular proliferation is observed between the nodules. Most cases occur in lower middle class families where nutritional deficiency was not obvious. The pre-cirrhotic symptoms complex is characterised by restlessness, irritability, excessive crying, disturbed sleep and sticky whitish bulky stool in the child. Mild hepatomegaly is present at this stage. Subsequently abdominal distension, fever and hepatosplenomegaly develop. Liver appears hard with sharp margin. Jaundice is seen in two-third of cases. As the disease advances, often rapidly, jaundice increases and ascites develops and death occurs from hepatic coma. Gastro-intestinal haemorrhage due to portal hypertension, features of severe hepatocellular dysfunction like gynaecomastia, spider nevi etc. are very rare. Varying grades of liver dysfunction is noticed in liver function tests, but nothing is characteristic. Liver biopsy provides confirmation of diagnosis. Treatment of the condition is mainly symptomatic. (Refer to special chapter on this subject.).

### Non-cirrhotic Fibrosis of Liver

Several conditions, either congenital or acquired may be associated with fibrosis of liver. Schistosoma mansoni infection may produce granulomatous and fibrotic lesions along the portal tracts. Non-cirrhotic portal fibrosis leading to obstruction of portal venules and portal hypertension occur in this condition. There is no regenerating liver nodule in the condition and hepato-splenomegaly occurs.

Non-cirrhotic portal hypertension associated with large splenomegaly has been noticed in India and other countries for many years. Non-cirrhotic portal fibrosis has been recognised as an important cause of this condition. The patient usually gives a long history of splenomegaly with or without repeated attacks of haematemesis and/or melena. They are frequently associated with hepatomegaly though ascites, jaundice or other clinical evidence of hepatocellular failure is uncommon. The liver function tests also do not reveal gross abnormality. Splenoportographic picture reveals frequently, a distinct pattern characterised by truncated appearance of large branches of portal vein having significant disparity between the large sized main intrahepatic branches of the portal vein and its branches of the second or third order. The histology of the liver shows periportal condensation of reticulin with or without spreading out of bands of condensed fibres thick or thin, straight or curved. Distal splenoportal shunt (warren) or graft interposition splenorenal shunt is ideal for prevention of death from gastrointestinal haemorrhage. Results of endoscopic oesophageal sclerotherapy have not yet been evaluated.

# INDIAN CHILDHOOD CIRRHOSIS

*G.C. MOOKERJEE*
*ML. SAPRA*

## Introduction

The title of Indian Childhood Cirrhosis (I.C.C) was coined by late Dr. S. T. Achar (1960) to include cirrhotic disease of liver in children which has been previously described in India under various names like—infantile cirrhosis, intercellular hepatic fibrosis and sub-acute toxic cirrhosis. Sen (1887) was the first to report this as "Infantile cirrhosis" of India. Hepatic cirrhosis is seen in infants and children, all over the world but the entity described as Indian childhood cirrhosis is encountered only in this country.

The Liver Disease Sub-Committee of ICMR (1955) defined this syndrome as "A disease peculiar to Indian infants and young children with a tendency to run in families and characterised by enlargement of liver (hard in consistency) in early stages. In the late stages splenomegaly, ascites and jaundice are superimposed. The onset is insidious with vague symptomatology. The course is variable, but generally slow and end usually fatal. It's etiology is unknown".

## Incidence and epidemiology

The disease is seen all over India but is more frequent along the Eastern Coast. The incidence is particularly high in strictly vegetarian castes like Hindu Brahmins and Baniyas. In Northern India, however, a particular caste amongst Hindus — the Agarwals are more commonly affected than others. It is uncommon in Muslim and Christian children. More than 30 per cent of children affected are first born. It is more often encountered in middle class families and is not particularly associated with poor socio-economic status. It appears that male children are affected more often than the females. The commonest age group affected is 1 to 3 years. Familial incidence is observed and more than one sibling may be affected.

## Etiology

The exact etiology of the disease is not known. The various factors considered are :

(1) *Climate :* No seasonal variations have been observed and no particular climate can be incriminated.

(2) *Diet and protein malnutrition* : Dietary factors have been blamed from time to time. There is no evidence, however, that the disease is due to protein malnourishment. Kwashiorkor does not lead to cirrhosis. Vegetarian diet has been blamed but no proof has been recorded. The prevalence of this disease in India and its absence in other countries, with similar climatic conditions and dietary deficiencies, is also against the possibility of malnourishment playing direct etiological role.

(3) *Viral hepatitis :* It is suspected that the condition may be a sequelae of viral hepatitis in infants because history of jaundice with fever suggestive of viral hepatitis may be obtained in a considerable number of cases. Therefore it was concluded in some uncontrolled observations that a few infants of viral hepatitis when followed up developed cirrhosis.

The points against viral hepatitis as the aetiological factor however are convincing :

(1) I.C.C. occurs more of less exclusively in India while viral hepatitis amongst children is common all over the world.

(2) The histological features of I.C.C. are distinct and do not resemble viral hepatitis at any stage.

(3) Epidemic of viral hepatitis in Delhi (1955-56) was not followed by any significant rise of childhood cirrhosis (Ramalingaswamy : Achar).

(4) The role of hepatotoxic agents : The histological picture of childhood cirrhosis resembles

alcoholic cirrhosis to a great extent except for absence of fatty change. It has been clearly demonstrated now that liver damage in alcoholic hepatitis is at least partly due to direct hepatotoxic action of alcohol and not due to induced malnutrition. In these children since there is no question of alcohol being the responsible hepatotoxic agent, some other hepatotoxic substances, yet unidentified, may be responsible for liver damage and cirrhosis. Toxic products in bush tea producing veno-occlusive disease and fungal toxins like aflatoxins have been considered but not proved.

(5) Genetic factors : The high familial incidence points towards the possibility genetic defect. No definite inherited metabolic defect or chromosomal abnormality has been demonstrated. Blood group incompatibilities, Rh-factor abnormalities, defect in maltose metabolism, ceruloplasmin abnormalities have all been excluded.

(6) Tuberculosis : Tuberculosis can lead to hepatomegaly but not Indian childhood cirrhosis. It should be remembered however, that there are more chances of 'drug' jaundice and serum hepatitis in tuberculosis. Tuberculosis may also be present coincidentally with Indian childhood cirrhosis.

(7) $\alpha$-Fetoprotein (AFP) : Nayak et at (1972) have demonstrated persistence or re-appearance of $\alpha$-fetoproteins in high percentage of cases of I.C.C. These proteins normally disappear from blood a few weeks after birth. Normally the foetal hepatocytes undergo transformation into adult type, just before or immediately after birth and stop further synthesis and secretion of AFP. So it is postulated that in infants who develop I.C.C., this transformation is defective and their hepatocytes are vulnerable. AFP however has been demonstrated previously in relation to hepatoma in a large number of cases.

(8) Autoimmunity : Prasad (1968) has demonstrated antibodies against liver tissue in 10 out of 12 cases of ICC and has postulated that it may be an autoimmune disease. Others have not found similar results.

(9) Defective cellular immunity : Attention on viral hepatitis as an etiological factor has been focused once again by the recent reports that a fair percentage of cases of ICC have Australia antigen in their serum. Chandra (1972) who found 20 per cent of his cases of ICC positive for Australia antigen has postulated that these cases have defective cellular immunity and are therefore more vulnerable to hepatitis virus. The reports regarding presenee of Australia antigen in cases of ICC are however, rather conflicting and the problem needs further research.

**Pathology**

Morbid anatomy : The liver is usually shrunken in size. It is firm and the surface is smooth, granular or finely nodular. The shape of the liver is maintained and the edges are sharp. The capsule is thickened. The cut surface is generally bile stained and greenish in colour. There is increase in fibrous tissue. The lobular markings may be exaggerated or there may be small nodules measuring 0.5-2 mm in diameter. The gall bladder and biliary passages are normal.

**Histology**

The histological findings at autopsy or on needle biopsy are characteristic and diagnostic of the disease. The main features are :

In the early stages —

(1) There are severe degenerative changes in the cytoplasm of hepatocytes. The nucleus remains intact while the cytoplasm shows vacuolar and granular dissociation.

(2) The cytoplasm shows irregular masses, indistinguishable from 'Mallory hyaline' characteristically seen in alcoholic hepatitis.

(3) There is no significant fatty change.

(4) Reticulin collapse and fibroblastic reaction are prominent giving rise to increase of intralobular connective tissue.

(5) Regeneration of hepatocytes is minimal or absent.

(6) The portal tracts are prominent and show round cell infiltration.

(7) There is no bile duct proliferation.

In late stages when the clinical disease is well established, the damage to liver cells goes on progressively increasing. The liver cells are disrupted and merge with each other. 'Mallory hyaline' is seen in large majority of cells and fibrosis is pronounced. Liver cell regeneration is inadequate and only small regeneration is inadequate and only small regenerating nodules may be seen here or there. Bile duct proliferation and biliary stasis may be seen at this stage.

**Clinical features**

For descriptive purpose, the clinical features are divided into 4 stages. It must be emphasized however that these stages merge into each other imperceptibly and it is not always possible to decide the stage of the disease in an individual case.

**Stage I (Early stage or stage or onset) :** The symptoms are vague, the appetite may be poor or rarely voracious. There may be diarrhoea or constipation, flatulence and abdominal distension. Low grade pyrexia is usually present. Irritability and peevishness may be present. Liver is enlarged and firm but there is no jaundice in majority of cases. Most liver function tests are not deranged much at this stage. Only liver biopsy may show evidence of hepatocellular necrosis.

**Stage II (Intermediate stage) :** In addition to the above features, there is now evidence of hyperdynamic circulation with tachycardia. Palmar erythema may be present. The liver enlarges further, is firm and has got a 'leafy' edge. Spleen may be slightly enlarged. There is still no jaundice and ascites. The liver function tests now show alteration of albumin globulin ratio.

**Stage III (Late stage) :** The child becomes extremely irritable; the abdomen is distended. Superficial abdominal veins are prominent. There is marked wasting with appearance of oedema and ascites. Spleen further increases in size. Liver may shrink but is still palpable and is hard with a sharp knife like edge. Icterus is present and the patient may develop epistaxis, haematemesis and melena. The stools are clay coloured.

The urine at this stage shows bile pigments, bile salts and traces of albumin. Liver function tests are markedly deranged. The flocculation tests become positive. SGOT, SGPT and alkaline phosphatase levels are raised. Liver biopsy reveals changes of well established disease. Splenic pressure is raised and splenoportogram shows evidence of portal hypertension and collateral circulation.

**Stage IV (Terminal stage) :** It is the end stage in which the condition of the child deteriorates progressively. The jaundice deepens, ascites increases, generalised anasarca may appear, fever persists and bleeding tendencies may be pronounced. Foetor hepaticus and flapping tremors appear and the patient passes into hepatic coma. The cause of death may be hepatic coma, gastrointestinal haemorrhage or secondary infection.

Progression from one stage to another varies from case to case. In some patients, the speed of evolution is very fast with rapid clinical deterioration leading to fulminant hepatic failure while in others the disease advances slowly with phases of remissions and exacerbations for years.

**Diagnosis**

The condition should be kept in mind and presence of an enlarged liver with a firm 'Leafy' edge in an Indian child between 1 to 3 years of age should arouse a strong suspicion. The diagnosis in early stages is rather difficult but once features like jaundice, splenomegaly, ascites and prominent abdominal veins appear, it is not difficult. The derangement of different liver functions has already been described under various stages.

A conclusive diagnosis of ICC can, however, be only established by a needle biopsy of the liver. The histological changes have already been described under histology. The procedure is simple and is safe in experienced hands.

**Treatment**

Since the exact etiology is not known, treatment is mainly symptomatic. The diet should be well balanced and nutritious. Vitamin supplements are required only when the child is not eating well or there is clinical evidence of deficiency. The activity should be moderately restricted. Hepatotoxic drugs and sedatives must be avoided. Corticosteroids have been tried but results are not satisfactory.

Complications should be treated as and when they develop. Ascites well require salt restriction, and oral diuretics. Mercurials are avoided. Potassium supplements must be given along with oral diuretics to avoid hypokalaemia which may precipitate coma. Abdominal paracentesis should be avoided as much as possible.

Bleeding from varices should be treated by supportive measures and blood transfusions. If the bleeding is not controlled within 12-24 hours, then one may consider use of Sengstaken — Blakemore tube (children size). It has got hazards of its own and is not recommended by many people. Pitressin has been tried and found useful by some workers but exact dosage schedule has to be modified depending on correct weight. Hypothermia has also been tried in some centres and found useful. If the bleeding cannot be stopped by above measures then emergency transthoracic ligation of varices or shunt surgery may be attempted. Definitive treatment for portal hypertension consists of decompression of portal venous system by shunt surgery. Management of hepatic coma is on lines similar to those in adults.

**Prognosis**

The prognosis is generally poor although it is claimed that a portion of cases may recover if diagnosed in early stages. Once jaundice and significant hepatomegaly appear, majority of cases end fatally.

---

[This chapter has been updated from the book on "Diseases of the liver by the authors originally published by Current Tech. Lit. Pvt. Ltd., Bombay, 1973].

## HEPATIC TUMOURS

*G.C. MOOKERJEE*
*M.L. SAPRA*

The only primary liver tumour which is common is primary hepato-cellular carcinoma. Haemangiomas are the only benign tumours encountered **frequently**. Metastatic tumours of the liver are however very common.

## HEPATOCELLULAR CARCINOMA (HCC)

**Incidence**

The incidence varies in different parts of the world. It is more common amongst males than females. It may be due to the fact that chronic hepatitis is due to virus B infection, alcoholism and hepatic cirrhosis are more frequently seen amongst males than females. The age incidence varies but the disease is prevalent even at relatively younger age group amongst African and Asian population.

**Aetiology**

The exact aetiology of the condition remains to be established. The disease is however seen more frequently in cirrhotics and cases with hepatitis B-virus infection. Other aetiological factors incriminated are plant and fungal metabolities like aflatoxins, contraceptive pills, androgenic-anabolic steroids, $alpha_1$ antitrypsin deficiency, irradiation and chronic liver disease with raised alpha-fetoprotein levels.

**Pathology**

There is usually marked enlargement of the liver. There are multiple nodules present throughout the liver and often one of the nodules is bigger than the others. The nodularity is partially due to tumour deposits and partially due to underlying hepatic cirrhosis. Sometimes a large tumour may be found replacing one lobe of the liver. At times there may be diffuse nodularity of the liver and it may not be possible to differentiate and portal vein is very common and tumour masses may spread to the inferior venacava and right atrium. Secondaries are common in the lungs and intraabdominal lymph nodes. Rarely, secondaries may develop in the brain, bones, kidneys and spleen.

Microscopically the characteristic pattern is trabecular although sometimes acinar, spindle cell, sclerosing or bizarre patterns may be encountered. The HCC cells always produce bile and these tumours are highly vascular.

**Clinical features**

The onset may be insidious or sudden. Generally the presentation is with right upper abdominal pain, weight loss and tender hepatomegaly. Fever is common often low grade and there is swelling of abdomen due to hepatomegaly and ascites. Jaundice may or may not be present in early stages. Deep jaundice is a late event.

Features of underlying chronic liver disease particularly hepatic cirrhosis may dominate the clinical picture and sudden deterioration in such cases may indicate development of HCC. A bruit is heard over the liver in a large number of cases and a friction rub over the liver may be heard due to perihepatitis. So an enlarged liver without obvious cause needs careful investigations (Fig. 16.8)..

**Differential diagnosis**

It is important to consider other treatable diseases in the differential diagnosis and diagnose them correctly rather than misdiagnosing them as HCC.

The common conditions to be considered in the differential diagnosis are hydatid cyst, amoebic liver abscess, tuberculomas and the storage diseases.

**Investigations**

Biochemical changes may abe due to underlying chronic hepato cellular damage only. There is increase in levels of globulin. Serum alkaline phosphatase and transaminase levels are raised.

Raised serum $alpha_1$ – fetoprotein levels although seen transiently in other conditions is virtually diagnostic of HCC if the values are sufficiently high (above 100 mg/100 dl).

HBsAg may be present in the serum. Hepatitis B-Virus (HBV) DNA are also detectable in

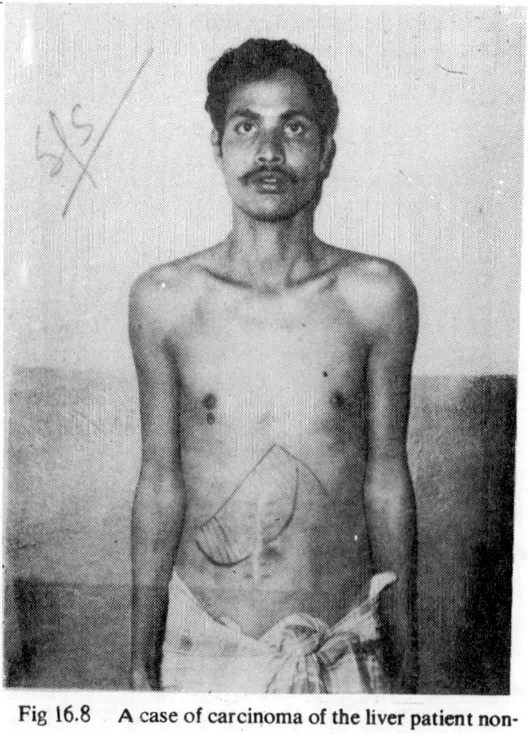

Fig 16.8 A case of carcinoma of the liver patient non-alcoholic; no history of jaundice *(Editor's case)* carcinoma confirmed by histopathology.

hepatocytes and cancer cells. There may be slight increase in leucocytic count and Hb levels.

Coagulation defects may be observed due to decreased fibrinolytic activity.

Localisation of liver tumours has become rather easy these days with the help of radioisotopic scanning, CT-Scan and ultrasonography. These techniques not only help in localising the hepatic tumours but also are useful in selecting liver biopsy sites and follow-up.

Hepatic arteriography is helpful in diagnosis as well as management of these tumours. Study of liver histology is absolutely essential for diagnosis and liver biopsy is therefore an essential investigation in all cases.

Biopsy can be taken under vision at laparoscopy or ultrasonogram from suspicious areas.

**Prognosis**

HCC is a highly malignant tumour and survival is usually a few months after diagnosis. Prognosis in Hbs Ag positive cases is particularly poor.

**Treatment**

Localized encapsulated tumours confined to only one lobe of the liver may be resected. Number of such cases is, however, very small. Transplantation of liver is being tried but results are poor. Majority of the patients have to be put on chemotherapy. Drug commonly used is Adriamycin (Daunorubicin). Response to therapy is monitored by plasma alpha-fetoprotein levels.

An alternative drug is 5-fluorouracil. Combination chemotherapy has not proved useful. Chemotherapy may be given intraarterially by selective catheterization of hepatic artery since the tumour is supplied blood mainly by this artery. This reduces systemic side effects. X-irradiation either alone or in combination with chemotherapy may reduce pain and decrease the size of the liver but is generally not used because of side-effects. In fact the results also are not consistent.

HBV is now available and its use should be a preventive measure.

## METASTATIC TUMOURS OF LIVER

Liver is involved in large number of cancers particularly when the drainage is by portal veins. The common sites for primary are stomach, pancreas, breast, lungs and colon. Prostate, thyroid, kidneys, oesophagus and gall bladder are other primary sites. The metastatic tumours of liver are much more common than primary HCC.

There may be one or two small nodules but generally the whole liver is full of metastases. The only physical sign may be hepatomegaly. Jaundice may or may not be present. It is particularly common when the primary is in the pancreas. Ascites is encountered very often but oesophageal varices are rare. Clinical features due to the primary tumour may dominate the clinical picture but quite often hepatic metastasis may be the first manifestation, of a malignant growth. "Occult" primaries are particularly common in the pancreas, stomach or lung. In some cases, however, there may be no symptoms due to hepatic involvement even when extensive metastasis are present in the liver. A good percentage of cases with hepatic metastases may die without hepatic symptoms and signs. A bruit or friction rub may be heard over the liver as in case of primary HCC.

The size, growth pattern, consistency and vascular pattern varies with the source of primary tumour. The whole liver may be involved or only a part of it may be effected. Complication due to necrosis and fibrosis is a helpful diagnostic feature because it is generally not seen in primary liver tumours. The histology depends upon the source of the primary and generally the features of the primary growth are retained. Majority of metastasis are adeno carcinomas or anaplastic carcinomas. Involvement of hepatic veins leads to abdominal pain, massive hepatomegaly, ascites and extensive spread to lungs. In a very small percentage of cases, calcification may occur although it is very rare.

The blood supply to metastatic tumours of the liver is mainly arterial as is the case in primary HCC.

Although involvement of periportal lymph nodes is quite common, this is the cause of icterus in only a small number of cases. Common causes of icterus in these cases are replacement of liver tissue by metastases and involvement of biliary ducts by the tumour.

The main diagnostic aids are liver biopsy, hepatic scan, ultrasonography and CT-scan. The liver biopsy may be done under vision on laparoscopy or ultrasonography. Aspiration cytology is as useful technique but is not practised much at present. A search for primary should always be made. At times even detailed investigations may not reveal the primary growth and it may be detected only at autopsy.

The biochemical tests are not of much use in diagnosis of hepatic metastases. The only abnormality frequently encountered is raised serum alkaline phosphatase. Th . however, is not seen in all cases.

**Prognosis**

It depends upon the site of primary malignancy and extent of hepatic involvement. Generally most of the patients with hepatic metastases die within one year.

**Treatment**

It is very unsatisfactory. Chemotherapy is used but the results are very unsatisfactory. The drug commonly used is 5-fluorouracil (5-Fu). Combination chemotherapy with cyclophosphamide, methotrexate, vincristine and 5-Fu gives no better results. The drugs may be given intra-arterially by catheter inserted into the hepatic artery to reduce systemic side-effects.

**Secondary Tumours** : Secondary metastatic tumours of the liver are 25-30 times commoner than primary tumours of the liver. The metastases may come from

a) Organs drained by the portal vein e.g. the gastro-intestinal tract, pancreas, gall bladder. Rarely tumours of uterus, ovaries, prostate and bladder may involve contiguous organs drained by portal vein and produce metastases in the liver.

b) Arterial emboli e.g. breasts, lungs, thyroid, adrenals, kidneys.

c) Direct spread from contiguous organs e.g. stomach, kidneys, gall bladder.

The incidence of secondary metastases is so high that about 30 per cent of all cases dying of carcinoma from any site, develop hepatic metastasis. The liver is markedly enlarged. It is hard in consistency and may be tender. The secondaries are usually superficial and it is possible in large majority of cases to palpate the umbilicated metastatic nodules. A friction rub may be heard over the liver. Jaundice is not marked unless secondaries in the porta-hepatis produce cholestasis, Malaise, lassitude and emaciation are usually present. Ascites and oedema may develop due to involvement of hepatic veins and inferior vena cava. Spleen may be enlarged although portal hypertension is generally not marked. Hepatic failure is rare.

Clinical features due to primary growth may at times be minimal and even difficult to diagnose.

Liver function tests are only mildly deranged. Serum bilirubin above 2 mg/100 ml indicates obstruction of major bile ducts. Alkaline phosphatase levels may be quite high (over 100 KA units).

Electrophoresis may reveal raised $\alpha_2$ and gamma-globulins. Leucocytosis is quite common.

The diagnosis may be confirmed by liver biopsy, peritoneoscopy or scintiscanning.

Special investigations depending upon the site suspected will be required to find out the site for the primary growth. In a patient with a known carcinoma, development of hepatomegaly abnormal BSP retention, raised serum bilirubin, aminotransferases and alkaline phosphatase and urobilinogenuria indicate hepatic metastases.

The treatment is only palliative because the metastases are generally multiple and resection is not possible. Analgesics and sedatives may be given to make the patient comfortable. Hepatic artery perfusion may be used to administer drugs like mitomycin – C for better local action. The response is however is however generally poor. Hepatic transplantation is still an experimental procedure in such cases.

## DISEASES OF GALL BLADDER

*G.C. MOOKERJEE*

Surgical textbooks should be consulted for details but important information essential for general practitioners is presented.

The gall bladder is a small egg-shaped (often described as pear shaped) organ with capacity of holding about 50 to 60 ml of bile. Its fundus is just behind the tip of right 9th rib. The liver has two hepatic ducts which come out at porta hepatis and join to form common hepatic duct. The common hepatic duct, the hepatic artery and portal vein lies intimately together, wrapped by the free edge of lesser sac. The common hepatic duct receives the cystic duct to form the common bile duct, which passes behind 1st part the duodenum finally opens in the inner aspect of the 2nd part of duodenal wall, where a muscular sphincter is present, known as sphincter of Oddi. In this area pancreatic duct also fuses with the common bile duct in the duodenal sub-muscosa. This forms a papilla like structure, known as ampulla of Vater. (Fig.16.9).

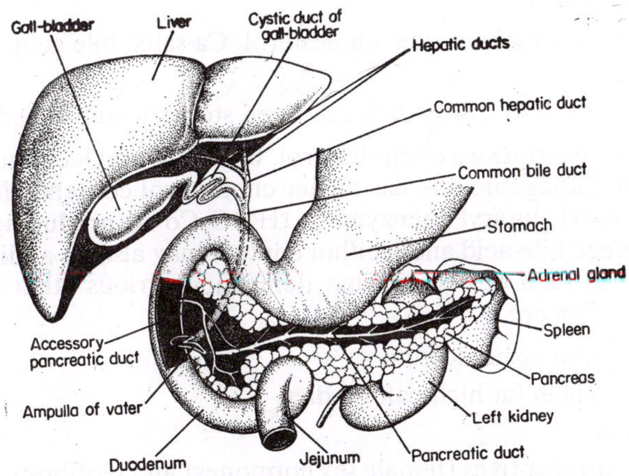


**Fig.16.9 : Diagramatic anatomy of the relations of gall bladder, duodenum and pancreatic head.**

The liver secretes about one to two litres of bile in 24 hours and it is stored in gall-bladder, where it is concentrated about 10 times. Gall bladder tone is chiefly controlled by cholecystokinin from duodenal mucosa, when the acid chyme enters duodenum from pyloric end of stomach. Drugs e.g. morphine, pethidine and pentazocaine causes contraction of sphincter of Oddi, while glyceryl trinitrate relaxes it.

### Congenital Disorders

Congenital anomalies of G.B. and bile ducts are not uncommon. These include anomalies of shape, size and position.

(1) Pharygena cap — A fold, separating GB into two parts (fundus from body)
(2) Rudimentary or giant G.B.
(3) Diverticula formation
(4) Floating GB — risk of torsion or volvulus
(5) Left sided G.B. — under left lobe of liver

**Anomalies of bile ducts**

(1) Congenital biliary stasis or hypoplasia of extra-hepatic ducts causing deep jaundice of newborn is due to obstruction. Stool is pale, jaundice very deep and progressive in the first few weeks of newborn's life. Treatment is expert surgical relief by entero-biliary anastomosis.

(2) Congenital choledochal cysts—chronic reflux of pancreatic juice into biliarv tree causing cholangitis. Treatment is surgical. Operations are difficult. The patients ultimately develop chronic cholangitis, hepatic fibrosis and portal hypertension.

**Gall Stones**

Gall stones are fairly common among elderly people above the age of 40 years more common in females who are obese. It is mentioned that one million new cases occur in U.S.A. every year (Harrison 1983). In tropics also it is fairly common disease, in elderly affecting both lean and obese but female sex predominating.

The most important clinical point to remember is that GB pain due to stones, may be confused particularly with coronary heart disease and vice versa. Both diseases may co-exist. Even chronic cholecystitis may behave in similar manner.

Gall stones are of two type :

(1) Mixed stones (80%) which contain cholesterol, Ca-salts, bile acid, pigments, proteins and lecithin etc.

(2) Cholesterol stones (20%) : Tiny dark coloured stones which may fill up the GB.

Normally relative concentrations of cholesterol, bile acids and lecithin are important to maintain healthy G.B. Lithogenic bile has higher cholesterol content which is due to increased activity of hydroxymethyl-glutaryl-coenzyme A (HMG-Co A) producing excessive cholesterol. On the contrary, reduced bile acid and lecithin content may also be additional factors. Bile acid synthesis may also be at fault due to enzyme deficiency various other factors predisposing to mixed gall stone formation are :

(1) Genetic factors — enzyme defects
(2) Obesity — due to high fat high caloric diet
(3) Diabetes mellitus
(4) Drugs—Oral contraceptives (female sex hormones) and clofibrate therapy
(5) Malabsorption syndrome
(6) Chronic GB disease

Pigment stones however may be due to genetic factors, chronic haemolysis and chronic GB disease. Symptom of cholelithiasis produce varied symptoms due to obstruction or inflammation of biliary passages. Though gall stone colic may be quite severe yet it is interesting that sometimes it remains silent or may produce mild upper gastro-intestinal symptoms (so called flatulent dyspepsia). Those are discussed in the chapter on chronic cholecystitis.

**Diagnosis of Gall-stones**

(1) Plain X-ray abdomen

(2) Oral cholecystogram — always successful if the stones are radiolucent. It can not be done if serum bilirubin is above 2 mg%. It is unsuccessful if there is defective absorption of dye tablets.

(3) Ultrasound study of G.B. – extremely valuable. Even small stones are detected. Facilities not available except in big cities.

(4) Radio-isotopic scanning – rarely required in routine practice.

### Treatment of Gall Stone

Patients who are having symptoms due to gallstone should undergo cholecystectomy. Treatment of silent gall stones may have to be decided on other factors e.g. age, general condition, presence of complications, e.g. I.H.D., diabetes mellitus, hypertension etc. Some patients may refuse surgery as medical treatment of gall stones is now a possibility but prolonged treatment is necessary. Stones may form again on cessation of therapy.

### Medical treatment

Oral therapy with chenodeoxycholic acid (CDCA) or urodeoxycholic acid (UDCA) may be successful in completely dissolving or partially dissolving radiolucent gall-stones in about fifty percent of patients. However it is not so effective in pigment stones, calcified (radio opaque) stones or in very large stones. Dose of CDCA should not be less than 15 mg per kg. day. It is expensive in the longrun as treatment may have to be continued for one to three years. Food & Drug Administration (USA) has not yet officially approved use of this drug till 1983. In India it is now available. UDCA is given in dosage of 5-10 mg/Kg of body weight. It is reported to act faster than CDCA. Now a days follow up is easy by ultrasonograms.

## ACUTE CHOLECYSTITIS

### Introduction

It is an acute inflammation of GB usually associated with obstruction of its outlet commonly due to stones, otherwise due to mucus plug or new growth. Diabetic patients are specially susceptible. Possibly it is initiated by chemical irritation from very concentrated bile, later organisms e.g. Esch coli or strep faecalis may be involved. Rarely gas-forming organisms are involved causing emphysematous cholecystitis.

The inflammation may be mild, catarrhal or severe in degree leading to pus formation i.e. empyema of the gall bladder.

### Clinical Features

The patients are usually fat but not necessarily sterile females. Age group usually above thirty but cases are occurring in twenties also.

The presenting feature is sudden onset of acute right upper abdominal pain also involving epigastric region. Patient is usually restless, with sweating; vomiting is common; fever develops varying from 37.8° to 39° C. High swinging temperature may occur in empyema of G.B. Mild jaundice may develop suggesting common duct obstruction.

Pain is usually continuous and not really colicky and may last for hours, till relieved by strong analgesics.

Increasing pain, high temperature, abdominal muscle guard tachycardia and high leucocytosis proclaims empyema of G.B. with risk of perforation or peritonitis. On examination abdominal tenderness and varying degree of rigidity is present. Deep breathing causes catch-like pain in the G.B. region (Murphy's sign). Sometimes G.B. is palpable.

### Laboratory Findings

(1) **Blood** – usually reveals polymorph leucocytosis. Serum bilirubin may be raised. Serum amylase level may be raised occasionally.

(2) Urine – may show bilirubinuria.

(3) Plain X-ray abdomen (Scout film) – taken in sitting posture may reveal gallstones.

(4) Ultrasonography – is extremely helpful in diagnosis.

**Diagnosis**

Diagnosis is clinical but in some cases laboratory findings are helpful, especially ultrasonography which can be easily done at bedside without any discomfort to the patients, but is not available in our rural practice.

Acute cholecystitis is to be differentiated from :

(1) Acute myocardial infarction — History along with SGOT (AST), SGPT (ALT) and E.C.G. are helpful;

(2) Acute pancreatitis — Serum amylase is very high. Vomiting a prominent feature. Common in alcoholics;

(3) Appendicitis — classical signs (Mc Burney's point) P.R. examination and development of symptoms are useful;

(4) Intestinal obstruction

History of coliky pain, vomiting, generalised abdominal discomfort, auscultatory findings and visible peristalsis (if present) are helpful.

(5) Right-sided renal colic will usually present abnormal urine (especially RBC's),plain X-ray abdomen may reveal the stone. Sonogram is very helpful.

(6) Pleurisy (right basal) may be confusing. Pleural rub - if detected helps in diagnosis.

(7) Acute intermittent porphyria — check urine for porphobilinogen.

**Treatment**

(1) Bed rest.

(2) Relief of pain by analgesics. Inj. pentazocaine 30 mg given by IM injection.

It is better than pethidine or morphine as these drugs cause spasm of sphincter of oddi.

(3) Naso — gastric tubal aspiration should be done initially and oral therapy discontinued.

(4) I.V. fluids are required to maintain fluid — electrolyte balance.

(5) Control of infection should be done by parenteral Co-trimoxazole or an antibiotic e.g. gentamycin or gabriomycin as bacteria involved are usually gram-negative, combination of drugs may be justified in severe cases. Chloramphenicol is usually avoided for its well-known though rare risk of bone marrow depression, but can be used if alternatives are not suitable.

Surgical consultation is recommended as ultimately surgery may be needed. Emergency cholecystectomy may be necessary if there is empyema or impending perforation. Otherwise cholecystectomy may be planned after a few weeks. Mortality of emergency cholecystectomy is higher, particularly in elderly with uncontrolled hypertensive, ischaemic heart disease and diabetic subjects.

## CHRONIC CHOLECYSTITIS

This is a common disease of the elderly which is almost always associated with gall-stones. It is better to refer these cases to surgical colleagues for operative treatment.

If not operated, a stone may be dislodged and cause obstruction of common bile-duct leading to obstructive jaundice.

It may also lead to acute pancreatitis. Very rarely a large stone may pass into small intestine and cause obstruction at the terminal ileum.

Those who continue to live with chronic cholecystitis suffer due to flatulent dyspepsia often called gall-bladder dyspepsia until one of the above complications supervenes.

*Non-calculous cholecystitis*

It may occur due to B. typhosum, Cl. Welchii, or in patients of diabetes mellitus and prolonged steroid therapy.

*Cholesterosis of G.B.*

This is due to lipoid deposits in mucosa of G.B. causing mucosal thickening known as cholesterosis, often detected during cholecystectomy; usually stones are present.

*Adenomyosis of G.B.*

It is hyperplastic condition of gall-bladder mucosa, usually detected by cholecystography. Gall-stone may be associated.

*Post-operative complications of G.B.*

In some cases symptoms of G.B. dyspepsia may persist even after cholecystectomy. These cases require thorough reinvestigation to exclude stricture or left over stones in common bile duct.

Some of these cases are considered functional. The term biliary dyskinesia is often awarded to this syndrome.

*Sclerosing cholangitis*

It is a fibrotic obliteration of larger bile ducts occurring after GB surgery of associated with ulcerative colitis or retroperitoneal fibrosis.

*Choledochal cyst*

A palpable mass is often felt in the right hypochondrium, jaundice or abdominal pain which calls attention to this rare condition. Treatment is surgical.

## CARCINOMA OF GB

Presentation is like that of a chronic GB disease, associated with rapid loss of weight anaemia and jaundice.

A mass is usually palpable, when the disease too advanced for useful surgery. Therefore all cases of suspected GB disease should be fully investigated early and surgical consultation is mandatory.

## DISEASES OF THE PANCREAS

*G.C. MOOKERJEE*

The pancreas is a glandular organ which secretes pancreatic juice, essential for digestion but it has a very important endocrine function which regulates carbohydrate metabolism. In addition to glandular acini which secretes pancreatic juice, it contains group of specialised cells called (1) Islets of "langerhans" (beta-cells) which secretes insulin and (2) alpha cells which secretes glucagon.

Both these hormones play important role in carbohydrate metabolism. These endocrine cells constitute about 10% of the whole glandular tissue. Their role in metabolic process has been discussed in the chapter on diabetes mellitus.

The exocrine secretion of pancreas is pancreatic juice which is alkaline (pH 7.5-8.5) containing trypsin, amylase and lipase as well as sodium, potassium and bicarbonates. About one litre of juice is secreted per day and its secretion is controlled by both vagal and hormonal control. Pancreatic disorders may be due to trauma, new growth, inflammation, cyst formation and fibrosis.

Islet cell tumours are special type of benign new growths which may cause severe hypoglycaemia due to hyperinsulinism. Malignant islet cell tumours may produce gastric and other polypeptides causing Zollinger-Ellison syndrome and its variants.

The following types of pancreatitis may be encountered :

(1) Acute pancreatitis

(2) Chronic pancreatitis
(3) Acute recurrent pancreatitis
(4) Chronic recurrent pancreatitis.

## ACUTE PANCREATITIS

### Introduction

An acute abdominal catastrophy which occurs due to autodigestion of the organ itself, due release of its own enzymes into pancreatic tissues.

Age group : Usually middle age and elderly people. Both sexes are affected but in India incidence in females is lower, possibly due to rare alcohol consumption.

### Aetiology

About 50% of the cases are with chronic biliary tract disorders, while 20% cases are associated with chronic alcoholic excess. No cause is often found in many cases. However, acute pancreatitis may be triggered in the following conditions : Abdominal trauma, severe bacterial infection, mumps, ascariasis, carcinoma (pancreatic head) diabetic ketosis, uraemia, hyperlipidaemia. SLE as well as during prolonged therapy with corticosteroids, chlorothiazides, oral contraceptives, azothiaprine and excessive vitamin D injestion. Even tetracylines and sulphonamides have been incriminated. Mechanism of the release of pancreatic enzymes it is not clearly understood.

Obstruction of sphincter of Oddi by stone, tumour, oedema and spasm causing reflex of bile activating pancreatic juice is an old theory which is no more accepted. Possibly varieties of precipitating factors enumerated above may activate the pancreatic enzyme system leading to digestion of cellular membrane and parenchymal cells. There is necrosis and interstitial haemorrhage (acute haemorrhagic pancreatitis). Auto digestion of the gland is due to activation of trypsin and lipase. Alcoholic cellular injury is a possible reason but many heavy alcoholics have lived full lives, dying due to hepatic cirrhosis or a stroke and never has any pancreatitis.

### Clinical Features

1. Onset is with epigastric pain more towards left epigastric region associated with retching, nausea and persistent vomiting.
2. Pain may be initially moderate in degree when the patient may get relief on bending forward ultimately pain becomes extremely severe, radiating to the back, scapular regions, lower abdomen.

   In some case pain is severe even at the onset.
3. Patient may soon develop signs of shock but in some cases shock is the predominant feature with less prominent abdominal pain.
4. Initially there is no abdominal rigidity but it gradually develops as peritoneal irritation supervenes, hence initially it may be mistaken with acute myocardial infarction because of upper abdominal pain, lack of muscle guard and signs of shock.
5. Once the picture is established it mimics any acute abdominal catastrophy. Haemorrhagic ascites may be present.
6. On examination patient looks toxic and pulse and respiration are rapid. Fever may be normal or subnormal with signs of shock. Abdomen distended but is not rigid in initial stage. It is tender all over. Peristaltic sounds are feeble or absent.
7. Left-sided pleural effusion may occur.
8. Cullen's sign is present, which consists of a zone of erythema and cyanosis around the umbilicus.
9. Gray Turner's sign is also noted in some cases which consists of echymoses in the loins. Both Cullen's sign and Grav Turner's sign are indicative of severe necrotic pancreatitis.

*Loewi's mydriatic test* — may be present which consists of dilatation of pupil by local instillation of adrenaline drops.

**Laboratory diagnosis**

BLOOD

1. Serum amylase : It is usually elevated within 48 hours. Normal values are 150 somogyı units (per litre) (or 340 I.U./litre).

   If the level is 1000 Somogyi units, diagnosis is certain. But the level quickly falls. Serum amylase creatinine ratio has no special advantage. Serum lipase also may be raised in 70% cases.
2. Leucocytosis may be present.
3. Level of blood glucose may be elevated.
4. Hypocalcaemia may be present.
5. Serum lipase may be elevated.
6. Serum electrolytes may be abnormal due to fluid-electrolyte imbalance.
7. Liver function tests may be abnormal characterised by :
   (a) Rise in serum bilirubin upto about 4 mg% in some cases;
   (b) Serum alkaline phosphatase and SGPT (ALT) may be increased in early stage;
   (c) Serum albumin may fall.

**Radiology**

Plain X-ray abdomen may show duodeno-jejunal ileus and absence of gas in transverse colon.

Presence of pancreatic calcification and gall bladder stones may be revealed.

A careful gastrografin X-ray of the duodenal loop may show duodenal oedema.

Ultrasonogram may not only reveal swollen pancreas but displaced stomach and duodenum. CT-Scan may show details of pancreatic mass and its surrounding relations but the cost is high. This test is routinely not required.

X-ray chest — may reveal atelectasis or pulmonary oedema.

**E.C.G.**

ECG may show ST — T abnormalities mimicking I.H.D., epigastric pain, shock and these ECG changes may be confused with acute myocardial infarction.

**Treatment**

As surgical consultation is mandatory in all cases of suspected acute abdomen, surgical colleagues should be kept in the picture. When in doubt laparotomy should be done and if the diagnosis is confirmed the abdomen should be closed with drainage. Pancreatic suppuration or pseudopancreatic cyst needs surgery.

The outline of management is as follows :

1) Stop all oral feeds and start continuous naso-gastric suction.
2) Parenteral antibiotics e.g. gentamycin, gabriomycin or chloramphenicol.
3) Inj. pethidine 100 mg or pentazocine 40 mg I.M.
4) Maintain fluid electrolyte balance and supply calories parenterally.
5) Supportive therapy : watch for complications.

# C H A P T E R – 17
# DISORDERS OF THE RESPIRATORY SYSTEM

## INTRODUCTION TO RESPIROLOGY

*G.C. MOOKERJEE*

Respiratory diseases may be classified as follows from the practitioner's view point :

(1) **Diseases of upper respiratory tract e.g. :**

Common cold or acute Naso-pharyngitis
Sinusitis
Tonsillitis
Pharyngitis
Laryngitis and other disorders including neoplastic growth

Some of them are very common in clinical practice while infections of upper respiratory tract are often self-limited but it is often forgotten that a badly treated sore throat may lead to a life-long disability, e.g. rheumatic fever or glomerulonephritis. Presence of $\beta$-haemolytic streptococci in particular may be serious. Children suffering from sore throat need special care.

(2) **Diseases of lower respiratory tract e.g. :**

Acute bronchitis
Broncho-pneumonia
Pneumonias
Lung abscess
Bronchiectasis
Chronic obstructive airway diseases (COAD)
Bronchial Asthma
Pulmonary eosinophilia
Tuberculosis
Disease of pleura
Pulmonary neoplasms
Pulmonary mycosis
Parasitic affections
Vascular disorders of lung, e.g. pulmonary-embolism & infarction.
Diffuse alveolitis and honey comb lung.

(3) **Disorders affecting the thoracic cage :**

Kyphoscoliosis, ankylosing-spondylosis, ascending paralysis, poliomyelitis causing ventilatory inadequacy.

(4) **Pulmonary affections due to diseases of other systems**

Pulmonary heart disease (cor pulmonale), collagen diseases, rheumatoid arthritis, sarcoidosis, developmental anomalies of lung.

(5) **Ventilatory problems**

These may be due to non-availability of adequate oxygen due to atmospheric pollution, oxygen lack or pulmonary disorders ultimately ending in respiratory failure. Causes may be :

High altitude
Deep-sea diving
Drowning
Laryngeal obstruction
Inhalation of vomit or food bolus (Dinner in wrong hole)
Neuromuscular weakness, e.g. poliomyelitis Landry's paralysis or myaesthenia gravis).
C.O.P.D. including industrial lung diseases.

(6) **Trauma :**

Blast injury of the lungs, shock-lung and A.R.D.S.

External injury and wounds due to violence, accidents and sports injury.

(7) **Therapeutic damage (Iatrogenic)**

Deep X-ray therapy, cobalt or super-voltage therapy.

Drug induced pulmonary disorders are becoming problems.

Many drugs may induce pulmonary damage via allergy, oedema or fibrosis. Anaphylaxis may also occur in some individuals due to injection of even a very small amount of horse serum or penicillin. Even oral drugs like aspirin, sulphonamides, broad-spectrum antibiotics, nitrofurans, phenytoins, procainamide, butazolidine etc. may produce mild to severe allergic reaction.

Bleomycin, myeleran and other anti-cancer agents, amitryptaline, methysergide, gold, practolol etc. are also capable of producing pulmonary damage.

Careful history taking may be useful to avoid such therapeutic accidents.

Paralysis of vocal cord or cords may produce significant problems. In unilateral paralysis, the paralysed cord is adducted to mid-line and the cause may be a mediastinal tumour or mitral stenosis.

## ANATOMY AND PHYSIOLOGY OF AIRWAYS

**The Airways**

Nose, nasopharnyx and larynx have mucosal cover with rich blood supply. Nasal air sinuses maxillary, frontal and ethmoidal, also have mucosal cover. They communicate through small openings, hence likely to be blocked due to mucosal oedema, producing persistent sinusitis. Atmospheric air gets warmed up while passing through nasopharynx and then enters larynx, trachea and finally into the bronchioles.

**Pharynx**

It is divided into upper nasopharynx and lower oropharynx by soft palate. Respiratory difficulty may arise due to greatly enlarged tonsils, adenoids, retropharyngeal abscess or falling back of tongue in comatose patients.

**Eustachian tube**

A communicating tube between pharyngeal cavity and middle ear, normally in apposition acts as a valve during yawning, eating and swallowing. A pressure of about 30 mm Hg is required to open the tube. Excessive adenoids, tenacious exudates, mucosal oedema can block the tube, causing middle ear pain due to in-drawing of tympanic membrane.

**Larynx**

Larynx is the voice-box which connects nasopharynx and trachea. Laryngoscopy is sometimes very useful in diagnosis. The left recurrent laryngeal (LRL) nerve goes down to thorax and winds round the aortic arch before reaching left vocal cord. Hence any local lesion in the zone of left hilum causes paralysis of left vocal cord. Right RLN also enters thorax but winds round right subclavian artery and returns to right side of larynx.

Trachea and main bronchi are supported by D-shaped cartilages. The convex part of the "D" forms anterior and lateral walls of trachea while flat part is posteriorly situated. The trachea is 10 cm in length and 14 to 22 mm in width and it divides into right and left main bronchi at the level of sterno-manubrial junction (4D vertebral body : upper border). Right lung has three lobar bronchi, while left has two. Each of them then subdivides into segmental bronchioles. Each segment has its own blood supply, lymphatics and venous drainage. (Fig.17.1).

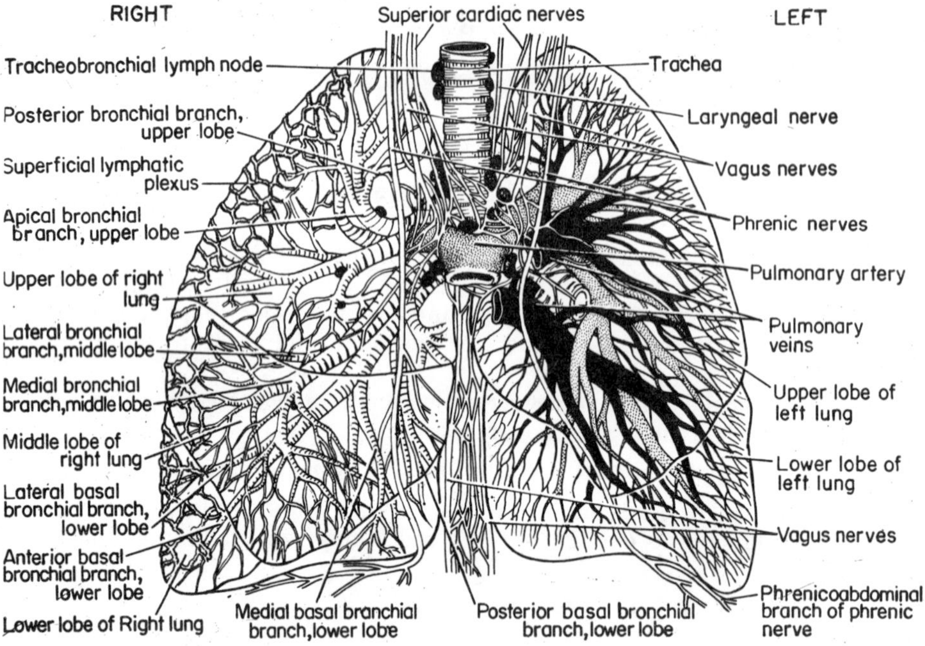


**Fig.17.1 : Showing trachea dividing into two main bronchi, etc.**

The right lobe main bronchus is slightly longer than the left and has less acute angle than left. Hence aspirated materials are easily inhaled in right middle and lower lobes.

The bronchial tree is just like an inverted tree and the anatomy of bronchial branchings and the lobes are illustrated in (Fig.17.2).

Bronchial tubes are lined by mucous membrane containing mucus secreting goblet cells and ciliated epithelium.

Right lung has three lobes and left has two, divided by fissures lined by pleural reflections. The five lobes are subdivided into 19 bronchopulmonary segments and each segment has its own blood vessels and lymphatics *(vide infra).* Anatomical variations, however, are sometimes encountered.

Large bronchi are also covered by ciliated epithelium. These go on branching and gradually form lobar, segmental to smallest bronchioles and finally terminal ones, i.e. respiratory bronchioles. Bronchial anatomy can be demonstrated up to small bronchioles in a good bronchogram.

Usually terminal bronchioles are reached after about 15 divisions by dichotomous branching but not symmetrical. These are the airways which ultimately end on terminal respiratory bronchioles (about 25,000 in number) and the alveoli, where gas exchange takes place. The terminal bronchioles are about 1.0 mm in length with diameter of 0.5 mm.

Blood vessels of each segment are branches of bronchial arteries carrying pure blood and branches of pulmonary arteries from right side of the heart, carrying venous blood for purification in the alveoli. Pulmonary veins carry purified blood from lungs to the left auricle. Venous drainage of lungs, however, is via bronchial veins.

Lymphatics are in two groups. One group follows peribronchial route while the other group is via subpleural plexus. These ultimately drain into pulmonary lymph nodes which are scattered

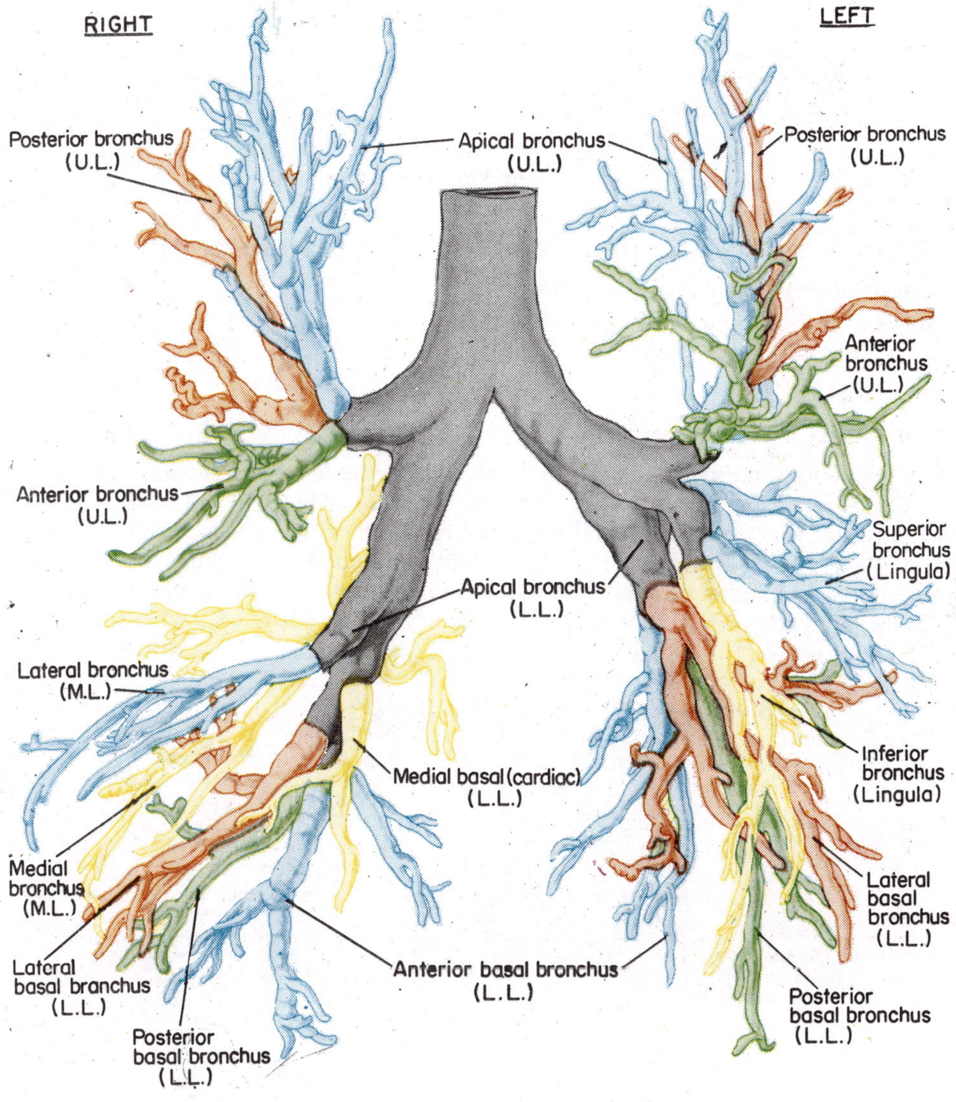


**Fig.17.2 : Segmental anatomy of bronchial tree.**

from the level of bronchial and tracheobronchial glands finally to drain into thoracic duct.

## THE LUNGS

Each lung has two distinct anatomical components :

(1) The conducting system starts with branches of bronchial tube (large bronchi) up to terminal bronchioles, alveolar duct and alveolar sac (Fig.17.2).

Through this conducting zone atmospheric air is inhaled into the alveoli. Air can communicate from one area of alveoli to another via intra-alveolar pores (Khon's pore) as well as through bronchio-alveolar canals and interconnecting respiratory bronchioles. This has been discovered by electron microscopy. These connections are used during diseased states helping ventilation in distal areas and preventing atelectasis.

(2) In the alveoli gaseous exchanges take place where air in alveoli and blood around the alveolar capillaries come into close contact. Exchange of gas takes place in these minute bubble-

like alveoli. Each alveolus is lined by two types of flattened epithelial cells. Type I cells are numerous and form the alveolar sac linings, while Type II cells are relatively a few which protrude into the alveolar space. These Type II cells contain osmophilic materials and are the source of lipoprotein substance covering the inner wall of the alveolar sac.

This acts as surface tension lowering mechanism known as 'surfactant'. It is due to the 'surfactant' that the tiny alveoli sustain their shape of bubble-like sacs, through which gas exchange occurs.

Each alveolus has the following structures as demonstrated by electron microscopy :

(a) Endothelial cell lining
(b) Epithelial cells Type I & II
(c) Endothelial cells of blood vessels (capillaries)
(d) Lymphatics

**Lower respiratory tract**

The trachea divides into right and left main bronchi at the level of sternomanubrial function (4-D vertebral body : upper border). Right lung has three lobar bronchi while left has two. Each of them then subdivides into segmental bronchioles. Each segment has its own blood supply, lymphatics and venous drainage (Fig.17.2). The right main bronchus divides into three bronchopulmonary branches and left into two the upper and lower lobar branches. These five lobar bronchi subdivide into 19 bronchopulmonary segments (Fig.17.3).

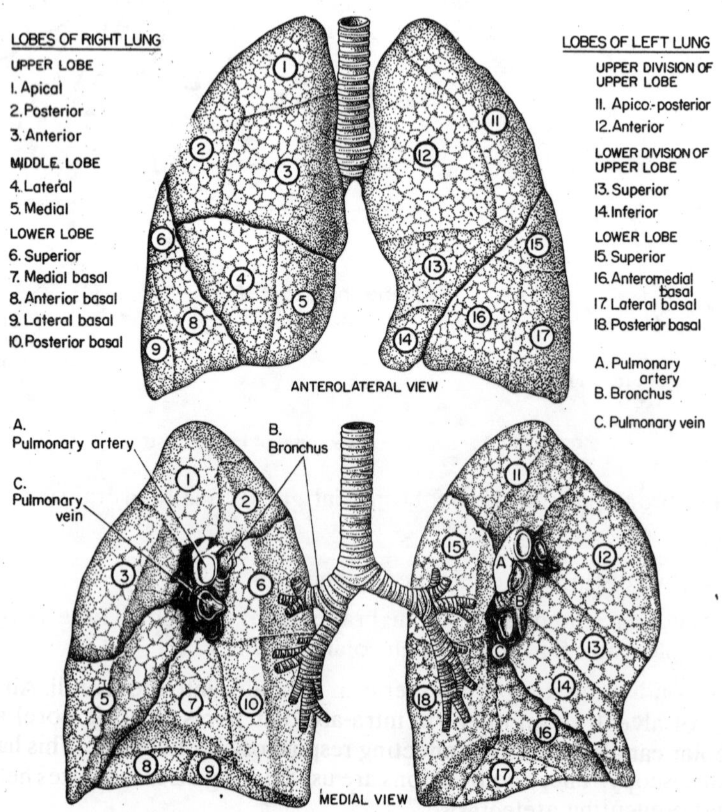


**Fig.17.3 : Showing trachea dividing into 'Lobar' bronchi and their lobes**

**Segmental branches**

| | |
|---|---|
| Right upper lobe | 1. Apical 2. Posterior 3. Anterior |
| Right middle lobe | 4. Lateral 5. Medial |
| Right lower lobe | 6. Apical 7. Medial basal (cardiac) |
| | 8. Anterior basal 9. Lateral basal |
| | 10. Posterior basal |

In the left lung there is no median or cardiac lobe (Fig.17.3) and nomenclature some what differs.

| | |
|---|---|
| Left upper lobe : | 1. Apical 2. Posterior (apico-posterior) |
| | 3. Anterior 4. Superior 5. Inferior (out of lingular branch) |
| | There is no middle lobe in left lung. |
| Left lower lobe : | 6. Apical 7. Anterior 8. Lateral |
| | 9. Posterior. |

The right main bronchus is about 2 cm. which first gives rise to right U.L. bronchus and subsequently divides into middle lobe and lower lobe bronchus. This portion between U.L. bronchus, till its further subdivision is called intermediate bronchus.

The left main bronchus is about 5 cm in length, which then divides into upper lobe and lower lobe bronchus. Each lobar branch subdivides into segmental branches.

The segmental bronchi are numbered according to international agreement. (after Brock & Foster-Carter). Lobar segments are clearly illustrated in Fig. 17.3.

Segmental anatomy is important in locating pathological lesions as well as surgically. When a patient in deep sedation or in coma lies on one side, aspirated fluid material may enter a particular segment or segments causing aspiration pneumonitis.

As a sequellae to segmental pneumonitis, bronchiectasis may occur in certain vulnerable segments. As segments are localised and unilateral, these can be surgically removed.

The middle lobe bronchus arises in a hook-shaped angle from right bronchus. Enlargement of local lymph glands in this angle may cause partial or complete obstruction of middle lobe bronchus resulting in atelectasis of the middle lobe, radiologically possible to diagnose. This may occur due to tuberculosis in children or bronchogenic carcinoma in adults. (Brock's middle lobe syndrome) Similarly an F.B. may be lodged in a segmental bronchus leading to atelectasis.

Segmental bronchus further subdivides into bronchioles and finally end up in terminal bronchioles. Though the segmental anatomy is more or less fixed anatomy and can be readily recognised in postero-anterior and lateral X-ray films, variations in segmental anatomy are not uncommon. This, however, is more important to the thoracic surgeons. For instance, the azygos vein looping over the apical segment of the upper lobe may produce an unfolding fissure in the upper lobe, presenting an isolated segment, the so-called azygos lobe.

The wall of bronchial tubes consists of mucosa, submucosa and fibrocartilagenous layer, including plain muscles. Mucosal lining of large bronchus consists of pseudo-stratified ciliated epithelium, as well as goblet cells, scattered in the superficial layer of ciliated cells. There are two or three rows of cuboidal cells in the larger bronchi. Over the carina at the tracheal bifurcation, squamous epithelium is present instead of ciliated epithelium with occasional goblet cells in the mucosa as well as submucosa. There are leucocytes, lymphocytes, and mast cells also.

Specially look for the following clinically and in X-ray films :

(1) Pulmonary agenesis — absence of one lung. Chest wall is asymmetrical.

(2) Pulmonary or mediastinal cysts. Large cysts may cause pressure symptoms and respiratory problems. Multiple small cysts form cystic-bronchiectasis.

(3) Hyperinflated lung or lobe which may cause tension lung, or pneumothorax.

(4) Arterio-venous fistula, single or multiple results in low resistance blood flow, increased cardiac output and may result in cardiac failure, cyanosis, finger clubbing and hypoxia will be noted. Haemoptysis may occur.

(5) Eventration of diaphragm – one side of cupola is elevated usually asymptomatic but in newborn it may cause respiratory embarrassment if too much elevation is present,resulting in displacement of abdominal viscera into thorax as well mediastinal shift. Urgent surgery is called for.

(6) Congenital diaphragmatic hernia – this also may cause urgent surgical problems of the newborn. Auscultation reveals characteristic intestinal sounds in the chest. X-ray chest settles the diagnosis.

There may be many other minor or major deformities of chest wall sternum, spine or ribs which should be noted. Pectus excavatum or funnel chest may cause displaced heart and even systolic murmur leading to wrong diagnosis. Pectus carinatum or pigeon chest may be associated with congenital heart disease. Gross kyphoscoliosis may lead to chronic respiratory problems.

## PHYSIOLOGY

Physiology of respiration is important to understand the diseases of the chest and their treatment. Applied respiratory physiology which deserves special mention is :

(a) Ventilation e.g. mechanism of breathing and its control.

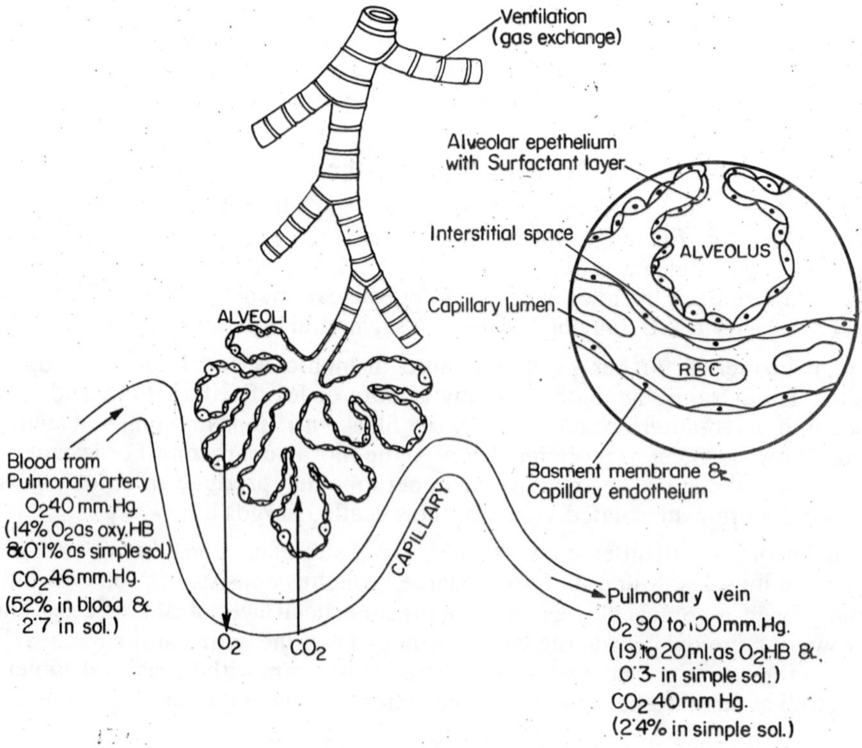


**Fig.17.4 : Showing alveolo-capillary gas exchange pathway.**

(b) Perfusion of the lungs by the output of the right heart.

(c) Distribution of ventilation and perfusion inside the lungs.

(d) Diffusion of oxygen and carbon dioxide between the terminal airways, the alveoli and the pulmonary capillary blood Fig. 17.4.

Ventilation involves movement of air in and out of the lungs. As the inspiratory muscles contract intrathoracic pressure falls and air flows into the lungs whereas expiration is a passive process and there the intrathoracic pressure rises due to elastic recoil of the lung. Alveolar ventilation is assessed by the arterial $PCO_2$ (36-44 mm Hg). Underventilation causes rise of $PCO_2$ and is found as a late consequence of chronic bronchitis and emphysema or when respiration is depressed by narcotics, anaesthetics, intracranial disease or in kyphoscoliosis which restrict thoracic or diaphragmatic movements. Over-ventilation causes fall in $PCO_2$ which occurs in bronchial asthma, interstitial lung disease, pulmonary embolism, salicylate poisonings, pontine lesions, metabolic, acidosis, anxiety states or hysteria.

Automatic rhythmic respiration occurs due to the Respiratory Centre situated in the medulla oblongata. Afferent impulses can be neural originating from receptors sensitive to stretch, bronchial irritation and pulmonary "inflation-deflation-reflexes". It is also due to chemical stimuli arising in chemosensitive cells present in the carotid sinus and aortic bodies. Ventilation is increased when the peripheral chemoreceptors are stimulated by arterial hypoxia, increase in hydrogen-ion concentration of arterial blood or when central chemoreceptors are stimulated by increased hydrogen-ion concentration of CSF.

Normally alveolar ventilation is uniformly distributed in different parts of the lungs and is matched by uniform distribution of blood flow and gas exchange in the lungs. The ventilation and perfusion ratio can have any values between infinity and zero. When infinity, the areas of the lung behave as dead space causing wasted ventilation and when zero, the lungs behave as a physiological right-to-left shunt resulting in wasted perfusion. The ventilation and perfusion is imperfect even in the normal lung because in the erect posture, gravity favour the distribution of blood flow to the lung bases and of ventilation in the upper zones. In most of the lung diseases, ventilation and perfusion of lung is impaired in certain degrees.

Just as water runs downhill, oxygen and carbon dioxide move across the blood-gas barrier by a process of diffusion from a region of high partial pressure to one of low. So in interstitial lung disease, diffusion of gases is impaired because of thickening of alveolar wall. Most of the conditions which may have this effect can also cause maldistribution of ventilation and blood flow. When the available area for gas exchange is reduced as in emphysema, the ability of the lung to transfer gases diminishes and this becomes significant during exercise causing hypoxaemia. Administration of oxygen may therefore be helpful.

Pulmonary function tests will indicate how the functional capacity of the airways may be impaired. This has been discussed in the next chapter.

It is probable that lungs are not just a respiratory organ for exchange of gases but experimental data on animals suggest that lungs also have metabolic and immunologic function. It may be actively concerned with metabolism of many biologically active substances like "peptides, amines, cyclic nucleotides and lipids" (Block E.R. & Stalcup S.A. — Chest : 81, 2 Feb. 1982).

## CLINICAL MANIFESTATIONS IN RESPIRATORY DISEASE

Clinical manifestations in respiratory diseases include cough, sputum, dyspnoea, stridor, haemoptysis, chest pain, hypoxaemia, hypercapnia, respiratory failure and clubbing of the fingers and toes. Some of these will draw attention to respiratory disorder. Fever may or may not be present. However, it should be understood that many of the above symptoms may occur due to extra-pulmonary disorders, hence careful clinical appraisal and appropriate investigations are essential to establish the aetiological diagnosis.

### Cough

Cough is an explosive expiration against closed glottis. Due to the explosive blast of air, glottis gets open suddenly. The cough may be physiological in order to clear the airways of mucus and in that case it is infrequent and occasional. When it is frequent and continued it usually denotes some pathological process in the respiratory passages. Sequence of events of cough and mechanism involved is depicted in Table-17.1.

**Table 17.1 — Sequence of events of cough**

**SEQUENCE OF EVENTS OF COUGH**

A DEEP INSPIRATION ---➤GLOTTIS CLOSED ---➤ HIGH INTRATHORACIC POSITIVE PRESSURE ---➤GLOTTIS FORCES OPEN ---➤BLAST (COUGH).

WHEN COUGH COMES IN BOUT, GLOTTIS ACTS AS SHUTTER.

**STIMULUS FOR COUGH**

↓

**GLOSSO–PHARYNGEAL & VAGAL**

Nerve endings, e.g. BLAST OF COLD AIR, IRRITANT GAS, FUMES, SMOKE OR LOCAL STIMULI DUE TO INFECTION.

COUGH HELPS MUCOCILIARY ESCALATOR ON DUTY

↓

(1) TO REMOVE EXCESS MUCUS

(2) TO REMOVE, DUSTS, BACTERIA & FB

COUGH IS A PHYSIOLOGICAL PROCESS, BUT IF CONTINUED OR RECURRENT IT PROCLAIMS RESPIRATORY DISEASE.

COUGH REFLEX PATHWAYS ⟶

(A) AFFERENT : SENSORY : VAGAL NERVE ENDINGS IN LARYNX, BRONCHI, BRONCHIOLES AND ALVEOLI.

(B) EFFERENT : ALL EXPIRATORY MUSCLES, ACTING VIOLENTLY AGAINST CLOSED GLOTTIS.

Though the cough reflex is caused by various stimuli within the respiratory tract, emotional factors, irritation of ear drum (via Arnold's branch of vagus), cold blast of air,etc., may also provoke cough reflex. However, generally cough will be provoked by an irritation of neuronal receptors of the respiratory tract between pharynx and bronchial tubes.

Careful assessment of the type of cough may give clue to the diagnosis in many cases.

(1) A smoker's cough is often a social nuisance. However, if there is change in the character of the smoker's cough, it may be a pointer to some underlying pathology, e.g. bronchiectasis or carcinoma of the lungs.

(2) Sudden occurrence of acute and violent cough may indicate F.B. in the lung.

(3) Cough with hoarseness denotes laryngitis.

(4) Brassy cough denotes involvement of trachea or bronchi.

(5) Cough with dyspnoea and wheeze denotes broncho-spasm (asthma or chronic bronchitis).

(6) Productive cough with mucopurulent sputum suggests suppurative pneumonia (lung abscess), bronchiectasis or tuberculosis.

(7) Cough with frothy, pink, blood stained sputum means pulmonary oedema (L.V.F.).

(8) Nocturnal cough or cough during accustomed exertion may be due to cardiac decompensation.

(9) Whooping cough is diagnosed by the nature of cough.

(10) In paralysis of vocal cord, cough is known as 'bovine cough'.

**Complications of cough :**

Violent bouts of cough may cause spontaneous pneumothorax, fracture of ribs and even strangulated hernia.

Chronic cough may produce emphysema as in cases of chronic bronchitis.

**Sputum**

Sputum is the spitted-out, mucoid or mucopurulent material which may come from any part of the respiratory tract, although it usually signifies expectoration coming from larynx and below it. Lung abscess and pneumonias are characterised by purulent sputum. Blood-streaked sputum may proclaim pulmonary tuberculosis, mitral stenosis, pneumonia or pulmonary infarction. Diagnostic value of sputum examination is presented as follows :

**Inspect and smell at the same time**

Note colour and consistency :

Foul odour denotes : lung abscess, bronchiectasis, chronic bronchitis, gangrenous lesion of lungs usually due to anaerobic infection or superinfection with fusiform bacilli, spirillum or fungal organisms. Breaking down carcinoma may also cause foetid sputum but often blood stained. Mucoid sputum is suggestive of overactive goblet cells, found in chronic tobacco smokers, chronic bronchitis, bronchiectasis and industrial lung diseases.

Mucopurulent sputum denotes secondary infection. If expectoration is profuse, it should be collected and kept in a conical glass, and it will separate into three layers after a few hours, suggesting bronchiectasis or lung abscess.

Purulent sputum : Large amounts of purulent sputum denotes suppurative pneumonia, ruptured lung abscess, advanced bronchiectasis and gangrene of the lung.

**Colour of sputum may also suggest diagnosis :**

Rusty tenacious sputum-early pneumonia.

Cream or yellowish-staphylococcal pneumonitis

Reddish brown tinge-Friedlander's (Klebsiella) pneumonia

Greenish-sputum — pseudomonas pneumonitis

Frothy-pink sputum-pulmonary oedema

Blood-tinged sputum : See haemoptysis

Sulphur granules — if present in sputum denotes actinomycosis. It is therefore evident that simple inspection and smell of sputum may give us many important clues to the diagnosis.

Culture may be contaminated, malignant cells may be misreported but inexpensive clinical observations are always rewarding.

**Microscopic examination of sputum**

The next important step is miscroscopic examination of sputum which will reveal the nature of infecting organisms, e.g. Gram-positive or Gram-negative cocci or bacilli, e.g. diphtheriae, tubercle bacilli, fungal spores and filaments can be recognised by proper staining. Eosinophils, malignant cells, bronchial epithelia, fungi, hooklets of hydatid, animal parasites, industrial dusts and materials, e.g. silica, asbestos, cotton flax etc. can also be recognised.

Culture of sputum is important, useful but usually not properly carried out. Physician must see the sample and preferably send the patient to laboratory or collect the sample himself in proper media. It is better to discuss with Pathologist when sensitivity tests are necessary.

**Haemoptysis**

Haemoptysis is spitting of blood derived from the lungs or bronchial tubes and is a common symptom in mitral stenosis, pulmonary tuberculosis, bronchiectasis, pulmonary infarction, bronchial carcinoma and acute or chronic bronchitis. Common and rare causes of haemoptysis are illustrated in Fig.17.5.

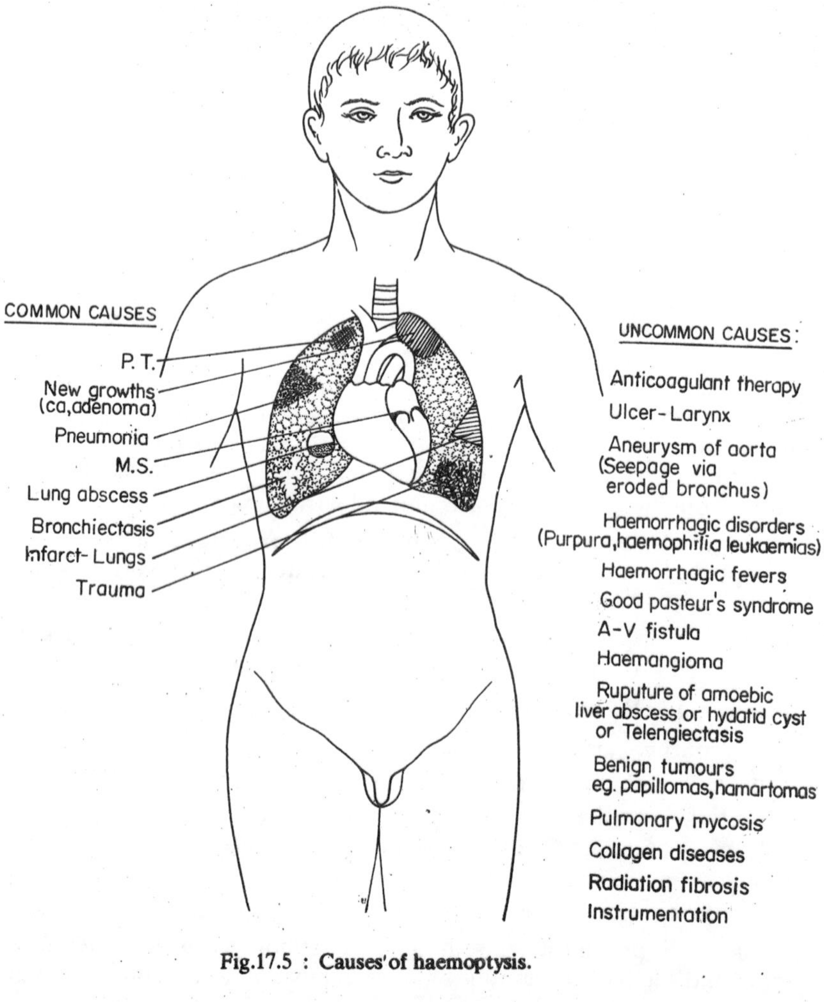


**Fig.17.5 : Causes of haemoptysis.**

Dyspnoea and pain chest pain problem has been discussed in the section on cardiovascular disease.

## SPECIAL INVESTIGATIONS OF RESPIRATORY DISEASE

History as well as clinical examination is of supreme importance. Besides sputum examination, respiratory disorders may be investigated by the following methods :

1) **X-ray chest and, if required, tomography or zonography are routine procedures. Tomo- or zonography is done to detect or localise suspected pathology not seen in routine films. Check menstrual date before radiological investigations in women.**
2) *Haemogram & ESR* – helps to differentiate pyogenic infection from tuberculosis and allergic aetiology to some extent.
3) ***Laryngoscopy*** – to exclude tuberculosis, new growth, syphilis or laryngeal palsy.
4) ***Fiberoptic bronchoscopy*** – Lesions of the bronchial tree can be visualised up to segmental bronchioles and biopsy can be taken.

5) *Bronchography* – Bronchial anatomy can be visualised, especially useful to study the extent of bronchiectasis.

6) *Skin tests* – The following tests are of value :

(a) Tuberculin test helps especially to exclude tuberculosis. Positive test may mean present or past infection.

(b) Allergy testing – very valuable to detect offending allergens.

(c) Kveim test – is useful in diagnosis of sarcoidosis.

(d) Cassoni's test – for hydatid disease.

7) *Biopsy* – Biopsy of glands, pleura and lung tissue can be done. It is useful for diagnosis of tuberculosis, chronic granuloma, secondaries from malignant growth reticulosis, Hodgkin's disease, sarcoidosis etc. Pleural fluid should also be investigated fully and therefore diagnostic aspiration, wherever possible, should be done if effusion is suspected.

8) Pulmonary angiography is a very useful investigation which can help in the diagnosis of vascular malformation, pulmonary embolism, new growth and cysts etc, but should be judiciously done. This is not without a little risk.

9) Pulmonary function tests – These are non-invasive investigations carried out by special instruments to study ventilation and ventilation-perfusion functions of the respiratory tracts. Along with blood gas analysis and pH studies, disorders of respiratory function can be well assessed.

10) Radioactive scanning of lungs is the most modern technique and so is ultrasonic imaging. A separate chapter has been included to explain these non-invasive methods.

11) *C.T. scanning* is sometimes necessary.

## LUNG FUNCTION TESTS

*N.C. DAS*

The functions of the lungs mainly depend upon two mechanisms, namely, (1) ventilatory function and (2) diffusion of gases across the alveolar membrane, that is transcapillary gas exchange. Perfusion of the lung bed is a combined function of heart directly and lungs indirectly.

**Ventilatory Function**

Ventilation implies the movement of air in and out of the lungs and for its accomplishment requires :

a) patent airways, right up to the bronchioles,

b) integrity and mobility of the thoracic cage and diaphargm,

c) normal compliance i.e. normal elasticity and distensibility of the lungs.

Defects in any one of these requirements will result in inadequate ventilatory function.

Patent airways is of utmost importance and is normally achieved by ciliary action, cough reflex, bronchial peristalsis and collateral respiration. Integrity and mobility of the thoracic cage and diaphragm account for the production of adequate pressure changes in the pleural space thereby assisting the airflow in and out of the lungs during respiration. Distensibility and elasticity of lung tissue allow the lung to distend during inspiration and to record during expiration. Elasticity is further necessary for the proper distribution of gases throughout the lungs.

**Assessment of adequacy of ventilation**

During ventilation,specific lung volume changes occur due to air flow in and out of the lungs. Measurement of those volumes may provide partial information about the ventilatory efficacy. Four specific lung volumes can be measured directly, namely :

1) **Tidal Volume** (TV) is the volume of air/gas inspired during each respiratory cycle. Average volume in adult male is 450-600 ml.
2) **Inspiratory Reserve Volume** (IRV) is the maximum amount of additional air/gas that can be forcefully inspired after a normal inspiration. Average volume is 2400 ml.
3) **Expiratory Reserve Volume** (ERV) is the maximum amount of air/gas that can be forcefully expired after a normal expiration. Average volume is 1200 ml.
4) **Vital capacity** (VC) is the maximum amount of air/gas volume that can be expelled from the lungs by forceful effort following a maximal inspiration. It is thus the sum of TV, IRV, and ERV. Average volume is 4200 ml.

A few other lung volumes are measured indirectly, namely :

5) **Residual Volume** (RV) is the amount of air still remaining inside the lungs at the end of the maximal expiration. This residual amount of air probably helps in preventing the collapse of the lung alveoli. Average volume is 1200 ml.
6) **Functional Residual capacity** (FRC) is the amount of air remaining in the lungs at the end of normal expiration. It therefore includes ERV and RV together. During normal respiratory cycle this combined amount of air remains inside the lung and takes part in the gaseous exchange ($O_2$ & $CO_2$) between the alveoli and blood in the pulmonary capillaries. Hence this amount of air is called 'functional' or Functional Residual capacity. In quiet respiration, this functional residual volume of air is almost static inside the lungs. The tidal air, being the dynamic volume moving in and out of the lungs, aids the exchange of gases by variable partial pressure/tension exerted by the various component gases, namely oxygen and carbon dioxide.

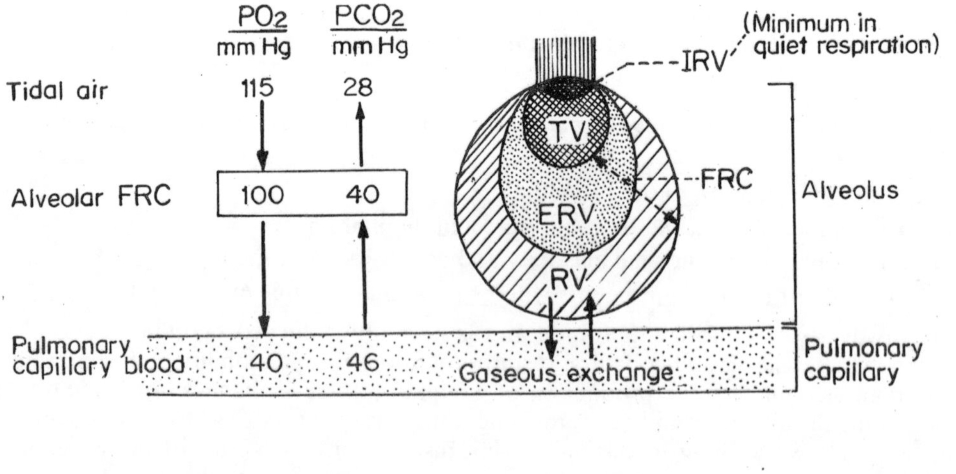


Fig.17.6 : In normal respiration, air movement in the FRC is negligible, hence no turbulence in that air. The gaseous exchange of $O_2$ and $CO_2$ between alveoli and pulmonary capillaries takes place due to difference in pressure gradient in those two compartments. Similar exchange of gases takes place between FRC and TV to eliminate $CO_2$ and add $O_2$ to FRC.

IRV as shown in the figure can be increased by forced inspiration. It actually adds to the tidal air, aiding rapid and large volume of gaseous exchange. However, it may create turbulence in the FRC, which will not be desirable ordinarily.

7) **Total Lung Capacity** (TLC) is the volume of air, the lungs can hold after forceful inspiration. It therefore means the sum total of IRV, TV, ERV and RV. In other words **vital** capacity plus **residual** volume constitutes total lung capacity.

Representing diagrammatically the approximate values of the various lung volumes and capacities in an adult male is as under :

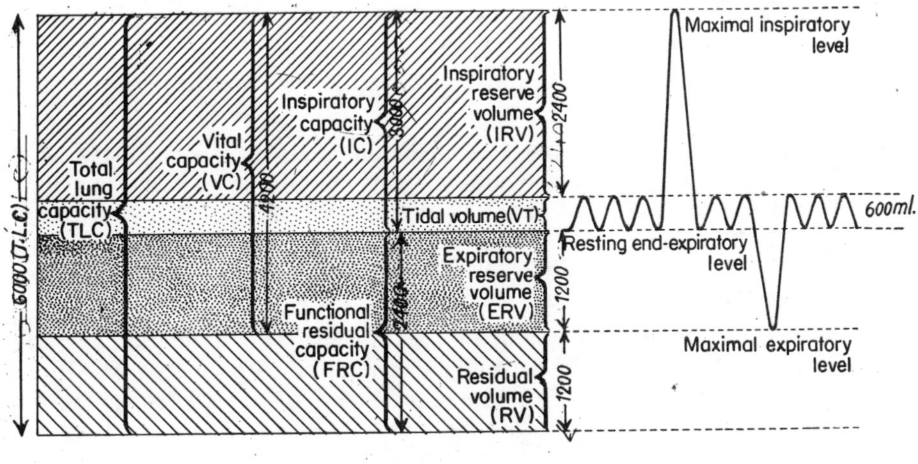


**Fig.17.7 : Measurement of ventilatory functions.**

**Volumes** are variable with efforts, except RV

**Capacities** are kept constant by anatomical frame of the lungs and their structures.

The normal values of all these volumes vary with age, sex, height, weight and size of the individual. Therefore, it will be fallacious to consider those values in absolute terms. It should rather be related in a proportion where it will become more apparent whether or not these values are abnormal. In the same individual the **vital capacity** is approximately 75 per cent of the total lung capacity, i.e. VC : TLC = 75%. It decreases with advancing age or in lung disease. Similarly, residual volume is only 30 per cent of the total lung capacity, i.e. RV:TLC = 30%. If this figure increases, it will usually indicate that some pathological process like emphysema is present.

## Minute Volume or Minute Ventilation

It means the amount of air moved by the lung in normal quiet respiration during one minute. Tidal volume multiplied by the number of breaths taken in one minute will give this figure. Normally a healthy male breathes about 12-14 times in one minute and the tidal volume is approximately 500 ml per breath. Thus the minute Ventilation is approximately 6 to 7 litres.

## Effective Alveolar Ventilation

The term implies the volume of air which takes part in the gaseous exchange between lung alveoli and the blood in pulmonary capillaries in one minute. Evidently it will be less than the minute ventilation, since the dead space air is to be subtracted. Usually the dead space volume in an adult male is 150 ml. Therefore, tidal volume minus dead space volume (500 - 150 ml) = 350 ml of air will actually take part in the gaseous exchange. This volume (350 ml) multiplied by number of breaths per minute, i.e. 4.2 to 4.9 litres approximately will be the effective alveolar ventilation.

The above two, namely minute ventilation and effective alveolar ventilation are often used, since normal respiratory ventilation is not a quiet regular process in respect to tidal volume and respiratory frequency, but frequent deep breaths are an integral part of the pattern of normal breathing. It has been demonstrated that a shallow constant tidal volume leads to a progressive collapse of the alveoli and that deep breaths reverse this trend by inflating the collapsed air space. Sighing mechanism is an integral part of normal respiration.

**Maximal Breathing Capacity (MBC)**

It means the maximum volume of air that can be breathed per minute. In other words, if the person breathes in and out maximally (i.e. his vital capacity amount of air) as fast as he can (say 30-40 times per minute), the total amount of air thus moved during one minute will indicate the MBC. Usually the person is advised to breathe maximally and fast for about 15 seconds and then expressed as flow per minute. Average values are between 120 and 150 litres per minute.

Two other measurements are occasionally considered to evaluate the ventilatory capabilities of a patient.

(1) **Breathing reserve,** which correlates the maximum breathing capacity (MBC) with minute volume (MV). Breathing reserve obviously means the difference between MBC and MV, e.g. if MCB = 150 litre per min and MV = 10 litre per min, then breathing reserve will be (150-10) = 140 litres per min. Therefore the **breathing reserve ratio** will be breathing reserve (140 L) : MBC (150 L/min) = 94%. Normal value of this ratio is between 90 and 96%. When it falls to 60% or lower, dyspnoea occurs.

(2) **Air velocity index,** which uses maximum breathing capacity in relation to vital capacity. It is the percentage of MBC of the patient in relation to predicted MBC, which is to percentage V.C. of the patient in relation to predicted V.C. Predicted values of MBC and VC are obtained from normograms. In patients with lung disease such as emphysema or asthma, the air velocity index becomes less than one because the maximum breathing capacity is decreased more than vital capacity. On the other hand, where there is a loss of the functional parenchymal tissue of the lung, e.g. in pneumothorax, thoracotomy etc., the index is above one because vital capacity is decreased more than MBC.

## LUNG FUNCTION TESTS

Most of the lung function tests are designed to estimate the ventilatory efficiency of the individual. The main idea is to make systematic study of the dominant functional abnormality in intrapulmonary airflow and thereby to establish the type of ailment the individual is suffering from, that is (i) Obstructive airflow pathology, (ii) Restrictive pathology, or (iii) Combined obstructive and restrictive pathology.

For this a spirometer is often used. Tests which involve forced expiration are the most practicable means of assessing ventilatory function, that is, case of movement of air in and out of the lungs. However, one must be aware that spirometric measurements require the full cooperation of the patient, and this may be a serious handicap in sick or psychologically handicaped individuals. The pulmonary function tests are most valuable when they are interpreted in the light of the clinical picture. Also the tests offer a useful check of estimates of the severity of pulmonary dysfunction.

All over the world dry bellow type spirometer is commonly used to do the lung function tests. VITALOGRAPH being most common, is described below :

**Vitalograph**

It is a dry-bellows-spirometer and is most widely used in all countries. The subject takes a maximal inspiration, applies the lips tightly round the mouthpiece and then makes a sudden forced expiration, continuing to expire until no further expiration is possible. As the air enters the bellows of the Vitalograph, the recording arm moves over a recording chart fixed on a platform which moves at a steady speed by servo-mechanism. The result is, an oblique line is described on the chart by the stylus. From the chart markings and this oblique line drawn, large amount of information to assess the ventilatory function is available.

The chart itself is like a graph paper, having vertical volume calibration in 50 ml, having recording in :

(i) ATPS – (air volumes at ambient temperature 20°C, normal barometric pressure of 760 mm of Hg and saturated with water vapour).

(ii) BTPS – (air volumes at body temperature 37° C normal barometric pressure and saturated with water vapour)

**The horizontal lines depict the time-scale, and numbers 1 to 6 seconds of continuous chart** travel time is available when the recorder runs non-stop. The time-scale is given in 0.1 sec increments and commensurate with the extraordinarily high recorder speed accuracy of the vitalography spirometer.

**The main spirometric indices available from the oblique line drawn are :-**

FVC (FORCED VITAL CAPACITY), in litres. Maximum volume of air which can be expelled as rapidly and completely as possible after maximum effort i.e. forceful.

FEVt (FORCED EXPIRATORY VOLUME TIMED) in litres. Volume of air, which can be expelled with maximum effort over a given time interval during a forced expiration after maximum inspiration. **(also called Timed Vital Capacity).**

FEV% (FORCED EXPIRATORY RATIO) i.e. FEV/FVC X 100%—Timed Forced Expiratory volume expressed as a percentage of the measured FVC (also called Timed Vital Capacity ratio).

MVV (MAXIMUM VOLUNTARY VENTILATION) **in litres per minute.** Maximum volume of air which could be exhaled by breathing deeply and rapidly with maximum voluntary effort for a short time, usually 10 to 15 sec; also called MBC-Maximum Breathing Capacity. In the vitalographic method, it makes use of the $FEV_1$ value multipled by a physiological frequency factor of 37.5 for one minute it is only a dynamic estimation of maximum ventilation possible by the individual (120/min).

FMF (FORCED MID-EXPIRATORY FLOW) in litres per sec or min; average rate of airflow during the middle two quarters of the volume segment of the forced expiratory spirogram (i.e. from $V_{25}$% to $V_{75}$% of the FVC).

FMFT (FORCED MID-EXPIRATORY FLOW TIME) in seconds; Time interval occupied by the airflow during the middle two quarters of the volume segment of the forced expiratory spirogram.

PEFR (PEAK EXPIRATORY FLOW RATE) in litres per min; It is measured by weight Peak Flow Meter or Mini Peak Flow Meter. In measuring peak flow, the subject takes a maximal inspiration and then gives a maximal expiratory blast through the instrument. The pointer sticks at the point of maximum excursion and the PEFR can then be read directly from the scale. At rest button returns the pointer to zero.

PEFR is reduced in the presence of airway obstruction and is a useful index of the severity of the obstruction. However, because the maximum rate of expiratory air flow is governed by lung volume and not on the pressure applied (i.e. high rate being achieved at high lung volume and low rates only at low lung volume). PEFR may also be reduced in restrictive disorders which reduce lung volume or vital capacity. This can be conveniently converted into percentage i.e. Forced vital **Restrictive air flow from the lungs.**

This parameter (PEFR) is probably most useful as a means of assessing severity and changes in severity of airway obstruction, when the type of ventilatory defect is not in real doubt. Normal adult males achieve values of the order of 400 to 800 litres per minute and females about 200 to 600/L per min.

The main advantage in using a spirometer (Vitalograph), rather than the peak flow meter, to assess ventilatory function, is the greater amount of information available to obtain an instant impression of the patient's ventilatory status from the appearance of the curve.

**Volume Measurements**

If we compare the Forced vital capacity of the patient with the predicted vital capacity of an identical healthy individual, we at once know the amount of restriction the patient has in his total lung volume or vital capacity. This can be conveniently converted into percentage i.e., Forced vital capacity/Predicted vital capacity × 100 to note the percentage of Restrictive ventilatory defect.

Predicted vital capacity can be obtained from Nomograms supplied, knowing the sex, age and height of the individual. (Nomogram by Kamburoff and Woitowitz 1972, in the book 'Lung Function Tables and Nomograms').

We also know that normally in a forced expiration after maximal inspiration, approximately 70 to 80% of the lung air volume is exhaled out in one second, i.e. $FEV_1/FVC \times 100 = 70$ to 80%. This is connected with the voluntary effort of the individual. If, however, the expiratory pressure is sustained, the remaining volume of air is exhaled out in next 3 to 4 seconds by the collapsing alveoli till closing-volume is reached. In obstructive lung disease,the amount of air that can be forced out within a certain time is reduced below normal. Thus, lowering of $FEV_1$% will indicate mathematically the magnitude of obstruction.

In chronic airway obstruction there is a linear relationship between the $FEV_1$ and the steady state of diffusing capacity. In patients with an $FEV_1$, below one litre especially if it remains unchanged after bronchodilatation, will indicate a reduced 'diffusing capacity' of gases (i.e. gas transfer) and the presence of pulmonary insufficiency, (T.T. Chapman *et al*).

**Flow Measurements**

From the curve of the vitalograph, the flow of the lung air in relation to time is easily obtainable and it gives a comprehensive idea of magnitude of obstruction and the site of obstruction to the air flow.

FEF (Forced expiratory flow) of the first litre is an index specifically sensitive to obstructive defects in the larger airways and/or to changes in the non-elastic components of airways resistance. It is effort dependent and particularly responsive to bronchodilatation. Normal mean values range from 6.5 to 9.0 litres per sec in male and 4.5 to 6.0 litres per sec in female (Comroe, 1962).

FMF (Forced mid-expiratory flow), i.e. the middle part of expiration is a more sensitive index of obstructive defects and is specified for obstructions prevailing in the smaller airways, being largely independent of effort. Normal mean values ranges from 3.0 to 5.4 L/sec in male and 2.8 to 4.0L/sec in females.

FEEF (Forced end-expiratory flow), i.e. the Vitalographic terminal part of curve is more sensitive in detecting smallest airway obstruction than FMF (Forced mid-expiratory flow). It compares closely to elaborate laboratory tests, such as (a) Closing lung volumes, (b) Flow-volume curves, (c) Body plethysmography, (d) Frequency dependence of compliance, and (e) Gas exchange, utilised for detecting early involvement. Spirometric standards for healthy adult males and females are given as 'Predicted values FEEF, 75 to 85%. If less than 75% of the predicted value it is indicative of early obstructive ventilatory defect or disease of the smallest airways.

**Differential Assessment Facilities of the Vitalograph**

In order to quickly assess the type of ventilatory defect the individual is suffering from i.e. (i) Obstructive. (ii) Restrictive or (iii) Combined and to determine the degree of defect, we commonly use MILLER's prediction quadrant.

The vertical scale of this indicates the Restrictive element of ventilatory defect, i.e., measured

FVC/Predicted FVC as per cents, and the horizontal scale depicts the obstructive element of the ventilatory defect, i.e. $FEV_1/FVC \times 100\%$. The bold lines divide the whole graph into four blocks (quadrant) with easy read out types of ventilatory defects mentioned. By plotting the above two parameters the type and degree of ventilatory defect can be easily judged.

## Gaseous Exchange

**Gaseous exchange between alveoli and pulmonary capillaries depends upon :**

**(1) An adequate pressure gradient of gas between the two compartments;**
**(2) Diffusibility of the gases;**
**(3) Uniform distribution of the gas and blood over the entire membrane surface;**
**(4) Permeability of the membranes through which the gas will diffuse and**
**(5) Efficient transport of blood and gas to and from the lung parenchyma. This mainly depends on the circulation.**

### Pressure gradient

Adequate movement of gases will depend on the partial pressure of the gases in the alveolar and the pulmonary capillary blood. We are mainly concerned with the movement of oxygen and carbon dioxide across the separating membrane between these two compartments, namely, alveolar epithelium and capillary endothelium separating alveoli (filled with air) and the capillary (filled with liquid, namely, blood).

**Gas transfer across alveolo-capillary membrane :**

| **Alveolar Air** | **Pulmonary Capillary Blood** |
|---|---|
| Alveolar air is fully saturated with water vapour, which exerts a fixed pressure of 47 mm Hg. | Blood entering the capillary bed through pulmonary arteries contains only part of $O_2$ **and $CO_2$ in physical solution, and the partial pressures exerted by the dissolved $O_2$ and $CO_2$ are –** |
| Therefore pressure exerted by other gases in alveoli, namely $O_2$, $CO_2$ and $N_2$ is (760-47) = 713 mm Hg. | |
| Alveolar air contains 14% $O_2$ Thus partial pressure of $O_2$ alone is 14% of 713 = 100 mm Hg i.e. $PAO_2$ = 100 mm Hg | $PO_2$ = 40 mm Hg |
| **Similarly, $CO_2$ being 5.5% by volume, $PACO_2$ = 5.5% of 713 = 40 mm Hg** | Hence. oxygen moves across and |
| Hence, carbon dioxide moves | $PCO_2$ = 46 mm Hg. |

**Alveolo-capillary membrane.**

If the separating membrane is normal, oxygen will move from the alveoli to the capillary blood due to high pressure gradient, and similarly carbon dioxide will move in the reverse direction, until gaseous equilibrium is reached. In the systemic arterial blood we thus find $PaO_2$ to be 100 to 97 mm Hg and $PaCO_2$ to be 40 mm Hg.

### Diffusibility of gases

The diffusibility of $CO_2$ is excellent, being approximately 20 times greater than that of oxygen. Therefore, the concentration of $CO_2$ in the pulmonary capillaries and alveoli reaches equilibrium very rapidly (40 mm Hg) and circulate in the systemic arterial blood. Any difference between the PA $CO_2$ (alveolar) and Pa $CO_2$ (arterial systemic) will therefore indicate alteration in the permeability of the alveolo-capillary membrane. However, ventilation perfusion incoordination must also be remembered.

**Since oxygen diffuses much more slowly across the membrane than $CO_2$, initial finding in** pulmonary disease may be a lowering of the arterial oxygen saturation, and in the late stage of alveolo-capillary insufficiency only the arterial $PCO_2$ will start rising.

**Diffusing capacity of the lung is best measured with carbon-monoxide which has great affinity** for haemoglobin but does not saturate the plasma, and whose rate of uptake by the pulmonary circulation is limited only by its rate of diffusion across the alveolo-capillary membrane. The diffusion capacity of carbon monoxide is then converted by formula to that of oxygen.

**Distribution of gas and blood over the membrane surface.**

Under normal conditions, there is uneven ventilation and perfusion of the lungs, with the **dependent** areas doing most of the work. With the stress of exercise the entire capillary bed is opened and most of the alveoli participate. As a result, there is an overall increase in the diffusing capacity.

**Ventilation-perfusion ratio**

The normal alveolar ventilation (VA) in an adult is approximately 4 litres per minute and the **total perfusion (Q) is about 5 litres per minute. Therefore, proportion of ventilation, to** perfusion is equal to (4 litres per min) : (5 litres per min) = 0.8. The ratio is known as ventilation — perfusion ratio i.e. V A : Q = 0.8 normal.

The ventilation perfusion of the whole lung is a composite of the ratios of each individual alveolus which are evidently different in different parts of the lungs.

Relative variations of ventilation and perfusion as seen in the lungs are :

1. **Normal unit** in which both ventilation and perfusion are relatively equal. Here VA : Q = 1:1 = 1 (Normal 0.8).
2. **Dead space unit** in which the alveolus is normally ventilated but there is no blood flow through the capillaries. Hence VA = Q = 1 : 0 = (Infinity).

(3) **Shunt unit** in which the alveolus is completely unventilated but blood flows through capillaries. Blood goes from right to left heart without undergoing gas exchange.

Here VA : Q = 0 : 1 = 0 (zero)

(4) **Silent unit** in which both alveolus and capillary are completely collapsed. Functionally as if these units are not there and has no effect on the VA/Q ratio. Here VA : Q = 0 : 0 = 0 (zero).

Any one of these absolute conditions may exist in the lungs at any time. Practically an indefinite number of ventilation-perfusion relationship exist between dead space units and normal units. The complexities of ventilation-perfusion (V : Q) ratio are primarily due to spectrum between the two extremes of dead space and shunt. The total alveolar ventilation is thus composed of two portions, namely, (a) dead space unit ventilation and (b) effective alveolar ventilation which physiologically exchange gases with pulmonary blood.

Uneven ventilation is common in various pulmonary diseases, such as infiltration, parenchymal destruction or obstruction. In such individuals poorly ventilated and hyperventilated areas may exist side by side and may lead to pulmonary insufficiency even though the minute volume of breathing is normal or increased.

The tests for uneven distribution of inspired air are based on the form of a "**nitrogen wash out**" using either a single or multiple breathing technique.

"**Single breath Xenon test**" may also be used. Here the patient is asked to breathe air containing $Xe^{133}$ and the distribution of Xenon in various zones of the lungs is scanned by stationary detector. The test is simple and quick, but requires expensive set-up. It not only gives an idea of distribution of the gas in different parts of lungs, but the rate of ventilation of each zone can be determined.

To determine the perfusion inequality isotope tagged Human Serum Albumin is administered intravenously and pulmonary circulation is then scanned by a detector. More recently Technetium is being used.

**Venous admixture**

The final value of arterial oxygen tension and saturation is due to mixing of fully saturated/oxygenated blood with blood from relatively under-ventilated parts of the lungs which is less saturated. This phenomenon is known as "Venous admixture" and is expressed as a percentage of cardiac output. In a man, the normal venous admixture is 1 to 5% of cardiac output. In other words, normally 50 to 250 ml of the blood passing through the lungs in one minute has never come in contact with oxygen at all due to maldistribution of ventilation-perfusion. A rise in the percentage of venous admixture will thus mean that more direct or anatomical shunt has occurred.

Shunts in excess of 30 per cent may be seen in congenital cardiac disease, lung trauma, fat embolism, pneumonia and gross obesity. In such cases having more than 30% shunts, compensation by increasing the inspired oxygen concentration is not possible to restore to normal. Changes in inspired concentration have almost no effect on $PaO_2$. Compensation by increasing the inspired oxygen concentration is effective up to a point only.

| Percent of existing shunt | Percent of inspired $O_2$ to restore normal $PaO_2$ |
|---|---|
| 10 | 30 |
| 20 | 57 |
| 30 | 67 |
| Beyond 30 | Not possible to restore |

**Permeability of the membrane**

Permeability of the membranes may decrease due to widening of the diffusing path between alveolar wall and pulmonary capillary by collagenous fibrous tissue, as seen in pulmonary fibrosis or destruction of parenchymal tissue. Oedema fluid in the interstitium in case of pulmonary oedema *per se* causes no significant barrier to any gas transfer.

In evaluating gas exchange impairment, one must exclude ventilation-perfusion abnormalities, such as congenital heart disease with right to left shunt. A right to left shunt with mixed venous blood getting to the systemic arterial circulation may either be (i) anatomical, such as intracardiac shunts or pulmonary arteriovenous fistula, or (ii) functional, when blood flows through an atelectatic non-areated portion of lungs. Any abnormality of gas exchange will increase the difference in the partial pressure of gases between alveolar air and arterial blood.

**Alveolar-arterial oxygen difference ($PAO_2$-$PaO_2$)**

In a normal person breathing atmospheric air containing 21% of oxygen, the $PAO_2$, i.e. alveolar oxygen tension is approximately 105-100 mm Hg. and $PaO_2$, i.e. systemic arterial oxygen tension is 97-95 mm Hg. Thus the difference between $PAO_2$-$PaO_2$ = 3 to 5 mm Hg approximately. The normal range of this value is between 5 and 15 mm Hg. If the $PaO_2$ falls below 90 mm Hg. further tests must be done to determine the cause of hypoxia. Since most of the hypoxia seen in pulmonary insufficiency is due to shunting, the administration of 100% oxygen is an essential test in evaluating and management of these patients. Administration of 100% oxygen for about 10 minutes will raise the alveolar $PAO_2$ to about 700 mm Hg and this will overcome any diffusion block by mass-action and will raise the systemic arterial oxygen tension ($PaO_2$) to about 640 mm Hg. This will eliminate hypoxemia. However, if there is an anatomical or functional right to left shunt, the 100% oxygen test will have no effect and arterial $PO_2$ will remain below 300 mm Hg.

**Alveolar-arterial Carbon dioxide difference ($PA\ CO_2$-$Pa\ Co_2$)**

In a normal individual there is no significant difference between alveolar and arterial $PCO_2$. Usually $PACo_2$-$PaCo_2$ is less than 1 mm Hg, since Carbondioxide diffuses so rapidly across the alveolar membrane that the limits of diffusion are not reached. If major differences are found between $PACo_2$ and $PaCo_2$, it is almost exclusive due to ventilation-perfusion in coordination. The alveolar $PACo_2$ is lower than the arterial $PaCo_2$ in all types of ventilation-perfusion dysfunction.

$PacO_2$ is primarily determined by alveolar ventilation and is nearly independent of blood flow. $PaO_2$ is primarily determined by cardiac output, pulmonary blood flow, and only secondarily by alveolar ventilation. Factors influencing the magnitude of alveolar and arterial $PO_2$ difference include — (a) magnitude of venous admixture, (b) actual alveolar oxygen tension, (c) cardiac output, (d) temperature, pH and base excess of the blood, (e) haemoglobin concentration and (f) alveolar ventilation.

The blood gas analysis is usually accomplished by putting in heparinised arterial blood in 'Micro-Astrup blood gas analysis' or by spectrophotometer or by other techniques.

**Alveolar and blood — gas values (tension)**

| Gas | Alveoli | Arterial blood | Venous blood |
|---|---|---|---|
| $O_2$ | 104 mm Hg | 95 mm Hg | 40 mm Hg |
| $CO_2$ | 40 mm Hg | 40 mm Hg | 46 mm Hg |
| $O_2$ Saturation | 100% | 97% | 70% |
| $O_2$ with 100% $O_2$ inhalation | 700 mm Hg | 640 mm Hg | — |
| $O_2$ Saturation | 100% | 100% | |

**Conclusion**

In case of respiratory inadequacy, we will have to find out where the fault lies. Is there any defect in the ventilatory function or in gas exchange or in perfusion of the lungs ? Abnormalities of ventilatory function can be easily detected by making a spirometric study, (Vitalograph) and corrected accordingly. If the various spirometric findings are within normal limits, gaseous exchange studies should be undertaken by using blood-gas analyses. The values of alveolar and arterial oxygen and carbon dioxide tension should be obtained.

Low $PaO_2$ and high $Pa\ Co_2$ are indicative of respiratory insufficiency. If it is not of ventilatory origin, give 100% of oxygen for 10 min with a mark and measure again the alveolar and arterial $O_2$ and $Co_2$ tension. If the $PaO_2$ rises to 600 mm Hg or above, there is no shunt effect from right to left. High $Pa\ Co_2$ value in such cases can be lowered by increasing ventilation. On the other hand, if the $PaO_2$ does not rise after giving 100% oxygen test, the high value of $PaCo_2$ is invariably due to some ventilation-perfusion incoordination.

To find out the exact nature of the defect in diffusion or in distribution of gas and blood over the membrane surface, more elaborate tests like (a) carbon monoxide inhalation test, (b) nitrogen wash out test, (c) single breath Xenon test etc. should be undertaken.

For the low $PaO_2$, circulatory and other factors must be properly assessed and corrected.

• [Updated and based on annual oration 1981 at the Society of Anaesthiology, published in Ind. J. Anaesth (30.1), 7.]

## INFECTIONS OF THE UPPER RESPIRATORY TRACT (URT)

*ANIL ADHYA*

The common infections of the upper respiratory tract are usually due to virus, but sometimes bacterial and rarely fungal affections may occur as follows :

**a. Viral Infections of U.R.T :**

I. **Common cold or coryza or croup —**

(a) Rhinoviruses
(b) Respiratory syncytial Viruses.
(c) Para-influenza Viruses
(d) Adeno-Viruses

II. **Pharyngo-laryngo-conjunctivitis –**
(a) Adeno-Viruses
(b) Influenza Viruses
(c) Para-influenza Viruses

**b. Bacterial Infections :**

I. **Acute –**
(a) Streptococcal sore throat and acute tonsillitis
(b) Pharyngitis : Acute catarrhal and septic pharyngitis
(c) Acute sinusitis
(d) Diphtheria

II. **Chronic :**
(a) Chronic pharyngitis
(b) Chronic laryngitis
(c) Chronic tonsillitis
(d) Chronic sinusitis

Acute affections of U.R.T. may be mild, or very serious. It may be due to virus or bacterial invasion, following viral damage. Sometimes it is a part of general infectious disease, e.g. measles, influenza, enteric fever, scarlet fever and German measles. The last two are rare in tropical zones. In serious septic pharyngitis, the whole oro-pharyngeal mucosa may be inflammed with brawny oedematous mucosa (Ludwig's angina). Sometimes retropharyngeal abscess or even peritonsillar abscess may be followed.

Therefore, the classification of the U.R.T. must be made on clinical grounds, while search should be made for causative organisms e.g. virus, bacteria, spirochaetal organisms (Vincent's angina), thrush (moniliasis) membranous lesions (diphtheria) as well as mycoplasma pneumonae affection of U.R.T.

## ACUTE NASO-PHARYNGITIS

This is generally known as coryza due to viral infection causing mild to moderate degree of fever, nasal discharge, sneezing, pain in throat and even laryngitis causing hoarse voice. Severe headache with aches and pain in the body may be present due to myalgia and arthralgia.

In small children, temperature may be high especially when it is forerunner of measles. Always look for Koplik's spot and if present measles can be predicted.

In septic pharyngitis,temperature may be high and there is always chance of aspiration of septic discharge into bronchioles, especially in children or aged people leading to aspiration pneumonia or lung abscess.

Look for retropharyngeal or peritonsillar abscess.

**Treatment :**

**(1) Prophylactic –**

A child habitually suffering from cold should be reviewed during free interval, when enquiry should be made regarding environment and habits especially to check the diet, clothing, exercise and ventilation. Too much carbohydrates in diet predisposes to catarrhal infection. The diet should be balanced with adequate vitamin supplements but this does not mean too much cream, butter, and sweets. A balanced mixed diet is all that is required to maintain good nutrition.

Clothing should be absorptive but not heavy. Exercise needs be regular but not beyond child's capability. Over-crowded environment is not satisfactory. Children often play in water and do not care to change wet clothing. Training to protect from inclement weather is essential. Vaccine administration in time, if not contraindicated, is beneficial. However, some children need individualised care.

**(2) Active –**

Treatment is supportive and symptomatic.

A child having severe cold, should be in bed even if there is no rise in temperature.

Plenty of fluids should be given, acetylsalicylic acid and antihistaminic drugs in adequate doses may be beneficial. Administration of antibiotics is to be kept reserved for complications and secondary bacterial infections, should the occasion arise bacteriolytic and not a bacterio-static antibiotics e.g. tetracyclines be used. Ampicillins or amoxycillins are quite effective. Tetracyclines should also be avoided for infants and children as these drugs given repeatedly or for long periods may cause discoloured teeth.

**Anatomy of Tonsils :**

Tonsils belong to epithelial group of lymphoid tissue. Larger collection of lymphoid tissues under pharyngeal mucous membrane is described in Waldeyer's ring.

The sub-epithelial collection of lymphoid tissue in pharynx is :

(1) **Nasopharyngeal Adenoid :** subepithelial lymphoid tissue collection situation on the roof of nasopharynx. Air passing through nasopharynx comes in contact with its enlarged surface.

(2) **Palatine or faucial** – The tonsils lie between anterior and posterior pillar of tonsils in the fauces of the pharynx.

(3) **Lingual tonsils** – At root of the tongue. Collectively the above structures form the Waldeyer's ring (imaginary).

The lymphoid tissue essentially consists of –

(1) A suporting framework and (2) a cellular mass.

(1) The framework is formed by –

(a) Reticulum fibre with cells.
(b) Collagenous and elastic fibres.
(c) A few muscle cells.

(2) The cellular mass is composed of large and small lymphocytes and their precursor cells.

The lymphoid tissues differ from lymph nodes in the following manner :

(a) These are subepithelial in situation.
(b) These have no afferent channel.
(c) They have no distinct cortex and medulla.

## ACUTE TONSILLITIS

Acute infection of the palatine tonsils may be a part of acute upper respiratory tract viral infections or due to streptococcal tonsillitis. Clinical types are follicular, parenchymatous, or membranous, all caused by bacterial invasion.

Initial viral invasion of the mucous membrane may have the path for secondary bacterial infection. The streptococci, staphylococci, and pneumococci may be present in a healthy mouth.

Liability and severity of tonsillitis is dependent upon general body resistance, tendency of local accumulation of debri in tonsillar crypts and incomplete resolution from an attack of tonsillitis.

Common tonsillar infection is caused by beta-haemolytic streptococcus. This may also occur in epidemics especially when overcrowding and inadequate ventilation facilitates bacterial invasion. Nasal obstruction necessitates greater or lesser degree of mouth breathing with consequent dripping of pharyngeal mucous membrane, also predisposes to tonsil infection.

The condition is common in children after the age of three or four and also occurs in years of adolescence and adulthood. This is rare in infancy and after the age of 50 years.

**Symptoms and Signs**

The disease may begin insidiously with systemic disturbance like dry throat, general malaise, fever and thirst. In children,sore throat may not always be complained of and diagnosis may only be apparent on inspection of the throat, during investigation of anorexia, unexplained fever, and even abdominal pain in some cases.

Onset of disease may also be sudden with typical primary tonsillitis with β-haemolytic streptococcal infection. There may be rise in pulse rate and temperature which may be as high as 40.5 degree Celsius (105°F). Pain may be acute in throat with difficulties in swallowing and radiating to ears. Voice may be thick and muffled due to progressive swelling to palate and pharynx. The glands at the angle of the jaw (mandible) become swollen and tender with stiff neck, headache, pain in the back and limbs.

On examination,the breath may be foetid and the tongue coated. Appearance of tonsils will, of course, vary with the progress of the disease. In mild cases the tonsils are red and swollen and the palate and pharynx also become inflammed (parenchymal tonsillitis).

In more severe cases there may be exudation of purulent yellow material from tonsil-crypts, giving spotted appearance to tonsils along with swelling of the palate and uvula (follicular tonsillitis).

In many many cases the purulent debri spread and coalesce and may finally invade the neighbouring areas and in this way a false membrane is formed (membranous tonsillitis). This membrane is soft and friable and does not adhere closely to underlying tissue in contradistinction to diphtheritic membrane, which bleeds on.

**Differential Diagnosis :**

1. **Diphtheria** –
   - (a) The onset is insidious associated with local discomfort and mild constitutional symptoms.
   - (b) Temperature is usually low grade rarely about 39°C unless there is complication.
   - (c) The membrane forms on the tonsils but may extend into the palate and other parts of pharynx and larynx.
   - (d) The membrane is usually dirty grey in colour which cannot be removed easily and when pulled out with forcep it causes bleeding.
   - (e) Identification of Klabs-Loffler bacillus in the membrane is diagnostic.

It must be emphasized that in case of doubt it is safer to treat the case as one of diphtheria without waiting for swab report, which may sometimes be misleading.

**Vincent's Angina** –

(a) This is subacute tonsillitis with ulcerations, usually limited to one side.

(b) Its onset is slow, sore throat is less and fever not usually high.

(c) A pseudomembrane usually forms on the ulcers due to necrosis of superficial layer of epithelium.

(d) It is soft and grey or greenish in colour and comes away in fragments leaving irregular ulcers with sloping edges.

The disease is common in children and young adults with debilitated health and low vitamin-C contents in blood. Decaying teeth predisposes to the condition.

The diagnosis is confirmed from a throat swab culture spirocheets denticola and Vincent's fusiform bacillus.

## GRANULOCYTOPAENIA AND LEUKAEMIA

This may present with acute sore throat and necrotising lesions of tonsils. Ulcers are usually present in mouth and elsewhere in oropharynx with less in inflammatory surrounding reactions; throat and pharynx may rather appear pale. A complete haemogram especially white cell count and morphology will clinch the diagnosis.

## INFECTIOUS MONONUNCLEOSIS (GLANDULAR FEVER)

The condition is common in Europeans and is caused by E-B virus. It is difficult to distinguish especially in initial stage, from severe attack of acute tonsillitis. This common in young adults, persists with fever in spite of antibiotic therapy, with severe local discomfort and swelling and membrane formation on pad of tonsils. Clinical enlargement of different group of lymph nodes, spleen, and liver in varying proportions is common.

The diagnosis of the condition is confirmed from —

(a) **Peripheral blood picture** with at least 50% lymphocytes of which significant number are atypical cells.

(b) **Paul-Bunnel-Davidson Test** — demonstration of presence of antibodies which will haemolyse ox red cells.

## APHTHOUS ULCERS

This is a very painful condition which may present as sore throat. Aetiology of the malady is uncertain, may be viral.

The ulcer is usually solitary, small and superficial and may appear any where in oral cavity and pharynx but is common on anterior pillars of fauces.

## SCARLET FEVER

This is streptococcal tonsillitis with erythematous petechial skin rash, stippled palate, strawberry tongue and tachycardia disproportionate to pyrexia. The condition is common in Europeans.

**Complications** : This may be local or systemic.

**Local Complications :**

(1) **Chronic Tonsillitis** — When tonsils do not return normalcy in spite of appropriate chemotherapy and recurrence of attack is frequent.

(2) **Peritonsillar Abscess (Quinsy)** — When infection and subsequent pus formation occurs in the aeriolar space between tonsil bed and capsule.

(3) **Acute Otitis Media** — Some children are specially prone to get otitis media following acute tonsillitis.

(4) **Cervical Adenitis** — Suppuration may spread to jugulodigastric group of lymph nodes. The condition is uncommon nowadays because of adequate antibiotic therapy.

(5) **Parapharyngeal Abscess** — When pus formation occurs between superior constrictor muscle and deep cervical fascia following tonsillitis or Quinsy.

**Systemic Complications :**

Chiefly associated with haemolytic streptococcal tonsillitis.

(1) **Rheumatic Fever** — Tonsils may be the portal of entry of organisms when acute tonsillitis associated with attack of rheumatic fever.

(2) **Acute Glomerulonephritis** — This is recognised by puffy face. Oedema, oliguria & Hypertension, Urine contains albumin, RBC's, casts, specific gravity is above 1024.

(3) **Sub-acute infective endocarditis** — Patients with valvular lesions of heart may develop endocarditis with vegetations on the damaged valves due to organisms from infected tonsils.

(4) **Sydneham's Chorea** — This rare condition may occur in patients with acute tonsillitis.

**Treatment**

Treatment of acute tonsillitis is essentially medical which may be divided into local and general.

**Local treatment :**

**Mouth wash and gargle** — Rinsing mouth with diluted antiseptic solution has a soothing effect and helps to keep the mouth clean. It is very doubtful whether gargle reaches the tonsils themselves.

Aspirin in suspension may be used for gargling to dissolve sticky mucus when there are no contraindications, e.g., drug sensitivity or peptic ulcer. Paracetamol or aspirin may be given orally one tablet two or three times daily to relieve pain.

**Local application of heat** — When cervical lymph-glands are swollen and tender application of warmed flannel or cloth-pad may be applied to neck.

These various local measures may be comforting but it is doubtful if they are of any real therapeutic value and should not be persisted into the point of tiring or annoying the patient.

**Lozenges** — Containing antibiotics are ineffective in true tonsillitis, moreover have added disadvantage of sometimes causing troublesome glossitis and even encourage overgrowth of monilia.

**General :**

**Symptomatic measure** — In acute tonsillitis patient is well advised to have rest in bed and to remain isolated. Pulse and temperature is recorded 6 to 8 hourly, and if possible a throat-swab should be taken for culture of organisms and sensitivity tests for antibiotics.

Patients should encouraged to drink more fluid and routine attention to bowel clearance should be forgotten.

**Antibiotic therapy** — Principles of antibiotic therapy should not be overlooked; these are not to be used for minor sore throats because of risk of development of organisms of resistant strains and allergic reactions on the part of patients. Further this may jeopardise successful therapeutic effect in the event of further major illness.

Antibiotic measure is to be withheld in early stages unless and until it is apparent that the patient has a major attack and not responding to symptomatic therapy or is known to have complications from previous attack.

When a decision is taken in favour of antibiotic therapy, this should be administered in proper dosage, initially by intramuscular route if necessary, then oral route may be used for maintenance of optimum blood level. The therapy should be continued, even after the patient is symptomatic, for three to five days.

Penicillin is undoubtedly most appropriate in majority of cases, should there be no history of drug sensitivity.

**Dose :** I.M. injection of procaine penicillin, 300,000 units and benzyl penicillin 100,000 units should be given in severe cases and the doses may be repeated in 12 hours in patients of all ages over 6 years of age, and are to be continued once or twice daily. Ampicillin, amoxycillin and co-trimoxazole are also usually quite effective and can be given orally.

Throughout the course of the disease test urine for albumen and watch for development of rashes, cardiac murmurs or joint lesions. Pain in the ears may point towards onset of otitis media or may be first symptom for peritonsillar abscess (quinsy). In later case the tympanic membrane will appear normal.

## ACUTE BRONCHITIS

*G.C. MOOKERJEE*

### Introduction

It is an acute inflammation of the tracheobronchial tree due to virus, bacteria or some bacterial super-infection on viral tracheobronchitis.

### Aetiology

Small children and aged are more susceptible, particularly if malnourished. Too much tobacco smoking is an important predisposing cause. Patients of chronic bronchitis, pulmonary fibrosis, CCF and chronic heart disease are also susceptible. Patients are also prone while on corticosteroid therapy or on immuno-suppressive drugs. Subjects with hypogamma-globulinaemia are extremely liable. Exposure to cold, dust, industrial gases and fumes, e.g. ammonia, sulphur dioxide, nitrogen dioxide and irritant factors. Many infectious diseases, e.g. measles, whooping cough, typhoid or typhus fever and toxaemic patients develop bronchial inflammation.

### Pathology

In acute pyogenic tracheobronchitis, the organism concerned was Str. pneumoniae, H. influenzae and staphylococcus pyogenes.

Infection due to viruses of measles, whooping cough, common cold, influenza virus, para-influenza virus, respiratory syncytial viruses etc. may damage the tracheobronchial tree, followed by secondary bacterial invasion.

The tracheobronchial mucosa becomes congested followed by acute submucous inflammation causing pouring out of mucus followed by polymorph cellular emigration. The inflammation may progress from catarrhal stage to acute purulent bronchitis, producing mucopurulent expectoration.

### Clinical Features

When it is preceded by common cold or pharyngitis or sinusitis, symptoms due to these conditions will be prominent. When it is a part of systemic infection e.g. due to infectious fever, other clinical manifestations will be evident.

Usual manifestations are as follows :-

(1) Retro-sternal pain or raw feeling

(2) Fever mild to moderate 38° to 39°C.

(3) Dry irritating cough later mucoid or mucopurulent expectoration.

(4) Wheezing due to bronchial inflammation. Bilateral rhonchi and coarse rales are heard. Expiration may be prolonged.

It may progress to bronchopneumonia if neglected or if patient's resistance is poor. Severe cause may have dyspnoea and cyanosis especially if chronic bronchitis, or emphysema, or heart disease is associated.

### Treatment

Great care should be taken if the patient is in geriatric or paediatric age group especially smaller children.

Patients should be given bed rest except in very mild cases. Antibiotics should be carefully chosen depending on the clinical background or severity of attack.

Sputum examination is often very helpful if examined under microscope by Gram's stain.

Haemophilus influenzae may be very serious, especially in patients of old age group. Ampicillin 2 to 3 gm daily or Amoxycillin 250 to 500 mg. thrice daily for 7 to 10 days usually adequate.

Parenteral penicillin or ampicillin may be prescribed if patient cannot take by mouth. Tetracyclines should be avoided in small children. Co-trimoxazole is also effective.

Supportive treatment consists of adequate fluid intake, proper diet and relief of cough. Numerous proprietary cough syrups are available and most of these contain anti-histaminics which can be useful to some extent but anti-histaminics may cause thick and tenacious sputum, causing further trouble. Simple expectorant mixtures should be prescribed containing codeine and syrup Vasaka. Oxymel scilla and syrup ipecuc may be included. Steam inhalation with tinc-benzoin may give relief. Trypsin and chymotrypsin orally help to reduce viscosity of sputum. If bronchospasm is troublesome salbutamol, ephedrine or aminophylline should be prescribed as indicated. When acute bronchitis supervenes in case of chronic bronchitis or bronchial asthma, great care is necessary in treatment, (vide chapters on chronic bronchitis and asthma). Cough suppressing drugs should be meticulously avoided in cases of C.O.P.D. with acute bronchial infection.

## PNEUMONIAS

*G.C. MOOKERJEE*

### Definition

Pneumonia signifies inflammatory diseases of the lung, affecting one or more segments, lobes. Patchy lesions involving both lungs denote broncho-pneumonia.

The term "pneumonitis" denotes inflammation of the pulmonary tissues but it is usually applied to segmental pneumonia.

### Classification

**A. Anatomical**

1) Lobar
2) Segmental
3) Lobular, which when bilateral is termed bronchopneumonia.

**B. Aetiological**

1) Specific
2) Non-specific

Specific, when a causative pathogen can be isolated from the sputum. Commonest of all is pneumococcal pneumonia.

The other group is known as "Aspiration pneumonias". These are due to aspiration of infected material from upper respiratory tract usually causing segmental pneumonitis due to mixed organisms.

SPECIFIC PNEUMONIAS may be due to the following :

1) **Bacterial pneumonias**

a) Pneumococcal (Commonest)
b) Streptococcal
c) Staphylococcal
d) Klebsiella pneumonia (Friedlander's bacillus)
e) Haemophilus influenzae
f) Mycobacterium tuberculosis
g) Leginonnaire's disease.

2) **Viral pneumonitis**
   a) Adenovirus
   b) Myxovirus : Influenza and parainfluenza virus and respiratory syncytial virus.
   c) Rhinovirus.
   (d) Psittacosis-ornithosis virus
   (e) Measles, variola, cytomegalovirus. Infectious mononucleosis picovirus etc.

3) **Fungal pneumonitis**
   a) Histoplasmosis
   b) Aspergillosis
   c) Candidiasis
   d) Coccidiomycosis
   e) Actinomycosis & Nocardiasis

4) **Pneumonitis**
   a) R. Burnetti (Q - fever)
   b) R. Prowazeki (Typhus) etc.

5) **Rickettsial pneumonitis**
   a) Entamoeba histolytica
   b) P. falciparum
   c) Pneumocystes carini.

6) **Pneumonias due to non-infectious causes :**

a) **Chemical pneumonias** — Due to toxic fumes, smokes and gases; nasal drops containing paraffin; domestic accidents due to kerosene, a quite common emergency, especially among small children.

b) **Drugs :** Cytotoxic drugs, particularly bleomycin may cause pneumonia.

c) **Radiation :** Supervoltage X-ray may cause radiation pneumonitis during therapy of malignant diseases.

d) **Miscellaneous :** Pneumonias may also be caused when immune mechanisms of the body are impaired, e.g. hypo or dysgamma-globulinaemia, leukaemias, lymphomas, myelomatosis and administration of steroids for long periods. Bacterial and fungal super infections usually supervene.

**Non-specific or Aspiration Pneumonias**

Likely to occur in very weak or malnourished patients, after oral surgery, dental extraction, too much alcoholic drinks, narcotic drugs in excess, comatose patients, after drowning etc. Patients in extremes of age are specially susceptible. Sputum smear examination or culture will show mixed organisms, usually commensal flora from oropharynx.

## PNEUMOCOCCAL PNEUMONIA

This is characterised by homogeneous consolidation of one or more lobes or segments of the lung due to pneumococcus which constitutes about 80% of all cases of pneumonias. Extremes of age group are more susceptible.

**Pathogenesis**

Pneumococci may be present in the nasopharynx of normal population. They may act as carriers and may cause pneumonia in others or sometimes in themselves, when resistance is low. The organisms go down the respiratory pathway in mucus blanket, especially when ciliary activity is depressed. Preceding viral affection may be an important factor in precipitation of pneumonia.

Pneumococci (types 1,2,3,6,7,14 & 19) are usually involved and due to their multiplication, bacterial toxins are liberated. This results in engorgement of the capillaries in the alveolar walls and large number of erythrocytes and leucocytes with fibrin exudate escape into the air-sacs (stage of red hepatisation). The affected alveoli become full of fibrinous network in which the lymphocytes and polymorphs are entangled (grey hepatisation). Subsequently the coagulum is replaced by large number of polymorphs which phagocytose the bacteria and eventually the exudation is absorbed from the air cells. (stage of resolution). Occasionally resolution may be delayed or fibrosis may occur if patient is not adequately treated. Associated pleural effusion may also occur (Syn-pneumonic effusion).

**Clinical Features**

The patient looks ill with flushed face. Temperature rises abruptly with chill and rigor and the patient is unable to take deep breath. There is pleuritic chest pain, mild cyanosis; the cough is dry, irritating and painful. Sputum is rust-coloured, may sometimes be blood stained as well. The rate of respiration is increased to 30-50/minutes with pulse and respiration ratio altered to 3 : 1 or 2 : 1. The alaenasi together with the accessory muscles of respiration, are active and herpes labialis is often present. Movement of chest during respiration over the affected lobe is diminished which is also dull on percussion with increased VF and VR. Bronchial breathing may be present over the whole or part of the lobe, sometimes together with whispering pectoriloquy. Crepitations are heard usually later in the illness and during resolution.

---

COMPLICATIONS OF PNEUMONIA
(Result of inadequate treatment or delay)

| | |
|---|---|
| SEPTICAEMIA | PERICARDITIS |
| CIRCULATORY COLLAPSE | MENINGITIS |
| PLEURAL EFFUSION | ARTHRITIS |
| or EMPYEMA | PERITONITIS (Children) |
| DEHYDRATION | |
| DELAYED RESOLUTION | |

(Look for obstructive pathology, e.g., F.B., gland or new growth)

---

**Diagnosis**

Initial rigor, herpes labialis, physical signs of consolidation together with polymorphonuclear leucocytosis and segmental radiological capacity establish the diagnosis but sometimes it is necessary to differentiate it from other types of specific and aspiration pneumonias, pulmonary infarction, pulmonary tuberculosis and tuberculous pleurisy with effusion, pulmonary collapse and acute bronchitis.

**Laboratory Diagnosis**

1. **Haematological** – Polymorphonuclear leucocytosis. Total count is often 20,000-30,000 cm. A low count carries bad prognosis.
2. **Radiological** – A hazy, uniform shadow is seen in the area corresponding to the anatomical situation of the affected lobe.
3. **Sputum** – Gram's staining and microscopical examination shows gram-positive diplococci. Culture of sputum may be done, but is usually unnecessary.
4. **Blood culture** – (usually unnecessary) 50% positive.

**Treatment**

a) **Specific** – Penicillin is the drug of choice but should not given orally. Crystalline penicillin G or procaine-penicillin 600,000 units should be given twice daily I.M. in mild cases. In severe cases up to one million units of crystalline penicillin may be given intramuscularly every six hours. The treatment is to be continued until the patient has been afebrile for 3-4 days.

If injections are not desired, ampicillin or amoxycillin may be used orally in dosage of 250-500 mg six hourly for 7-10 days. Although most cases usually respond well to penicillin or penicillin derivatives, penicillin-resistant cases are being reported (Douglas and Crofton). In such cases or in cases of penicillin allergy, co-trimoxazole, tetracylines, demethocycline, lincomycin, cephalosporins may be used. In severe cases or if the patient is not responding, antibiotic sensitivity should be carried out. Cefazolin 4.0 g I.V. daily injections have been reported useful in severe cases. Also be cautious to investigate underlying bronchial obstruction due to a growth or F.B., especially if there is delayed resolution.

**Supportive therapy**

Absolute bed rest is important in severe cases. Humidified oxygen to be used in the initial stages. Avoid narcotic cough suppressants especially in children and old. Paracetamol may be used judiciously for hyperpyrexia. Diazepam or nitrazepam at night gives good sleep and is also useful if there is restlessness. Codiene phosphate 15 to 30 mg is used for relieving pleural pain. In old people, watch carefully for CHF and digitalise if necessary. Anti-histamine containing syrup be better avoided.

Ensure adequate fluid intake and provide proper nutrition, High protein food supplements and multivitamin supplements should be used. A polyvalent pneumococcal vaccine is available in USA for protection of high risk subjects especially children or old with heart or kidney disease.

## STAPHYLOCOCCAL PNEUMONIA

Rare about 2 to 5% of all pneumonia. Common during influenza epidemics and can be very severe causing fatalities especially in young and old.

Abscess formations are common, which look like thin-walled cavities in radiograph.

Pneumothorax or pyopneumothorax may occur especially in children.

A simple sputum smear and microscopy after Gram's staining will establish the causative organism.

Inj. penicillin is recommended in 20 million daily dose. I.M. if organisms are sensitive, which is usually not so nowadays. It may be treated with erythromycin 500 mg. six hourly orally.

In cases of severe infection,cloxacillin, naficillin, clindomycin,vancomycetin or cephalothin may be required in appropriate doses. Co-trimoxazole may also be effective singly or in combination. Sensitivity test is desirable as possibility of resistant strains always exists, especially in hospital infection.

## HAEMOPHILUS INFLUENZAE PNEUMONIA

Usually complicates chronic bronchitis and bronchiectasis. During influenza epidemics it can be a secondary invader. Ampicillin, amoxycillin and co-trimoxazole are effective in high doses. Sensitivity tests may be done before starting treatment with any of these agents. Recently moxalactum has been used with good results.

## STREPTOCOCCAL PNEUMONIA

Very rare. Usually complicates influenza, especially during epidemics. Streptococcus pyogenes broncho-pneumonia should be treated as in case of pneumococcal infection. Rarely Str. Viridans may cause segmental pneumonitis. Sensitivity test is usually necessary in these cases.

## FRIEDLANDER'S PNEUMONIA

Friedlander's pneumonia is due to klebsiella pneumoniae and is usually serious. Sputum is like red current jelly. It causes massive consolidation of mostly upper lobes. It may cause leucopenia instead of leucocytosis. It may also be mistaken for tuberculosis.

Since this is usually sensitive to streptomycin and chloramphenicol, Inj. streptomycin 1.0 gm. twelve hourly is given I.M. together with chloramphenicol 500 mg. six hourly orally for about a week or two.

Alternatively, co-trimoxazole orally or gentamycin intramuscularly in divided doses may be used. More recently cefotaxime or cephalosporins have been used successfully.

## TUBERCULOUS LOBAR PNEUMONIA

Details of pulmonary tuberculosis have been discussed in a separate chapter but it should be stressed that all patients clinically diagnosed and treated as pneumonia, should have sputum checked carefully to exclude tuberculosis especially in developing countries.

## VIRAL PNEUMONIAS

Viral affection causes diffuse inflammation of the lung in the form of broncho-pneumonic patches rather than localised consolidation and is characterised by general malaise, anorexia, remittent fever and dry, hacking cough. The disease is usually self-limited and usually settles down within about two weeks. But the influenza viruses may cause very severe broncho-pneumonia often aggravated, due to associated secondary organisms. The treatment is symptomatic. Antibiotics are given to control secondary infection. Very young and old people may develop severe types and require careful treatment. Microscopic examination of sputum smear after Gram's staining, will show presence of secondary organisms and suitable antibiotics can be chosen. Antibiogram may be done wherever indicated.

## ASPIRATION PNEUMONIA

Aspiration of vomit may cause an acute haemorrhagic pneumonia characterised by pulmonary oedema, haemoptysis, marked bronchospasm and shock. Recurrent aspiration of milk feeds, liquid paraffin etc. may give rise to lipoid pneumonia characterised by cough, sputum, haemoptysis and chest pain.

### Treatment

**A) Specific**

Inj. Benzyl-penicillin one mega unit 6 hourly I.M. In penicillin-sensitive persons, tetracyclines 500 mg. six hourly orally or 100 mg. six to eight hourly I.M. may be given. In severe cases, cloxacillin or methicillin one gm. stat intravenously followed by 0.5 gm. six hourly or Inj. Gentamycin IM should be used.

**B) Supportive treatment**

i) Rest in bed.
ii) Oxygen inhalation may be very useful in severe cases.
iii) Catheteric suction, to relieve accumulated pulmonary secretion.
iv) Tracheostomy in critically ill patients, to avoid irreversible hypoxia.
v) Anti-tussives. Avoid narcotics in extremes of age.
vi) Analgesics — e.g. paracetamol better than aspirin.
vii) Respiratory failure and shock should be treated energetically.

Peripheral circulatory failure is sometimes very severe when high doses of steroids and careful fluid therapy are desirable.

## RARE PNEUMONIAS

Besides the specific pneumonias described above, many serious diseases may be terminally complicated by pneumonias or broncho-pneumonias. If this is not treated with proper antibiotics and supportive therapy fatalities may result due to toxaemia and pulmonary failure.

More recently proteus, pseudomonas and serratia are being noted in pneumonias occurring in old debilitated people, alcoholics or those who required tracheal suction or intubation etc. during respiratory care. Cephalosporins or tobramycins are useful.

Pneumonias can occur in patients of smallpox, chicken-pox and other infectious fevers, e.g. enteric fever, typhus fever, etc. Brucellosis can however produce specific pneumonitis and pleural effusion. Influenza virus and other viruses can cause bronchopneumonias but secondary invaders soon are added. In epidemics, severe influenzal pneumonitis may cause high mortality.

Protozoal pneumonias may occur due to malaria (MT infection) and pneumocystis carini. Pneumocystis carini pneumonia often affects patients who are suffering from leukaemic disease or patients under treatment with high dose of steroids or anti-cancer drugs.

Pneumonia may also occur due to overdose of radiotherapy used for treatment of malignant diseases. In this situation, local pathology consists of thickening of alveolar walls and infiltration of alveoli with lymphocytes, macrophages and ultimately resulting in fibrosis.

The radiological appearance somewhat resembles pulmonary oedema.

The treatment is unsatisfactory but steroids may be helpful in acute stage. Associated secondary infection should also be treated.

## CHEMICAL PNEUMONIA

Chemical pneumonia occurs usually due to industrial gases or metal fumes. There may be broncho-spasm, pneumonitis associated with pulmonary oedema. Acute cases should be treated with humidified oxygen and steroids.

In comatose patients, regurgitation of acid gastric contents may be inhaled causing chemical pneumonitis. This is known as "Mendelson syndrome". It may also occur during anaesthesia or in achalasia cardia, oesophageal strictures or hiatus hernia. Prevention is more important but the treatment consists of respiratory toilet, aspiration of irritant materials, oxygen inhalation steroids and antibiotics.

## LIPOID PNEUMONIA

Inhalation of mineral, animal or vegetable oils may cause lipoid pneumonia. Kerosene or diesel oil may also cause serious pneumonitis. Excessive use of nasal drops containing mineral oil may cause localised lipoid pneumonia.

Radiological picture is very characteristic consisting of Rosette-like nodular shadows. There may be interstitial fibrosis and small bullae formation. Sometimes aggregated inhaled material may form segmental collapse and fibrosis and radiological appearance may look like a picture of new growth.

Prevention is the best method of treatment because once the damage has been done, it cannot be reversed. However, steroids and antibiotics are used in early stage.

## MYCOPLASMA PNEUMONIA

During World War II, a kind of pneumonia was noted which was associated with myalgia, lymphadenopathy, skin rash and sometimes arthritis. This syndrome was then known as primary atypical pneumonia. Positive cold agglutination tests in serum were noted in 60% of the cases. In X-ray chest, ground glass opacities were noted in lower zones of one or both lungs, mostly right-sided. It is now known that the causative organism is a mycoplasma, which are the smallest free-living-organisms, capable of reproduction like bacteria. Tetracyclines and erythromycins are generally used but many patients have recovered without any antibiotic therapy.

## RICKETTSIAL PNEUMONIA

This is also known as Q. fever and the name is derived from "Query fever". Interestingly enough, the disease was described for the first time in Queensland. It is caused by a rickettsia known as Coxiella Burneti, discovered by Burnet and Cox, independently from Australia and U.S.A. respectively. Besides, transmission by ticks and mites, humans can be infected by dusts from stored hides of cattle and sheep. Incubation period is from 2 to 3 weeks. The disease has influenza-like onset, associated with bradycardia and sometimes hepatosplenomegaly The treatment consists of supportive therapy and use of tetracycline or chloramphenicol.

## LEGIONNAIRE'S PNEUMONIA

The disease resembling atypical pneumonia was recognised in July 1976, in an explosive outbreak which occurred mostly among delegates of an American legion convention. Out of 220 cases, 34 ended in fatalities.

The clinical feature resembles influenza-like onset gradually becoming worse. Physical signs may be unremarkable while chest roentgenogram shows extensive lesions. Respiratory failure and hypotension are serious complications.

This is due to Legionella pneumophilia, a coccobacillus, often causing severe respiratory infection associated with gastroenteritis and toxic nephritis.

Tetracyclines, doxycycline, erythromycin and rifamycin are effective. Erythromycin is drug of choice, given orally 0.5 g six hourly for 2-3 weeks. In severe cases I.V. administration is desirable initially. Rifamycin is given 10-20 mg/kg per day.

## LUNG-ABSCESS

(Syn : Suppurative pneumonia)

*G.C. MOOKERJEE*

Suppurative lesions of the lungs including necrotic abscesses and gangrene of pulmonary tissues, are related in terms of degrees. Abscess is rather localised to a segment or lobe while gangrene is more diffuse involving wider areas.

### Aetiology

Obstruction of a bronchus and infection of lungs distal to it is the basic pathology. The organisms may be commensals of the throat, aspirated into the segment of a lobe or sometimes blood borne. Anaesthetics, narcotics, alcohol and coma may encourage suppurative or aspiration pneumonitis.

Pyaemia is also an important cause causing multiple pyaemic lung abscesses.

Extremes of age, e.g., infants and octogenarians are most susceptible. Obstruction of a bronchus may also be due to :

Tuberculous glands, tumours, bronchostenosis and F.B.

Amoebic liver abscess may burst into pleura and lungs but primary amoebic lung abscess may also occur.

A new growth may become necrotic in the centre and may look like a lung abscess in the radiograph.

**Pathology**

The local lesion depends upon the aetiology. The abscess may be single or multiple or even scattered in both lungs.

Aspiration abscesses are segmental in distribution. As the right bronchus is more vertical than left, aspiration is more common in the right side.

The posterior segment of upper lobe and the apical segment of the right lower lobe being most vulnerable.

A bronchogenic carcinoma may break down centrally giving impression of an abscess. The walls are thick and saggy, located anywhere in midzone or base :

Staphylococcal lung abscesses are multiple and are then walled, giving multiple soap-bubble appearance.

Organisms should be isolated by culture and sensitivity tests as it is helpful in choice of treatment. Usually streptococci, haemophilus influenzae, staphylococci, Friedlander's bacilli, anaerobic organisms, Vincent's spirochaetes and fusiform bacilli are involved.

**Clinical features**

Most cases have an abrupt pneumonic onset but in some cases of aspiration pneumonitis, onset may be insidious, hence initially it is neglected as minor illness. Later high temperature, chest-pain, dyspnoea and toxaemia supervene to disclose the diagnosis. Haemoptysis may also be present.

It may follow a dental extraction or a bout of late night boozing party, especially in elderly people.

Initially there is not much expectoration but within a few days, mucopurulent sputum or blood-stained sputum is noted.

**PHYSICAL SIGNS**

These depend on the size, situation and nature of abscess :

(a) If the abscess is not large and deep seated — no physical signs.

(b) If multiple small and bilateral, broncho-pneumonic signs may be present.

(c) If superficial near pleura, signs of pleurisy proclaimed by pleural rub. If effusion has occurred signs of pleural effusion will obscure the presence of abscess.

(d) If abscess is large, signs are restricted chest movement, dullness on percussion, diminished air entry and possibly transient pleural rub.

(e) Once the abscess cavity has started draining out, signs of cavity e.g. cavernous breath sounds and cracked pot sounds may be elicited.

If the lesion is not resolved for a few weeks abscess may become chronic, temperature is continued with toxaemia and clubbing of fingers becomes evident.

**Complications**

Empyema, pyaemia, brain-abscess, and amyloidosis

**Laboratory Findings**

(a) Leucocytosis is evident WBC being above 20,000 cmm. Microscopic examination of sputum reveals pus cells and organisms, already mentioned.

(b) Amoebic pus is classically described as chocolate or anchovy sauce coloured but it may be otherwise, e.g., greenish or yellowish with faint chocolate shades.

(c) Sometimes blood-culture is positive.

**Radiology**

Chest X-ray may show a localised opacity, segmental pneumonitis or pleural effusion.

Always PA and lateral view of chest should be taken.

Once the abscess has started draining and if pleural effusion is not present, a local circumscribed oval or round shadow may be seen with fluid level.

Tomography may be very helpful.

Staphylococcal suppurative pneumonitis presents multiple soap-bubble appearance.

Hydatid cyst may be confused with lung abscess which also has a fluid level round or oval outline in chest radiograph. Look for water-lily appearance.

A bronchogenic carcinoma may present as a circumscribed round or oval shadow or a mass with central necrosis presenting an abscess like appearance. The walls of abscess are typically thick and shaggy in appearance. These are usually squamous celled carcinoma. However, occasionally cavitated carcinomas may also have thin walls. Timely bronchoscopy and sputum cytology are helpful.

Infected lung cysts or bullae or large tuberculous cavity may also be confused with septic lung abscess.

Actinomycosis or other deep mycosis may sometimes sometimes simulate lung abscess.

Careful sputum examination and bronchoscopic aspiration will settle the diagnosis.

**Prognosis**

If properly treated prognosis is always good, provided diagnosis is not delayed. Prognosis is bad if diagnosis is delayed, proper facilities of antibiogram are not available and if there are background diseases, e.g., uncontrolled diabetes mellitus, carcinoma or advanced tuberculosis or mycosis.

**Treatment**

The treatment will depend on correct aetiological diagnosis. Hence most useful point is proper examination of sputum, its culture and antibiogram. If antibiotic sensitivity reports are not available, examination of sputum-smear by Gram's staining is a cheap and simple method to obtain ideas regarding the type of organisms involved.

(a) Use of appropriate antibiotic or anti-amoebic agent or antifungal drug.

(b) Postural drainage and physiotherapy.

(c) Bronchoscopy : Besides its great value as a diagnostic agent, flexible fiberoptic bronchoscopy used for aspiration of tenacious secretions and carrying out bronchial toilet, is often life-saving.

(d) Surgical treatment is rarely necessary if proper medical treatment is carried out. If the abscess is large, it has to be drained externally or a in case of bronchiectatic suppuration, lobectomy may be necessary.

Customarily, the antibiotic therapy is started with high dose of parenteral crystalline penicillin, e.g., one to two mega units, three to six hourly, depending on the clinical severity; later on suitable changes are made depending on the clinical progress or nature of offending organisms detected by sputum examination and antibiogram.

Supporting therapy, e.g., oxygen, fluids, diet and symptomatic treatment is continued to relieve cough and promote sleep. Anaemia is often marked and one or two units of fresh blood transfusion may be useful.

Sometimes surgical help is necessary, especially if abscess is thick-walled and large, not draining well or chronic abscess.

## BRONCHIAL ASTHMA

(Allergic airway obstruction; Idiopathic airway obstruction)

*G.C. MOOKERJEE*

### Definition

Bronchial asthma should be defined as a syndrome where there is recurrent and episodic breathlessness associated with wheezing expiration, lasting for hours and days with varying severity, caused by variable degrees of bilateral broncho-spasm. The attacks may spontaneously cease and may recur without warning. Hence this condition must be differentiated from cardiac asthma and pulmonary oedema due to any cause.

The narrowing of bronchial airways is usually due to –

(1) Broncho-spasm with contraction of smooth muscles of the bronchial tree;

(2) Oedema of bronchial mucosa membrane and submucosa;

(3) Presence of mucus within the lumen of bronchial tree resulting in further narrowing of bronchioles. Mucus also becomes thick and sticky.

During any attack of asthma usually the first two are always present and the third factor makes the situation desperate.

### Aetiology and Pathogenesis

The exact aetiopathology of bronchial asthma is still not clearly understood. Although allergy and infection are both well-known causes to precipitate broncho-constriction, it is not clear how the numerous agents, e.g., pollens, animal-fur, house-dusts, mould-spores, chemicals, fumes and obnoxious gases produce asthmatic attacks. Possible triggering factors may also be psychological and environmental, including infection. Physical exertion is also known to be a potent factor. Before we discuss the aetio-pathogenesis of bronchial asthma any further, it should be remembered that "bronchial asthma" is different from "cardiac asthma" or asthma-like attacks of acute or chronic bronchitis. It is felt that the term "cardiac asthma" be abolished and replaced by acute left ventricular failure or acute pulmonary oedema.

The pathological changes in well-established asthmatic patients are as follows :-

(1) Broncho-constriction of all grades of bronchi or bronchioles;

(2) Oedematous submucosa with congestion;

(3) Much plugging of bronchioles in almost all branches of bronchial tree which may also contain eosinophils;

(4) Denudation of ciliated epithelium usually due to viral or bacterial infection. In this situation pus cells also may be present in the sputum;

(5) There may also be thickening of the basement membrane and great increase in the number of goblet cells, in chronic cases.

### Immuno-pathology of allergic asthma

Researches in immunopathology during the last decade have proved the importance of enzyme – cellular response as a result of hypersensitivity reaction.

Gell and Coombs have classified the immunopathologic reactions into four types (Types I to IV).

Type I – Immediate anaphylactic response. i.e. atopic asthma.

Type II – Cytotoxic response as seen in Goodpasture's syndrome and certain drug reactions.

Type III – Immune complex disease e.g. pulmonary vasculitis (SLE & other collagen diseases) and serum sickness.

Type IV — Cell mediated, e.g., pulmonary eosinophilia. Parasites may be responsible.

In the case of acute allergic asthma, immediate hypersensitivity reaction (Type I of Gell-Coombs) occurs due to an agent to which the patient has become hypersensitive to the inhaled or ingested antigen which gets attached to the specific antibody on the cell surface culminating in release of agents resulting in asthma. This variety is called atopic or extrinsic type.

In extrinsic or atopic asthma the offending agent (antigen) produces immediate wheal and flare on skin testing. Immunoglobulin type IgE antibody is carrier of reagenic activity. In this type IgE having affinity for mast cells and basophil granulocytes cause antigen-antibody reaction. The allergen-IgE complex acts on the bronchial mucosal cells releasing chemical mediators, e.g., histamine slow reacting substances (SRS-A), bradykinins, prostaglandins and eosinophilic chemotactic factor of anaphylaxis (ECF-A).

In non-atopic type of asthma, skin tests usually do not produce any reaction. The bronchial tree becomes involved in acute infection or due to chemicals or industrial fumes and gases. Immunoglobulins are not raised. Immediate Type-I reaction is related to antibodies which belongs to IgE type of immuno-globulin, while in the delayed hypersensitivity (Type-II) or arthus type is related to IgE or IgM. Recent researches also suggest that IgG may also play some important role. Clinically asthma may be divided into extrinsic and intrinsic types on the following basis, which is easy to appreciate in clinical practice.

**Table — 17.2 : Types of bronchial asthma**

| Factors | Extrinsic asthma (atopic) | Intrinsic asthma |
|---|---|---|
| 1. Age | Childhood or teenaged | Adults from 20 to 40 years |
| 2. Family history | Usually present | Negative |
| 3. Causes | Usually specific antigens | Infection or exercise |
| 4. Skin test | Usually positive and IgE level is usually raised IgG may also be involved | Negative. No rise of immuno-globulins |

In certain cases besides the chemicals mentioned above, pollens, spores of fungi, house-dusts, mites, aspergillus fumigatus and various items of food such as cow's milk, prawn, shrimps, rotten fish, snails, etc. may cause allergic asthma. Many industrial gas and chemicals may also cause asthmatic attacks. Drug sensitivity causing asthma is also well-known.

Extensive research is being carried out to work out the immuno-pathological basis of asthma. The clinical problems of treatment still remain unsolved.

**Clinical features**

On clinical grounds, bronchial asthma can be divided into two groups, e.g., extrinsic and intrinsic asthma. The differential features of these two types are presented in Table-2 (vide *supra*).

**Clinical features of an attack**

Dyspnoea may be mild or severe depending on the attack of broncho-spasm and mucosal oedema-cough is present with scanty jelly-like mucoid expectoration.

There may be associated feeling of oppression in chest, leading to respiratory distress in severe cases. Patient cannot remain lying in bed and usually sits up and leans forward trying to get more air as he feels suffocated. Wheezing of broncho-spasm can be heard even without a stethoscope. Patient may become cyanosed with cold perspiration and the clinical feature may be mistaken for acute left ventricular failure.

On auscultation, plenty of rhonchi can be heard with variable rales.

In very severe cases, pulmonary ventilation may be so reduced that only few bilateral rhonchi may be heard. Blood pressure may be raised normal or low, pulse rate is always high with or without cyanosis. Perspiration with cold extremities is often the presenting feature of myocardial infarction in old patients and chest pain may be lacking. In such cases morphine or pethidine is life saving while in bronchial asthma a single dose of morphine or pethidine may cause fatality.

When severe attack continues for hours without responding to emergency treatment is termed as "Status asthmaticus" (nowadays being renamed "Acute severe asthma").

During acute attack, the patient becomes so apprehensive that he feels that death is impending. He is unable to talk and finds great difficulty in throwing out the inhaled air out of his lung. Even larynx may become partially obliterated leading to stridor and sometimes it may be necessary to do laryngoscopy or bronchoscopy to exclude local cause.

The duration of attack varies from time to time and unless it is controlled by proper treatment it may last for days. Therefore a patient is unable to eat and drink leading to nutritional and particularly hydration problems.

However, it is interesting to note that the patient may remain free from attacks for days and weeks and in some cases the attack comes two or three times a year.

**Precipitating Factors**

(1) *ALLERGENS* — There are so many possible allergens that it is extremely difficult to enlist them. Allergens may come from food, pollens, fungi or their spores. Among the food items, shellfish, crab meat, prawns, shrimps, sometimes rotten fish or even vegetables may be reponsible.

Aspergellus fumigatus is often a responsible agent which requires careful recognition. Presence of mites in house-dust or quilts is also not uncommon.

House-dusts, animal furs and droppings of birds, cats, dogs and horses even drugs may also be responsible for allergy.

(2) *INFECTION* — Respiratory tract infection may precipitate asthma in patients of all age groups. It is therefore important to eradicate the infection at the earliest possible stage, because in all known asthmatics, prevention of infection may prevent a severe attack.

(3) *PSYCHOLOGICAL FACTORS* — Although some physicians doubt the influence of psychological factor in the causation of attack, it is felt that psychological stress definitely may precipitate or exacerbate attacks in asthmatic patients. However, this is not a very major factor in most cases at least among Indian patients.

(4) *DRUGS* — Drugs like aspirin, penicillin and prostaglandins may cause asthmatic attack. Many organic chemicals, industrial fumes also may induce asthmatic attack.

(5) *EXERCISE* — Sometimes patients remain free from attacks while leading a sedentary life but even mild or moderate exertion may result in asthmatic attack. In some cases, it is curiously seen that asthma may improve after graduated exercise, the cause is not very clear. Possibly "Yoga" also helps in a similar way.

**Nature of Allergic Asthma**

Allergic asthma associated with Type-I allergy is most probably due to antibody known as Allergens which become fixed to the cells of bronchial mucosa. The fixation of allergens with fixed antibodies in the cells results in a series of enzymatic reactions. These end-products may affect bronchial muscles, blood vessels and goblet cells. The antibody which is responsible for Type—I allergic reaction is a type of gamma globulin known as IgE. In this Type-I asthmatics inhalation as well as prick tests are immediately positive while in patients with Type-III (Arthus type) allergic cases, the prick tests or provocative allergic reaction occurs after 4 to 8 hours. In these Type-III cases, the antibodies are not IgE but are IgG or IgM.

### Atopic Asthma

In atopic asthma offending antigens produce immediate skin reaction characterised by wheal and flare due to IgE induced allergic reaction. The chemical mediators concerned may be any of the following :-

Histamine and histamine-like substance

Prostaglandins

Bradykinin

SRS — A (Slow-reacting substance)

ECF — A (Eosinophilic chemotactic factor)

PAF — Platelet activating factor from mast cells.

In non-atopic subjects, the skin tests are mostly negative. In the case of these patients the upper respiratory tract infections are usually the triggering factor. Drug induced asthma may sometimes be so violent as to produce severe asthmatic attack as soon as the minute quantity of allergen comes in contact with the patient. The best example is violent and anaphylactic reaction due to serum injection (ATS or ADS). In the case of confirmed asthmatics however, even cold air, some exercise or psychological trauma may evoke an attack. Finally it is difficult to understand the exact aetiology, because pathogenesis of asthma is not fully understood. Although considerable advances have been made to clarify the nature of antigen-antibody reactions, the role of immuno-globulins especially in atopic asthma is not fully understood.

### Physical Signs

Sign during an attack is particulary that of overinflated lung. The patient is usually sitting and patient with the extraordinary muscles of respiration working maximally. The neck veins may appear full with or without cyanosis. The wheezing respiration can be heard from a distance. The expiration is prolonged with inability to speak.

In severe attack only wheezing is heard with hardly any audible breath sound. Pulse rate is usually above 120 per minute but regular.

Occasionally pulsus paradoxus may be present. Peak flow rate is much below normal and if it is less than 100 litres per minute there is risk of ventilatory failure.

Blood gas analysis shows reduced $PO_2$ and rising $PCO_2$. When the attack is not severe, the patient usually is dyspnoeic only on exertion. He may have slightly barrel-shaped chest and auscultation may show prolonged respiration.

Asthma induced by infection (non-atopic asthma) will have some different clinical picture. They may be evidence of upper respiratory tract infection, nasal congestion or even a nasal polyp.

### Investigations

Blood examination — Eosinophils may be increased which may sometimes be over 30% or 40% in case of typical eosinophilia which may present as typical asthma syndrome.

### Skin Tests

This is a very complicated method in which allergy experts are greatly interested. However, local allergens must be available which is not easy to organise unless a special allergy clinic is available. When properly performed it helps to identify atopic subjects and it is then possible usually, to discover specific allergens. Food challenge or inhalation challenge is also an alternative method and by which allergy experts may help in difficult cases.

### Diagnosis

In the young age group diagnosis of asthma is not difficult but in older people, chronic bronchitis and acute LVF (so-called cardiac asthma) should be excluded.

Aetiological diagnosis is, however, not easy. In our centre routine skin testing is adopted by preparing extracts from house dusts or suspected allergens. Allergens available, from imported ones may not be so useful in our areas as allergens may be different.

However in clinical practice good history taking and careful clinical assessment helps a lot. The following points are helpful :-

1) Family history of allergy;
2) Presence of asthma and childhood eczema in family. Sometimes same individual suffers from both in episodic manner. One may improve while the other appears;
3) Precipitation of asthma during house cleaning drives (dust allergen);
4) Exposure to animals — cats, dogs and horses;
5) Attacks occurring during visit to a particular house or garden (pollens);
6) Drugs and industrial gases and fumes causing attack.

Having noted these points much information may be obtained to help the patients without elaborate skin-testing. However, selected cases may be referred to allergy experts for skin tests as well as provocative challenge with suspected allergens.

**X-Ray Chest**

Chest X'ray usually is not of much help except that it may reveal evidence of emphysema in lung and may occasionally reveal undetected pneumothorax.

**Pulmonary Function Tests**

These tests may help us to determine the degree of airway obstruction and to compare the effects of therapy such as bronchodilator or steroid therapy. Not possible to do in acute asthma.

**Differential Diagnosis**

1) Chronic bronchitis with acute exacerbation
2) Tropical pulmonary eosinophilia
3) Left ventricular failure commonly known as 'cardiac asthma'
4) Spontaneous pneumothorax
5) Laryngeal bronchial obstruction (unilateral wheeze) or mediastinal obstruction.

The chief aim is to relieve the patient's distress and if possible to prevent further attack. With the drugs currently available it is not difficult to relieve the patient's symptoms but it is a problem to prevent or predict future episodes.

**Treatment of Moderate Attack**

Most cases of bronchial asthma respond well to ephedrine, adrenaline, orciphrenaline, terbutaline and isoetherine. All these drugs except adrenaline and ephedrine have $\beta_2$-selective activity without much adverse effect on heart. The other useful drugs are theophylline compounds such as aminophylline and choline-theophyllate. Atropine and its derivatives being anti-cholinergic may be useful but rarely used nowadays.

**Management**

Sherwood Jones classified asthmatics in the following grades (Asthma 1977, Ed Clark J.H. & Godfrey S) :

1A — Able to do sedentary duty with moderate difficulty. Sleep occasionally disturbed.
1B — Able to do light domestic duties; sleep disturbed
2A — Bed-ridden, able to go to toilet
2B — Bed-ridden, unable to sleep. Pulse rate remaining less than 120

3 — Totally bed-ridden. No sleep. No relief with inhaler

4 — Patient immobile and completely exhausted.

The first two groups require continuous drug therapy with oral ephedrine and aminophylline and sometimes other combinations e.g. salbutamol, and terbutaline. Sometimes antibiotics are essential when infection precipitates the attack. Once spasm is relieved, patients sleep well with or without sedatives. All others require intensive care **preferably** in hospital or respiratory care unit.

It may be noted that the above classification does not include patients who are liable to get episodic asthma but remain quite well in between.

**Complications**

1. Recurrent bronchitis and patchy pneumonitis due to infection
2. Atelectasis due to mucus plugs in bronchioles
3. Bronchiectasis — patchy bilateral; due to mucus plugs and infection
4. Respiratory failure due to ventilation — perfusion defect
5. Cor pulmonale a late complication due to RVH
6. Pneumothorax due to rupture of emphysematous bullae
7. Rib fracture due to distressing cough
8. Sudden death may be due to ventricular arrhythmias precipitated by too much isoprenaline inhalations.

The following principles are to be followed for proper treatment :

1. Relief of bronchospasm
2. Removal of mucus plugging
3. Control of infection, if any
4. Control of allergic factors
5. Prevention of precipitating factors.

Treatment will depend on the severity of the attack. The following simple classification may be helpful.

1. Acute episodic attacks occur suddenly but usually respond to treatment within a few hours
2. Hyperacute and continuous asthma for hours, even days, being refractory to usual antispasmodics i.e. status asthmaticus
3. Chronic mild to moderate attacks, varying in degree during hours of the day, relieved by antispasmodics and/or inhalers
4. Seasonal

Numerous factors are involved e.g. food, drugs, house-dust, pollens, industrial or agricultural dust, fumes etc. Psychological stress, pregnancy, physical exertion and exposure to cold and rain also may be primary or aggravating factors. All these multiple factors have to be taken into account for planning treatment. Another syndrome causing asthmatic attacks, is known as tropical eosinophilia, which has been separately dealt with.

**Drugs Available for Treatment :**

1. **Aminophylline** — oral, IM or IV route. Rarely per rectum at night.
2. **Ephedrine hydrochloride** — Oral 30 mg four to six hourly
3. **Adrenaline hydrochloride** — 1/1000 sol. by subcut/IM route
4. **Tab. Terbutaline** — 2.5 or 5.0 mg, oral, 4-6 hourly
5. **Tab. Orciprenaline** — 20 mg, oral 6-8 hourly
6. **Tab. Salbutamol** — 2 to 4 mg, oral, 4-6 hourly

7. **Tab. Isoprenaline** — 20 mg given sublingually in acute attacks but should not be given frequently as indiscriminate use may cause cardiac dysrhythmia.

8. **Adrenergic inhalations** (per dose)

| | | |
|---|---|---|
| Isoprenaline | : | Special inhalers are used to give 0.1 to 0.5 ml. of 1/200 soln. |
| Orciprenaline (Alupent) | : | Metered quantity per inhalation (100-200 ug.) |
| Salbutamol 0.1 mg (Ventorlin or Asthalin) | : | Check regarding tendency to overdosage during self-administration |

Nebulised Isoetharine (Bronkosol) 0.5 ml in 3 ml. of half normal saline, four hourly.

For effective bronchodilatation, two puffs are taken from the inhaler. It is better to inhale a puff deeply and hold the breath for five seconds; wait for 3 to 5 minutes, then take a second puff, if required. Do not take any more for 3 to 4 hours. If it does not help, consider change of drugs..

In many cases patients do not properly inhale leading to treatment failure.

9. **Corticosteroids :**

Among the available drugs, prednisolone is the drug of choice. Cortisone produces water and sodium retention. Betamethasone is likely to cause muscular weakness. Methyl-prednisolone is most expensive.

ACTH is more suitable for children requiring steroids but has to be given parenterally. Any steroid drug given for prolonged period causes adverse side-effects which should be carefully watched for. Intermittent therapy of two or three weekly doses may be tried. If the dose can be kept at 5 to 10 mg per day side-effects are minimum.

a) Prednisolone : oral or intravenous route
b) Inj. ACTH given IM usually 20 - 40 units 8 hourly. Long acting preparation,e.g. ACTH acthergel is given 40 - 80 units once daily.
c) Beclomethasone dipropionate : dose is usually 420 mcg daily in 3 to 4 divided doses. It should never exceed 840 mcg (0.84 mg) in 24 hours. Betamethasone—17 valerate is also used in dosage of 800 mcg in 3 or 4 divided doses.

These are delivered as metered puffs through special inhalers.

10. **Sodium chromoglycate :** It is a kind of organ specific preventive therapy, which acts at the level of mast cells (type I allergic reaction). It inhibits release of allergens from sensitised mast cells. It is given by inhalation by a special spin-cap inhaler supplied by the manufacturers. It is of no use once attack has started.

Dose — One cap given q.d.s. The therapeutic response is achieved within first four weeks of regular therapy, hence expensive and not so popular in this part of the world. But once the patient can be stabilised on this regime, long-term steroids are not necessary, a special advantage in the management of childhood asthma. However, during severe attacks, surgery or stress, corticosteroids may have to be reintroduced. It is non-toxic but occasionally reports of respiratory tract irritation, laryngeal oedema and severe bronchospasm have been recorded.

11. **Mucolytic agents :** old drugs e.g. potassium iodide, ammonium chloride, glyceryl guaicholate once popular, are now being replaced by cysteine derivatives (Mucomist) given by inhalers.

Bromhexine may also be useful given orally. Other newer drugs are Ambronol and Farrerol (flavone derivatives) are under clinical trials.

12. **Prostaglandins :** Prostaglandins $E_1$ and $E_2$ also have antiasthmatic properties and are still in the realm of clinical research.

13. **Desensitisation or hyposensitisation :** It is useful in cases of seasonal or pollen induced asthma. In other types of asthma desensitising therapy is rarely successful.

14. **Control of infection** : Essential with appropriate antibiotics, where infection is present.
15. **Psychotherapy** : It is of limited value but useful in some cases where psychological factors play any role.
16. **Supportive therapy** : (a) Control of acidosis, (b) Adequate hydration, (c) Attention to electrolyte balance, (d) Maintenance of nutrition, (e) Proper nursing case, (f) Promotes sleep.
17. **Ventilation** : This is a very important problem during acute attacks especially in status asthmaticus. Intermittent oxygen inhalation through nasal catheters or preferably by ventimask gives relief. Watch for progressive anoxaemia as well as carbon dioxide narcosis. Blood gas and pH studies are extremely useful in severe cases as clinical judgement has limitations.

    Assisted ventilation may be necessary when $PCO_2$ is rising above 50 mm Hg. in spite of treatment. Acidosis is controlled by IV sodium bicarbonate, given in dosage of 50 to 100 mEq. Repeat if required. Bronchoscopic bronchial lavage with normal saline is sometimes necessary to clear thick mucus plugs.

    These procedures can only be performed by experts in fully equipped respiratory care units with updated laboratory.
18. Yoga-therapy is also useful in chronic cases.

**Treatment of severe attack (Status Asthmaticus) :**

1) Patient should be allowed to take his own position of comfort. Usually he sits in the bed with a cardiac table or pillows to support him.
2) Oxygen inhalation through a ventimask or nasal catheter may be helpful.
3) If there is no contraindication Inj. adrenaline 0.5 ml of 1/1000 solution is injected SC or IM. This may be repeated after 10 to 30 minutes if relief is not achieved.

   Alternately, one ml of 1/1000 sol. of adrenaline may be charged in a syringe and is given very slowly in five minutes. Pulse and B.P. should be checked carefully.
4) If still the attack continues or if adrenaline is contraindicated, give aminophylline 250 to 500 mg usually 5 mg/kg) as an intravenous bolus but slowly in 3 to 5 minutes. Most acute attacks should respond to these two drugs but if the patient is still unresponsive it is called 'status asthmaticus' nowadays renamed as acute severe asthma and further aggresive therapy must continue.
5) In such situation give a bolus dose of Inj. hydrocortisone 3 mg/kg or its equivalent preparations (dexamethasone or betamethazone) as bolus dose and repeat 100 - 200 mg 2 to 4 hourly till there is definite improvement and then reduce the dose gradually. Relief can be achieved within a few hours to 24 hours after giving 600 to 1000 mg of hydrocortisone. The dose then can be reduced and be tailed off within 2 to 3 days but it may be necessary to continue oral glucocorticoids after 48 to 72 hours up to a week in some cases.
6) Inj. Salbutamol should be given simultaneously and in many cases its action is excellent along with steroids and aminophylline. Weights flow-meter can be used at bed-side to measure pulmonary ventilation to assess further therapy. $PO_2$ and $PCO_2$ may also be measured. If there is tendency of $PO_2$ to fall and $PCO_2$ is rising, it is a danger signal and it is essential to use mechanical ventilation aid as well as arrange for bronchoscopic lavage to wash out thick mucus from smaller bronchioles. In such situation, if respiratory support is not available, sudden death may occur. Severe metabolic acidosis also is likely to be present in such cases, therefore IV sodium bicarbonate 50 to 100 m.Eq. over 5 to 10 minutes slowly should be given to correct acidosis. Once this is done patient becomes more responsive to adrenergic drugs.
7) It is needless to say that nutrition and hydration must be looked into to keep a check on

urinary output. Use sedatives and give enough assurance that patient will be well once again.

8) Antibiotics may be given if underlying infection is suspected. Sputum may be sent for microscopic and bacteriological tests but if evidence of infection is present, broad spectrum antibiotics should be started but without waiting for the results.

9) Mucolytic agents are also helpful e.g. acetyl cysteine (Mucomist) given as aerosols. Bromhexine is given orally as tablets but this is more useful in chronic cases.

10) Beclomethazone spray may also be useful and may reduce parenteral dose of glucocorticoids. Its role is more effective in recurrent acute asthmatic attacks, where it is not safe to use parenteral steroids continuously in high dosage.

11) It should be remembered that severe cases of status asthmaticus can be treated efficiently in a respiratory care unit, hence the practitioner should decide to treat his patient up to a certain limit and arrange to send the patient to a properly equipped hospital whenever possible as medical emergency.

12) Acute anaphylactic attacks due to serum injection (ADS or ATS) or drugs e.g. penicillin can produce severe bronchospasm with hypotension and shock. These patients also will require energetic first-aid emergency therapy including treatment of shock with intravenous fluids, pressor agents, steroids and supportive therapy. Hence it is a rule that while giving serum or a new drug parenterally, an emergency anti-anaphylactic-shock-tray (AAST) should be available containing adrenaline, aminophylline, hydrocortisone or its equivalent, a bottle of 5% glucose solution,antihistamine e.g. phenergan ampoule plus sterile syringes and I.V. giving set.

**Chronic Asthma**

Chronic asthma or recurrent asthma patients require individualised therapy.

1) Mild cases are usually IgE mediated. The attacks are sometimes exaggerated according to season. Usually they can be well-controlled by one to three tablets of ephedrine 30 mg or terbutaline (2.5 to 5 mg) or metaproternol (20 mg); some require additional salbutamol orally or by inhaler per day.

2) Additional aminophylline tablets can be given, if necessary. Many proprietary drug combinations are available containing ephedrine, aminophylline plus phenobarbitone (in low dosage), patients usually get to know and buy them across the table of pharmacist's shop. This is not to be encouraged, as over-drugging is usual. Liquid preparations of aminophylline, e.g. choline theophyllate in alcoholic base is often very useful, as the drug is quickly absorbed and rapidly effective.

3) If there is no contraindication isoprenaline inhaler or tablet may be used sparingly but Patients use these tablets indiscriminately resulting in cardiac arrhythmias or even myocardial infarcts.

4) Disodium-chromoglycate (DSCG) can be used to prevent attacks in patients who are liable to get frequent attacks. One small capsule is used through spin-inhaler specially provided as an outfit by the manufacturer. One spin cap may be used 3 to 4 times daily.

Occasionally irritation of respiratory mucosa may occur due to DSCG inhalations. Sometimes isoprenaline is combined with (DSCG) but it is not a good practice and frequent use of isoprenaline is harmful.

5) If DSCG is found unsuitable beclomethasone spray can be used (20 mcg) 3 to 4 times daily.

6) Hyposensitization can be attempted in selected cases by allergy experts. However, avoiding exposure offending substances is also a simpler way of preventing attacks if offending agents are known.

Gammalergen, a combination of histamine and immunoglobulin marketed by Cure Well (India) is sometimes useful in allergic asthma.

Dose — 2.0 ml given S.C. at interval of four to seven days. The course may be repeated after one, three and six months to obtain good results.

Another freeze dried drug Inj. Histablock (Histamin and human immunoglobulin complex) is also available.

Dose — 2.0 ml given S.C. at 4-7 days interval. Booster doses at one, three, six and 12 monthly interval are recommended. Later yearly dose may be necessary.

7) Psychotherapy is always useful.

8) Breathing exercises are essential. Yogic exercises have helped many patients, as this has both psychotherapeutic and muscle relaxing effects. Moreover, subcortical or hypothalamic centres are somehow influenced by yogic methods.

9) Anti-histaminic drugs do not very much help routinely but some patients do get relief after a night dose before going to bed.

10) Glomectomy, once in vogue, has gone out of fashion.

11) Long-term corticosteroids may rarely be required but should be avoided as far as possible. If it is essential to recommend it, give minimal dose of the drug. Sometimes it can be given as one or half tablet of prednisolone, betamethasone or dexamethasone, 2 to 3 times daily or even on alternative days. Never to be given in empty stomach, preferably with milk and antacids. Side-effects and complications should be looked into carefully.

**Conclusion**

While treating bronchial asthma with various drugs remember the possible side-effects especially due to :

(i) Aminophylline — gastric irritation, gastritis (oral use). Cardiac arrhythmias, hypotension and convulsion (large I.V. dose given rapidly).

(ii) Corticosteroids — Cushingoid effects due to hypercortisonism. When both oral aminophylline and steroids are used over long periods, gastric ulcer may occur. Other complications should be watched for.

(iii) Sympathomimetic drugs — Cardiac arrhythmias or ischaemic episodes.

(iv) Disodium chromoglycate — Bronchial irritation and asthma.

(v) Long-term steroid therapy or even local beclomethasone spray may cause pulmonary mycosis.

Recent researches relating to cylic AMPs and cylic GMPs may open new line of therapeutics in relieving asthmatics.

## PULMONARY TROPICAL EOSINOPHILIA

(Syn : Eosinophilic lung : Pulmonary eosinophilosis)

*G.C. MOOKERJEE*

**Introduction**

Loeffler (1936) described a condition termed pulmonary eosinophilia, clinically characterised by cough, mild febrile reaction and slight bronchospasm. This syndrome was known as Loeffler's syndrome or simple pulmonary eosinophilia. This syndrome was considered due to allergic response to drugs, e.g. sulphonamide, nitrofurantoin or PAS etc.

Wingarten (1943) published reports on 'Tropical Pulmonary Eosinophilia' (TPE), as an asthma-like syndrome, of moderate to severe degree, associated with high eosinophilia, which dramatically responded to arsenic therapy. The radiological picture usually presented the appearance of miliary mottling.

In India, Frimodt-Moller and Barton (1940) noted miliary mottling in some cases of pulmonary tuberculosis, where high eosinophilia was noted along with miliary lung-mottling. They coined the name 'Eosinophilic Lung'.

Weingarten (1943) presented a comprehensive definition of the condition and introduced neoarsphenamine as a therapeutic agent. Carter *et al* (1944) and Jhatakia (1946) postulated mite infestation as the aetiological factor. The filarial infection theory as the causative factor was put forward by Dhanaraj *et al* (1957). Diethyl carbamazine (Hetrazan) was introduced for successful treatment of the disease by Ganatra and Lewis in 1955.

Since then many reports were published especially from India. Sri Lanka and other countries describing the aetio-pathogenesis of TPE and its difference with other syndromes like prolonged pulmonary eosinophilia, asthmatic pulmonary eosinophilia, panarteritis nodosa and Wagner's granulomatosis etc.

All these conditions produce pulmonary symptoms of varying severity associated with raised eosinophil count usually above 20% except in simple pulmonary eosinophilia it is not very high. The typical absolute eosinophil count in TPE is above 800 cu mm.

Generally the aetiology is not clear but multiple agents, e.g. microfilaria, ascaris lumbricoides, fungi (aspergillus fumigatus), drugs e.g. aspirin, butazolidine, chlorpropamide, nitrofurantoin, PAS etc. have been blamed.

Dhanraj (1957) demonstrated very high level of positive complement fixation test in patients with an antigen prepared from microfilaria imitis. Role of filarial infection was raised by Webb (1960) but does not appear to be an important factor.

In India most valuable studies were done by Viswanathan (1949). Udwadia (1966), Jaggi and Viswanathan (1976), to clarify the pathogenesis.

The disease is chiefly seen in India, Sri Lanka, Burma, Malaysia and Indonesia. The maximum number of cases in India are from West Bengal, Bihar, Tamil Nadu, Maharashtra, Uttar Pradesh, Rajasthan and Madhya Pradesh.

PATHOLOGY :

Initially there is exudation of histiocytes and lymphocytes in the interstitial tissues of the lungs. This is followed by Type I hypersensitivity reaction and eosinophilic reaction. It may be so intense that eosinophilic pneumonitis may occur and microabscesses may form. Later on, histiocytic reaction and fibroblastic proliferation may occur, including granulomatous changes and foreign body type of giant cell reaction with monocytic infiltration. Long-standing cases may develop pulmonary fibrosis.

**Clinical Features**

Cough is mostly the first symptom. Persistent dry cough or sometimes with sticky mild expectoration may continue. Mild haemoptysis is rarely noted.

The attacks of mild to moderate bronchospasm lead to dyspnoea. Sometimes attacks of severe bronchial asthma may be stimulated with wheezing rhonchi and prolonged expiration.

Temperature varies usually from 37° to 38°C, rarely it may be higher. Fatigue, chest pain, abdominal muscular pain due to continued cough may be troublesome. Patient may become anaemic and lose weight gradually, if not treated properly.

**Diagnosis**

Signs of asthmatic bronchitis, *scanty,dry,tenacious sputum* with or without fever, sometimes splenic enlargement and generalised lymphadenopathy suggest the possible diagnosis. Blood picture and radiological findings are supportive of clinical diagnosis. IgM and IgG levels in blood may be raised.

**Blood Examination**

Leucocyte count may be raised from 10,000 to 80,000 cumm with eosinophils as high as 20% to 80%. Absolute eosinophil count is also very high. In most cases it will above 200 to 3000 cmm.

W.R. is sometimes positive due to altered A:G ratio.

**Filarial Complement Fixation Test :-** Some of the cases of tropical eosinophilia show a positive complement fixation test with 1% alcoholic extract of microfilaria immitis. The titre may fail even if the test becomes negative after treatment.

**Microfilaria in the blood :-** They can be rarely demonstrated in the peripheral blood.

**Sputum Examination :-** Eosinophils may be plenty.

**Stool Examination** may show evidence of ascariasis.

**Radiology :**

Bilateral miliary mottlings or ground glass opacities may be present. Sometimes prominent linear streakings are seen radiating from hilar zone to periphery.

In long-standing cases, there may be increased reticulation of mid and lower zones, of the lungs or even well-marked fibrosis of the lungs. Filarial complement fixation test may be positive.

**ECG**

Non-specific ST-T changes may occur in long-standing cases, occasionally premature beats may also occur.

**Pulmonary function tests :**

Obstructive airway patterns are often noted and initially it is reversible. In long-standing cases both obstructive and restrictive changes may be demonstrated.

**Treatment**

In cases of microfilarial aetiology, diethyl-carbamazine (DEC) is nowadays the standard treatment along with supportive therapy. The drug is given orally in dosage of 100 mg. three times daily for 10 to 20 days.

Sometimes DEC may not be well-tolerated and, if so, antihistaminics or sometimes short course of corticosteroids may have to be added.

The course of treatment may have to be repeated if there is tendency to relapse. Even two to three courses may be necessary within six months to a year. Ascariasis or filariasis (if any) should be eradicated meticulously.

In refractory cases, pentavalant arsenicals may be considered which was the standard treatment before DEC was introduced. However, risks of arsenic therapy must be weighed against benefits expected in a given case.

Symptomatic treatment to relieve fever, bronchospasm and cough should be given as in cases of bronchitis and asthma.

Some cases resistant to therapy described above may require corticosteroid therapy along with DEC.

Drug-induced cases will usually improve after discontinuing the drug followed by symptomatic treatment with or without corticosteroids.

# BRONCHIECTASIS

*G. C. MOOKERJEE*

## Introduction

Bronchiectasis denotes permanently localised or generalised dilatation of the bronchi associated with chronic cough and expectoration due to recurrent bronchopulmonary infection.

Clinically it is recognised by indirect evidence but can only be diagnosed with certainty by bronchography or at autopsy..

## Types

(A) **Morphological**

Depending upon the pattern of dilatation, bronchiectasis is classified into the following types :

(i) Saccular
(ii) Fusiform
(iii) Cylindrical
(iv) Moniliform

(B) **Clinical**

(1) **Common —** characterised by copious foetid expectoration and recurrent haemoptysis, associated with intermittent episodes of fever.

(2) **Dry or silent bronchiectasis** (Bronchiectasis sicca) — characterised by recurrent bouts of haemoptysis without foetid expectoration.

(3) Symptomless type — only recognised at autopsy.

## Aetiology

Incidence is becoming less due to use of effective antibiotics of modern age. Bronchial obstruction and bronchial infection are the factors that cause bronchiectasis. Bronchopneumonia, whooping cough, smallpox, and measles in childhood result in bronchial obstruction by stenosis as an after-effect causing patchy atelectasis.

In adults, tuberculous hilar lymph node enlargement may cause lobar or segmental collapse and hence bronchiectasis. Pulmonary tuberculosis of the upper lobes when healed by fibrosis may also result in bronchiectasis.

It can also develop in a collapsed segment or lobe of the lung caused by obstruction of a bronchus by a foreign body or neoplasm.

Industrial fumes and toxic gases are also possible causes, by causing chronic bronchitis.

Bronchiectasis may also have a congenital origin e.g. (a) Kartagener's triad comprising of paranasal sinusitis, transposition of viscera and bronchiectasis, (b) agenesis or lung tissue, (e) sequestrated lung, (d) unilateral pulmonary emphysema, (e) congenital cystic condition, (f) mucoviscidosis, and (g) congenital hypogamma-globulinaemia.

## Pathogenesis

Bronchiectasis results when the bronchial wall is weakened and a dilating force acts upon it. There is traction effect on the bronchial wall due to fibrosis around. The bronchial wall may remain weakened since birth or may be acquired due to infection. The dilating force is provided by the exaggeration of the inspiratory pull. In consequence of obstruction of a large bronchus by a foreign body or neoplasm the portion of the lung which it supplies collapses and infection sets in there.

Accumulation of secretions distal to obstruction causes weakened bronchi to dilate. In case of small bronchial obstruction as in acute respiratory tract infection, bronchial lumens obstructed by secretions cause collapse of the lung distally and result in greater transmural pressure in the bronchi above the obstruction and a subsequent dilatation of the bronchi proximal to the obstruction. The part of the bronchial tube distal to the obstruction is also completely obliterated due to collapse and infection leading to weakening of the wall, resulting in dilatation.

In some instances thick viscid mucus plug acts as obstructive agent in segmental bronchiole, associated infection resulting in atelectasis and collapse. If these patients are promptly treated, bronchiectasis becomes reversible. When, however, infection persists due to unrelieved obstruction bronchiectasis becomes permanent. In one word 'obstruction, infection and collapse' are the *sine qua non* of bronchiectasis.

**Clinical Features**

The disease is insidious in onset and is characterised by early morning postural cough and copious foetid expectoration of yellowish or greenish sputum. Associated findings are low grade fever, fatigue, anorexia, anaemia and recurrent haemoptysis, which at times may be severe. Dyspnoea and chest pain may also be complained of in advanced cases. Localised course rales indicate the site of bronchiectasis.Classical symptoms and signs are summarised in Table 17.3.

Many cases may show signs of associated lung collapse and fibrosis in the form of retraction of chest wall, mediastinal shifting to the same side and bronchial breath sounds. Compensatory emphysema may be seen in unaffected parts of the lung as well as on the opposite side. In long-standing cases clubbing of the fingers and toes is seen.

**TABLE 17.3 : CLASSICAL SYMPTOMS AND SIGNS OF BRONCHIECTASIS**

± Chronic cough

± Sputum output exceeds 60 ml in 24 hours, sputum may be mucopurulent, purulent, offensive and copious.

± Blood-tinged sputum or frank profuse haemoptysis — sometimes alarming

± Fever not always present

± Dyspnoea when it is bilateral and extensive

= Recurrent pneumonitis (spill over mechanism)

= Coarse rales in affected zones

= Clubbing in established and advanced cases. Cyanosis and respiratory failure in final stages

**Clinical Diagnosis**

History of persistent or recurrent cough, particularly with purulent copious sputum of long duration is very suggestive of bronchiectasis and is reinforced if coarse rales are heard in a particular area of the chest, at repeated examinations over a period of months or years. Clubbing, if present, suggests an advanced stage. But bronchiectasis at times may have to be differentiated from chronic bronchitis, although both the diseases may co-exist. A new growth may be associated. When haemoptysis is the presenting symptom it has, of course, to be differentiated from other causes of haemoptysis like pulmonary tuberculosis, carcinoma of the bronchus, mitral stenosis, lung abscess, etc. **Therefore, bronchiectasis is not a complete diagnosis.**

**Laboratory Diagnosis**

1. Polymorphonuclear leucocytosis and high ESR may be seen if active infection is present. Anaemia is often noted.
2. **Sputum** — Plenty of pus cells and gram positive or gram negative organisms are seen under the microscope. Culture yields pyogenic organisms. Commonly H. influenzae is the causative

organism, with which mixed organisms including anaerobes are also found. A simple gram's stain may be helpful for choosing antibiotics in rural settings with inadequate laboratory facilities.

Sensitivity tests, however, are often necessary to choose proper antibiotics.

3. **Chest radiograph** – X-ray chest may look normal or may be associated with :
   (a) Atelectasis
   (b) Patchy opacities (pneumonitis)
   (c) Hypertranslucent areas (emphysema)
   (d) Cystic areas or honey combing
   (e) Ring shadows with fluid levels.
4. **Bronchography** – When surgical treatment is planned in unilateral or local bronchiectasis, bronchography should be done.

**Bronchoscopy**

Bronchoscopy may be considered especially where new growth is suspected and with modern fiber-optic bronchoscope openings of segmental bronchus can be seen and specimen can be taken for biopsy.

**Respiratory Function Tests**

Especially vital capacity and $FEV_1$ may be measured along with $PO_2$ levels.

**Complications**

1. Pneumonia
2. Dry pleurisy
3. Pleural effusion with or without empyema
4. Sinusitis
5. Haemoptysis – often severe
6. Cerebral abscess
7. Splenomegaly
8. Amyloidosis

**Treatment**

(A) **Medical** – It aims at ensuring an adequate drainage of the bronchi and control of the infection.

(i) **Postural drainage & physiotherapy** – Since upper lobes will drain naturally by gravity when the patient is in erect posture, postural drainage aims at draining one or both lower lobes. The patient is so advised that he leans over the edge of the bed with head well below the level of the body which is supported by placing pillows suitably for comfort. The patient is advised to vigorously cough out the sputum. For elderly and weak patients, the foot-end of the bed may be raised instead. Physiotherapist may assist by light massage and percussion of chest and encourage bronchial drainage.

(ii) **Antibacterial drugs** – These should be prescribed whenever there is an acute exacerbation of infection, Sputum-culture report and antibiogram will decide the therapy. Yellowish greenish sputum suggests presence of infection. If the sputum is purulent and foetid, tetracycline, ampicillin or amoxycillin may be started in full doses.

Penicillin once in vogue is less useful due to resistant organisms, hence is not the first choice nowadays. Oral preparations should not be used even if the organisms are sensitive to penicillin.

Co-trimoxazole, erythromycin, ampicillin or cloxacillin preparations may be necessary. The same antibiotic may not be effective during recurrences. Ideally culture of organism and sensitivity tests are rewarding. Prolonged use of antibiotic may also be required in some cases when there is recurrent infection, twice a week antibiotic administration over weeks may be useful, given together with intensive postural drainage. The treatment should be continued until the sputum is no more mucopurulent. Thereafter posture drainage alone should be continued.

Whenever possible organisms should be cultured from sputum and antibiotic sensitivity be done for choice of antibiotics. Prolonged antibiotic cover may sometimes be necessary in long standing cases. Patients should be warned not to take antibiotics only for three or four days and stop it as soon he feels better.

(B) **Surgical** — It aims at eliminating the bronchiectatic area and is indicated in young patients with recurrent haemoptysis, without associated bronchitis or asthma and in patients who are not medically cured yet the disease is sufficiently limited so as to permit lobectomy without seriously affecting the respiratory function.

**Prophylaxis**

This includes complete and prompt treatment of pneumonia in childhood and adolescence, treatment of chronic sinusitis and removal of the causes of bronchial obstruction like neoplasms and foreign body etc. leading to lung collapse.

**Cystic Fibrosis**

A hereditary disease associated with abnormal viscid bronchial secretion due to yet undetermined cause. Bronchiectasis is associated with abnormal glandular secretion chiefly affecting pancreatic secretion. Sweat sodium is high (above 70 m.mol/l) and is diagnostic.

The newborn continues to have meconium ileus and develops malabsorption syndrome, cystic bronchiectasis, clubbing of fingers; even lung abscess and cirrhosis of liver at the end stage.

Treatment consists of antibiotics, pancreatic enzymes, vitamins A and D, low fat and high protein diet. Better to refer these children to special paediatric centres once diagnosis is suspected.

## ATELECTASIS

*G.C.MOOKERJEE*
*P.N.BISWAS*

The term 'atelectasis' is used to denote air-less or collapsed state of the lung. Atelectasis literally means "imperfect expansion" of the lung which may be noted at birth, i.e. congenital condition. However, the whole lung or a lobe or a segment of normal lung may become airless or collapsed due to local pathology. This type of atelectasis of collapse is therefore acquired.

**Classification of Atelectasis**

1. Congenital — atelectasis of the newborn, usually premature babies.
2. Acquired — (A) Due to pressure on the lung from outside compression collapse
   - a) Pleural effusion
   - b) Pneumothorax
   - c) Diaphragmatic hernia
   - d) Extensive thoracoplasty

(B) Due to obstruction of the lumen (Absorption collapse)
  a) Foreign body in the lumen
  b) Mucous plug or secretions
  c) New-growth protruding into lumen of a bronchus
  d) Pressure of enlarged glands on a bronchus
  e) Stricture

3. Massive collapse (post-operative)

**Congenital Atelectasis and Atelectasis of Newborn**

Failure of initial alveolar expansion of the lungs commonly seen among the premature infants, dying shortly after birth.

**Causes :**

a) Immaturity of the diaphragm and other respiratory muscles.
b) Brain injury – damage to respiratory centre, over-sedation of the mother before delivery.
c) Congenital abnormality of bronchioles, alveolar ducts, and alveoli.

Some preventive measures are possible, e.g. proper care of premature labour and avoiding neonatal anoxia etc.

**Acquired Collapse**

The conditions are due to compression of the lung or absorption of air as a result of obstruction to some part of the bronchial tree. Besides the clinical feature of the primary condition, signs of collapse will be present. Signs of collapse will depend on the size of collapsed zone. If there are small and multiple areas of atelectasis, physical signs will be hardly possible to elicit. If a lobe or a few segments are collapsed, the following signs may be evident on the affected side depending on the size of collapsed area :

a) Diminished chest movement
b) Poor breath sound
c) Impaired P.N.
d) Reduced V.F. & V.R.

If the collapse involves larger areas or the whole of one lung the physical signs are remarkable. This may occur post-operatively or follow severe trauma, foreign body (e.g. bolus of food, large blood clot, a small marble swallowed by playing child.

The clinical findings are sudden dyspnoea, cyanosis, high fever and shock. The chest on the affected side is immobile, heart and trachea displaced to the same side. Air entry almost absent with tubular or bronchial B.S.

Obstruction due to mucus plug may lead to infection distal to obstruction and atelectatic pneumonitis proclaimed by sudden rise of temperature about 39.4°C (103°F). This is common in very young and very old people. X-ray chest shows segmental area of collapse seen as linear shadows; when right middle lobe is affected a triangular shadow may be, best seen lateral picture.

Occasionally pressure from outside on the middle lobe bronchus caused by lymph node or blockage of the bronchus by a mucus plug may result in chronic infection, bronchial obstruction and atelectasis. It may pass into bronchiectasis (middle lobe syndrome).

**Acute massive collapse**

Massive collapse of the whole lung or whole lower lobe occasionally develops following an upper abdominal operation commonly seen in smokers aged obese people, debilitated patients, patients suffering from chronic bronchitis. Sudden onset of chest pain in the lower part of thorax, severe dyspnoea with cyanosis in a patient who is looking seriously ill are usual presenting symptoms. Cough may be present usually unproductive.

Pulse and respiration rates are rapid, often rise of temperature occurs with circulatory collapse.

On clinical examination there is diminished or little respiratory movement on the affected site. The apex beat and trachea are displaced towards the affected site. Affected side is dull on percussion, breath sounds diminished or absent. There may be tubular or bronchial breathing over the affected area.

Findings of the X-ray chest are characteristic. If the whole lung of one side is affected there will be a homogeneous opacity, with deviation of trachea and cardiac shadow to that side. If one of the lobes is affected there will be a triangular shadow. The apex of the triangle will point towards hilum.

Surrounding area usually shows compensatory emphysema. In these cases skiagrams of anterior and lateral views will be helpful in diagnosis. The clinical state may have to be differentiated from lobar pneumonia,embolism, pneumothorax and pleural effusion.

**Treatment**

Preventive measures should be taken to avoid post-operative massive collapse. The patient undergoing any planned operation should be free from respiratory infection. The patient should be taught deep-breathing exercises and should continue these exercises before and after operation. Smoking should be stopped permanently. Tight abdominal binder must not be used after a major abdominal operation. The patient should sit as soon as possible. Drugs depressing respiration should be used carefully.

In the patient who has already developed atelectasis treatment is to promote cough and expectoration, which helps to establish ventilation in the collapsed lung.

The patient should lie flat on his back and gently roll side to side, several times a day. The chest may be forcibly tapped over the affected lung. The affected lung should be uppermost. This may be repeated several times. Failing this bronchoscopic aspiration may be life-saving. To control infection suitable antibiotics should be used.

## CHRONIC OBSTRUCTIVE PULMONARY DISEASE

*D.BANERJEE*

**Introduction**

Chronic bronchitis and emphysema are referred to as chronic obstructive pulmonary disease. Chronic asthma is sometimes included in this broad group. They are all charactērised by dyspnoea, cough and wheeze and signs of obstruction to expiratory airflow. In chronic asthma, airway obstruction is usually reversible, partially reversible in chronic bronchitis and irreversible in emphysema.

Airways obstruction in chronic bronchitis is due to swelling of bronchial mucosa and accumulation of tenacious mucus within the air passages. In emphysema it is due to bronchial compression and collapse due to overdistended alveoli which may be aggravated by bronchitis. In chronic asthma obstruction is usually paroxysmal, associated with broncho spasm, mucus swelling and plugging.

Commonly a mixed state of chronic bronchitis and emphysema occurs. However, emphysema does not always follow chronic bronchitis nor does chronic bronchitis always accompany emphysema. Hence the two conditions are discussed as separate disease entities.

## CHRONIC BRONCHITIS

Chronic bronchitis is a long-standing disease of the bronchial trees associated with chronic inflammatory changes in the mucosa, causing excessive secretion of mucus, recurrent cough and expectoration in the absence of any specific cardiorespiratory disease, the criterion laid down for chronicity is that cough and sputum must be present on most days of three months in a year for at least two consecutive years. It may be 'simple' with mucoid expectoration, 'mucopurulent' with present or intermittent mucopurulent expectoration or 'obstructive' with persistent widespread narrowing of airways and increased resistance to airflow during expiration. Aggravation of obstructive bronchitis by infection or irritation causing severe dyspnoea and wheeze is called 'asthmatic bronchitis' or 'chronic infective asthma'.

### Aetiology

Chronic bronchitis occurs most commonly in adult males. It is often seen in those belonging to lower socio-economic class. It affects city dwellers, factory and mine workers. It is more common in smokers than non-smokers. Bronchial irritation is caused by environmental atmospheric pollution due to smoke or fog, dust and fumes, household air pollution from kitchen smoke and personal habit of smoking. All these may act as initiating factors in hypersecretion of mucus in the bronchial tree.

Clinical and pathological studies have revealed a close relation between cigarette smoking and chronic bronchitis. Excessive cigarette smoking impairs ciliary activity of bronchial mucosa and bactericidal action of macrophages thus exposing the bronchial tree to the direct effects of inhalants and infection. It produces bronchial spasm resulting from irritation of bronchial mucosa.

Atmospheric pollution, smoking and viral infections lower the resistance of the bronchial mucosa, thus paving the way for infections. The commonest infecting organisms are H. influenzae and pneumococcus. Both appear during acute infections, but H. influenzae persists for long periods.

### Pathology

There is excessive secretion of mucus. Normal secretion is 60 to 100 ml in 24 hours. Its main function is humidification of inspired air and removal of particular material from it in conjunction with ciliary mechanism.

The excessive mucus arises from hypertrophied mucous membrane produced by the 'goblet' cells in the bronchial epithelium and dilated mucus glands in the bronchial wall. The severity of the bronchitis can be correlated with the increase in size of mucus glands by the Reid index which is the ratio of bronchial gland to bronchial wall and is normally one-fourth.

Increased secretion results in obstruction of airways providing a good nidus for infection. The mucus membrane is infiltrated with inflammatory cells with oedema and abscess formation. On healing ciliated columnar epithelium is replaced by squamous epithelium. Infection may extend downwards with narrowing, distortion and destruction of bronchioles. It may extend to the alveoli causing fibrosis without disturbing alveolar structure. These patients become respiratory cripples from severe airways obstruction but do not exhibit structural emphysema.

About 25% of patients develop mild to moderately severe emphysema. Recurrent microabscesses at the junction of the bronchioles and alveoli project into the lumen and together with viscous infected sputum clog the bronchioles. Air is 'trapped' in the alveoli during expiration when the calibre of the airways is less than in inspiration. Alveoli become permanently overdistended with rupture of walls leading to emphysema. This may be irregular or centrilobar in distribution but panacinar emphysema is usually seen.

The capillary bed is destroyed in the process.

The disability is great when the condition affects small airways. Secretions, infection and bronchospasm cause great disability in these sites unlike the disease confined to the larger airways. The onset of emphysema leads to a progressive reduction in effective alveolar surface.

**Clinical features**

The disease usually manifests with cough and expectoration which is later followed by dyspnoea and wheeze. Initially, it is believed to be smoker's cough which is dry and lasts for months or years without causing much disability. It begins to worsen during winter, increasing in severity with successive years till it persists throughout the year. Cough is then accompanied by mucoid sputum. There is tightness in the chest. The patient begins to cough out large quantities of sputum (bronchorrhoea) in the morning and at night on lying down. Sputum may even be blood-tinged.

The amount of sputum increases during exacerbations and infections and becomes mucopurulent or purulent in character. Colour of sputum may be yellowish or greenish. As the disease advances, the patient becomes more breathless and gets wheezing while breathing. Worsening of these features may confine the patient to bed.

Physical signs due to narrowing of airways are prolongation of expiration more than inspiration. This is because the bronchi dilate during inspiration and the effect of narrowing will be more marked during expiration. Rhonchi, mainly expiratory, may be localised, or wheezing rhonchi may be heard all over the chest along with fine and coarse crepitations. Signs of emphysema may be detected when it develops.

**Radiology**

There are no radiological abnormalities in the early stages of chronic bronchitis. In 25% of cases there is evidence of emphysema. Over inflation of the lungs with increased retrosternal space and low diaphragm is seen. Later there may be increase in size of the cardiac shadow with dilatation of the pulmonary trunk and prominent hilar vessels due to rise of pulmonary arterial pressure. Lung fields may show 'inflammatory shadows'. Bronchography shows marked distortion, dilatation and irregularity of the bronchial tree. Bronchial lumen is narrowed with peripheral poor filling ('sawn-off tree' appearance). In chronic bronchitis,bronchography is not advised due to marked airways obstruction.

**Pulmonary Function Tests**

There may be no abnormality at the onset. Later, airways obstruction may be detected by measurement of FVC (forced vital capacity), FEV, (forced expiratory volume in 1 second) and PFR (peak expiratory flow rate). $FEV_1$ as percentage of observed FVC is greatly reduced but is reversible with bronchodilators. PFR shows corresponding reduction and both show further decline with progress of the disease. Airways obstruction is considered severe if the FEV is less than 50 per cent of FEV. The onset of small airways obstruction is better detected by measurement of MMFR (maximum mid expiratory flow rate) and closing volume.

When emphysema supervenes RV (residual volume) is increased and RV/TLC and TLC (total lung capacity) are increased due to over-inflation. Diffusing capacity is not affected and $PaO_2$ is near normal. But hypoventilation results in alveolar $CO_2$ retention and rise of $PaCO_2$. During exacerbation of the disease, there is a fall in $PaO_2$ and further rise in $PaCO_2$ accompanied by respiratory acidosis.

A simple test of airways obstruction, without any special apparatus is FET (forced expiratory time). A stethoscope is placed on the trachea and patient is asked to expire forcefully and fully. Normally it is possible to expire fully in 4-5 seconds. With airways obstruction FET is prolonged and this corresponds to decrease in $FEV_1$.

**Complications**

*Ventilatory failure :* As a result of widespread airways obstruction there is diminished ability to move air in and out of the alveoli and alveolar $CO_2$ concentration rises and $O_2$ diminishes.

Haemoglobin has greater affinity for oxygen and in the absence of diffusion defect can take up all available oxygen. $PaO_2$ thus remains near normal. $CO_2$ in blood is however proportional to alveolar $CO_2$ concentration and thus $PaCO_2$ is raised quite early. During acute episodes there is collapse of small areas of lung which are not ventilated but perfused with blood. Blood is then shunted from pulmonary artery to pulmonary vein without gas exchange. This causes oxygen desaturation of blood, hypoxaemia and cyanosis ('blue'). A normal person responds to raised $PaCO_2$ by hyperventilating, but, in this disease, chronic $CO_2$ retention does not produce hyperventilation as the respiratory centre becomes less sensitive and responds only to higher levels of $PaCO_2$ and the chemoreceptors do not respond to anoxia. These patients do not have dyspnoea ('puffing') in spite of hypoxaemia and hypercapnoea. Besides central cyanosis the patient may have tachycardia, collapsing pulse and warm hands. In severe hypercapnoea there may be muscle twitchings and tremors, headache, drowsiness, confusion or coma associated with narrow pupils, depressed tendon reflexes and extensor plantar response. Fundoscopy may show engorged veins and sometimes papilloedemas. Reabsorption of bicarbonate and sodium from renal tubules to compensate for acidaemia may lead to sodium retention and peripheral oedema.

**Cardiac failure** – Pulmonary hypertension, resulting right ventricular hypertrophy (cor pulmonale) and ultimate failure is due to several factors. There is (1) reduction in the pulmonary capillary bed due to extensive destruction of parenchyma of the lung, (2) 'air trapping' raises intra-alveolar pressure with consequent compression of capillaries, (3) hypoxia, which causes pulmonary arteriolar vasoconstriction, (4) increased pulmonary blood flow and (5) increased blood viscosity with polycythaemia which accompanies extreme hypoxia.

The advent of pulmonary hypertension is recognised by the following signs : accentuation of pulmonary second sound, atrial presystolic gallop rhythm due to augmented atrial contraction, sometimes signs of tricuspid incompetence. With right ventricular failure, the jugular veins are engorged. The liver which may be palpable due to descent of diaphragm becomes enlarged and tender and oedema of feet appears, which may be disproportionate to the degree of cardiac failure.

ECG shows clockwise rotation of heart, right axis deviation, RS pattern in chest leads, peaked P waves, QR pattern in AVR and V1, ratio of R/S is less than 1 in VS with prominent S wave in $L_1$ and incomplete RBBB. (Fig.17.8).

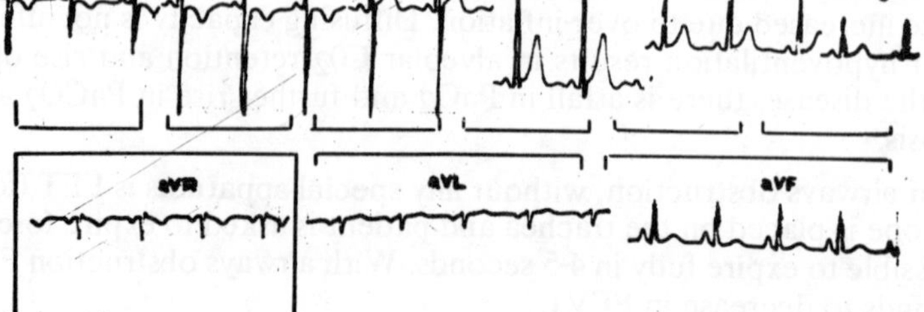


Fig.17.8 : Electrocardiogram in right ventricular hypertrophy. Right axis deviation RS pattern in chest leads, incomplete right bundle branch block and peaked P waves in leads 2 and 3 (P pulmonale) are seen.

As a result of respiratory and right ventricular failure, both of which appear early in the course of chronic bronchitis, the patients are cyanosed (blue) and oedematous ('bloated'). Hence they are referred to as 'blue bloaters'. They do not usually have dyspnoea (or 'puffing') as in emphysema.

**Course and prognosis**

Chronic bronchitis is a progressive disease, with acute exacerbations and remissions, eventually causing ventilatory and cardiac failure. Some patients die within 5 years of onset of symptoms while others survive for 20 to 30 years, with gradually diminishing respiratory reserve.

**Treatment**

*Preventive measures :*

The disease is preventable. This involves total stoppage of smoking and control of atmospheric pollution. Some patients are benefited by moving out of a polluted environment or change of occupation. As infections cause exacerbations and further decline in the disease, vigorous treatment at the earliest opportunity is essential.

**Control of infection :**

Pneumococci and H.influenzae are highly sensitive to chloramphenicol, tetracycline, ampicillin, amoxycillin and co-trimoxazole. Penicillin is effective against pneumococci, less so against H. influenzae. The patient should be advised to observe the colour of his sputum every morning and report immediately if it becomes turbid. Penicillin G one mega unit 12 hourly, tetracycline or ampicillin 250 to 500 mg 6 hourly for 5-7 days may be prescribed. Amoxycillin 500 mg, 8 hourly or co-trimoxazole (trimethoprim 80 mg and sulphamethoxazole 400 mg.) 12 hourly are also advocated. Doxycycline has an advantage over tetracycline. It needs single dose in a day and can penetrate respiratory tract secretion better than tetracycline. it can be given 200 mg. stat, then 100 mg. once daily. Chloramphenicol, 250 mg. 6 hourly, is extremely effective but should be reserved for severe infections when other antibiotics fail.

If response to antibiotics is unsatisfactory, sputum culture should be undertaken and treatment amended by the result.

In early stages of the disease, intermittent therapy is sufficient. For advanced disease with impaired defence mechanism, it has to be continuous for long periods. Complete eradication of infection is difficult due to stagnant secretions and blockage of small airways. Continuous suppressive treatment throughout the winter or round the year is not favoured because of the likelihood of emergence of resistant strains.

**Symptomatic Treatment** is required for relief of cough and to control bronchospasm.

An expectorant containing potassium iodide 300 mg. or glyceryl guacolate 100 mg. 3 times daily is useful. Water intake must be high as it reduces the viscosity of sputum and facilitates expectoration. A hot water drink in the early morning relieves cough. Steam inhalation, heated nebulisers and ultrasonic equipment are used to humidify the airways by delivering liquid to mobilise mucus and clear sputum. Mucolytic aerosols with n-acetyl cystine are beneficial in patients with thick mucus.

**Relief of Bronchospam :** Bronchodilator drugs, ephedrine hydrochlor 15-30 mg 2 or 3 times daily or long acting ephedrine resinate 125 mg twice daily are effective orally. Theophylline derivatives, choline theophyllinate 200 mg. hydroxytheophyllin 100 mg. and beta-2 adrenergic stimulants, salbutamol 4 mg. or terbutaline 5 mg. 3 times daily are also used.

[Refer to chapter on Bronchial Asthma]

**Physical Measures :** Postural drainage is used to relieve obstruction by clearing the secretions. It is necessary because the normal mechanism of cough reflex and bronchociliary action are depressed in this disease. Positions are adopted in bed for gravitational flow from different lobes of the lung aided by tapping or clapping of the chest rhythmically with cupped hands to dislodge the secretions.

**Breathing exercises :** Patients breathe in an incoordinated manner in this disease. In place of chest and diaphragmatic movements, abdominal and accessory muscles are active. The patient can achieve a coordinated deep breathing pattern by 'pursed lip' breathing. A full deep inspiration with abdomen moving outwards is followed by a prolonged slow expiration through pursed lips, augmented by active contraction of diaphragm and abdominal muscles. Such slow expirations do not cause 'air-trapping' as may occur with ordinary forcible breathing exercises. While expiring, the patient presses his hands placed on lower ribs and upper abdomen inwards and upwards so as to contract the abdomen and push the diaphragm up to expel the trapped air. Intermittent positive pressure breathing is used in acute respiratory failure. A cuffed endotracheal tube is introduced and connected to a ventilator (Bird, Monoghan, Bennet, Ohio). The inspiratory process is done by the machine with peak pressure at beginning of inspiration. Bronchodilator aerosols delivery and humidification may be done simultaneously. The procedure is used for better distribution of inhaled gas to poorly ventilated areas of the lung by opening collapsed airways and alveoli. The treatment is given intermittently several times a day.

**Oxygen therapy :** During exacerbations of chronic bronchitis with hypoxia and hypercapnoea, altered consciousness, confusion and drowsiness, controlled oxygen therapy (2 litres per minute continuous) is of great value. Hypoxia is a stimulus to ventilation. Uncontrolled oxygen abolishes hypoxic stimulus and results in hypoventilation, respiratory acidosis and $CO_2$ retention. Oxygen must therefore be given with monitoring of blood gases, so as to raise arterial oxygen tension without inducing respiratory depression. Sedatives and hypnotics are dangerous. Morphine is contraindicated as it depresses the respiratory centre. Tracheobronchial suction and mechanical ventilation in intensive care units are required in critical condition. Right ventricular failure is often precipitated by acute exacerbation of the disease. Besides antibiotics and controlled oxygen therapy, diuretics, thiazides and frusemide 40 mg, once or twice daily, are used to relieve oedema. If failure is not reduced, digoxin 0.125 to 0.25 mg as maintenance dose with potassium supplement is used. As tachycardia is a feature of hypoxia, assessment of exact requirement of digoxin is difficult.

## PULMONARY EMPHYSEMA

In a broad sense, emphysema means unnatural distension of lungs with air. For instance, a collection of air under the skin is called subcutaneous emphysema. Pulmonary emphysema refers to the structural changes in the lung characterised by localised or generalised overdistension of air spaces (acini) distal to the terminal bronchioles due to dilatation or destruction of the alveolar walls.

**Pathology :** Pulmonary emphysema has been classified into 4 groups depending on the portion of the acinus involved; centriacinar (centrilobular), panacinar, periacinar (paraseptal) and irregular.

The respiratory bronchioles which arise from the terminal bronchioles, continue into alveolar ducts and sacs. All of these have alveoli on their walls and constitute the 'gas-exchange' area of the lung. Each group of respiratory bronchioles and branches constitute a discrete lobule or acinus. Emphysema may occur in the whole or part of the acinus. Centriacinar (centrilobular), emphysema involves the centre of the lobule and converts them into air-filled spaces surrounded by less affected lung. This occurs typically in dust disease, in which the centrally situated respiratory bronchioles are loaded with dust causing destruction of their walls. Several such bronchioles fuse together and form a large air-filled space in the centre of the lobule surrounded by normal alveoli. Such a condition is also called 'focal' emphysema.

In panacinar (proximal acinar) emphysema all the alveoli in the lobule or acinus are involved. This type occurs in chronic bronchitis. Due to extension of infection from bronchioles, there is 'air-trapping' during expiration, rupture of alveoli due to constant coughing and damage by irritants (cigarette smoke and air pollution) along with 'avascular necrosis' due to interference with blood supply consequent to raised intra-alveolar pressure. The condition is also termed 'diffuse obstructive emphysema'. Panacinar emphysema without airways obstruction occurs in compensatory emphysema and is a benign condition.

In *periacinar* emphysema (paraseptal, distal acinar) the condition develops near the periphery of the acini, adjacent to the pleura or fibrous septa. It presents with emphysematous bulla or spontaneous pneumothorax and is hence termed as 'bullous emphysema'.

In *irregular* emphysema, changes develop irregularly around scar tissue resulting from inflammation, infection or collapse.

'Panacinar diffuse obstructive emphysema' which occurs in chronic bronchitis, with widespread airways obstruction, is the most crippling and important type of emphysema. In 'focal centriacinar emphysema' of dust disease, localised airways obstruction is present. There is no airways obstruction in 'periacinar bullous emphysema' and in 'panacinar compensatory emphysema'.

Besides these classical varieties, certain other conditions are also included under the broad term 'emphysema'. These are :-

*Interstitial* emphysema occurs due to escape of air from bronchi or alveoli due to some violent respiratory effort as in status asthmaticus or whooping cough. The air tracks along vascular sheaths towards the hilum and mediastinum producing 'mediastinal' and 'subcutaneous emphysema' in the neck.

*Surgical* emphysema is caused by injuries which penetrate both pleura and lung. Air escapes into the subcutaneous tissue.

*Compensatory* emphysema is a result of expansion of a portion of the lung which compensates for destruction or collapse of the remaining portion of the same lung or opposite lung.

*Senile* or *atrophic* emphysema is associated with dilatation of alveolar ducts and sacs in the aged (duct ectasia).

### Aetiology

The vast majority of cases are secondary to chronic bronchitis; cigarette smoking, air pollution and repeated bronchial infection are the main contributory factors. Primary emphysema occurring in young adults in the third or fourth decade and mainly affecting the lower lobes is associated with genetically determined alpha 1 antitrypsin deficiency. This can be recognised by the serum electrophoretic pattern which shows absence of normal alpha 1 globulin peak. Antitrypsin is the chief component of alpha 1 globulin and is capable of inhibiting the action of proteolytic enzymes. It thus protects the lung from such substance released by disintegrating neutrophils and alveolar macrophages associated with infection. The deficiency is through an autosomal recessive gene.

### Clinical features

The condition starts in middle age and breathlessness is noted first. It increases gradually and becomes troublesome. If the individual is a smoker there may be cough and sputum. Otherwise they are absent. On examination the following signs of hyperinflation of the lung may be observed, symmetrically diminished expansion of the chest wall; increased resonance on percussion; diminished (distant) breath sounds with prolongation of expiration; there are no adventitious sounds but rhonchi and crepitations may be due to associated bronchitis; reduced cardiac and liver dullness. In advanced cases accessory muscles of respiration are active. The sternomastoid, scalenus anterior and trapezius muscles contract to move the chest upwards and forwards during inspiration. The typical 'barrel shaped' or 'Square' chest, with increased antero-posterior relative to lateral diameter, develops as the ribs are held in a horizontal position. Even though there is obvious dyspnoea, the chest movements are markedly reduced and the thorax is held in an inspiratory position. Jugular veins remain filled during expiration due to positive intrathoracic pressure. With onset of cardiac failure they become engorged during inspiration. The supraclavicular and suprasternal fossae are followed out during inspiration due to excessive fall in intrathoracic pressure in an attempt to draw in more air through narrowed airways. The costal margin is drawn inwards (costal paradox) during inspiration due to inward traction from the low flat diaphragm. There is a reduction in the length of the trachea palpable above the sternal notch because of elevation of the sternum. Trachea descends during inspiration due to traction of the low flat diaphragm.

**Radiology**

The lungs are abnormally translucent. The ribs appear more horizontal. Antero-posterior diameter of the chest is increased. Normal retrosternal translucent area is increased in width. The diaphragm is low and flat reaching below the anterior end of the seventh rib or lower. The heart is narrow and vertical with normal or prominent hilar vessels and loss of peripheral vascular markings. Complete loss of vasculature in a well demarcated hypertransradiant zone is seen in bulla or bullous area.

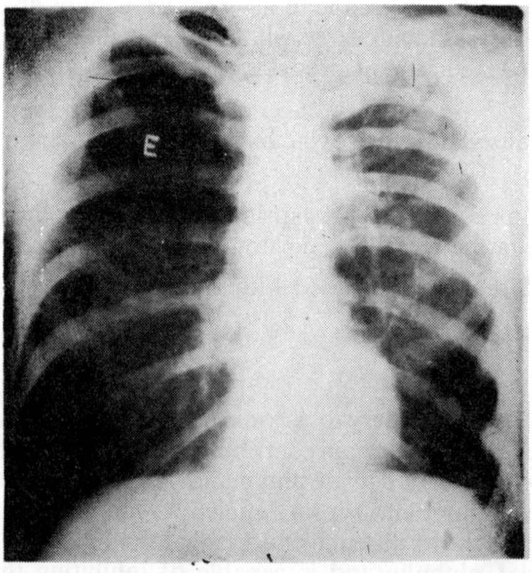


**Fig.17.9 : X-ray of the periacinar emphysema of right lung with large bulla (E) at apex. Tubercular infection of left lung and pleural adhesion has held up the left diaphragm. The inflated right lung has pushed the mediastinum out and caused descent of right diaphragm to a low flat position. Large bulla was the cause of dyspnoea in this patient.**

Such bullae are generally seen at the apices of the lungs or along the margins (Fig.17.9). Should they occur at the base the diaphragm outline may appear blurred. There is a marked reduction in the excursion of the diaphragm during breathing on fluroscopy.

**Pulmonary function tests :** Functional abnormalities may not always reveal the structural change that occurs in emphysema. Early emphysema is difficult to detect. In the absence of airways obstruction $FEV_1$ and FEV per cent are normal but RV is always increased. RV/TLC ratio and TLC are both increased. Diffusing capacity is diminished due to disorganisation of peripheral gas exchange areas. There will be some areas getting adequate ventilation and others too little. (Refer to chapter on Respiratory Function Tests).

### Complications

**Respiratory failure :** Mild to moderate hypoxaemia occurs early in emphysema but $PaCO_2$ remains normal. The medullary respiratory centre responds only to alternations in $PaCO_2$ but peripheral chemoreceptors in the carotid and aortic bodies and intracranial central receptors are sensitive to anoxia. Anoxia, by stimulating these receptors, produces an increase in the depth and rate of respiration and thereby increases the diffusing capacity to restore the $PaO_2$ level to normal. Thus the oxygen saturation of the blood is kept normal by deep and rapid breathing which constitutes dyspnoea. Patients with emphysema have no airways obstruction and are not cyanosed (i.e. pink) but are usually dyspnoeic (i.e. puffing). They are referred to as 'pink puffers'.

**Pulmonary hypertension and right ventricular failure :**

Develop later due to the same factors as in chronic bronchitis.

**Pulmonary bullae :** Single or multiple, large or small, may develop. Bullae are inflated thin – walled spaces created by rupture of the alveolar walls. They are usually situated subpleurally and are commonly found along the anterior wall of the lung. A small bulla may rupture causing spontaneous pneumothorax. Bullae may also increase in size and become so large that they interfere with ventilation of the lung.

### Treatment

There is no specific treatment. The patient may benefit from treatment of associated chronic bronchitis and asthma. Preventive measures, such as cessation of smoking, avoiding dusty environment and antimicrobial treatment of respiratory infections are important. With these measures persons who exhibit alpha –1 antitrypsin deficiency can be protected from further development of the disease.

Obesity must be avoided and corrected since excess weight is an extra burden on the reduced cardiorespiratory reserve. Gentle exercises should be encouraged. Breathing exercises of yogic type which induce relaxation of cervical muscles and encourage movement of the diaphragm are advocated. The patient should exhale slowly through pursed lips.

Advanced cases of emphysema with profound hypoxia benefit from continuous oxygen therapy at home (domiciliary oxygen).Oxygen is administered through nasal canula at a rate of 2 litres per minute up to 16 hours a day. Administration is begun at night as the hypoxaemia worsens in reclining position and during sleep.

### Chronic Obstructive Pulmonary Disease

A condition is which there is chronic obstruction to air flow due to chronic bronchitis and/or emphysema is called chronic obstructive pulmonary disease (COAD). It is also called chronic obstructive airway disease (COAD). Although the degree of obstruction may be less when the patient is free from respiratory infection and may improve somewhat with bronchodilator drugss, some obstruction is always present.

There are distinctive features of the two broad categories, chronic bronchitis and emphysema. In bronchitis there is marked involvement of airways without anatomical changes. There is hypoventilation, retention of $CO_2$ and early development of pulmonary hypertension and cardiac failure. In emphysema there is marked destruction of the lung tissue and early hypoxaemia. The patient hyperventilates and thus keeps $CO_2$ in the blood at normal level until late in the disease. During the course of the disease, the patient may progress in one or other direction between these two forms, or may remain in an intermediate state with overlapping features of both conditions.

Bronchitic patients are often obese, plethoric and do not appear obviously short of breath. They develop cyanosis cardiac failure and oedema quite soon in the disease and are termed 'blue bloaters'. In emphysema, patients are breathless from the start but do not have cyanosis or oedema and hence are termed 'pink puffer'. They are often thin in build. Ventilatory failure and cardiac failure are late developments.

The distinguishing features of chronic obstructive pulmonary disease with predominance of bronchitis and of emphysema are given in Table 17.3

**Table 17.3 – Chronic obstructive pulmonary disease**

| | Predominant bronchitis | Predominant emphysema |
|---|---|---|
| Appearance | blue bloater | pink puffer |
| Age | above 40 | above 50 |
| Sex | males more than females | rare in females |
| Build | heavy | slender |
| Cough | Severe | mild or absent |
| Bronchial infections | frequent | occasional |
| Sputum | copious and purulent | Scanty and mucoid |
| Duration of exertional dyspnoea | short (2-5 years) | long (5-20 years) |
| Central cyanosis | moderate or severe | slight or absent |
| Rhonchi | numerous | few |
| Polycythaemia | present | absent |
| $PaO_2$ | slightly reduced | moderately reduced |
| $PaCO_2$ | always increased | normal or slightly increased. |
| Airways obstruction | always present | generally absent or slight |
| Residual volume | moderately increased | markedly increased |
| Diffusion | normal | decreased |
| X-ray | emphysema nil or slight. Occasional inflammatory shadows. | emphysema marked inflammatory shadows rare. |
| ECG | right ventricular hypertrophy | normal |
| Right ventricular failure | early onset | late onset |

## OCCUPATIONAL PULMONARY DISEASES

*D. BANERJEE*

In certain occupations, the inhalation of dusts, fumes and other noxious substances for varying periods of time leads to development of pulmonary diseases. Involvement of the respiratory system by non-living particle contaminants, mineral or organic, in the atmosphere is called **dust disease.** Pulmonary fibrosis due to inhalation of mineral dusts for prolonged periods is termed **'pneumoconiosis'.** Fibrogenic capacity of mineral dusts varies. They are :

a) Dust capable of producing gross fibrosis : silica and silicates (mica, asbestos, talc and beryllium);

b) Dust capable of producing fibrosis on intense and prolonged exposure : coal dust, graphite;

c) Inert dusts producing mineral fibrosis : iron, tin.

Development of pneumoconiosis depends on the dose of the inhaled dust, size of the particles, duration of exposure and degree of response in the tissues. Only dust particles of 1-3 microns size reach the peripheral gas exchange portions of the lungs and initiate the changes. Bigger particles are cleared away by the mucociliary mechanism of the respiratory epithelium.

Dust particles from the alveoli are carried by macrophages to foci of lymphoid tissues in the lungs. Irritation produced by solution of the particles in tissue fluid initiates widespread pulmonary fibrosis.

Inhalation of organic dusts of vegetable or animals can produce hypersensitivity reactions in bronchioles and alveoli. Irritant gases and fumes may cause acute pulmonary oedema, bronchitis and asthma.

Diagnosis is based on occupational history, with details of nature and duration of exposure. Persons may change their occupation and hazards to which they may have been exposed in previous occupation must be carefully sought for. Radiology and pulmonary function tests are required to assess the disability.

The disease is preventable by taking adequate precaution to reduce the dust in the working environment, a function of the industrial hygienist. Periodic clinical and radiological examination of workers should be made and change of occupation advised if abnormal shadows or symptoms appear.

Details of occupational pulmonary diseases are given in **Table—17.4.**

Important occupational lung diseases are considered below :

## COAL WORKERS PNEUMOCONIOSIS

The disease is due to prolonged inhalation of coal dust. It may affect coal miners, loaders, transport workers, stokers and trimmers of engines and furnaces. About 10 per cent of miners are affected in the coal mines in Bihar.

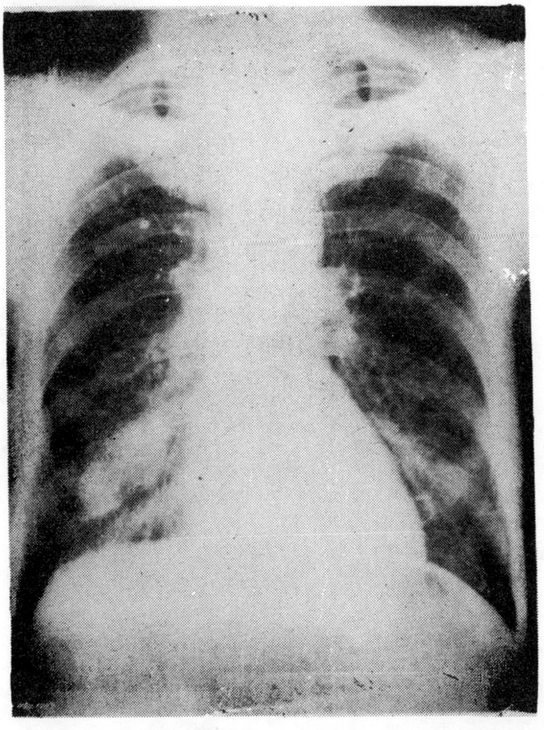

Fig.17.10 : X-ray of coal worker's pneumoconiosis. Besides the calcified spots of healed tuberculosis, fine nodular opacities and reticulation are seen in both lung field mainly in the upper and mid zones. Enlarged hilar glands, particularly on the right, vascular shadows and emphysema are noted.

**Table : 17.4 Occupational pulmonary disease**

| **Condition** | **Cause** | **Name of disease** | **Occupation** |
|---|---|---|---|
| Pulmonary fibrosis and emphysema. | Coal | Coal workers pneumoconiosis. | Coal mining, loading, transport, stoking and trimming of engines and furnaces. |
| —do— | Silica | Silicosis | Fire-brick, ceramic, steel, foundry, metal grinding, boiler scaling, stone quarrying and dressing, mining mica, gold, tin and copper. |
| Pneumonitis and fibrosis. | Asbestos | Asbestosis, | Mining, manufacture of brake lining, electrical insulation, fire-proofing. |
| —do— | Talc | Talc pneumoconiosis | Various industries. |
| —do— | Beryllium | Beryliosis | Radio tube, neon tube, aircraft, atomic energy industries. |
| Minimal fibrosis | Iron Oxide | Siderosis | Arc welding |
| —do— | Tin Oxide | Stannosis | Mining. |
| Bronchiolitis alveolitis | Cotton, flex, hemp dust | Byssinosis | Textile. |
| —do— | Bagasse | Bagassosis | Paper |
| —do— | Mouldy hay | Farmer's lung | Agriculture |
| Asthma | Vegetable grains, animal products — feather, wool and fur. | — | Various occupations |
| —do— | Chemical — Toluene diisocyanate. | — | Plastics and Rubber |
| Cancer | Arsenic, asbestos, chromate, nickel, tar, radioactive ore. | — | Various Industries. |
| Chronic bronchitis, Emphysema. | Cadmium | — | Welding, electroplating. |
| Acute pulmonary | Ammonia, chlorine, phosgene, sulphur — dioxide and trioxide. | — | Accidental exposure in various industries. |

The dust is deposited in the respiratory bronchioles and alveolar ducts where they produce 'dust foci'. Narrowing of the airways and erosion of bronchial wall leads to focal emphysema which are the characteristic changes in coal workers' pneumoconiosis (Fig.17.10). The retention of the coal dust is more in the upper and middle lobes than in lower lobes and they have a mottled black appearance.

**Simple pneumoconiosis :** Since a small amount of silica is present in coal dust, minimal fibrosis develops. Dust laden macrophages disintegrate in the lung tissue and stimulate formation of reticular and collagen fibres, around the coal deposit ultimately forming star-shaped 'Coal macules'. These are enlarged to form nodules of simple pneumoconiosis.

**Progressive massive fibrosis :** If the coal dust contains higher concentration of silica, dense fibrosis is stimulated, tuberculosis and other infections may be associated causative factors. Collagen fibres are laid down to form fibrotic masses (progressive massive fibrosis) located in the upper lobes, which gradually enlarge. Softening and necrosis with formation of cavities may occur in the fibrotic masses either due to ischaemia or tubercular infection. Fibrotic lesions may involve bronchi and pulmonary vessels resulting in chronic bronchitis, bronchiectasis, pulmonary hypertension and right heart failure (complicated pneumoconiosis) Silica content is low in Indian coal mines and massive fibrosis is uncommon (Fig.17.11).

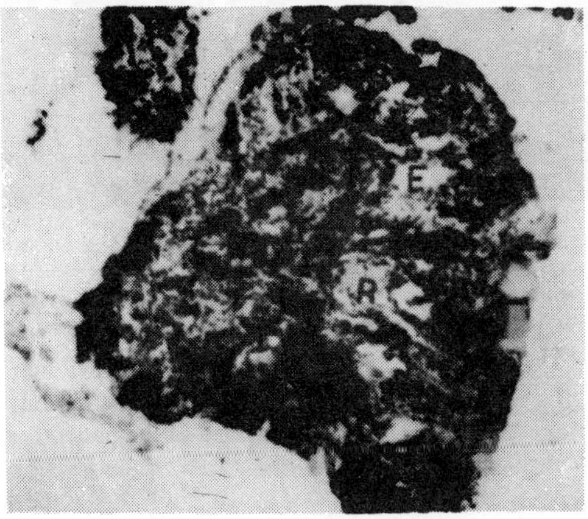


Fig.17.11 : Histology of coal worker's pneumoconiosis. Black coal dust has filled the respiratory bronchioles (R) and spread to surrounding lung tissue, appearing as linear strands. Focal emphysema (E) is seen. Section is from lung biopsy specimen of the patient in Figure 3.

## CAPLAN'S SYNDROME

A rheumatoid disease may appear on the background of pneumoconiosis with appearance of clearly defined round opacities in both lungs especially at the periphery (Caplan's syndrome). Pneumoconiosis may appear along with, before or after arthritic manifestations develop. Antinuclear and rheumatoid factor may be present in the blood in some cases.

**Radiological findings :** Even before the appearance of symptoms coal workers may exhibit radiological changes. Initially a granular or fine reticular pattern (Fig.17.12) is seen in the lung fields. Small circular punctiform shadows appear later and correspond to formation of coal nodules and focal emphysema. The shadows are relatively less opaque than in silicosis. Hilar glands are enlarged. Radiological opacities in the lung fields due to inhalation of mineral dusts are categorised in accordance with an international classification. Categories numbered 1 to 3 indicate the profusion of the opacities (extent and density of distribution). In Category 1 the opacities occupy about one-third of the total area of the lung fields, in Category 2 most of both lung fields and in Category 3 they are very numerous. The size of the opacities is indicated by letters, p (punctiform) indicates nodules up to 1.5 mm, m (micronodular) indicates nodules 1.5 to 3 mm, and n (nodular) nodules 3-10 mm in size. The letters A,B and C indicate the extent of

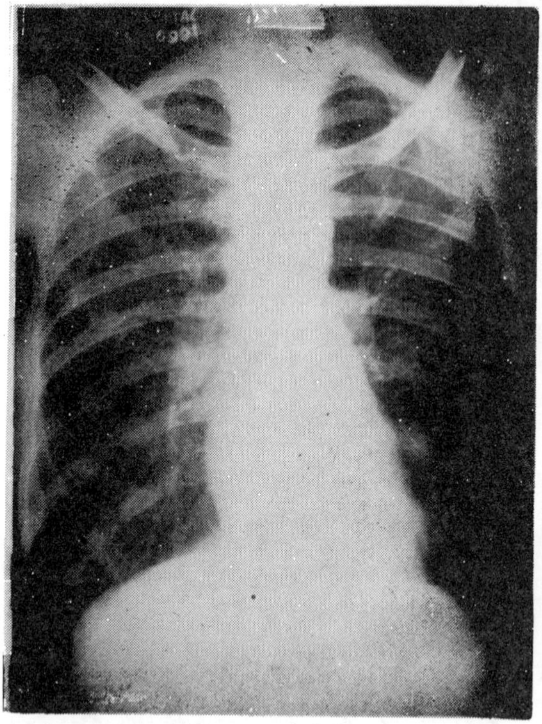

FIG.17.12

Fig.17.12 : X-ray of silicosis in a fire brick worker — nodular opacities and fine reticulation are seen mainly in the upper and mid zones 'Ground glass' opacity of upper lung fields is due to thickened pleura. Hilar glands are enlarged. Emphysema is present.

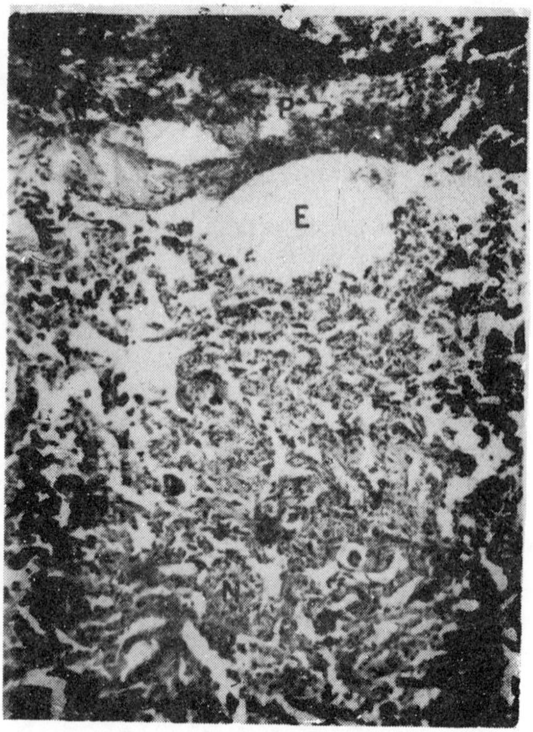

FIG.17.13

Fig.17.13 : Histology of silicosis. Cellular fibrous tissues arranged in islets in whorl-like fashion (N) are seen. There is subpleural emphysema (E) and pleural layer (P) in thickened. Section from lung biopsy specimen of the patient.

massive fibrosis; the letter D indicates distortion of any thoracic structure (mediastinum), lung fissures, diaphragm or pleura) by the fibrosis of complicated pneumoconiosis. Commonly punctiform opacities (size of miliary tuberculosis) are seen in Indian miners.

**Clinical features :** Develop after many years of exposure and follow appearance of radiological opacities. Such opacities may be seen after 10-20 years of underground work. Initially there may be no signs or symptoms. Dyspnoea appears gradually and progressively increases. In massive fibrosis it is disabling. Cough is a late symptom. It may be associated with mucoid or inky black sputum (melanoptysis). Chest pain and haemoptysis may occur. Cyanosis is absent and the patient may be classed as a 'pink puffer'.

**Functional abnormalities :** Are not seen in the early stages. With increasing fibrosis there is reduction of $FVC_1$ & TLE with lowered gas diffusion. Reduction of $FEV_1$ is progressive and correlates with years of occupational exposure. $FEV_1$ less than 1.5 litres indicates total disability. Reduced FEV per cent occurs if there is associated chronic bronchitis and emphysema.

**Preventive measures and prognosis :** Suppression of dust and periodic radiological examination of workers is necessary.

Simple pneumoconiosis does not deteriorate once dust exposure ceases, but progressive massive fibrosis cannot be halted by leaving the occupation.

## SILICOSIS

Silicosis is a chronic fibrosis of the lungs due to prolonged exposure to free silica (silicon dioxide). Silica occurs in pure crystalline form in quartz and in a combined form in clay, mica and other silicates. Quartz is a common mineral constituent of rock, granite and sandstone.

The disease occurs as an occupational hazard in mining mica, gold, tin, copper and coal, in those engaged in sandblasting, quarrying and fire-brick manufacture. It affects boiler scalers, steel and foundary workers. High prevalence rates are reported in mica miners (34%) and fibre brick workers (15%). It is common in steel workers.

The disease is liable to develop in those who inhale the dust particles of 2 micron size in high concentration over a long period (20-40 years). Fine dust deposited in the alveoli and bronchioles is engulfed by macrophages ('dust cells') and transported along peribronchial and peri-vascular lymph channels to hilar glands and lymphoid tissues in the lungs. Some also remains in the peribronchial spaces and stimulates a fibrotic reaction at these sites. In the early stages a fibroblastic reaction appears in the aggregate of 'dust cells', later islets of cellular fibrous tissue are seen. The tissue is arranged in a whorl-like fashion in concentric layers and is often hyaline. Pleural thickening of varying degree is seen (Fig.17.13). The classical *silicotic nodule* usually develops in relation to a respiratory bronchiole. It comprises of acellular fibrous material enclosed by a zone of concentrically arranged cellular fibrous tissue. Nodules enlarge and coalesce leading to widespread fibrosis and pleural thickening. A diffuse interstitial fibrosis with round cell infiltration occurs with a mixed dust of silica, coal and iron in steel and foundry workers.

The exact mechanism of production of silicotic nodules is still a matter of speculation. The original theory of **mechanical irritation** by hard quartz particles has been discarded. **Silica solubility** theory, according to which, polymers of silicic acid liberated by solution of silica in tissue fluid, is the cause of cell necrosis and fibrosis is also now abandoned. An **immunological** mechanism is now postulated for production of silicotic hyaline which resembles amyloid. The silica particles are coated with protein in the lung and act as antigens stimulating the formation of collagen fibres. Dead macrophages contributed polysaccharides and lipids to silica and initiate the deposition of collagen around the particles. Morphologically the lesions are greyish black and are prominent in the upper lobes and hilar lymph nodes.

**Clinical features :** The disease is slowly progressive. Extensive lesions may be seen in some patients without symptoms or signs. Mild to moderate degress of the disease are compatible with good health. The main symptom of advanced silicosis is dyspnoea on exertion, which steadily worsens until the patient becomes a respiratory cripple. There may be cough and expectoration due to associated chronic bronchitis and emphysema. Cor pulmonale is a frequent development and the patients go on to be 'blue bloaters'. There is increased susceptibility to tuberculosis which manifests with fever, cough, haemoptysis and loss of weight.

**Radiology :** Is the basis of diagnosis. Punctiform or nodular opacities are seen mainly in upper and mid zones (Fig.17.12). They may coalesce with fibrotic contraction of upper lobe. Enlarged hilar nodes in some cases show 'egg-shell' calcification. There may be associated emphysema and pleural thickening. In complicated silicosis (silico-tuberculosis) coalescing nodules with breakdown are seen (Fig.17.10).

**Functional abnormalities :** Restrictive ventilatory defect with reduced FVC,$FEV_1$ and TLC is seen due to fibrosis. If airway obstruction is superimposed FEV per cent is diminished along with diffusion defect.

**Prognosis :** The condition progresses even when the exposure has stopped. Hence the great necessity to keep down the dust in the working environment by improved ventilation, use of wet techniques and dust masks. There is great susceptibility to tuberculosis which needs specific therapy.

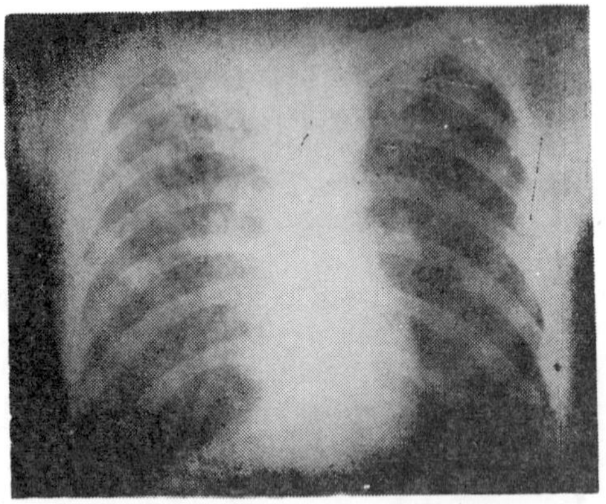

Fig.17.14 : X-ray of silico-tuberculosis in a fire brick worker. Large nodular opacities with massive consolidation and cavitation are seen particularly in right upper zone.

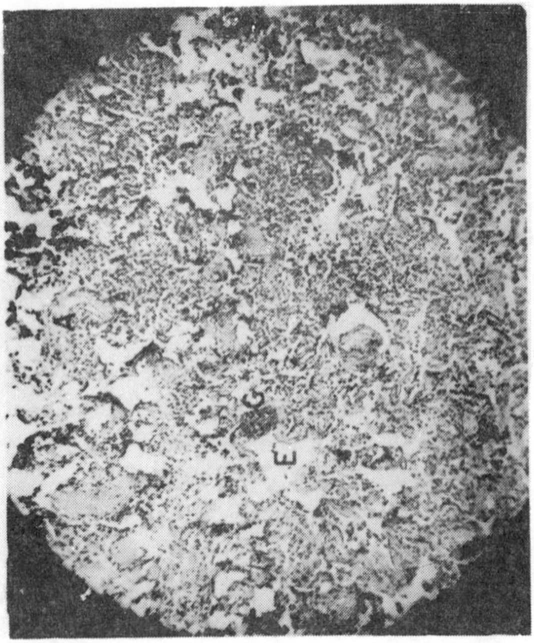

Fig.17.15 : Histology of extrinsic allergic alveolitis. Alveolar spaces are filled with polymorphs, lymphocytes and plasma cells. Collagenous thickening of alveolar walls (A) and few giant cells (G) are seen. There is irregular emphysema (E) *(Section is from a lung biopsy specimen).*

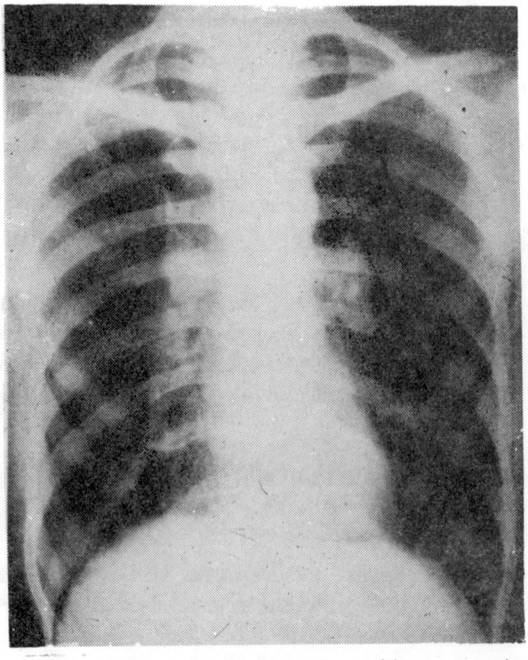

Fig.17.16 : X-ray of a female patient with cryptogenic fibrosing alveolitis. Coarse mottlings are present on both sides particularly in the lower zones. Diaphragm is raised.

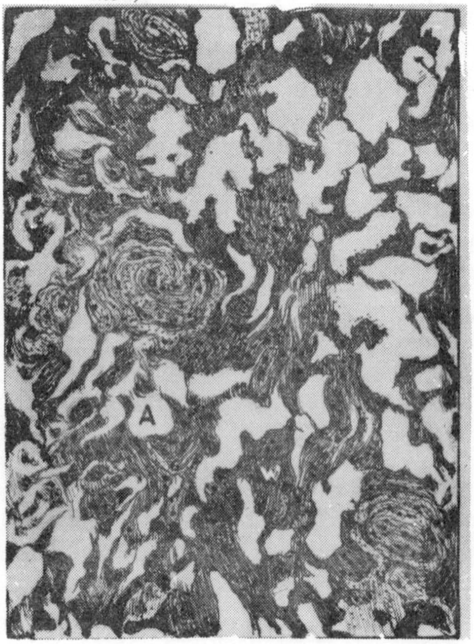


Fig.17.17 : Histology of cryptogenic fibrosing alveolitis Diagramatic sketch from a lung biopsy specimen showing fibrous thickening of alveolar walls (W) with empty alveolar spaces (A).

## ASBESTOSIS

Asbestos or hydrated calcium-magnesium silicate is an indestructible fibrous mineral which is mined in Canada, South Africa, Rhodesia and U.S.S.R. It occurs in three forms : white (chrysolite) blue (crocidolite) and brown (amosite) asbestos. It is a silky material which can be woven into fire proof fabrics. Because of its soft texture and high resistance to heat and chemicals it is used extensively in the manufacture of insulating boards, electrical insulation, brake linings, cement plaster and paint.

The dust is inhaled during mining and manufacturing process. Prolonged exposure leads to diffuse pulmonary fibrosis and varying degree of pleural thickening. The fibres of varying size, some as long as 200 microns, get caught in the terminal bronchioles where they stimulate intra alveolar deposition of fibrous tissues which form fibrous nodules together with thickening of the alveolar walls. Short fibres are removed by macrophages through the alveolar walls into the lymphatics resulting in interstitial fibrosis and pleural thickening, plaques and calcifications. Pleural affection is bilateral, localised or generalised, but usually confined to the lower parts of the lung. Bronchial carcinoma and mesothelioma of pleura and peritoneum may develop.

The characteristic lesion is the 'asbestos body'. These are found in clumps within the fibrous tissue alveoli and sputum. Each asbestos body contains a central core of asbestos fibre, surrounded by a layer of iron-containing protein material derived from haemoglobin.

**Clinical features :** The onset is insidious and the disease develops very slowly over a period of 5 to 10 years. The main symptoms are cough, dry or with expectoration, exertional dyspnoea, and loss of weight. Dry crepitations are audible in the bases, but there are no ronchi. Clubbing of fingers and toes is seen. Sputum shows 'asbestos bodies'.

**Radiology :** Is diagnostic. There may be diffuse nodular or linear opacities or honeycombing mainly in lower two-thirds of the lung fields which may be covered by a 'ground glass' appearance due to pleural thickening. Pleural plaques may appear as axillary shadowing taking the form of a line or band-like shadow parallel to the thoracic wall. The outline of heart and diaphragm appears shaggy.

**Pulmonary function :** Shows a restrictive ventilatory defect, reduced lung volumes and impaired diffusion with absence of airway obstruction.

**Prognosis :** Bronchiectasis, pleural mesothelioma commonly due to blue asbestos and bronchial carcinoma are frequent complications. Indications of bronchial carcinoma is 10 times higher in patients suffering from asbestosis. Death may result from respiratory failure, congestive heart failure or complicating bronchial carcinoma or malignant pleural effusion.

Asbestosis can occur in people who live in the neighbourhood of asbestos mines, mills or waste dumps. There is no specific treatment and further exposure to dust should be stopped immediately whenever the diagnosis is made.

## BERYLLOSIS

It is an occupational hazard affecting those engaged in the production of beryllium alloys, fluorescent and radio tubes, aircraft and atomic energy industries. In contact with skin or beryllium can produce ulcers or granulomas.

Acute and chronic respiratory involvement can occur. The acute form is due to inhalation of a large dose of the dust and occurs soon after exposure. Alveoli are filled with fibrin, red cells and a few polymorphs and alveolar walls are infiltrated with lymphocytes and plasma cells. This chemical pneumonia manifests clinically with dry cough, breathlessness and discomfort in the chest. Patient is afebrile. It may resolve completely or pursue a fulminating course to a fatal termination or progress to the chronic type. Radiological examination shows miliary mottling. Corticosteroids are useful to control the condition.

The chronic form follows exposure to a low dose over a long time or after a latent period following acute exposure. The manifestations are due to a hypersensitivity reaction. It is characterised by epitheloid cell granuloma with giant cells and monocytes in the alveolar wall and a granulomatous lesion in the hilar lymph nodes due to passage of beryllium througn the lymphatics. Diffuse fibrosis simulating sarcoidosis occurs later.

The onset is insidious with progressive dyspnoea, weakness, fatiguability, loss of weight, cough with mucoid sputum. There may be clubbing and cyanosis. **Radiological** examination shows a granular or reticular pattern which progressed to a 'ground glass' appearance over both lung fields. The hilar nodes are enlarged.

**Pulmonary function** shows impaired diffusion capacity.

**Complications :** Spontaneous pneumothorax and right heart failure may develop.

**Patch test :** With 2% beryllium nitrate or sulphate is diagnostic but there is a danger of flare-up of the underlying disease. Beryllium excretion in urine can be tested.

**Steroids :** Can control progress of the disease.

## BYSSINOSIS

It is an occupational hazard resulting from inhalation of dust of cotton, flax or hemp. It affects 8 to 16% of cotton mill workers in Maharashtra but has not been confirmed in jute mill workers.

It commonly occurs in those who work in the dusty blowing and carding room of cotton mills It is a hypersensitivity reaction due to some factor in cotton dust which releases a histamin-like substance causing bronchial spasm.

**Clinical features :** After working in the mill for 10 years or more, the patient notices tightness in the chest and wheeze on Monday after returning to work following his weekend holiday. The symptom appears in the late afternoon and subsides the same evening. It is called "Monday feeling". The condition may persist and occur on all days. Later the features of chronic bronchitis and emphysema are added. An acute form called 'mill fever' occurs in some persons who arrive newly or after a long period of absence at the cotton mill. There are general symptoms like fever, chills, coryza or cough within 6 hours of exposure. The manifestations subside gradually within a few days when the individual develops tolerance and there are no further attacks.

**Radiology :** There is no specific radiological abnormality. Vascular markings are prominent, emphysema and, in advanced stage, diffuse pulmonary fibrosis may be seen.

**Pulmonary function :** Airway obstruction is seen with reduction of $FEV_1$. This is noted from the initial stage of Monday fever throughout the week even when there is no tightness in the chest. Reduced $FEV_1$ is initially reversible but becomes irreversible in advanced stage.

Presence of IgE antibodies can be detected.

**Prognosis :** Progress of the disease can be halted by removing the worker from exposure to high concentration of cotton dust.

## BAGASSOSIS

Bagassosis is caused by inhalation of heavy concentration of overheated mould (sugarcane fibre) dust. Bagasse is used as raw material for the manufacture of paper in India.

**Clinical features :** The manifestations are due to a Type 3 hypersensitivity reaction caused by inhalation of a fungus contaminant of mouldy bagasse (Thermoactinomyces vulgaris). The disease may present in acute and chronic form. In the *acute type* there is high fever, extreme dyspnoea and cough after heavy exposure to bagasse dust for some weeks. If the patient is removed from the place of work, the symptoms subside spontaneously. The *chronic type* ia a milder but progressive respiratory illness. Cough with expectoration and exertional dyspnoea develop after exposure to the dust for 2 years. Rhonchi and crepitations may be heard in auscultation.

**Radiology findings :** Miliary or punctiform mottlings are seen in the lung fields or there may be inflammatory shadowing due to bronchopneumonia.

**Pulmonary function :** Ventilatory insufficiency with reduced diffusing capacity is observed.

**Prognosis :** The acute form subsides after removal from dust exposure. The chronic form may lead to emphysema and respiratory failure. There workers should be removed from the dusty areas of the factory.

## FARMER'S LUNG

Clinical and pathological manifestations are due to type 3 hypersensitivity reaction to the antigen of phylum actinomyces group present in mouldy hay.

Farmer's lung, bagassosis, mushroom worker's disease, maple break disease are all due to hypersensitivity to similar inhaled antigens and are grouped under the term 'extrinsic allergic alveolitis'. Tissue changes are characteristic and in the acute stage comprise a cellular exudate consisting of polymorphs, lymphocytes and plasma cells in the alveoli and small epitheloid granulomata (tubercles). Alveolar septa are infiltrated with lymphocytes and plasma cells. In the chronic form interstitial fibrosis without granulomatous reaction is observed.

*Histological* changes and the finding of precipitins in the serum suggest that allergic alveolitis is a Type 3 hypersensitivity reaction but the occurrence of small granulomata indicates that a Type 4 eaction may also be implicated.

**Clinical features and radiological findings** are similar to those of bagassosis. Farmer's lung occurs among agricultural workers due to inhalation of dust from mouldy hay or other vegetable products, containing fungal spores. When the hay is stored in wet conditions, heat is generated facilitating growth of thermophilic actinomyces. The *acute* form is characterised by fever, chill cough, dyspnoea and occasional haemoptysis occurring 4 to 8 hours afer exposure. Signs of pneumonic consolidation with polymorphonuclear leucocytosis are seen. Some cases go into the *chronic* form (due to repeated exposure) which chronic cough and increasing dyspnoea. Radiological examination shows fine miliary mottling or nodular shadows in the lower zone with extensive fibrosis in the later stages. Pulmonary function shows restrictive defect with diminished diffusing capacity and hypoxaemia. Precipitins against hay antigen can be demonstrated in the serum.

The condition is preventable. Drying of hay before preservation minimises the growth of actinomyces. Corticosteroids (Prednisolone 20-40 mg daily) is useful for acute manifestation.

# RARE PULMONARY PROBLEMS

*D. BANERJEE*

## PULMONARY FIBROSIS

Pulmonary fibrosis is not a single disease entity but the end result of number of aetiologically different diseases (Table 17.3).

There are 3 main types of pulmonary fibrosis :-

1. **Replacement** fibrosis : Fibrous tissue replaces lung damaged by infection or other destructive process, e.g., in pulmonary tuberculosis, abscess, bronchiectasis or following radiation therapy

2. **Focal** fibrosis as in pneumoconiosis.

3. **Interstitial** fibrosis which is the end result of disease affecting primarily the interstitial tissue of lung rather than bronchi and blood vessels.

In general, focal and interstitial fibrosis show minimal physical signs and radiological changes but they are associated with symptoms of hypoxia in the form of exertional dyspnoea. On the other hand, physical signs and radiological changes are more conspicuous in replacement fibrosis, which produces gross localised abnormalities on physical and radiological examination and minor systemic effects.

**Aetiological Classification of Pulmonary fibrosis Table 17.5**

**Chronic infections :**

Pulmonary tuberculosis, abscess, bronchiectasis, fungal and parasitic diseases of lungs.

**Dust and physical agents :**

Coal workers pneumoconiosis, silicosis, asbestosis, siderosis, beryllosis, industrial fumes, radiation therapy to chest.

**Chronic venous congestion :**

Mitral stenosis, left ventricular failure.

**Collagen diseases :**

Rheumatoid arthritis, scleroderma, systemic lupus erythematosis, polyarteritis nodosa.

**Granulomatous diseases :**

Sarcoidosis, Wagner's granulomata.

**Neoplasms :**

Alveolar cell carcinoma, lymphangitic carcinomatosa, leukaemia.

**Histiocytosis :**

Histiocytosis X, Letterer Siwe's disease.
Hand Schuller Christian disease.
Eosinophilic granuloma.

**Mesodermal dysplasia :**

Tuberose sclerosis

**Hypersensitivity :**

Extrinsic allergic alveolitis.

**Toxins :**

Paraquat, busulfan.

**Idiopathic :**

Cryptogenic fibrosing alveolitis, honeycomb lungs, idiopathic pulmonary haemosiderosis, Goodpasture's syndrome, alveolar proteinosis, alveolar microlithiasis.

**Interstitial lung disease :** Is a group of disease, caused by different pathological processes, all of which have similar symptoms, physical signs, radiological changes and disturbances of pulmonary function. They have the following features in common : thickening of the alveolar wall by oedema, cellular exudate or fibrosis, increased stiffness of the lung (reduced compliance) associated with exertional dyspnoea; maldistribution of pulmonary ventilation and perfusion and defective gas diffusion leading to hypoxia, hyperventilation and hypercapnoea.

Tuberculosis, recurrent bacterial infections, chronic pulmonary oedema, mineral dust pneumoconiosis, extrinsic allergic alveolitis due to inhaled organic dusts, ingestion of toxic substances (paraquat, busulfan) and unknown causes without any external stimulating agents such as cryptogenic fibrosing alveolitis, sarcoidosis and other uncommon diseases may produce diffuse interstitial fibrosis of lungs.

**Chronic pulmonary oedema :** As a result of mitral valve disease or left ventricular failure there is a rise in pulmonary venous and capillary pressure (pulmonary hypertension). This causes oedema and thickening of alveolar walls leading to diffuse fibrosis. The condition is suspected when there is excessive dyspnoea in a cardiac patient.

## EXTRINSIC ALLERGIC ALVEOLITIS

It is a hypersensitivity reaction occurring in the bronchioles and alveoli response to exposure to finely particulate organic dust of wide variety. Fungal spores, vegetable, avian porcine, bovine or insect material may act as allergens. Farmer's lung and bagassosis result from exposure to mouldy hay and bagasse respectively. Other such conditions are due to mouldy mushroom compost (mushroom picker's lung), mouldy barely or malt (malt worker's lung), mouldy maple-bark or redwood sawdust (maple break disease), mouldy oak or cork dust (suberosis), pigeon or turkey-pigeon (budgerigar) droppings (birdfancie's lung) and posterior pituitary extract, porcine or bovine, snuff used in diabetes insipidus (pituitary snuff taker's lung). Fungal contamination of air-conditioners and humidifiers may have identical results.

**Pathology :** Due to antigenic stimulus of organic dust a hypersensitivity reaction develops with systemic and pulmonary reactions. This results in inflammation of the alveolar walls (alveolitis) and ultimate fibrosis. There is cellular thickening of the alveolar walls with infiltration and alveolar exudation of lymphocytes,polymorphs and plasma cells along with histiocytic granuloma (tubercles) with giant cells. Finding of granuloma is characteristic and is not seen in fibrosing alveolitis. Collagen deposition in the alveolar walls and conversion of granulomas into scars produces gross fibrosis.

**Clinical features**

The condition should be suspected when a person who is regularly exposed to heavy concentration of organic dust complains, after re-exposure to the same dust, of dry cough and dyspnoea without wheeze. Repeated exposures cause further aggravation of symptoms and they become continuous. The patient may be febrile, cyanosed and dyspnoeic at rest. Coarse crepitations without rhonchi are heard all over the chest. Clubbing is not common. There may be diffuse micronodular mottling mainly in the upper zones of chest X-ray. $FEV_1$ and FVC are both reduced but $FEV_1/FVC$ ratio is normal indicating a restrictive ventilatory defect without airway obstruction. $PaO_2$ is reduced and $PaCO_2$ is slightly below normal due to hyperventilation.

**Diagnosis :** is confirmed by a positive precipitin test in serum or a provocation test in which inhalation of an aerosol containing the suspected antigen is followed after 3 to 6 hours by pyrexia and other symptoms along with a reduction in FVE.

**Treatment :** Mild forms rapidly subside when exposure to the dust ceases. In severe cases a corticosteroid should be given 3 to 4 weeks. In severe hypoxia oxygen is administered in high concentration.

## CRYPTOGENIC (IDIOPATHIC) FIBROSING ALVEOLITIS :

(Hamann-Rich Syndrome)

Fibrosing alveolitis is a chronic inflammation of the lungs of unknown aetiology with predominant involvement of the alveolar walls. It is characterised by inflammatory cellular thickening of the alveoli with a marked tendency to fibrosis and exudation of mononuclear cells in the alveolar spaces. The original description of diffuse interstitial fibrosis by Hamman and Rich is a variant of this disease having an acute course with rapid fatal end.

**Pathology :** Two histological patterns are seen, mural and desquamative. In the *mural* pattern there is a fibrous thickening of the alveolar walls with scanty exudation into the alveolar space of polymorphs, lymphocytes and plasma cells. Granulomas are not seen as in allergic alveolitis. Alveolar structure is distorted in an irregular manner and there is absence of hyperplasia of lymph follicles. In the *desquamative* pattern alveolar spaces are filled with mononuclear cells of alveolar origin in a uniform manner with minimal thickening of the alveolar walls. Alveolar structure is maintained and there is prominent hyperplasia of lymph follicles. A varying combination of both patterns is seen in many cases. Both patterns result in diffuse fibrosis affecting the peripheral gas exchange areas leaving a few spaces with cells and honeycomb changes from dilated bronchioles. (Fig. 17.16 and Fig.17.17).

**Clinical features**

The disease affects middle aged and elderly individuals equally in both sexes. The clinical picture may be divided into 3 types, acute, subacute and chronic according to the rapidity of progress of dyspnoea. Duration of illness is less than 6 months in the *acute* type, 6 months to 2 years in *subacute* type and above 2 years in *chronic* type. Progressive exertional dyspnoea is usually the presenting symptom often accompanied by persistent dry cough. In most cases there is cyanosis and gross clubbing of fingers and toes due to hypoxaemia. Chest expansion is poor, but hyperventilation is a striking feature. Coarse crackling crepitations at the end of inspiration, persisting after cough (basal rales), are heard mostly at the bases. Radiological examination shows widespread fine or coarse mottling bilaterally, predominant in the lower zones. In the mural type small round opacities or ring shadows may lead to honeycomb appearance. In the desquamative type the opacity is irregular with patchy shadowing at the lung bases. The diaphragm is elevated due to contraction of the lower lobes, and the lungs appear. Small $FEV_1$ and FVC are reduced proportionately, a restrictive pattern without airway obstruction, there is poor gas diffusion, with hypoxia and hypocapnoea. Diagnosis may be confirmed by lung biopsy. Serological tests for antinuclear and rheumatoid factor may be positive even in the absence of arthritic manifestations.

**Prognosis :** is uncertain and may vary from death in a few months to survival with minimal symptoms for many years.

**Treatment :** with corticosteroids is effective in 30 per cent of the acute cases but not in others. It may have to be maintained for several years or even for life.

## HONEYCOMB LUNGS

It is a condition characterised by existence of numerous small cysts throughout both lungs. It occurs as a late development in fibrosing alveolitis. but may occur as a part of rare systemic diseases such as histiocytosis tuberose sclerosis, and Marfan's syndrome.

**Pathology :** Cysts vary in size upto 1 cm. in diameter and are thin-walled and occupy a wide area in the lungs. They are located in the terminal parts of the bronchial tree, which are separated by fibrous septa and they do not take part in the exchange of gas. Though some may have a developmental origin, the majority appear to be due to an acquired inflammatory condition. The peripheral parts of the bronchial tree are affected by inflammatory thickening, hyperplasia of smooth muscle or fibrosis. The bronchiole dilates and forms cystic sacs and a check valve obstruction increases their size.

**Clinical features**

It is commoner in males and occurs in all age groups. It manifests with progressively increasing dyspnoea. There is a great predisposition to infection presenting with fever, cough and sputum in children. In the younger age group there is a tendency for cysts in contact with the pleura to rupture, with recurrent pneumothorax which may be bilateral. In adults the condition progresses slowly leading to right heart failure.

**Radiological** examination shows existence of numerous cysts distributed bilaterally along with reticulation or fibrosis throughout the lung. On bronchography, the bronchogram is normal and the radio-opaque material does not enter the cysts even after coughing.

**Treatment :** There is no specific treatment. Infections, pneumothorax and heart failure are to be treated when they occur. To prevent recurrent pneumothorax, pleurodesis or pleurectomy is done. Radiotherapy is dangerous as it induces fibrosis.

## SARCOIDOSIS

**Sarcoidosis** is a granulomatous condition of the body. Besides the lungs, it can involve the skin, eyes, liver, spleen and central nervous system. The cause is unknown. Apart from the absence of caseation and tubercle bacilli, the lesions are histologically similar to tuberculous follicles, but there is no evidence to support the view that the disease is caused by any of the mycobacteria. Though pulmonary tuberculosis is very common in India, sarcoidosis is very rare.

**Pathology :** The mediastinal and superficial lymph nodes, lungs, liver, spleen, skin, eyes, parotid glands and phalangeal bones are most frequently involved. The characteristic histological finding is of non-caseating epitheloid follicles. These may restore spontaneously, but in some cases they stimulate the production of fibrous tissue, the disease is seldom fatal except when it affects vital organs such as lungs, heart or central nervous system.

**Clinical features :** It occurs commonly in women. In the USA it is commoner in blacks than in white people. In India cases are often missed due to lack of proper investigation. In 50 per cent of cases there are no symptoms and they are detected on routine radiography. Principal symptoms are cough with mucoid expectoration, fever, polyarthralgia and loss of weight. Dyspnoea is related to the extent of fibrosis. General examination may show evidence of erythema nodosum iritis, bilateral parotid swelling, superficial lymphadenopathy and hepatosplenomegaly, Chronic pulmonary sarcoidosis may lead to development of interstitial fibrosis, pulmonary hypertension and cor pulmonale.

**Radiology :** Shows pulmonary infiltration with bilateral symmetrical hilar node enlargement. The infiltration consists of nodular shadows 1 to 3 mm in size but may be bigger or smaller. Pulmonary fibrosis may be present.

**Pulmonary function :** Shows diminished FVC and $FEV_1$ and impaired diffusion.

**Diagnosis :** is confirmed by demonstration of the sarcoid nodule on biopsy of lymph nodes or liver, in cases with clinical history of generalised systemic involvement. Typical chest X-ray and finding of circumscribed 'punched out' areas in the diaphysis of the phalanges is also suggestive. There is increase of gamma globulin in the serum associated with hypercalcaemia. The tuberculin skin test is usually negative (negative Mantoux reaction). Kveim Test makes use of a crude suspension of affected tissues containing sarcoid granuloma. This is injected subcutaneously and a biopsy is made at the site of injection 3 to 6 weeks later. If typical sarcoid granuloma is seen, the result is positive. Sputum and gastric lavage should be carefully examined to exclude tuberculosis. The disease has to be differentiated from aspergillosis, carcinoma, occupational lung disease, diffuse interstitial fibrosis, leukaemias, tuberculosis and beryllosis.

**Treatment :** Many cases resolve without treatment. The drug of choice is corticosteroids. This has to be continued for many years and the dose must be kept at the minimum required to suppress the manifestations of the disease. (Details also discussed in P.112).

## IDIOPATHIC PULMONARY HAEMOSIDEROSIS

It is a rare disease of unknown aetiology. Spontaneous haemorrhage into the lungs causes recurrent episodes of pyrexia, haemoptysis and iron deficiency anaemia. Haemosiderin derived from blood is released by macrophages into the interstitial tissues of the lung and stimulate development of fibrosis. The patient may die from haemorrhage, respiratory failure or cardiac failure due to pulmonary hypertension. Pulmonary haemosiderosis associated with acute glomerulonephritis is called Goodpasture's syndrome.

## PULMONARY ALVEOLAR PROTEINOSIS

It is characterised by filling of alveoli by proteinaceous material derived from sloughing of alveolar walls. This rare disease affects young women. There is sudden onset of fever associated with hoarseness, cough and purulent sputum, progressive dyspnoea and cyanosis. Fine crepitations are audible on examination of the chest. Radiological examination shows diffuse linear shadows radiating bilaterally from the hila or nodular opacities. Pulmonary function shows impaired diffusion. The diagnosis may be confirmed by lung biopsy.

Chymotrypsin a proteolytic enzyme is the drug of choice.

**Pulmonary alveolar microlithiasis :** is characterised by intra-alveolar calcified laminated concretions throughout the lungs. The aetiology is unknown. There is shortness of breath with cyanosis and clubbing. There may be a few scattered coarse crepitations on auscultation. Radiological examination shows minute calcified circles throughout the lungs, less marked at the apices (onion peel appearance). Diagnosis may be confirmed by lung biopsy.

## PULMONARY TUBERCULOSIS

*G. C. MOOKERJEE*

### Introduction

Robert Koch discovered the acid and alcohol fast bacilli (AFB) as the causative agent of tuberculosis in the year 1882 but the disease was known even in ancient times. It is a world-wide disease though in the present decade, it is chiefly a problem of the developing countries. WHO estimates that there are about 10 to 12 million cases in the world out of which 75% are in the developing countries. About three million tuberculosis cases end in fatality every year.

Though developing countries suffer more due to tuberculosis, the chances of contact have increased considerably with other countries due to international movements and sputum + ve cases are also treated outside hospitals.

Since the discovery of modern anti-tuberculous drugs after 1948 and programme of BCG vaccination as well case finding programme by Mantoux testing etc. the facilities of world-wide control have become greater. Mass miniature radiography in industries, schools, among workers, and labourers should be encouraged in all countries, but this facility is still lacking a great deal, especially in this part of the globe. Sources of infection and risk factors of tuberculosis are illustrated in **Table 17.6)**

**Table showing sources of tuberculosis and risk factors**

**SOURCES**

| | |
|---|---|
| KISSING ESPECIALLY SMALL CHILDREN | FOMITES |
| COUGHING IN THE OPEN ESPECIALLY TOBACCO, BETEL CHEWING & SPITTING-ANYWHERE HABIT | EATING HOUSES ESPECIALLY MILK & ICECREAM VIA ANIMALS : CATS, DOGS & COWS. |

**RISK FACTORS**

GREAT-RISK FACTOR IS VIRULENCE OF ORGANISMS BUT OTHER FACTORS ARE :

| | |
|---|---|
| GENETICS | ALCOHOL, TOBACCO |
| AGE & SEX | GASTRECTOMY |
| YOUNG & OLD | MALABSORPTION |
| MALNUTRITION | STEROIDS & IMMUNOSUPPRESSIVE DRUGS |
| DIABETES | SEVERE MENTAL DISEASE |
| FEMALES : REPEATED PREGNANCY | POOR LIVING CONDITION |

**OCCUPATION**

SOME OCCUPATIONS ARE PARTICULARLY LIABLE

| | |
|---|---|
| HOSPITAL STAFF, | BUS CONDUCTORS, |
| COAL MINERS, | CASHIERS & SHOP ASSISTANTS, |
| INDUSTRIAL WORKERS | SCHOOL TEACHERS, |
| FOOD-HANDLERS | YOUNG SCHOOL-GOING KIDS. |

**HOST-DEFENCE**

| | |
|---|---|
| GOOD NUTRITION | NATURAL IMMUNITY |
| GOOD LIVING CONDITION | PROPER CARE OF INFECTED SUBJECTS. |
| BCG VACCINATION. | |

Tuberculosis may affect almost all organs of the body but the commonest of all forms of tuberculosis is respiratory tuberculosis. Thoracic tuberculosis includes pulmonary tuberculosis (primary and post-primary) as well as pleural disease and mediastinal tuberculosis. Pulmonary tuberculosis is most common.

Other forms of tuberculosis are : Miliary tuberculosis, tuberculous meningitis, renal tuberculosis, and abdominal tuberculosis. Diagnosis of abdominal tuberculosis is often missed.

It also affects bones, joints, skin and pelvic organs. Non-respiratory tuberculosis has been discussed elsewhere in this book excluding tuberculosis of pelvic organs, bones and joints, being surgical subjects.

**Bacteriology**

There are four types of mycobacterium tuberculosis, but humans are affected by human and bovine types. Avian type very rarely may cause human disease. The human type usually causes respiratory tuberculosis while bovine type usually affects G.I. tract, tonsils, glands etc. i.e. depending on route of entry. Due to miliary spread any organ may be affected. Human type is inhaled while bovine type is usually milk borne.

The organisms are highly susceptible to sunlight but may remain alive for months even years in darkness. They may resist 5% phenol for a few hours but 1% hypochlorite solution rapidly kills it. The organisms are rapidly destroyed by heat. If patients use paper handkerchief, these can be easily burnt, otherwise boiling or steam-disinfection is best. Woollen garments and blankets should be sterilised by dry heat, but cotton materials are sterilised by boiling. Open sunlight, however, is a cheap and good substitute.

The tubercle bacillus (mycobacterium) belongs to the genus mycobacteriae, of the order of actinomycetes. It is a slender organism which does not take Gram's stain easily, hence it is stained by Zeel-Nielsen method, by pouring hot carbol fuschin, over the slide smeared with sample to be examined. Once it is stained the slide is washed with acid and alcoholic reagent and acid fast bacilli are seen under the light microscope. Its detailed structure can be seen by electron microscope for research purposes. For routine clinical diagnosis Zeel-Nielsen's method and culture of the acid fast bacilli (AFB) in the Lowenstein Jensen medium is adequate. The culture takes four to six weeks to grow in anaerobic condition.

**Classification of tuberculosis :**

American Thoracic Society has classified tuberculosis for clinical assessment (American Lung. Association 1974 : as quoted in the monograph on Tuberculosis : CHEST VOL. 76, 6,1979). Table 17.4 shows the classification.

Table 17.6 Classification of Tuberculosis (1974)

| Class |
|---|
| 0 No TB exposure, not infected (no history of exposure, negative tuberculin skin test). |
| 1. TB exposure, no evidence of infection (history of exposure, negative tuberculin skin test). |
| 2. Tuberculous infection without disease (positive tuberculin skin test; negative bacteriologic studies, if done), no roentgenographic findings compatible with TB, no symptoms due to TB. |
| 3. TB : infection with disease |

On the basis of this classification, appropriate treatment can be correctly recommended.

## PRIMARY PULMONARY TUBERCULOSIS

The first infection by the tubercle bacilli is called primary tuberculosis. The organisms most frequently reach the pulmonary alveoli through inhalation and there is a local reaction followed by affection of the regional lymph glands. This first local lesion and glandular component is the primary complex'.

Similar reaction may occur in small intestine or tonsils by bovine tubercle bacilli, when source of infection is milk of infected cow.

In majority of individuals it heals completely with or without calcification. In some others the lesion is walled off by collagenous tissue and the tubercle bacilli stop multiplying so as to remain dormant. In a few others, the lesion may be acutely progressive or develops haematogenous spread resulting in miliary tuberculosis or tuberculous meningitis.

### Pathology

The primary lesion is subpleural. It may occur in any part of the lung in children though in adolescents and young it tends to occur towards the upper zones. Primary lesion can as well be multiple.

With the deposition of tubercle bacilli in an alveolus, serous or serofibrinous exudate appears containing neutrophils; the neutrophils are soon replaced by macrophages which engulf the tubercle bacilli. The tubercle bacilli are now either destroyed gradually or become less virulent or may multiply. After 3-8 weeks the individual develops hypersensitivity to tuberculoprotein. When the macrophages rupture, the tubercle bacilli are released to produce classical pathological picture of tuberculosis, consisting of a granulomatous lesion, containing epitheloid cells derived from macrophages. Langhan's giant cells are derived also from macrophages, lymphocytes and varying degrees of fibrosis. As a result of hypersensitivity, necrosis may also occur to varying degrees. These changes result in production of cheesy materials in the centre of the lesion which may eventually become calcified.

The glandular components also may produce local pressure effects, if they enlarge due to tuberculous lesion. It can obstruct a bronchial tube and produce collapse of a segment or even lobe.

This may lead to tuberculous pneumonia, termed as epituberculosis (Elisberg and Neuland). This may occur in right middle lobe causing collapse of whole middle lobe (Broeck's syndrome). In a child such atelectasis of middle-lobe may occur due to tuberculosis or a F.B., but if a similar picture occurs in adults possibility of a new growth should be considered. The primary complex may also produce the following complications :

1. Involvement of tracheal and paratracheal glands, often quite large
2. Erosion into above leading to tuberculous tracheo-bronchitis
3. Pleural effusion
4. Bronchiectasis
5. Obstructive emphysema
6. Tuberculous pneumonia
7. Bronchostenosis.

**Clinical features**

The children may experience a brief febrile episode at the time of tuberculin conversion which is usually treated as short-term febrile illness or influenza etc. Sometimes the child may have reduced appetite, fretfulness and failure to gain weight. Cough, though unusual, may sometimes be paroxysmal mimicking whooping cough. Sometimes children continue to get low grade fever and poor general health. On examination, no detectable abnormalities can be seen. The child may be thin, pale and may develop a few local crepitations over the affected lung with the primary complex.

**Clinical diagnosis**

History of contact with a patient of tuberculosis, vague ill-health, positive tuberculin test should always arouse suspicion. Respiratory signs may be insignificant. Sometimes it may be mild bronchitis or patchy pneumonitis. Presence of erythema nodosum is supportive evidence but it may also occur in sarcoidosis, streptococcal infection, coccidioidomycosis and due to sulpha-drug. This lesion is a non-specific allergic reaction and histologically does not show tuberculous pathology. It occurs commonly in the skin of shin bones or rarely in medial aspect of thighs.

Mantoux test also becomes strongly positive. If the pulmonary component caseates or caseating gland breaks into a vein, there is acute miliary spread, causing tuberculous meningitis or miliary tuberculosis.

**Fate of Miliary Spread**

From the site of primary complex the tubercle bacilli may go anywhere in the body, e.g., CNS, bones, kidneys, liver, spleen, mesenteric glands or skin and lodge there for years and may flare up infection when resistance is poor. The result is miliary tuberculosis.

In abdomen (usually bovine type) it can cause small intestinal tuberculosis, ileocaecal tuberculosis, strictures and obstruction of gut, mesenteric lymphadenitis (tabes mesenterica).

**Laboratory Diagnosis**

BLOOD PICTURE : Haematology may be unremarkable but usually there may be lymphocytosis; raised ESR is highly suspicious. Initial polymorphonuclear reaction may sometimes occur.

TUBERCULIN TEST : 0.1 ml. of glycerinated purified protein derivative (PPD) is injected intradermally over the anterior aspect of the forearm and the extent of induration is read after 72 hours. The reading exceeding 10 mm. is indicative of positive reaction and signifies infection with the virulent tubercle bacilli. It indicates tuberculous disease in the following :

(a) Patient under 2 years of age
(b) Patient under 6 years of age, provided the child is exposed to a known case of tuberculosis.
(c) Recent conversion from negative to positive.

| | |
|---|---|
| TINE TEST : | It is easier to perform than tuberculin test as it is done by multi-puncture method. The appearance of a papule more than 5 mm. in diameter during the first 24 to 72 hours indicates a positive test. It may be a good screening test, but cannot replace time-honoured Mantoux test. |
| RADIOLOGY : | It has a very important place in diagnosis of adult pulmonary tuberculosis. In primary complex, the pulmonary component may be insignificant or sometimes unremarkable. Glandular component consists of well-marked hilar adenopathy. |
| ANIMAL INOCULATION : | Has no place in diagnosis at least in India. Our guinea-pigs are also very resistant to T.B. |
| DEMONSTRATION OF BACILLI : | From sputum, gastric lavage, laryngeal swab. Sputum culture or culture of suspected body fluid should be done wherever feasible. This will, however not delay begining the treatment in suspected cases. Fluorescent microscopy is a very useful method in diagnosis. |

## POST-PRIMARY PULMONARY TUBERCULOSIS

### Pathology

Types of histopathological lesions occurring in the lungs vary from case to case as well as in different areas of the same lung. The typical forms are :

1. Exudative lesion
2. Caseating lesion
3. Productive lesion
4. Cavity formation
5. Fibrosis
6. Calcified lesion.

### Exudative Phase

Initially there is vasodilatation and alveolar epithelial damage (pre-exudative phase of Canetti) due to multiplication of tubercle bacilli and liberation of toxin.

Bacilli are present in the cells and outside the cells. This is followed by local oedema, fibrinous exudate, collection of histocytes, lymphocytes, and polymorph cells to fight the battle with the tubercle bacilli (hypersensitive phenomena).

### Caseation

The exudative battle in most cases ends in caseation. The infiltrating cell mass and local tissue become shapeless homogenous cheesy mass along with dead and dying bacilli.

### Productive lesion

If all goes well around the caseating lesion, there is giant cell formation and epitheloid cell aggregation to form classical tubercles. A few bacilli may also be present in the tubercle.

The giant cell of Langhan's type has large pale nucleus (the epitheloid cell) and multiple nuclei distributed peripherally. There is lymphocytic infiltration around it and tendency to fibrosis (process of healing). If the process continues favourably the whole lesion heals by fibrosis and finally calcification.

### Cavity formation

However, if the lesion is progressive, the caseous material liquefies and finally erodes into a bronchus and the materials are discharged leaving behind a cavity. The wall of the cavity is lined by caseous substance and large number of tubercle bacilli.

There may be many small cavities or a few large ones. These may get distended if the draining bronchiole gets partially obstructed resulting in check valve mechanism. Air goes into cavity but cannot exist. This results in a distended thin-walled cavity.

The cavity is a potential source of haemoptysis as well as a source of spread of the disease locally in the lung tissue (secondary lesions). It may also cause haematogenous dissemination.

Bronchiectasis, bronchial cold abscess and emphysema may occur in neglected cases.

Rapidly progressing lesions may cause acute tuberculous bronchopneumonia. On the other hand, persons with high resistance may harbour the disease in chronic fibrotic stage, with or without cavity for months or years, disseminating infection to others.

### Post-Primary Tuberculosis

*This is the adult form of tuberculosis and is the major problem. Most of these cases are sputum positive, hence are responsible for spread of the disease in the community.*

*P.P. Tuberculosis occurs in the following ways :*

*a) Direct progression of the primary complex*
*b) Reactivation of the dormant primary lesion*
*c) Haematogenous return of bacilli from a gland or distant organ to the lung.*
*d) Reinfection from exogenous source due to contact.*

### Classical Presenting Features

- Evening rise of temperature
- Progressive loss of weight
- Dry cough, later mucopurulent expectoration
- Haemoptysis
- Night sweat
- Lymphadenitis
- Pleurisy
- Pleural effusion
- Pneumothorax.

PATHOGENESIS OF POST-PRIMARY LESION

**1. Progressive Primary Lesion**

*a) When primary complex occurs in adults, it may progress to P.P. lesion,, as seen in European adults.*

*b) In Indians and Africans even childhood primary complex may progress to P.P. tuberculosis.*

**2. Reactivation of Primary Lesion**

*Possible any time during adult life till old age (original lesion, however, small).*

Especially when defensive factors are poor.

*In children strongly positive test is of particular risk even if radiologically negative.*

**3. Haematogenous Spread**

*From primary focus (lymphatic spread) tubercle bacilli enter blood stream and redistribute by pulmonary arteries, resulting in bilateral scattered lesions, evenly distributed. Bacilli also may get lodged in many organs.*

**4. Exogenous Infection**

*Once the primary complex heals enough, resistance develops to prevent endogenous super infection.*

**A Rare Occurrence**

Note : Most post-primary tuberculosis are reactivations of dormant lesions.

*However, drug resistant organism may cause super infection in patients. This is extremely rare.*

**Varied Symptomatology :**

- Recurrent cough and colds
- Fatigue
- Anorexia or dyspepsia
- Influenzal onset with continued fever
- Continued pyrexia (P.U.O.)
- Pneumonic onset/not resolving with treatment
  Diabetes mellitus not responding to therapy

**Asymptomatic Type :**

Detected by chest radiography

**Physical Signs in the Chest :**

These will vary according to the extent and stage of the disease as well as on the site of pulmonary lesion. However, the following guidelines should be remembered :

1. Early lesions may not be detected by stethoscope, only radiology may reveal.
2. Post-tussive crepitations may be detected at the apices of one or both lungs or localised wheeze may be heard.
3. Signs of fibrosis-chest flattened, displaced cardiac apex/trachea V.F. reduced, if pleura is thickened or may be increased if lungs are consolidated with patent bronchi.
4. Signs of patchy consolidation with impaired resonance and bronchial breath sounds.
5. Signs of cavity-impaired or tympanitic percussion note i.e. cavity is large-sized. B.S. may be bronchial, cavernous or amphoric. Crackling rales may be heard.

**Treatment**

Treatment should be planned according to the stage of infection or possible exposure. Nowadays most cases, especially early disease can be treated as outdoor cases. It is necessary to screen the contacts, especially all children in contact should be examined and both X-ray chest and Mantoux testing must be done. American Thoracic Society and American Lung Associations have classified stages of tuberculosis as follows for purposes of therapy

**Category-I**

Patients exposed to infectious case but has not developed any evidence of tuberculous infection.

If tuberculin skin test is not yet positive, prophylactic therapy may be given only to children especially below 5 years of age and particularly neonates. For others consider treatment on individual merits.

Drug : INAH for 3 months

At present it is difficult to ensure this in developing countries.

**Category-II**

**Tuberculous infection but no evidence of disease :**

Mantoux-positive cases without any other evidence i.e. fever, loss of weight, infiltration, adenopathy, with negative bacteriology.

These cases up to 35 years of age should be given one year's therapy with INAH. Above this age group, consider cases on their own merit especially if,

1) General health is poor
2) On corticosteroid therapy
3) On immunosuppressive drugs.

There is, however, no general agreement on this point. Therefore, cases should be considered on their own merit.

**Category-III :**

**When disease is evident**

These cases should be given full chemotherapy with at least three anti-tuberculous drugs to start with. Hospital admission is not necessary unless there are complications, e.g., high fever, anaemia, severe haemoptysis, massive pleural effusion or tuberculous meningitis etc. Mild cases may even continue sedentary jobs, provided they are sputum negative.

It is ideal to send the sputum for culture and sensitivity test before starting treatment, but these facilities are very limited in this part of the world at present, especially in rural areas.

A decade ago the standard regimen of treatment was adequate doses of Inj. streptomycin with isoniazid and PAS or thiacetazone. Later on, ethambutol was being used more often, as PAS is often not well tolerated and thiacetazone, though cheap, tends to be toxic.

Duration of treatment was 18 months to two years. In cases with cavities, duration may be longer.

During the last decade Inj. streptomycin is being gradually replaced by oral rifampicin. Pyrazinamide is another useful addition, during first two months of therapy.

When streptomycin is used, it is given initially for three months only subsequently any two drugs are used, one of the two being INH. The modern regime of rifampicin, INH and ethambutol appears to be excellent and the duration of treatment is also reduced to about nine months, except in extrapulmonary tuberculosis and patients complicated by diabetes, silicosis etc.

In Madras, several other regimens were carried out by giving two or three weekly injections of streptomycin along with INAH and PAS to treat large number of cases with reasonable success, however it is far from ideal though this may suit the requirement of developing countries for the present, where lack of drug supply and communication difficulties are often supreme. Considering the cost of travel to hospital and expenses in private clinics and cost of injections (if taken at home) and duration of treatment in months, rifamycin, INH and ethambutol combination should be considered ideal in all respects. More recently pyrazinamide is replacing ethambutol, during the first two months or all the four may be used in some cases.

**Modern therapy**

Combination drugs is most important. Inj, streptomycin is not routinely used nowadays because of its oto-toxicity. It should be avoided also in elderly people especially above 50 years and if there is renal insufficiency.

In cases of tuberculous infection there are millions of organisims, some of them being resistant to one drug or the other. Therefore, initial regimen of three drugs is most effective way of treating tuberculosis. In those where resistance is suspected even four drugs may be used. With adequate treatment most organisms will die but a few organisms may still survive, who have slow metabolism and infrequent multiplying capacity. To control these organisms prolonged drug therapy is essential.

Of the available drugs rifampicin, INAH and pyrazinamide are the most effective agents in killing rapidly dividing organisms. Rifampicin has very rapid effect and persister-organisms are quickly killed, pyrazinamide is particularly effective against bacilli within macrophages. Isoniazid is strongly bactericidal against rapidly mutltiplying organisms.

Therefore, these three drugs are of supreme importance in controlling pulmonary tuberculosis and it is most likely that even six months' therapy may be successful if these three drugs are used. The role of pyrazinamide is most important in the first two months and may be replaced by ethambutol, if there is no renal insufficiency. Ethambutol may affect visual acuity and colour vision, so it is safer to test visual acuity and colour vision before starting ethambutol and periodically check up regarding visual problems during ethambutol therapy.

Rifampicin and pyrazinamide both are hepatotoxic and may cause hepatitis. Rifamycin particularly induces hepatic enzymes and hence helps in active metabolism of contraceptive pills, steroids, barbiturates and anticonvulsants.

However, it is essential that every case has to be assessed on its own merits and choice of appropriate drugs can only be made after due consideration of clinical data.

Physicians in developing countries should be more alert and resourceful in treating their cases depending on the economic facilities available. General scheme for treatment should be as follows :

## PRIMARY TUBERCULOSIS

1) **Symptomatic cases :**

*Either,*

A—1) Streptomycin 20 mg./kg./day. for the first 2 months of the therapy if there are no contraindications;

2) Isoniazid 5-10 mg./kg. upto a maximum of 300 mg. per day;

3) PAS 300 mg./kg./ day,

Thiacetazone 4 mg./kg. upto a maximum of 150 mg. per day may be given as alternative to PAS;

*or, if the patient can afford.*

B—1) Isoniazid as above;

2) Rifampicin 20 mg./kg./day up to maximum of 600 mg. per day; and

3) Ethambutol 15 mg./kg./day.

Pyrazinamide-1500 mg may be more effective than ethambutol which can be added later instead of pyrazinamide, (given for 2 months initially)

2) **Asymptomatic cases :**

(a) Children under 5 years of age with positive Mantoux test only : prophylactic Isoniazid 5 5 mg/kg./day for 6 months.

(b) Children with positive radiological findings :

(i) Isoniazid 5 mg./kg./day and

(ii) Thiacetazone 4 mg./kg./day

OR

PAS 300 mg./kg./day

OR

Rifampicin 20 mg./kg./day for a period of 12 months.

3) Infants exposed to infection :

i) BCG Vaccination

ii) Isoniazid 5 mg./kg./day (ideally difficult to achieve in developing countries).

### Post-Primary Tuberculosis

(A) **Specific treatment**

Use any three drugs to start with, depending on the situation. If Inj. Streptomycin is used, it is given daily (or sometimes alternate days) for three months, then two drugs are usually given but INH should be included unless there is some definite reason.

Rifampicin can be used in lieu of Streptomycin, it is given usually for six months, with due precautions.

Inj. Streptomycin should be avoided in elderly patients as it may cause vestibular damage in elderly age group.

## ANTI-TUBERCULOUS AGENTS IN USE

*Streptomycin* : It interferes with normal protein synthesis of the bacilli, probably by disturbing the function of the genetic code. The recommended dosage is 15 mg./kg. up to a maximum of 1.0 gm. intramuscularly daily for an average adult. It is given for a total period of 3 months, sometimes for a longer period even. It should be avoided in persons above 50 years of age as it often causes vestibular damage. For elderly patients rifamycin is now available as a good substitute.

Side-effects of Streptomycin include giddiness, exfoliative dermatitis reaction, haematological disturbances and sometimes renal damage. Should giddiness occur, which is often the case in about 30% of the patients who are specially elderly, the drug may be temporarily withdrawn and then lower dosage, e.g., 0.5 g daily may be tried in the evening if an alternative drug cannot be used.

In Madras, trials with two or three injections have been used with reasonable success but it is better to change the drug and prescribe rifamycin in these cases.

**Isoniazid (Isonicotinic acid hydrazide — INH)** — It possibly acts by interfering with bacterial respiration. The generally recommended dose is 5-10 mg./kg. up to a maximum of 300 mg. per day. It is a companion drug for most of the anti-tuberculous drug combinations. Although it is least toxic, it may produce hypersensitivity with fever, drug rash, jaundice lymphadenopathy, peripheral neuropathy, rarely convulsions. Reports of psychiatric complications are also on record. Optic neuritis is rarely reported. So watch for any visual symptoms carefully. Neuropathy can be prevented by simultaneous administration of pyridoxin 10-20 mg. per day.

Dose for children under four years is 10 mg/kg per day. In tuberculous meningitis and miliary tuberculosis, the dose is 10-15 mg/kg daily, for chemo-prophylaxis it is given in dosage of 5 mg/kg daily.

Isoniazid injection contains 100 mg/ml.

**PAS** — The dose is 150 mg/kg. subject to a maximum of 12 gms./day in three divided doses. The drug causes a variety of side-effects like anorexia, nausea, dyspepsia, diarrhoea, skin rashes, hepatic dysfunction and rarely leukaemoid reaction, lymphadenopathy, splenomegaly and thyroid enlargement. The drug is unable to exert its maximal antibacterial effect on the organism within macrophages thereby limiting its antitubercular activity, it is no longer considered "first line" drug and has been replaced by ethambutol especially in Western countries. Most patients also do not like it.

**Thiacetazone** — It is given in the dosage of 3-5 mg./kg./day up to a maximum of 150 mg. daily. Its side-effects include anorexia, nausea, jaundice and bone-marrow depression. It is a bacteriostatic drug and owing to its cheapness it has been used specially in developing countries.

**Ethambutol** — Although considered as a second line drug it is being used nowadays as an important therapeutic agent. Primary resistance to this drug is not yet reported. It acts by inhibiting RNA synthesis and phosphate metabolism. The recommended dose is 25 mg./kg. to start with, preferably 20 mg./kg./day for 2 months and afterwards 15 mg./kg./day. Except for a few reported cases of retrobulbar neuritis its toxicity is minimal. But then it occurs with high dosage (25 mg./kg.) and usually after 2-3 months. The patient complains of blurred vision or decreased visual acuity or sometimes colour blindness. No abnormality, however, can be detected on ophthalmoscopy and these side-effects are all reversible. However, it is important to closely watch the patients while on this drug.

**Rifampicin** — It acts by inhibiting RNA polymerase. The dose is 8-12 mg./kg. or 450-600 mg. daily. The side-effects include orange or red colouration of the urine, anorexia, nausea and elevation of hepatic enzymes. The incidence of jaundice with hepatitis is less than 1 per cent. Thrombocytopenic purpose is to be withdrawn. Induction of hepatic enzymes has been mentioned already.

**Cycloserine (Themiserine)** — It is a bacteriostatic drug. It is given orally in 500-100 mg. daily dose. It is neurotoxic and may cause tremors, muscular twitchings, convulsions and suicidal tendency. The drug should be avoided in epileptics, psychotics and in presence of renal damage. Undoubtedly it is the most important drug now, which has reduced the course of treatment to about six to nine months.

**Pyrazinamide** — It is a highly effective bactericidal drug and the dose is 40 mg./kg./day. But it has potent side-effects in the form of hepatic damage, renal damage, disturbances of plasma concentrations of prothrombin, albumin and globulin. But its use in first two months of therapy has many advantages.

**Ethionamide** — It is chemically related to isoniazid. The recommended dose is 15-20 mg./kg./day. Side-effects include nausea, vomiting, salivation, hepatic damage and peripheral neuritis.

**Isovin** : It is a hydrozone derivative and chemically known as P-hydroxym m-methoxy-benzal dehyde isonicotinyl hydrazone. This drug has been widely used in Russia, Australia, and recently in India.

Dose : 1 to 2 g. daily. Tablets are available of 500 mg. Toxic effects are reported to be rare.

**Viomycin, Kanamycin, Capreomycin** — These are antibiotics and may be thought of it if streptomycin is not tolerated.

Viomycin is given as sulphate usually in a dosage, in adults, of 1 gm, twice daily, twice a week. But its antituberculous action is poor and toxicity is high like vertigo, deafness, renal damage, skin rashes, etc.

Kanamycin is similar to viomycin in efficacy and also in toxicity. The usual dosage is 15 mg./kg. not exceeding 1 gm. daily. Capreomycin is administered intramuscularly in a daily dosage of 1.0 gm. Toxicity includes allergic reactions with skin rashes, auditory or vestibular dysfunction and evidence of renal damage. These drugs are very rarely used and, when prescribed, will require expert supervision.

**Recent Trends**

The modern concept of treatment, however, is showing considerable changes, with the object of reducing duration of therapy. In the West, patients are receiving short course chemotherapy with rifamycin, ethambutol and INAH. The present position is well summarised by Joseph H. Bates (International Conference on Tuberculosis : CHEST : 26, Dec. 1979 supplement) quoted as follows :

"Regarding short-course chemotherapy and the extensive discussion that followed, indicate that this form of treatment is almost certain to be adopted by most physicians attending the conference. A number of highly effective and safe regimens have been described. The drugs most useful for short-course treatment are isoniazid, rifamycin, streptomycin and pyrazinamide. At this time the most effective regimens for patients with smear-positive pulmonary tuberculosis are those that extend over a nine-month treatment period, although it is probable that most smear-negative culture-positive patients, as well as those that never have positive cultures can be treated for a total duration of only four to six months. Therapy regimens of even shorter duration were described that are reasonably effective, but the results are not as satisfactory as those obtained with the nine-month or traditional 18-24 month regimens".

Finally, it may be recommended that in severe cases rifamycin, INH, ethambutol and pyrazinamide should be used for best result. Pyrazinamide may be discontinued after two months. The remaining drugs should continue and drugs may be required up to six or nine months depending on the case. The alternative regime may be rifamycin (or streptomycin when rifamycin is contraindicated or not tolerated), INH and pyrazinamide. Pyrazinamide may be replaced after two months by ethambutol. This regime may also be successful in six to nine months.

Various centres are still using different regimes with varying degrees of success depending on economy, socio-economic status and tolerance.

**Supportive Treatment**

Besides symptomatic treatment for fever, cough, insomnia etc., the following points are relevant :

(1) **Rest and graduated exercise :** Should be planned depending on the stage of disease, febrile state and presence of complications.

(2) **Adequate diet :** Calorific adequacy with good mixed diet and supplement of vitamins should be enough. Possibly high protein content and additional milk content in the diet may accelerate weight gain quickly.

However, our vitamin supplement is all that is necessary. Monthly weight record is a good index of adequate nutrition.

(3) **Follow-up :** The most important point in successful therapy is continuous drug therapy and periodic regular follow-up. INH is always the most important drug and choice of companion drugs depends on other factors including tolerance, drug resistance and availability. The patient should be indoctrinated in the beginning to impress that irregular drug therapy is dangerous.

In India, lack of patient's co-operation is the most important cause of relapse and development of drug resistance due to irregular drug intake.

Relapse cases may require more careful therapy by ascertaining drug sensitivity, changing the drug combinations and isolating them cautiously to avoid spread of resistant-organisms. In these cases four-drug combination may be required.

## PREVENTION

**Case finding**

(1) Routine health examination and medical paramedical personnel.

(2) Sputum examination

(3) Tuberculin testing

(4) Mass-miniature X-ray.

II. **Isolation of open cases :**

(1) Often difficult due to poverty, lack of accommodation, inadequacy of hospital beds.

(2) Effective treatment, co-operation of patients most important. Lack of facilities in certain remote areas causes failure.

III. Control of diseases among cattle and proper sterilisation of milk by diseased kitchen staff.

IV. Good nutrition, balanced diet, fresh air, avoid overcrowding (not always available for the poor of the developing countries).

V. **BCG Vaccination**

Especially in the developing countries.

VI. **Chemoprophylaxis**

Mantoux positive children in particular.

# DISEASES OF THE PLEURA

*G.C. MOOKERJEE*
*J. RAYCHOUDHURI*

Each lung is covered by a double-layer serous membrane with a potential space between the two layers. The outer or parietal layer covers the inside of chest wall and superior surface of diaphragm and is sensitive to pain; the inner or visceral wall covers the lungs and its fissures but is insensitive to pain.

The parietal layer is supplied by blood vessels, lymphatics and nerves from the intercostal spaces while visceral layer is supplied by bronchial vessels and it has sympathetic nerve supply only. Parietal layer of the superior diaphragmatic surfaces is supplied by phrenic nerve from the neck but peripheral areas of diaphragm are supplied by intercostal nerves. Normal intrapleural pressure varies with phases of respiration. During inspiration it is 4 to 8 cm of water pressure and -2 to -4 cm at the end of expiration. The pleural space contains a thin film of pleural fluid which functions as lubricant.

The pleural cavity may be affected due to the various causes, **(Table 17.7)**.

When there is fibrinous inflammation it is called dry pleurisy, **but when there** is collection of fluid between pleural layers, it is called pleural effusion. Pleuro-**pericarditis** may sometimes occur due to contiguous affections from pericardial disease.

**Inflammation :** Viral, bacterial or mycotic infections.

**Trauma** (With or without injury to thoracic cage) usually presents as hydropneumothorax or haemothorax.

**New growth** — Carcinoma of lung, or pleural malignancy e.g. mesothelioma of pleura presents as large pleural effusion, may be haemorrhagic.

**Secondaries due** to malignancies elsewhere.

**Diseases of heart & kidneys** — causing anasarca (usually bilateral).

**Sub-diaphragmatic** affections e.g. liver abscess or subdiaphragmatic suppuration : pleurisy or pleural effusion.

**Pulmonary infarction :** pleurisy or haemorrhagic effusion; usually not large.

**Collagen disorders** causing pleurisy or pleural effusion.

**Renal failure** — uraemia causes pleurisy and pleural effusion.

**Table — 17.7 : Causes of Pleural Disease**

*Inflammation* — Viral, bacterial or mycotic infections.

*Trauma*- (with or without injury to thoracic cage) usually presents as hydropneumothorax or haemothorax.

*New growth* — Carcinoma of lung, or pleural malignancy e.g. mesothelioma of pleura : presents as large pleural effusion. May be haemorrhagic.

**Secondaries due** to malignancies elsewhere.

*Diseases of heart and kidneys* — causing anasarca (usually bilateral).

*Sub-diaphragmatic* affections e.g. liver abscess or subdiaphragmatic suppuration : pleurisy or pleural effusion.

*Pulmonary infarction* — pleurisy or haemorrhagic effusion; usually not large.

*Collagen disorders* — causing pleurisy or pleural effusion.

*Renal failure* — uraemia causes pleurisy and pleural effusion

## ACUTE FIBRINOUS PLEURISY

*(Syn : Dry pleurisy or pleuritis)*

### Introduction

It is an inflammation of pleural layers almost always due to one of the causes mentioned above. However, tuberculosis is the most common cause of pleurisy, especially in developing countries.

### Clinical features

Sudden onset of pain in the chest wall aggravated by coughing or deep breathing, with or without fever and chill usually heralds the episode. Pressure on chest wall may cause considerable discomfort. Diaphragmatic pleurisy causes pain referred to the tip of shoulder (via phrenic nerve supply) or upper abdomen via lower intercostal nerves.

**Classical signs are :**

(a) Diminished movement of affected side of chest

(b) Pleural friction rub.

### Treatment

(a) Rest in bed is essential along with analgesics, sedatives and codiene syrup to control cough. Specific therapy depends on underlying aetiology.

(b) Kaolin poultice may give relief.

(c) Strapping of chest wall is occasionally required if pain is severe in spite of the above measures.

## PLEURAL EFFUSION

### Introduction

Pleural effusion is a collection of fluid in the pleural cavity most commonly due to tubercular aetiology in our country, but other causes should also be excluded (Table 17.6). The tubercular focus may be either due to primary complex, or post-primary.

In children and adolescents a pleural effusion may be the only manifestation of primary tuberculosis, without any warning sign of chest pain or fever. Sometimes it follows primary tuberculosis, due to hypersensitive reaction of the pleura to the primary infection. In infants and children below three years pleural effusion as a manifestation of primary complex is rare, it is found usually after 3 years, and mostly in the age group of 10 to 12 years. Pleural effusion in this age group demands more attention as it may lead to secondary dissemination by blood-stream. Many patients of adult tuberculosis give past history of pleural effusion treated inadequately.

In elderly and heavy smokers possibility of new growth should be suspected, but still in developing countries tuberculosis may be the cause.

### Clinical features

It usually starts with pleuritic pain if the volume of fluid is small but with further collection of fluid, visceral and parietal pleura are separated and the pain subsides as pleuritic pain is caused by rubbing together of the two layers of pleura. The symptom depends largely on the amount of fluid collected resulting in collapse of the underlying lung, and the rate of accumulation of fluid. Large collection of fluid may occur insidiously over a course in the presence of other symptoms like ill-health, weight loss, night sweats or protracted pyrexia of the remittent type for a period of 2 to 3 weeks.

But in case of large collection or rapid collection of fluid, the presenting feature is dyspnoea on slight exertion or even at rest.

**Physical examination**

**Inspection**

Interspaces are fuller and expansion of chest-wall is sluggish on the affected side.

**Palpation**

Apex beat of heart and trachea are displaced to opposite side, if the effusion is large, V.F. and V.R. are both diminished. However, the mediastinal shift may not occur if the lung is atelectatic due to presence of underlying new growth. It may even shift to the side of effusion.

**Percussion**

Dull percussion note is quite impressive and it is called stony dullness.

**Auscultation**

Inaudible breath-sound, diminished vocal resonance (V.R.) and sometimes bronchial breathing are found above the level of fluid. Aegophony and whispering pectiroloquy may be heard.

**Radiological examination**

When accumulation of fluid is less than 300 c.c., it may not be detected even by X-ray film. The earliest radiological sign is obliteration of costo-phrenic angle and loss of sharp outline of posterior part of diaphragm in the lateral X-ray film. With accumulation of more fluid, a dense and uniform opacity is found in the lower and lateral part of hemi-thorax, tapering off above in the axilla, and medially. During resolution, the upper border may be slightly curved. Heart and trachea may be shifted by a large effusion. However, if there is collapse of a lobe, mediastinal shift is not well marked.

**Diagnosis**

Thoracentesis should be done in all cases to establish the aetiological diagnosis unless the fluid is too small. Chemical, bacteriological and microscopic examination of the fluid is necessary.

**Laboratory tests**

Routine tests consist of estimation of protein content, cytology search for AFB and culture of organism. Presence of blood suggests trauma, neoplasm or infarction.

Lymphocytosis favours tuberculous aetiology. Malignant cells may be searched for in suspicious cases. Special tests are often done, e.g., glucose and amylase estimation. Glucose is less than 40 mg in empyema, tuberculosis and rheumatoid arthritis.

Amylase is raised in pancreatitis. Triglycerides are raised in chylous effusions. Lactic dehydrogenase level is less than 200 I.U. in transudates.

In case of large collection of fluid with dyspnoea, at least a litre of fluid should be aspirated slowly to relieve symptoms. Fluid of tubercular pleural effusion, usually clots on standing, specific gravity more than 1015, protein content more than 3 g. per 100 c.c. of fluid, and cells are chiefly lymphocytes. At least 30 ml. of fluid should be collected in a sterile test tube for bacteriological and chemical tests and about 50 to 100 ml. in a citrated container to detect the presence of malignant cells.

Rapid aspiration of large quantities of fluid should not be done as it may cause pulmonary oedema on the opposite side. Purulent fluid should be surgically drained.

Repeated aspiration may be necessary if reaccumulation continues.

If frank blood is found in the pleural fluid, possibility of trauma, malignancy and pulmonary infarction is to be considered. It is only by diagnostic aspiration that presence of blood or chyle can be detected. Damage to thoracic duct results in chylo-thorax. It may occur due to blunt injury, intra-thoracic malignancy, filariasis or after thoracic surgery.

Chemical analysis confirms the presence of true chyle. Pseudochylous effusion may be due to cholesterol-rich fluid occurring in long standing effusion.

Chemical examination of fluid gives additional help, e.g. higher pleural fluid amylase than blood in pancreatic effusion, lower fluid glucose (less than 12 to 16 cm) in effusion of rheumatoid origin or higher lactic dehydrogenase (L.D.H.) in exudative effusion, if protein content is not decisive. It is to be kept in mind, however, that negative findings in X-ray, sputum, pleural fluid do not exclude the aetiology of pulmonary tuberculosis in young adults. To clinch the diagnosis pleural biopsy from the parietal pleura should be taken when there is presence of fluid to avoid injury to the lung. Abraham's or Cope's needle is generally used.

### Differential diagnosis

Pleural thickening, pneumonic consolidation, atelectasis should be carefully excluded. If collection of fluid is massive and very rapid after aspiration, one should remember malignancy, especially in persons over 40 years of age.

### Treatment

Treatment depends on aetiological diagnosis. If aetiology is uncertain pleural aspiration is necessary. If fluid is too small, pleural biopsy may also be considered.

### Tuberculous effusion

This should be treated as a case of pulmonary tuberculosis. Inadequate therapy may lead to pulmonary tuberculosis within five years or even later on.

Removal of available fluid by repeated aspirations (500 to 1000 ml per day) in two or three sitting prevents adhesions. However, careful use of corticosteroids for four to six weeks, along with A.T.T., often gives complete resolution. In developing countries especially in rural areas, this method of therapy is preferred by many as risk of empyema due to repeated aspiration can be avoided.

In malignant effusion repeated aspiration may be necessary as fluid reaccumulates quickly causing dyspnoea.

Radiotherapy of the hemithorax and cytotoxic drugs (discussed in a special chapter) should be used.

## EMPYEMA THORACIS

When the pleural effusion is purulent the diagnosis is empyema thoracis. The pus may be thin opalescent fluid or it may be so thick that it is difficult to draw it out with aspirating needle. Sometimes the empyema is loculated i.e. encysted empyema.

### Aetiology

Similar to the causes of pleural effusion. Rupture of sub-diaphragmatic abscess, amoebic liver abscess, bacterial pneumonias advanced bronchiectasis, penetrating injury of chest wall and tuberculosis are common causes.

### Pathology

Both parietal and visceral layers of the pleura are inflammed. The shaggy, rough surface is covered with purulent exudate and, if not properly and quickly treated, there is progressive fibrosis leading to collapsed lung which cannot expand at all.

The empyema may become communicated with bronchus leading to broncho-pleural fistula. Thus air enters into the pleural space containing pus and some pus is coughed out. The result is pyopneumothorax.

### Clinical features

The clinical features are similar to pleural effusion but the patient has high swinging temperature, sweating, rigor and toxaemia.

Physical signs are not different from pleural effusion. Small encysted effusion can be detected by radiology.

**Diagnosis**

1. High polymorph leucocytosis.
2. Thoracocentesis-aspiration of purulent fluid establishes the diagnosis.

**Treatment**

Acute cases will require supportive therapy, proper intensive antibiotic therapy and drainage of pleural space by intercostal tube connected to water seal collecting bottle, as done in cases of tension pneumothorax. The intercostal tube is introduced in the most dependent part.

Sensitivity test of organisms cultured from aspirated pus is the best guide to decide antibiotic therapy.. Till the report is at hand, high doses of penicillin, ampicillin or amoxycillin may be started parenterally. Watch carefully the amount of drainage and the consistency of the pus, as well as the general condition. If progress is not satisfactory within a week, surgical drainage must be considered, i.e. rib resection and drainage may be necessary. (Fig.17.18).

Chronic empyema is purely a surgical problem.

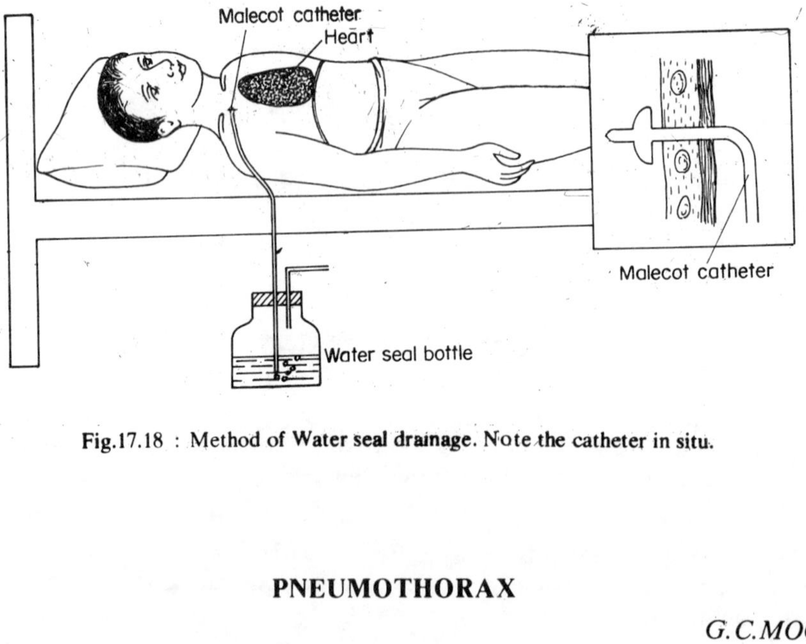


Fig.17.18 : Method of Water seal drainage. Note the catheter in situ.

## PNEUMOTHORAX

*G.C.MOOKERJEE*

**Definition**

Pneumothorax means accumulation of air in the pleural space.

**Aetiology**

Pneumothorax may be :

(i) Spontaneous
(ii) Traumatic
(iii) Artificial

*Spontaneous pneumothorax* develops when the air gets entry into space through the visceral pleura by rupture of the subpleural emphysematous bullae or tubercular focus or cysts of the lungs or lung abscess etc. It may also develop through the mediastinum, by rupture of the oesophagus due to its disease (sometimes pregnancy vomiting) or during its surgical instrumentation or operative procedure in this area. In such case it is usually bilateral pneumothorax.

**Traumatic pneumothorax** results following injury through the chest wall whereas deliberate introduction of air induces *artificial pneumothorax.* Causes of pneumothorax are enumerated in as follows.

**Causes of pneumothorax**

1. Emphysema usually associated with chronic bronchitis,bronchial asthma & bronchiectasis.
2. Tuberculous fibrosis and adhesions, especially subpleural focus.
3. Chronic non-tuberculous disorders, e.g., pneumoconiosis, interstitial fibrosis, congenital cystic disease of lungs.
4. Mechanical stress :

(a) Penetrating injury
(b) Rib fracture
(c) Thoracic surgery
(d) Instrumentation
(e) Mechanical ventilators
(f) Hyperbaric oxygen therapy
(g) High altitude or deep-sea diving

Artificial pneumothorax is rarely performed nowdays.

**Types :**

1) **Open** – when the air moves freely in and out of the pleural space during respiration.
2) **Closed** – when the air is locked in the pleural space.
3) **Valvular** – when the air enters during inspiration and is prevented from escaping during expiration (tension pneumothorax).

It tends to enlarge progressively causing eventually cardio-respiratory embarrassment, hence it is termed *tension pneumothorax.*

**Clinical features**

If the pneumothorax is large and rapidly developing, there is sudden pain with severe dyspnoea simulating acute myocardial infarction. The symptoms will depend upon rapidity of occurrence, amount of air and degree of mediastinal shift.

**Diagnostic Signs**

Immobile hemithorax with hyper-resonance and absent breath sound if collection of air is large.

The following signs should be looked for :

1. Diminished movement of affected side, even bulging of chest wall.
2. Displaced trachea and apex beat to opposite side.
3. Vocal fremitus – reduced or absent.
4. Hyper-resonance on percussion of chest causing obliteration or cardiac dullness in left-sided lesion or reduced hepatic dullness in right-sided pneumothorax.
5. Breath sounds diminished or absent and metallic or amphoric sounds may be heard.
6. In left-side pneumothorax, a crunching sound may be heard with each heart beat if there is air in the mediastinum (Homan's sign).
7. **Succussion splash** is heard if there is fluid in pleural space.

## TENSION PNEUMOTHORAX

Valvular opening allows air to enter during inspiration but is unable to escape during expiration, resulting in increasing pressure causing mediastinal shift, there will be increasing cyanosis with dyspnoea, gross mediastinal shift, even displacement of liver downwards (if right-sided) and positive coin test.

### Diagnosis

The sudden onset of dyspnoea with acute chest pain especially following some physical effort or a bout of cough is strongly suggestive. Presence of dyspnoea and characteristic physical signs clinch the diagnosis but it may have to be differentiated sometimes from acute myocardial infarction, massive pulmonary embolism or perforated peptic ulcer. Chest radiograph settles the diagnosis in most cases.

Skiagram of chest reveals radiotranslucent area not traversed by any bronchovascular markings with border of the collapsed lung and shifting of the apex of the heart and trachea to the opposite side. Features of the lung lesion may also be present.

### Treatment

(1) Symptomatic treatment includes oxygen inhalation, analgesics, e.g., combination of acetylsalicylic acid with phenacetin and codeine given in dosage of one tablet twice or Inj. pethidine hydrochloride 100 mg intramuscularly. Analgesics which depress respiratory centre are not recommended.

(2) Small pneumothorax occupying less than 30% of hemithorax and if there is no dyspnoea, does not require any active interference except rest and supportive treatment. If any underlying pathological lesion e.g. emphysema or tuberculosis is present, it requires attention.

(3) Pneumothorax with dyspnoea needs aspiration of air. Relief of pressure is urgent and is of great importance in case of tension-pneumothorax and it is done with a wide bore needle, connected to a long narrow rubber tubing, the free end of which is kept under water seal in a bottle at lower level than the chest. The needle is introduced through the second intercostal space in the mid-clavicular line.

(4) Tension pneumothorax is a medical emergency. A wide bore needle is introduced in the second inter-costal space, to relieve compression of great veins by releasing air pressure. **Then a water-seal drainage is used. (Fig.17.19).**

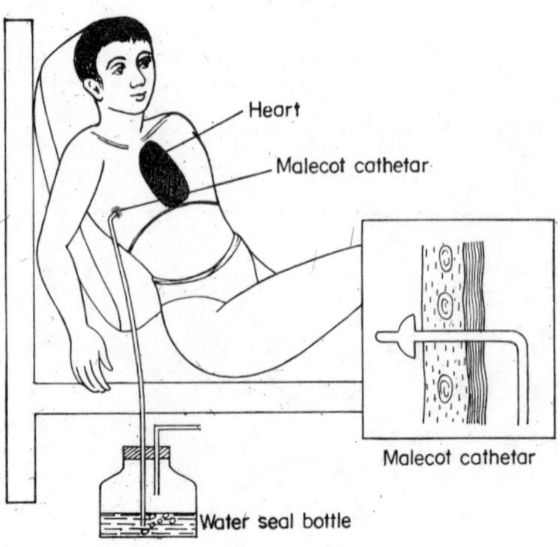


**Fig.17.19 : Water Seal Drainage.**

FIG 17.19 Showing **method of** water-seal drainage of pleural space containing air. The water seal prevents **air from** returning back into chest but allows exit of air due to raised intrapleural **pressure and** causes re-expansion of lungs.

(5) Recurrent pneumothorax is treated surgically by pleurectomy or some form of chemical pleurodesis to induce adhesions. Iodised talc, kaolin emulsion or camphor in olive oil have been used. Risk of carcinogenic effect cannot be ruled out.

Haemopneumothorax requires surgical drainage to prevent fibrosis and calcification Large emphysematous bullae may also require attention of thoracic surgeon.

## BRONCHOGENIC CARCINOMA

(Syn : Carcinoma of the Lung; Bronchial Carcinoma; Bronchial Malignancy *

*G.C. MOOKERJEE*

### Definition

Bronchogenic carcinoma originates from the epithelial lining of the bronchial tree. Therefore, some of them arise from larger branches and are situated nearer the hilum, while others arise from smaller bronchioles and are peripherally situated.

### Aetiology

The incidence of carcinoma has been steadily rising in all countries. However, in India it is not as common as in the western world. Possibly lack of facilities of investigations in rural areas is one of the factors responsible for lower incidence. In rural practice where even radiological investigations are not easily available to the poverty-stricken people, many such cases are possibly diagnosed as tuberculosis. However, data available from Indian Cancer Hospitals suggest that mortality from lung cancer may be around one-fourth of all deaths from carcinoma.

Among the aetiological factors the most important cause is considered to be cigarette smoking. In heavy smokers, bronchial carcinoma is about 10 times more common than among non-smokers. People who smoke more than 30 to 40 cigarettes a day are at a much greater risk of dying due to bronchial carcinoma after 50 to 60 years of age.

As men smoke more cigarettes than women, women are at a lesser risk. In western countries the increase of smoking habits among women makes them more susceptible.

Filter-tipped cigarettes are possibly less harmful and smoking through "Hucca" as practised in India, Bangladesh and Pakistan is also probably less harmful.

In Iceland, smoking was practically unknown before World War II but with the increasing smoking habits among them, it will be interesting to note its incidence in future.

Other important aetiological factors are pollution of air due to industrial fumes and smoke as well as occupational exposure to asbestos, arsenic, bichromates, haematites, nickel, silica and uranium etc.

* Table 17.20 shows the list of occupations which are at special risk of developing malignancy of respiratory organs :

* Occupation and malignancy of larynx, trachea and bronchogenic carcinoma

- Construction workers.
- Food, drink and tobacco workers.
- Glass and ceramic makers.
- Warehousemen, storekeepers, packers,
- bottlers.
- Electrical and electronic workers.
- Furnaces, forge and foundry rolling mill workers.
- Painters and decorators.

* Table 17.20 occupational risks of respiratory malignancy (Adopted from the Registrar General's Occupational Mortality Tables, publication of H.M.S.O., London, (1971).

Incidence of carcinoma is not more in coal-workers, rather presence of anthracosilicosis may retard the local spread of new growth due to massive coaldust-induced fibrosis.

In air pollution the carcinogen appears to be hydro-carbons, particularly 3 : 4 benz-pyrines which is a hydro-carbon. Repeated or too much exposure to ionising radiation are also carcinogenic.

**Pathology**

Bronchogenic carcinoma arises from the epithelial lining covering bronchus, bronchioles, mucus glands of the airways and possibly also alveolar epithelium.

Three types are recognised :

(i) Squamous celled carcinoma
(ii) Adeno-carcinoma
(iii) Undifferentiated carcinoma

W.H.O. has classified bronchogenic carcinoma into the following types

1) Epidermoid carcinoma
2) Small celled carcinoma
(includes polygonal, fusiform, lymphocytic type etc.)
3) Adenocarcinoma (includes acinar, papillary and bronchiolo-alveolar).
4) Large-cell carcinoma (includes solid tumours with or without mucin giant cell and clear-cell tumours).
5) Combined epidermoid and adenocarcinomas.

**Squamous Celled Carcinoma**

They form about 50% of the bronchial carcinomas which histologically show typical cell-nests, epithelial pearls, fibrous stroma as well as keratinization. The cells are flattened squamous type which can be easily recognised. This type of carcinoma is more often associated with cigarette smoking, these have a tendency to break down and may present as lung abscess.

**Adeno-carcinoma**

Incidence less than 10% of lung carcinomas and are more peripherally situated. They have tendency to early metastasis. They appear tubular or glandular in type under microscope and may contain mucin. A small percentage of cases are alveolar-cell or bronchiolar carcinoma. These may be related to chronic lung diseases particularly fibrosing alveolitis.

**Oat-celled carcinoma**

(Anaplastic Carcinomas)

The remaining 40% are undifferentiated or oat-celled type which contain typically pleomorphic cells. Supporting stroma is very little while deeply stained large nucleated cells fill up this space. This variety may ocur anywhere in the lung and is most malignant.

The malignant cells may spread locally as well as via lymphatics and blood stream. The metastasis may occur in the brain, liver, kidneys, adrenals, bones, skin or any other organ. About 25% of all brain tumours are metastasis from pulmonary carcinomas. Hence possibility of cerebral metastasis should be remembered when lung carcinoma is present.

Metastasis via lymphatics may travel along peri-bronchial and peri-venous lymphatics draining into hilar and paraaortic glands. When lymphatics are heavily crowded by malignant traffic, it is radiologically seen as streaky shadows in both lungs described as lymphangitis carcinomatosis.

**Clinical picture**

Symptoms and signs will depend at the stage when the patient comes to the doctor. Early diagnosis is only possible if periodic health check-up is made, as in Defence Services or in industrial executives.

In early cases there are NO SIGNS at all. Rather when signs are detected the lesion is too advanced.

Roughly I feel patients usually delay their diagnosis by about two or three months, as they may be treating themselves with cough mixtures and home remedies for some time. It is also probable that doctors may dealy the diagnosis by not ordering a routine chest X-ray. The "sine qua non" of early diagnosis is to order an X-ray chest as early as possible, although small lesions of less than 5 millimetres will not be picked up even by routine chest radiography.

The presenting features usually consist of the following :

(1) Progressive loss of weight and anorexia.

(2) Undue fatigue and/or breathlessness on accustomed exertion.

(3) Persistent cough not relieved by treatment. In smokers there may be change in the nature cough and expectoration.

(4) Haemoptysis especially in elderly people.

(5) Unexplained low-grade fever, with or without purulent sputum.

(6) Chest pain which is persistent; unexplained vague pain in shoulder joints or pulmonary osteoarthropathy.

(7) Aches and pains in muscles and joints in the elderly smokers-brachial neuralgia.

(8) Hoarseness of voice (recurrent laryngeal nerve palsy).

(9) Difficulty of swallowing.

(10) Epileptic fits, hemiparesis or features of cerebellar degeneration.

(11) Hepatomegaly.

(12) Skin nodules.

(13) Endocrine changes *(vide infra)*

### Physical signs

Signs also depend on the stage of the disease as well as complications due to spread of the growth and metastatic effects. The following presentations are usually met with :

**In early stage :** No detectable physical signs, as the growth usually in the bronchial tube is too small to produce any local effects. If the growth enlarges into the bronchial tube there may be signs of collapse and pneumonitis. Pneumonitis may be partially cured by antibiotics and radiological signs of unresolved pneumonia may be evident.

### Pancoast tumour

It is also known as superior pulmonary sulcus tumor. The syndrome is due to bronchogenic carcinoma in the upper lobe infiltrating local soft tissues, bones and lower brachial plexus. Presenting features are severe pain shoulder and arm (ulnar nerve distribution) wasting of muscles, destruction of the first rib and Horner's syndrome.

Pleural effusion is often a presenting feature which, however, means that the lesion is quite advanced.

Pressure effects due to enlarged glands in the mediastinum will cause obstruction to superior vena cava and compression of left bronchus, recurrent laryngeal nerve or oesophagus. Respiratory stridor difficulty of breathing, oedema and cyanosis of face with engorged neck veins are the clinical features. This is however very advanced stage (inoperable)

Bronchogenic carcinoma produces signs and symptoms due to

**1) Pulmonary involvement :**

Collapse of a lobe or the whole lung
Consolidation due to pneumonitis of the partially obstructed lobe
Pleural effusion
Mediastinal pressure effects (mediastinal syndrome)

**2) Local spread :**

a) Pressure on nerves : e.g. left recurrent laryngeal nerve (hoarseness)
Cervical sympathetic (Horner's syndrome)
Phrenic nerve-paralysis of diaphragm (unilateral)
Brachial plexus-shoulder pain and muscular wasting due to pressure on $C_8$ $D_1$ roots (brachial plexus).
Intercostal nerves-local pain.

b) **Pressure on local intrathoracic structures :**

| | | |
|---|---|---|
| Oesophagus | : | Dysphagia |
| Ribs | : | Erosion causing severe bone pain |
| Heart | : | Pericarditis or pericardial effusion, rarely arrhythmias. |

**3) Metastasis :**

It can be anywhere in the body but about 25% of intracranial S.O.L are due to bronchogenic carcinoma.

Metastasis may be blood-borne or lymphatic-borne.

Intracranial metastasis may cause headache, convulsions, hemiparesis, dysphasia, cerebellar degeneration etc.

Metastasis may occur in bones, liver, kidneys, skin and opposite lungs.

**4) Non-metastatic manifestations : (toxic, hormonal)**

- Pulmonary osteoarthropathy and finger clubbing
- Peripheral neuropathy
- Cerebellar degeneration
- Dermatomyositis and polymyositis
- Myasthenic syndrome (Eaton-Lambert syndrome)
- Endocrine syndromes
  - Cushing's syndrome
  - Hyper-calcaemia
  - Hyponatraemia (dilutional)
  - Hyper secretion of hormones from malignant cells : Excess ACTH, ADH, oestrogens and parathormones.

## Diagnosis

Early diagnosis is possible if timely investigations are made in suspicious cases. Not only routine skiagram is necessary but early bronchoscopy should not be avoided. When physical signs are present, the growth is usually inoperable. Mass miniature radiography detects some early cases, provided these are carefully interpreted. Common mistake is to attribute pulmonary opacities to tuberculosis and treat this by anti-tuberculous drugs till the growth becomes inoperable (Fig.17).

In some cases both tuberculosis and carcinoma both may co-exist. In some others unfortunately the primary growth may be missed and diagnosis is made due to metastasis.

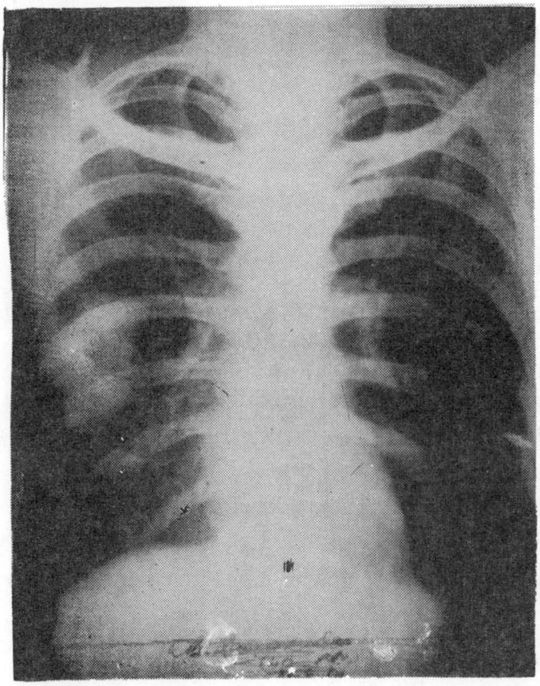

Fig.17.20(a) : Carcinoma lung : Initially treated as Tuberculosis. When patient presented with a coin shadow one year ago.

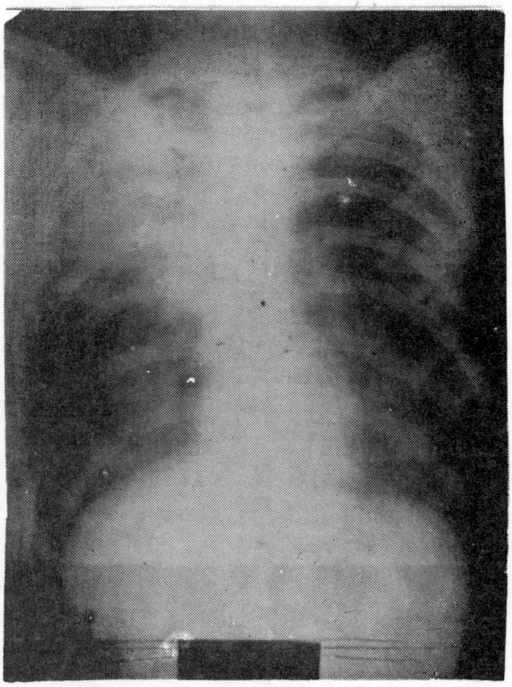

Fig.17.20(b) : Pancoast tumor : Initially mistaken as tuberculosis when typical findings were lacking 9 months ago.

It is stressed again that the important point in diagnosis is strong clinical suspicion and early radiological examination of patients at risk, especially the middle-aged people who are particularly exposed to industrial pollution or cigarette smoking. Important tests are discussed in detail as follows :

**Radiography of Chest**

X-ray should be taken in full inspiration and after expiration which may reveal evidence of air-trapping. The following radiological features are usually encountered :

i) An area of segmental atelectasis.
ii) A round shadow (coin lesion) seen in postero-anterior chest X-ray is highly suspicious.
iii) Evidence of unexplained shadows in chest X-ray also requires thorough investigation.
iv) Unresolved pneumonia or chronic lung abscess may conceal the new growth. Large pleural effusions are also suspicious although it is commonly due to tuberculosis.
v) Pleural effusion, unless very small, should always be aspirated so that the aspirated fluid can be investigated to establish the aetiology.

Sometimes progressive development of atelectasis in serial pictures may be mistaken for resolution of opacity. Apical lesion may be mistaken for tuberculosis, while it may be the 'Pancoast' tumour. Round-shadows or coin-shadows require thorough scrutiny.

**Biopsy**

Pleural biopsy may also be helpful. When the radiological shadow is peripheral, lung biopsy should be considered when bronchoscopy is non-contributory. A barium meal oesophageal radiography may declare that secondary deposits have occurred in the mediastinum, so it is inoperable. Thoracoscopy is useful in the same way.

**Cytology of Sputum**

Mass sputum cytology is not a practical solution but whenever a smoker or a patient of chronic bronchitis or bronchiectasis has exacerbation of respiratory symptoms or haemoptysis, he should be reinvestigated for sputum cytology.

"Sputum cytology is a valuable investigation in skilled hands". In one series of 2545 patients, 48% was positive by sputum cytology and only 32% by bronchoscopy (Crofton & Douglas).

**Bronchoscopy**

This is today one of the most valuable instruments for diagnosis of pulmonary neoplasms. The modern fiberoptic flexible instruments may reach up to segmental branches and bronchial nylon brush catheter can take samples of epithelial layer for cytology. It can also collect biospy material for histopathology. But the patient should be referred to the surgeon early enough for bronchoscopy. 75-80% tumours can be diagnosed by bronchoscopy.

**Mediastinoscopy**

This is a useful method practised in suspected cases of bronchogenic carcinoma not only as an aid to diagnosis but also to decide if thoracotomy is justified.

Thoracoscopic lung biopsy using diathermo-coagulating device is being tried by modern surgeons.

Investigations for diagnosis of bronchogenic carcinoma are summarised as follows :

**Investigations for Diagnosis**

1. Clinical background e.g., history of smoking, age and strong clinical suspicion.
2. Chest X-ray – Very important single test which may show :

   Hilar alterations areas of pulmonary shadowing, small coin shadow, lung abscess, unresolved pneumonia, peripheral mass, lymphangitis carcinomatosis or pleural effusion.
3. Tomography or zonography are additional radiological tests.
4. Cytology of sputum but negative result does not exclude.
5. Bronchoscopic examination and biopsy.
6. Pleural biopsy or thoracoscopic lung biopsy.
7. Examination of pleural fluid.
8. Radioisotopic scanning of lung,
9. Ultrasonography – especially where fluid is present.
10. Pulmonary angiography especially vascular tumours.
11. C-T Scan (computerised axial tomography).

Radioisotopic or radionuclide studies are not routinely required but are valuable in the diagnosis, detection of metastasis as well as pre-treatment assessment of the case., Ventilation scanning with isotopes Kr determines effective and expected lung function after surgery. Various other materials e.g. 67 Ga or 99 Tcm labelled albumin are used depending on the case.

**Prognosis**

Unless early diagnosis is made surgical treatment cannot be of real benefit. When metastasis is present the prognosis is poor. In advanced cases only palliative chemotherapy or radiotherapy can be done to relieve suffering. Radical surgery i.e., lobectomy or pneumonectomy followed by radiotherapy or chemotherapy is the only hope of success in selected cases.

In anaplastic carcinoma, radiotherapy is very effective.

**Management**

The most important point is to decide, whether radical surgery i.e. lobectomy or pneumonectomy is possible. During operation surgeons may have to resect some mediastinal glands which appear involved. Pre-treatment evaluation of the patient (performance status) and stage of disease are both important.

If too much local spread is noted, possibly it is better to abandon the operation and consider radio-therapy and/or chemotherapy. When the chance of success is very little, it is no use going for a mutilating operation making the end stage a miserable existence.

In most published series, five year survival is rarely more than 30% in operated cases. If all cases are analysed (operable or non-operable) the overall 5 years' survival is not above 10%.

Before surgery is considered, patient's fitness for surgery should be carefully assessed. Advanced age, poor nutrition, severe anaemia, distant metastasis, poor lung function, presence of pleural effusion, pancoast tumour, pre-existing emphysema, poor cardio-vascular reserve, hypertension and I.H.D., poor liver function (alcoholic liver) and poor renal function, are definite contra-indications to surgery.

*Radiotherapy*

If surgery is not possible, radiotherapy helps in relieving distressing symptoms, e.g., intractable cough and chest pain. The compression effect of expanding new growth superior vena cava obstruction also may be relieved, pressure on a large bronchus or oesophagus can be reduced. Modern super-voltage or mega voltage radiation has reduced local tissue reactions in skin and adjoining organs. Modern mega voltage machines can deliver larger dose in a minute or two, which would require 15 to 20 minutes' exposure with older deep X-ray therapy machines.

However, radiotherapy cannot replace surgery but sometime it may be useful after radical operation in some cases. Hazards of radiation, e.g., damage to skin and oesophagus, airway obstruction, local oedema, systemic reactions, fever, nausea, vomiting etc. should be carefully watched for. Sometimes combined chemotherapy and radiotherapy helps to minimise these reactions. Prednisolone cover is also helpful to relieve unpleasant symptoms. Chemotherapy has also some important role to promote palliation with or without radiotherapy. In pleural effusion, radiotherapy is contraindicated, where chemotherapy can be used. A separate chapter on chemotherapy for malignant disease has been included in this book.

**Prevention**

It should be noted that :

(1) "Bronchial carcinoma is largely a preventable disease" (Davies DF (1966) — J. Chronic Disease 19, 819 as quoted by Crofton & Douglas : Respiratory Disease 2nd Ed, Blackwell Sci. pub. 1975).

(2) On the basis of studies in doctors, Doll Hill (Brit. Med. Jour. (1964) 1,1399, 1460) calculated that 90% of the cases could be prevented, if tobacco smoking were abolished.

(3) Atmospheric pollution and exposure to industrial and occupational hazard areas are also at risk.

## BRONCHIAL ADENOMA

*G. C. MOOKERJEE*

**Definition**

Bronchial adenoma is a benign tumour arising from the glands of bronchial mucosa but they may sometime become malignant.

**Pathology**

The tumour occurs in two forms e.g. carcinoid type about 90%; cylindroid type and mixed types about 10% of cells looking like argentiffinoma.

In cylindroid type the cells are arranged in glandular form cylindrically.

The importance of histological diagnosis lies in the fact that though these are benign tumours, they may become malignant, a point which is very important in choice of treatment. The tumour is more common in females and 50% of the cases may occur in child-bearing age.

**Clinical features**

Sudden unexpected haemoptysis is often the presenting symptom. As it has bronchial as well as pulmonary component it may sometimes cause bronchial obstruction and infection distal to the obstructed bronchus. In such a situation the patients may present with typical signs of pneumonitis.

Pneumonitis may clear up as a result of antibiotic therapy but the tumour remains and may grow slowly producing episodes of haemoptysis.

**Diagnosis**

Although radiological opacity may be present when there is pneumonitis with collapse of a segment of lobe of the lung, diagnosis can only be confirmed by bronchoscopy.

Rarely the tumour produces carcinoid substances in which case large quantities of 5-hydroxyindole acetic acid may be detected in the urine.

**Treatment**

The only correct treatment is surgical excision of affected lobe. If the operation is delayed the tumour may infiltrate locally and further surgery may become difficult and extensive resection may be required.

## PULMONARY METASTASIS

Secondary carcinomatosis of the lung may present as a primary lung disease while the actual primary growth may be in any of the following organs :

| | |
|---|---|
| Thyroid | Uterus |
| Breast | Ovary |
| G. I. tract | Testes |
| Kidney | Prostate. |

Malignant melanomas may also cause metastasis in the lungs

**Clinical features**

The chief presenting features may mimic bronchitis, pneumonia or tuberculosis when metastasis becomes extensive but in early state it can only be discovered by a chest radiograph. Sometimes primary growth may remain undiscovered, while the presenting feature may be due to pulmonary metastasis.

Initially secondary deposits are often symptomless and may be accidentally discovered by chest X-ray. Sudden haemoptysis may be the first symptom.

Pulmonary lymphatic carcinomatosis may also occur due to carcinoma of bronchus itself or due to lymphatic metastasis from breast, stomach and pancreas.

In these cases there is progressive dyspnoea and rapid deterioration.

**Diagnosis**

Though there is possibility of detecting malignant cells in the sputum yet radiography is the chief diagnostic method. The usual findings are of the following types :-

(a) Single or multiple round opacities.

(b) A large round shape-like a ping-pong ball (suggestive of hypernephroma).

(c) Miliary tuberculosis-like shadowing in both lungs.

(d) Carcinomatous lymphangitis which is extremely typical in appearance. The hilar region is enlarged with radiating and exaggerated lymphatic striations spreading out to the surface of the lung bilaterally.

It is a clinical rule that before attempting surgical removal of any extrapulmonary new growth, a chest X-ray must be taken. Lastly, needle biopsy of the lung may sometimes be helpful in establishing the histopathology of the tumour.

## PULMONARY NEOPLASTIC METASTASIS

(Metastatic tumours)

Primary malignant growth anywhere in the body can produce secondary metastasis in the lungs. The following malignancies may produce metastasis in the lungs :

| | |
|---|---|
| Thyroid | Breast |
| Stomach | Ovaries and Testis |
| Pancreas | Uterus |
| Kidneys | Oesteogenic sarcomas |
| | Malignant melanomas. |

Sometimes primary growth may be undiscovered while the presenting feature may be pulmonary metastasis.

Initially secondary deposits are often symptomless and may be accidentally discovered by chest X-ray. Sometimes these may be sudden haemoptysis.

Pulmonary lymphatic carcinomatosis may also occur due to carcinoma of bronchus itself or due to lymphatic metastasis from breast, stomach and pancreas.

In these cases there is progressive dyspnoea and rapid deterioration.

### Treatment

No surgical treatment is possible but palliative chemotherapy, radiotherapy and symptomatic treatment should be given depending on the chemical background.

## SARCOIDOSIS

(Boeck's Sarcoid)

*G.C. MOOKERJEE*
*D. BANERJEE*

### Introduction

The cause of sarcoidosis is still unknown. However, it is agreed internationally that sarcoidosis is a non-caseating granulomatous disease chiefly involving hilar, mediastinal as well as peripheral lymph glands, while almost any organ, e.g., lungs, liver, spleen, eyes, phalangeal bones, myocardium, skin and nervous system may be involved. The hilar glands and the lungs are most commonly affected.

Basnier (1889) called it 'Lupus Pernio' while Tenneson (1892) demonstrated its histopathology for the first time. The name 'Sarcoid' was introduced by Boeck (1899) due to its superficial resemblance with sarcomatous tissue. Schaumann (1914) described the systemic nature of the disease in his article on 'Surle lypus Pernio'.

During and after World War II, introduction of mass miniature radiography has revealed many cases around the world. Though rare, it occurs in all countries and many international conferences were held to discuss this interesting disease. Due to its protean presentation, patients may go to various specialists, depending on the initial symptomatology. Most commonly it is discovered in X-ray films by noting bilateral hilar lymphadenopathy. Keratoconjunctivitis, glaucoma or even Sjogren's syndrome may occur. Pulmonary heart disease or conduction disorders of heart may also be a presenting feature.

## Aetio-Pathology

Various aetiological agents are blamed, e.g., tubercle bacilli, atypical mycobacteria, Epstein Barr virus, pine pollen, beryllium, genetic factors etc. Immunologic deficiency of cell-mediated type (T-lymphocyte) is blamed but food B-lymphocyte immunity has also been observed. This alveolitis gradually progresses into non-caseating epitheloid granuloma which may end in fibrosis in course of time or may be resolved spontaneously.

The histopathological appearance resembles a tubercle which does not caseate; there is also no evidence to support the view that the disease is caused by any of the mycobacteria. Though pulmonary tuberculosis is very common in India, sarcoidosis is rare. The mediastinal and superficial lymph nodes, parotid glands, lungs, liver, spleen, skin, eyes and phalangeal bones may be involved. The characteristic histological findings are non-caseating epitheloid follicles, consisting of multinucleate giant cells, epitheloid cells and lymphoid cells. These may restore spontaneously, but in some cases they stimulate the production of fibrous tissue.

## Clinical Features

It occurs more commonly in women. In the USA it is commoner in black than in white people. It is not so common in Indians, Chinese and Negroes in Africa. Fifty per cent of patients have no symptoms and they are detected on routine radiography. Principal symptoms are cough with mucoid expectoration, fever, polyarthralgia and loss of weight. Dyspnoea is related to the extent of fibrosis. General examination may show evidence of erythema nodosum, iritis, superficial lymphadenopathy, hepatosplenomegaly and bilateral parotid swelling. The disease is seldom fatal except when it affects vital organs such as lungs, heart or central nervous system.

Some cases of sarcoidosis run an acute course but most cases are mild and usually self-limiting. Initially there is mild fever, erythema nodosum, polyarthritis and bilateral hilar enlargement.

Some cases run subacute course and in these cases the prognosis is usually very good.

Chronic form is more damaging as it insidiously damages the involved organs. Parotid swelling, eye involvement, cranial nerve palsy or peripheral neuropathy may occur. In lungs it leads to pulmonary fibrosis and ultimately respiratory failure. Cardiomyopathy leads to arrhythmias and cardiac failure. Neurological involvement may be progressive presenting with cranial nerve lesions, polyneuropathy and arachnoiditis. Eyes, joints, multiple lymph nodes are involved. Bone cysts may develop in phalanges of hand and feet. Skin lesions, e.g., lupus pernio (Chilblain-like purple patches) are often seen.

Skin lesions in sarcoidosis may occur in 50% of cases. In some cases symptoms are minimal in other organs.

There are varieties of lesions, e.g., papules, nodules, lupus pernio and erythema nodosum. Skin lesions should be differentiated from other granulomatous conditions, e.g., tuberculosis, leprosy, F.B. granuloma, leishmaniasis and rosacea. There is a tendency of skin lesions to erupt in old scar tissues.

*Pulmonary function* : Shows diminished FVC and $FEV_1$ and impaired diffusion in advanced cases due to progressive pulmonary fibrosis.

**Laboratory Diagnosis**

**Blood** — Normocytic anaemia of mild to moderate degree may be observed. Sometimes eosinophilia may be present, ESR is usually raised. Hypercalcaemia is noted in 25% of cases. If this is progressive, metastatic calcification, renal calculi and nephro-calcinosis may occur. In some reported cases latex fixation test (done in rheumatoid arthritis) is positive.

There is hypergamma globulinaemia with increase in serum immunoglobulins, (IGM, (IgM, IgG). Hypercalcaemia may be observed.

There is complete or partial anergy to skin tests. The tuberculin (Mantoux) skin test is usually negative. Sputum and gastric lavage should be carefully examined to exclude tuberculosis. T-lymphocyte sub-population is decreased.

Diagnosis is confirmed by demonstration of the sarcoid nodules in the lymph nodes or liver biopsy tissue in patients with clinical history of generalised systemic involvement. Whatever be the tissue examined, a non-caseating tuberculoid granuloma is not by itself sufficient for histological diagnosis of sarcoidosis and is described as "consistent with the diagnosis of sarcoidosis". Clinical features, radiological appearance and some laboratory findings are used as supporting evidences.

*Kveim Test* is carried out with crude suspension of ground-tissue containing sarcoid granuloma. The antigen obtained from human sarcoid tissue is injected subcutaneously and a biopsy is made from the local tissue-reaction occurring at the site of injection three to six weeks later. If typical sarcoid granuloma is seen the result is positive.

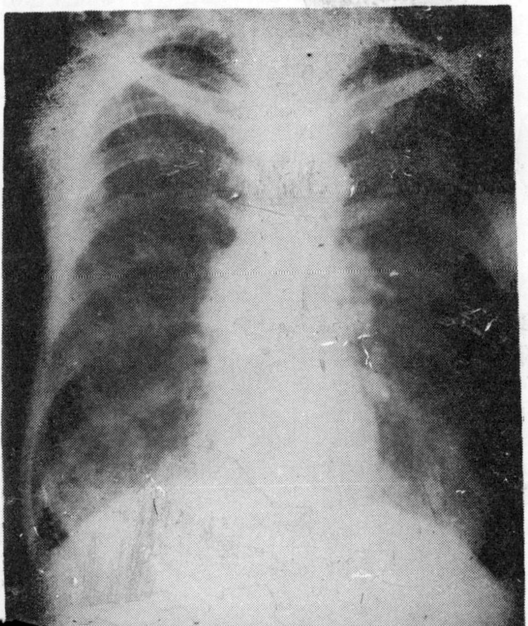

*Chest radiography* may show hilar adenopathy (Fig.17.21). Small nodular shadows may show hilar adenopathy. Fluffy confluent patches may be noted in both lung fields. In advanced cases fibrosis may be present. Small nodular shadows may appear in upper and mid-zones of both lungs. In progressive cases pulmonary fibrosis may occur. Honeycomb lung may result and sometimes eggshell calcifications of hilar glands are seen.

*Tomography* may be required to distinguish the nature of nodal enlargement from other possible causes, e.g. tuberculosis, lymphoma and malignancies. Nodular and micronodular shadows are to be differentiated from miliary tuberculosis, pulmonary eosinophilia, carcinomatosis, pneumoconiosis, fibrosing alveolitis, histoplasmosis and histiocytosis — X.

Increase in serum angiotensin-converting enzyme (SACE) may be a possible biochemical marker of the disease. This enzyme catalyses the conversion of angiotensin I to angiotensin II. High levels are found in active sarcoidosis. This test is particularly helpful in assessing response to treatment and in detecting relapse.

(Progress in Clinical Medicine — Vol.8, p.107, Churchill Livingstone. Chest-Vol 82, p.557, 1982).

More recently bronchial secretions obtained by bronchoscopic lavage have been immunologically investigated to study the role of T-lymphocytes and monocytes.

Gallium scanning ($Ga^{67}$) has been very useful too to study sarcoid tissue in the lungs as Ga tends to localise in the alveolar macrophages.

**Differential Diagnosis**

Sarcoidosis has to be differentiated chiefly from tuberculosis malignancy, mycosis and collagen disorders. However, it may mimic many disorders and syndromes, due to its tendency to involve multiple organs including skin, heart and central nervous system.

**Treatment**

Many cases resolve without treatment. But cases which run a progressive course will require corticosteroids. Some good reports of methotrexate, chlorambucil and chloroquine affecting its course are also available.

The chief difficulty to decide the indications of instituting corticosteroid therapy is that many cases run a benign course and may spontaneously resolve or burn out without any of these drugs.

However, anterior uveitis, hypercalcaemia, pulmonary and myocardial involvement are definite indications of steroid therapy. Skin involvement of the face may cause permanent disfigurement, hence early steroid therapy is necessary. It is also difficult to predict how long treatment should be given because response is variable. But in any case one to two years' treatment may be essential.

**Steroid-therapy**

Initial dose to start is about 40 mg daily for about four weeks and watch the result. If there is improvement reduce the dose gradually to about 20 mg daily and continue for four to six weeks closely watching its effect till the dose can be further reduced and finally discontinued.

If there is no improvement within first four weeks the drug can be gradually tailed off and discontinued.

Symptomatic treatment should be given depending on the [illegible] of the disease.

## MEDIASTINAL TUMOURS

*G.C. MOOKERJEE*

These tumours may originate in any intrathoracic organ as well as from the thoracic wall and spinal cord. Some of the lesions are not really new growths but are enlarged organs, e.g., aneurysm of aorta, oesophageal dilatations, hiatus hernia, eventration of diaphragm etc., which may simulate intrathoracic neoplasms. The mediastinal tumours may be classified as follows :

**Classification :**

1) Developmental tumours and cysts, e.g. dermoids, teratomas, bronchogenic and pleuro-pericardial cysts.
2) Connective tissue tumours, e.g. fibroma, lipoma and sarcoma.
3) Tumours of the lymph nodes, e.g. secondary carcinoma, usually from bronchus or breast; lymphomas including Hodgkin's disease and leukaemias.
4) Neural tumours, e.g. neurofibroma.
5) Thymic tumours, e.g. malignant thymoma.
6) Parasitic growth e.g. hydatid cyst.

**Benign Tumours**

Dermoids and teratomas are usually anteriorly located while neuro-fibromas occurs in the posterior mediastinum. Thymus and intrathoracic goitres are located in the superior mediastinum. Small benign tumours rarely produce any symptoms and are often accidentally discovered by routine chest radiograph.

Larger tumours produce pressure effects usually by compressing superior vena cava. They very rarely can compress trachea, bronchus or mediastinal structures, unless very large.

**Malignant Tumours**

These new growths, primary or metastatic, not only produce compression of intrathoracic structures but also invade the organs. They may produce varieties of symptoms, depending on the organs involved.

The common features are as follows

**(1) Obstruction of the superior vena cava :**

Presenting with cyanosis and oedema of head and neck, extending to upper limb. Anastomotic veins appear in the anterior chest wall with distended external jugular vein.

**(2) Compression of trachea :**

Brassy cough, stridor and dyspnoea.

**(3) Compression of bronchus :**

Atelectasis of a lobe or whole lung causing dyspnoea.

**(4) Compression of oesophagus :**

Dysphagia

**(5) Pressure on nerve trunks :**

(a) Left recurrent laryngeal :

Hoarseness due to paralysis of left vocal cord.

(b) Phrenic :

Diaphragmatic paralysis.

(c) Sympathetic trunk :

Horner's syndrome, i.e., constricted pupil, enophthalmos and ptosis of the affected side.

**(6) Extension into the pleura or pericardium :**

Pericarditis or pleurisy. May cause pleural effusion.

## Diagnosis

Besides clinical features due to compression or invasion of tissues and organs diagnosis is confirmed chiefly by radiology and tomography. Additional aids are ultrasonography radio-isotopic gamma camera scanning and CT-scan which may be required in some cases. Biopsy of suitable tissues and mediastinoscopy may be helpful.

## Treatment

Depends on the nature of the lesion. For instance, aneurysm of aorta may now be tackled by surgery using prosthesis, in suitable cases.

Leukaemias are treated medically. Lymphomas and Hodgkin's diseases are treated by radiotherapy and chemotherapy. Advanced presssure symptoms and dyspnoea can be temporarily managed by radiotherapy if the growth is radio sensitive. Benign tumours can be removed by surgery.

# MYCOTIC DISEASES
(Deep Mycosis)

*G.C. MOOKERJEE*

## Introduction

Mycotic diseases (mycosis) are rare but their importance in clinical medicine is very important. They not only cause systemic and local diseases but some of the fungi are sources of many antibiotics.

Fungi are present in the soil as well as found in the skin, dental crepts and gastrointestinal tract. They may invade skin, mucous membrane or deep tissues under special circumstances, e.g., gross malnutrition, severe infection, advanced malignancies and during prolonged antibiotic or steroid therapy.

Mycotic infection may affect the skin, mucosa as well as deep tissues. In India dermatomycosis is quite common. Among mucosal and deep mycosis, actinomycosis, moniliasis, aspergillosis, maduramycosis are not rare. Rhinosporidiosis, sporotrichosis, blastomycosis, histoplasmosis and cryptococcosis are very rare in India.

The most important character of fungi is dimorphism. Histoplasmosis, sporotrichosis and blastomycosis produce yeast-like forms in tissues while they assume mycelial form and produce asexual spores in Sabouraud's medium. However, cryptococcus neoforman does not change its character in tissue and culture media. Actinomycosis is actually a transitional organism between bacteria and fungi.

Actinomyces Israeli, an anaerobic Gram-positive organism which occurs in filaments and becomes segmented breaking into rod-like bacteria. At the same time they produce spores and vegetative branching mycelia only in tissues but not in artificial culture media. In the affected tissues these filaments form compact mass called sulphur granules. Therefore, these are nowadays considered as an intermediate form between true fungi and bacteria. Its response to treatment by anti-bacterial drugs and antibiotics also suggest its bacterial nature rather than fungal. Its name ray-fungus still remains, hence its inclusion in this chapter.

Hypersensitivity sometimes plays an important role in some fungal infections and sometimes marked local or even systemic reaction may occur after intradermal infection of extract of the fungus.

# ACTINOMYCOSIS

## (Syn : Ray Fungus Disease)

### Introduction

It is a chronic infection of deep tissues caused by Actinomycosis Israeli, causing suppurative inflammation with tendency to sinus formation. It is caused by Actinomycosis Israeli and anaerobic gram-positive branching filamentous organism, closely resembling bacteria than fungi. An aerobic type known as nocardia asteroides is however rarely known to affect man. Actinomycotic pus has minute visible granules, (also called sulphur granules) which under microscope appear multifilamentous, arranged in radial striations usually ending in club-shaped bodies. This is why it was named as 'Ray-fungus'. Actinomycosis and nocardiasis infections are not nowadays considered as true fungal infections but has been included here for convenience.

### Pathology

Human infection may occur in oral cavity in association with gingivitis or chronic tonsillitis. The lesions, though usually localised, may spread into contiguous tissues without being limited by anatomical barrier. They are characterised by multilple indurated abscesses and sinus tracks presenting as dermal, oral, cervico-facial, pulmonary and abdominal actinomycosis.

Actinomycotic granules in the pus measuring 12 mm in diameter are known as "sulphur granules". Microscopically these granules are composed of gram-positive staining hyphae.

### Cervico-Facial Actinomycosis

The oro-cervico-facial variety spreads from carious teeth or infected tonsillar crypts following trauma. The lesion may present as indurated swelling over the angle of the mandible, face or the neck. This breaks into single draining sinuses with pus containing "sulphur granules" Pain is minimal or absent and regional lymph nodes are not enlarged, a point in differential diagnosis. Bone involvement can be detected by X-ray.

### Thoracic Actinomycosis

Thoracic actinomycosis are of three types e.g. pleuropulmonary broncho pulmonary and mediastinal.

The onset is usually insidous. The patient complains of cough, mucoid, mucopurulent or blood stained expectoration, low grade pyrexia and gradual loss of weight. Clinical picture may be confused with tuberculosis, bronchiectasis, or malignancy.

Chest X-ray presents diffuse coarsely nodular shadows or dense circumscribed tumour-like opacities, consolidation, pleural thickening with or without osteitis of the ribs.

### Abdominal Actinomycosis

It may invade caecum, appendix or any other abdominal structure. An indefinite mass may be felt in ileocaecal region or elsewhere. Clinical diagnosis is difficult unless sinus formation has occurred and usually the diagnosis is confirmed during laparotomy.

### Diagnosis

In pulmonary mycosis sputum may show sulphur granules. The granules should be crushed and seen under the microscope. Associated cells are plasma-cells, lymphocytes and Russet's hyaline bodies.

Differential diagnosis is to be made from tuberculoma, chronic suppuration, osteomyelitis, gummatous lesions, and neoplasms. Anaerobic culture of organisms is done to differentiate Israeli from Nocardiasis.

### Treatment

Penicillin is the drug of choice though the organism is also sensitive to erythromycin, ampicillin and amoxycillin. Broad-spectrum antibiotics and streptomycin are useful in cases of penicillin allergy.

Ten to twenty mega units of penicillin may be required, which is given IM for four to six weeks.

Injection of streptomycin and/or sulpha group of drugs may be required especially to control associated gram-negative organisms. Some recent reports claim very good results with tetracyclines given in dosage of 500 mg six hourly for four to six weeks.

Empyema should be treated with antibiotics, aspiration, drainage and surgery. Sometimes thoracotomy and partial resection may be required. Plastic surgery may be needed in some cases.

## NOCARDIASIS

(Syn : Nocardia estroides and brasiliensis)

### Introduction

N. astroides and brasiliensis are filamentous soil bacteria which can cause deep mycosis. Abscess formation is usual but there is less sinus formation as in ray-fungus disease. Pulmonary nocardia involvement consists of patchy consolidation, cavity formation and pleural invasion. Ribs may be affected. Metastasis in brain, meninges and other viscera may occur.

### Clinical

Pulmonary lesion may be single or bilateral and multiple, so it may be mistaken for tuberculosis.

### Diagnosis

Pus or sputum should be examined by Gram's method as well as for acid-fastness. Aerobic culture may also be done.

### Treatment

Sulphadiazine used to be drug of choice, but recently trimethoprim-sulfamethoxazole combination two to eight tablets twice daily has been found useful. The drugs should be continued for weeks or months till complete remission has occurred. Surgical treatment in addition may be required as in case of actinomycosis.

## MYCETOMA

(Syn : Madura foot, Maduramycosis, Maduromycosis)

### Introduction

Mycetoma is a localised fungal lesion, usually on a foot or hand, less often elsewhere associated with history of local trauma.

It is characterised by swelling, induration, suppuration and sinus formation.

The fully developed mycetoma is a chronic suppurative, granulomatous lesion with multiple abscesses and sinus formation with fistulous tracts communicating with each other. Fungal cells may be seen microscopically in pus or within the macrophages or giant cells.

### Clinical picture

Commonest site of the lesion is the foot. Initial manifestation consists of a papule, small nodule which forms an indurated, area with a vesicle or an abscess which ruptures with sinus formation.

### Diagnosis

Diagnosis is confirmed by the demonstrating characteristic granules containing the fungi. Maduramycosis should be differentiated from diabetic foot, tuberculosis, elephantiasis or neoplasm. Culture of organism is Sabouraud's agar may confirm the clinical diagnosis.

### Treatment

Besides local treatment, e.g., dressings and antiseptics, electrocoagulation and amputation of the foot may be necessary, sometimes Amphotericin—B should be used. Trimethoprim-sulphamethoxazole or sulphonamides and sulphones are also recommended. Dapsone is given in dosage of 100 mg twice daily for several months.

A new antibiotic Hamycin (Hindusthan Antibiotics) has been found useful in dosage of 125 mg three times daily for 8-10 days. Two or three courses may be required but dramatic recovery has been claimed in India.

## CANDIDIASIS

(Syn : Thrush or Moniliasis)

### Introduction

The common variety causing human infection is C. Albicans. It is an acute or chronic fungal disease essentially involving superificial tissues of skin and mucous membranes. Very rarely systemic haematogenous dissemination has been reported. Candida albicans may be present in normal individuals in yeast-like form as a saprophyte, in the mouth, respiratory passages, gastro-intestinal tract, vagina and peri-anal skin. Malnutrition, diabetes, prolonged antibiotic or steroid therapy, leukaemias and malignant diseases promote candidiasis.

### Pathology

Systemic lesions may be acute and suppurative with multiple abscess formation or chronic with granuloma formation. Heart, lungs, kidneys, liver and central nervous system may be affected.

Fungus can be seen on a slide stained with haematoxylin and eosin or periodic-acid. Schiff staining. It can be also grown in Sabouraud's glucose media.

### Clinical features

Symptoms depend on the site of involvement. Various types are as follows :

### Candidiasis of mucous membrane (Thrush)

The classic lesion of thrush appears as multiple, sometimes confluent white or creamy patches of exudate mostly on buccal mucosa, tongue and gums. It may rarely occur on palate, fauces and tonsils spreading downwards.

### Candidiasis of skin

Skin lesions are usually formed in the contiguous folds and are reddish macerated and oozing. Onychia and paronychia may also occur.

### Disseminated Candidiasis

The superficial or endogenous lesion may disseminate by contiguous or haematogenous spread. Septicaemia is followed by shock, renal failure ending in coma and death but fortunately rare.

Pulmonary involvements simulating chronic bronchitis. asthma, bronchopneumonia, pleural effusion mav occur. Splenomegaly and peticheal rash may occur. Monilial endocarditis is now well-known and is indistinguishable from the bacterial variety. Infection may be introduced during cardiac catheterization or cardiac surgery. Since the valvular vegetations are thick and fragile, emboli formed are unusually large, blocking medium and large-sized arteries. Monilial meningitis may also occur.

### Treatment

For oral lesions, mouth washes with nystatin solution two to four ml (200,000 units/ml) four to six hourly is useful. For vulvo-vaginal infection suppository (100,000 units) is useful intravaginally two to three times in a day. One per cent gentian violet was used in the past but clotrimazole and miconazole are also being used recently.

For systemic candidiasis, amphotericin is used. Inj. amphotericin (Fungizone) usually available in 50 mg. vials as 5 mgm/ml Initial dose should be 5 mg dissolved in 250ml of 5% glucose solution and given as I.V. drip for 4 to 6 hours. If there is no reaction, the dose should be increased to 10 mg in 500 ml of 5% glucose to be given I.V. The dose is to be increased by 10 mg daily to a maximum of 50 mg per day. Subsequently 50 mg per day can be given on alternate days. Total dose should not exceed 2.0 gm. To ensure preservation of veins and avoid thrombophlebitis, heparin should be added (10-20 mg) in each bottle of glucose solution. Chlorpromazine 25 to 50 mg should be given orally half an hour before each infusion.

If CNS is affected, the intrathecal dose is 0.5-1.0 mgm daily. Hepato-renal damage is contra-indication to amphotericin therapy. Antihistaminics, salicylates and steroids are likely to reduce the side-effects of therapy. Steroids should not be used. Amphotericin—B has been used with flucytocin (Ancolon) given orally. It is claimed that dosage of amphotericin may be reduced if this combination is used.

A new antibiotic saramycetin is reported to be useful which is administered subcutaneously. Dose is saramycetin 4 to 7 ml/kg daily in four divided times for 4 to 6 weeks.

## ASPERGILLOSIS

### Introduction

Aspergillus fumigatus may affect patients with poor resistance as in case of moniliasis. It is usually a bronchopulmonary disease which affects lung tissue previously damaged by disease like pneumonia, bronchiectasis, tuberculosis, lung abscess, pulmonary infarction, pneumoconiosis or carcinoma. Proliferation of branching filaments may produce a mass called 'Aspergilloma'.

The alternative form of pulmonary aspergillosis is allergy due to the fungus, characterised by transient pulmonary infiltration and manifested with fever, wheezing and eosinophilia.

Disseminated aspergillosis is very rare. Haematogenous dissemination from pulmonary lesion causes metastatic abscess in brain, myocardium, kidney, skin and bone. Endocarditis with vegetations over valves due to the fungus may cause mural endocarditis.

### Clinical features

Three types of bronchopulmonary aspergillosis are encountered :

1. **Saprophytic type :** Minor infections hardly producing any symptoms. With extensive infection, fever, cough, purulent expectoration and haemoptysis may occur. Aspergilloma usually occurs within an existing cavity in the upper lobe of lung.
2. **Allergic type :** It presents with recurrent attacks of fever, wheezing and cough. Sputum is mucoid and tenacious. Skin hypersensitivity and eosinophilia are associated.
3. **Disseminated type or invasive form :** This form occurs as superinfection in patients who are suffering from Hodgkin's disease, carcinoma, leukaemias, having prolonged steroid or continued antibiotic therapy. This form presents as pneumonitis, mediastinitis, meningitis, endocarditis, myocardial and cerebral abscesses.

### Diagnosis

Presence of fungus alone does not establish the diagnosis. But clinical picture, X-ray finding and sometimes skin tests with aspergillus antigen may be of value.

### Treatment

Intravenous Amphotericin B-therapy is recommended. Average dose : 1.0 mgm/kg of body weight to be given for several weeks. Flucytocine (ancobon) may also be added as for moniliasis. In cases of recurrent haemoptysis or empyema surgical treatment may be needed.

In allergic type of aspergillosis, inhalation of aerosols containing nystatin, and systemic corticosteroids may be used. Concurrent cytotoxic drugs may be used if necessary. Recently an aerosol containing pimaricin in 2.5 per cent suspension has been used with benefit (Edward and La Touche).

## TORULOSIS

(Syn : Cryptococcosis, Busse-Bussehke's disease)

### Introduction

Torulosis is caused by cryptococcus neoformans which has special tendency to affect pulmonary tissues. Skin, viscera,central nervous system and bones may also be involved.

The main source of fungus is pigeon-manure but it is also found in soil, skin and G.I. tract of human beings. The pathological lesions in the lungs resemble tumour-like formations, so named as torulomas CNS and other organs are involved by dissemination from the pulmonary lesion. The yeast-like organisms grow freely to produce tumour-like masses but there is hardly any true inflammatory reaction.

In CNS it may behave like a tumour in the brain or produce meningo-encephalitis.

### Clinical features

Pulmonary symptoms are due to bronchitis, pneumonitis or pleurisy. Radiologically it may show localised or diffuse areas of infiltration. Lower lobes are usually affected but there is no hilar involvement. Multiple, coarse or miliary mottling and peribronchial infiltrations may occur.

Encapsulated tumour-like formations resemble pulmonary new-growths. Lung biopsy may be required to confirm the diagnosis of pulmonary cryptococcosis.

Symptoms of CNS involvement are severe headache, nausea, vomiting, vertigo, ocular manifestations. It may mimic tuberculous meningitis or intracranial SOL. Examination of C.S.F. reveals budding yeast-like cells during microscopy with a drop of Indian ink. The organisms can be cultured in Sabouraud's medium.

Torulosis may supervene in patients of Hodgkin's disease, carcinoma, leukaemia and diabetes mellitus.

### Treatment

Amphotericin-B (Fungizone) in slow I.V. drip is recommended as for other fungus infections. Combination with flucytocin (Ancobon) is more effective. Usually six weeks treatment may be required. Oral ketoconazole plus glucytosine are being recently tried in non-meningeal torulosis. In meningo-encephalitis or cerebral torulosis it should be given intrathecally or by intracisternal route in addition to intravenous administration. Intrathecal dose is 0.5 mgm on alternate days.

## HISTOPLASMOSIS

(Syn : Darling's disease)

### Introduction

Histoplasmosis caused by histoplasma capsulatum (a dimorphic fungus) which affects chiefly the reticulo-endothelial system. The clinical manifestations vary from a mild respiratory infection to a widespread disseminated disease causing fever, anaemia, pulmonary lesions, hepato-splenomegaly, ulcerations of the G.I. tract.

It is particularly endemic in certain areas of America, with low incidence in Great Britain, Africa and Asia. The fungus is present in soil, dust and animal excreta (especially bird droppings). It occurs in yeast-like forms in tissues as well as in filamentous form with spherical spores-chlamydospore). It assumes yeast-like form in tissues as well as in culture media at 37°C. Occasionally filamentous form is also found in pulmonary cavities.

Histoplasmosis may occur as a mild and benign pulmonary disease and may only be detected radiologically as multiple pulmonary calcifications after the active disease is over. Sometimes, however, reticulo-endothelial system is affected. Granulomatous lesions occur in the liver, spleen lymph nodes and bone marrow. Central necrosis of the granulomata may also occur simulating tuberculosis. Healed lesions also get calcified.

### Clinical features

All age groups are susceptible but it occurs mostly in extremes of age.

Three clinical types encountered :

(a) Acute type

(b) Disseminated type

(c) Chronic type (Cavity formation occurs).

It is often found in association with tuberculosis, Hodgkin's disease, diabetes mellitus and leukaemias.

Sometimes it is detected by routine chest radiography presenting calcifications in the lungs.

**Acute Form :** It generally runs a benign course. Patients may have mild respiratory illness, e.g. influenza, bronchitis or atypical pneumonia. Radiologically diffuse, or round opacities may be noted along with hilar lymphadenopathy. The lesions may be calcified later, hence mistaken and treated as tuberculosis.

**Chronic type :** It occurs usually in older adults. It is characterised by chest pain, low grade fever, cough, dyspnoea, haemoptysis, and loss of weight. Therefore it mimics tuberculosis.

**Disseminated type :** It is very rare. In this type there is haematogenous dissemination affecting reticulo-endothelial system. Clinically it is characterised by fever, loss of weight, splenomegaly and hepatomegaly, generalised lymphadenopathy, anaemia and leucopenia. Endocarditis, pericarditis, adrenal insufficiency and meningitis may occur.

### Diagnosis

In acute primary disease urine, sputum or bronchial aspirates and gastric lavage material should be examined. The stained smear of the infected material may show small, oval mostly intracellular yeast cells. In disseminated disease, bone marrow and lymph node biopsy may be of help. Culture in Sabouraud's media will grow mycelial forms. Culture in blood sugar will, however, demonstrate yeast forms thus proving dimorphic nature of the fungus.

### Treatment

In mild forms sulphonamides, e.g., sulphamezathine may be useful. But in acute progressive histoplasmosis, Amphotericin—B should be used in usual dosage for 4 to 6 weeks or longer.

## GEOTRICOSIS

Geotrichum candidum is usually secondary to other existing infection but it is so commonly found in respiratory or G.I. tract that mere isolation of the fungus does not establish a diagnosis.

Clinically it is characterised by tracheitis or acute or chronic bronchitis or pneumonitis. X-ray chest has no characteristic picture. Sputum examination may show organisms, which may be cultured by suitable method.

Potassium iodide, nystatin, sulphonamides, hamycin, or colistin have been recommended.

## SPOROTRICHOSIS

Sporotrichosis is a chronic mycosis caused by Sporotrichum Schenckii. The fungus is present in the soil and agricultural lands and therefore farmers and gardeners are often affected. Cutaneous sporotrichosis should be suspected if a skin lesion does not heal easily. Disseminated lesion may also be associated with skin lesions, hence the diagnosis of cutaneous sporotrichosis is a pointer to diagnosis. The skin lesion may form an indolent ulcer or a nodule following a foot injury. It does not heal easily and the lesion may last for months or even years. Generalized lesion is rare, but may occur due to spread via lymphatics or by haematogenous route :

Lungs, kidneys, breast, testicles, bones, joints and even central nervous system may be involved.

Diagnosis is confirmed by demonstration of the fungi or by histopathology.

**Treatment**

Potassium iodide in 1% solution is given orally in dosage of 1.0 ml. three times daily. Gradually the dose is increased by 0.5 ml daily to limit of maximum tolerance up to about 10 ml daily. To be continued 3 to 4 weeks. Patient should be watched for signs of iodide intoxication. Locally skin lesions should be treated with tincture of Iodine.

Amphotericin-B or Saramycetin may have to be used in difficult cases.

## COCCIDIOIDOMYCOSIS

**Introduction**

It is a mycosis caused by coccidioides immitis, which affects bronchi and lungs and sometimes widespread dissemination may occur in multiple organs. It has not been reported in India but chiefly seen in USA, Mexico and Argentina.

**Clinical features**

Fever, cough, pain chest with or without expectoration and occasional haemoptysis. Thin walled cavities with patchy infiltrations are seen radiologically. Pleural effusion with erythema nodosum may occur. ESR is also raised,hence may be mistaken with pulmonary tuberculosis.

**Diagnosis**

Positive skin test and demonstration of fungi from sputum, pleural fluid, biopsy material or CSF may be useful to settle the diagnosis.

**Treatment**

Amphotericin-B (Fungizone) is given I.V. up to total doses of 5 mg in usual manner as previously described. Therapy should be continued for 4 to 6 weeks. I.V. hydrocortisone may be used to combat severe toxic reactions. Flucytocin combination orally may be tried.

## RHINOSPORIDIOSIS

**Introduction**

Rhinosporidiosis is characterised by production of hyperplasia of mucous membranes and polypoid growths. Mycosis is common in India and Sri Lanka but sporadic cases are found all over the world. The disease may be acquired by bathing in infected water. Polypoid vascular growth containing endospores, red cells, inflammatory cells and giant cells is seen microscopically. Polypoid growth may occur in the nasal cavity, conjunctival, pharyngeal or bronchial mucous membranes. Nasal obstruction of especially bronchial obstruction may cause serious problems. These growths may be surgically removed.

# RESPIRATORY FAILURE

*G. C.MOOKERJEE*

*P. N.BISWAS*

**Definition**

Respiratory failure (RF) is defined as impairment of respiratory function resulting in inadequate oxygenation of blood with or without $CO_2$ retention. The diagnosis of RF can be confirmed by gas analysis of arterial blood. When partial pressure of arterial oxygen $PaO_2$ falls below 60 mm of Hg (8 K Pa) or partial pressure of $PaCO_2$ (7 KPa) is above 52 mm Hg. respiratory failure is said to be present.

Normally in young people arterial $PO_2$ is 95 mm of Hg (12.7 KPa) and arterial $PCO_2$ is not more than 45 mm Hg (6 KPa) and arterial pH is 7.39 — 7.42. In acidosis due to respiratory failure it will be 7.2 or less. In old people around 60 years and above, the arterial $PO_2$ tends to be below 82 mm Hg (11 KPa). In geriatric age group it may be as low as 72 mm Hg (9.7 KPa).

Abnormal blood gas level may however occur in other conditions without respiratory insufficiency, e.g. congenital heart disease (L to R shunt). It should also be noted that in early respiratory failure there may not be any dyspnoea at rest.

**Types of RF**

RF may be acute or chronic. The causes of RF are presented in Table-I. However, mechanism of development of RF may be broadly classified into two types.

In Type I-RF the $PaO_2$ is reduced (i.e. hypoxaemia is present) while $PaCO_2$ is normal or even low. Hypoxaemia occurs due to hypoventilated alveoli as ventilation is not adequate, hence blood following through alveoli remains inadequately oxygenated.

If hypoventilation continues in alveoli, $PCO_2$ may start rising (Type II-RF).

In high altitudes, alveolar ventilation is normal ,it gets exaggerated (dyspnoea) but oxygen tension of the air breathed is low. RF in these situations will improve with oxygen therapy.

Hypoxaemia due to shunting of blood (venous to arterial side) due to congenital heart disease or vascular anomaly will not be fully reversed by oxygen therapy. Similarly, anaemia or co-poisoning may also cause hypoxaemia. though ventilation and perfusion is normal.

**Physio-pathology**

It should be realised that usually there are three factors involved in respiratory failure :

1. Hypoxia
2. Hypercarbia
3. Acidosis

Hypoxia usually results from inadequate alveolar ventilation (air) and perfusion (blood flow) in the lungs. The amount of blood following through alveolar capillaries is not adequately oxygenated, due to hypoventilated alveoli. This occurs in :

1. Airway obstruction
2. Atelectasis
3. Fluid filled alveoli.

This process results in fall in arterial $PO_2$ but usually $CO_2$ level is not raised. Hypoxia is also aggravated if anaemia or CCF is present in addition.

Rise of $CO_2$ or hypercarbia results when $CO_2$ produced in tissues is not adequately eliminated, due to over-production of $CO_2$ in relation to alveolar ventilation capacity.

In respiratory failure, therefore, acid base balance is also impaired which can be diagnosed by pH studies.

**Causes**

Causes of respiratory failure are too many and can be classified into three broad groups :

**1) Pulmonary Causes**

Practically all severe lung diseases may be responsible e.g. :

| | |
|---|---|
| Chronic bronchitis | Pulmonary oedema |
| Emphysema | Pulmonary fibrosis |
| Atelectasis | Pulmonary thromboembolism |
| Pneumonias | Granulomas |

**Type II — RF**

This is also called ventilatory failure. In this state arterial $PCO_2$ is raised above 45 mm Hg (6 K pa) even in resting condition. When alveolar gas exchange is unable to cope with the $CO_2$ production in the tissues, $PCO_2$ gradually rises. Raised $PCO_2$ also causes some disturbances of function of respiratory centre and causes acidosis due to $CO_2$ retention.

**2. Thoracic cage defects :**

| | |
|---|---|
| Kypho-scoliosis | Thoracic surgery |
| Chest injury | Ankylosing spondylosis |

**3. Neuro-muscular disorders :**

| | |
|---|---|
| Strokes | Myasthenia Gravis |
| Head injuries | Botulism |
| Poliomyelitis | Tetanus |
| | Sedatives and narcotic drugs |
| Guillan-Barre syndrome | Anaesthetic agents |
| Muscle relaxants | Muscular dystrophies |

**Pathogenesis**

Depending upon blood gas alterations respiratory failure may have the following :

Biochemical characteristics :

| **Hypoxaemic** | **Hypoxaemic with hypercarbia** |
|---|---|
| $PaO_2$ — low | $PaO_2$ — low |
| $PaCO_2$ — normal or low | $PaCO_2$ — raised |

**Hypoxaemia : (Low $PaO_2$ with normal or low $PaCO_2$)**

The ventilation/perfusion disturbance is found in diseases affecting alveolar wall and interstitium e.g. :

**Hypoxaemia with hypercapnia (low $PaO_2$ and raised $PaCO_2$)**

When the ventilation is not adequate, alveolar carbon dioxide tension rises, and oxygen tension falls.

**Causes of alveolar hypoventilation :**

1. Condition associated with improper distribution of inspired air i.e. chronic bronchitis.
2. Condition where responsiveness of the respiratory centres to $CO_2$ is depressed.
3. Gross reduction of functioning tissue of the lung, e.g., emphysema, atelectasis, massive pleural effusion.
4. Muscular and neuro-muscular junction disorders : Myasthenia gravis and polyneuritis. Ventilatory capacity is assessed by measuring the FEV and FVC.

**Clinical features :**

**Hypoxaemic Symptoms**

| | |
|---|---|
| Fatigue | Dizziness |
| Central cyanosis | Visual failure |
| Muscular incoordination | Tachycardia |
| Mental confusion | Hypertension |

**Hypercapnic Symptoms**

| | |
|---|---|
| Warm extremities | Dilated retinal vessels or |
| Mental confusion | Papilloedema |
| Drowsiness to coma | Exaggerated reflexes |
| Bounding pulse & small pupils | Extensor plantar response |

**Acidotic Symptoms**

| | |
|---|---|
| Headache | Tremors |
| Dyspnoea | Muscular rigidity |
| Tachycardia | Polycythaemia |
| Mental confusion | Cardiac arrythmias, cardiac arrest |

**Management**

Acute ventilatory failure in a serious medical emergency needs careful treatment. A middle-aged or old patient suffering from chronic bronchitis and emphysema suddenly develops an infection. He may come to his doctor with mild manifestation of respiratory failure such as dyspnoea and cyanosis or in comatose condition i.e. in carbon dioxide narcosis. Increasing difficulty to cough out, shortness of breath and increasing cyanosis are usual presenting symptoms of impending respiratory failure.

The therapeutic approach to these cases is :

1. To clear the air passage of secretion and to prevent accumulation of mucous in airways.
2. To improve alveolar ventilation.
3. To increase the oxygen content of the inspired air.
4. Treatment of complications and associated causes of respiratory failure.

**Impending ventilatory failure**

At this stage the patient is conscious and co-operative. The patient may be cyanosed and capable of coughing. The process which precipitates respiratory failure has to be controlled at this stage. Arterial oxygen tension is usually less than 60 mm Hg. The following measures are necessary to increase and maintain alveolar ventilation.

**Supervised coughing**

The patient should be encouraged to cough and try to bring out sputum. Help of physiotherapist may be necessary. The patient should be under continuous care of a nurse or physiotherapist.

**Oxygen**

A careful controlled oxygen therapy must be given. Oxygen must be given continuously by ventimask, Edinburgh mask or nasal canula. Concentration of oxygen in the inspired air may be about 30%. If this causes drowsiness, concentration should be around 24%. If there is hypercapnia, ventilation is less responsive to carbon dioxide and in such situation ventilation depends more on hypoxic stimulus to respiratory centre. Correction of hypoxia therefore eliminates anoxic drive to adequate ventilation. Hence uncontrolled oxygen can be harmful.

The drugs which depress respiratory centre should be avoided. Narcotics and too much sedatives must be avoided.

**Moderately severe ventilatory failure**

The patient is drowsy and confused but may respond to question and stimuli. Cyanosis is marked, with shallow breathing, thick mucus secretion and ineffective cough.

Arterial $CO_2$ tension is usually above 60 mm of Hg. Urgent treatment is mandatory, which can be best done in respiratory care unit in collaboration with an anaesthetist.

1. Cleaning the airways by aspiration through bronchoscope or through a catheter passed inside trachea and bronchi or through laryngoscope. Improvement of ventilation and oxygenation restores the patients.
2. Controlled oxygen therapy : This may begin with 24% concentration or intermittently.
3. Respiratory stimulus like Inj. Nikethamide may be given in 2 ml doses hourly to 4-hourly.
4. I.V. aminophyllin one bolus dose to be followed up by continuous drip in 5% dextrose solution.
5. Corticosteroids are given where it is indicated, e.g. in severe bronchial asthma.
6. Respiratory infection should be energetically treated with appropriate antibiotics.
7. Dichlorphenomide is a carbonic anhydrase inhibitor which stimulates respiration. It is potentially dangerous but occasionally of value, hence should be used with proper judgement.

**Severe respiratory failure**

It is a serious medical emergency. The patient is semi-comatose or in comatose state, deeply cyanosed, incapable of coughing. He gets drowned in his own secretions.

Arterial $CO_2$ is above 80 mm of Hg. Hence mechanical, ventilatory and respiratory toilet in a respiratory care unit is essential to severe life.

## ADULT RESPIRATORY DISTRESS SYNDROME (ARDS)

*J.S. BHALLA*

The term 'Adult Respiratory Distress Syndrome' (ARDS) is used to describe a severe life-threatening respiratory failure, which appears in individuals with previously healthy lungs, after damage to the lung from diverse conditions. Since the clinical feature, the lung shadows in the radiographs and the pathological changes seen in the lungs of those who died was common to all, irrespective of the type of initial lung insult, that a comprehensive term was essential. The present title was introduced by Ashbaugh in 1967 because of morphological similarity to the neonatal respiratory distress syndrome and it has replaced other synonyms of the past i.e. "Shock Lung", "Pump Lung" etc.

This condition is being recognised more frequently and better understanding of the pathogenesis has led to early detection (based on high index of suspicion for the condition and its antecedent events) but drawback is that it leads to usage of the term without any reference to aetiological cause that may influence management.

The single important feature of the syndrome is pulmonary oedema without concomitant increase in left atrial pressure and there is increasing tendency to include in this all the causes of non-cardiogenic pulmonary oedema.

There is an ever-increasing number of disease entities or diverse aetiological causes (non-cardiogenic which are associated with ARDS) — more important ones can be listed as below :-

(i) Shock (Hypovolaemic).
(ii) Trauma with hypertension — thoracic or non-thoracic.
(iii) Infections — pulmonary infections, e.g., bacterial, viral, fungal and pneumocystis, and extra pulmonary (septicaemia).
(iv) Inhalation of gases, viz, chlorine, nitrous dioxide, smoke, ozone. oxygen in high concentration.
(v) Aspiration of gastric contents, water (e.g. in drowning).

(vi) Drugs (over-dosage) including heroin, morphine, Mathadone, aspirin, dextropropoxyphene (proxyvon etc.), nitrofurantoin.

(vii) Post-cardio-pulmonary bypass ("Pump Lung", "Post Perfusion Lung").

(viii) Embolism, e.g., fat embolism, amniotic embolism and embolisation from cellular aggregates.

(ix) Immunologic response to host antigens (Good Pasteur's syndrome, S.L.E.).

(x) Associated with systemic reactions to processes originated elsewhere, e.g. Gram negative septicaemia, haemorrhagic pancreatitis.

(xi) Neurogenic — cerebral oedema, intra-cranial haemorrhage.

(xii) Metabolic-diabetic coma, uraemia.

Incidence is apparently increasing because of more effective resuscitative measures having been made available for the critically ill. Estimated 1.5 lakh cases occur annually in USA. No definite estimate is available in India.

**Pathology and Pathophysiology**

A constant feature of ARDS on autopsy is increased fluid in the lung — it is pulmonary oedema in the absence of any increase in pulmonary capillary hydrostatic pressure, a distinguishing feature from cardiogenic pulmonary oedema.

Histopathologically two distinct phases can be described :-

(i) Acute exudative phase where in damage of capillary endothelium and alveolar Type I epithelial cells is accompanied by interstitial oedema. Platelet aggregates present in the capillary and clumps of leucocytes over the damaged endothelium. At a later stage oedema spreads to peribronchial and intra-alveolar region and focal haemorrhages may be there. Characteristic hyaline membrane (consisting of damaged Type I alveolar epithelial cells, fibrin and other plasma proteins), lines the alveoli and may extend into some respiratory bronchioles.

(ii) Chronic proliferative phase — In this the damaged Type I alveolar cells are replaced by cuboidal and granular Type II cells. There is regeneration of the capillary endothelium and alveolar epithelium, infiltration of interstitial space by lymphocytes and fibroblasts, thus resulting into thickening of the whole interstitium. The normally present surfactant (produced by Type II alveolar cells) is absent. Patchy alveolar collapse is present.

Initial injury to the alveolar capillary membrane leads to the leakage of fluids, cellular components of blood into interstitial space and at later stages into the alveoli. Alveolar collapse occurs secondary to the effect of alveolar fluid affecting surfactant activity. Later, even the production of surfactant is hampered due to injured granular Type II alveolar cells. This results in patchy alveolar collapse and non-homogenous regional dysfunction (ventilation-perfusion imbalance and physiological right-to-left shunt). Because of decreased compliance of lungs work of respiratory muscles increases markedly. Any condition resulting in increased capillary hydrostatic pressure, altered plasma oncotic pressure, lymph drainage and even capillary permeability would lead to what may be ARDS. In this, role of complement component, viz. C5a (elevated plasma level of which may predict the likelihood of onset of ARDS) and metabolism of arachidonic acid liberated from membrane phospholipids in the lung by activated platelets, mast cells and leucocytes, are being recognised. There are two separate, yet interlinked metabolic pathways involved in production of certain prostaglandins and leuketrines which lead to pulmonary capillary hypertension, broncho-constriction (through SRS—A) and increased pulmonary capillary permeability (through C5a).

**Clinical Features**

Development of ARDS varies in intensity and time of appearance since it follows varying direct or indirect lung insults.

Initially the individual may be free of respiratory symptoms of signs — this is the time when the individual is under treatment for infection and is being resuscitated from shock as the case may be. Radiograph of chest at this stage may be normal (if no primary respiratory disease or injury is there), pain of any type may produce hyperventilation and respiratory alkalosis.

For another two days also the individual has no obvious respiratory distress except tachypnoea (investigation may reveal alveolar and arterial oxygen tension difference and depressed $PO_2$ despite decreased $PCO_2$). It may be mentioned here that neonate respiratory distress syndrome shows increased $PCO_2$, instead and also metabolic acidosis is present due to marked muscular activity.

If condition is not recognised, it progresses further, there is worsening of hypoxaemia, alveolar and arterial oxygen tension difference widens. Clinically cyanosis appears and dyspnoea develops. Examination of chest reveals crepitations which keep on increasing to crackling rales. Patient is restless and disoriented, his renal functions are also suppressed. X-ray chest reveals classical widespread intra-alveolar and interstitial infiltrates. Finally, the individual slips into gross hypoxaemia, hypercapnoea, metabolic acidosis and becomes comatose. Death results from hypoxic myocardial failure or fatal arrhythmias.

**Management**

The hallmark of management of ARDS is early diagnosis and appropriate management of the existing conditions which lead to direct or indirect lung insult. There is no simple method of diagnosing pulmonary interstitial oedema and even lung radiograph may be normal in early stages. Closing volume is abnormal in early stages but it is not simple to assess that, routine lung functions being normal. It is, therefore, very important to have a high index of suspicion in cases suffering from conditions known to be associated with ARDS. Unexplained tachypnoea *must not* be ignored. Syndrome may be prevented in some cases by prompt treatment of shock, avoiding fluid-overload; preventing aspiration, use of oxygen inhalation where essential, antibiotics and corticosteroids in selected patients.

Sheet-anchor of treatment is proper ventilatory support for correction of tissue hypoxia. Principles of therapy are :

(i) Oxygen, initially through nasal catheter on suspicion and later on through ventilators (if diagnosed late). It is necessary to remember that by concentration oxygen can produce adverse effects on the lungs. It is also known that severity of oxygen toxicity is dependent on oxygen concentration and duration of flow. From oxygen-dissociation curve it is clear that concentrations of more than 50 to 60 per cent do not give much advantage by way of increase in tissue oxygenation. It is, therefore, safe to use 50 per cent oxygen in ventilatory support in order to give IPPV (Intermittent Positive Pressure Ventilation) through volume preset ventilator when patient is in coma. Positive End-Expiratory-Pressure (PEEP) is more desirable if hypoxaemia persists. Normally level of PEEP is kept below 20 cms of water (safer is 10 to 15 cms of water). Higher pressures are likely to jeopardise cardiac filling and pumping which is monitored through Swanganz catheter for assessment of pulmonary capillary wedge pressures. Continuous positive airway pressures are used if work of breathing is required to be decreased.

Recently high frequency positive pressure ventilation (HFPPV) with consequent decreased tidal volume has received attention and this forestalls the risk of barotrauma since low levels of PEEP and efficient alveolar gas distribution and blood gas exchange are achieved.

Extra-corporal membrane oxygenation (ECMO) in severe ARDS could prolong life, however long-term survival rate is not altered. Low frequency positive pressure ventilation (LFPPV) with extra-corporal $CO_2$ removal (ECCO2R) has helped in removal of $CO_2$ through veno-venous bypass using large surface area membrane lungs with low inflation pressure, low ventilatory rate and low intra-alveolar oxygen tension are useful as iatrogenic adverse effects of IPPV and PEEP. Its long-term evaluation in ARDS is awaited.

Attempts are made to reduce high oxygen requirement by heavy sedation (if not otherwise contraindicated). Hypothermia increases amount of oxygen in solution; however alteration in dissociation curve in hypothermia lessens the benefits thus expected.

Fluid therapy : Great care should be observed in early resuscitative measures as well as in acute phase of ARDS since volume overloading may aggravate pulmonary oedema. Monitoring pulmonary capillary wedge pressure (PCWP) through flow-directed balloon catheter, judicious use of diuresis, properly regulated flow of fluids. Infusion of colloid solutions such as purified protein fraction or 25% albumin is indicated. Other respective therapeutic indications of crystalloides or colloids remain unchanged.

Corticosteroids : Their use is controversial; however detection of predictors, viz. C5a in the plasma may warrant heavy dosage (30 mgm/kg methyl-prednisolone 6-hourly for first two days).

Antibiotics : Since majority of the cases of ARDS have infective focus as a triggering mechanism, use of appropriate antibiotics (regulated by antibiogramme on cultures of sputum or endoscopic aspirates in cases of respiratory infection) is necessary. Antibiotics may even be used prophylactically.

Nutrition : Patients suffer from nutritional depletion and if it continues, muscular weakness including respiratory muscles might appear. Therefore nutrition parenterally and through intragastric tube is essential.

**Prognosis :** Mortality rate remains very high (more than 50% cases, even in intensive care units). These patients may require many days' ventilatory support and other management as above, before they show any sign of recovery.

## PULMONARY MANIFESTATIONS OF SYSTEMATIC DISEASE

*G.C. MOOKERJEE*

Many systematic diseases may have dominant pulmonary manifestations and this may be mistaken for primary lung disease. These important disorders are enumerated for quick reference.

(I) **Infectious diseases :**

Many viral, bacterial, mycotic or parasitic pulmonary affections may present with pneumonitis, bronchopneumonia and pleurisy, e.g., typhus fever, Q-fever, anthrax, pneumonic plague, blastomycosis etc.

(II) **Collagen diseases :**

Polyarteritis nodosa may present with pneumonitis, eosinophilic asthma and pleural disease. SLE may have recurrent pleural effusions, pulmonary vasculitis and fibrosing alveolitis. Scleroderma may have progressive pulmonary fibrosis. Nonatopic asthma may occur in giant cell arteritis.

(III) **Rheumatoid arthritis :**

Pulmonary manifestations may sometimes occur before typical arthritis is established. Pulmonary manifestations are pleural effusions, pleuropericarditis and rheumatoid pneumonitis.

(IV) **Wegener's granuloma :**

It is a systemic and pulmonary disorder which may chiefly present as a respiratory disorder and sometimes mistaken for tuberculosis.

(V) **Leukaemias :**

Acute leukaemia may often present with sore throat and respiratory manifestations.

**Iatrogenic causes**

(i) **Bronchial asthma :**

Aspirin and many nonsteroidal analgesics, penicillin, antitetanus and antidiphtheric sera, may be responsible for bronchial asthma.

(ii) **Pulmonary fibrosis :**

It may occur due to cytotoxic drugs e.g., busulphan, bleomycin, gold therapy, nitrofurantoin, methysergide and practolol.

Radiotherapy may also cause pulmonary fibrosis due to too much radiation.

(iii) **Pulmonary eosinophilia :**

Sulphonamides, penicillins, and nitrofurantoins.

(iv) **SLE like syndrome :**

It may occur due to hydralazine, procainamide and phenytoin.

# CHAPTER – 18
# CARDIO-VASCULAR SYSTEM

## INTRODUCTION TO CARDIOLOGY

*G.C. MOOKERJEE*

Symptoms of heart disease may be dyspnoea (breathlessness), cough with or without haemoptysis, chest pain, palpitation, fainting, hepatic pain, oedema legs, undue fatigue or even sudden coma or convulsions. Though these symptoms are not diagnostic of heart disease yet these symptoms are important pointers to cardiac pathology. Therefore, heart disease should only be diagnosed with other supportive evidences.

### Dyspnoea

Dyspnoea is subjective discomfort of breathing. For the patient, it may be slightly uncomfortable if dyspnoea is mild, but distressing, if there is severe difficulty in breathing. In health, respiratory movements are not felt except during physical exertion. Sometimes during emotional stress, respiratory movements may become exaggerated or patient may sigh from time to time and even may feel choked due to emotional outburst.

Once the patient complains of dyspnoea it requires serious evaluation. Patient usually will say "Doctor, I get easily breathless nowadays", or "Suddenly I wake up at night and cannot get enough breath" or "My physical capacity is becoming worse due to shortness of breath." This is probably cardiac dyspnoea. But if the patient says to doctor suddenly "I get choked, cannot breathe properly and there is wheezing in the chest", it is probably bronchial asthma. This comes like a bolt from the blue even at rest.

Sudden onset of dyspnoea while lifting a heavy weight or during a bout of cough (especially in emphysematous patient) suggests pneumothorax.

Dyspnoea with high fever suggests acute respiratory infection. It is also important to remember that a chronic bronchitic may develop heart failure (cor pulmonale).

Therefore, when a patient complains of dyspnoea, it is essential to take a good history at first and mentally assess whether it is likely to be due to cardiac, respiratory, metabolic, endocrinal, psychogenic or mechanical cause.

Anaemia and cyanosis can be excluded by inspection. A pregnant lady, an obese person or a patient of non-cardiac ascitis (i.e. due to cirrhotic liver or tuberculous ascitis) may also be dyspnoeic. The pregnant lady, however, may become worse due to respiratory infection in advanced state of pregnancy, while one must be sure that she has no mitral valve lesion. Mediastinal tumours present typical clinical picture, which cannot be mistaken.

Cardio-respiratory dyspnoea is due to pulmonary congestion while dyspnoea of congenital heart disease is due to hypoxia (right to left shunt).

Dyspnoea occurring during accustomed exertion is often the first warning of heart disease. Dyspnoea may be clinically graded as follows (New York Heart Association) :

**Class I – (mild) :** Dyspnoea occurring on usual exertion, e.g. walking in level ground at normal pace.

**Class II – (moderate) :** Dyspnoea on moderate exertion e.g. running, scrubbing, climbing stairs etc.

**Class III – (severe) :** Dyspnoea on slight exertion e.g. attempt to walk or getting down from bed or getting up from chair and attending to personal routine activities e.g. shaving, defaecation etc.

**Class IV – (emergency) :** Dyspnoea even at rest. Occurrence of nocturnal dyspnoea should be considered as a danger signal. These patients require emergency medical attention.

**Special types of Dyspnoea :**

**Orthopnoea :** It is a type of dyspnoea, which is noted when the patient lies flat in bed. The patient is more comfortable, i.e. less dyspnoeic when he is elevated with pillows or a back rest.

**Paroxysmal Nocturnal Dyspnoea :**

This is another form of dyspnoea which occurs suddenly during sleep, due to severe pulmonary venous congestion and may lead to acute pulmonary oedema. It is strongly suggestive of L.V.F. due to disease of left side of heart. Patient feels suffocated and sits up panting for breath. The breathlessness is associated with cyanosis and wheezing in both lungs and pink frothy sputum may be brought out, if attack is not terminated by treatment. Sometimes change of posture from lying to sitting position may relieve the attack spontaneously in a few minutes. This type of attack usually occurs in patients of mitral stenosis or acute left ventricular failure (cardiac asthma). Pressure in pulmonary veins is raised above 40 mm Hg and osmotic pressure of plasma is exceeded causing leakage of fluid from pulmonary capillaries into alveoli. Rupture of capillaries produces pink expectoration.

Dyspnoea is an unpleasant respiratory symptom, but it may occur due to many causes other than heart disease.(Table 18.1) Cardiac dyspnoea is not specific for any cardiac lesion, but it may indicate some form of heart failure. Acute pulmonary oedema is usually due to advanced mitral valve disease, aortic valve disease, severe hypertension or I.H.D.

**Cheyne-stoke breathing or (Periodic breathing) :** May be noted in cases of cardiac failure. This is due to anoxia of respiratory centre in medulla. Mild form of apnoea alternating with hyperventilation may also occur in very old people during deep sleep.

Small children often appear breathless due to bilateral nose block or due to nasopharyngeal catarrh.

**Stridulous respiration :** Is due to pressure upon trachea or larynx or F.B. causing obstruction or laryngeal diphtheria. In-drawing of the lower chest wall and epigastrium is a typical finding.

**Table-18.1 : Causes of Dyspnoea**

| COMMON CAUSES | | RARE CAUSES |
|---|---|---|
| **Pulmonary :** | Acute Bronchitis<br>Pneumonias and Bronchopneumonias<br>Bronchial asthma<br>Chronic bronchitis and emphysema | **Pulmonary**<br>Occupational and industrial lung diseases<br>Pulmonary fibrosis<br>F.B. in a major bronchus.<br>Carcinoma |
| **Cardiac :** | Mitral and aortic Valvular heart disease<br>Hypertensive H.D. and Coronary heart disease causing heart failure | Sarcoidosis.<br>Hammon Rich syndrome<br>Pulmonary alveolar proteinosis<br>Pulmonary granulomatosis. |

*Table contd. to next page.*

*Table continued from previous page (Table — 18.1)*

| COMMON CAUSES | | RARE CAUSES |
|---|---|---|
| **Abdominal :** | Large ascitis<br>Severe obesity | |
| **Physiological :** | Advanced pregnancy specially hydramnios or twins.<br>Obesity | **Cardiac**<br>Congenital heart disease |
| **Psychogenic :** | Severe emotional and hyperventilation syndrome. | **Miscellaneous**<br>Renal failure<br>Metabolic acidosis (e.g. diabetic ketosis).<br>Neuromuscular weakness of thoracic cage. |

**Note :**

An infant may be dyspnoeic at birth due to congenital defects of the heart, acute respiratory disorder or diaphragmatic hernia. The last condition is easily repairable by surgery with total restoration to normality. The diagnosis can be made at bed-side by hearing tinkling intestinal sounds in the chest. X-ray chest will be confirmatory.

**Palpitation**

Palpitation is subjective awareness of heart beating. It is often a symptom of heart disease, but it may also occur due to physical exercise, emotional stress, fever, anoxia, thyrotoxicosis, shock and haemorrhage. It also can occur due to sympathomimetic drugs. In various types of heart disease, rapid action of the heart may occur sometimes regularly or even irregularly. Sinus tachycardia may be regular as in hyperdynamic circulation, CCF and all other conditions described above. Tachycardia may be due to atrial flutter, atrial fibrillation, ventricular tachycardia and ventricular flutter. However, in atrial fibrillation it is irregularly irregular. Sudden onset and abrupt end of regular but very rapid heart rate above 140 pm. suggests paroxysmal tachycardia.

Hence it is to be realised that analysis of symptoms in relation to history, mode of development of symptoms and physical signs present, along with appropriate investigations, will give clue to the underlying disease. Patient's attitude, subjective tolerance may confuse the issue, if not properly interpreted.

A young patient may complain of palpitation, difficulty of breathing (hyperventilation) and pain in chest without any heart disease and may be relieved by proper psychotherapy along with sedatives, tranquilisers and assurance, while an elderly man complaining of 'gas' in the stomach after a heavy dinner may develop severe heart attack before midnight.

Hence considerable care and judgement is essential in interpretation of symptomatology. (Refer to the chapter on Arrhythmias).

**Bradycardia**

Though bradycardia is not a symptom of heart disease, yet some patients detect it accidentally. It may due to viral infection, toxic carditis and heart block. It should, however, be noted that well-trained atheletes may have heart rate around 50 to 60 per minute.

**Chest pain**

Anterior wall chest pain may be due to ischaemic heart disease (IHD) causing inadequate coronary circulation; other causes of similar pain are enumerated in chapter on IHD. Additional investigations, i.e. resting as well as post-exercise ECG and radiological investigations may be required. True cardiac pain which is due to hypoxia of myocardium is felt in front of the chest like heavy load or pressure or sense of constriction or crushing. It may also be mild, annoying type of discomfort, often mistaken for 'gas' in stomach. Usually retrosternal in nature, it may be felt elsewhere in the precordium and may spread along one or both arms, neck, jaw, back of chest and abdomen.

It is aggravated by physical exercise, emotion or heavy meals and it is relieved by rest, relaxation or by chewing glyceryl trinitrate tablets. Cause of pain is myocardial oxygen lack, accumulation of metabolic products irritating myocardial nerve endings causing pain (Refer to the chapter on I.H.D.).

**Syncope**

Syncope is not a specific symptom of cardiovascular disease. Most commonly it is due to non-cardiac causes, e.g. vasovagal attack and inadequate venous return, causing reduced cardiac output. This may also occur due to prolonged standing (military parade), especially in hot humid climate; high intrathoracic pressure may also prevent adequate venous return, e.g. Valsalva manoeuvre, bouts of severe cough (cough syncope), too much straining to urinate (micturition syncope) especially on getting up from sleep. Lowering of cardiac output affects cerebral blood flow, which may be due to low cardiac output or vagal effect (slowing of heart) or heart block or cardiac arrest.

Syncope may also be due to power failure, i.e. failure of pace-maker of heart or defective conduction of cardiac impulse; cardiac syncope causing cessation of cerebral blood flow may occur in the following conditions :

(1) I.H.D. (acute myocardial infarction)
(2) Complete heart block
(3) Severe aortic stenosis, VSD or Fallot's tetralogy
(4) Carotid or vertebro-basilar insufficiency
(5) Severe tachycardia or bradyarrhythmias
(6) Left atrial thrombus (ball valve type) or myxoma.

**Squatting**

A typical posture assumed by children when breathless, specially noted in Fallot's tetralogy or other forms of cyanotic congenital heart disease. Though exact mechanism is not clear, possibly squatting improves oxygen saturation.

**Oedema**

Cardiac oedema is minimum in the morning, but first noticed as ankle oedema in the evening but if the patient is in the bed, oedema is noted in the sacral region. Renal oedema is worse in the morning but is initially noted in the face. Hormonal disorders as well as contraceptive pills may cause dependent oedema. Nutritional oedema is due to hypo-proteinaemia due to malnutrition. Oedema of hepatic cirrhosis is diagnosed with associated signs of liver cirrhosis.

Fluid may accumulate in the peritoneal cavity (ascitis) and in pericardial cavity (pericardial effusion) or as a part of generalised oedema (anasarca). Cardiac or renal oedema pits on pressure. Renal oedema initially affects the face in periorbital region and then spreads downwards in other parts of the body. Ankle swelling and hepatic pain should draw attention to congestive heart failure; the diagnostic points are :

(a) Engorged neck veins — due to raised J.V.P.
(b) Pulmonary congestion — basal crepitations
(c) Enlarged tender liver and rarely splenic enlargement

(d) Dependent oedema and weight gain (starting with ankle swelling and sacral oedema)

(e) In advanced cases, ascitis, pleural and pericardial effusion may occur.

The D.D. of pitting oedema in legs consists of :

(1) Congestive heart failure
(2) Hypoproteinaemia as in malnutrition
(3) Cirrhosis of liver
(4) Constrictive pericarditis
(5) Beri-beri (wet type)
(6) Obstruction of venous return from lower limbs (deep vein thrombosis)
(7) Collagen disorders
(8) Gross obesity
(9) Premenstrual tension.

If the oedema is non-pitting, often called solid oedema, it is due to obstruction of lymphatic vessels or severe obesity.

### Cough

Cough is often an early symptom of cardiac decompensation. Two types of cough are noted :

1. Dry cough, especially on exertion
2. Cough with expectoration and wheezing with or without haemoptysis.

In cardiac disease cough is due to raised pulmonary venous pressure. Cough associated with blood tinged or pink frothy sputum suggests L.V.F. causing pulmonary oedema.

### Haemoptysis

Haemoptysis may occur in mitral stenosis, L.V.F. or due to pulmonary emboli. Other causes are tuberculosis, pneumonias, lung abscess, bronchiectasis, trauma, pulmonary-instrumentation or blood disorders. Details are discussed in the chapter on respiratory diseases.

### Cardiac cachexia

In advanced chronic cardiac failure, wasting occurs, due to chronic malnutrition as a result of poor appetite, restricted diet and malabsorption. Children fail to grow, when the disease is present in early childhood or during infancy, as in congenital heart disease.

### Cardiac psychosis

Psychiatric symptoms may occur due to poor cerebral perfusion in cardiac disorders due to reduced cardiac output.

### Cerebral symptoms

Cerebral symptoms are due to inadequate cerebral circulation leading to hypoxia of the brain. The patient may be confused, delirious or excitable if the cardiac output falls to precarious level, syncopal attacks, convulsions and coma may occur.

### Cyanosis

It is a physical sign, but usually patients will complain about it. It is blue discolouration of skin and mucous membrane noticed when reduced haemoglobin is more than 5.0 g per 100 ml of blood. It may occur on exertion while a child is crying or undergoing physical exertion. It may not be present at rest in some cases. Cyanosis may be central or peripheral (Table 18.2). Central cyanosis is suggestive of congenital heart disease, especially in children, but other causes of central cyanosis are :

1) Pulmonary disorders causing hypoventilation of lungs
2) Broncho-pulmonary arterial anastomosis shunt

3) Pulmonary A-V-Fistula
4) Large diaphragmatic hernia.

Peripheral cyanosis is caused by low cardiac output or vasoconstriction, e.g. due to extreme cold climate.

**Table-18.2 : Differentiating features of**

| Central Cyanosis | Peripheral Cyanosis |
|---|---|
| (a) When blue venous blood is shunted from right chambers of heart to the left side or if there is defective oxygenation due to pulmonary disorders.<br>Cyanosis due to inadequate oxygenation of alveoli will improve by oxygen inhalation, but cyanosis due to shunting of blood will hardly improve by oxygen inhalation. | (a) If it is due to extreme vasoconstriction, e.g. exposure to cold climate or if the circulation is too poor, e.g. low output states. |
| (b) Bluish colouration is seen in mucous membranes and lips (warm situations) | (b) It is not associated with clubbing or polycythaemia. |
| (c) Usually clubbing is present with cyanosis. If haemoglobin (Hb) level is too low (below 5g%), then cyanosis will not be seen as 5.0 g% of reduced HB, should be present in blood for cyanosis to be evident. | (c) Cyanosis is seen is exposed areas, in peripheral parts e.g. fingers, nails, nose, lobes of the ear and exposed lips. |
| (d) It may be associated with polycythaemia. | (d) The blood being in prolonged contact due to slow circulation in tissues deprived of more oxygen and thus reduced haemoglobin content is high. |
| | (e) It disappears when part is warmed up. |

Cyanosis and clubbing of fingers are typically seen in Fallot's tetralogy. Squatting helps in increasing flow of more blood to pulmonary vessel for improving oxygenation in Fallot's tetralogy.

**Malar flush**

In chronic low output states, a dusky mauve flush may be noted in fair-skinned people. This is due to dilated capillaries in the dermis, in which circulation is sluggish. It is most typically found in mitral stenosis with pulmonary hypertension.

**Nocturia and oliguria**

Both these symptoms may occur in heart disease, but frequency of urine may occur due to diabetes mellitus, cystitis, diabetes insipidus or psychological reasons. Oliguria may occur due to renal disease, dehydration or hypovolaemic shock. Frequency of urine of cystitis is associated with pain or dysuria.

**Fatigue**

Finally, it is essential to stress that fatigue, general weakness, tiredness with accustomed exertion is often a very important pointer to incipient or early cardiac failure or coronary insufficiency. Such symptoms may also be due to:

| | |
|---|---|
| Anaemia | Diuretics in excess |
| Insomnia | Potassium depletion |
| Heat exhaustion | Emotional strain |
| Too much sedatives and tranquilisers | Addison's disease |

**Abdominal symptoms**

In congestive heart failure (C.H.F.) due to venous congestion, stretching of liver capsule may cause considerable pain in right upper abdomen and even this may be mistaken for hepatitis.

Mild jaundice also may occur in this state. Urobilinogen may be increased in the urine.

In C.H.F. the patient may complain of flatulence, lack of appetite, nausea and even vomiting. These symptoms are due to congestion of gastrointestinal mucosa and may result in malabsorption.

Digitalis toxicity may also cause anorexia, nausea and vomiting, even before cardiac arrhythmia is noted.

## CARDIOVASCULAR DIAGNOSIS

**History**

The most important part of the clinical examination is *history taking.* This is a very special art which cannot be learnt by reading books only, but this has to be mastered in the hospital wards and from seniors and expert clinicians during periods of clinical clerkship and housemanship.

Even sophisticated instruments may fail to give a correct diagnosis if history, clinical findings are not properly evaluated. History not only pertains to the patient's symptoms but his age, sex, country, climate, environment, occupation, perinatal situations, milestones of growth in childhood, addictions and family background are all very important. Student must always try to take good history before he proceeds to make physical examination. But while attending any life-saving emergency, history may have to be taken in several stages while emergency treatment is in progress.

**Physical examination**

During examination of a cardiac case, firstly note the skin colour and observe the respiratory movements, (dyspnoea, orthopnoea, irregular respiration). Also make a note whether there is anaemia, dehydration, cyanosis,puffiness of face or abnormal pulsations is neck. Arterial pulse can be felt but venous pulse cannot be felt but easily seen especially by using a back rest.

Examine the extremities,if skin is warm and moist (peripheral vasodilatation), severe thyrotoxicosis, anaemia and high fever might be the causes.

Skin may be cold and pale in peripheral vasoconstriction. When cardiac output is less this phenomemon is observed as in primary cardiac diseases.

The importance of good inspection cannot be over emphasised. The body configuration is an important clue to many diseases. In Marfan's syndrome the patient is tall, slim, with long extremities. His arm span is longer than head and torso (head to pubis). It is associated with congenital heart disease.

A patient with hypertension may have trunkal obesity with slim limbs, denoting Cushing's syndrome. Extreme obesity may be a case of Pickwickian syndrome.

Squatting and cyanosis are classical features of Fallot's tetralogy. Muscular dystrophies may be associated with heart disease.

Facial characteristics of Mongol, Down's syndrome, Morquio's syndrome and Hurler's syndrome are well-known.

**Clubbing**

It is due to thickening and expansion of the terminal phalanges. In early stage the skin at the root of nail appears shiny and angle between the nail and skin fold may get obliterated and some spongy sensation is felt at the root of nail. It occurs in cyanotic congenital heart disease, SBE, bronchogenic carcinoma, bronchiectasis, lung abscess, cirrhosis of liver, chronic diarrhoea, e.g. ulcerative colitis and malabsorption syndrome. It may also be congenital and be present in childhood.

Skin and mucous membranes become blue if arterial oxygen saturation is below 85%. Cyanosis may be central or peripheral.

**Pulse**

Arterial pulse is a wave due to pressure changes affecting its wall due to flow of blood. Therefore it has two components, i.e. :

1) Pressure-effects with each systole of heart
2) Volume and velocity of blood flow.

During clinical examination of arterial pulse both radials, carotids, femorals, popliteals, posterior tibialis and dorsalis pedis should be palpated. Femoral pulse is weak and delayed in coarctation of aorta. Peripheral vessels of the leg are obliterated in Buerger's disease.

**Examination of Radial pulse**

Feel both the radial pulses and note if there is any difference. Sometimes there is anomalous course of one radial artery, hence it is not felt. An emboli on the other hand may cause obliteration of a radial artery. Similarly, aortic aneurysm, a large mediastinal growth, cervical rib, pulseless disease (Takayasu's syndrome), scalenus anticus syndrome may cause inequality of pulses or obliteration of one radial pulse.

The qualities to be assessed during examination of pulse are as follows :

**Rate**

Usually pulse rate varies with age. Generally, the range lies between 60 and 90 per minute at rest.

There are wide variations between the individuals. If above 90 per minute, it is called tachycardia. If below 60 per minute, it is called bradycardia. Neither tachycardia nor bradycardia is essentially a sign of heart disease. When pulse is irregular, compare it with heart rate and note the difference. Infants and children have high pulse rate than adults. Pulse rate in newborn is about 140 and up to one year 120 pm. It slows down by third year to 100 pm and in school age to about 90 pm. In old people it is around 80 pm.

(2) **Rhythm**

Normal pulse has a regular rhythm. In disease it may become irregular. Irregularity might be irregularly irregular. Pulse rate might quicken during inspiration and slow during expiration. There might be an extra beat (ectopic) or a beat might be missed (dropped beat). For details refer to chapter on arrhythmias.

(3) **Character or quality**

Difference between systolic and diastolic pressures, is called pulse pressure which determines amplitude or volume. When stroke-volume is large and there is diminished peripheral resistance, collapsing pulse occurs. This is best appreciated by holding up the patient's hand. The examiner's hand will feel a slap of radial pulse (rapid rise and rapid fall). It is also known as Corrigan's pulse. Special types of pulse should be recognised at bedside for clinical diagnosis.

(4) **Volume :**

The volume is related to cardiac output. It corresponds to amplitude of the movement of arterial wall. A low volume or so-called hypokinetic or weak pulse, e.g. mitral stenosis, aortic stenosis, acute myocardial infarction, shock CCF, cardiac tamponade, constrictive pericarditis. toxic myocarditis and coarctation of aorta.

*A large volume pulse is due to high output state or hyperkinetic pulse* e.g. fever, anaemia, thyrotoxicosis, cor pulmonale, high blood pressure, cirrhosis of liver, arterio-venous fistula, beri-beri and Paget's disease.This may occur to some degree during physical exercise and pregnancy.

(5) **Tension**

It gives a rough idea of diastolic pressure. When tension is low the artery is easily compressible without much resistance. If diastolic pressure is high the arterial pulse remains more or less palpable during systole and diastole.

**Nature of arterial wall**

'Wear and tear' phenomenon occurs in aging arteries. In younger people arterial wall is so elastic that it cannot be distinguished from the adjacent structures. In older age artery gets hardened and even calcified and can be felt like a hard rope. Loss of elasticity may lengthen the arteries to be tortuous. Tortuosity is easily observed on brachials and sometimes in the neck. Condition of the retinal vessels can also be visually assessed by ophthalmoscopic examination of fundus oculi. Every medical student who aspires to be a good physician should master the technique of ophthalmoscopy.

**Arterial blood pressure**

Method of recording arterial blood pressure (B.P.) has been discussed in detail in the chapter on systemic hypertension.

**Special types of pulse**

1. **Water hammer or collapsing pulse**

It is also called Corrigan's pulse after the name of Dominic Corrigan. It is found in aortic incompetence, P.D.A., aortopulmonary window, rupture of sinus of Valsalva into ventricle, as well as in all high output states already described earlier.

2. **Anacrotic pulse**

A slow sustained rise of the pulse is felt in severe aortic stenosis. The anacrotic notch may also be felt best in carotids. A slow rise and slow fall also may occur in aortic stenosis which is called pulsus parvus tardus.

3. **Dicrotic pulse**

As if there is double beat during diastole, the second wave is smaller.

4. **Pulsus bisferiens**

The first peak of the pulse (percussion wave) is followed by a second peak (tidal wave). This is felt in aortic incompetence with stenosis and in hypertrophic subaortic stenosis.

5. **Pulsus alternans**

An alternate strong and weak pulse usually present in LVF or toxic myocarditis. It has a bad prognosis but in a healthy person, sometimes it may occur in association with paroxysmal tachycardia, the latter having no adverse prognosis.

6. **Pulsus bigeminus (coupling of pulse)**

Pulse beats occurring in couples with a pause. This may be noted in digitalis toxicity, ischaemic heart disease, rheumatic heart disease etc. A.V. block with ventricular escape or block in atrial flutter (2 : 1, 3 : 1 or 4 : 1) may mimic this.

**Pulsus paradoxus**

The pulse volume to be lower during inspiration as found in massive pericardial effusion and chronic constrictive pericarditis.

**Jugular venous pulse (J.V.P.)**

Examine the patient is semirecumbent position usually at an angle of 45°. Sometimes it can be seen at 30° or may be necessary to elevate the patient above 60°. The idea is to see the upper level of venous pulse. The light should be enough and neck should be relaxed by turning the head slightly to the right side and by placing a pillow under the neck. Expose the whole area above

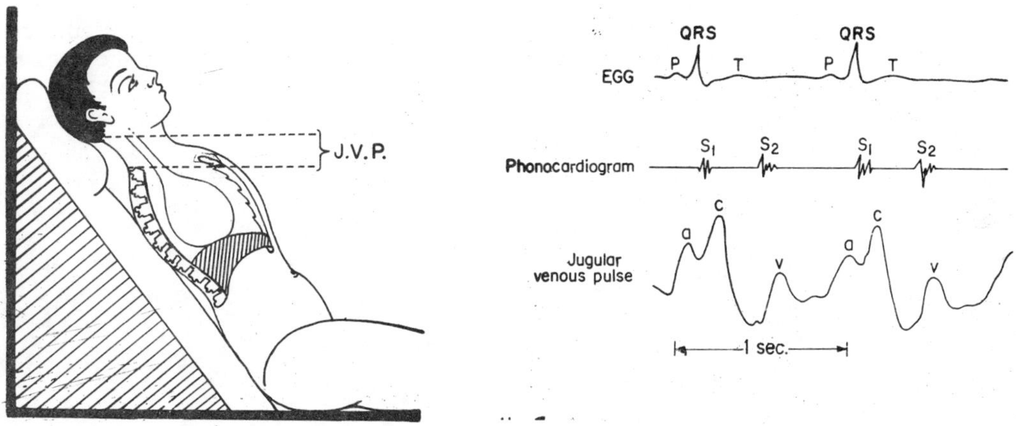


Fig.18.1 : Showing method of watching J.V.P., E.C.G., phonocardiogram and jugular venous pulse illustrate the relative timings.

the clavicle by removing the clothes. In this position, venous pulsation (internal jugular vein) may be visible just above the clavicle. Sternal angle is taken as reference point because it is always 6 cm. above mid-point of right atrium in lying, sitting or standing position. Normal jugular venous pulse is shown in Fig.18.1.

Vertical height of jugular venous pulse is normally 0-2 cms. above the sternal angle. A venous pressure of +4 cm or more is taken as abnormal. If pulsation is not seen, gentle manual pressure over the right subcostal area makes it visible (hepatojugular reflux), JVP is raised in right ventricular failure and obstruction to superior vena cava. In non-cardiac cases, though jugular veins are engorged, they are not pulsatile.

Level of JVP rises during expiration and falls with inspiration when intrathoracic pressure decreases. Persistently elevated JVP is always pathological.

Mean JVP is raised in the following conditions :

1. R.V. failure
2. High output states
3. Superior vena cava obstruction (distended veins do not pulsate as in raised venous pressure).
4. Constrictive pericarditis
5. Tricuspid stenosis
6. Right atrial myxoma
7. Emphysema, pleural effusion and pneumothorax (due to loss of negative pressure in/the thorax).

The normal JVP has three positive (a,c, and v) and two negative waves (x and y). These waves denote intracardiac pressure events and helps in bed-side diagnosis. Along with ECG tracings and heart-sound recording (phonocardiography), many cardiac disorders can be diagnosed (Fig.18.1).

The first heart sound ($S_1$) is synchronized with the end of a wave i.e. where also c wave begins a wave is due to right atrial systole and c wave is due to the beginning of ventricular systole. During v-wave right atrium gets filled by blood from venous side.

The period c and v is period of ventricular systole. Y descent occurs in diastole. When there is resistance to flow, waves are exaggerated.

**Cannon waves**

High venous pressure waves synchronous with carotid pulse are produced by auricular contractions against closed tricuspid valve. It therefore means auricular contraction coinciding with ventricular systole.

**Abnormal "a" waves**

**Large 'a' waves**

1. Pulmonary stenosis (or atresia)
2. Pulmonary hypertension
3. Tricuspid stenosis (or atresia).

**Absent 'a' waves**

Auricular fibrillation.

**Abnormal "v" waves**

**Large "v" wave**

Tricuspid incompetence (due to reflux of blood in right atrium during ventricular systole).

**Accentuated 'x' descent**

1. Constrictive pericarditis
2. Cardiac tamponade

**Slow 'Y' descent**

When there is obstruction of flow in the right atrium, e.g. tricuspid stenosis or myxoma in the auricle.

**Palpation**

**Apex-beat :**

First find out the position of the apex beat furtherest to left and downwards. When the finger feels the impulse it is the apex beat (cardiac impulse). Start palpating from axillary side towards sternum by finger-tips. Describe position of the apex beat from left sternal line and note whether it is inside or outside the midclavicular or midaxillary line and in which intercostal space it is located. Do not forget to note the position of trachea. Shifting of trachea denotes mediastinal shift.

Precordium should be carefully palpated to find out —

1. Cardiac enlargement
2. L.V.H.
3. R.V.H.
4. Thrills
5. Palpable heart sounds
6. Palpable friction rub.

In L.V. hypertrophy, the apex beat moves downwards and outwards and is sustained and thrusting.

In R.V. hypertrophy, the apex beat moves outwards but not downwards and sustained heave is felt near left border of sternum. This is called left parasternal heave.

**Heart Sounds :**

Tapping apex beat due to loud $S_1$ is felt in mitral stenosis. Pulmonary valve closure ($P_2$) may be felt in third left interspace.

**Thrill**

Press the hand over the chest and you may feel a vibrating sensation. This is called thrill. The thrills may be systolic, diastolic or systolo-diastolic (continuous) thrills at apex are better felt if the patient lies flat and half-turn on his left side. Basal thrills are best felt if the patient leans forwards and holds the breath in expiration.

**Percussion**

Radiology is a better guide than percussion to assess cardiac border, still it must be practised as it is quite useful. Its main importance lies in patients with pericardial effusion. Here the area of dullness is absolute and increases both sideways and upwards. Cardiac dullness may be found to the right of sternum in dextrocardia or to left of sternum in lung collapse or fibrosis (left). In the latter case, a band of resonance can be percussed on left of sternum.

**Auscultation**

It is essential to have a good stethoscope which has diaphragm and bell, with well fitting earpiece, with elastic tube not too long. Modern electronic stethoscopes are not for general practice and have special advantages over the classical ones, provided the user knows how to auscultate. A rigid diaphragm should be used. St. George's style stethoscope is locally available. In a busy street-side room, auscultation is never satisfactory. A quiet room, a relaxed patient and well-trained ears are the triads of good auscultation.

Firstly, it is essential to appreciate normal heart sound. Important heart sounds are illustrated in (Fig.18.2).

There are two major sounds 'lub' and 'dup'. These are called first and second sounds.

Between the second and first there are minor sounds and clicks not always present in normal heart and are quite important, e.g. third and fourth heart sounds, ejection clicks and opening snaps (O.S.). Besides these, there are murmurs which should be recognised clinically and all these require repeated and properly guided bed-sidework under a 'Guru'. Presence of a murmur does not always indicate heart disease. Wrong interpretation leads to unnecessary waste of time and money and also cardiac neurosis.

**First heart sound**

It is longest of all four heart sounds and is heard at the apex, caused by closure of the mitral and tricuspid valves. Echocardiography recorded with phonocardiography will be helpful. As contraction of left and right ventricles is not always synchronous, splitting of first sounds may occur and gives the clue. Mitral valve closure is best heard at the apex of L.V. (mitral area) while tricuspid has a softer note, heard best at the lower left sternal area (tricuspid area). Wide splitting (not changing with respiration) suggests right bundle branch block (RBB) due to delayed contraction of right ventricle. First sound may be weak (valves not closing properly), in mitral regurgitation, myocarditis, ischaemic heart disease and due to calcified mitral valves. It is loud in tachycardia and ASD but loudest in mitral stenosis. Variations of intensity of first sound may occur in complete AV dissociation, e.g. heart block.

## Second heart sound

It is caused by closure of aortic ($A_2$) and pulmonary valves ($P_2$); the two components are almost synchronous in expiration but are heard separately as two distinct sounds in full inspiration, due to increased blood flow into right ventricle and decreased in left ventricle at this point of time. When $P_2$ is louder than $A_2$, pulmonary hypertension is suspected as in atrial septal defect (A.S.D.).

Delayed $P_2$ suggests RBBB. In ASD there is wide and fixed splitting of $A_2$ and $P_2$. In advanced right heart failure also $P_2$ is delayed as well as loud (due to pulmonary hypertension). In complete HB also there will be wide splitting of first and second sounds. Shortened L.V. systole will also produce wide splitting of second heart sound ($A_2$ before $P_2$) and will be heard in mitral incompetence and VSD.

Prolonged L.V. systole as in LBB and aortic stenosis will result in $P_2$ occurring before $A_2$ in expiration (L.V. contracting late). However, sounds will come closer or splitting disappears in inspiration (called reversed splitting).

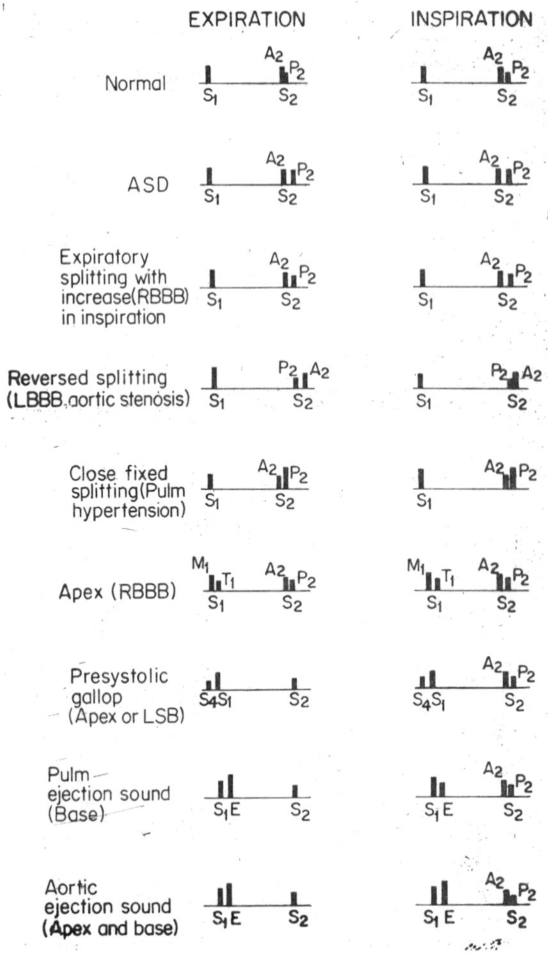


Fig.18.2 : Showing various heart sounds, which should be recognised and learnt at the bedside only.

Similar phenomena may also occur in severe hypertension.

## Diastolic sounds

There are several sounds (besides murmurs) which should be recognised in diastolic phase. These are to be carefully mastered at bed-side during clinical clerkship as they have great diagnostic significance.

## Third heart sound

It is a sound produced at the beginning of the left ventricular filling and is often heard normally in young age group. In older patients it usually signifies abnormal ventricular flow as may occur in mitral incompetence or ischaemic heart disease (I.H.D.), due to altered left ventricular compliance. It is best heard by the bell of the stethoscope.

## Systolic click

An early systolic click occurs at the point of opening of the semilunar valves i.e. just at the onset of ejection often present in hypertensive heart disease or stenosis of semilunar valves (aortic or pulmonary). A mid systolic click may be heard in prolapse of the mitral valve.

**Fourth heart sound**

It is a low frequency sound produced due to atrial systole and is always abnormal, and is best heard by the bell of the stethoscope. Normally atrial systolic sound is not audible. It is heard in left ventricular hypertrophy (LVH), I.H.D. or cardiomyopathy (CMP) and is related to hypertrophied or diseased left ventricle.

**Opening snap (O.S.)**

It follows $P_2$ (i.e. $A_2$, $P_2$ and US) and is heard in mitral stenosis unless the mitral valve is calcified. It is more high-pitched than 2nd sound and well heard in the left border of sternal area nearer to apex beat by the diaphragm of the stethoscope.

**Gallop Rhythm :**

When additional sounds, e.g. $S_3$ (third heart sound) or $S_4$ (fourth heart sounds) are heard it is called gallop rhythm. It may be triple gallop or quadruple gallop (See Fig.18.2).

$S_1 - S_2 - S_4 - S_1$ — Triple Rhythm —
$S_1 - S_2S_3 - S_1$ — " " —
$S_1 - S_2S_3 - S_4S_1$ — Quadruple Rhythm

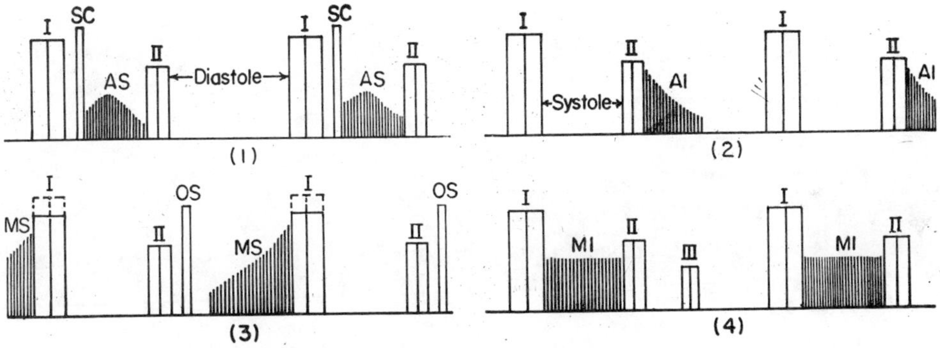


Fig.18.3 — showing the first and second heart sounds and timings of systolic and diastolic murmurs :
(1) Aortic stenosis (2) Aortic incompetence — early diastolic murmur (3) Mitral stenosis — diastolic murmur ending in loud 1st heart sound. (4) Mitral incompetence — pansystolic murmur.

**Sites of auscultation**

Sites of auscultation —

A — Aortic area
A 2nd right costal cartilage
P — pulmonary area
2nd Intercostal space just left to sternum
T = Tricuspid area — Lower end of sternum
M = Just medial to apex beat — mitral area

**Cardiac Murmurs**

Cardiac murmurs are continuous vibrations which vary in length, intensity, pitch and quality.

They may be classified as systolic and diastolic, systolic murmurs are heard between $S_1$ and $S_2$, while diastolic murmurs are heard between $S_2$ and $S_1$ (Fig.18.3)

Diastolic murmurs indicate organic heart disease while systolic may or may not. Diastolic murmurs are fainter and little more difficult to recognise.

Murmurs have to be graded according to their intensity, i.e. Grades 1 to 6 as follows :

Grade 1 — Very faint (audible only in quiet room)
" 2 — Faint murmurs
" 3 — moderately loud
" 4 — loud
" 5 — Very loud
" 6 — loudest possible.

Murmurs are conducted towards the direction of blood flow, causing the sound.

Murmurs produced in the left side of heart are better heard during expiration while in right side of heart are better heard during inspiration.

Thus a murmur is described as per timing (systolic or diastolic), intensity (Grade), conduction and relation with phases of respiration.

Systolic murmurs are further divided into :

(a) Mid-systolic or ejection
(b) Pansystolic
(c) Flow.

Diastolic murmus are further divided into :

(a) Early diastolic murmur
(b) Mid-diastolic murmur
(c) Pre-systolic or late diastolic murmur.

Further details of abnormal cardiac murmurs are discussed under respective diseases.

**Pericardial friction rub**

When pericardium gets inflammed, movements of the parietal and visceral layers during each heart beat produce harsh creaking noise, the pericardial rub. When fluid separates two layers of pericardium (pericardial effusion) friction sound disappears, and rub may still be audible in a small area of precordium unless the effusion is large. When diaphragm of the stethoscope is pressed on precordium both layers of pericardium come still nearer, and the friction sound is intensified.

**Approach to cardiac auscultation**

You should ausculate your own heart daily and as many normal individuals as possible.

(1) Auscultate over 4 classical areas.
(2) Beginners should make a habit of drawing auscultatory events.
(3) When you listen by stethoscope, ask yourself the following questions.
  (a) Do I hear normal heart sounds $S_1$ and $S_2$ ?
  (b) Are there other sounds $S_3$, $S_4$, Os, EC ?
  (c) Are there any murmurs ?
  (d) Is there a friction rub ?
  (e) Are there sounds which are non-cardiac ?
(4) Get your finding confirmed by your teachers.

Cardiac auscultation is rewarding after long experience at the end of which one recognises the music of heart disease. Auscultation is better recognised rather than listened to.

**Lung Bases**

Listen over posterior part of lower lobes. If crepitations are present, they indicate pulmonary congestion, pneumonitis or bronchiectasis. If any doubt, ask the patient to cough twice and then listen again.

**Inspection of the Chest**

Following observations should be made :-

| | |
|---|---|
| 1) One side more prominent than the other | Scoliosis or congenital heart disease<br>Large pleural effusion |
| 2) Prominent or depressed sternum | Pigeon breast or funnel-shaped chest |
| 3) Visible pulsation at the apex beat | Thin chest wall or cardiac enlargement |
| 4) Pulsations in left 2nd and 3rd I.C. space | Dilated pulmonary artery |
| 5) Pulsation at the root of neck | Dilated aorta |
| 6) Collateral vessels on the scapulae behind | Aortic coarctation |
| 7) Epigastric pulsations | R V enlargement, hepatic congestion, aneurysmal abdominal aorta or thin nervous subject |
| 8) Pectus excavatum | May cause shifting of apex beat to left. |

**Hepatomegaly**

Central venous pressure is further reflected by palpation of liver firmly. The transmission of venous pulse may be felt and seen in presence of passive liver congestion as in congestive heart failure and hepatomegaly. In tricuspid stenosis, liver may pulsate with each heart beat and if varicose veins are present pulsation may be transmitted to them also.

**Oedema**

When in subcutaneous tissues excess fluid is present, it is called oedema. Firm pressure with a finger or thumb for at least five seconds produces a depression in swollen area, (pitting oedema) which takes some minutes to disappear when pressure is released *(vide supra)*.

Oedema is usually elicited over ankles, tibia and sacrum.

Legs should be observed for :

(a) Oedema;
(b) Varicose-veins and ulcers;
(c) If one leg is more oedematous than the other, if superficial veins are distended or if calf muscle is tender, suspect deep venous thrombosis of leg.

In this chapter important and practical considerations for bed-side diagnosis have been highlighted. However, the student must refer to textbooks of clinical diagnosis for further details.

## NORMAL ELECTROCARDIOGRAM

*G.C. MOOKERJEE*

**Introduction**

The electrocardiogram (ECG) is a graphic record of electrical events of the cardiac cycle i.e. heart beat. The cardiac impulse is spontaneously generated in the sinus node and this spontaneous rhythmic contractility is a unique property of cardiac muscle. This electrical impulse is formed in the sinus node at regular intervals at the rate of 60 to 90 beats per minute in a healthy adult and the cardiac muscle contracts at the rate generated by the sinus node. The cardiac impulse traverses the auricles, the bundle of His and ultimately the ventricles and then contraction of heart takes place i.e. systole. This is followed by diastole when heart muscle remains relaxed as well as electrically refractory at the onset of diastole. As the heart is situated within the body in fluid medium containing electrolytes, the path of cardiac impulse can be recorded by applying electrodes in specific positions of body surface.

The impulse formation and its transmission in the myocardium, produces weak electrical currents, which are magnified by the ECG machine and recording can be made in moving graph paper. The recording paper has graphic inscription of large and small squares and it moves at 25 mm/sec. or 50 mm/sec. for recording of ECG. Each small square is 0.04 sec (1/25 sec) and each large square is 0.2 (1/5 sec).

**Standardisation :** E.C.G. has been standardised in relation to deflection caused by one milli volt. One milli volt causes deflection of the stylus by 10 milli meter. Only properly standardised E.C.G. should be read.

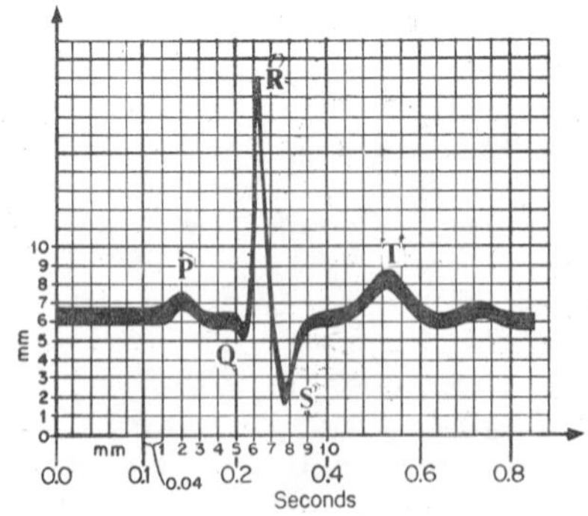


**Fig.18.4(a) — A normal Complex of E.C.G. showing P-wave followed by Q, QRS, T-wave.**

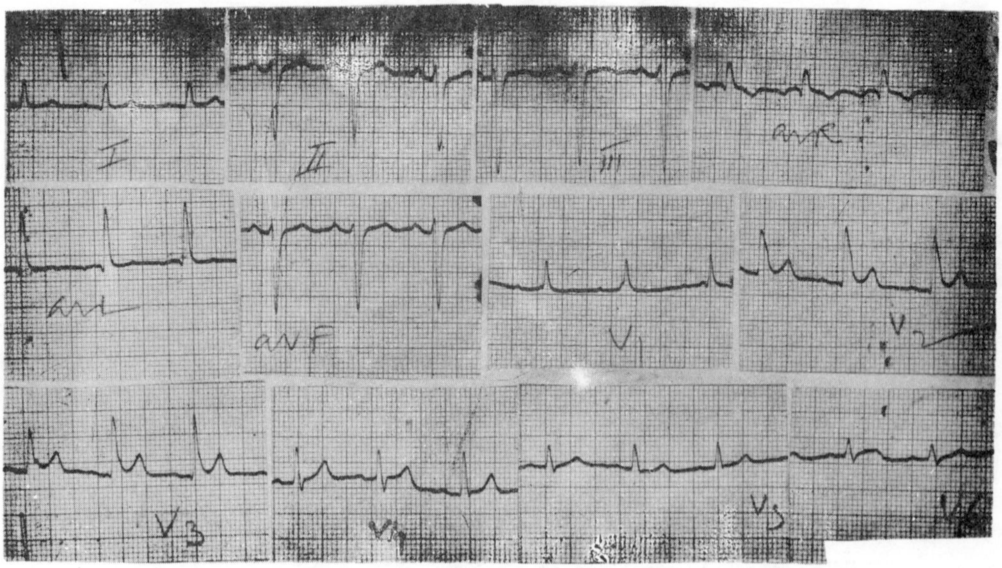


**Fig.18.4(b) — showing E.C.G. of a symptomless "Sadhu" (vegeterian) in good health aged 108 years. E.C.G. shows rate of 90 p.m.; R.A.D.; R.B.B.B. No obvious heart disease.**

**Voltage measurements :** The voltage measurements are made with reference to base line. The deflection above base line is considered positive, while below the base line is negative.

Fig.18.4(a) shows a diagram of ECG complex depicting different parts of ECG i.e. P, QRS and T waves and intervals.

**How to read ECG**

In any ECG the following points should be assessed (Fig.18.4)

1. Rhythm and rate
2. Standardisation
3. Voltage
4. P - wave
5. P - R interval
6. QRS interval
7. QRS complex
8. ST segment
9. T and U wave
10. QT interval

For routine purposes a 12 lead ECG is taken but more elaborate studies can be made in special circumstances and special leads e.g. esophageal lead or His-bundle ECG can be taken.

In order to properly read an ECG at least 4 to 5 complexes should be recorded for each lead and one long lead of 8 to 10 complexes should be recorded specially to study the cardiac rhythm, for routine work. For special purposes continuous monitoring may be necessary by using cardiac monitoring device.

The ECG is specially helpful in the diagnosis of the following conditions :

1. Arrhythmias
2. Atrial and ventricular hypertrophy
3. Bundle branch block and conduction defects
4. Ischaemic heart disease – Routine ECG as well as exercise testing and Holter monitoring methods may be required.
5. Myocardial diseases, cardiomyopathy and pericarditis
6. Drug induced ECG changes especially due to digitalis, quinidine, electrolyte abnormalities especially hypo or hyperkalaemia.

**Rhythm :** Proceed as mentioned below :

1. Regular or irregular.
2. If normal P waves precede every QRS complex, rhythm is sinus.
3. If deformed P waves precede QRS complex, rhythm is junctional or nodal.
4. If there are no P waves preceding QRS complex, rhythm is junctional if QRS interval is normal. If QRS interval has increased duration, the rhythm is ventricular.
5. Mention if QRS complexes are grouped or not, and also if they are dropped or not.

**Rate :** The distance between two vertical lines (small square) on ECG paper = 0.04 seconds. Count the number of squares between two consecutive QRS complexes. Divide 1500 by this number. If this number is 15, the heart-rate is 1500 divided by 15 = 100 per minute. If distance between two consecutive QRS complexes is not uniform, count at three places, take the average of it and use this average number for dividing 1500. ECG-calipers are also available for direct measurement of rates.

Normally the auricular and ventricular rates do not differ, but they should be counted individually as these may vary in some disorders of rhythm e.g. complete heart block (i.e. third degree heart block), AV block or some cases of second degree AV block. In auricular fibrillation, only wavy lines are seen, hence auricular rates cannot be properly counted.

**Intervals :** PR intervals (A-V conduction time) : normal value 0.12 to 0.2 sec. It is measured from the beginning of P-wave to the onset of QRS complex. Strictly speaking, therefore, it is P - Q and not PR which has become accepted by usage. The PR interval should not exceed 0.2 second but possibly 0.21 sec. may also be considered normal. The age, body build and heart rate are actually important.

Nomogram produced by Ashman R & Hull, E : *Essentials of Electrocardiography,* Macmillan, 1937 shows that at heart rate of 70 p.m. for large adults PR interval may be 0.21 which for small adults is 0.20. At heart rate of iii - 130 p.m., PR interval for large adults is 0.18 which for small adults it is 0.17. Similarly for children the PR interval is shorter than in adults.

**PP interval :** If the rhythm is regular, PPinterval, RRinterval should be equal. If the ventricular rhythm is irregular or if auricular and ventricular rates are different but regular, PP interval and RR intervals will differ. The auricular contraction rate should be measured from counting between two successive P waves.

**QRS interval :** It measures ventricular depolarization time. It is measured from the beginning of Q wave (or R wave where Q is absent) up to the end of S wave. The QRS interval is normally within 0.1 sec. but in $V_2$ and $V_3$ up to 0.11 sec may be considered normal.

**RR interval :** Will vary according to heart rate. It is the interval between two successive R waves, In regular rhythm RR interval in seconds (peak to peak of two successive R waves divided by 60, will indicate the heart rate. However, this can also be found out by a nomogram. If the ventricular rhythm is irregular, count the number of R waves in 10 seconds interval and calculate the rate per minute. If fifteen R waves are present in 10 seconds interval, the ventricular rate is 15 × 6 = 90 per minute.

**QT interval :** QT should be less than 35 mm. — It is the electrical systole measured as distance between beginning of Q wave and end of T wave. It varies with heart rate and therefore it is corrected for purpose of standardisation, which is known as corrected QT interval (Q-Tc). It is computed from a nomogram which gives Q-Tc. At the heart rate of 60 p.m. Q-Tc adult males sh[illegible] t exceed 0.42 sec and for females 0.43 second.

**VAT (Ventricular activation time) :** VAT is the time interval taken for the electrical impulse to travel from endocardium to pericardium i.e. it is the distance between onset of Q to the peak of R wave. Measured from a surface ECG, it cannot be very accurate as thickness of chest wall differs causing errors. It can be accurately measured by direct electrodes placed over the surface of heart and endocardium. Normally VAT should be within 0.03 sec in $V_1$ - $V_3$ and 0.05 sec. in $V_5$ - $V_6$.

**P - wave :** P - wave is the electrical activation of atrium. Normally upright in leads I, II, aVF and inverted in aVR, it has not a constant configuration in other leads. Normally its duration is less than 0.1 sec and amplitude less than 2.5 mm. If P is taller in lead I than in lead III and is wide and notched, it is called P-mitrale which is characteristic of mitral stenosis. If P is taller in lead III than in lead I and is pointed, it is called *P-pulmonale,* which is characteristic of *cor-pulmonale.* (See : Pulmonary embolism — Fig.18.32).

**PR segment and S - T Junction (J junction) :** PR segment is the portion of complex which begins from the end of P wave to the onset of QRS complex, which is normally isoelectric.

**S - T segment :** This RS - T segment which starts from where QRS ends and ST begins or the J - junction. The ST segment is usually isoelectric. It may be elevated or depressed above or below the base line (i.e. the time from end of T - wave to onset of next P - wave (T-P segment).

**T - wave :** ST segment is followed by T - wave. Normally T-waves are upright in leads I, III, AVL, AVF, $V_3$ to $V_6$ and inverted in aVR. In all the other leads it may vary. Height of T wave should not be more than 5 mm in limb leads and more than 10 mm in chest leads. If it is more than this its cause needs evaluation. However, it must be remembered that T wave is the most vulnerable portion of the ECG and it may be affected by many factors. T - wave may be tall due to hyperkalaemia or even exposure to hot environment, while T - waves may be flattened or inverted due to hypokalaemia, myxoedema, extreme cold exposure, toxic myocarditis or cardiomyopathy. Tall T may also occur in I.H.D. (especially inferior wall infarction).

T - waves are variable in shape and direction on III, aVL, aVF, $V_1$ and $V_2$. Interpretation of T-wave should be very cautiously done to avoid cardiac neurosis.

The most common causes of ST elevation are acute myocardial injury (infarction) or pericarditis.

Depression of ST segment (horizontal or significant down-sloping) may be due to ventricular strain, ischaemia or digitalis effect.

**U-wave :** T-wave may or may not be followed by a small wave called U-wave. Usually it is upright. When inverted, it indicates either myocardial ischaemia, ventricular stress or electrolyte imbalance.

**Q - U interval :** It is the distance between onset of Q wave to the end of U wave (when present). It measures the time of total ventricular repolarization including purkinje fibres in the myocardium.

**POINTS TO REMEMBER :**

1. Abnormal looking ECG may sometimes be seen with normal hearts.
2. ECG may be normal even though heart might be abnormal.
3. ECG should be assessed along with history and clinical background.
4. To be more conclusive, study of serial ECG's is essential.
5. Do not read too much from an ECG.

A technician recording an ECG should not make any comments to the patient. If there are some abnormalities requiring immediate attention, the technician should urgently inform the physician concerned. A case report published in the Guy's Hospital Gazette, London is a classic example of wrong interpretation about ECG relating to heart.

A patient's ECG showed some minor abnormalities and his doctor diagnosed him as a case of I.H.D. The man lost his job and finally committed suicide. On post-mortem his coronary arteries were normal.

A good history, clinical findings, follow-up of the case, proper medication and exercise tests including echocardiography, coronary angiography, Holter monitoring and modern radioisotopic investigation wherever possible may be undertaken in controversial cases.

## ECHOCARDIOGRAPHY

*SANJIB K. MUKERJEE*

### Introduction

The use of ultrasound in the diagnosis of heart disease is called echocardiography. The ultrasound is so named because it is beyond the reach of human hearing. The sound waves, when passed in an homogenous medium, travels in a straight line. If, however, any object of different density (called accoustic impedance) seems to come on its way, the sound will reflect mostly and refract partly. These reflected sound waves, called echoes, during their onward and return passage, can be converted into electrical wave patterns which can be seen in the television screen and recorded in a graphic paper.

When the high frequency sound waves are travelling along tissues of two different types e.g. muscles and blood, an echo is generated; which returns to the transducer. The time taken for this echo to return is a measure of distance of the reflective structure from the transducer.

The basic circuit of the echocardiography instrument allows one transducer, which is responsible to transmit a known amount of ultrasound and then it acts as a receiver, for the returning echoes. When the returning echo takes the form of a spike it is called A-mode. When these spikes were converted to a dot (brightness), it is called B-mode. One can then sweep the oscilloscope in order to introduce a time axis. It is useful in detecting echoes on a moving object, such as heart and hence called M(Motion)-Mode display. Initially M-Mode echocardiography was used for all diagnostic purposes.

However, with the advancement of technology in ultrasound two-dimensional echocardiography was introduced. The later further enhanced the diagnostic capability of the instrument. Finally, Doppler was added which bridged few loop holes in echocardiographic diagnosis.

The ultrasound equipment is a complex instrument. The transducer contains a piezo-electric crystal, which when stimulated electrically can vibrate at a very high frequency, producing a burst of ultrasound, which it transmits. During the receiving cycle, the same piezo-electric crystal responds to the reflected sound and vibrates which is converted back to electric signal and can thus be amplified and appropriately displayed and also recorded.

**Methods :** In echocardiography no special preparations of the patient are necessary. The patient lies in the comfortable bed with semi-inclined (30° inclination) position and turned towards the left. The operator sits comfortably by his side and puts a small transducer in the left precordium between 2nd and 4th left intercostal space near the sternal edge. The transducer is directed perpendicularly on the chest wall. Initially the mitral valve is identified and then by turning the transducer either towards the apex or towards the base, the other cardiac structures are identified. One can scan to and fro, from base to apex frequently. Usually 4 different views are taken as follows :

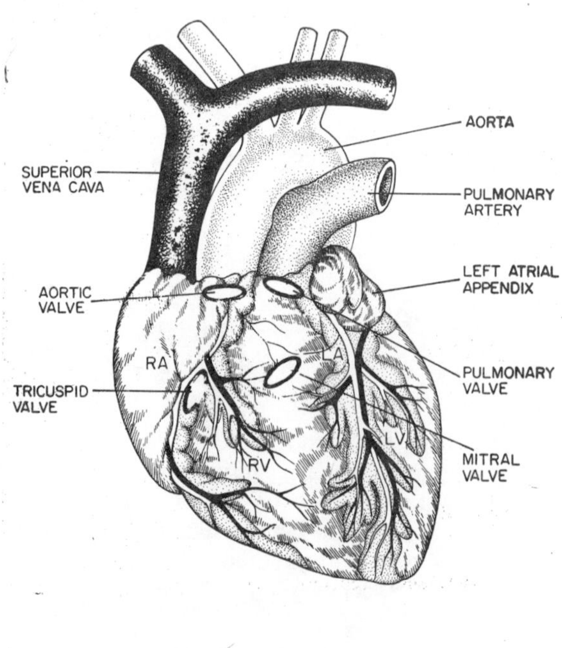


Fig.18.5(a) : showing valve positions; Echo transducer is placed perpendicularly on the chest wall at different levels (See text).

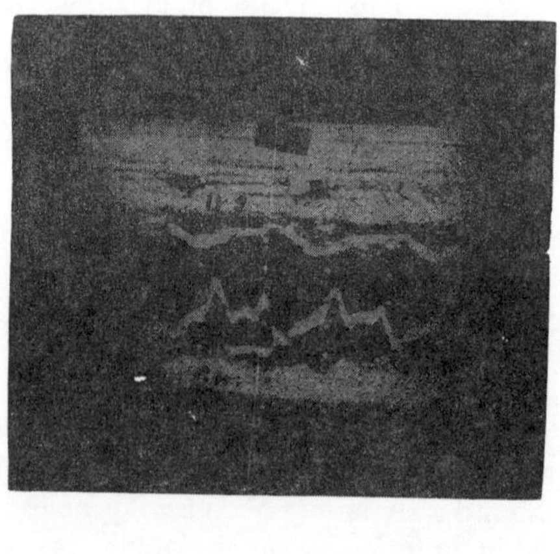

Fig.18.5(b) — Normal M-Mode Echocardiogram

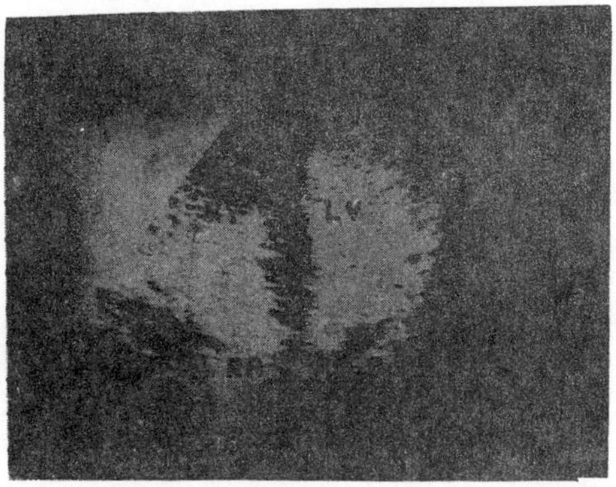

Fig.18.6(a) — Normal 2D-Echocardiogram showing four chambers

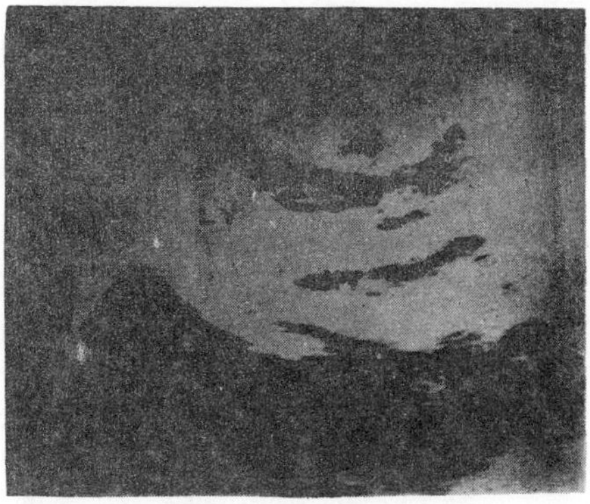

Fig.18.6 (b) — 2D — Normal-long axis view showing mitral valve in diastole

(1) At the level of apex
(2) At the level of mitral valve
(3) At the junction of left atrium and left ventricle containing the anterior leaflet of the mitral valve
(4) At the level of the aorta and left atrium.

With M-mode only ice pack view of the heart showing these 4 views can be seen. However, with two dimensional transducer, a larger area of the heart can be seen and by rotating the transducer, long axis, short axis, apical, two chamber and four chamber views, subcostal views, suprasternal views are taken. This technique can document the whole of cardiac silhouette.

**Indications for performing echocardiography**

An echocardiography helps in identification of cardiac structures and any abnormality can be detected. However, it is valuable in identifying following diseases :

Mitral stenosis, mitral valve prolapse, flail mitral valve, aortic stenosis and regurgitation.

Vegetations in any valves and pericardial effusion.

Left ventricular function, hypertrophic cardiomyopathy, restrictive cardiomyopathy and congestive cardiomyopathy.

**Congenital Heart Diseases :**

Atrial septal defect, co-arctation of aorta, pulmonary stenosis, and bicuspid aortic valve,
Endocardial cushion defect, truncus arteriosus, tetralogy of fallot, tricuspid atresia, pulmonary atresia,
Ebstein's anomaly, some forms of ventricular and septal defects, double outlet right ventricle and single ventricle etc.

**Mitral Valve Disease**

**Echo** characteristic of normal mitral valve M-mode :

In M-mode study, mitral valve looks like a 'M' and 'W' pattern. The anterior leaflet looks like capital 'M' and posterior leaflet looks like 'W'. The leaflets have the following points which is to be remembered as it signifies important cardiac events. Mitral valve opens widely during diastole : Its initial opening is labelled as D-E point, then there is sudden closure, which is labelled as E-F slope, then there is a short period of diastasis during which time nothing is happening and finally there is atrial contraction which is manifested by a point and then the two leaflets meet at systole, labelled as C-D following that cycle repeats itself. (Fig.18.7 (a), (b) & (c) : Mitral stenosis).

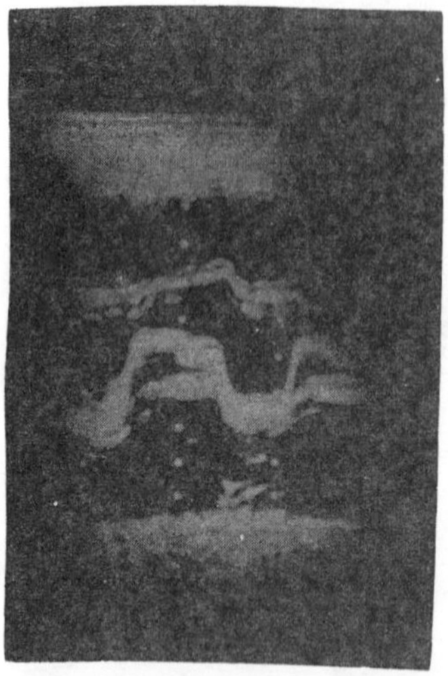

Fig.18.7(a) : Echocardiogram of mitral valve showing significant mitral stenosis : Both anterior and posterior leaflets are thicker than normal E-F slope is flat, Posterior leaflet is moving anteriorly — (See text)

AML = Ant. Mitral Leaflet
PML = Post Mitral Leaflet
PW = Post wall L.V.
RV = Rt. Ventricle

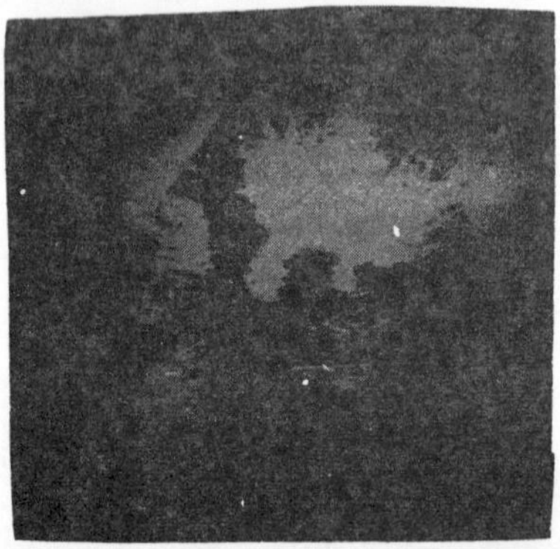

**Fig.18.7 (b) — 2D - apical four chamber view showing mitral stenosis**

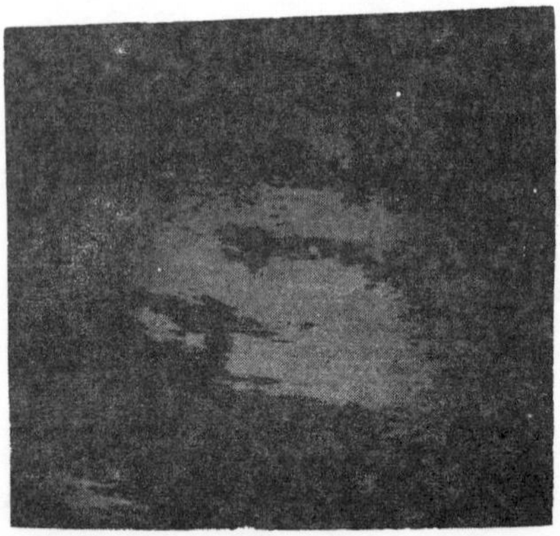

**Fig.18.7(c)** — 2D-view of long axis showing mitral stenosis

## MITRAL STENOSIS

Historically, mitral stenosis was first diagnosed through echocardiography. In mitral stenosis, the two leaflets of mitral valve are thickened and E-F slope is significantly reduced because the stenotic valve remains open during diastole. The posterior leaflet of the mitral valve is moving anteriorly, instead of being a virtual mirror image motion of the anterior leaflet. The E-F slope can be measured and accordingly, semiquantitative assessment of degree of stenosis can be made. There are some exceptions to this rule. With two dimensional echocardiography, the characteristic "bowing" of the anterior leaflet, can be seen. The posterior leaflet either is immobile or moving anteriorly, the leaflets ends are thickened and there is little separation between the two leaflets seen on long axis view. In the short axis view, irregular surface area of the reduced mitral valve can be seen and the actual surface area of mitral valve can be determined.

Four chamber apical view also shows characteristic doming of the mitral valve, with large left atrium and normal or smaller than normal sized left ventricle. The right ventricle comparatively appears more enlarged.

In mitral regurgitation however, if it is of rheumatic origin, one can still see the thickened mitral valve. E-F slope is still reduced and abnormal posterior leaflet motion is seen. Indirect evidence of severe left atrial enlargement and left ventricular enlargement can seen. In two dimensional study one can sometimes document inadequate co-aptation of the mitral valve leaflets during systole. With added Doppler techniques, further information regarding severity of mitral regurgitation can be made.

A common clinical mimicar of mitral stenosis is left atrial myxoma. Left atrial myxoma has similarities with mitral stenosis. They both have reduced E-F slope but in left atrial myxoma there is definite a line of separation between the edge of tumour and the mitral valve leaflet. Moreover, there are clouds of echoes behind the mitral valve must be shown through repeated scanning from aortic root to left ventricular apex. With two dimensional study, not only the left atrial myxoma can be seen, but also the right atrial myxoma can be seen too. It shows the characteristic to and fro movement of the tumour like a Ping Pong ball, moving in and out of the left atrium.

**Mitral Valve Prolapse**

This is a common disease and with echocardiography increasing number of such cases are being diagnosed. Here, the normal echo pattern of mitral valve is seen during diastole but during systole, either the posterior leaflet are pouching downwards or the whole of both leaflets are pouching downwards (Hammocking). Phonocardiogram can be taken at the same time, showing the click, occurring at the same time with mitral valve prolapse. Again one should be very careful in diagnosing this mitral valve prolapse, as it can be produced artificially through irregular positioning of transducer. The transducer must be in perpendicular to mitral valve and both anterior and posterior leaflets of the mitral valve must be shown and repeated scanning should be done. Sometimes one can use amyl-nitrate to document this mitral valve prolapse. Again with two dimensional study mitral valve prolapse can be better demonstrated and it can be seen at long axis view where either the posterior leaflets are pouching towards the left atrium or both leaflets are pouching towards left atrium. Mitral leaflets are sometimes thickened and in four chamber apical and two chamber apical views, the mitral valves in systole can be demonstrated occupying a position 2 mm below the line drawn from mitral annulus. However, one cannot fairly assess the amount of mitral regurgitation directly. The Doppler technique will help in these cases.

Besides mitral valve prolapse, non-rheumatic mitral regurgitation can occur in papillary muscle dysfunction, flail mitral valve, where echocardiography can also help. Mitral valve can be the seat of sub-acute bacterial endocarditis and vegetations can be seen over the mitral valves. It consists of dense fuzzy echoes over the anterior and posterior leaflets of the mitral valves, together or independently and being mobile it has a characteristic to and fro movement during systole and diastole.

Fluttering of the mitral valve is seen in aortic insufficiency.

**Tricuspid Disease**

M-mode echocardiography cannot see tricuspid valve, in its entriety unless the tricuspid valve comes to be placed more anteriorly, as in young children in corpulmonale or atrial septal defect, Ebstein's anomaly etc. However, with careful transducer angulation one can see tricuspid valve in systole most of the times. With added two dimensional study, one can confirm or exclude M-mode findings. Tricuspid stenosis has the same echo findings as mitral stenosis. Prolapse of the tricuspid valve has same echo characteristics as with mitral valve and tricuspid vegetation can be detected in a similar way. However, tricuspid regurgitation is difficult to detect and with contrast echocardiography and annular measurement technique and Doppler study will help in detecting the tricuspid regurgitations.

In Ebstein's disease one can clearly diagnose through echocardiography. Here one can record mitral valve and tricuspid valve simultaneously, there were increased tricuspid valve excursions. The tricuspid valve closure occurs 60 milli-seconds or more after mitral valve closure. However, with M-mode sometimes it is difficult to document delay in tricuspid valve closure. In two dimensional study, however, one can see unusual position of the tricuspid valve attachment which is nearer to the apex and thus a fair amount of distance seen from mitral valve leaflet attachment and tricuspid valve particularly in the 4 chamber apical view. The large right atrium, small right ventricle with wide excursion of the tricuspid valves are very characteristic.

Right ventricular myxoma has similar echo findings as described under left atrial myxomas. Tricuspid vegetations of subacute bacterial endocarditis seen in heroin addicts can be seen better through two dimensional study. In M-mode, it is not only difficult but may sometimes be misleading.

### The Aortic Valve Disease

The aortic valve has 3 cusps, right coronary, left coronary and non-coronary cusps. In M-mode only two cusps are documented. In two-dimensional study all three cusps can be seen.

In M-mode, one can see two walls of the aortic root moving parallel to each other, showing up as two bright lines, as a box like configuration during systole. These boxes represent the opening of the leaflets, as initial separation, of two leaflets, then it remains separated and finally close forming a single line occupying the mid posterior during diastole. The anterior echo is formed by the right coronary cusps and the posterior echoes by the noncoronary cusps.

If aortic root is measured during systole, normally it is less than 35 mm. Dilatation of the aortic root seen in Marfan's disease, aortic aneurysms. The leaflet-separation of the aortic valve can also be measured at its middle and if it is less than 1 cm. then aortic stenosis is likely. The aortic valve is thickened and can be documented as two or more layers during diastole. Various measurements, related to determine the severity of aortic stenosis has been postulated. It correlates with gradients and surface area of the aortic valve in children but not in adults, due to thickening of the valves, calcification, rheumatic affection etc. However, with two-dimensional study one can further document bicuspid or unicuspid aortic valve with doming and to and fro movements of the domed stenotic valves during systole and diastole, characteristic of congenital aortic stenosis. Though in bicuspid aortic valve, one can see the eccentrically placed aortic leaflets during diastole but the later can be artifactual. Hence, two dimensional study must be done. Now with added Doppler technique, one can assess the flow velocity and give some idea about the severity of the stenosis.

### Aortic Regurgitation

When aortic regurgitation is associated with aortic stenosis, the echo features of aortic stenosis, as described above will be seen, in addition fluttering of the mitral valve can be documented. It looks like fine tremor-like motion of anterior or sometimes both anterior and posterior leaflets of mitral valve. In simple aortic regurgitations, the aortic valve may be normal. Sometimes only thickening of the aortic valve can be seen. Aortic root may be dilated. Indirect evidence of left ventricular volume overload will be seen and recently it was claimed that by measuring the systolic dimensions of left ventricle, one can determine, suitability of aortic valve replacement. Left ventricular systolic dimension of 55 mm is the key figure, as above that figure usually causes increased mortality. With two dimensional study, one can see prolapse of the aortic valve leaflets and inadequate apposition of the two aortic valve leaflets during diastole. With added Doppler technique, further direction velocity of blood flow can be determined both during systole and diastole, thus enhancing the accuracy in the diagnosis (Aortic valve disorders).

Aortic valve vegetation can be detected fairly accurately both in M-mode ,and two dimensional study. In M-mode one can document, fuzzy echoes attached to either leaflets of the aorta. In two dimensional view, one can see echo-refractile mass, mobile, attached to either anterior or posterior cusp of the aortic valve. It has a characteristic to and fro motion which once seen cannot be forgotten sometimes, the vegetation mass could be detached, causing embolism to distant areas and that also could be documented through echocardiographic study.

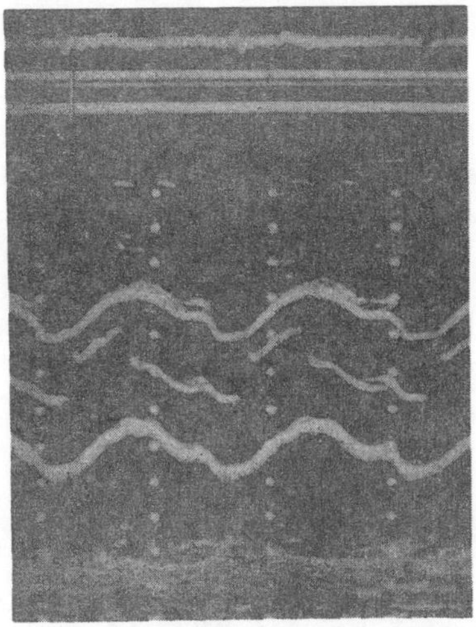

Fig.18.8 : Normal Echo at aortic valve level
M-mode Echo Aortic valves aortic root level. Aortic root has undulating motion in systole and diastole. The Aortic Cusps (AC) have box-like configuration in systole.

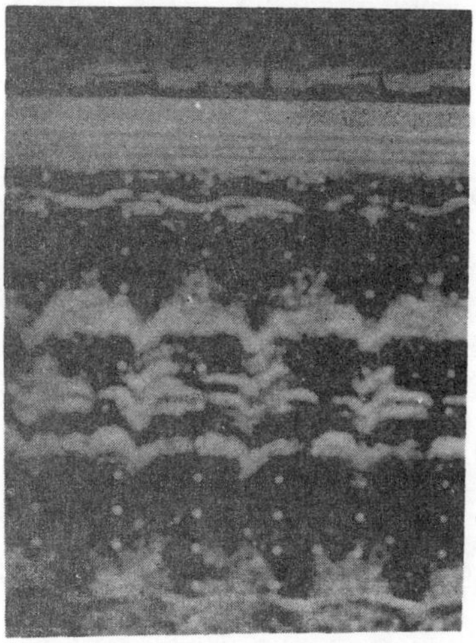

Fig.18.9(a) : M-mode Echo showing significant Aortic stenosis.

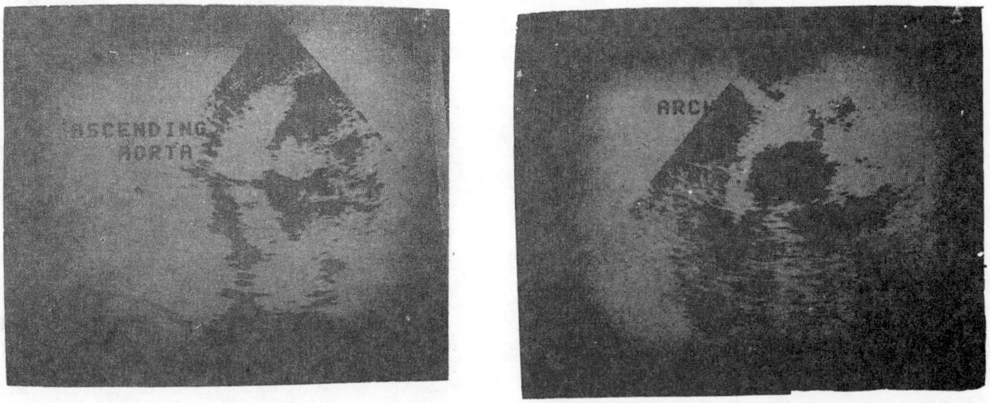


Fig.18.9 (b) & (c) — showing ascending and arch of aorta openings of major branches can be seen clearly.

## DISORDERS OF CARDIAC RATE AND RHYTHM

*G.C. MOOKERJEE*

### Introduction

The heart normally contracts at a regular rhythm and the rate varies according to age and state of physical activity. Irregularity of rhythm or heart-rate too fast or too slow beyond physiological range is called cardiac arrhythmia or dysrhythmia. The muscular contraction of the heart is initiated by electrical impulses spontaneously generated by a specialised group of cells situated in the sino-atrial node (SA node). Impulses generated at SA node are transmitted through the auricular wall to the bundle of His, which consists of A V node and its branches. The right bundle divides into branches in the wall of right ventricle while the left bundle divides into two fascicles anterior and posterior and then branches in the left ventricular wall. The terminal branches of the bundle of His are called Purkinje fibres. More recent researches show that the intraventricular conduction system is more complex. The right bundle branch is more or less a continuation of bundle of His, entering right ventricle. The left branch actually divides into three fascicles in most people — anterior, posterior and anteroseptal. There is intricate intercommunication between anterior and posterior divisions. Autonomic-impulse-forming-tissue is present in SA node, coronary sinus. His-Purkinje system and in the A V node. This area of SA node and the top of bundle of His is called junctional tissue. The S.A. node is controlled by both sympathetic and parasympathetic nerves, hence its impulse formation is under nervous influence. But autonomic nervous control of A.V. node is not so well marked. It is also thought that A.V. junction may have two separate pathways of conduction, one being faster route and the other slower (Marriot). This may explain re-entry phenomenon.

If sinus node (SA node) fails to generate impulses, the cells of A.V. node and bundle of His can generate impulses but at a slower rate.

Normally depolarization starts at the SA node and the impulse travels through the auricular walls towards auriculo-ventricular junction. This is the 'P' wave of the ECG. As SA node is the master-controller of cardiac rhythm, normal rhythm is known as sinus rhythm. Each P wave is followed by the PR interval, i.e. the time taken for the impulse before ventricles receive the order to contract and at the end of PR interval 'QRS' wave form is depicted denoting electrical activity of the ventricles.

It is sometimes seen that the heart rate is increased during inspiration, while decreased during expiration. This is due to vagal effect and this periodic change of rate and rhythm is called sinus arrhythmia. The normal rate of impulse formation of SA node is 60 to 80 per minute in adults while the A.V. node can beat only at slower rate of about 50 per minute. So the AV node can only originate a beat when SA node is silent. If AV node is silent ventricular conducting cells can beat only at 30 to 40 per minute.

**Sinus Tachycardia**

Tachycardia means rapid heart action. Normal heart rate at birth varies from 120 to 140 per minute. As the age advances heart rate goes on diminishing and is between 70 and 80 per minute by the age of 18. In adults, the rate may be as low as 60 per minute especially in atheletes, while in adults, pulse rate more than 90 per minute is abnormal.

Underlying causes of tachycardia are emotional outburst, anxiety, fever, thyrotoxicosis, carditis, heart failure, constrictive pericarditis, large haemorrhage and shock. Sympathomimetic drugs or any disorder stimulating sympathetic nervous system will cause sinus tachycardia. Rapid heart rate may be observed in otherwise normal ECG and should be interpreted against clinical background. Whenever a patient complains of palpitation, aetiological basis should be searched for carefully.

**Sinus Bradycardia**

Bradycardia or slow heart rate by itself is not abnormal. It is due to increased vagal tone. Healthy adults (especially atheletes) may have a slow heart rate but usually not less than 60 per minute. Slow heart rate may also be due to jaundice, myxoedema, raised intracranial pressure and cardiac depressant drugs, e.g. digitalis, quinidine, verapamil, lidocaine, $\beta$-receptor blockers e.g. propranolol, also phenylamine lactate.

If heart rate falls below 60 per minute careful evaluation is indicated especially to exclude heart block. Slow heart rate is either due to sinus bradycardia or heart block.

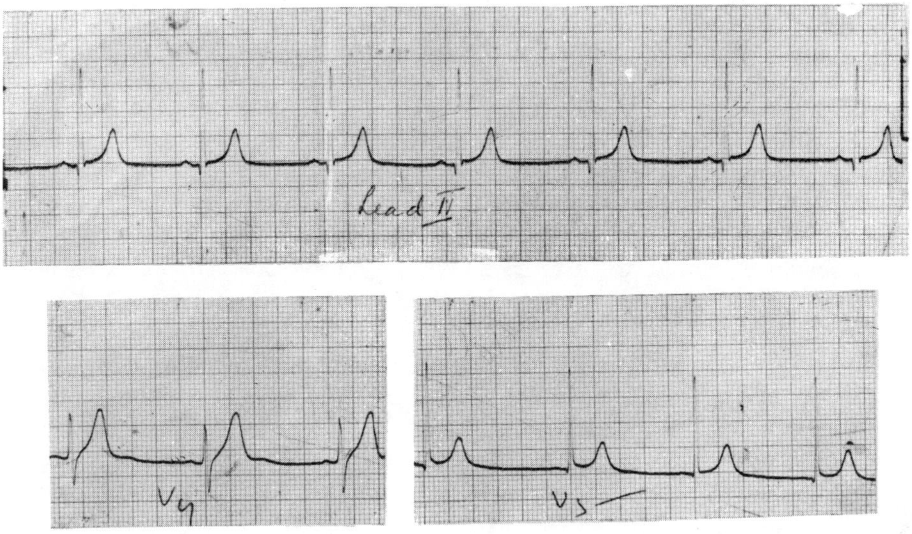


Fig.18.10 : Sinus Bradycardia

**Re-entry**

This is a phenomenon which can occur in the heart muscle if conduction of some part is depressed than the remaining portion. Normally, wave of depolarization spreads equally in the muscle wall, but if one region becomes transiently less conductive, a normal impulse already travelling the normal part (non-depressed area) of the myocardium can pass in a retrograde manner. This may lead to abnormal rhythm, due to passage of the impulse going round and round.

The re-entry phenomenon may cause tachycardias of atrial, AV nodal and ventricular origin. An excellent account of this subject is given in Marriot's Practical Electrocardiography.

**Sinus Arrhythmia**

As already mentioned inspiratory quickening of heart rate and expiratory slowing is called sinus arrhythmia. This is due to changing vagal tone. Sinus arrhythmia can be exaggerated by drugs which increase vagal tone e.g. digitalis. It can be abolished by exercise or atropine. Sinus arrhythmia is often noted in children and adolescents and is otherwise normal. It is related to rhythmic variations associated with impulse formation at the respiratory centre.

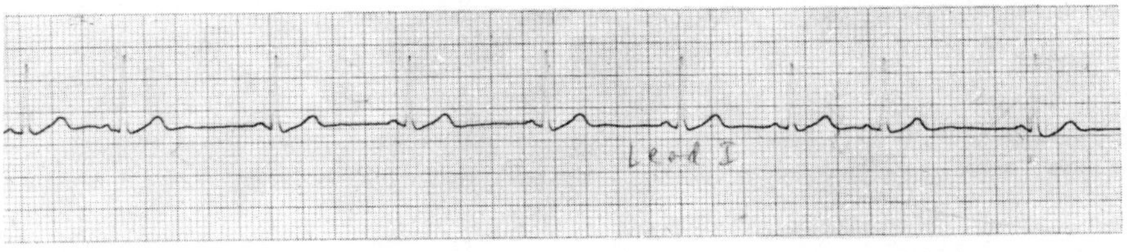


Fig.18.11 : Sinus Arrhythmia.

## ECTOPIC RHYTHMS

Cardiac impulse normally originates in the SA node but when it arises elsewhere in the myocardium, it is called ectopic rhythm. Ectopic focus may be in atrial, junctional or ventricular tissue. Broadly speaking, if the focus is above the ventricles, it is supraventricular and if it is in the ventricle it is ventricular. Supraventricular arrhythmias are atrial fibrillation, atrial flutter, atrial or nodal tachycardias. Extrasystoles or premature beats may originate from atria, A.V. node or the ventricles. The intricate path of transmission of cardiac impulse from SA node to AV node still remains controversial.

As ectopic beats are premature, the interval between ectopic beat and preceding normal beat (coupling interval) is shorter than the interval between any two normal beats.

This fact is most important in management because treatment to control the ectopic beats may be desirable, while suppression of escape beats and beats due to intermittent BBB may be dangerous. Remember all beats with abnormal confirguration are not to be designated as ectopic beats.

The origin of ectopic beats is not always easy to determine and not only long strips of ECG recording is required but also it may be necessary to record simultaneous records of two leads.

## ATRIAL EXTRASYSTOLE (ECTOPICS)

The focus of extrasystoles (ES) or premature beats may be in the auricular wall or AV node. An ectopic beat is a premature beat and as a result the next regular sinus impulse is delayed. The ectopic beat is felt earlier at the wrist (or may not be felt at all if the ventricular contraction is weak) and the next beat is delayed. ECG will show deformed or inverted P but QRS is normal in shape and direction but the PQRST complex occurs early and there is a pause till next normal beat, which is not fully compensatory (Fig.18.12). The distance between the two normal sinus beats is actually less than two cycles.

In auricular or nodal ES, QRS complex may not be normal,looking if there is bundle branch block.

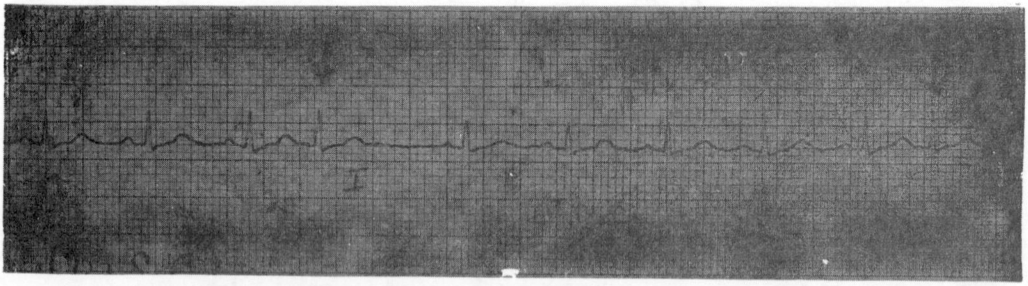

Fig.18.12 : Atrial ectopics

If the atrial ectopic beat occurs too early it may get blocked either at AV node or in bundle branch (still remaining refractory) leading to prolonged PR interval and atrial ectopic beat. This may appear in ECG as partial or complete BBB (functional partial or complete RBB). As the resulting QRS complexes are broad, this can be mistaken for ventricular ectopic beat.

Atrial ectopics can occur in healthy young people and are then benign but they may occur in all kinds of heart disease as well as during anaesthesia or after cardiac surgery.

Treatment depends on the cause.

## NODAL EXTRASYSTOLE

(AV junctional beats)

The impulse may originate from the AV node or bundle of His. This is called nodal extrasystole.

The impulse spreads upwards in the atria (retrograde) and downwards (antegrade) in the ventricles. The QRS complex is normal and is supraventricular type.

The timing of P wave is uncertain, its configuration is abnormal. It may precede or may merge, with, or follow, QRS complex. Discharge of sinus node again does not allow full compensatory pause. Cardiac muscle being inherently irritable subnormal cardiac impulses are created due to undue excitation.

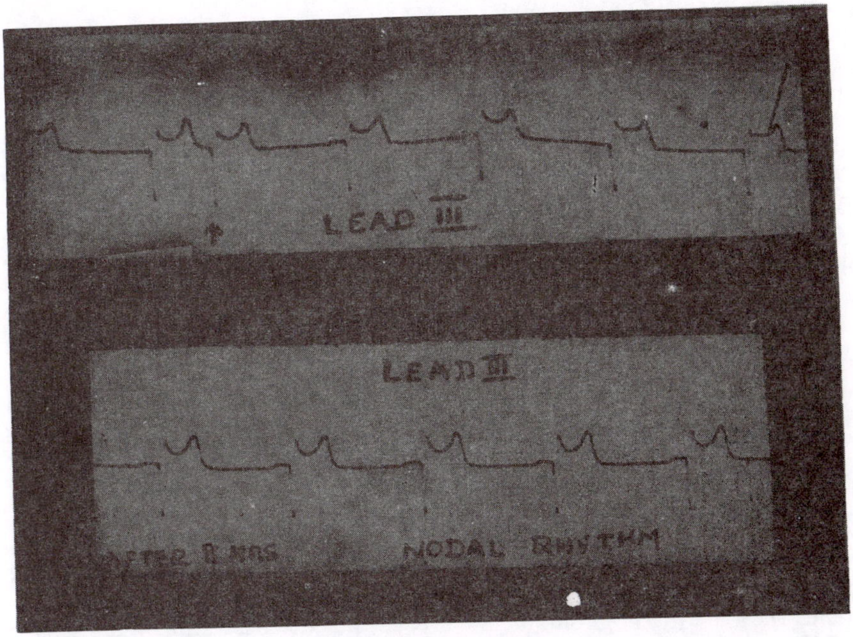


Fig.18.13 : Nodal Rhythm

## VI TRICULAR PREMATURE BEATS OR EXTRASYSTOLE (VPB)

( entricular ectopic beats)

PB may arise from either of the two ventricles, the QRS complex is wide and T-wave is in op osite direction of major component of QRS complex. The subsequent normal impulse re hes ventricular muscle in its refractory pause and does not result in a contraction. So there is co pensatory pause after the ventricular extrasystole. The total duration between the previous an the subsequent normal beat is equal to two beats. Extrasystoles may be unifocal or multifocal; th unifocal beats are similar in appearance while multifocal beats are different in contour and coupling intervals.

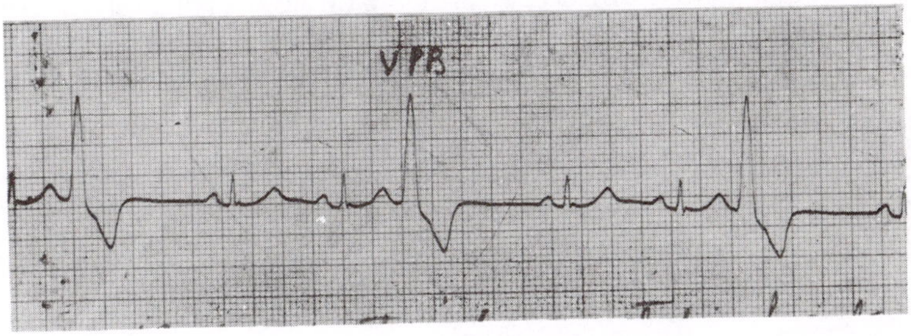


Fig.18.14 : Ventricular extrasystoles

If ventricular extrasystole occurs earlier in diastole, the next normal impulse may produce a contraction which is interpolated between two normal beats. Extrasystoles may produce coupling of beats, known as pulsus bigeminus.

When ventricular ectopics occur too early in the cardiac cycle, it may almost come nearest to T-wave and this is called 'R on T' ventricular ectopics. In these situations sudden ventricular tachycardia or ventricular fibrillation may be precipitated, hence requires close watch and treatment.

Similarly late ventricular ectopics may occur immediately following normal wave and therefore the normal impulse depicting the normal P wave will not be able to initiate a normal QRS. The ectopic ventricular beat may also have a slurred up-stroke, hence may be mistaken for a delta wave of Wolff-Parkinson-White syndrome.

## PARASYSTOLE

In this type the ectopic, ventricular focus discharges in between two normal beats without disturbing the normal sinus rhythm. Occasionally ventricles may be simultaneously activated by both ectopic and normal impulses, then the resulting beat is a fusion beat.

U-wave in ECG represents supranormal recovery phase. Subthreshold stimuli can activate ventricles during this phase. Any stimulus can form parallel pacemaker competing for control. This phenomenon is known as parasystole. Sinus impulse and parasystolic impulse may overlap to produce a fusion beat. Though prognosis is not bad, parasystole may mask underlying ventricular tachycardia. Parasystolic rhythm, more often than not, is unresponsive to anti-arrhythmic therapy.

## AETIOLOGY OF EXTRASYSTOLES

Though it may occur in healthy individuals, these may be associated with myocardial disease. Tea, coffee and tobacco in excess may be responsible. In elderly people these should be more seriously considered especially when they are frequent. They arise from many sites i.e. when they are multifocal, they are pathognomonic of myocardial disease, and/or digitalis toxicity. In patients of I.H.D. occurrence of frequent E.S. often heralds an impending infarction, though some cardiologists do not agree to this view.

### Clinical features

Ectopic beats are sometimes forceful and the patient complains of palpitations and becomes apprehensive. Increased volume of post-extrasystolic normal beat may be felt as a thrust. Sometimes anxious patient becomes panicky. Flutterring sensation occurs due to irregularity. Patient may also have a sinking feeling.

### Treatment

Infrequent extrasystoles require no therapy especially in the young. The background is important. If there is no adverse history and clinical findings are normal, reassuring the patient usually suffices. Aggravating factors like excessive tea, coffee, alcohol, tobacco should be banned. However, when they are associated with some cardiac pathology or digitalis intoxication, they will need proper treatment.

Injudicious use of drugs may be more harmful. Most drugs often used indiscriminately have some side-effects. In young people without heart disease, remove possible exciting factors and keep watch.

When there is a background myocardial disease, close watch is more important. Ventricular E.S., coupled beats, multifocal E.S and unusual premature beats (so called R on T-wave) are more serious. In olden days quinidine used to be given to suppress these EB's but suppression serves no useful purpose. Now we have newer drugs but none of them are free from side-effects.

Beta-adrenergic agents may be used carefully orally but are contraindicated in heart failure, bronchial asthma, diabetes mellitus and peripheral vascular disorders.

Disopyramide orally in dosage of 100 to 150 mg 3 to 4 times daily may be useful. The side-effects are anticholinergic in type e.g. dry mouth, urinary retention (in elderly) and dangerous in presence of glaucoma. A special chapter is included on the use of 'Drugs in Cardiology' which should be carefully mastered.

## ATRIAL FIBRILLATION

### Pathophysiology

Atrial fibrillation is observed in many cardiac disorders. Atrial ectopic rate is 350 to 600 per minute. There is varying degree of atrioventricular block. Ventricular response being totally irregular. It was believed formerly that circus movement may cause this irregular rhythm. Atria might have several discharging sites, which may form irregular impulses.

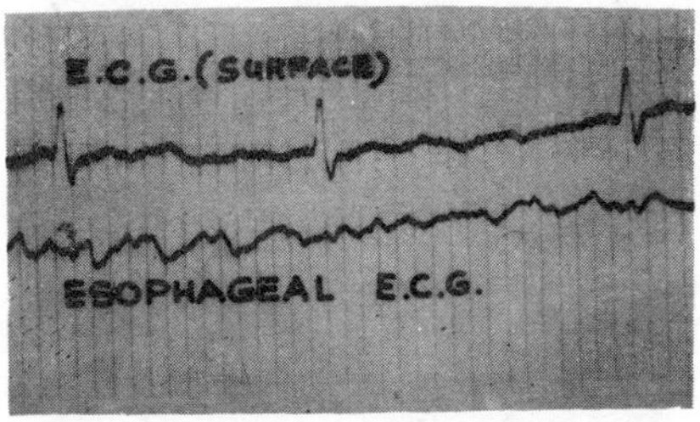


Fig.18.15(a) : Atrial fibrillation noted in surface ECG and oesophageal lead ECG.

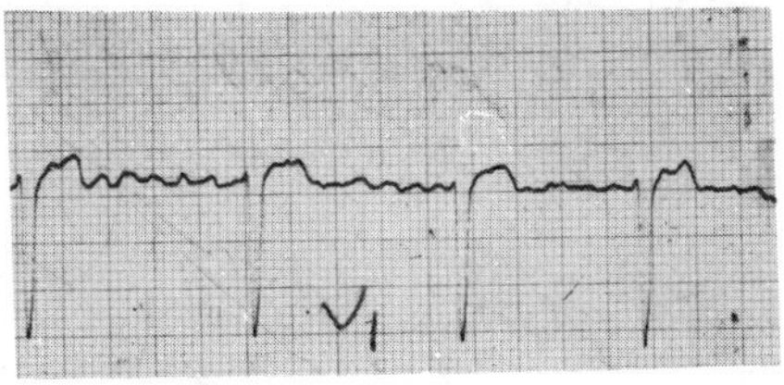


Fig.18.15(b) : shows lead $V_1$ with atrial fibrillation.

### Aetiology

Atrial fibrillation is observed with undermentioned conditions :

(1) Rheumatic heart diseases especially mitral stenosis
(2) Ischaemic heart disease
(3) Hypertensive heart disease
(4) Thyrotoxicosis
(5) Pericarditis
(6) Cardiomyopathy
(7) Idiopathic or lone fibrillation
(8) Miscellaneous conditions like chronic lung disease, or mediastinal tumours.
(9) Post-operatively — after thoracic surgery
(10) Congenital heart disease like A.S.D.

### Pathophysiology

Atrial fibrillation is observed in many cardiac disorders. Atrial ectopic rate is 350 to 600 per minute. There is varying degree of atrioventricular block. Ventricular response being totally irregular. Usually AV node prevents ventricular rate to go higher than 200 min, generally much slower than auricular rate. However, ventricular rhythm will be slow and regular during atrial fibrillation, if there is pre-existing complete AV block. It was believed formerly that circus movement may cause this irregular rhythm. Atria might have several discharging sites, which may form irregular impulses.

### Clinical features

The pulse is irregularly irregular. Though usually fast, it may be slow depending upon degree of

AV block. On auscultation heart rate is irregular and faster. Many weak contractions cannot produce radial pulse and there is a difference between heart rate and pulse rate. This is called pulse deficit. In jugular veins, there is no evidence of atrial contractions i.e. 'a' waves are not seen. First heart-sound varies in intensity. Second sound may or may not be heard. In mitral stenosis systolic murmurs are heard but presystolic rumble of mitral stenosis is absent because of ineffective atrial contractions, ECG shows :

(1) Normal P waves are absent;

(2) Fibrillary waves are seen, replacing 'P' waves;

(3) Irregularly placed QRS complexes have varying 'R' amplitude.

**Diagnosis**

Pulse-apex deficit is usually diagnostic, Multiple extrasystoles may mimic atrial fibrillation. Here though pulse-apex deficit is present it is not usually high, multiple ectopic beats may disappear after exercise. Atrial flutter needs to be ruled out. Jugular veins show flutter waves.

In partial heart block, dropped beats may create confusion but 'a' waves can be observed in jugular veins. ECG is diagnostic.

**Treatment**

Aetiological factor e.g. thyrotoxicosis if discovered should be treated. However, main intention should be to control ventricular rate by digitalisation. However, if adequate digitalisation fails to control heart rate, beta-blocker or calcium channel blocker in small dose can be administered. Good old drug quinidine is replaced nowadays with recently available calcium-blockers or beta-blockers. In chronic rheumatic heart disease, if there is persistent auricular fibrillation, anticoagulants should be used to prevent embolism. When above mentioned drug regimen fails electrical defibrillation is attempted. Due to risk of embolism, anti-coagulants are given before 'electroversion'.

## ATRIAL FLUTTER

In atrial flutter, atrial contractions are both co-ordinated and regular. The ventricles are discharged by every second, third or fourth impulse, thereby producing varying types of block e.g. 2 : 1, 3 : 1, or 4 : 1.

**Aetiology**

Aetiological factors are more or less the same as in atrial fibrillation. Sometimes it is idiopathic as no cause can be detected.

**Clinical features**

The heart rate is faster and regular. Atria may contract around 300 times a minute. But due to varying degrees of block at A.V. level, ventricular contractions may be 75 to 150 per minute, depending upon the degree of block. Carotid sinus pressure may reduce the rate to half but effect is temporary. Flutter waves may be seen in jugular venous pulse. In ECG 'saw-tooth' appearance of atrial waves with ventricular response at alternate or every third or fourth beat settles the diagnosis of atrial flutter.

When there is 2 : 1 conduction in atrial flutter, it may be mistaken for sinus tachycardia. Leads II, AVF, $V_1$, $V_2$ and $V_6$ should be carefully inspected to detect F waves,

**Treatment**

Treat the aetiological factor. Ventricular rate should be controlled by digitalisation which converts atrial flutter into fibrillation. Withdraw digitalis at this stage abruptly and sinus rhythm may be restored or flutter may continue with increased degree of AV block.

More rapid and safe way is direct-current QRS-synchronised shock, when electroversion is planned, anticoagulant should be administered one week before cardioversion to minimise chances of embolism.

Propranolol may be used to control rapid rate after digitalisation. In some selected cases atrial pacing is done.

## PAROXYSMAL TACHYCARDIA

Paroxysmal tachycardia may be supraventricular or ventricular. Supraventricular tachycardias are :

(1) Paroxysmal atrial fibrillation and flutter (vide supra)

(2) Paroxysmal atrial tachycardia

(3) Paroxysmal nodal tachycardia or AV-junctional tachycardias.

Definite differentiation between supraventricular and ventricular tachycardia must be done by E.C.G., to discover where the ectopic focus is situated i.e. atrial, nodal or ventricular as treatment of ventricular tachycardia is entirely different.

### PAROXYSMAL ATRIAL TACHYCARDIA (PAT)

PAT may be idiopathic. It is mostly seen in young healthy individuals. Excessive tea, tobacco or coffee may be the cause. It may occur in healthy adult without any heart disease. However, digitalis toxicity is also an important cause.

The onset is abrupt and also it terminates abruptly, justifying the title 'paroxysmal'. Duration is variable from a few seconds to hours or even days. The termination of attack is also sudden. Palpitations frighten the patient, who becomes anxious and depressed mentally. Patient complains of precordial discomfort or anginal pain. Polyuria occurs at the end of attack unless the attack is brief. In diseased heart, prolonged paroxysms may produce syncope or Stoke Adam's syndrome and cardiac failure.

**ECG shows usually a normal** QRS complex with upright or **inverted** P-waves (Fig.18.17).

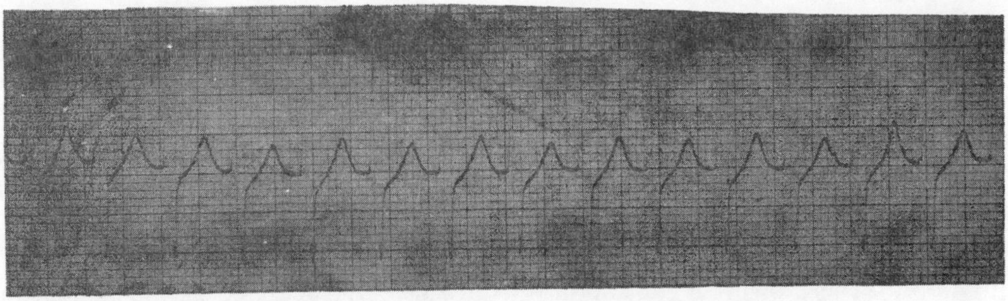

Fig.18.16 : Supraventricular Tachycardia. Note : 'P' waves not visible in the ECG.

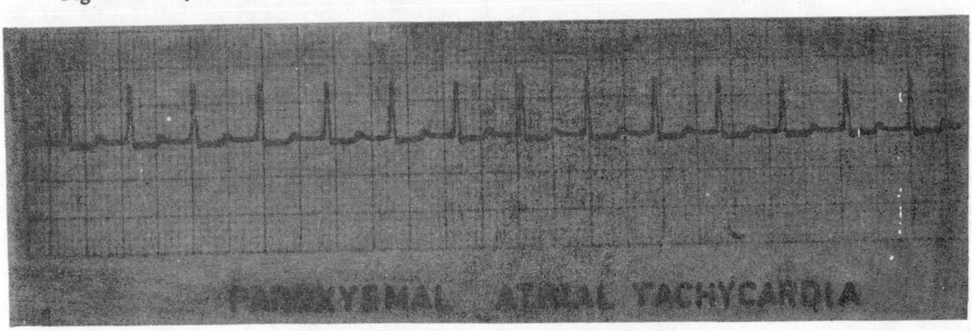


Fig.18.17 : Paroxysmal atrial tachycardia

**Paroxysmal nodal tachycardia**

It is very rare. The ECG is diagnostic. QRS complex is normal; inverted P waves may precede, may get buried in or may follow QRS complex.

**Paroxysmal ventricular tachycardia (PVT)**

The commonest cause of PVT is advanced heart disease, though also observed in digitalis toxicity. Patient has similar complaints like paroxysmal atrial tachycardia. Jugular venous pulse may show cannon waves (high amplitude 'a' waves). First heart sound may be occasionally heard loud. ECG shows wide and bizarre QRS complexes usually at a very high rate.

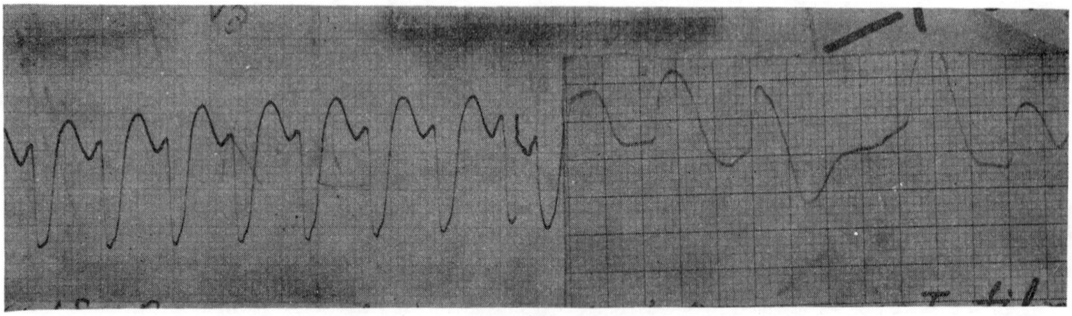

Fig.18.18 : Paroxysmal Ventricular tachycardia going to fibrillation

**Treatment**

Transient symptomless tachycardias do not require any special treatment except "assure and watch".

**Atrial tachycardia**

(1) Assure the patient and use tranquilizers.

(2) Vagal tone can be increased by mechanical means :

(a) Drink a glass of ice-cold water;

(b) Induce vomiting by putting finger in oropharynx;

(c) Perform Valsalva manoeuvre. Forcible expiration with glottis closed;

(d) One can hold the breath as long as he can;

(e) Ice-cold bag may be applied on one side of face;

(f) Carotid sinus pressure is gently done on one side of the neck. Be careful in old people. Right-sided massage is usually more effective.

The patient should have no pillow. He must lie flat on the bed. Turn the head to one side. Locate carotid sinus which lies near the upper border of thyroid cartilage and opposite the angle of jaw. It lies on transverse process of the vertebra. It is massaged up and down firmly for about 5 to 10 seconds. During carotid massage heart rate must be constantly watched lest patient should develop asystole.

If mechanical measures fail, I.V. verapamil 5 to 10 mg given very slowly taking 2 to 5 minute. Disopyramide usually terminates the attack especially in WPW syndrome. Digoxin is also useful but check if it is digitalis-induced or not.

If required, electrocardioversion is attempted after discontinuing digitalis. However, in some patients where anaesthesia cannot be given or if taking digitalis from a long time, atrial pacing is attempted.

**Treatment**

Drugs used to control supraventricular tachycardia may be used judiciously. These are beta-blockers, digoxin, verapamil, disopyramide, procainamide or quinidine.

It is necessary to be cautious in using these drugs, as combination may be harmful e.g. combination of verapamil and $\beta$- blockers may be dangerous. (Refer to the chapter on drugs in cardiology). In auricular fibrillation of W-P-W syndrome digitalis should not be used. The new drug amiodarone deserves trial in refractory cases.

In some cases drugs may not produce the desired effect so pacing or surgical division of bundle of Kent may be required.

It is, however, true that most cases of WPW syndrome have a benign course.

**Treatment of ventricular tachycardia**

(a) Electrical cardioversion is the method of choice.

(b) If due to myocardial infarction, I.V. lidocaine (xylocaine) is first choice. Alternatively, procainamide I.V. can be used. Nowadays, oral tocainide also has been found to be very useful.

In digitalis toxicity, electrical cardioversion is usually avoided and propranolol is used. Phenytoin sodium is also useful.

Mexiletine hydrochloride, disopyramide and amiodarone are nowadays used in refractory cases. Mexiletine resembles lignocaine but can be orally used. Disopyramide has quinidine-like action. Amiodarone is Ca-channel blocker.

Recently many drugs have been tried including disopyramide and the latest is amiodarone but these drugs should be cautiously used by the experienced. Surgical division of re-entrant circuit has been attempted by experts, when drugs fail to control.

If bradycardia is interspaced with ventricular tachycardia, some cardiologists have used I.V. atropine as drug of first choice in dosage of 0.3 mg I.V. The dose may be repeated at five-minute intervals two or three times. However, general practitioners should refer those cases to cardiology units whenever possible.

Surgical techniques are being developed to dissect abnormal focus to abolish recurrent ventricular tachycardia. Electrophysiological instruments are also developed for pin-pointing pathological tissues.

## HEART BLOCK

**(1) Sino-Atrial Block (S.A. Block)**

In S.A. block the cardiac impulse is initiated from the S.A. node, but there is a block between the S.A. node and the atrium. So a complete PQRST complex is omitted. It is usually due to vagal overactivity in a hyperactive carotid sinus. Digitalis overdose and inferior wall myocardial infarction sometimes cause S.A. block.

*E.C.G.* – PQRST-complex is completely missed and P.P. interval is twice the normal length. Treatment is directed towards the cause. Sometimes asystole is continued. Stokes-Adams attacks occur and pacing may be needed in these cases.

**(2) Atrio-Ventricular Block (A.V. Block)**

When an impulse travelling from atrium to ventricle is blocked or delayed, A.V. block occurs in varying degrees. When atrial contraction exceeds ventricular, partial A.V. block is present. The common causes of A.V. block are idiopathic fibrosis and I.H.D. This can also occur due to digitalis toxicity, drugs like verapamil, rheumatic fever, collagen diseases, including rheumatoid arthritis, diphtheria, dystrophia myotonica, congenital heart diseases and cardiac surgery.

A.V. block may be of three types e.g. first degree, second degree or third degree block (complete heart block). The first two types are also called partial heart block.

(a) **First-degree block**

Here P-R interval is prolonged and is more than 0.2 seconds. E.C.G. is diagnostic.

(b) **Second degree block (partial heart block)**

1) Mobitz type I (Wenckebach type) — In this variety P.R. interval gradually increases and then a beat is dropped.

2) Mobitz type II — In this type QRS complex is dropped without any antecedant lengthening of PR inerval.

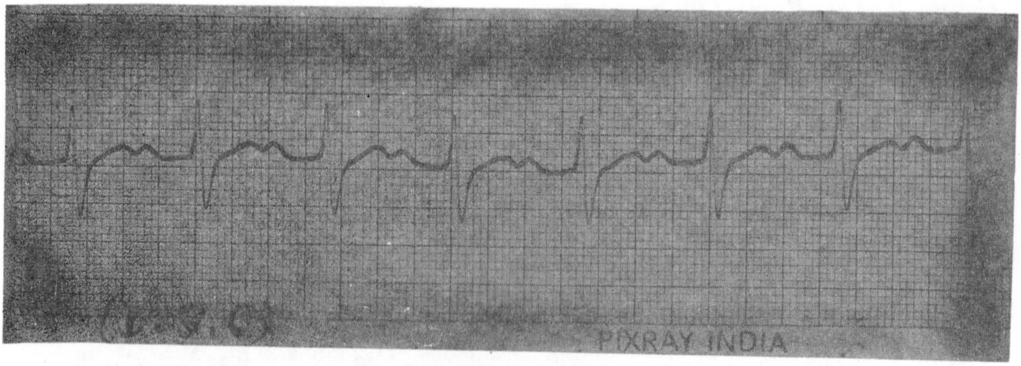


Fig.18.19 : 1st Degree A.V. Block showing prolonged P.R. interval

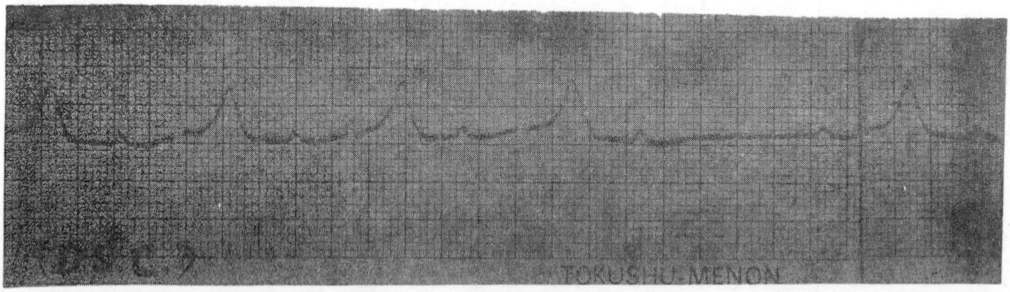


Fig.18.20 : Wencke-back type A.V. Block

(c) **Third degree of complete heart block**

In complete HB the atria and the ventricles contract independently. Ventricles beat at much slow rate and the rhythm is known as idioventricular rhythm. PR interval varying erratically is the clue.

**Aetiology of heart block**

Heart-block usually indicates significant pathology in heart. It has been observed in ischaemic heart disease, rheumatic heart disease, valvular heart disease like aortic stenosis and digitalis overdose. Heart-blocks have been also documented in diphtheria and syphilis. Heart block may be present at birth so it is known as congenital heart block. In congenital heart block the

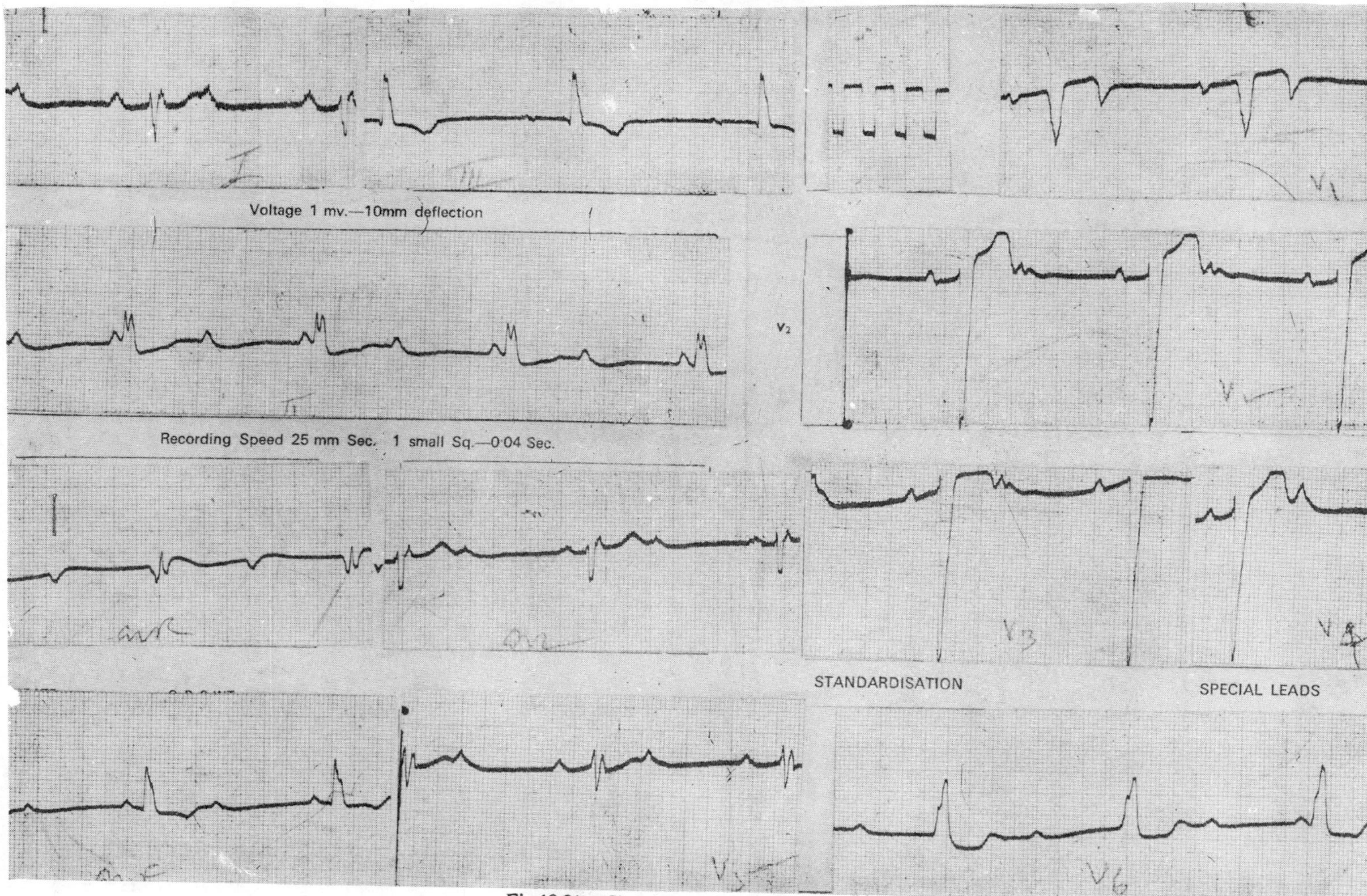


Fig.18.21 : Showing complete heart block

ventricular rate is not very slow. Heart block has also been noted in cardiomyopathy, collagen disorders and following cardiac surgery. Atrial fibrillation and flutter may be complicated by complete heart block.

**Clinical diagnosis**

The following signs have to be observed in bed-side assessment. Note the 'a' waves in the J.V.P., heart sounds, the pulse and effect of exercise in bed. In partial heart block, some 'a' waves are not followed by heart-sounds. Atrial waves ('a' waves) are more than ventricular rate. Exercise slows the heart rate. In complete heart block, atrial activity revealed by 'a' waves in the neck and ventricular activity revealed by heart-sounds with pulse have no normal relation. Heart-rate is usually less than 40/min but in type congenital it is around 50/min; 'a' waves are seen irregularly. If atria and ventricles contract simultaneously, a large 'a' wave (Cannon waves) are seen and loud first heart sounds are heard on auscultation with muffled atrial sounds during diastole. In complete heart block, heart-rate does not vary with the exercise. If asystole is prolonged, Stokes Adams syndrome may occur.

**E.C.G. :** The P waves and QRS complexes lose their normal relation. The P-waves are many more than QRS complexes which are slower.

**Treatment**

Aetiological factor should be treated, whenever identified. Isoprenaline and belladonna group of drugs have been used. Sustained release oral isoprenaline 30 mg × Q.I.D. may help. Sometimes corticosteroids are useful. If Stoke Adams attacks occur artificial pacemaker should be implanted. In heart blocks, if physical activity becomes severely limited or congestive failure occurs, pacing should be considered. However, function of condition of myocardium should be taken into account, as pacemakers can generate impulse but cannot cure myocardial damage. Congenital H.B. may not require pacemaker unless symptomatic.

**AV dissociation**

This is a situation where atria and ventricles are independently beating but it is not same conditions as third degree of heart block. It is important to recognise it, as in heart block it may be necessary to implant a pacemaker, which is not required in AV dissociation. In AV dissociation some of the atrial impulses may block and produce a premature ventricular contraction before the ventricular focus discharges. (Refer to Marriot's Practical Electrocardiography 7th Ed. P.304)

## STOKE-ADAMS SYNDROME

When cerebral circulation stops more than a few seconds, consciousness is lost and convulsions may follow. Such a situation arises in complete heart block, leading to cerebral anoxia. Similar situation occurs also in ventricular tachycardia or fibrillation.

During cardiac asystole cerebral circulation also ceases. If this continues for more than two seconds convulsions occur and if more than two minutes death may follow. During attack the face becomes pale and peripheral cyanosis occurs. When heart resumes activity a characteristic flush spreads from below upwards up to the neck and face. History is very helpful in diagnosis.

**Treatment**

There may be spontaneous termination of the attack. Adrenaline 1 in 1000 (0.3 to 0.5 ml.) may be given I.M. or I.V. depending upon gravity of situation. Long-acting adrenaline — in oil may be given for prolonged effect. If cardiac asystole continues, cardiopulmonary resuscitation should be started without any delay. Once the patient is resuscitated, need for pacemaker should be considered. Digitalis is contraindicated unless the patient is in failure.

## BUNDLE-BRANCH BLOCK

When there is block in bundle-branch, excitation is delayed. Depending upon the situation of the block, ECG pattern is characteristic. Right bundle branch block (RBBB) is usually benign in most cases but it is also observed in ischaemic heart disease, hypertensive heart disease and congenital heart disease especially A.S.D.

Left bundle branch block (LBBB) is usually associated with organic heart disease.

Left bundle has two fascicles, hence block may appear either in left fascicle or right fascicle or in both. In some individuals three fascicles may be present. In left anterior hemiblock, the block is situated in left fascicle and in left posterior hemi-block, posterior fascicle is blocked.

Bundle-branch-blocks are difficult to diagnose clinically. ECG pattern is diagnostic.

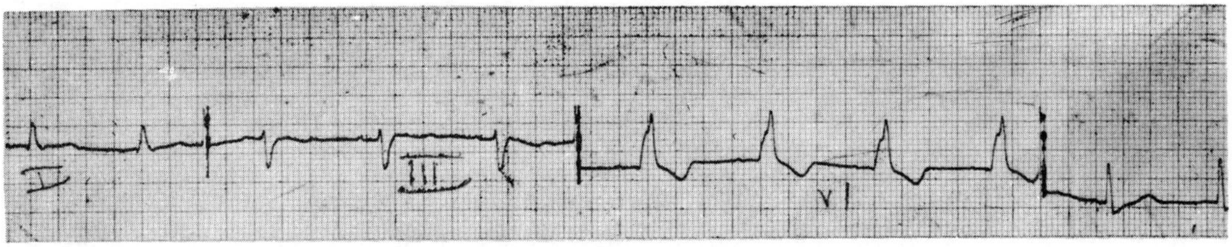

Fig.18.22(a) — showing right bundle branch block

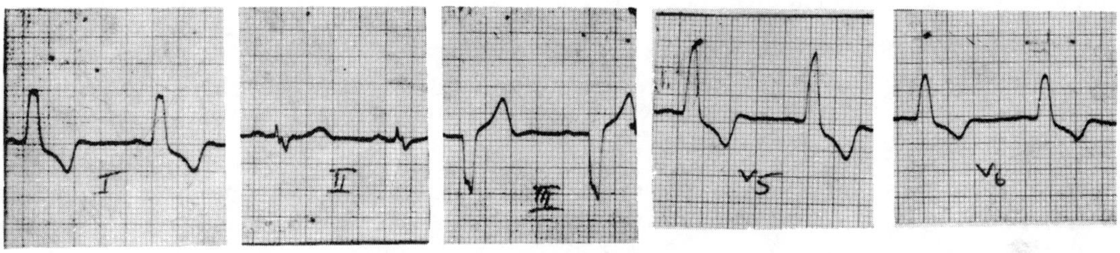

Fig.18.22 (b) — showing left bundle branch block.

Recognition of BBB is important as it may mimic corresponding ventricular hypertrophy and strain pattern, from which it must be differentiated. Ventricular extrasystoles also should not be mistaken for BBB. The important features of BBB are as follows :

| Leads | RBBB | LBBB |
|---|---|---|
| I | Wide S wave | No. Q; monophasic R |
| $V_1$ | M-Shaped QRS, variants of RSR' or QR, wide R | QS or rS |
| $V_6$ | Early intrinsicoid deflection and wide S wave | No Q; late intrinsicoid deflection; monophasic R |

## HEMIBLOCKS

### Axis deviation and fascicular blocks

The left bundle of His has two fascicles, the anterior and posterior supplying the anterosuperior and posterosuperior surface of the left ventricle. Most hearts may have an additional fascicle of left bundle called "centriseptal" branch. Some bundle consists of fan-like distribution of its terminal parts so there are no clear-cut anterior, superior or centripetal branches.

However, for practical purposes the hemiblocks are of two types involving anterosuperior or anterior hemi-block and posteroinferior or posterior hemi block.

Study of axis deviation is important to diagnose hemiblocks.

**Hexaxial reference system**

The precordial or chest leads of ECG reflect the electrical activity of horizontal plane while limb leads reflect the electrical activity of frontal plane. This is the hexaxial representation system.

By the hexaxial reference system it is possible to calculate the mean QRS axis and its position, In the frontal QRS axis, left axis deviation (LAD) has Lead I as dominant positive waye and both II and III are negative. In lead II if R wave remains larger than S, LAD is unlikely. In RAD the QRS in lead I is negative while in II and III it is positive.

Normally the mean frontal QRS axis is between AVL and AVF (i.e. $-30°$ to $90°$).

If the axis shows counter-clockwise rotation (i.e. to the left of AVL) i.e. less than $-30°$ it is abnormal LAD while if it is more than $+90°$ it is RAD.

It is also possible to express the exact mean frontal QRS axis in degrees fairly accurately but for clinical purposes such precision is not required (for details of the controversies, reference may be made to Marriot's Practical Electrocardiography).

**Anterior hemiblock**

In this situation left ventricle is activated via posterior fascicle of left bundle resulting in upright dominant R in lead I & AVL and deep S in leads II, III & AVF. The mean frontal axis will show abnormal LAD.

As LAD may also occur in inferior myocardial infarction care must be taken to interpret anterior hemiblock. Note the presence of initial r-wave in II, III and AVF and initial Q in leads I and AVL.

**Posterior hemiblock**

In posterior hemiblock there will be initial positive small r in leads I and AVL and an initial negative q in leads II, III and AVF along with abnormal RAD. The lead II and III will have upright R and lead I predominantly negative. Other causes of RAD e.g. RVH should be excluded to make a diagnosis of posterior hemiblock.

**Bifascicular and Trifascicular block**

When RBB as well as the fascicles of LBBB are blocked, there will be complete HB. Bifascicular block commonly occurs in RBB plus anterior fascicle block (i.e. left side). Posterior fascicle is rarely involved with RBB as posterior fascicle usually has very good blood supply.

When both fascicles are involved (left side has two or three fascicles) there is complete HB.

**Sick Sinus Syndrome**

It is a sino-atrial disorder in which the sinus node (chief pacemaker of heart) fails to produce an impulse or fails to transmit the impulse from sinus node to atria, resulting in asystole or bradycardia. Sometimes tachycardias may be associated with this condition, hence it is also called 'Trachy-brady' syndrome.

**Causes**

(1) Idiopathic fibrosis of the sinus node
(2) I.H.D.
(3) Cardiomyopathy

(4) Drug like digitalis or quinidine and some modern anti-dysrhythmic agents
(5) Cardiac surgery especially repair of A.S.D.

**Clinical features**

It may occur in young or old, usually in the old people.

Symptoms are dizzy spells, syncope or sometimes palpitations. It should not be mistaken for sinus arrhythmias.

**E.C.G.**

(1) Sinus bradycardia — heart rate may be 30 to 40 beats per minute.
(2) Absence of sinus node activity i.e. no P waves can be seen or may occur intermittently (dropped P waves). The intervals between recorded P waves in ECG are arithmetical multiples of original cycle length.
(3) Escape beats may occur from subsidiary pacemakers. Atrial ectopics also may occur.

Paroxysmal tachycardias, auricular fibrillation and flutter may also occur.

**Diagnosis**

The diagnosis is confirmed by ECG but as it is not usually possible to take ECG during the attack, 24 to 48 hours ambulatory monitoring may be done.

**Treatment**

Anti-arrhythmic drugs may worsen the situation, hence the ideal treatment is implantation of pacemaker. Therefore, suspected cases sick sinus syndrome; tachybrady syndrome or A.V. junctional disease should be referred to specialised cardiac centres.

**Post-tachycardia syndrome**

ST-T changes are sometimes due to tachycardia. Tachycardia shortens diastolic interval and therefore curtails coronary blood flow which occurs during the diastole. If there is pre-existing symptomless coronary atherosclerosis ST-T changes may occur during tachycardia consisting of depression of ST-T segment and inversion of T-wave. ST-T wave changes and may persist for hours or days after the tachycardia is over. This has been called post-tachycardia syndrome (Marriot). It is felt that this phenomenon may be renamed as "Threatened Infarction".

## WOLFF-PARKINSON-WHITE SYNDROME

In the Wolff-Parkinson-White syndrome (WPW syndrome), one ventricle may get activated earlier. This is supposed to be through an accessory bundle (bundle of Kent). As conduction is accelerated, so also it is known as accelerated conduction syndrome or pre-excitation syndrome. Though usually benign, it forecasts the possibility of on-coming atrial arrhythmias, especially paroxysmal tachycardia, predominantly affecting males in all age groups; diagnosis is only by E.C.G. (short PR interval, lengthened QRS duration with initial delta wave).

The syndrome is classified into two types :

Type A and type B depending on the shape of $V_1$, complex. In A type, ventricular complex is prominently positive where the bundle of Kent is on the left side of the heart and in type B it is on the right side and ventricular complex is negative. This explanation, however, is not accepted by all.

Two types of arrhythmias may occur in W-P-W syndrome i.e. :

(1) Paroxysmal supra-ventricular tachycardia
(2) Atrial fibrillation.

It should be remembered that digitalis though useful in atrial fibrillation is dangerous in W-P-W syndrome as the bundle of Kent will allow rapid contraction of auricular impulse to ventricle causing dangerous ventricular tachycardia.

## LOWN-GANONG-LEAVING SYNDROME

The typical picture also consists of short PR in interval with normal QRS without any slurring. There is tendency to paroxysmal tachycardia. In this syndrome also there is a duplicate path of conduction between atrium and bundle of His, a by-pass of AV node. As the by-pass directly goes to Bundle of His, QRS has no delta wave as in WPW syndrome. (Refer to the chapter on Drug Therapy in Cardiology and anti-arrhythmic drugs).

# SYSTEMIC HYPERTENSION

*K.K. DATEY*
*NARENDRA KUMAR*
*A.A. HINGORANI*

### Introduction

Blood pressure (BP) is defined as the lateral force which the column of blood exerts against the walls of the vessels through which it flows. BP is regulated mainly by peripheral resistance and cardiac output.

The average normal at birth is about 65/40 mm Hg and between 5 and 10 years, 90-110/50-70 mm Hg. Ideally, in adults the BP should be 100-120 mm Hg systolic and 70-80 mm Hg diastolic. There is no unanimous agreement on the arbitrary cut-off point between normal and high BP though 140/90 mm Hg and above is accepted by many as hypertension. However, it has been shown by Life Insurance statistics covering millions of lives that figures higher than 120/80 mm Hg increase morbidity and mortality and, therefore, in adults the ideal blood pressure should be 120/80 mm Hg. Many physicians believe that only elevated diastolic pressure is of serious consequence. However, newer data have clearly indicated that the risk of high systolic BP is equally, if not more, important than diastolic B.P., in causing cardiovascular catastrophy.

Hypertension in fact poses a great threat to life at all ages and for both sexes, and the relative risk is not reduced with advancing age. It is a misconception that blood pressure necessarily rises with age, as this is neither inevitable nor innocuous. There are several communities in Chile, Ester Island, Pukapuka, Tokelav, Papua,New Guinea, and certain parts of South Africa and Asia in whom there is little or no increase in systolic or diastolic blood pressure with age. These communities are usually small and isolated. They have high level of physical activity and low salt intake, four grams or less per day. However, due to our present-day life-style and diet, the incidence of hypertension increases with age.

*Casual blood pressure*

Contrary to prevailing notions, casual blood pressure readings are not misleading. Readings many years apart correlate well, and the Framingham evidence reveals that the risk of cardiovascular event was strikingly related to casually determined blood pressure.

Again, the lowest blood pressure recorded in a patient should not be the basis for deferring the treatment of the average of a series of reading is high.

*Labile blood pressure*

Greater lability of blood pressure is definitely not innocuous. Blood pressure is labile, and as the pressure gets higher it also becomes more labile. Hence, the lability should not be a reason for not treating a patient with high blood pressure.

In the early stages, hypertension is usually labile, showing an inappropriate transient rise in response to stress, emotion, cold, or physical exertion. The labile prehypertensive state later

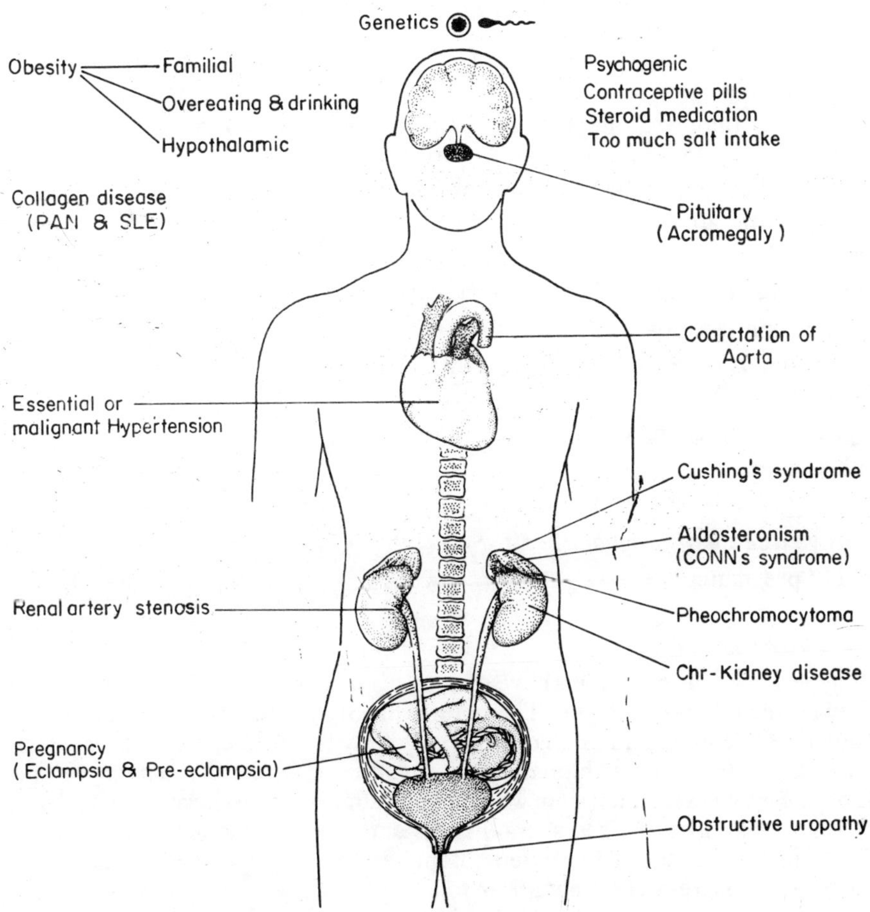


18.23 : Important factors in the aetiology of hypertension. Many drugs (P.24) are also responsible — *(Editor)*

becomes established and the BP is then persistently elevated. The incidence of hypertension in India is between 5 and 15% in the adult population (it is about 25% in the West), and accounts for about 20% of cardiovascular patients admitted to a hospital.

**Aetiology and pathogenesis**

Hypertension is a manifestation and not a disease by itself. In about 90 to 95% of the cases no cause can be found and, therefore, it is called essential, primary, idiopathic, or benign. The remaining 5 to 10% of the cases are secondary hypertension in which an underlying cause can be detected, and in these, hypertension is usually present before the age of 30 years. (Fig. 18.23).

**Classification of hypertension**

(A) Essential hypertension

(B) Secondary hypertension

Important and common causes of secondary hypertension are Fig. 18.23 :

1. *Organic diseases* :
   (a) Coarctation of aorta
   (b) Renal diseases (glomerulonephritis; pyelonephritis; renal tuberculosis; polycystic disease; hydronephrosis; renal tumour; renal artery stenosis)
   (c) Diseases of the adrenal medulla (pheochromocytoma)
   (d) Diseases of the adrenal cortex (Conn's syndrome; Cushing's syndrome; adrenogenital syndrome)
2. *Hypertension due to drugs* : (This is often reversible.)
   (a) Hormonal contraceptives
   (b) ACTH and corticosteroids
   (c) Ephedrine
   (d) Tricyclic antidepressants
   (e) Amphetamine
   (f) Licorice and carbenoxolone
3. *Hypertensive disease of pregnancy*
   Toxaemia of pregnancy

**Essential Hypertension**

Essential hypertension is common above the age of 40 years, and the incidence increases with age. Heredity plays an important role. The natural history of essential hypertension is variable, complex, and unpredictable, and as it contributes greatly to cardiac, cerebrovascular, and renal diseases, and takes a heavy toll of human life, *it is a misnomer to call it a benign disease.* These individuals have a labile vascular system which reacts abnormally to nervous stimuli as a result of excitement, emotional disturbances, mental stress and strain of modern life, etc. It is believed that these stressful events lead to increased adrenaline and cortisone secretions which act upon the renin-angiotensin system and play a key role in primary and secondary hypertension. The renin produced in the ischaemic kidney acts with angiotensinogen (a substance produced in the liver) to produce angiotensin I (hypertensin I). This is a mild vasoconstrictive substance and is enzymatically converted in plasma into angiotensin II (hypertensin II) which is a powerful vasoconstrictor and is responsible for increased peripheral resistance including that in the arterioles of the kidney. This further aggravates hypertension and a vicious cycle is established.

Recent studies indicate that hypertension may be associated with high, normal, or low plasma renin activity. *Those with high plasma renin activity have a more severe course and unfavourable prognosis (higher incidence of cardiac complications).* They usually respond to renin lowering agents like beta-blockers. Those with low plasma renin activity have better prognosis and they often respond to diuretics.

Hypertension accelerates atherosclerosis in the coronary, cerebral, and peripheral arteries. In hypertension the left ventricle has to work against increased blood pressure. This leads to hypertrophy of the left ventricle and ultimately results in its failure. On the other hand, the hypertrophied heart needs more blood which the atherosclerotic coronary arteries are not able to provide and this may manifest as ischaemic heart disease (angina, myocardial infarction, etc.).

*Hypertension in infancy and childhood*

BP should be recorded with the correct size cuff. Children with even transient increases in blood pressure are more likely to develop hypertension in later life.

*Hypertension in the elderly*

Hypertension in the elderly is of two types — classical hypertension, i.e. diastolic BP more than 95 mm Hg., and pure systolic hypertension with systolic pressure of 160 mm Hg. or more with diastolic BP less than 95 mm Hg. In pure systolic hypertensive patients, the incidence of ECG abnormalities is more than in non-hypertensive elderly patients. Control of hypertension in both the types is essential as it reduces morbidity and mortality. However, treatment in the elderly should be less aggressive, and *drugs should be selected taking into consideration the associated diseases, e.g. coronary artery disease, cerebrovascular and obstructive airways diseases.*

Moreover, renal and autonomic nervous functions are depressed in the elderly hypertensive patients and, therefore, excretion of antihypertensive drugs is slow and these patients are more prone to postural hypotension. Therefore, smaller doses of the antihypertensive drugs are usually adequate.

**Hypertensive disease of pregnancy**

The hypertensive disease of pregnancy (also termed as pre-eclampsia, toxaemia of pregnancy, etc.) is an important cause of perinatal mortality and premature birth. It also accounts for high maternal morbidity and mortality. The cause of hypertension in toxaemia of pregnancy is not known and many theories have been postulated.

The presence of two or more of the triad components, viz. *hypertension, proteinuria, and oedema confirms the diagnosis of toxaemia or eclampsia of pregnancy.* Other symptoms may be blurred vision, generalised or occipital headache, nausea, vomiting, and oliguria. Toxaemia of pregnancy is more common in the first pregnancy, especially in those with pre-existing essential hypertension, hydatidiform mole, diabetes mellitus, or Rhesus incompatibility.

The significance of level of blood pressure during pregnancy differs from that in the non-pregnant state, and it is erroneous to extrapolate data from non-pregnant to pregnant women. Even slight elevations of diastolic arterial pressure are of significance in pregnancy. A *diastolic blood pressure recording of 85 mm Hg or more, irrespective of systolic blood pressure, should be considered abnormal,* and if encountered in the third trimester indicates urgent need for special medical attention. If pre-pregnancy recording or sequential BP recording during pregnancy is available, a rise of 15 mm Hg. or more in the diastolic reading should be considered abnormal.

**Method of blood pressure recording**

The width of a standard BP cuff (rubber bag) is 12 cm. Cuff sizes for infants and children should be : under 8 years, 8-9 cm; under 4 years, 5-6 cm; and under 1 year, 2.5 cm or less; and for the obese it should be 16 cm. *If BP of an obese person is taken with a standard cuff, the systolic reading will be higher by about 10-30 mm Hg.* However, a near accurate reading with the standard 12 cm cuff can be obtained by placing the cuff on the forearm and palpating the radial artery. The patient should be relaxed and calm. A few successive readings should be taken at interval of a few minutes. In some, the initial reading may be very high due to excitement and one should not be surprised if in a few minutes the BP drops considerably, at times to within the normal range. However, these high readings should not be ignored, and these patients should be closely watched.

**Blood pressure recording in lower extremities**

It is important that the proper size of the cuff should be used. Firstly, the patient is made to lie in the prone position. A deflated cuff is applied evenly and snugly around the thigh. The lower edge of the cuff should be one inch above the point at which the bell of the stethoscope is to be placed on the popliteal artery, in the popliteal fossa. *The cuff should never be placed over the joint.* When the cuff is inflated it should neither bulge nor get displaced. If veins in the lower extremity are congested, the limb should be elevated to promote venous drainage and the cuff applied in this position. Palpatory and auscultatory readings are taken in the same way as in the upper extremity. If the cuff is too small for the size of the thigh it can be applied over the cuff, and BP taken by palpating and auscultating over the posterior tibial artery.

At the first examination, BP should be recorded preferably in all the four limbs. If BP in the lower extremities is lower than in the upper limbs it suggests coarctation or obstruction in the aorta. Difference in BP in the two arms is normally less than 10 mm Hg, but in the elderly with arteriosclerotic narrowing at the origin of great vessels, the BP difference may be much greater. The higher BP is the correct reading and for follow-up the arm with the higher pressure should be used for recording BP.

**BP recording in the standing position**

When a patient is on antihypertensive drugs it is necessary to record the BP in the standing position also. The subject should stand up with his arms relaxed by his side and the blood pressure recorded exactly in the same way as in the sitting or supine position. While recording BP, the upper level of the mercury column should be at the level of the eye of the observer.

**Diagnosis**

Early diagnosis is essential so that treatment can prevent complications, and this is possible only if BP is taken in every case routinely. Diagnosis of high BP is easy and physical examination and laboratory investigations will help in finding the cause and complications of the disease.

**Investigations**

Complete urine examination, X-ray chest, and an ECG are desirable in every new case.

*Urine examination* may point towards a renal cause by the presence of protein, casts, RBCs and pus cells. Alkaline urine indicates alkalosis suggesting Conn's syndrome (hyperaldosteronism).

**X-ray chest** may show enlargement of the left ventricle, early left ventricular failure, and unfolding of the aorta. Notching of lower borders of ribs (particularly 3rd to 6th) suggests coarctation of aorta.

**ECG** may be normal. LVH with strain may be seen in severe cases and this tends to regress in a few months after the BP is reduced.

**Serum creatinine** should be done as it gives an idea of the kidney function.

**Urine culture and sensitivity** is indicated when urinary tract infection is suspected.

**Intravenous pyelography (IVP)** is indicated in all young patients or when kidney disease is suspected. Difference in the length of the two kidneys by more than 1.5 cm suggests unilateral renal dysfunction. In chronic pyelonephritis, the pattern is characteristic (serrated borders). If BP is severe and of recent origin, IVP with rapid sequence study (taking serial films at one minute intervals for the first five minutes and later at 20 minutes intervals), is taken so that initial delayed appearance of the contrast media may be detected in the ischaemic kidney which would have gone undetected in the standard five, ten, and twenty minute exposures.

**Renal scanning and isotope renography**

These are safe, non-invasive screening tests for patients of renal and renovascular hypertension, and are superior to IVP.

**Aortography**

When a renovascular cause such as renal artery stenosis, middle aortic block or coarctation of aorta is suspected, an aortogram is indicated to confirm the exact location and extent of the lesion before resorting to surgery. When renal arterial narrowing is demonstrated, to establish that the condition is responsible for the hypertension, one should determine renal vein renin activity from both renal veins.

**Renal vein renin activity**

If the ratio of renal vein renin activity from the blood of the affected to the unaffected side is more than 1.5 to 2, the patient can be expected to benefit from surgery for the renovascular lesion.

**Secondary causes of hypertension and their differential diagnosis**

The following are common causes of secondary hypertension and should be considered when hypertension is present before the age of 40 years.

1. *Chronic pyelonephritis* : This is the most common renal cause of hypertension and should be suspected, especially in a child or young female, and in male patients with evidence of obstructive uropathy due to calculus, enlarged prostate, etc.

There is usually a past history of recurrent urinary tract infections, evidenced by fever with rigor and pain in the loin, and urine examination shows pus cells, WBCs and casts which are the hallmark of the disease. IVP shows asymmetric irregularity of kidney outline, blunting of calyces which later become clubbed with thinning of the cortex overlying the dilated calyces.

2. *Chronic glomerulonephritis* : Past history of acute nephritis may be present; urine shows protein and casts and the specific gravity is low and fixed. Creatinine clearance is reduced and serum creatinine may be raised. Kidney biopsy can confirm the diagnosis.

3. *Coarctation of aorta* : Femoral pulsations are feeble and delayed, or absent, and the BP is higher in the arms than in the legs. Visible and palpable collaterals in the interscapular region and a murmur at the back due to the narrowing of the aorta are distinctive. X-ray chest may show rib notching and post-stenotic dilatation of the aorta. Aortography is confirmatory.

4. *Renal artery stenosis* : This possibility should be considered in severe hypertension of recent onset with a bruit (systolic, extending into diastole) around the umbilical area. IVP, renal vein renin studies, and aortography are diagnostic.

5. *Middle aortic syndrome* : This is a non-specific stenosing aortitis presenting as hypertension, especially in young females. History of intermittent claudication, absence of radial pulse, and a murmur over the upper abdomen or inter-scapular region are suggestive of this condition. Aortography confirms the diagnosis (discussed under vascular diseases).

6. *Pheochromocytoma* : This is due to an adenoma of the adrenal medulla manifesting as hypertension which may be paroxysmal or persistent. During an attack, the BP shoots to over 200/120 mmHg. Profuse sweating is often prominent during an attack. Other features are headache, palpitation, pallor, nausea, tremor, weakness, anxiety, epigastric or chest pain, flushing, paraesthesia, visual disturbances, dizziness, convulsions, etc.

Twenty-four-hour urinary catecholamine content is determined and, if it is more than 130 ug, it confirms the diagnosis of pheochromocytoma (normal 130 μg). When BP is normal, histamine test causes a rise of blood pressure in 75% of the cases of pheochromocytoma, but not in normal individuals. In the presence of hypertension, I.V. phentolamine (Regitin) lowers the blood pressure in patients with pheochromocytoma, but not in normals.

7. *Conn's syndrome (Primary aldosteronism)* : Nocturnal polyuria and muscular weakness are striking features. Sometimes extreme muscular weakness may be complained of as soon as diuretics are administered. Unprovoked hypokalaemia (in a patient who is not on diuretics and salt restricted diet) is an important clue. Urine is alkaline. Non-suppressibility of plasma aldosterone

levels after rapid infusion of saline (2 litres in 4 hours) and low plasma renin activity after sodium depletion are confirmatory.

8. *Cushing's syndrome* : This syndrome, in the majority of cases (70%), is due to bilateral hyperplasia of the adrenal cortex. Adrenocortical adenoma and carcinoma of the adrenal gland account for the remaining. Hypertension occurs in 80% of the cases, but is the presenting feature in only 10%. Hypertension is severe and may sometimes progress to the malignant phase.

Diagnosis can be confirmed by determining urinary excretion of 17-hydroxycorticoids in 24 hours' urine and by estimating plasma cortisol. Intravenous pyelography, perirenal gas insufflation, selective angiography, and adrenal venography are used to outline the adrenal tumour. C.T. scan also will clearly show the enlarged gland or tumour.

**Complications**

If hypertension is not treated or is inadequately treated, complications are prone to occur. The incidence of this will depend on the severity and duration of the disease and the effectiveness of the treatment. With treatment, complications can be controlled and even reversed. Those with high plasma renin (facility for this test is available in only a few laboratories) are more prone to develop complications.

1. *Cardiac complications* such as left ventricular failure and ischaemic heart disease are common. LVF is due to an increased load on the left ventricle as it has to work against elevated BP. Ischaemic heart disease is caused by accelerated atherosclerosis in the coronary arteries brought about by hypertension and hypertrophy of the left ventricle. Sooner or later, cardiac complications occur in about 60% of the cases. At times, acute pulmonary oedema may be the first manifestation of hypertension.

2. *Neurological complications* such as transient ischaemic attacks, stroke, cerebral or subarachnoid haemorrhage, and hypertensive encephalopathy can occur in about 20% of the cases. These are brought about by cerebral atherosclerosis and may be precipitated by sudden elevation of BP.

3. *Renal complications* : Kidneys are always affected. Renal failure is a late manifestation, but nocturnal polyuria, albuminuria, and urine of fixed specific gravity are early indications that the kidneys are affected. Initially, serum creatinine and blood urea are normal, but they increase in later stages. Renal complications account for approximately 15% of the deaths in hypertensive patients.

4. *Malignant (accelerated) hypertension* : This is defined as an accelerated phase of hypertension having a number of clinical manifestations, the hallmark being papilloedema with diastolic BP usually 130 mmHg or more. It is common between the ages of 30 and 50. Males are more frequently affected than females in a ratio of 3 to 1. Malignant hypertension can occur in any patient during the course of essential or secondary hypertension. The cause of malignant hypertension is not known. However, it is more common in renal than in other forms of hypertension. It is at least ten times more frequent in chronic glomerulonephritis than in essential hypertension. In India, probably not more than 0.25 per cent of cases of essential hypertension becomes malignant. It may also occur in patients without any previous history of hypertension. The full-blown picture includes manifestations of hypertensive encephalopathy such as severe headache, vomiting, visual disturbances, transient paralysis, convulsions, stupor, and coma. There is usually impairment of the renal function and in the late stages patients invariably develop uraemia. Cardiac failure is not uncommon in malignant hypertension.

In this phase of hypertension there is progressive damage to the blood vessels in the vital organs, particularly the kidneys. The pathological hallmark of malignant hypertension is 'fibrinoid necrosis' in the arterioles of many organs, and especially the kidney.

With the availability of effective antihypertensive drugs, mortality in cases of malignant hypertension, which used to be 85-100% in 18 months to three years, has been reduced to less than 50%.

5. *Eye complications* : Fundus examination shows evidence of retinopathy in almost all cases except the very mild and recent ones. Narrowing and tortuosity of the retinal arteries is the earliest change. Later, arterioles compress the veins causing arterio-venous nipping. In severe cases cotton wool exudates and haemorrhages may be seen. Papilloedema is the hallmark of malignant or accelerated hypertension. Although a few cases with accelerated hypertension may not have papilloedema, almost all do have retinal haemorrhages and exudates.

**Prognosis** : Life Insurance Corporation records covering millions of lives have shown that a BP of 130/90 mm Hg in a male aged 35 years, who is otherwise healthy, decreases his life expectancy by about four years, a BP of 140/95 mmHg decreases it by nine years, and a pressure of 150/100 mmHg, by 16 years. Women tolerate hypertension better than men. The level of BP, complications, and adequacy of treatment influence the prognosis. Malignant hypertension, if not treated appropriately, may prove fatal in about a year. Outlook at any stage is greatly improved with proper treatment.

**Treatment**

*Hypertension, systolic or diastolic, labile or fixed, symptomatic or asymptomatic, complicated or uncomplicated, must be treated.* In the past, physicians did not think it necessary to treat pure systolic hypertension (with normal diastolic BP) and were hesitant to treat hypertension in the presence of renal failure or those with a past history of stroke. Now it is generally agreed that such patients should also be treated, but special precautions should be taken while lowering the BP.

Presistent elevation of BP above 140/90 mm Hg should be treated. In the asymptomatic stage, the main aim is to prevent complications of hypertension. Therefore, treatment should be started early. If complications have already occurred, the need for treatment is still greater. Not only is there amelioration of symptoms of angina or CCF, but even complications, e.g. LVH, retinopathy, etc., may regress and disappear. Even if this does not happen, at least their further progression is halted. Conditions such as encephalopathy, intracranial haemorrhage, dissecting aneurysm, acute pulmonary oedema, eclampsia of pregnancy, and malignant hypertension constitute a medical emergency. In these, anti-hypertensive treatment must be immediate and aggressive to save the patient's life.

Before embarking upon treatment, it is necessary to find out if the hypertension is secondary to some correctable condition. In 90 to 95% of the cases there is no cause, but in about 5 to 10% a cause can be detected. Some of the conditions e.g., unilateral renal disease, coarctation of aorta, renal artery stenosis, etc., can be treated surgically and the hypertension is permanently cured in about 2% of the cases, provided the surgery is performed before irreversible changes have taken place. If the patient refuses to undergo surgery or irreversible changes have occurred, he can be given the same treatment as for essential hypertension but in smaller doses and often with combination of drugs.

The aim of treatment is to normalise the BP to about 110-140/70-80 mm Hg which is possible in most cases. In severe or complicated cases when this is neither possible nor desirable, or when by doing so side-effects are encountered, one can reduce BP in an individualised way, consistent with safety. Even if BP is not normalised, a moderate reduction will help to a great extent.

In all cases (except in emergencies), BP reduction should be gradual. This is especially important in elderly individuals with borderline cerebrovascular insufficiency and in those with renal failure. The BP is often controlled in a few days, but the treatment should be continued life-long. The maintenance dose in many cases is small.

There can be no doubt that successful therapy of hypertension must start with reorientation of the patient, of his habits and ways of living, and of his outlook towards life. It is seldom possible to change his occupation. The physician can inspire confidence in his patient, enable him to deal with life as it comes and encourage him not to revolt against the inevitable. Here the family doctor can play an important role, by talking to the patient and giving him the necessary advice.

**General Management**

In mild to moderate uncomplicated cases, BP can be controlled with self-regulation techniques, modification of life-style, change in diet, and reduction of weight.

*Rest and relaxation*

The patient should learn the art of relaxation to modify his reaction to mental tension, and to develop a new philosophy of life.

There are various self-regulation techniques : (1) Shavasana, (2) Biofeedback, (3) Trascendental meditation, (4) Autogenic training, (5) Zen, etc. Of these, we found Shavasana simple, useful, and most acceptable to a majority of the patients.

*Shavasana (Yoga) :* In India, from time immemorial Yoga has been advocated for physical fitness and mental relaxation. Since Shavasana and Yoga modify the maladaptive response to the environment, these are useful in stress-linked diseases. Shavasana and Yoga training is extremely useful, play an important role in modifying the effects of stress, and has a favourable influence on psychosomatic diseases which are so prevalent in the modern world. By practising Yogic exercises, particularly Shavasana, is many cases blood pressure can be normalised and in others, the drug requirement can be considerably reduced.

*Technique :* This asana should be practised on an empty stomach, preferably in the morning after evacuating the bowels. The patient is allowed a light breakfast about an hour or two before this asana. He should wear light and loose clothes while performing the asana.

The patient should lie in the supine position, with the lower limbs 30 degrees apart and the upper making an angle of 15 degrees with the trunk, the forearms in the midprone position and fingers semiflexed. The eyes should be closed with the eyelids dropping. He should feel comfortable and fully relaxed in this position. He should take slow, rhythmic diaphragmatic breathing (abdomen going out during inspiration and coming in during expiration), with a short pause (fraction of a second) after each inspiration and a longer one at the end of each expiration. This pause is essential so that concentration is not lost. After establishing this rhythm, he should attend to the sensation at the nostrils, the coolness of the inspired air, and the warmth of the expired air. The procedure helps to keep him inwardly alert and to forget his usual thoughts, so that he becomes less conscious of the external environment, thereby attaining relaxation. He should relax the muscles so that he feels the heaviness of different parts of the body. This is achieved automatically once he learns the asana. The asana is to be performed for 30 minutes. An experienced supervisor can check that there is no movement of any part of the body, except rhythmic abdominal movements. Physical relaxation can be checked by an observer from time to time by lifting the extremities and letting them go, to observe their flaccidity. The limbs should drop like a dead weight. Most persons learn the asana correctly in three of four weeks.

After he learns the asana correctly, the respiratory rate comes down and is usually between 4 and 10 per minute, the heart rate comes down from 80/minute to about 60/minute, and BP is lowered considerably if it is high, but by only a few millimetres if it is normal. This asana, if practised correctly, will help him to relax, change his reaction to tension, give him a feeling of well-being and keep him physically fit, and mentally alert and happy (Refer to chapter on "Yoga and medicine").

*Biofeedback :* Biofeedback is feedback of any biological information about oneself. If hand temperature is transmitted through a sensitive pick into a polygraph and read on a meter, the information is conveyed through the eyes to the cerebral cortex. This completes the biocybernetic loop. Visually perceiving hand temperature on the meter, one can train onself to increase or reduce the temperature.

Similarly, with the help of other instruments, e.g. the G.S.R. (galvanic skin resistance) or EMG (electromyogram) attached to the body, one can get information regarding muscle tension, and with reduction of muscle tension,blood pressure can be reduced.

Any of these self regulation techniques can be used depending upon the availability of training and the choice of the patient. These can be used alone or with antihypertensive drugs, depending upon the severity of hypertension.

Adequate rest at night is necessary and for this one may use in the beginning diazepam or chlordiazepoxide. After learning Shavasan, sedatives and hypnotics will not be required. Relaxation at weekends, and enjoying holidays once or twice annually are good ways of avoiding mental tension.

*Diet*

Excess salt in diet and obesity play a very important role in the development of hypertension. Salt restriction compatible with palatibility is advised. Obesity should be controlled and optimal body weight maintained (see chapter on Obesity). Fat content of the diet should be low and saturated fats in particular should be reduced.

Smoking should be avoided. Alcohol intake should be reduced to a minimum, if it cannot be avoided altogether. Excessive use of tea and coffee can aggravate hypertension and, therefore, should be curtailed.

*Exercise*

Exercise which is recreational and of moderate intensity may be encouraged. Exercises, particularly isometric, involving the upper limbs, elevate BP. The same applies to carrying heavy weights. Competitive sports should be avoided. Yogic postures are very valuable and will help considerably. However, hypertensives should avoid Shirshasana and Sarvangasana Yogic exercises.

*Drugs to be avoided*

Corticosteroids, oral contraceptives, nasal decongestants, tricyclic antidepressants, amphetamines, antihistaminics, and sex tonics tend to aggravate pre-existing hypertension and should be avoided. Anticoagulants may involve the risk of haemorrhage in cases of hypertension, and it is desirable to avoid them.

## 'MODIFIED STEP CARE' APPROACH FOR HYPERTENSION'

— Discontinue drugs, if any, which are likely to raise BP
— Modification of diet
— Modification of life-style
— Reduction of weight (if overweight)
— Self-regulation techniques
+
— A diuretic on alternate morning
and
Reserpine or propranolol or
Methyldopa or clonidine

Step 3 +
— Prazosin or hydralazine

Step 4 +
— Captopril or minoxidil or guanethidine

**Principles of drug therapy**

Before starting medication the patient should be educated on the need for antihypertensive therapy as it would reduce morbidity and mortality. This is especially necessary if the patient is a asymptomatic prior to treatment, because the treatment is life-long and the patient's compliance is essential.

Whatever drug regimen is employed, the critical issue is to control BP. It is desirable to select drugs which are safe and relatively free from side-effects, particularly impotence and postural hypotension. Drug selection also depends upon accompanying symptoms, associated diseases, severity of hypertension, and the presence of complications. The patient should be asked if he has taken any antihypertensive agent, and if so, its response and side-effects, if any. This will help in planning treatment. Many authors have advocated a diuretic as the first step and, if the response is inadequate, add an antihypertensive drug. We do not advocate this, because diuretics, when given daily, result in hypokalaemia, hyponatraemia, hyperuricaemia, hypocalcaemia, hyperglycaemia, haemoconcentration, platelet aggregation, etc. We prefer to start with an antihypertensive drug to the sympathetic inhibitor group (methyldopa, serpasil, etc.) or a beta-blocker and add a diuretic on alternate mornings to overcome the sodium and water retention. In India, reserpine is preferred because of its low cost and easy availability. Whatever drug is used, first a small dose is given to determine if it has any side-effect. The dose is then increased gradually till the desired effect on the blood pressure is obtained or there are side-effects. As an ideal anti-BP drug is not available, a combination of drugs is preferred to counteract any undesirable side-effects. Table 18.3 will be of help in selecting the correct combinations.

In all cases who are on a sympathetic inhibitor, a diuretic on alternate days is added. The use of diuretics has a three-fold purpose. Firstly, diuretics wash away sodium which is retained by a sympathetic inhibitor (almost all antihypertensive drugs retain sodium and if diuretics are not given, pseudotolerance develops. Secondly, diuretics add to the antihypertensive effect of sympathetic inhibitors. Thirdly, diuretics have a specific antihypertensive effect by volume depletion, particularly in the low renin group which volume depletion, particularly in the low renin group which constitutes about 30% of the hypertensive population.

In patients in whom the response to a sympathetic inhibitor and a diuretic is not satisfactory or in those with severe hypertension of long duration, a vasodilator is added. It constitutes a very good third-line drug. The main advantage of a vasodilator is that it potentiates the action of other drugs and counteracts the side-effects of sympathetic inhibitors, mainly bradycardia and negative inotropic effect, particularly encountered with propranolol. The sympathetic inhibitor-diuretic-vasodilator regimen has received wide popularity. Treatment failure is often due to the following factors : (i) insufficient dose (ii) excess salt in diet, and (iii) failure to add a diuretic. In chronic cases treatment failure may be due to secondary hyperaldosteronism (for which an aldosterone antagonist may be added), or renal arteriolar changes (for which a vasodilator should be added). Lastly, in all therapeutic failures, secondary causes of hypertension should again be looked for.

During follow-up, BP should be checked both in supine and standing positions and also after a little exercise to discover if there is any postural hypotension. Sympathetic inhibitors interfere with baroreceptor reflexes which may lead to orthostatic hypotension and postural giddiness. For this very reason the patient should be advised to avoid prolonged passive standing, e.g. waiting for a bus, standing in a telephone booth, etc.

**Antihypertensive drugs** (Table-18.3 : Commonly used antihypertensive drugs, their doses, side-effects, merits and relative or absolute contraindications) :

Anti-hypertensive drugs fall into the following four major categories according to their site of action, but there is considerable overlap :

**Table-18.3 : Anti-hypertensive drugs : Doses, side effects, merits and contraindications**

| Drugs | Doses | Common side effects | Merits | Contraindications (Relative or absolute) |
|---|---|---|---|---|
| I. **Drugs acting on sympathetic Nervous system** | | | | |
| A. **Central and Peripheral inhibitors** | | | | |
| Rauwolfia Serpentina<br>Active Alkaloid Reserpine | Inj. 1-5 mg (IM)<br>0.1 - lmg TDS (O) | Lethargy, depression, insomnia, bradycardia, nasal congestion, dreams, impotence, parkinsonism. | Low cost | obesity, depression. |
| Alpha Methyldopa | 250-500 mg TDS (O)<br>500-1000 mg IV | Lethargy, depression, somnolence, drowsiness, postural hypotension, impotence. | | Depression. |
| Clonidine | 0.15 mg - 1.5 mg TDS (O)<br>Inj. 0.1 mg - 0.45 mg (IV, IM) | Dryness of mouth, drowsiness, general weakness.<br>If withdrawn abruptly, overshoot of BP and tachycardia. | Migraine, menopausal flushing | Patients on tricyclic anti-depressants, $\beta$-blockers; brady-cardia. |
| B. **Adrenergic Receptor Blocking agents** | | | | |
| **Beta-Blockers** | | | | |
| Propranolol | 40-80 mg BD or TDS (O) | Bradycardia, bronchospasm, CCF, dizziness, depression, nausea, lethargy, weakness, cold extremities. | IHD, Labile hypertension, Pts. on antidepressants, gout, high renin hyper-tension, BP fluctua-tions with emotion, exertion; pts. with palp-itation, tachycardia, arrhythmia. | COPD, CCF, heart block elderly pts., diabetes, peripheral vas. disease. |
| Newer drugs include Metoprolol | 50 - 100 mg OD (O) | | | |
| Atenolol | 50 - 100 mg OD (O) | | | |
| Pindolol | 10 - 30 mg BD (O) | | | |
| **Alpha-Blockers** | | | | |
| Phentolamine Mesylate<br>OR<br>Phentolamine Hydrochloride | 50 mg QDS (O)<br>Inj. 5 mg adults (IV)<br>Inj. 1 mg children (IV) | Tachycardia, cardiac arrhythmia | Useful in Pheochromocytoma, clonidine withdrawal hyper-tension, hypertension from MAO inhibiting drugs. Now becoming popular drug except in pregnancy. | |

| Drugs | Doses | Common effects | Merits | Contraindication (Relative or absolute) |
|---|---|---|---|---|
| **Combined alpha & Beta blockers** | | | | |
| Labetalol | 100-200 mg TDS | Postural hypotension, skin, rashes, dry eyes, headache, tiredness, epigastric pain, nausea, vomiting, tingling sensation. | Renal hypertension | Chronic digitalis resistant heart failure, A.V. block, COPD. |
| C. **Ganglion Blockers** | | | | |
| Guanethidine | 5-100 mg OD (O) | Postural hypotension, sexual dysfunction. | | Elderly hypertensives, recent MI, cerebrovascular insufficiency, pheochromocytoma. |
| II. **Vasodilators :** | | | | |
| (a) Hydralazine | 25-100 mg TDS (O) | Drug fever, palpitation, tachycardia, headache, skin rashes, postural hypotension, depression, dizziness, SLE. | Useful in bradycardia. | Angina. |
| (b) Prazosin | 2-5 mg TDS (O) (start with 0.5 to 1 mg) | Giddiness, postural, hypotension, weakness, dryness of mouth, abdominal cramps. | Can be used when hypertension associated with angina, CCF. | |
| (c) Minoxidil | 2.5-5 mg OD, BD (O) | Reflex tachycardia, change in hair colour, itching of eyes, intractable oedema. | Renal hypertension, resistant hypertension | Angina, elderly hypertensive. |
| (d) Diazoxide | 5 mg/kg body weight 100-300 mg IV (ampoule 300 mg) | Giddiness, Postural hypotension, angina, and MI. | Malignant hypertension, hypertensive crisis. | Cardiac failure, angina, MI, dissecting aortic aneurysm, coarctation of aorta. |
| (e) Sodium Nitroprusside | Hypertensive crisis 10-200 mcg/min IV drip (6-120 drops/min) | Nausea, retching, headache, muscle twitching, dizziness, palpitations, tachycardia, flushing of face, sweating, abdominal pain. | Angina, MI, aortic dissection, intracranial haemorrhage, cardiac failure, during anaesthesia. | Hypothyroidism, severe renal failure. |

| Drugs | Doses | Common effects | Merits | Contraindication (Relative or absolute) |
|---|---|---|---|---|
| III. **Drugs that interfere with Renin - Angiotensin mechanism** | | | | |
| Captopril | 25-100 mg TDS | Light headedness, drug rash. | High renin Hypertension. | |
| Seralacin | IV infusion 0.1 ug/kg/min. | If normal renin then increase in BP. | Effect only when high renin or sodium depleted. | |
| IV. Diuretics | | | | |
| A. **Potent Diuretics** | | Hyponatremia, Hypokalaemia, Hypomagnesaemia, Hyperglycaemia, Hypercalcemia. | Effective in renal insufficiency, systemic acidosis or alkalosis when urgent diuresis e.g. pul. oedema; resistant oedematous state. | |
| Furosemide | 40-80 mg (O)<br>20-400 mg (IV, IM) | ,, and hearing loss | —do— | |
| Ethacrynic acid | 50-150 mg (O)<br>50 mg (IV) | ,, ,, | —do— | |
| Bumetanide | 1-5 mg (O)<br>0.25 - 2 mg (IV, IM) | ,, ,, | —do— | |
| B. **Thiazide Group** | | Hypersensitivity reaction e.g. purpura, dermatitis, photosensitivity, depression etc., hypokalaemia, hyperuricaemia, nausea, vomiting. | | |
| Chlorothiazide | 250-500 mg OD, BD (O) | —do— | | |
| Hydrochlorothiazide | 25-50 mg OD, BD (O) | —do— | | |
| Chlorthalidone | 100 mg OD (O) | —do— | | |
| C. **Potassium sparing diuretics** | | | | |
| Spironolactone | 25-50 mg TDS, QID (O) | G.I. disturbances, gynaecomastia, rarely agranulocytosis | Secondary hyperaldosteronism | Avoid in renal failure and hyperkalaemia |
| Triamterine (Dytide — Triamterine 50 mg) Benzthiazide 25 mg) | 1-2 tabs. OD or BD | Hyperkalaemia, nausea, vomiting, diarrhoea. | —do— | —do— |
| Amiloride | 5-20 mg (O) | Hyperkalaemia, G.I. disturbances. | —do— | —do— |

I. Sympathetic inhibitors, agents which interfere with the activity of the sympathetic nervous system.

II. Vasodilators, which relax vascular smooth muscles.

III. Drugs, which interfere with the renin-angiotensin system.

IV. Diuretics.

**1. Sympathetic inhibitors :**

**A. Central and Peripheral Inhibitors**

**Rauwolfia group of drugs**

These are useful in mild to moderate hypertension. Rauwolfia serpentina is used in the form of dried extract, total alkaloids and active alkaloids. Although many alkaloids have been isolated, reserpine is the most potent and is commonly used. The rauwolfia group of drugs are popular in India because of the low cost and easy availability. Reserpine is also available in various drug combinations, viz. adelphane, terbolan, etc. Injection serpasil is available for hypertensive emergencies. This drug has a tendency to produce mental depression, and therefore, should be avoided in cases with a history of depression. A careful watch of the patient is necessary from time to time to detect this depression.

**Action**

This drug depletes the stores of catecholamines centrally as well as peripherally at the sympathetic nerve endings. It has a central sedative as well as a vagotonic effect. This drug also lowers plasma renin.

**Dose**

The oral recommended dose of reserpine varies from 0.1 to 0.1 mg daily in two or three divided doses. Higher doses usually do not lower BP further, while side-effects are more frequent. Injection serpasil can be given intramuscularly in a dose of 1-5 mg in hypertensive emergencies. The injection may have to be repeated every four to six hours.

The disadvantages of this drug, in cases of hypertensive emergencies, are : It takes from a half hour to two hours to act, and it may be unsafe to wait so long in an emergent situation, and it is also not suitable in hypertensive neurological complications because the drowsiness produced by this drug masks the neurological manifestations.

**Side-effects**

The common side-effects are nasal congestion, fatigue, dreams, drowsiness, impotence, and insomina. Depression and parkinsonism induced by this drug are serious and take several weeks to disappear even after stopping the drug, particularly when the drug is not discontinued at the earliest indication of the side-effect. Vagotonic effect gives to bradycardia and may lead to diarrhoea, hyperacidity, and even peptic ulceration. Recently, breast carcinoma in a few female patients has been reported after prolonged use of this drug, but this has yet to be corroborated.

**Alpha-methyldopa**

It can be given in all grades of hypertension and can be used in the presence of CCF and pheochromocytoma and in patients on tricyclic anti-depressants. It can also be used in hypertensive patients with renal failure.

**Action**

The mechanism of action of alpha-methyldopa is not definitely established, although it was supposed to be a dopa-decarboxylase inhibitor.

It is now hypothesised that the drug acts as a false neurohumoral transmitter. Alpha-methyldopa enters the brain where it is converted into alpha-methyldopamine and alpha-methyinordrenaline. The latter displaces noradrenaline from granule stores. Alpha-methylnoradrenaline is less potent than noradrenaline and is capable of functioning as a false neurohumoral transmitter and its potency produces the relative hypotensive effect.

This drug also directly inhibits the central vasomotor centres and suppresses the renin release from the kidney.

**Dosage**

The usual effective dose is 250-500 mg thrice daily. It has a tendency to retain sodium and water and hence it is best used with an oral diuretic agent. Injectable alphamethyl dopa is available (not in India) for hypertensive emergencies and the dose in 500-1000 mg/IV, to be repeated every 4-6 hours.

**Side-effects**

These are infrequent with dosage up to 1 g a day. The common side-effects are lethargy, depression, and somnolence which usually disappear after a few days. Impotence and postural hypotension are usually seen with higher doses. Fortunately hepatitis and haemolytic anaemia are rare.

**Clonidine**

It is the drug of choice when hypertension is associated with migraine. It can also be used in malignant hypertension.

The drug should be avoided when the patient is on tricyclic antidepressants. It should also be avoided when the pulse is slow. The patient should be cautioned not to stop clonidine suddenly, but to reduce it gradually over four or five days before stopping it as there may be rebound phenomena resulting in hypertensive crisis due to sudden withdrawal, especially if the dose administered is above 0.5 mg per day.

**Action**

It stimulates the alpha adrenergic receptors in the brain stem with decreased sympathetic discharge to arterioles. It also decreases plasma renin, peripheral resistance, heart rate and cardiac output.

**Dose**

The dose varies from 0.15 mg a day in three or four divided doses. In cases of severe or malignant hypertension, it can be given I.V. or I.M. in doses of 0.1 to 0.45 mg. However, there may be a transient initial rise in BP after IV administration, which is followed by a rapid fall of BP.

**Side-effects**

Prominent side-effects are : dryness of mouth and eyes, drowsiness, and general weakness. These tend to diminish with continued use. Bradycardia and constipation are some of the other side-effects.

B. **Adrenoreceptor blocking agents**

**Alpha receptor blocking agents** such as phentolamine, phenoxybenzamine, and hydrogenated ergot alkaloids are only mild antihypertensive agents and, therefore, are of limited value, except phentolamine. Phentolamine is indicated in situations associated with excessive amounts of circulating catecholamines, e.g. exogenously administered catecholamines, and for conditions viz. pheochromocytoma, clonidine withdrawal hypertension and hypertension resulting from MAO inhibiting drugs. MAO inhibitors are both hypotensive and mood elevators. However, with these drugs there is danger of acute exacerbation of the hypertensive state if certain drugs, e,g, sympathomimetics or tryamine-containing substances (cheese, yoghurt, broad beans, yeast extracts, wine, beer etc.) are taken.

**Beta receptor blocking agents**

These drugs are useful in the management of hypertension but their mode of action is as yet imperfectly understood. The commonly used beta-adrenergic blocking agent is propranolol.

Propranolol is a useful drug in the treatment of hypertension and has the following *advantages* : (1) Postural hypotension and impotence do not usually occur (these are most objectionable side-effects with sympathetic inhibitors). (2) It does not cause sodium and water retention and, therefore, the drug does not lose its efficacy. Yet, it is a good practice to add a diuretic as diuretics potentiate its action. (3) BP fluctuation in response to exertion, emotion, and tachycardia is minimised by propranolol and therefore, this drug is most useful in labile hypertension. (4) It is useful for hypertensive patients who in addition have palpitation, tachycardia, arrhythmias, or angina. (5) The drug is safe in renal failure and is also effective in malignant hypertension.

However, this drug has *many drawbacks* : It is contraindicated in (1) CCF (overt or impending), (2) heart block, (3) obstructive pulmonary airway diseases (Cor pulmonale or COPD), and (4) should be avoided in the presence of cardiomegaly, sinus bradycardia and peripheral artery disease, and in diabetics who are on antidiabetic drugs, as propranolol masks the warning signs of hypoglycaemia in diabetics. In our experience in the city of Bombay we have found that about 15% of the hypertensive patients have some degree of obstructive airway disease. In these subjects beta-blockers may aggravate their respiratory symptoms. About 10% of patients cannot tolerate the drug. All these limit the usefulness of this drug.

**Action**

It is believed that the action of propranolol is a direct one on renal juxta glomerular cells thereby suppressing renin release. It causes beta-blockade in the heart and thereby decreases heart rate, cardiac output, and stroke output.

**Dose**

The usual dose of propranolol is from 40 to 320 mg a day in two or three divided doses. However, higher doses up to 2000 mg have been used. It is desirable to start with smaller doses (20 mg twice daily) and to increase it gradually according to response and/or side-effects. Heart rate should not fall below 55 per minute. It is desirable not to stop the drug suddenly as it may produce tachycardia, arrhythmia, or angina, or may even precipitate myocardial infarction.

**Side-effects**

Side-effects are seen in 15 to 20% of the cases. In about five to 10% it may become necessary to discontinue the drug. The main side-effects are bronchospasm, fatigue, headache, vivid dreams, insomnia, dizziness, unsteadiness, undue bradycardia, nausea, vomiting, flatulence, skin rashes, etc. Patients may complain of cold extremities as a result of constriction of the vessels due to unopposed action of the alpha receptors.

**Combined alpha and beta receptor blocking agents**

**Labetalol Hydrochloride** (Normadate, Tab. 50 mg, 100 mg, and 200 mg.)

**Action**

This most modern drug lowers the blood pressure, by blocking the alpha adreno-receptors in peripheral arterioles, thereby reducing peripheral resistance, and also by its beta adreno-receptor activity, which protects the heart from the reflex sympathetic drive normally induced by peripheral vasodilatation. Cardiac output is not significantly reduced at rest or after moderate exercise. Increase in systolic pressure during exercise is reduced after Labetalol, while corresponding changes in the diastolic pressure are essentially normal. All these effects can benefit the hypertensive patient. As the alpha and beta blockade are incomplete, the barostatic reflexes remain sufficiently active to prevent postural hypotension in most patients. However, postural hypotension may occur with higher doses.

**Dose**

The drug should be started with a dose of 50 mg two or three times a day and gradually increased to 200 mg two or three times a day. Severe cases may require a dosage as high as 2 gms daily. Patients can usually be maintained on twice daily regime.

**Precautions**

Labetalol should not normally be given to patients who are in chronic digitalis resistant heart failure or atrioventricular block, and to those who are prone to bronchospasm.

It is not necessary to discontinue Labetalol in patients requiring anaesthesia, but they should be given intravenous atropine prior to induction. Avoid in pregnancy.

**Side-effects**

Postural hypotension may occur if the initial dose is too high or the dose is increased too rapidly or when the daily dose is high. The patient may get skin rashes, dry eyes, headache, tiredness, epigastric pain, nausea, and vomiting. A tingling sensation in the scalp may occur, but this is usually transient. Blurring of the vision, eye irritation, cramps and lichenoid rash have been reported.

Labetalol does not adversely affect renal function and is particularly suitable in hypertensive patients with renal disease. Metabolites of the drug are excreted in the feces and urine and so the drug is unlikely to accumulate in blood even in renal failure.

**Ganglion blocking agents**

Guanethidine, bethanidine, debrisoquine, pentolinium, trimethaphan, and hexamethonium are also sympathetic inhibiting agents. They are potent but cause severe side-effects, such as orthostatic (postural) hypotension, sexual dysfunction, etc. Of these, guanethidine and trimethaphan are sometimes used. When guanethidine 5-10 mg a day is given in addition to an alphamethyldopa-diuretic-vasodilator regimen, some hypotensive effect can be achieved with minimal side-effects. These drugs should be prescribed with caution in the presence of renal failure, cerebrovascular insufficiency, or angina, and are also contraindicated when a patient has pheochromocytoma or is on tricyclic antidepressants or phenothiazines. Guanethidine gives rise to marked postural hypotension, sexual dysfunction, and other side-effects. Therefore, this drug has hardly any place in the management of hypertension, more so as many better drugs are available.

**Treatment** is used in hypertensive emergencies and the indications for this drug are similar to sodium nitroprusside. It is favoured in patients of acute aortic dissection because aortic flow and ventricular ejection are minimally increased. It is administered in concentration of 1 mg/ml (0.1%) intravenously at a rate of 1.0 to 4.0 mg/min. Reduction in BP is achieved within minutes, and as soon as the drop is discontinued BP starts rising. Thus it is a rapidly acting drug and the duration of action is also brief.

**II. Vasodilators**

These are commonly used as part of a three-drug regimen in combination with serpena or methyldopa or propranolol and a diuretic. They are mainly indicated in chronic and severe cases and in the presence of renal failure. Besides synergistic effect with propranolol, these increase adrenergic activity and counteract bradycardia produced by propranolol and other drugs.

All vasodilators act by lowering the peripheral resistance. The vasodilators in common use are hydralazine, prazosin, sodium nitroprusside, minoxidil, and diazoxide.

**Hydralazine :** The only dose of hydralazine is from 25 to 200 mg thrice daily. Side-effects during a triple drug regimen using hydralazine are unusual. Although headache, palpitation, and tachycardia can occur due to increased adrenergic activity, these are minimised by concomitant use of propranolol. Sodium and water retention is counteracted by the diuretic in the triple regimen. A delayed but serious side-effect, lupus erythematosus-like syndrome may occur with large doses (more than 400 mg/day). Tolerance to hydralazine may be acquired rapidly. This drug should be avoided in angina and AMI.

**Prazosin :** The hypotensive effect of prazosin is due to the vasodilator action mainly on the arterioles. It also interferes with the peripheral sympathetic function at a site distal to the alpha adrenergic receptor, without blocking it, a diuretic greatly enhances the action of prazosin. The side-effects of this drug include giddiness, weakness, dryness of the mouth, postural hypotension, and abdominal cramps. These are not common and are usually not serious enough to require discontinuation of the drug. In some cases, the initial response is abnormal and there is a marked fall of BP. However, the abnormal BP response usually does not recur. The addition of a beta blocker helps in counteracting some of the undesirable effects and also helps to further reduce BP. The dose is from 1 to 60 mg a day (average, 5 to 10 mg/day) in three divided doses. Always start with 0.5 to 1 mg/day as postural hypotension may occur with the first dose.

**Minoxidil** (Tab. 5 mg) : Minoxidil is an orally effective, direct acting peripheral vasodilator which reduces elevated systolic and diastolic pressure by decreasing peripheral resistance. It is rapidly absorbed from the gastrointestinal tract and is mainly excreted by the kidneys. It does not interfere with the vasomotor reflexes and, therefore, dose not produce orthostatic hypotension. The drug does not affect CNS function in man. It usually increases renin secretion.

With an oral dose, blood pressure starts decreasing within 30 minutes, maximum fall occurs within two to three hours, and the total duration of action of a single dose is approximately 75 hours. The drug can be administered once or twice a day.

The side-effects are reflex tachycardia, intractable oedema and right-sided failure, change in the colour of hair, itching of eyes, etc. It is desirable to counteract the reflex tachycardia with drugs which produce bradycardia, e.g. propranolol, reserpine, etc. Diuretics are necessary to counteract the water retention.

The dose of minoxidil varies from 2 to 40 mg per day in divided doses.

**Sodium Nitroprusside :** It is a vasodilator drug which relaxes both arteriolar and venous smooth muscles. Thus, it reduces the pre-load and after-load. It is available as a reddish brown lympholized power in a vial. 50 mg or 100 mg of the drug should be dissolved in 2-3 ml of dextrose. The bottle should be promptly wrapped in aluminium foil or some opaque material to prevent degradation to cyanogen by light. The freshly prepared solution has a very faint brownish tint; if it is high coloured it should be discarded. If possible, it should be given by an infusion pump microdrip regulator. The rate of administration should be adjusted according to BP, the usual rate of administration is 6-120 drops/min. (10-200 mcg/min).

Since the end product of sodium nitroprusside metabolism is thiocynate, it is extremely important to estimate blood thiocynate levels as frequently as possible. The blood thiocynate level should not be allowed to go beyond 10 mg/100 ml. As thiocynate inhibits the uptake and binding of iodine, the drug should be used with caution in patients with hypothyroidism and severe renal impairment.

Minor adverse reactions such as nausea, retching, headache, muscle twitching, dizziness, palpitation, tachycardia, flushing of face, sweating, and abdominal pain may occur, but these symptoms disappear rapidly on slowing the rate of infusion or by temporary discontinuation of infusion. Methemoglobinaemia following nitroprusside infusion has also been reported.

**Diazoxide :** It acts directly on the smooth muscle producing relaxation. Although related chemically to chlorothiazide, it causes sodium retention and, therefore, diuretics should be used with it. It is especially useful in cases of malignant hypertension and hypertensive crisis. When given intravenously (5 mg/kg body weight), there is a fall of BP, within a few minutes. The pressure remains low for a few hours. The drug should be injected rapidly since it binds with circulating albumin in the blood and thereby loses much of its hypotensive and vasodilating effect. Injections may be repeated every 6-8 hours during the acute phase. *Administration of diazoxide to patients with hypertensive crisis can cause an angina-like syndrome and even myocardial infarction* as shown in a recent study of this drug. Some patients who are refractory to treatment with oral drugs respond to intravenous injection of diazoxide, and the BP can then be controlled with oral antihypertensive drugs.

If the drug is not injected properly into the vein it gives a severe local reaction in the tissues. It also produces sodium retention and hyperglycaemia.

Diazoxide should not be used in the treatment of compensatory hypertension such as that associated with coarctation of aorta or arterio-venous fistula. It should be avoided in patients with cardiac failure, angina pectoris, myocardial infarction, and dissecting aortic aneurysm.

**Verapamil :** If the above drugs are not available, verapamil could be used in hypertensive emergencies. The dose of verapamil is 300 mg added to 200 ml of 5% dextrose and is given by a slow IV drip and the rate of drip should be regulated according to the fall of BP. Within a few hours BP can be reduced to moderate level. Orally, verapamil has only a mild antihypertensive action.

III. **Drugs which interfere with the renin-angiotensin mechanism : Captopril :** This orally effective agent inhibits the enzyme responsible for both conversion of the inactive angiotensin I to the potent vasopressor angiotensin II and the breakdown of vasopressor bradykinin. The beneficial effect of this drug is due to elimination of angiotensin II and accumulation of bradykinin. Initial dose is 10 mg a day which can be gradually increased at intervals of 48 hours. Captopril can be safely given up to 1 gm/day.

**Seralcin :** It is a potent antihypertensive agent and is administered by IV infusion. It is used in malignant (accelerated) hypertension and as a diagnostic agent to determine the angiotensin component in hypertension. It was believed to be angiotensin II antagonist, but probably it is rather a weak competitive agonist. There is no hypotensive response until there is high renin activity or sodium is depleted. During high rates of seralacin infusion or after injection of a large bolus, there may be rise of BP in hypertensive subjects with low renin activity. In such hypertensive patients with low renin activity BP can be reduced by depleting sodium with a diuretic.

IV. **Diuretics**

As can be seen from Table II almost all the antihypertensive drugs have sodium and water retaining properties (as seen by increase in plasma volume) which can be counteracted by diuretics. Diuretics are also indicated in the presence of increased intravascular volume as seen in renal failure and congestive cardiac failure. The choice of the diuretic is of little importance if renal function is normal, but when creatinine clearance is reduced to 20-30% of normal, furosemide, bumetanide, or ethacrynic acid are mainly used as potentiating agents with other antihypertensive drugs.

When diuretics are used on alternate days (two or three days a week), usually it is not necessary to supplement potassium chloride, but when used daily the patient should be advised to take potassium chloride orally or encouraged to take orange juice, tomato juice, coconut water, and bananas as these foods are rich in potassium (see Table-18.3).

Potent (loop) diuretics in comparison with the thiazide group are more effective and retain their effectiveness even in the presence of serum electrolyte imbalance.

If secondary hyperaldosteronism, induced by diuretics, has occurred, aldosterone antagonist (spironolactone) is administered in addition to thiazides or potent diuretics. These should also be given when the patient complains of weakness which is often due to hypokalaemia.

**Precautions**

It is essential to evaluate renal function by estimating serum creatinine. When creatinine is elevated, serial values should be estimated every two or three days while the blood pressure is being regulated. If increase in creatinine is observed, the BP should be allowed to increase slightly by reducing the dose of the anti-hypertensive and diuretic agents until the creatinine again returns to the pre-treatment level.

**Hypertensive emergencies**

The aim of treating hypertensive emergencies is : prompt recognition and rapid reduction of blood pressure, though not necessarily to normotensive levels and not with the same urgency in every case.

An outline of the drug treatment of hypertensive emergencies is given in Table-18.4. However, these drugs have already been described in detail *vide supra.*

**Table-18.4 : Outline for parenteral drug treatment of hypertensive emergencies**

| Emergency | Preferred drugs-Inj. | Drugs less effective and use with caution-Inj. |
|---|---|---|
| Acute hypertensive encephalopathy | Sod. nitroprusside<br>Diazoxide<br>Trimethophan | Reserpine<br>Methyldopa<br>Verapamil |
| Acute left ventricular failure | Furosemide with<br>Sod. nitroprusside<br>Diazoxide<br>Trimethaphan | Hydralazine<br>Verapamil |
| Intracranial haemorrhage | Sod. nitroprusside<br>Trimethaphan | Reserpine<br>Methyldopa<br>Verapamil |
| Acute coronary insufficiency and myocardial aneurysm | Sod. nitroprusside<br>Trimethaphan<br>Propranolol | Reserpine<br>Hydralazine<br>Diazoxide |
| Malignant (accelerated) hypertension | Sod. nitroprusside<br>Diazoxide<br>Trimethaphan<br>Reserpine | |
| Pheochromocytoma and hypertensive crises associated with MAO inhibitors, cardiovascular catheterization | Phentolamine<br>Sod. nitroprusside | All others |
| Pre-eclampsia of pregnancy Hypertension with dissecting aortic aneurysm | Serpasil<br>Trimethaphan | |
| Clonidine withdrawal hypertension | Phentolamine<br>Beta blocker | |
| Hypertension with acute glomerulonephritis | Hydralazine<br>Methyldopa<br>Reserpine<br>Clonidine | |

There is no ideal antihypertensive agent which can be selected as the first choice. In fact, the choice of an antihypertensive drug to be used for a particular emergency would depend upon various factors :

1. Aetiology of the hypertension
2. Complicating diseases such as ischaemic heart disease.
3. Age of the patient

4. Rapidity of onset, duration of action, and antihypertensive potency of the drug.

In patients with a history of angina pectoris or myocardial infarction, lowering of BP to normotensive or hypotensive levels might precipitate a myocardial infarct or a cerebrovascular episode. Therefore, in these patients the diastolic BP should be reduced to 100-110 mmHg. initially and subsequently reduced further.

If there is undue reduction of blood pressure while treating with antihypertensive drugs, a direct pressor agent such as levarteranol bitartrate (4 mg/litre) or mephantine (15 mg) may be employed.

In hypertensive emergencies, oral antihypertensive drugs should be started with parenteral drugs, so that subsequently the patient may be controlled only with oral drugs.

## ISCHAEMIC HEART DISEASE

*G.C. MOOKERJEE*

*(Syn : Coronary heart disease, Coronary artery disease, atherosclerotic heart disease)*

### Introduction

Ischaemic heart disease (I.H.D.) is a syndrome caused by inadequate blood supply to the heart muscles chiefly due to coronary artery disease (spasm or occlusion of the coronary arteries). Occlusion of coronary vessels may be commonly due to atherosclerosis but also may be caused by local thrombosis or embolism, syphilitic narrowing of coronary ostium, collagen disease or arteritis.

The following conditions should be looked for :

- Left ventricular hypertrophy
- Severe anaemia
- Thyrotoxicosis or myxoedema
- Syphilitic aortitis — obliterating coronary ostia
- Collagen diseases
- Infective or non-specific arteritis
- Anomaly of coronary vessels — by angiogram.

All these pathological changes may insidiously or suddenly cause impaired blood flow of the myocardium. Inadequate vascular supply to the heart results in inadequate oxygen supply to the heart muscles for its metabolic requirement. Acid metabolites may accumulate in the myocardial tissues which stimulate nerve-endings, causing pain in the distribution of segmental nerve supply. This pain may be short-lasting, variable, recurrent or prolonged and is known as *angina pectoris.*

Recent researches suggest that coronary artery spasm is certainly an important cause of angina pectoris. It may occur at rest. Angiographic as well as radioisotopic imaging studies have shown, that ischaemia of myocardium leads to abnormal left ventricular function and nitroglycerine wonderfully relieves spasm. Role of prostaglandin and thromboxane $A_2$ are to encourage platelet aggregation. Hyperlipidaemia also inhibits the protective effects of prostaglandins. Therefore a complex mechanism seems to operate to keep proper physiological balance. One most important extraneous factor also adversely affects this process, i.e. cigarette smoking, which encourages platelet aggregation.

### Myocardial Circulation

Heart is supplied by the first two branches of the aorta, i.e. right and left coronary arteries, though a small amount of blood may enter myocardial tissues via veins of the Thebases, from the endocardial surface. The anatomy of the coronary arteries can be studied by coronary angiography, which is now a safe procedure in expert hands.

It is to be realised that heart muscle gets its blood supply during the diastole, because in systole the muscles are contracted, compressing the coronaries. Hence during tachycardia, there is precarious blood supply to the heart, as tachycardia reduces diastolic interval time hence coronary filling is also reduced.

Coronary atherosclerosis occurs with advancing age but why it occurs more extensively in some people, than others, is not yet clearly established. Young healthy soldiers who were killed during combat action also had evidence of atherosclerosis discovered during autopsy.

Similarly young people in their twenties and thirties also may show evidence of atherosclerosis during medicolegal autopsy.

There are many risk factors of I.H.D. and quite a few of these are avoidable (Table 18.5).

**Table 18.5 : Risk factors in the aetiology of I.H.D.**

1) *Genetic Factors : (Family history and blood group)*
2) *Dietary animal fat — in excess (specially saturated fat)*
3) *Essential fatty acid deficiency in diet*
4) *Too much sugar and too much carbohydrate in diet has also been incriminated.*
5) *Obesity — especially endomorphic types — more fatty and less muscular.*
6) *Hypertension (especially diastolic)*
7) *Diabetes Mellitus*
8) *High cholesterol and triglycerides (serum lipid profile showing low HDL : High LDL and VLDL)*
9) *Tobacco smoking (even moderate degree)*
10) *Excessive alcohol consumption*
11) *Thyroid disorders hypothyroidism and hyperthyroidism*
12) *Emotional stress of severe type (due to stress hormones). Ambitious and highly conscientious (personality type I).*
13) *Old age :* Although middle age group and even young are susceptible.
14) *Doubtful factors : Magnesium deficiency.*
15) *Racial and Geographical factors : may be important*
16) *Occupational factors :*

Top level business executives, politicians, lawyers, doctors, engineers are more susceptible, GP's suffer more than consulting physicians. Technical workers suffer more than labourers and farmers.

In this country, people with normal lipid profile as well as poor industrial workers also suffer. More data are required to find out importance of diet and environmental factors.

### Symptomatology

When ischaemia is extensive or if there is sudden occlusion of a major branch of the coronary artery myocardial infarction (M.I.) may occur associated with severe pain in chest with or without various complications.

Gradual narrowing of the blood vessels supplying the heart muscles, results in deficient supply of oxygen more gradually; therefore, initially it may not cause much symptoms at rest, excepting that chest pain occurs during physical exertion.

Coronary artery spasm or gradual narrowing of coronary vessels may cause anterior chest-wall pain especially on exertion which is known as 'syndrome of angina pectoris' or 'Coronary insufficiency'.

William Heberden published his classic paper on angina pectoris long before the discovery of microscope and ECG machine and when the morbid anatomists did not know much about the pathological changes in the coronary arteries.

**Pain of Cardiac Ischaemia (I.H.D.)**

Classical chest pain of I.H.D. usually starts as angina pectoris, which may be mild or severe. It may be felt as slightly annoying discomfort over and around the sternal area but in severe form it may be unbearable pain or distressing pressure in front of the chest. It may radiate along the inner side of arms, forearms and little fingers on both sides more commonly on the left. It may also radiate to the neck, jaw and even epigastrium. (Fig.18.24(a).. Sudden death may occur after a few minutes of severe precordial pain due to ventricular fibrillation and cardiac arrest.

Various types of pain as experienced by patients may appear as follows :

(1) Some discomfort in anterior chest wall or upper abdominal discomfort or gas pressing on the heart.
(2) Crushing pain across the chest.
(3) Heavy load over the anterior chest wall.
(4) Sensation of heart is being squeezed in vice.
(5) Some annoying feeling over the precordium.
(6) Uncomfortable heart burn related to food.

Localised pricking or stabbing pain over a small coin-sized area near apex of the heart is usually typical of anxiety state (pseudo-angina). Various other causes of chest pain which may be confused with cardiac pain are shown in table 18.6.

**Clinical Syndromes of I.H.D.**

Three clinical types are generally recognised :

(i) Syndrome of angina pectoris.
(ii) Acute coronary insufficiency or unstable angina (pre-infarction syndrome).
(iii) Myocardial infarction.

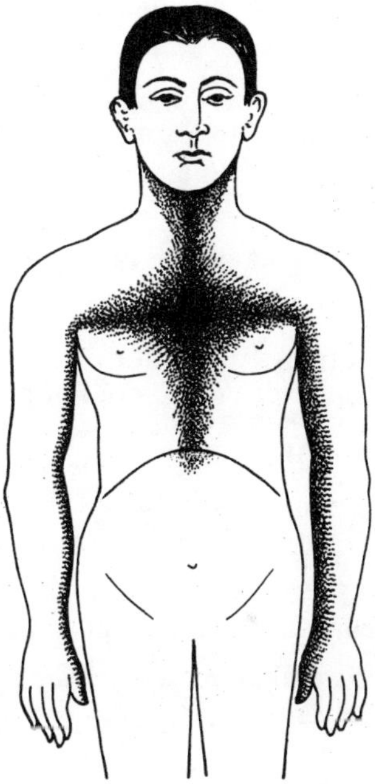

Fig.18.24(a) : Classical distribution of anginal pain

## SYNDROME OF ANGINA PECTORIS

Angina pectoris is a clinical manifestation of inadequate coronary blood supply which in the past was given many names, e.g. angina of effort, decubitus angina, nocturnal angina, intractable angina, Prinzmetal angina etc. but it is now proposed (Masari et al; 1975) that if the angina is due to coronary vasospasm it should be called primary but if it is due to an established lesion it should be called secondary. But in actual fact both factors may operate specially in elderly people.

When it occurs suddenly at rest or by disturbing the sleep, it is called angina of decubitus or "nocturnal angina". When it is brought about by effort it is named 'angina of effort'. Sometimes it occurs without exercise, but associated with ST elevation in ECG as in Prinzmetal's angina. These attacks are attributed to coronary spasm and may even end in myocardial infarction.

Older people may get attacks in toilet or during shaving. Raising the arms during shaving often precipitates the attack while more strenuous efforts may not do it (Harrison 1983). Emotional outburst is a notorious precipitating agent.

**Clinical types of angina pectoris**

Angina pectoris may be clinically classified into two groups :

(i) Stable angina

(ii) Unstable angina.

**Stable Angina**

This is commonest form of angina pectoris. The pain usually occurs during physical exertion or severe emotional stress, often during bathing or defecation. It is usually relieved by chewing or sucking a tablet of glyceryl trinitrate. The pain may recur again and similar episodes may continue for months or years unless properly treated. These recurrent episodic angina is termed chronic intractable angina.

**Unstable angina**

This is a new name of the well-known syndrome of "acute coronary insufficiency" also known as intermediate coronary syndrome, pre-infarction syndrome, acute coronary failure, threatened myocardial infarction and status angiosus etc.

To avoid further confusion W.H.O. has included all these into a group called "unstable angina", which may be of two types e.g. Type-I and Type-II.

Type-I is recent onset of angina which has increased in severity.

Type-II attacks occur at rest due to various triggering factors e.g. emotional upsets, exertion, heavy meals, exposure to cold or sexual activity.

**Atypical Angina**

(1) Sometimes anginal pain may have no radiation from precordium to periphery or it may have radiation in the reverse direction.

(2) The precordial pain may be very mild or even non-existent but pain may be felt in inner forearm and arm and mistaken for neuritis or fibrositis.

(3) Precordial pain may only be felt at rest or only a choking sensation associated with pain in throat or jaw.

(4) Sometimes it is associated with tachycardia with or without lone auricular fibrillation, pain being mild or minimal.

(5) Prinzmetal described a type, in which attacks occur in similar time and situation each day. In E.C.G. there is elevation of S.T. segment instead of depression but there is no evidence of myocardial infarction. This type is also known as 'angina pectoris inversa'. In this Prinzmetal-variant-angina, E.C.G. changes disappear as pain subsides. Prinzmetal's angina may sometimes precipitate ventricular fibrillation.

**Clinical Findings**

In angina pectoris, physical signs are usually lacking. In coronary insufficiency,clinical features vary considerably, sometimes it is only local pain with tachycardia or bradycardia. B.P. may rise or fall.

In MI the signs may be plentiful. Usually there is tachycardia, pulse rate reaching over 120 p.m. or even bradycardia, various types of heart block, severe hypotension, signs of shock, collapse even unconsciousness. Gallop rhythm may be heard proclaiming left ventricular dysfunction.

In many instances of anginal attacks patients initially may not have severe symptoms. They may attribute the discomfort to gas due to indigestion or rheumatism. The pain is often felt as pressure or load on the chest or some kind of compression in the anterior chest wall. The clinical picture of a classical myocardial infarction may be as follows :

(a) Sudden onset of acute anterior wall chest pain with or without radiation to the periphery.

(b) Sweating and cold extremities and cardiogenic shock
(c) Rapid pulse rate
(d) Ectopic beats, tachy, or brady-arrhythmias
(e) Signs of L.V.F. and pulmonary oedema

Sudden death may occur in severe AMI within a few minutes, usually due to **ventricular fibrillation.**

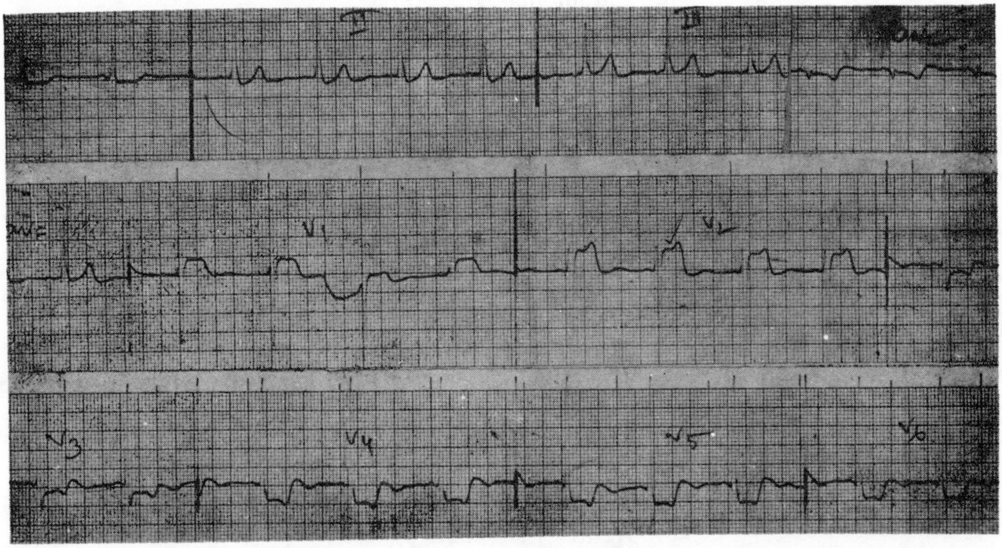

Fig.18.24(b) : ECG of a patient of severe chest pain showing acute myocardial ischaemic pattern with elevation $V_1$ & $V_2$ and depression of ST segment in $V_3$ to $V_6$.

## Diagnosis

If ECG is taken during pain of angina pectoris, ST-T changes or depression of S.T. segment may be noted, ECG taken soon after an attack or angina may or may not show any abnormality.

Differential diagnosis of anterior chest pain is presented in Table 18.6.

However, various new methods have been developed for diagnosis of early I.H.D. and angina pectoris which may have to be done in doubtful cases discussed in subsequent pages.

*Exercise stress test*

This test can be carried out in the doctor's clinic, where the patient is asked to do Master's step-test. The patient with normal ECG, who is a sufferer of anginal pain, may show a typical horizontal ST depression during exercise. Sometime it is difficult to interpret borderline ST-T changes.

More sophisticated tests consist of E.C.G. monitoring during exercise on a tread-mill. During the tread-mill exercise ECG monitoring can be carried out along with automatic recordings of pulse and B.P. These special investigations are discussed in the next chapter.

**Table 18.6 : Differential Diagnosis of Precordial Pain**

| | |
|---|---|
| (A) **C.V.S.** | (1) Ischaemic heart disease<br>(2) Pericarditis<br>(3) Aneurysm of Aorta<br>(4) Dissecting Aneurysm |
| (B) **Lungs** | (1) Pleurisy<br>(2) Pneumonitis<br>(3) Pulmonary embolism<br>(4) Carcinoma<br>(5) Spontaneous pneumothorax |
| (C) **Chest Wall and Spine** | (1) Fibrositis/Neuritis/Tietze's syndrome<br>(2) Bornholm's Syndrome<br>(3) Disc Syndrome<br>(4) Caries Spine<br>(5) Trauma to ribs, sternum and spine<br>(6) Impending herpes zoster |
| (D) **Mediastinum** | (1) Hiatus hernia<br>(2) Mediastinal tumour or carcinoma<br>(3) Mediastinitis<br>(4) Oesophageal spasm or oesophagitis |
| (E) **Abdomen** | (1) Peptic Ulcer<br>(2) Gall bladder and hepatic pain<br>(3) Splenic flexure syndrome<br>(4) Acute or subacute pancreatitis |
| (F) **Others** | (1) Anxiety state<br>(2) Ischaemic abdominal vessels<br>(3) Herpes Zoster<br>(4) Tabes dorsalis-gastric crisis<br>(5) Epigastric fatty herniation<br>(6) Malingeering |

But sometimes even after routine ECG, X-ray studies, enzymes estimations,etc., it may not be possible to pinpoint the cause of anterior chest wall pain. In such cases coronary angiography may be very useful. It will also show the vessels affected and the degree of narrowing due to the obstructive lesions.

Depending on the findings one can decide if coronary by-pass surgery may be necessary, provided the patient can afford. Facilities of coronary angiography are becoming gradually available in big cities and teaching hospitals in India and hence it may not be necessary to refer these cases to UK or USA.

### Treatment

#### Drug therapy

Many drugs are now available for treatment of acute angina pectoris, but nitroglycerin (glyceryl trinitrate) is still the drug of first choice. It acts within a minute or so and relieves anginal pain by decreasing arteriolar and venous tone as well as relieves preload and after load. One tablet (5 mg) should be placed under the tongue and is allowed to be dissolved. In urgency it can be chewed for almost immediate action. The side-effects are headache and hypotension. Headache rarely may be so disturbing that patient wants alternative drugs. Hypotensive patients may even faint after taking a tablet of trinitrate under the tongue, which passes off in a short time. Patient should be warned about these possibilities or the first dose may be given under supervision. As an alternative nifedipine can be used.

Usually isosorbide dinitrate or tetranitrate are used. Initially five and ten mg are given orally. These may be given every four or six-hourly.

Nitroglycerin ointments are now available which provide continuous cover for some hours. Transdermal nitroglycerin can give continuous release of the drug up to 24 hours.

The patient should also be taught to ward off the attack by rest, when attacks come after walking some distances. Window shopping or bird watching is a good method to avoid embarrassment in public. Trinitrate tablets should be in hand. Crush the tablet in mouth.

*Diet*

Smaller meals five or six times in a day is better than large conventional breakfast, lunch and dinner. Mental relaxation, prayers, musical evenings, religious meetings, good friendly atmosphere and card playing may be quite helpful. However, modern civilised life and high-tempo-action-packed occupational hazards may cause real problems. A good family doctor may be of great assistance to tide over problems than *Cath-lab specialists.*

Hence judicious use of tranquilizers and practice of detached attitude are useful. The family doctor should be the guide to decide when specialist consultation is necessary.

*Alternative drugs*

(1) *Beta-adrenergic-blocking agents* :

Quite a few new anti-anginal drugs are now available (Refer to the chapter on Drug therapy in cardiology and anti-arrhythmic drugs). These drugs reduce heart rate and relieve angina by reducing oxygen consumption of myocardium. But their effect on coronary vasculature is controversial.

However, all these drugs should be used with caution. Contraindications are CHF, AV-block, resting bradycardia, hypotension, arrhythmias and W-P-W syndrome. It should not be used in cases of bronchial asthma and Raynaud's disease. Side-effects vary on the type of $\beta$ blocker used. Beta-I blockers are less harmful in precipitating asthma or in masking hypoglycaemia symptoms in diabetics. Hence use of $\beta$-blockers-like propranolol in diabetics may be risky. Usual side-effects must also be carefully watched.

**Table 18.7 : Nifedipine and Verapamil**

| Action / Dose | Nifedipine | Verapamil |
|---|---|---|
| Vasodilatation | +++ | ++ |
| Sympathetic block (reflexly) | o ↓ | + ↓ |
| Dosage (TID) | 30 - 120 mg | 8 to 16 mg |
| Side effects | Nausea, flushing Hypotension, Palpitations | Nausea flushing, Hypertension, palpitation |
| Danger | Oedema | LVF |

**Calcium — entry blockers**

These drugs control calcium-influx into the myocardial cells and vascular smooth muscles. These drugs chiefly act by reducing tone of vascular smooth muscle and reduce oxygen demand. Myocardial oxygenation is also improved and coronary vasospasm is also reduced. However, atherosclerotic vessels may have little scope for the action.

The two drugs commonly used are Nifedipine and verapamil. The third drug Diltiazem is also available in India now.

Table 18.7 gives the relative merits of these two drugs.

In spite of some risks in using these drugs they are very useful in treating cases of unstable or variant angina and even stable angina, who do not tolerate nitrates or ß-blockers. Both these drugs are also useful in controlling hypertension.

**Platelet inhibitor drugs**

Anti-platelet aggregating agents have come into vogue since recent researches stressed the importance of prostaglandin-synthesis and role of thromboxane (the platelet aggregating agent). Prostacyclin diminishes platelet aggregation and helps vasodilatation. Drugs generally used are aspirin, sulphin-pyrazone and dipyridamole.

However, its possible role in preventing heart attacks and its long-term value has not been fully evaluated.

**General measures**

In all cases of I.H.D., it is important that life style of the patient may have to be readjusted as follows :

(1) Smoking must stop permanently.
(2) Reduce weight in obese patients.
(3) Diet has to be adjusted depending on body weight and lipid profile.
(4) If lipid profile is still normal, one egg for breakfast may be allowed if patient likes it. Animal fat, red meat and butter should be avoided.
(5) Alcohol : if patient is in the habit of taking alcohol regularly and is not prepared to give up, he may be allowed 30 to 60 ml of whisky or brandy to drink slowly in the evenings.
(6) Sedatives and tranquilizers are to be used as and when required.
(6) Diabetic patients with angina must be more careful regarding follow-up. Even minor chest pain if continued should be evaluated. Diabetes may cause cardiomyopathy and silent myocardial infarcts may occur. ß-blockers be better avoided.
(7) Anaemia, if present, should be treated as well as its cause should be determined.
(8) Associated endocrine disorders if any, need thorough investigation. Thyroid disorders whether thyrotoxicosis or myxoedema, both may cause or aggravate angina pectoris.
(9) Graduated exercise programme should be organised. In the author's experience, place of yoga is supreme in achieving mental tranquillity and relaxation.
(10) Proper sex-life depending as cardio-vascular status is also very important. Role of wife is supreme in this direction.

**Anticoagulants**

Anticoagulants in unstable angina is still a controversial subject. As treatment of unstable angina is unsatisfactory and drugs therapy with newer drugs also are not always rewarding, it is worthwhile giving a trial of anticoagulant therapy provided facilities are available, especially when patients cannot afford coronary by-pass surgery. Heparin is best drug to use as it is short acting and rapid in action. Oral anticoagulants can be convenient for the patient. In author's personal experience in the Armed Forces Hospitals both methods, produced satisfactory results, while in many large civil hospitals where facilities do not exist, there are many problems in prescribing anticoagulants, hence it is better to avoid.

*Role of Surgery*

(Coronary artery bypass)

Recent reports of the results of coronary artery bypass surgery is certainly encouraging. Selection of cases is most important. Good coronary angiography and left ventricular function assessment are the most essential steps. Anginal pain is usually relieved and many home-ridden patients are going to lead active life after bypass.

Those with good left ventricular function are better candidates even when three vessels are affected. Patients with unstable angina are the most difficult cases and require very expert handling. These patients are at the risk of developing sudden acute myocardial infarction, unless treated continuously. Aspirin therapy in addition to antianginal drugs, is helpful. Aspirin however will not relieve anginal pain, so long acting nitrates, $\beta$-blockers and calcium channel blockers should be judiciously used. When these measures fail, complete bed rest may relieve angina to recur again on resuming activity. These patients need careful handling to decide whether they should go for bypass surgery. Some patients are also becoming better with anticoagulants and antiplatelet therapy.

Percutaneous transluminal coronary angioplasty is also being done in recent times with good results and it is probable ,that angioplasty will become more popular than by-pass surgery.

## MYOCARDIAL INFARCTION

**Introduction**

In myocardial infarction (MI) there is necrosis of cardiac muscle due to inadequate coronary circulation. Sudden death may occur when obstruction to coronary flow is precarious. Most deaths occurring within 24 hours of the onset of attack are due to ventricular fibrillation.

**Anatomy of Coronary arteries**

There are three main sources of coronary arterial blood supply :

(1) The anterior descending branch of left coronary artery

(2) Circumflex branch of left coronary artery

(3) Right coronary artery.

The areas supplied by these arteries have their E.C.G. characteristics easily recognised.

(1) Anteroseptal

(2) Anterolateral

(3) Inferior wall or posterior

S.A. node and A.V. node are usually perfused through branches of right coronary artery. E.C.G. mapping can also be done by special techniques. Coronary angiography has now become a perfected technique in specialised centres and which can clearly reveal diseased vessels so that proper therapeutic measures can be selected.

**Pathogenesis**

Coronary occlusion occurs due to atherosclerosis of the coronary vessels in 90% of instances but coronary insufficiency can also be due to syphilitic narrowing of coronary ostium, embolic or inflammatory lesions. Thrombotic lesion in the atheromatous vessels may or may not be present. Emboli may come from vegetations on the mitral or aortic valve (infective endocarditis) or from left auricular thrombus. Polyarteritis nodosa is a very rare cause. The ultimate result of a major occlusion is myocardial infarction.

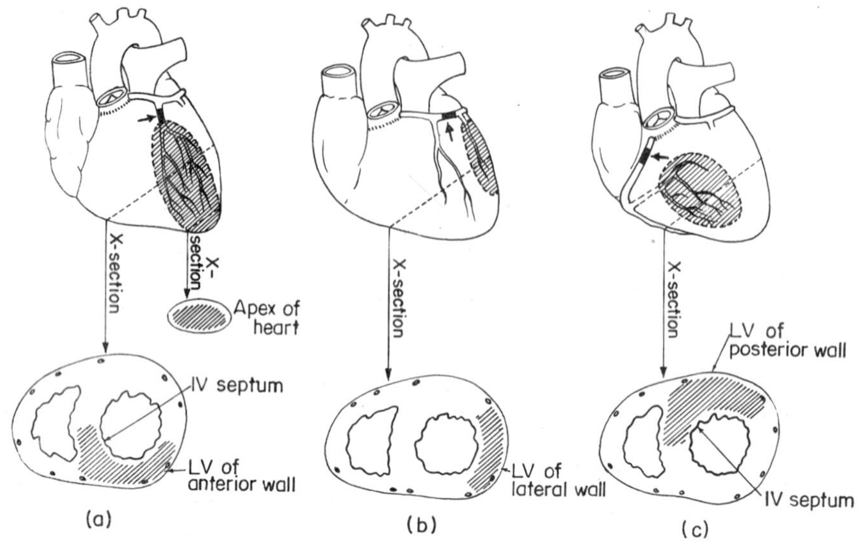


Fig.18.25 : Common sites of myocardial damage

Myocardial infarction pathologically means that there is microscopic and macroscopic damage to cardiac muscle, due to lack of oxygen supply. The cardiac muscle however may not become necrotic immediately or within a few hours. Detectable histological changes take about six hours to develop. So if the patient suddenly dies of coronary occlusion, due to severe atherosclerosis, myocardial necrosis may not be pathologically detected at autopsy.

If however patient dies after 24 hours or more, the cardiac muscles look pale, yellowish and later haemorrhagic.

Hence the relationship of atherosclerosis, thrombus formation and embolic lesions to myocardial infarction may be apparently clear but what triggers the episode is not yet well understood. Instances are recorded that patients dying of road accidents or due to war casualties, may show severe atherosclerosis, while there has been no history of angina pectoris during life-time.

Pathologists during medico-legal autopsies have demonstrated presence of scars of infarction in heart muscles in persons, who never complained of anginal pain in life.

In tropics and developing countries, under-weight people with low fat diet as well as having normal cholesterol levels also develop myocardial infarction. Data on their lipid profile are inadequate in developing countries. Hence much more studies are required before we can specify how a so-called heart attack is precipitated. Most attacks occur at night or early in the morning or while in the toilet but rarely during physical exertion.

**Symptoms**

Occurrence of MI is signalled by precordial pain in most cases though rarely it may be painless especially in very old people or diabetics.

Pain similar to anginal distribution may occur in 80% of cases. The degree of severity may vary. In old people painless MI may occur and the symptom may be only a fainting episode. Diabetic patients may sometimes develop myocardial infarction quite silently or without much pain.

Pain of angina pectoris is usually relieved with rest or rest plus glyceryl trinitrate (GNT), but once MI is established, GNT does not relieve pain but it may sometimes be more harmful causing further fall of B.P. which may be already low due to shock. GNT may be useful in the state of coronary insufficiency (pre-infarction angina) but once infarction has occurred it may cause "steal phenomena" and not resolve the infarction. In coronary artery spasm, it is undoubtedly of great value. Long-term therapy, high dose therapy, low dose therapy with beta-blockers are all recommended.

There may be evidence of L.V.F. without much frank physical signs. Careful assessment, however, may reveal evidence of orthopnoea and radiograph taken in bed may show perihilar congestion.$S_3$ and $S_4$, gallop rhythm can be heard and even a systolic thrust may be palpable over left parasternal area (left ventricular wall dysfunction).

Pericardial rub may occur in some cases after 24 to 48 hours. There may also be some low grade fever within 24 hours which returns to normal within five days.

Various presenting symptoms with or without chest pain are due to vasomotor instability, e.g.

(1) Sudden orthopnoea
(2) Fainting
(3) Tachycardia, bradycardia or irregular action or heart (dysrhythmias)
(4) Cold sweats with cold extremities following dyspnoea
(5) Symptoms of upper abdominal discomfort which may be attributed to 'gas' in stomach by the patients.

**Clinical findings**

In angina pectoris,physical signs are usually lacking. Hypertension may be associated.

In coronary insufficiency,clinical features vary considerably; chest pain may be associated, with tachycardia, bradycardia or some arrhythmias; B.P. may rise or fall.

In MI the signs may be plentiful. Usually there is tachycardia, pulse rate reaching over 120 pm or there may be bradycardia, various types of heart block, severe hypotension, signs of shock, collapse, even unconsciousness. Stoke-Adam's syndrome may occur. Gallop rhythm may be heard proclaiming left ventricular dysfunction.

In many instances, patients initially may not have severe symptoms. They may attribute the local discomfort to gas, due to indigestion or rheumatism. The pain is often felt as pressure or load on the chest or some kind of compression across the anterior chest wall. The clinical picture of a classical acute attack may be as follows :

1) Sudden onset of acute anterior wall chest pain with or without radiation to the periphery.
2) Sweating and cold extremities.
3) Rapid pulse rate.
4) Ectopic beats tachy-, or brady-arrythmias
5) Signs or L.V.F.

Sudden death may occur in severe AMI within a few minutes, which is usually due to ventricular fibrillation.

**Diagnosis**

The diagnosis is chiefly clinical, as E.C.G. changes may occur later on, after some hours and serum enzyme changes proclaiming myocardial injury are also not immediates. Anticipation is very important. The clinical judgement is the *sine que non* of early diagnosis and the 'G.P.' (family physician) is the supreme commander to decide the treatment, at home or hospital. Immediate hospitalisation in rural setting is not usually possible.

If E.C.G. is taken during pain of angina pectoris, ST-T changes or depression of S.T. segment may be noted, ECG taken soon after an attack of angina may or may not show any abnormality.

In acute MI, ECG changes occur within a few hours but almost always, characteristic changes are seen within 24 to 36 hours of infarction. The ECG changes are as follows :

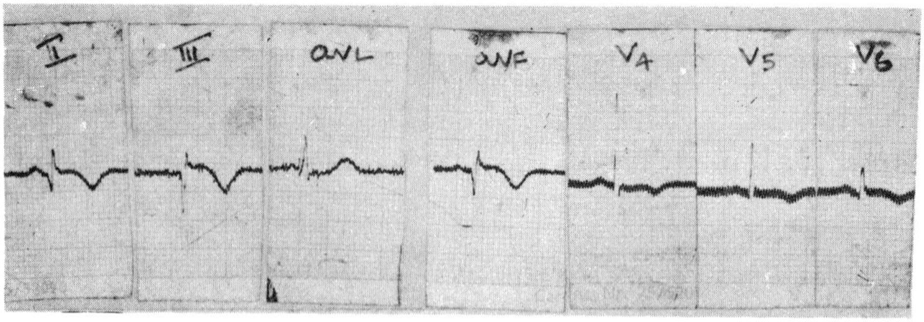


**Fig.18.26**(a) : Inferior wall infarction, also ischaemia lateral wall, possible subendocardial infarction. Patient aged 44, recovered and returned to active job.

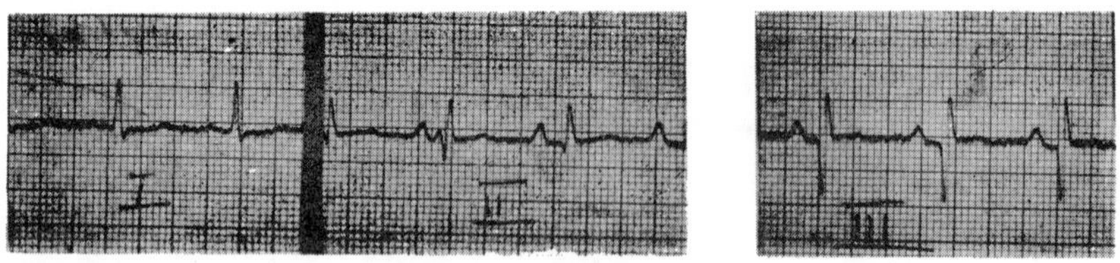


**Fig.18.26(b)** : Patient aged 62 years old case of COPD & Pulmonary tuberculosis (Healed). ECG shows old healed inferior wall infarction and V.P.B.

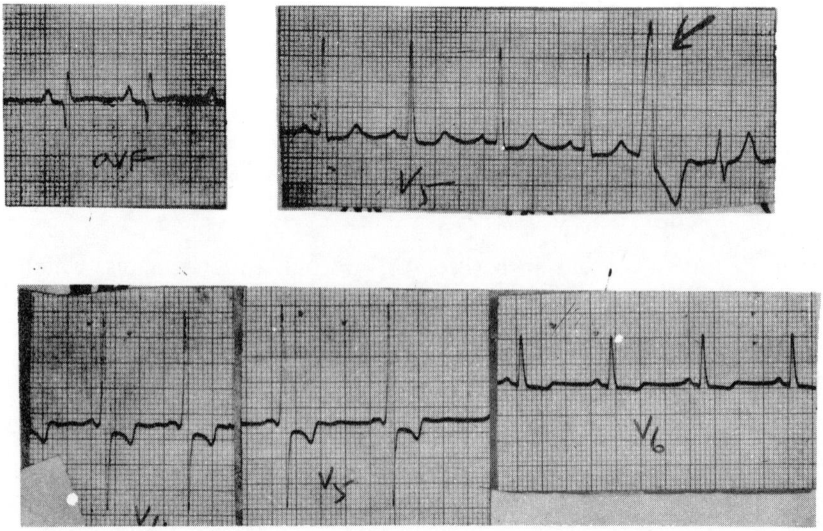


**Fig.18.26(c)** — **Patient aged** 57 years has hypertensive heart disease. ECG shows L.V. stress,ST (↓) and well marked T wave inversion. Suffers from recurrent anginal pain relieved by Isordil..

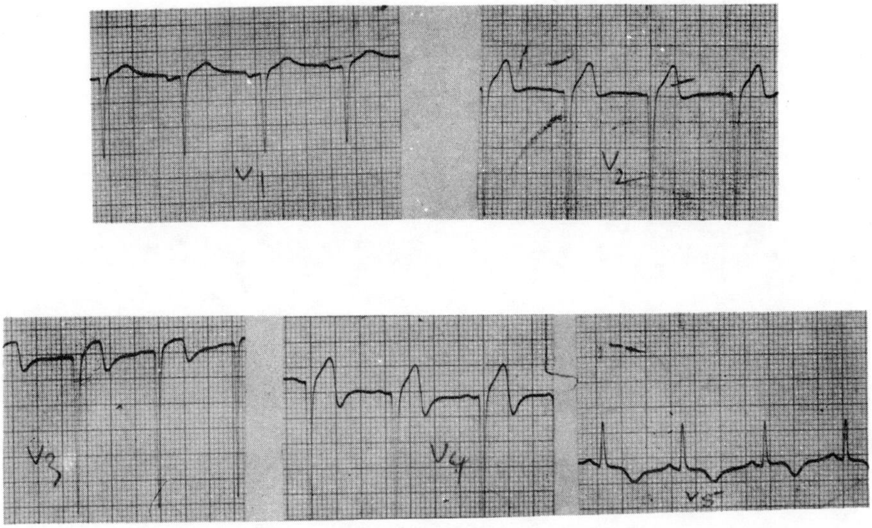


Fig.18.26(d) – Acute myocardial infarction showing well **marked** S.T. elevation in $V_3$ and $V_4$. Clinically acute chest pain over sternal area. No history of previous heart disease.

Fig.18.26 – *Showing ECG changes in acute myocardial infarction* :

1) **Extensive anterior wall infarction**

(Left coronary artery occlusion)

Q waves in leads I, II, AVL, $V_1$ to $V_6$ with ST elevation.

2) **Anteroseptal infarction**

(anterior descending branch of left coronary occluded)

Q in leads I, AVL, $V_2$ to $V_4$ with ST elevation

3) **Anterolateral infarction**

Q in leads I, AVL, $V_4$ to $V_6$ with ST elevation.

4) **Inferior wall infarction**

(right coronary artery occlusion)

Q in leads II, II & AVF with S.T. elevation.

As the damaged myocardium heals the Q waves regress elevated ST segment reverse and finally T-waves becomes inverted in the opposite direction. ECG may gradually improve but rarely becomes entirely normal.

The earliest change may be elevation of ST segment in some leads depending on the site of infarction, which are later on followed by T-waves inversion. If the infarction is transmural Q waves appear. Otherwise, if the whole thickness of muscle is not involved, Q waves may not appear but the R-wave amplitudes may be low.

The important points to note are :

(1) Elevated S.T. segments, in leads facing area of damage and reciprocal S.T. depression in opposite leads. ST elevation is due to the 'current of injury'.

(2) Inversion of T-waves.

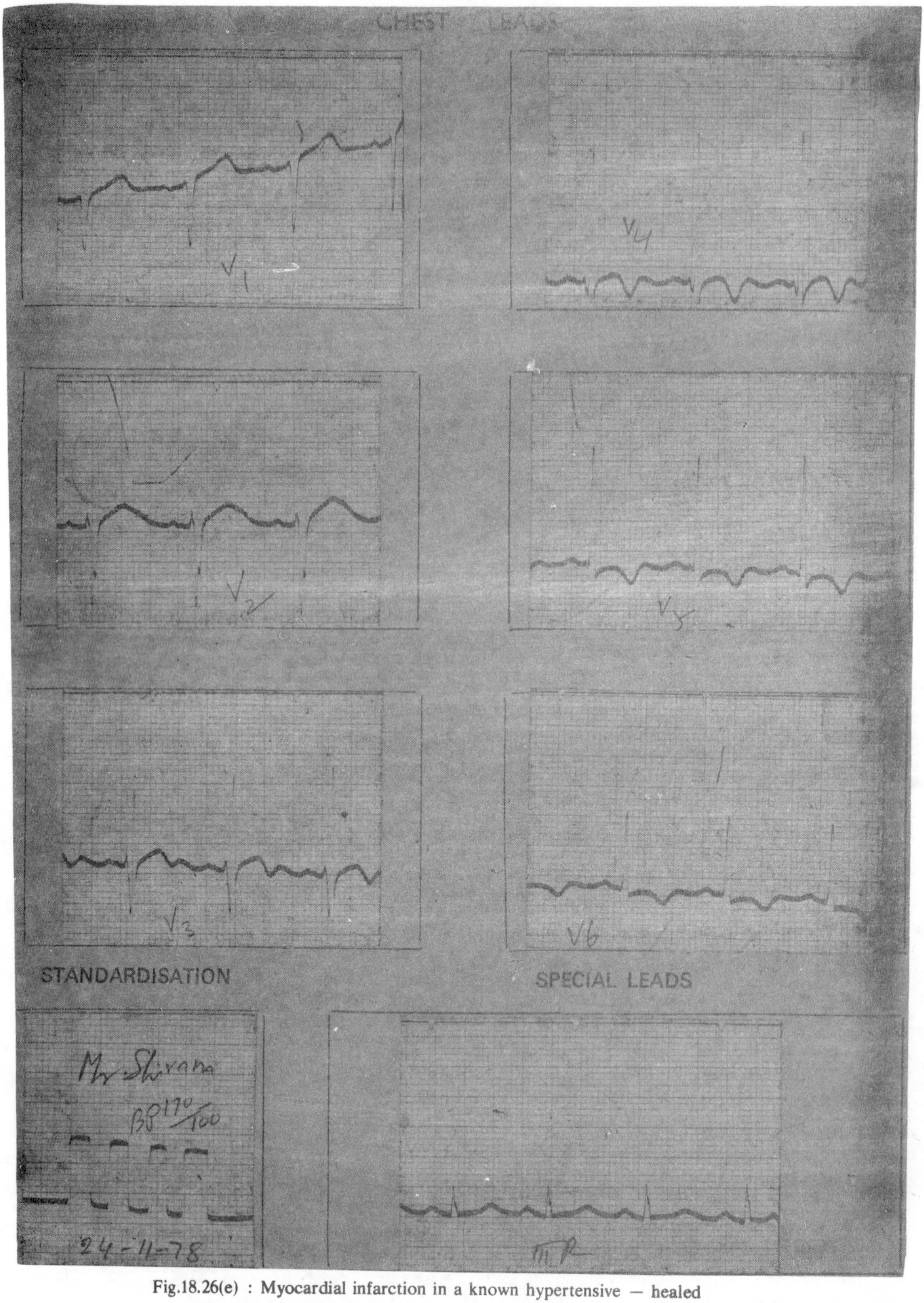


Fig.18.26(e) : Myocardial infarction in a known hypertensive — healed pattern antero-lateral wall. Patient race-horse trainer, in active job.

(3) Appearances of deep and wide Q-waves in appropriate leads, which indicates through and through infarction in this area of myocardium.

(4) S.T. segment elevation gradually becomes normal in a few days or weeks but sometimes may remain elevated for a long time or even permanently (possible aneurysm of the heart).

Figures 18.26(a) to 18.26(e) show some typical patterns of ECG changes commonly encountered.

Anatomically the following points are important. Left coronary involvement may present as follows depending on the area of damage :

(1) Antero septal $V_1$ to $V_3$

(2) Antero lateral $V_5$ to $V_7$

(3) Anterior wall $V_1$ to $V_5$

(4) High lateral I, AVL

Right coronary artery :

(1) Inferior wall — II, III, AVF

(2) Posterior wall — $V_1$ & $V_2$ — very tall T waves

The important points to note are :

(1) Elevated S.T. segments, in leads facing areas of initial damage and reciprocal ST depression in opposite leads. Pathological Q waves proclaim presence of myocardial necrosis when only ST changes are present without Q waves appears, it suggests that there is coronary occlusion without real pathological necrosis. Highly peaked tall T waves are also suspicious in this clinical setting.

(2) Inversion of T-waves.

(3) Appearances of deep and wide Q-waves in appropriate leads.

(4) ST segment elevation gradually becomes normal in a few days or weeks but sometimes may remain elevated for a long time or even permanently. Persistent elevation of ST-segment denotes myocardial dyskinesia but not necessarily dilatation.

**Investigations**

(1) Blood examination within 24 and 48 hours may show leucocytosis with raised E.S.R. Serum bilirubin may show a little elevation sometimes.

(2) Urine may show excess of urobilinogen in the early stage.

(3) Serum enzymes are also elevated within 24 to 48 hours.

(4) Serum enzymes are also elevated within 24 to 48 hours. Three types of enzymes are noted to rise within a few hours of attack. These enzymes are liberated from damaged myocardial cells.

**Serum enzyme levels**

Myocardial enzymes are released from myocardial cells after myocardial necrosis has occurred.

Three enzymes are usually measured i.e. SGOT, CPK and LDH.

In this part of the world facilities of SGOT estimation are commonly available, while CPK and LDH are often more useful, provided its enzymes are measured and serial observations are made.

**SGOT** — (Serum aspartate transaminase)

This enzyme starts rising from 6 to 24 hours after the onset of infarction and reaches its peak in 24 to 48 hours to return to normal within three to five days.

SGOT is also present in the liver and lungs, so some elevation of SGOT may also occur in pulmonary infarction and hepatocellular injury. The test is easily done in most laboratories and hence a reliable test for cardiac infarction in proper clinical setting.

**CPK (or CK)** – Creatine phospho-Kinase has three plasma isoenzymes, MM, MB and BB. *Elevated MB-CPK activity is almost specific of myocardial infarction.* It is elevated within 4 to 6 hours and reaches its peak in 12 to 48 hours and returns to normal level within 36 to 48 hours. The value of rising MB-CPK level between 24 and 36 hours of chest pain is highly specific. It also gives some idea of the extent of myocardial damage. Hence becoming more popular among cardiologists.

These enzymes can be measured in serum within 12 hours of chest pain and reaches its peak in 24 to 48 hours.

These enzymes, however, remain high even up to one to two weeks. The value of elevated LDH level is less specific because these enzymes are also present in RBC, brain, kidney, and gastric tissues. However, $LDH_1/LDH_2$ ratio of greater than 1.0 is suggestive of myocardial injury.

Serial estimations are valuable.

*However, none of these tests are useful within first 3 to 4 hours after the heart attack, which is the most critical period after the attack.* Even typical ECG changes may not occur soon after the attack, hence clinical diagnosis still remains the most valuable method. These sophisticated and expensive enzyme tests are not of much use to our rural patients.

The clinical diagnosis should not be difficult when typical features are present along with abnormal ECG findings. But in some cases diagnosis may be difficult in the most critical stage i.e. within first one to three hours of infarction. ECG change may not be always present and serum enzyme levels take time to be elevated and results also are not available at once. The clinician's role is therefore supreme.

Hence careful and critical evaluation of symptomatology and history is essential. Perforation of peptic ulcer and acute pancreatitis are the two most difficult problems.

In a large general hospital of Calcutta with 1500 beds about 500 to 600 cases are usually admitted annually. Most large hospitals have 6 to 8 beds in a CCU, hence it is not possible to admit all cases in C.C.U.

## Management

### Rest & nursing care

When attack is severe, patient must be kept in bed and should receive continuous nursing care, if possible in a C.C.U.

There is always some risk during transporting patient from the place of occurrence to hospital but proper supervision of treatment is hardly possible at home, except, in special circumstances. If the patient is in shock he should be kept in bed without a pillow in supine position but if there is L.V.F., he should be supported by a back rest at about 40° to 45° angle with oxygen line. The number of days of bed-rest depends on the seriousness of the attack. It may be a few days to two or three weeks depending on clinical situation, complications and E.C.G. findings.

Some patients often do not tolerate morphine and pethidine so well and suffer from nausea and vomiting. Pethidine with Phenergan may be helpful.

### Relief of pain

Morphine or pethidine are the best drugs to relieve pain. It is best to give 10 to 15 mg. of morphine sulphate or 50 to 100 mg of pethidine slowly I.V. depending on body weight and severity of the pain.

Nitrites which are always helpful in angina pectoris, do not relieve pain if infarction has occurred. Rather if too much nitrites are taken by the patient, there may be fall of B.P., hypoperfusion of myocardium and possible development of arrhythmias. "Occasionally in desperation, patients consume large quantities of nitrites over a short period of time producing hypotension and sometimes syncope" (Oxford Textbook of Medicine 13.175, 1983) However, if the patient is in I.C.U. and if there is no hypotension, GNT may be tried sublingually or by I.V. route, to find out if any useful result can be derived.

In order to relieve pain most important factors are adequate oxygenation and judicious use of analgesics. Second dose of morphine or pethidine may be required in a few cases who continue to have pain but if the pain is milder, milder analgesics like codeine phosphate 10 mg 2-3 times a day be given along with tranquilisers like diazepam 5 mg. two to three times daily.

**Oxygen**

Administration of oxygen by nasal catheter or by a suitable mask is useful and may give relief from chest pain, shock or pulmonary complications. Somehow most of our patients do not like masks.

Oxygen inhalation by nasal catheter is only alternative. Some patients feel better with intermittent oxygen inhalation which may ensure considerable self-confidence and security. As these patients get much psychological relief with an available oxygen supply at bed-side. There is no harm, as it gives him confidence and good night's sleep.

**Anticoagulants**

Although there is no uniformity of opinion about the usefulness of anticoagulants, it is advisable to use it in all severe cases of myocardial infarction or if it is a second attack. Frequent angina is also an indication but old age, presence of peptic ulcer or bleeding diathesis are contraindications (Vide previous chapter).

**Ambulation**

On theoretical basis it takes a transmural infarction to heal about 5 to 8 weeks so that a good scar is formed. Extent of myocardial damage can be studied by radionucleotide method but such facilities will not be available to most of us for many more years to come. Therefore, clinical assessment and easily available laboratory tests will beour guide in most circumstances. However, the sophisticated methods being used nowadays have been discussed in the next chapter.

Early ambulation is now encourged in most centres but has occasionally caused fatalities, as response of patients is not always predictable. Many formulae and indices are available and among these Peel's index is mentionable. It is, however, well-known that sometime not-so-serious a case may suddenly die due to arrhythmias, while very serious cases survive and recover very nicely. However, the following points are important in judging a patient's capacity to start ambulation.

(1) Subjective feeling of being well.

(2) Resting heart rate less than 90 pm.

(3) Systolic B.P. not less than 100 mm of Hg.

(4) Normal heart sound and heart size.

(5) Absence of signs of cardiac failure.

(6) Absence of orthostatic hypotension.

If systolic B.P. falls below 90 mm always be very cautious, especially if the lying B.P. is also low.

(7) Absence of arrhythmia and conduction defects.

ECG findings should not be given supreme importance but patient's clinicial status and psychological background have greater role to play than ECG changes. Rapid pulse rate, too low B.P., undue fatigue, dizzy spells, nocturnal breathing problem (not sighing or hyperventilation), recurrence of chest pain are the adverse signs requiring close clinical evaluation.

**Diet**

For shocked patient or if there is pulmonary oedema or CCF, he may only require sips of water or a little fruit juice with sugar but no salt. Once the patient's pain is relieved and there are no complications, start with 800 calorie diet, to be gradually increased. Fruit juice or milk without cream, barely water, artificial milk preparations with low fat content should be tried initially. Diet has to be amended depending on other factors like obesity, diabetes, hypertension or renal disease, if any.

Diet should then be built up depending on patient's previous food habit starting with light meals at breakfast, lunch and dinner.

Eggs, red meat, butter, ghee, fried food, rich fatty food are not permitted. Reduce the salt content of the food from this stage. Too much sugar intake is also harmful.

If the patient was a smoker, this is the time to force him in strong language to give up smoking permanently. If the patient was in the habit of taking alcohol, one drink (30 ml) of whisky or brandy may be allowed with plain water, which gives the patient confidence, psychological satisfaction of good progress and possibly good night's sleep. This is the time to reform hard alcoholics who can be educated to learn how to drink alcohol for good health. Literature on ill-effects of alcohol and smoking must be provided for his information.

**Management of complications**

It is important to very carefully watch for the complications. Assess manifestations of pump failure. Associated with weakness of the pump there may be signs of reflex neurogenic shock, arising from injured myocardium. Clinical features of shock are recognised by sweating, cold extremities, severe fatigue, confusion and reduced urinary flow. Pulse is rapid with low volume with marked fall of both systolic and diastolic blood pressure. Low B.P. alone is not shock. Management of cardiogenic shock is fully discussed in a subsequent chapter.

**Arrhythmias**

Arrhythmias are dangerous complications and therefore it should be treated carefully as soon as they tend to appear. These arrhythmias may be heralded by occurrence of a few supra-ventricular or ventricular ectopic beats but sometimes sudden rapid tachycardias may precede serious arrhythmias. Various degrees of heart block may also result in Stoke-Adam's syndrome, leading to loss of consciousness and even death. Modern monitoring facilities in C.C.U. or even home monitoring have completely changed the mode of treatment.

Arrhythmias which are more frequent in first 24 hours (most vulnerable period) can be detected easily and treatment can be instituted properly. Previously arrhythmias were not easily recognised, as continuous monitoring was not possible. Hence many unexpected deaths occurred due to ventricular fibrillation.

Presence of a few supraventricular ectopics needs further watching. Possibly it is better to watch them to prescribe some anti-arrhythmic drugs at once as most drugs also have their adverse side-effects. Ventricular ectopic beats (VEB's) are not uncommon and are dangerous if they come frequently or in turns of three or more. They are treated with I.V. lignocaine-drip. However, it may be pointed out that VEB's are due to myocardial damage and lignocaine is also a myocardial depressant. Therefore its use should be carefully recommended.

Sinus tachycardia is a reflex action due to sympathetic overdrive,due to pain or cardiac failure. Hence treatment of pain, cardiac failure or shock should receive urgent attention.

Sinus bradycardia is due to vagal over-activity but escape rhythm occurs, treat this with atropine. Heart block requires careful scrutiny and sometimes electrical pacing may be necessary as a life saving measure.

However, it is wise to remember that do not treat the ECG but take the total clinical features and condition of the patient. It is also to be noted that all antidysrhythmic drugs are myocardial depressants. A special chapter on 'Arrhythmias' has been included discussing their detailed mode of action.

**Shock**

This is a dreadful complication which must be treated with great care. This is dealt with in a special chapter in this book.

Treatment of cardiogenic shock is an extremely difficult problem in general practice. For proper assessment it is essential to assess the cardiovascular status by monitoring the following factors :

(1) State of consciousness and clinical data e.g. B.P., pulmonary congestion, pulse rate, arrhythmias, gallop, renal function (urine output) and metabolic acidosis.

(2) B.P. record can only be correctly in measured by direct arterial needle as routine clinical method can be fallacious.

(3) Oxygen, $CO_2$ level and pH should be measured but in any case oxygen inhalation must be ensured.

(4) Central venous pressure (C.V.P.) should be measured. The best method is to measure pulmonary wedge pressure (P.W.P.) by Swan-Ganz balloon catheter. If the P.W.P. is high, patient has volume overload and will require diuretics and inotropic drugs and if it is lower than normal (14 to 18 mm Hg), I.V. fluids should be given.

(5) If no such facilities are available and if hypovolaemia is clinically suspected, 5% glucose I.V. drip can be started and after infusing 200 to 300 ml, clinical condition be watched. If pulmonary congestion or breathlessness increases stop the I.V. drip and start diuretics and watch renal function.

(6) Vasopressor agents e.g. noradrenaline and mephentermine were used in the past. The modern opinion is going against it. It is argued that in cardiogenic shock there is already existing severe vasoconstriction and these drugs may be harmful.

Dopamine however is considered useful as it has inotropic effect on the myocardium and appears to improve cardiac output. It also has renal vasodilating action but constrictor action on muscular and cutaneous vessels. Hence it is recommended to infuse 200 mg of dopamine (5 ml ampoule) in a bottle of 5% dextrose to be given as I.V. drip at the rate of 20 to 40 drops per minute and carefully watch the effect.

If a pressor agent e.g. nor-adrenaline or mephentermine is used on a short-term basis when dopamine is not available, it should not be given as bolus-dose. Put 2-4 mg. of noradrenaline in a bottle of 5% glucose saline and ensure flow rate of 10-15 μg/min. As it produces intense vasoconstriction it should better be avoided in cardiogenic shock. Mephentermine sulphate 15 to 30 mg I.M. may tide over a desperate situation in rural setting and slow I.V. drug containing 150 mg of mephentermine in bottle of 5% glucose has saved many lives in the past although cardiologists working in ICU need not use these two drugs. It is reported that these drugs may increase the infarct size also. But it is also true that we have salvaged many patients in severe cardiogenic shock using one of these two drugs before Dopamine was available. These drugs were also reinforced with I.V. hydrocortisone in dosage of 200 mg bolus dose and then in I.V. drip up to 400 to 600 mg in first 24 hours.

There are also controversies in the use of steroids in cardiogenic shock but I will recommend its use in shocked patient of myocardial infarction in above dosage as I have salvaged many dying patients by using this drug.

*(Refer also to the chapter on cardiogenic shock).*

**Embolic manifestation**

Sudden pulmonary embolism is a very important cause of unexpected death due to a thrombus coming from clots in deep leg veins. Systemic arterial embolism from an intracardiac mural thrombus is not so common. The risk of embolism remains for two to three weeks, i.e. as long as the patient is in bed, receiving sedatives and tranquilisers. Leg movement and light physiotherapy are helpful in initial stages. Deep vein thrombus in legs can be detected early, by checking tenderness in calf-muscles every day. Calf muscles must be checked daily for any evidence of deep tenderness (Hoffman's sign for phlebothrombosis).

*Acute left ventricular failure* is another important complication and this is often manifested by sudden development of dyspnoea due to pulmonary congestion. Gallop rhythm and pulsus alternans are warning signs. Left ventricular failure may ultimately result is congestive heart failure recognised by enlarged tender liver and peripheral oedema. In a lying patient sacral region should be examined for oedema. The legs should also be daily inspected for oedema.

**Pericarditis**

Presence of pericardial rub over precordium proclaims pericarditis. This is often easily heard if the patient can sit up and lean forward. It may occur within a few days of heart attack or after a few weeks, there may be associated pleurisy (Dresslar's syndrome). It usually responds to analgesics but rarely corticosteroids are required especially where pleuro-pericarditis is present.

**Left ventricular aneurysm**

When myocardial infarction is through and through and if considerable area is involved the firbrous tissue formed in the infarcted area may distend to form an aneurysmal dilatation. If it causes left ventricular failure, surgery should be considered. Overall mortality is still about 15%.

**Mitral regurgitation**

Mitral valve prolapse may occur due to damaged papillary muscles. Mild cases can be treated with diuretics while severe cases should be surgically managed by mitral valve replacement.

**Cardiac rupture**

The damaged myocardium may suddenly rupture causing sudden death. Other injuries due to infarction may cause rupture of the I.V. septum resulting in pansystolic murmur as in VSD. Pansystolic murmur may also occur due to rupture and papillary muscle resulting in mitral regurgitation.

**Other Complications**

Other less acute complications are muscular wasting as well periarthritis, particularly of the shoulder-joint (Frozen shoulder).

Anxiety neurosis and depression state (melancholia) are sometimes quite troublesome. Attention to patient's mental rehabilitation is as important as cardiovascular rehabilitation.

Proper physiotherapy from the beginning usually prevents frozen shoulder or arthritic problems. Once frozen shoulder develops it is a difficult problem to tackle. Physiotherapy, ultrasonic heat and sometimes intra-articular steroids may be required.

**First-aid management acute attack**

1. Set up an IV drip of 5% glucose solution, if not already done.
2. Oxygen administration should be started.
3. Connect the patient to the scope (if available) and read the ECG to come to a diagnosis about the site of the myocardial infarction, the state of cardiac rhythm, presence of the arrhythmias etc. Inform your senior.
4. Inj. morphine 10-15 mg I.M. for relief of pain, if not already given and then repeat this as and when considered essential. Pethidine also can be given in dosage of 50 to 100 mg. Either pethidine or morphine can be combined with Phenergan 2.5 mg to ensure relief of pain as well as sedation. Those steps can be done even in coronary care ambulance including oxygen administration.
5. A thorough clinical examination should be done with the particular emphasis on the state of shock, CHF and arrhythmia.
6. Charts for the pulse. B.P., temperature, respiration should be meticulously maintained.
7. Chart for the intake/output of fluid and the drugs administered should be maintained.

8. Inj. Hydrocortisone or Dexamethasone may be useful in some cases, who are in shock.
9. Anticoagulants should be considered in all severe cases of myocardial infarction if there is no contraindication. Give Inj. Heparin 7500 units I.V. and then repeat 5000 units I.V. six hourly. BT-CT should be done before giving the next dosage so that the adjustment can be done. Heparin should be continued for 48 hours. Tab. Sinthrom (4mg) — start with four tablets stat then give two tablets on the second day and again two tablets on the third day. Prothrombin time should be done daily to adjust the dosage of Sinthrom. Vitamin K and Protamin should be available for emergency.
10. Introduction of intracoronary streptokinase is another new method in making attempts to revascularize the ischaemic heart.
11. Infarctectomy is too heroic with very limited success.
12. Rupture of heart is always fatal but rarely slow leak may result in formation of pseudoaneurysm. The aneurysm can however be diagnosed by echocardiography and may be surgically excised in rare cases.

## CARDIOGENIC SHOCK

*I.M. AHUJA*

### Definition

Cardiogenic shock may be defined as the clinical state resulting from inability of the heart to pump sufficient blood for the perfusion need of the vital organs. The most common cause of cardiogenic shock is acute myocardial infarction. Oligaemic shock is not included in this definition.

### Clinical signs and pathogenesis

Insufficient blood flow through the skin, skeletal muscles, kidneys and brain and excess secretion of catecholamines give the clinical signs of shock. The skin is pale, cold and moist because of vasoconstriction and sweating under the influence of excess catecholamines. There is profound muscular weakness as enough blood does not flow through the skeletal muscles. The resulting metabolic acidosis causes 'air hunger'. There is oliguria or anuria because of reduced renal blood flow. Mental confusion, or coma result from cerebral hypoxia. Excess secretion of catecholamines causes anxiety and fear of death. If the patient survives the acute episode, results of hypoxic damage of the kidney, lung, liver and brain may manifest as acute renal tubular necrosis, 'shock-lung', jaundice and cerebral oedema respectively.

In acute myocardial infarction, cardiac output goes down. To compensate for this, peripheral vasoconstriction and tachycardia occur under the influence of catecholamines. Blood pressure generally falls after acute myocardial infarction. Occasionally, there is disproportionate vasoconstriction and there is transient rise of blood pressure. In a few cases there is bradycardia instead of tachycardia. This is attributed to vagotonia. One should not therefore insist on finding low blood pressure and tachycardia before making a diagnosis of shock. If there are clinical signs of tissues under perfusion as detailed above, the patient may be said to be in shock.

It is to be noted that nowadays emphasis has shifted from blood pressure to blood flow. The aim of circulation is to maintain tissue perfusion and not any specific 'normal' blood pressure. Therefore, if the patient's skin is warm, his urinary secretion is normal and he is mentally clear, one does not need to give any vasoconstrictor drugs even if the blood pressure falls to 80 or 90 mm Hg systolic and 50-60 mm Hg diastolic. If the blood pressure falls below these figures, coronary and renal circulation may suffer.

**Management**

(a) **Intravenous line** : The first step is to establish a good intravenous line and to secure it well. Percutaneous introduction of a cannula into a major vein is preferable to a venesection in a small peripheral vein.

(b) **Intravenous fluids** : Most cases are in negative fluid balance because of sweating, vomiting, restricted fluid intake and loss of fluid into interstitial space. Even those not in a negative balance seem to improve with I.V. fluids because of increased filling pressure which improves cardiac output. Glucose 5% is the most commonly used fluid and is usually readily available. Dextran, plasma or even blood may be given and these are preferable because they stay longer in the vascular compartment. Fluid is given in increments of 100 ml at a fairly rapid rate while effects of circulatory improvement are observed, e.g. rise of blood pressure, fall of heart rate, skin becoming warm and resumption of urine output. Careful watch is kept on signs of overhydration, i.e. increase in respiratory rate, onset of cough and appearance of moist sounds in lungs. Jugular venous pressure may be allowed to rise to 5-7 on above sternal angle. Monitoring of left atrial filling pressure ('wedge' pressure) is desirable but is usually not feasible in general practice.

(c) **Inotropic drugs** : If the administration of fluid results in appearance of signs of overhydration without improvement of circulatory state, one should slow down the drip rate to a minimum and give drugs which will strengthen myocardial contractility. Dopamine in a dose of 2-5 microgram/kg/min (200 mg in 500 ml of 5% glucose given @ 5-12 drops/min) given as an intravenous drip increases myocardial contractility and increases renal blood flow. Drip rate should be carefully adjusted by repeated blood pressure readings and a careful record of urine output which is best measured by putting in an in-dwelling catheter.

Isoproterenol was in use before dopamine became available. It causes increase of myocardial contractility and heart-rate and peripheral vasodilatation. It may cause cardiac arrhythmias and increased myocardial oxygen consumption. Increase of vascular bed capacity necessitates administration of more I.V. fluids.

Digoxin is a potent inotropic drug but its action is too slow in onset for use in this acute emergency. Cardiac arrhythmias may arise because the myocardium is ischaemic.

(d) **Vasodilator drugs** like sodium nitroprusside, glyceryl trinitrate and hydralazine have been used in well-equipped hospitals with facilities for continuous monitoring of arterial, central venous and pulmonary capillary pressures. Their use in the setting outside a hospital does not appear practical.

(e) **Vasoconstrictor drugs** like noradrenaline and mephentine have been going out of favour because they increase peripheral vascular resistance and thus the mechanical work of the heart. Tissue perfusion may actually go down, with resultant metabolic acidosis. These drugs tend to cause cardiac arrhythmias. They may however be needed if blood pressure falls below critical pressure levels. These drugs should be given as an intravenous drip, the drip-rate being titrated to maintain the systolic pressure at about 90 mm Hg. They should not be given as a bolus.

(f) **Sedatives** like morphine should be given in minimal doses, just enough to relieve pain and restlessness. Morphine 2-5 mg I.V. may achieve this without causing respiratory depression. Drugs given intramuscularly are absorbed erratically in patients in shock.

(g) **Oxygen** should be administered to these patients as it may help to relieve pain and to reduce infarct size.

(h) **Antiarrhythmic drugs** : Ectopic beats do not produce effective forward flow and consume scarce oxygen. On the other hand, most antiarrhythmic drugs have a depressant action on the myocardium. Ectopic beats up to 5/min need not be treated. More frequent ectopic beats should be treated with xylocaine drip. This drug causes minimal myocardial depression. Marked bradycardia (below 50 beats/min) should be treated with atropine.

## PROGNOSIS

Mortality rate remains very high in cardiogenic shock in spite of all treatment. Tissue hypoxia for any length of time encourages irreversible circulatory failure. Energetic treatment should therefore be started as soon as signs of shock are recognizable. Those who survive the acute attack may succumb to acute renal tubular necrosis, shock lung or cerebral oedema. As the condition carries a high mortality rate, the patient should be admitted to a hospital as soon as feasible.

## RECENT ADVANCES IN INVESTIGATION AND TREATMENT OF CORONARY ARTERY DISEASE

*I.M. AHUJA*

### Introduction

Over the past decade a number of newer forms of investigation and treatment of coronary artery disease have been introduced. It is essential for a general physician to become familiar with their pros and cons so as to be able to select appropriate cases for referral to specialised centres or to initiate appropriate therapy in a given case.

In the field of investigation, advances have been made in exercise stress testing, radionuclide studies, coronary arteriography and echocardiography. These investigations are expensive in terms of specialised equipment and time spent by trained personnel and some of these carry a degree of risk to the patient. One has therefore to be careful about the type patient one refers for these investigations. The general principle of minimal discomfort/risk and maximal benefit to the patient should be followed. Investigations for mere "completeness", academic interest or prognostic stratification should be generally avoided as these give no benefit to the individual patient. Such investigations may be justified in recognised research institutions as parts of properly vetted research projects in which the expenses are not paid by the patient.

In the field of treatment, the newer forms of therapy are thrombolytic drug therapy, percutaneous transluminal coronary angioplasty, coronary artery bypass surgery, use of betablockers in the immediate post-infarction period, antiplatelet drugs, calcium channel blockers and transcutaneous nitroglycerine therapy. The capabilities and limitations of these forms of therapy need to be understood.

### Advances in Investigation

### Exercise stress testing

Exercise stress testing which was started by Masters as a simple office procedure, using his well-known double-step has been refined much further. Now it is carried out in an exercise stress testing laboratory (usually air-conditioned) on a tread-mill, in which the rate and inclination of the conveyor belt can be adjusted in order to give an exactly measured amount of exercise. The ECG traces are monitored either through telemetery or through a patient cable, the ECG morphology is monitored on a cathode ray oscilloscope and print-outs can be obtained while the patient is undertaking exercise. Artefacts due to patient movement or respiratory or muscle tremors are eliminated by suitable filtering or display/print-out of computer averaged ECG complexes. The computer also measures and records ST deviation, and occurrence and frequency of ectopic beats, and amplitude of R waves. Blood pressure is measured intermittently during the exercise, as its failure to rise with exercise indicates the presence of poor myocardial function. These laboratories are equipped with cardiac resuscitative drugs and equipment like defibrillators, oxygen and endotracheal intubation. This form of investigation has therefore become safer, more reliable and more expensive. Large number of studies in numerous centres have resulted in better awareness of the pitfalls in interpretation and the possibilities of false positives. The main conceptual advance has been the application of Baye's theorem to the interpretation i.e. if one applies the same yardstick (e.g. 1 mm ST depression) to two groups of patients, one in which the incidence of coronary artery disease is high (e.g. males above 50 years with chest pain on effort) and the other in which the incidence of IHD is low (e.g. females below 25 years with chest pain on effort), the same test, with same diagnostic criteria will produce more false positives and therefore be less reliable in the second group in which the incidence of IHD is low.

Exercise stress testing is a very useful tool in the diagnosis of angina pectoris in which physical examination usually yields negative results and resting ECG is normal. It is also useful in excluding myocardial ischaemia as a cause of chest pain. One must however be aware of causes of false positive results or of conditions which will give results which are difficult to interpret. These conditions include digitalisation, bundle branch block, hypokalaemia, Wolffe-Parkinson-White syndrome, mitral valve prolapse, hyperventilation, anxiety state and vasoregulatory asthaenia. One has therefore to interpret the results in the light of clinical history, physical examination and findings in the resting ECG.

Lately a number of patients have been subjected to exercise stress testing a few days following acute myocardial infarction with a view to be able to prescribe the amount of exercise that a patient can safely undertake following infarction, to pick up likely candidates for coronary arteriography and coronary artery surgery and for prognostication. The last of these can safely be left to a "jyotishi" or an astrologer. Facilities for coronary artery surgery are available to a very minute fraction of our population, and therefore this indication would be applicable only to those who can afford this form of surgery should it be indicated, and for prescription of correct amount of exercise it is cheaper to make the patient walk or go up a flight of stairs and note his symptoms, pulse-rate and occurrence of extrasystoles. One does not need measure the exact METS of exercise to give this simple advice.

In a very few cases,acute myocardial infarction has been precipitated by exercise testing and rarely deaths have occurred. It is therefore necessary to take an "informed consent" so that one is legally covered should anything goes wrong.

**Radionucleid Studies**

These are useful in studying myocardial perfusion, detection of infarction and evaluation of myocardial function :

(i) *Myocardial perfusion* can be studied by intravenous injection of thalium-201. Its flow through the coronary arteries and myocardium can be detected with suitable equipment. Poorly perfused areas of myocardium will appear "cold".

(ii) *Myocardial infarction* can be detected by injecting 99 mm Tc pyrophosphate which is taken up by infarcted muscle. The affected area therefore appears "hot".

(iii) *Myocardial function* is studied by giving an injection of technetium labelled red blood cells or albumin and studying its progress through the chambers of the heart with a gamma camera. Pictures roughly resembling a cinecardangiogram are obtained. One can calculate the ejection fraction and detect areas of akinesia or dyskinesia from these pictures.

These are useful forms of investigation and have the advantage of being non-invasive except for the intravenous injection. There are almost no side effects. The disadvantages are the very expensive equipment required and the fact that facilities for radionucleid studies are available in very few centres in India. These studies do not provide the anatomical details required for surgery which can be given only by coronary arteriography. These investigations are therefore more in the nature of screening to pick up cases of ischaemic heart disease which would need further investigation by coronary arteriography.

**Coronary arteriography**

Selective coronary arteriography is carried out by advancing a catheter up the femoral or brachial artery to the mouth of the coronary artery and injecting radio-opaque material into it. Pictures are taken in various projections to visualize the sites and extent of obstruction. The patient has to be admitted in a hospital. The procedure is moderately uncomfortable. Repeated injections of radio-opaque material cause flushing and rarely cause allergic reactions. Local complications like blockage of the femoral or brachial artery occur in a few cases. The procedure carries a mortality rate of about 0.1%.

Selective coronary arteriography is essential to outline the severity and location of coronary artery narrowing, to study the distal run off beyond the obstruction and presence of collateral circulation. Left ventriculography is done at the same sitting to detect areas of akinesia and dyskinesia and to study the ventricular ejection fraction which is a good indicator of left ventricular function. Cases with multivessel disease and obstruction of the left main coronary artery carry a poor prognosis and are therefore candidates for early coronary artery bypass surgery. Those with a very poor ejection fraction ($<$30%) are usually considered poor risks for surgical treatment. Resection of dyskinetic areas or aneurysms may be taken up at the same time as coronary artery bypass grafting. The procedure costs Rs.10,000/- or more. It is a prelude to surgery in patients with coronary artery disease. It is therefore not indicated in those who are not likely candidates for bypass graft operation because of mildness of symptoms, associated disease, advanced age or because of financial reasons. In a very few cases the procedure may be indicated to exclude the diagnosis of ischaemic heart disease.

### Echocardiography

This investigation has been very useful in the diagnosis of congenital and rheumatic heart disease and in disease of the pericardium, but its utility in the diagnosis and management of ischaemic heart disease has been limited. Two dimensional echocardiography is useful in studying the size of cardiac chambers, ventricular ejection fraction and to detect areas of akinesia. In the rare cases of rupture of ventricular septum following myocardial infarction, 2D echocardiography has been useful in detecting the defect in the septum.

Other forms of medical imaging like CT scan, nuclear magnetic resonance and digital subtraction angiography are for the present not very useful in the diagnosis and management of ischaemic heart disease.

## Advances in treatment

### Coronary artery bypass grafting

The operation consists of grafting a vessel, usually the saphenous vein into the root of the aorta at one end and into the coronary artery at the other, bypassing the obstruction. Three, four or more grafts may be required to bypass the blockages in the major coronary artery branches. Good quality coronary arteriograms are essential before undertaking surgery. The major indications for surgery are angina pectoris which is not adequately controlled with optimum drug treatment and multivessel and left main coronary artery disease with a view to preventing myocardial infarction and sudden death and thus prolonging life. After a lot of controversy, most people now agree that this form of surgery prolongs life and improves its quality. The main measure of improvement of quality of life would be the ability of the patient to return to his preferred life-style which might have been limited by symptoms of angina or left ventricular dysfunction. The greater the age of the patient, less there will be to gain in terms of added longevity. One must weigh these facts before recommending surgery as the expense on this operation is pretty high. If one counts the cost of investigation, hospitalisation, surgery, drugs and follow up and adds to its the expense on travel, lodging, food and loss of earning of the patient and one close relation, the total cost may be atleast one lac of rupees in India and Rs.2.5 lacs or more abroad. A very small percentage of families in India can afford such amounts. It is the physician who can take a detached view of the gains and losses. The affected family is usually emotionally too involved to make an objective decision. The physician should consider not only the cost of the operation but also the personality of the patient, likelihood of his getting back to productive work and the expertise of the surgical team, nursing facilities, incidence of infection in the hospital etc. before advising surgery. If surgery is not considered feasible or advisable for any of the above reasons, coronary arteriography should also not be advised as this investigation is of no use to a patient who is not a candidate for surgery.

**Percutaneous transluminal coronary angioplasty**

In this procedure a catheter with a balloon on its tip is advanced into the lumen of the partially obstructed coronary artery. The balloon is inflated to break up the obstructing atheromatous plaque to increase the internal diameter of the coronary artery. Exact positioning of the balloon and the results achieved by its inflation are checked by coronary arteriography. This is a much lesser undertaking than coronary artery bypass grafting, which requires open-heart surgery. Results are good in selected cases with significant localized obstruction of a major coronary artery. The vessel may gradually get narrowed again over the next months or years by deposition of atheroma. The procedure can then be repeated. Not all patients have lesions which are suitable for this type of treatment. There is a risk of precipitating myocardial infarction. A well-equipped catheterization laboratory and trained staff are essential pre-requisites.

**Thrombolytic therapy for acute myocardial infarction**

The outcome of acute myocardial infarction depends upon the quantity of muscle mass which undergoes necrosis due to loss of its blood supply. If a thrombus blocking the coronary artery can be dissolved soon (say within 6 hrs) of its occurence and blood flow restored it may be possible to salvage a proportion of ischaemic myocardium which would otherwise have become necrotic. With this aim, thrombolytic agents like streptokinase (cheaper, more side effects) or urokinase (more expensive, fewer side effects) have been perfused directly into the affected coronary artery or given systemically intravenously. Selective coronary arteriography before and after treatment has demonstrated the reopening of the affected vessel. Intracoronary perfusion of thrombolytic agents can only be carried out in a well-equipped cardiac catheterization laboratory. Intravenous administration does not require such specialised facilities. One has to give large doses of drugs and thus risk a higher incidence of side-effects. Reopening of the blocked arteries is not demonstrated directly in such cases. The occurrence of reperfusion arrhythmias and improvement of E.C.G. changes of infarction is taken as evidence of reopening of the blocked coronary artery. Anticoagulant therapy is commenced simultaneously and is continued for the six weeks to prevent recurrence of thrombosis. Cases in which anticoagulant therapy is contraindicated (e.g. those with a peptic ulcer) are not suitable candidates for this therapy. Fever and allergic reactions are the side-effects. The most important factor in determining the beneficial effects of this therapy is the time interval between onset of acute myocardial infarction and institution of thrombolytic therapy. Ideally it must be given not later than 6 hours after the onset of symptoms. The proportion of cases who receive such therapy is therefore low.

**Drug therapy after AMI**

*Beta-blockers* : It was at one stage considered that beta-blockers should not be used after acute myocardial infarction as they may precipitate cardiac failure. More recent studies have however shown that their use in the post myocardial infarction phase reduces the incidence of sudden death and reinfarction. This effect is not merely due to the antiarrhythmic properties of these drugs but may be related to the reduction of myocardial oxygen requirement and therefore relief of ischaemia. In many units, the administration of beta blockers after AMI is routine. The administration of timolol 10 mg BD or propranolol 60-80 tds commencing 5-7 days after AMI and continued for the next 12-24 months is recommended.

**Antiplatelet drugs :** Aspirin, dipyridamole and sulfinpyrazone have been used in the post-infarction period with the aim of reducing platelet stickness and thus recurrence of infarction. Unfortunately dipyridamole has not been used singly in any trial, therefore its contribution has not been clearly evaluated. Similarly the role of the other drugs in reducing recurrence of infarction has not been proved beyond doubt. The recommended dose of aspirin is 300 mg once a day. Being the cheapest and most easily available of these three drugs it is the most commonly used.

**Hypocholesterolaemic drugs** like clofibrate have been of doubtful value in preventing myocardial infarction except in the rare cases of familial hypercholesterolaemia. In the usual run of cases the marginal gain is counterbalanced by the increased incidence of gall-bladder disease and possibly intestinal malignancy which follow administration of these drugs. Routine administration of these drugs is not recommended.

**Calcium channel blockers** are being used more widely for the treatment of angina pectoris following AMI. The two drugs most easily available and commonly used in India are verapamil and nifedipine. Verapamil slows the heart, reduces myocardial contractility and thus its oxygen requirement and slows electrical conduction. It is therefore useful in cases of angina with a relatively high heart-rate and no conduction defects. Constipation is the main side-effect. Nifedipine on the other hand increases the heart-rate, reduces myocardial contractility and does not materially affect conduction. This will be useful in cases with slow heart-rate or those with conduction defects. It is said to be particularly useful for atypical (Prinzmetal) angina which is characterised by pain at rest and ST segment elevation during pain. Coronary artery spasm is an important factor in these cases. Calcium channel blockers lower the blood-pressure and are therefore contraindicated in those with marked hypotension.

**Transdermal nitroglycerine** — Specially designed water-proof adhesive patches containing measured amounts of nitroglycerine are now available. These have a special membrane between, the drug depot and the skin, which regulates the release of drug across it, so that it is absorbed at a constant slow rate. One patch is usually effective for 24 hours, thus avoiding the necessity of repeated doses. Blood levels of the drug remain fairly constant giving relief of symptoms and avoiding side-effects like headache which result from higher blood levels of nitrates. The patient is able to bathe with the patch in position. Other drugs can be combined with the therapy as required.

## REHABILITATION AFTER A HEART ATTACK

*I.M. AHUJA*

Acute myocardial infarction is life-threatening and dramatic. Its management is discussed in all text books of medicine. The fate of the survivor of the acute attack and his management are, however, not discussed in any detail by many books. Treatment of this phase of illness is equally important as mismanagement can cause much unnecessary disablement and unhappiness. In addition to the physical disability, which may vary from negligible to considerable, the patient suffers from psychological problems. Adjustment at home and at work may need the help of the physician.

### Pathology

To begin with, one should picture to oneself the underlying pathology as the management and expected gains would depend upon one's perception of the basic problems. In the vast majority of cases there is significant and fairly widespread atheromatous obstruction of the coronary arteries, the atheroma obliterating nearly 75% of the lumen at places. During the early stage after infarction, there is necrotic material and polymorphonuclear infiltration of the infarcted area. There is gradual replacement of polymorphs by red blood cells as new capillaries invade the area. Necrotic material is replaced by collagen tissue over the next few weeks. Six weeks after the infarct, the time by which most patients are discharged from hospital, the scar is not yet firm and avascular. Firm healing takes from 3 to 6 months. Most post-discharge deaths occur within one year of the acute attack, the majority being within the first six months. One should keep these facts in view when advising treatment, return to work and exercise. In this article, the management of an uncomplicated case of myocardial infarction, commencing about six weeks after discharge, will be discussed.

### Symptoms

An unhurried interview is essential. One should let the patient talk, asking the minimum number of questions. This gives one a good insight into the patient's personality. Questions should be worded simply, e.g. "How much can you walk ?" Most patients are up and about by this stage. Some are too weak to walk. Others have been prevented from walking by an overcautious doctor. One has to build up physical activity from this baseline. A question about sleep may bring forth information about worries about his illness or about the family. Some patients are woken up by nocturnal dyspnoea or angina. A few will have early morning wakefulness typical of depression. Constipation is not an uncommon symptom because of restricted diet and drugs like verapamil. This will need looking into, as straining at stools is known to cause cardiac arrhythmias. Some patients complain of excessive weakness or fatigue. This too may be due to dietary restriction or excessive use of drugs like diazepam. It is not often realized that diazepam has a long half-life and tends to accumulate if given daily. One should enquire into smoking and drinking habits. If this is the first interview with the patient, this may not be the appropriate time to enquire too deeply into the family circumstances and financial matters, but this information will require to be gathered. The exact nature of work, mode of reaching the work place and location of residence (upstairs or downstairs) are other relevant facts which one should find.

**Clinical examination**

On general examination one looks for evidence of obesity and cardiac failure. Pulse-rate and its response to mild exercise is noted. Persistent or undue tachycardia on exercise may indicate impaired myocardial function or anxiety. The presence of ectopics and their response to exercise should be noted. On auscultation one particularly looks for third or fourth heart sound as evidence of diminished myocardial compliance and for systolic murmur of mitral incompetence due to papillary muscle dysfunction. Blood pressure is taken and the patient is asked if he had hypertension earlier. Chest radiograph is taken for evidence of cardiomegaly and left ventricular failure. Electrocardiogram serves as a base-line and documents the presence and nature of ectopics. Persistent elevation of ST segment may suggest the development of ventricular aneurysm. Blood sugar and cholesterol are estimated to see if their levels are raised and would require therapy. Lipid profile is asked for by many physicians, but rarely leads to any specific therapeutic action.

**Aims of further management**

One should define in one's mind, the aims of further management and what one expects to achieve keeping in view the underlying pathology. There will be no argument that angina and cardiac failure require treatment. Associated disease like hypertension, diabetes and obesity will require appropriate therapy. Is there any form of treatment, diet or exercise which will prevent recurrence, cause regression of atheroma, encourage development of collaterals or reopen clogged arteries ? These aspects remain controversial and will therefore be discussed in some detail.

**Diet**

Restriction of caloric intake to treat or prevent obesity is essential. Diet should be constructed out of what the patient eats normally and what is usually cooked in his home. He can simply reduce the quantity eaten and avoid rich fatty foods. Crash diets and special diets do not usually work out as the problem is life-long. There is some controversy about the use of saturated and unsaturated fats. Those consuming a lot of saturated fats usually have higher blood cholesterol levels and these in turn are related to higher incidence of atheroma. Whether consumption of unsaturated fats after myocardial infarction will prevent further infarction is doubtful. However, a change to unsaturated fats (which do not solidify at room temperature) seems prudent. If this change does not help the patient, it may at least help his children, as atheromatous deposits commence at a fairly young age.

There are similar doubts about cholesterol intake. The endogenous production of cholesterol is approximately 2,000 to 3,000 mg/day and the endogenous production is said to be cut down by the amount one consumes in one's food. Yet, the standard advice is to reduce daily intake of cholesterol to below 300 mg/day. Eggs (cholesterol content approximately 250 mg each yolk) should be avoided. An egg without its yolk does not taste like an egg, but like slime. There is nothing sacrosanct about egg for breakfast, one can get the same amount of protein from a cup of skimmed milk. One hears about white meat being superior to red meat after a heart attack, but there is little difference between the cholesterol content of chicken (60 mg/100 g edible protein), fish (70 mg) and mutton (65 mg). Fish has more unsaturated fats and may therefore be preferable. Red meat, pork and lard should be avoided.

A word about social eating may not be out of place. At times one sees patients who have withdrawn from this pleasant pastime because the food might have been cooked in "dalda" or that the custard may have yolk of egg in it. This seems like carrying things too far, and doing without an evening out to avoid such "poisonous" stuff may be too high a price to pay for the doubtful gains. One does not need to bore one's friends and hosts with one's heart attack. One should pick up from the table a little bit of everything, avoiding what one considers too rich in calories, fat or cholesterol. An occasional indiscretion is not likely to make any significant difference to the atheroma which has collected over the previous few decades.

**Smoking**

The evidence against smoking is too strong to be ignored. Not only are heart attacks more common among smokers, the incidence of reinfarction is higher in those who continue to smoke and lower in those who give up smoking after the episode. One's advice should therefore be quite unambiguous, consistent and repeated. Missionary zeal should however be kept out of one's advice, as there are patients who are genuinely unable to give up smoking and they will either tell lies or go to another doctor. If the doctor smokes himself, his advice is not likely to be of any use.

**Alcohol**

If anyone thinks that a bit of brandy in the evening will make his heart stronger, he is fooling himself. The vast majority of our patients do not drink to an extent which would be directly toxic to the heart muscle (approximately half a bottle of spirit per day), but even social drinking would add its quota of calories (approximately 150 cal/large peg) and may make one eat a little more than one would otherwise and this creates problems in weight control. The patient must count these extra calories. The recent news that small amounts of alcohol (3-4 small pegs) may increase the high density lipoproteins and protect the heart against future heart attacks has gladdened those who enjoy a "chhota" in the evening. A prudent doctor should await more evidence before advising his patients to start drinking for this purpose.

**Exercise**

The amount of exercise must be individualized and essential work must get the first priority. This seems like starting the obvious, but every now and again one sees a patient with cardiac failure or frequent ectopics going out for his prescribed 3-5 km walk and coming back exhausted, because the doctor said that he must. This does not make sense as there is no proof that physical exercise opens up the clogged arteries or prevents recurrence of heart attacks. Physical training does make the body more efficient, reducing the oxygen requirement of work, improves morale and confidence and helps return to normal life-style and work. Gains in terms of improvement of underlying disease are questionable. Physical work and exercise within limits of anginal pain, excess breathlessness, faintness and exhaustion should be encouraged and may be essential for the patient to earn his living. He should avoid sudden severe physical exertion for which he is not conditioned e.g. running after a bus or carrying loads upstairs. Exercise with breath held, e.g. pushing a car, weight lifting or underwater swimming are known to cause marked rise of blood pressure and should therefore be avoided. Free-breathing exercises like jogging specially walking are good, but one should not overlook the risk of getting run over in the traffic conditions of our cities. Golf is an expensive way of walking in a safe area. Yoga is a good relaxation technique. The exercise is insufficient to increase mechanical efficiency or to open up coronary collaterals.

Sex is a topic which most of our patients do not bring up although it is always in their mind. A mature physician should discuss it freely and frankly with his patient, perhaps not in the very first interview. The amount of exercise involved in a sexual intercourse has been measured and amounts to about the exertion involved in going up two flights of stairs. If the patient can undertake this much exertion, he can return to his normal sexual activity. Whether the man or the woman plays the active role makes little difference in the oxygen consumption. "Will I die during the sex act ?" Very few such incidents have been recorded, the usual setting being partner other than wife and place other than home and usually after excessive eating and drinking. "But doctor, you said I should avoid sudden, severe exertion". Yes, but most of out patients are 50 years plus and married for 20 years plus and usually living with their own wives. Sex is neither sudden nor severe under these circumstances.

**Drugs**

Angina pectoris, cardiac failure, hypertension, cardiac arrhythmias, diabetes and any other associated disease will require appropriate treatment. Nitrates, including transdermal nitroglycerine, beta blockers and calcium channel blockers are the drugs commonly required.

Lipid lowering drugs like clofibrate have been out of favour lately because there is no evidence that they reduce the frequency of heart attacks or the mortality rate. Advantage, if any, is counteracted by the increased incidence of gall-stones and small intestinal disease including malignancy. Anti-coagulants are now rarely used for long-term prevention. Low dose heparin has not quite caught on. Antiplatelet drugs have been more fashionable recently. The subject was reviewed by Mitchell (1983) and the evidence for aspirin, sulphinpyrazone and (Dipyridamol) was carefully weighed. The verdict was "not proven" for all three drugs in spite of their wide-spread usage and "pushing" by their manufactures and protagonists.

Evidence in favour of beta blockers preventing recurrence of heart attacks is fairly strong now and many centres are using these drugs as a routine, starting about a week after the acute infarct and continuing for 1-2 years (Pratt and Roberts, 1983). Propranolol (80 mg t.d.s) and metroprolol are probably as effective as timolol which was used in the best known trial. The author has no first-hand knowledge of the use of these drugs for the specific purpose of preventing recurrence of infarction. These drugs are commonly indicated for the treatment of post-infarction angina, arrhythmias or hypertension. Patients on these drugs may be deriving the additional benefit of their protective action. Calcium channel blockers have also been used for the same purpose, but there is not enough evidence in their favour at present.

Some patients will require tranquilizers, although a sympathetic physician who has time to listen to and answer the patient's questions is often an effective tranquilizer. A few patients may require anti-depressant therapy. One should be aware of the possibility of these drugs causing cardiac arrhythmias.

Are there any specific drugs which will cause regression of atheroma ? The answer is negative for the present.

**Return of work**

The patient should generally return to his previous job except if specifically disabled for it, e.g. jobs involving hard physical work or airline pilots. Return to the same organization generally ensures a more sympathetic attitude and return to shorter hours and less strenuous work initially. During this phase the patient should be called up for review more frequently, possibly every week or 10 days, to check his response to work, to answer the many questions which arise in the patients mind and generally to encourage him to get back to his normal life-style, possibly full stream ahead in about six months after the acute infarction. The frequency of reviews can then be reduced to once in 3 to 6 months or once a year, with the assurance that he is welcome anytime that he has any problem.

**Surgery**

The question of surgery will be raised by most patients as more and more people are learning about coronary artery bypass grafting from the lay press. The expected gains from surgery are relief of angina and probable improvement of myocardial function and longevity. On the negative side is the operative, mortality rate of about 5% in India, perioperative infarction (2-3%) and the cost. In India the operation will cost Rs.60,000 to one lac. This amount includes cost of initial investigations, including coronary arteriography, drugs, hospitalization, surgeons fees, travel expenses and cost of a close relation staying with the patient. One must consider all these overheads because this is what the family finally ends up paying and not just the surgeon's fees. Getting operated in USA will similarly cost not less than Rs. 250,000. Not many families are able to afford these amounts and if in one's opinion the financial condition of the family does not permit such expense, it may be more kind not to mention surgery if the patient does not ask about it.

**Miscellaneous**

Patients may ask if they can travel abroad. All aircrafts are pressurized, air travel is therefore no problem. But falling ill abroad can be very expensive, therefore it is better to be covered by adequate insurance or financial backing. Air travel also may involve carrying hand baggage over long distances in cold weather. Customs clearance delays and formalities are bad enough to give a heart attack to a perfectly normal person. One should therefore advise these patients not to carry back gifts and things from abroad.

Driving is also known to cause rise of blood pressure and to cause ectopic beats. One should advise against driving in the early stages of convalescence, especially in case of people who want to reform the habits of all other drivers, cyclists and pedestrians. Some people are, however, more tense in the rear seat than in the driver's seat.

In the organization of day-to-day activity one should advise relaxation and avoidance of impatience, hurry and temper. Getting ready a few minutes before the time of departure can help.

Interpersonal relations in the family need adjustment. The wife often takes up the attitude, "He never listens, I told him to give up smoking 20 years ago". or "I should have looked after him better". The children, who are often grown up by now, take on a more protective attitude. "Daddy doesn't pick up that bucket of water" which the daddy resents because he likes to retain his position as the strong and dependable head of the family. The physician is able to help only if he knows the family well and has a good rapport with them. If the wife is understanding and educated enough, it helps if she can accompany the patient during the reviews.

The fact that the patient has greater chance of getting another attack, especially within the first year post-infarction, should not be emphasized. One should however advise about settling one's financial affairs and making out a proper will on the basis of "anyone of your age should". In the Armed Forced we have the experience of rehabilitating cases of acute myocardial infarction after very stringent resting. Many of them are back on fully duty and are holding positions of responsibility. This experience shows that the outlook of a "heart-case" may not be that bleak after all. Functional recovery is excellent in many patients with good motivation.

Finally, a bit of philosophy. One must put the heart-attack in its proper perspective. Above the age of 65 to 70 years the remaining longevity may not differ significantly with or without dont's. One can thus be less stringent in this group of patients. Heart attack is after all only one of the numerous causes that people die of. If we busied ourselves with precautions against all known causes of death, we would be left with little time to live. Let us not forget that life is for living.

# VALVULAR HEART DISEASE

*D.C. GHOSH*

## Introduction

Mitral valve disease is the commonest form of chronic rheumatic valve disease, the valve being affected in about 85 per cent of cases. The affected valve may be either stenosed offering obstruction to the flow of blood from the left atrium to the left ventricle or the valve may be incompetent resulting in regurgitation of blood from the left ventricle to the left atrium during ventricular systole. Mitral stenosis with some degree of incompetence is however very common.

## MITRAL STENOSIS

There is usually a period of silent interval between the onset of rheumatic fever and the appearance of the signs and symptoms of mitral stenosis as the valve gradually narrows. Although in western countries, signs of mitral stenosis becomes apparent in the twenties and disability appears in late thirties or forties, however, juvenile mitral stenosis is fairly common in India, and the Middle East.

### Aetiology

The commonest cause of mitral stenosis is chronic rheumatic valvulitis; although a definite history of rheumatic fever may not be available in about 50 per cent of cases. Viral and rickettsial infection have rarely been incriminated. Congenital mitral stenosis is a rare entity and is often associated with coarctation of aorta or endocardial fibroelastosis. The association of mitral stenosis and ostium secundum type of atrial septal defect is referred to as Lutembacher's syndrome, but the mitral valve lesion is almost invariably of rheumatic aetiology.

### Pathology

As a result of rheumatic endocarditis, there is thickening of valve leaflets, fusion of the chordae tendinae and fusion of the commissures. The end result is a funnel shaped deformity with a button-hole shaped orifice of the valve. The normal mitral valve which has an area of about 4.5 $cm^2$ is gradually reduced. Symptoms appear when the valve area is reduced to 2.5 $cm^2$ although signs may be discernible much earlier. When the valve area is reduced to less than 1 $cm^2$, the narrowing is said to be critical.

The left ventricle is usually normal or small in size in isolated mitral stenosis. The left atrium is characteristically enlarged. The wall of the left atrium is histologically normal or there may be disruption of muscle fibres. Mural thrombosis may be seen in the free wall just above the posterior leaflet. This is known as McCallum's patch. In the lungs one may notice changes of pulmonary venous congestion, pulmonary hypertension. Pulmonary haemosiderosis may develop in very late stage of the disease. The right ventricle dilates and there may be dilatation of the tricuspid valve ring.

Congenital mitral stenosis may take the form of a parachute valve or there may be commissural fusion like that seen in rheumatic mitral stenosis. The abnormal insertion of the chordae into a single papillary muscle produces the parachute valve.

### Haemodynamics

The underlying defect in mitral stenosis is obstruction to the flow of blood from the left atrium to left ventricle during diastole, resulting in a rise of pressure proximal to the obstruction. There is rise of pressure in the left atrium which dilates. The extent to which the left atrium dilates depends on its internal pressure and the state of atrial myocardium. As the pressure in the left atrium rises there is consequent rise of pressure in the pulmonary veins. In order to maintain blood flow through the lungs, pulmonary arterial pressure starts rising in a linear relationship initially but this relationship is no longer maintained after some time and pulmonary arterial pressure rises rapidly due to arteriolar constriction — (Vasoconstrictive or active pulmonary hypertension).

The left atrial pressure in health does not exceed 12 mm Hg. In mitral stenosis the left atrial pressure progressively increases. A rise of pressure in left atrium is a good evidence of the mitral valve obstruction, but the only certain method of determining obstruction at the level of mitral valve is to estimate the diastolic pressure gradient across it by simultaneous measurement of left atrial and left ventricular pressure (Oram). The smaller the valve area, the higher will be the pulmonary venous pressure and consequently higher will be pulmonary vascular resistance and lower will be the cardiac output. In mitral stenosis, blood flows normally from the left ventricle to the aorta, but during diastole a pressure gradient exists between left atrium and left ventricle due to continuing effort of the left atrium to force blood through the narrow mitral valve producing a turbulence during diastole.

**Clinical features**

*Dyspnoea* is the commonest presenting symptom in patients with mitral stenosis. Shortness of breath on exertion is complained of by about 80 per cent of patients. The dyspnoea is due to pulmonary congestion resulting from elevated left atrial pressure. The increased stiffness or decreased compliance of the lungs increases the work of breathing. Any factor that increases the heart rate is likely to aggravate dyspnoea in mitral stenosis.

*Acute pulmonary oedema* may be precipitated by emotion, infection, physical exertion, pregnancy, atrial fibrillation and anaesthesia. Anaemia and thyrotoxicosis are also likely to precipitate acute pulmonary oedema.

*Paroxysmal nocturnal dyspnoea* is not uncommon. A patient who usually complains of shortness of breath on exertion may go to bed in his usual state of health. After about an hour or two he gets up from sleep with an intense sense of suffocation accompanied by cough. He sits up or tries to proceed to go near an open window in an attempt to get some relief. The dyspnoea intensifies and he brings up pink frothy sputum.

*Haemoptysis* is an important presenting symptom if carefully enquired of. It may be the result of frank pulmonary haemorrhage from rupture of pulmonary veins. Pink frothy blood stained sputum may occur during an attack of acute pulmonary oedema. Infarction of lung is another cause for haemoptysis. Bronchitis in patients with mitral stenosis may cause blood streaking of the sputum.

*Recurrent bronchitis* — Bronchitis often associated with wheeze results from mucosal oedema caused by congestion in the bronchial veins which drain into pulmonary venous system.

*Embolism* — Both systemic and pulmonary embolism may occur. Systemic embolism is more common in patients with atrial fibrillation. A fifth of the patients with mitral stenosis develop this complication sometimes during their lives. Hemiplegia or loss of use of a leg are recognised complications of systemic embolism. An unexplained incidence of epilepsy or hypertension in patients with mitral stenosis has been attributed to cerebral or renal infarction (Stevens).

*Palpitation* — It is rare in pure mitral stenosis unless atrial fibrillation is present.

Symptoms due to raised pulmonary vascular resistance include fatigue, angina pectoris, coldness of the extremities. Abdominal discomfort, anorexia, swelling of the ankles and feet become the presenting features when right heart failure sets in.

*Fatigue* — Results from low cardiac output and is sometimes the presenting feature.

Angina results from low cardiac output in patients with raised pulmonary vascular resistance. As dyspnoea is the dominant symptom in mitral stenosis, a history of angina may not be obtained unless carefully sought.

**Physical signs**

The physical signs vary with the degree of severity of lesion and also on the amount of increase in pulmonary vascular resistance.

General appearance of the patient is unremarkable. The so-called "mitral facies" is not so common in our patients. It is classically seen in white people when there is severe pulmonary hypertension and low cardiac output. The characteristic physical signs of mitral stenosis may appear much earlier than symptoms. The physical signs are often so insignificant that mild exercise is necessary to elicit signs. Patient is told to sit up and down from the lying posture for about 8 to 10 times and careful auscultation is done in left lateral posture.

*Pulse* — In a classical case the pulse is usually normal but may have small volume. Atrial fibrillation is common.

The jugular venous pulse is usually normal but a prominent 'a' wave appears with the development of pulmonary hypertension and a 'v' wave when tricuspid incompetence occurs.

The apical impulse described as 'tapping' is not due to right ventricular enlargement but results from forceful closure of the mitral valve. When pulmonary vascular resistance becomes established with consequent enlargement of right ventricle, a palpable thrust in the left parasternal region become evident. This thrust may also be the result of forward displacement of right ventricle by the enlarged left atrium. A diastolic thrill may be palpable over the apex. Pulsation of the pulmonary artery may be left in the left second intercostal space when pulmonary vascular resistance is very high. The closing sound of the pulmonary valve may be felt as a shock.

Auscultation will reveal the classical signs if the patient remains in sinus rhythm. These are — (1) loud first heart sound, (2) more or less normal second sound, (3) an opening snap, and (4) Mid-diastolic and/or presystolic murmur.

In diastole, the mitral valve leaflets are held widely open and because of the pressure difference between left atrium and left ventricle valve closure is delayed. At the onset of systole the valve leaflets have to travel a relatively long distance in order to close the valve. Rapid closure with abrupt checking of the valve leaflets by the chordae produces the loud first heart sound. The second heart sound is audible and followed by high frequency sound the "opening snap (OS)". This is produced by abrupt opening movement of the stenosed valve as the left ventricular diastolic pressure falls below the raised left atrial pressures. The interval between the second sound and the opening snap reflects the degree of stenosis and is certainly wider than the true splitting of the second (up to 40 milliseconds). In severe stenosis — the OS comes very close to the second sound ($S_2$) whereas in mild stenosis $S_2$-OS interval increases up to 120 milliseconds. The OS is best heard in the left fourth interspace. The loud first heart sound and opening snap are not heard when fibrosis and calcification of valve occur.

The characteristic findings in a case of pure mitral stenosis are the presence of a rumbling mid-diastolic murmur due to turbulent flow through narrow mitral orifice. Since the closure of the valve is delayed and there is some diastolic flow as the mitral valve is closing the flow across a diminishing valve orifice, produces the presystolic murmur. Atrial contraction in the later part of the ventricular diastole perhaps also contribute to the presystolic accentuation. The length of the diastolic murmur also reflects the degree of the severity of the stenosis. The diastolic murmur is often best heard in a localised area located near the apex of the heart.

In presence of low cardiac output and large right ventricle it may be necessary to listen lateral to the apex with the patient lying on his left side. When atrial fibrillation develops, the presystolic accentuation may disappear. With the onet of raised pulmonary vascular resistance, the physical signs tend to be different. The patient usually has peripheral cyanosis with cool extremities and small volume pulse. Systemic venous pressure starts rising and auscultatory signs become less florid. Pulmonary incompetence secondary to pulmonary hypertension may produce an early diastolic murmur at the pulmonary area (Graham Steel murmur) with accentuated second heart sound. With the development of tricuspid incompetence a pansystolic murmur becomes audible over the tricuspid area. This murmur usually becomes more pronounced during inspiration. A prominent systolic 'V' wave in the neck and enlarged pulsatile liver and common accompaniments of tricuspid incompetence.

Assessment of severity of stenosis based on auscultatory signs alone is not of sufficient accuracy; the degree of pulmonary vascular changes shown in chest X-ray and cardiac catheterisation are more reliable indices of severity of stenosis.

**Complications** — Atrial fibrillation, pulmonary hypertension, congestive cardiac failure, systemic pulmonary embolism are recognised complications of mitral stenosis. Hoarseness of voice and dysphagia are far too rare. The rapid ventricular rate at the onset of atrial fibrillation (AF) is a serious complication of mitral stenosis, because the time available for diastolic filling of the left ventricle is drastically reduced, pulmonary venous pressure raises sharply and pulmonary oedema may be precipitated. AF also contributes to the development of left atrial thrombus and systemic embolism.

Pulmonary hypertension develops gradually over the years. About 20 per cent patients show reactive pulmonary hypertension with diffuse pulmonary arteriolar narrowing, thus exchanging pulmonary congestion for right heart failure.

**Electrocardiogram** — In presence of sinus rhythm the ECG shows presence of left atrial enlargement. The 'P' wave is bifid in lead II and has a wide late negative component in $V_1$. Evidence of right ventricular enlargement, i.e. a tall R wave in lead $V_1$ and tall peaked P wave in leads II, III and avF will suggest pulmonary hypertension. Atrial fibrillation is quite common.

**X-ray examination** — The chest X-ray provides useful information about cardiac silhouette and the lung fields in mitral stenosis. Fig.18.27 (e).

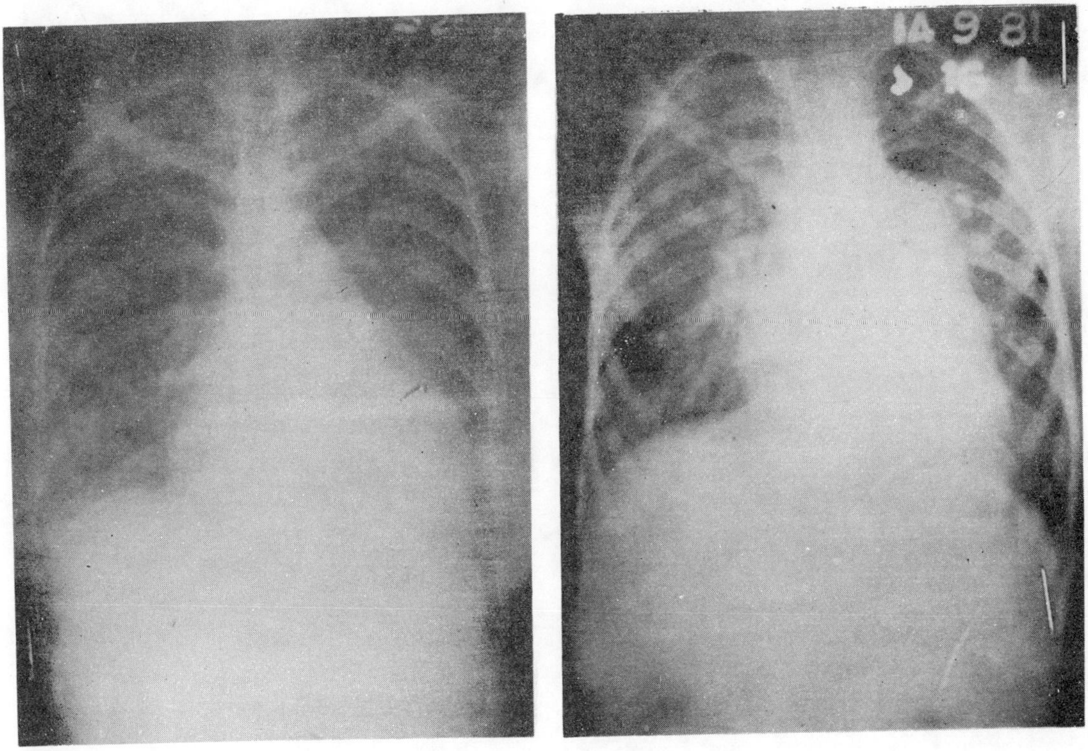

Fig.18.27(a) — Early M.S.

**Fig.18.27(b) — Note the left auricular bump**

Fig.18.27 : Radiographic pictures in Mitral stenosis.

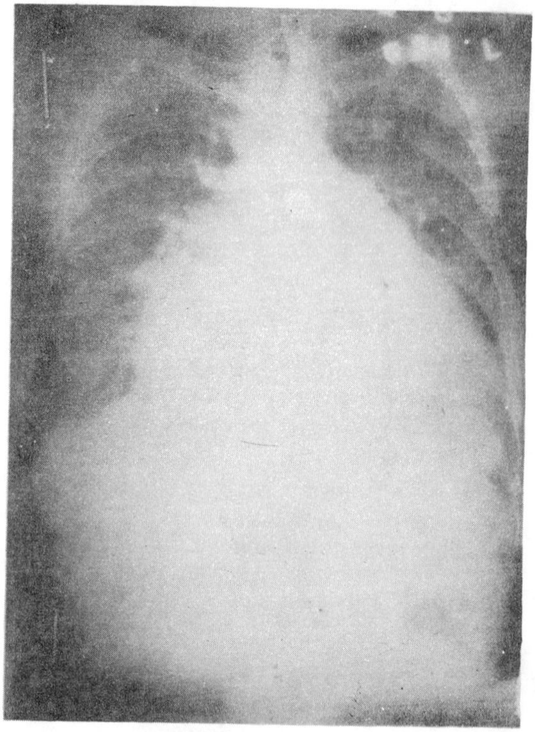

Fig.18.27(c) : Giant auricle

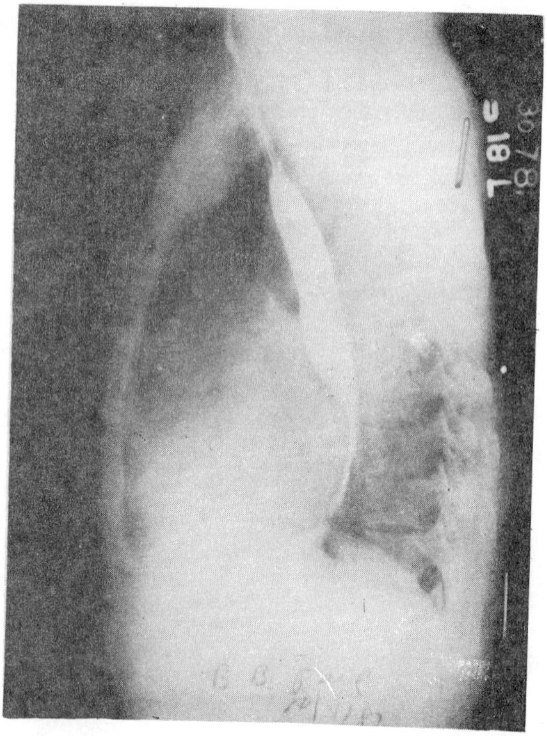

Fig.18.27 (d) — Left atrial impression in barium swallow picture.

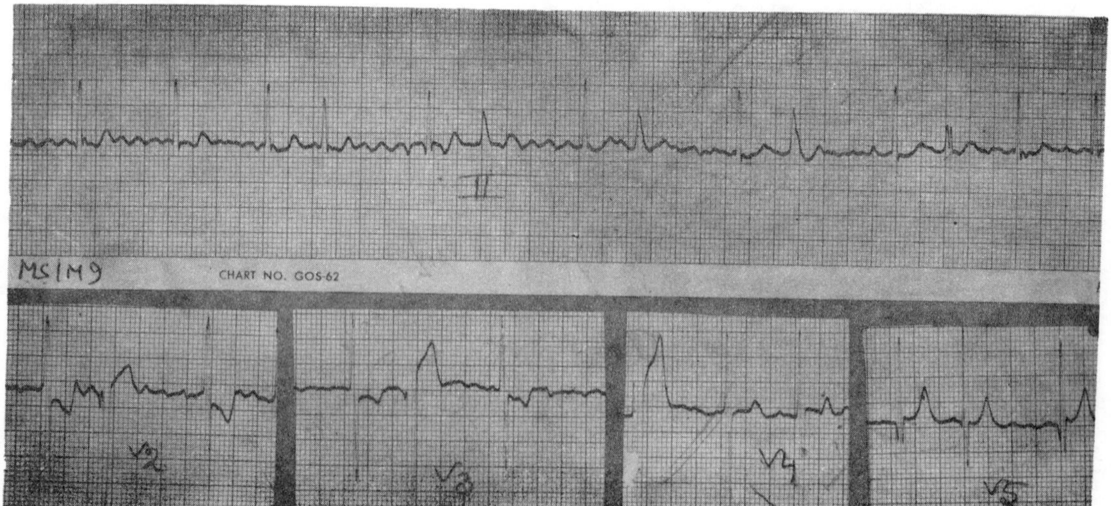


Fig.18.27(e) — A case of M.S./M.I. showing atrial fibrillations with several ectopics.

**Cardiac Silhouette**

The heart is usually not enlarged.

Left atrial enlargement gives rise to –

(1) Double contour of the right border of the heart.

(2) Elevation of the left main bronchus with splaying of the carinal angle.

(3) Straightening of the left border of the heart (mitralisation) by the enlarged left atrial appendage may also produce a localised bulge immediately below the pulmonary artery.

(4) Posterior displacement of the barium filled oesophagus in the lateral view of the chest following barium swallow.

(5) Enlargement of main pulmonary artery when pulmonary hypertension is well established.

(6) Calcification of the valve or of left atrium.

**Lung fields**

A good correlation has been observed between the left atrial pressure and changes in the lung fields. With left atrial pressures of 15 mm. Hg. there is diversion of blood to the upper lobes with dilatation of pulmonary veins. When the left atrial pressure exceeds 20 mm. Hg. oedema of interlobular septa are seen as Kerley 'B' lines, associated interstitial oedema. Left atrial pressure above 30 mm. Hg. results in alveolar oedema and perihilar haze and collection of fluid in the pleural space. When pulmonary hypertension sets in, pulmonary venous congestion is replaced by dilatation of the proximal part of the pulmonary arteries with peripheral pruning of distal vessels. Long-standing cases may demonstrate miliary mottling resulting from pulmonary haemosiderosis.

**Cardiac catheterisation and cine angiogram** – are not usually necessary for diagnostic accuracy since the echocardiogram provides useful information and is an important non-invasive diagnostic tool.

**Echocardiogram :** It characteristically demonstrates reduced closure rate of the anterior leaflet of the mitral valve with loss of significant reopening of the valve with the atrial systole. (Refer to Chapter on Echocardiography).

**Differential diagnosis**

The two important conditions which resemble the physical findings of mitral stenosis are left atrial myxoma and cor triatrium. Features suggestive of myxoma are :

(a) Absence of history of rheumatic fever.

(b) Short history of illness.

(c) Syncope on change of posture.

(e) Constitutional symptoms – fever, arthralgia, raised ESR and abnormal globulins.

(f) Female male ratio as high as 10 : 1. On auscultation the diastolic murmur changes with change of posture.

(g) Echocardiogram is very helpful in confirming the diagnosis.

In cor triatrium, the left atrium is divided by a septum separating the pulmonary veins from the mitral valve orifice. The opening in the septum produces a pressure gradient. Cardiac catheterisation and angio-cardiogram are necessary for diagnosis.

**Management of mitral stenosis**

Ideal treatment of mitral stenosis is essentially surgical. Therefore medical treatment is almost entirely symptomatic.

Mild dyspnoea generally responds to diuretics and measures to prevent recurrence of rheumatic activity is all that is necessary. Atrial fibrillation (AF) can usually be controlled by digoxin. In some cases if tachycardia cannot be controlled by digoxin alone small dose of a beta-blocker

(Propranolol) may help, provided cardiac failure has been excluded. Electrical cardioversion after preliminary anticoagulation may be considered in young patients with atrial fibrillation, but is generally unhelpful as the underlying conditions continue to remain. When AF becomes established, in absence of any definite contraindication, anticoagulants can be used.

Surgical treatment comprises of mitral valvotomy or commissurotomy. It usually gives good results if the valve is pliant but mitral incompetence may occur if the valve is less narrowed than usual and is operated too early.

Indications for mitral valvotomy –

(1) Presence of significant symptoms, limiting activity.

(2) If pulmonary oedema develops without precipitating cause or if it develops during pregnancy

(3) If atrial fibrillation is causing deterioration of the clinical condition.

(4) If an episode of embolism has occurred.

The following criteria are to be carefully considered for selecting patients for operation –

(1) Presence of significant symptoms.

(2) Valves must be pliant.

(3) Absence of mitral incompetence.

(4) Absence of calcification of the valve.

In absence of these criteria, mitral valve replacement should be considered.

A second or even a third mitral valvotomy may have to be performed when restenosis occurs or when the first operation has failed to relieve the mechanical block. Raised pulmonary vascular resistance is not a contraindication for surgery and a satisfactory reversal of pulmonary vascular disease can be achieved after operation.

**Prognosis**

With the introduction of mitral valve surgery the prognosis of patients with mitral stenosis has certainly become good. Although the lesion cannot be cured and myocardial involvement cannot be reversed by surgery, relief of dyspnoea and prevention of attacks of pulmonary oedema can be assured.

## MITRAL REGURGITATION

Mitral regurgitation or mitral incompetence usually results from rheumatic valvulitis and unlike mitral stenosis is more common in males than in females and it occurs as both an acute and a chronic lesion. Pure rheumatic mitral incompetence is rather uncommon and there may be associated mitral stenosis or aortic or tricuspid valve lesions.

**Causes of Mitral incompetence –**

1. Rheumatic fever
2. Non-rheumatic –
   (a) Congenital –
   - Ostium primum type of atrial septal defect
   - Marfan's syndrome
   - Endocardial fibroelastosis
   - Hurler's syndrome
   - Pseudoxanthoma elasticum
   - Ehlers Danlos syndrome

(b) Acquired —

- Degenerative
- Ischaemic heart disease and acute infarction
- Subacute infective endocarditis
- Mitral valve prolapse
- Papillary muscle dysfunction
- Hypertrophic obstructive cardiomyopathy
- Systemic lupus erythematous
- Rheumatoid arthritis.

**Rheumatic mitral valve disease**

**Pathophysiology —**

During the stage of acute rheumatic fever carditis may cause mitral incompetence but in two-thirds of cases this murmur is lost within a period of one to six months. In the remaining the mitral incompetence becomes established. The valve mechanism is disorganised as a result of scarring and thickening of valve cusps, thickening and shortening of the chordae and dilatation of the valve ring.

**Haemodynamics**

Because the valve is incompetent, during ventricular systole blood will leak back into left atrium. Left atrium will therefore slowly dilate to accommodate the regurgitant stream of blood. Although the left atrial pressure increases during ventricular systole, it quickly falls during diastole, so the mean left atrial pressure is not so high as in mitral stenosis. During diastole there is no obstruction at the level or mitral valve so that left ventricle fills rapidly. But the work of the left ventricle is increased as it has to pump the forward flow, i.e. the usual quota of blood received from the pulmonary circulation as well as the regurgitant amount. The left ventricular stroke volume is thus increased and the left ventricle undergoes hypertrophy and dilatation.

**Clinical features :-**

**Symptoms —** Many patients remain free from symptoms, the condition being discovered during the course of routine examination. In others dyspnoea, palpitation and chest pain are the presenting symptoms. Dyspnoea is less severe than in case of mitral stenosis, because pulmonary venous congestion is less impressive. Dyspnoea is however a predominant feature in acute mitral incompetence because of sudden increase in left atrial pressure due to acute regurgitation of blood into a small left atrium. *Acute pulmonary oedema is, therefore, uncommon in rheumatic mitral regurgitation.*

Palpitation due to ectopic beats is a common feature. Embolic manifestations are far less common.

**Signs :-**

The arterial pulse is often normal, but has a quick upstroke. In the elderly patients, atrial fibrillation may be present. The venous pulsation in the neck is normal until pulmonary hypertension becomes established.

The apical impulse is displaced downwards and outwards and is hyperkinetic. A systolic thrill may be palpable over the apex. A left parasternal lift caused by left atrial expansion may be felt and on occasions the third heart sound may be palpable.

On auscultation, the first heart sound is not usually accentuated. A pansystolic murmur starting with the first heart sound and going up to or even beyond the second sound is audible. The murmur is harsh blowing in character and is conducted up to posterior axillary line. A third heart sound may be audible during diastole. It is caused by rapid ventricular filling. This is followed by a short mid-diastolic murmur caused by rapid flow. The second sound is often widely split because of shortened left ventricular ejection time.

**Electrocardiographic findings :** The electrocardiogram is usually normal. In some cases 'P' mitrale atrial fibrillation or left ventricular hypertrophy may be seen.

**Chest radiograph :-** In mild mitral incompetence the cardiac silhouette is ordinarily normal. With increasing severity, the heart enlarges and left atrium dilates. Aneurysmal dilatation of the left atrium may occur, and a systolic expansion of the left atrium may be seen on fluroscopic examination. There may be calcification of the valve or of the left atrium in long-standing cases. The changes in the pulmonary vascularity depends on the pulmonary venous and atrial pressures.

**Special investigations**

(1) Non-invasive

In echocardiogram an increased excursion of the mitral valve is seen. The echocardiogram is much more helpful in differentiating other cases of mitral incompetence, e.g. mitral valve prolapse and hypertrophic obstructive cardio-myopathy. In the former late systolic posterior movement of prolapsing mitral valvular tissue can be seen whereas in the latter, systolic anterior motion (SAM) of the anterior leaflet of the mitral valve and increased thickness of the interventricular septum can be demonstrated.

(2) Invasive

At cardiac catheterisation, no pressure gradient is observed across the mitral valve during ventricular diastole. In pure mitral incompetence the left atrial pressure is not as high as in mitral stenosis. Selective left ventricular angiogram in a lateral position will demonstrate position of mitral valve and regurgitation of the dye in the enlarged left atrium.

**Complications**

(1) Atrial fibrillation

(2) Subacute infective endocarditis

(3) Pulmonary hypertension

(4) Systemic embolism

**Differential diagnosis**

A pansystolic murmur over the mitral area may be produced in ventricular septal defect. The murmur of tricuspid incompetence is audible more internally, more pronounced during inspiration and is not conducted towards the axilla. Increase of systolic 'v' wave in the neck, an enlarged pulsatile liver and evidences of pulmonary hypertension are features which are helpful in the diagnosis of tricuspid incompetence.

**Management**

Management will depend upon the severity of the condition and presence of complications :-

(1) Mild and asymptomatic mitral incompetence requires no treatment. But as these lesions are susceptible of developing infective endocarditis, antibiotic prophylaxis is necessary before dental treatment, cystoscopy and other surgical or gynaecological procedures likely to produce bacteraemia.

(2) Chronic disease and those presenting with features of cardiac failure can be managed with digoxin and diuretics with potassium supplements. When the symptoms are severe and medical management has proved to be ineffective, mitral valve replacement is to be considered.

(3) Acute mitral incompetence irrespective of its cause will require emergency valve replacement.

(4) Mitral incompetence complicated with atrial fibrillation.

Whereas use of anticoagulants is advocated in atrial fibrillation complicating mitral stenosis, opinions differ on the routine anticoagulation of patients with mitral incompetence, as the risk of embolism is comparatively less in the latter.

**Mitral valve replacement**

Usually a mechanical prosthesis consisting either of caged ball or discs or tilting discs are used. The operative mortality varies from 5 to 10 per cent. Mechanical prosthesis have the problem of giving rise to emboli and patients with these prostheses need life-long anticoagulant treatment. This complication tends to occur more frequently during the early months and becomes rare after four years or so. An overall incidence is about 5-10 per cent.

Biological tissue valves prepared from homografts and heterograft are less likely to produce emboli, but they suffer from the problem of mechanical failure.

**Dysfunction of a replaced valve**

It is easy to identify the presence of a ball valve if one carefully looks for opening and closing clicks. The tilting disc will not produce an opening sound, but a short diastolic murmur may be heard. Biological valve with no opening or closing sounds may produce a short diastolic murmur. Appearance of unexplained symptoms such as dyspnoea, chest pain, tiredness, sudden paralysis of limbs, yellow colouration of urine due to haemolysis or any change in the auscultatory signs will suggest valve dysfunction or dehiscence.

## TRICUSPID VALVE DISEASE

As in mitral valve disease, the tricuspid valve may be either stenosed or incompetent or both stenosis and incompetence coexist.

**Tricuspid stenosis**

(a) Rheumatic fever is by far the commonest cause of tricuspid stenosis. It is almost invariably associated with rheumatic mitral valve disease.

(b) Congenital tricuspid stenosis-tricuspid atresia, is rare.

(c) Carcinoid tumours and rarely a right atrial tumour may produce obstruction at the level of tricuspid valve.

**Clinical features**

Females are more often affected than males. The following signs are helpful in diagnosing tricuspid stenosis :-

JVP — When sinus rhythm is present, a giant 'a' wave is visible in the jugular venous pulse, with an insignificant 'v' wave and slow 'y' descent.

On palpation of the precordium, there is no left parasternal or right ventricular heave. Rarely a diastolic thrill is palpable over the tricuspid area. On auscultation, the pulmonary second sound is not accentuated but a low-pitched presystolic or mid-diastolic murmur is heard at the left fourth intercostal space close to the lower end of sternum. This murmur is more pronounced during inspiration. An opening snap and low tricuspid component of the first heart sound are occasionally audible. Liver is usually enlarged and ascites and oedema are common accompaniments.

**ECG :** Will show tall peaked 'P' wave in lead II indicating right atrial enlargement.

**Chest X-ray**

Cardiac silhouette — a large right atrium is almost always present. This may be associated with features of mitral valve disease which usually co-exist. But unlike mitral stenosis, the lung fields look unduly clear in pure tricuspid stenosis.

**Echocardiogram :-** Will show delayed closure of the tricuspid valve, this being situated anterior to the mitral valve.

**Differential diagnosis from mitral stenosis** :—

Since tricuspid stenosis spares the lungs,symptoms of elevated left atrial pressure, e.g. acute pulmonary oedema, haemoptysis and bronchitis are usually absent. The lung bases appear clear on auscultation and in spite of engorgement of neck vein, oedema of feet, the patient can lie flat in bed or is able to sleep on one pillow.

**Treatment**

Either closed or open valvotomy of the tricuspid valve may be performed but the risk of producing a tricuspid incompetence is considerable. Open heart surgery and valve replacement is therefore preferred.

## TRICUSPID INCOMPETENCE

**Aetiology**

(1) **Functional :** Because of its anatomical pattern tricuspid incompetence is commonly functional in origin and functional tricuspid incompetence secondary to right ventricular enlargement with dilatation of the valve ring is commoner than organic tricuspid incompetence.

(2) **Organic — Congenital :** This usually takes the form of Ebstein's anomaly. This is caused by downward displacement of the abnormally formed tricuspid valve ring and leaflets into the cavity of the right ventricle. Symptoms vary from mild degree of cardiac disability to severe heart failure with central cyanosis. Cyanosis resulting from right to left shunt across a patent foramen ovale, elevated jugular venous pressure with prominent 'V' wave, a quiet precordium on palpation and scratchy systolic and diastolic murmur over the tricuspid area, a bizzare RBBB pattern in electrocardiogram and cardiac silhouette resembling pericardial effusion (globular enlarged heart) are diagnostic.

**Acquired —**

(1) Rheumatic — Almost invariably seen in association with mitral valve disease.

(2) Traumatic — Blunt chest injury resulting in rupture of papillary muscles, chordae and avulsion of valve leaflets may cause tricuspid incompetence.

(3) Infective endocarditis — Right-side endocarditis amongst "main lining" drug addicts.

(4) Carcinoid syndrome.

Organic rheumatic tricuspid incompetence is suspected if features of tricuspid stenosis are present and those of pulmonary hypertension are absent. Symptoms and signs include upper abdominal pain due to hepatic enlargement, oedema, jaundice, a large 'V' wave in jugular vein, a right ventricular heave, a pansystolic murmur at the lower left sternal edge. Characteristically, the murmur increases with inspiration. This variation with inspirations may not be detectable in presence of very high venous pressure.

**Management**

Functional tricuspid incompetence secondary to mitral valve disease usually responds to surgical correction of the mitral valve lesion. Organic cases will require annuloplasty or tricuspid valve replacement.

## AORTIC VALVE DISEASE

Next to mitral valve disease, aortic valve is the common form of valvular heart disease and accounts for about 35 to 40% of patients with significant valvular lesions. Haemodynamically significant aortic valve disease has been classified into predominant aortic stenosis and predominant aortic incompetence.

**Pathology**

As a result of outflow obstruction in aortic stenosis the left ventricle becomes overloaded and undergoes concentric hypertrophy. The wall of the left ventricle becomes thickened at the expense of left ventricular cavity. The septum which is also involved bulges into the cavity of the right ventricle. In aortic incompetence, on the other hand, left ventricle becomes overloaded during diastole and both dilatation and hypertrophy occur. The size of the left ventricle becomes very large. The appearance of the valve depends upon the aetiology of stenosis or incompetence.

## AORTIC STENOSIS

### Aetiology

**Rheumatic** — Chronic rheumatic endocarditis may cause fusion of the commissures of aortic valve resulting in stenosis.

**Congenital** — It is also a common cause in adults, the valve being bicuspid in most instances. Physical signs are trivial in childhood and adolescence. Subsequent calcification and distortion in middle age produce significant symptoms.

**Degenerative** — In the elderly, degenerative changes in the aortic valve with sclerosis and calcification may produce signs of aortic valve stenosis in absence of significant obstruction.

**Hyper-lipoproteinaemia (Type II and III)** is a rare cause of aortic stenosis.

In addition to stenosis at the level of the valve there may be obstruction above the level of the valve i.e. congenital supravalvular stenosis or below the level of valve i.e. subvalvular stenosis. In subvalvular stenosis, a localised fibrous ring produces the obstruction or the obstruction may arise from septal hypertrophy in hypertrophic obstructive cardiomyopathies (IHSS).

### Haemodynamics

Haemodynamic consequences occur when the orifice of the aortic valve which is normally above 3 $cm^2$ is reduced to around 50 per cent of its size. The stenosis causes pressure load on the left ventricle which undergoes hypertrophy (concentric hypertrophy). The end-diastolic pressure in the left ventricle increases because of reduced myocardial compliance with consequent rise of pressure in the left atrium. Pulmonary congestion then begins to appear. In course of time the stenosed valve calcifies irrespective of the aetiology. Calcification may involve coronary ostia. Although in the majority of cases calcification is confined to the aortic valve, it may spread downwards to involve the anterior leaflet of the mitral valve or A-V node. The latter condition may give rise to prolonged A-V conduction or even complete A-V block. As a result of ejection of blood through a stenosed orifice like a jet, there is dilatation of ascending aorta.

### Clinical features

**Symptoms** — (1) Breathlessness may not be an early symptom. It results from elevated left atrial pressure consequent upon increased left ventricular end-diastolic pressure. It starts as shortness of breath on exertion and may progress to orthopnoea. Paroxysmal nocturnal dyspnoea occurs in the late stage of the disease.

(2) Angina pectoris is a common symptom and may occur even in presence of normal coronary arteries. It is, however, clinically indistinguisable from angina resulting from coronary arterial disease. Angina in aortic stenosis has been attributed to (a) low mean aortic pressure, (b) jet effect which interferes with coronary filling, (c) discrepancy between the flow and needs of the hypertrophied left ventricle, and (d) rarely coronary embolism.

(3) Syncope — Occurs in about 20 per cent of cases. It results from exercise induced vasodilatation in presence of a fixed cardiac output. It may be the result of transient episode of A.V. block or the result of locking of the valve due to calcium deposit.

(4) Dizziness — It is most frequent when the patient is standing. Poor cerebral perfusion caused by low cardiac output and orthostatic mechanism, contributes to this symptoms.

(5) Sudden death — May occur due to combination of above mechanism.

### Physical signs

Pulse is of small volume and in severe cases may be plateau in form. Anacrotic notch is not always felt in radial pulse. The carotid pulse in the neck is slow rising with a reduced amplitude and an early notch in the upstroke may be felt. A thrill may also be palpable over the carotid.

The jugular venous pulse and pressure are normal but a small 'a' wave may frequently be seen. It probably results from Bernheim effect, the hypertrophied septum reducing the cavity of the right ventricle.

The apical impulse is sustained heaving in type due to left ventricular hypertrophy. A thrill is usually palpable over the aortic area. On auscultation, the first sound is normal and is occasionally preceded by an $S_4$ (fourth heart sound) due to atrial contraction. The second sound is single when the valve is calcified due to loss of the aortic component. In young patients, where the cusps are mobile, aortic component is audible but delayed. This is described as 'reversed splitting'. The characteristic murmur of aortic valve stenosis is a rough ejection systolic murmur audible over the base. The murmur is conducted along the carotid and is also audible over the apex. The ejection murmur cannot start until aortic valve opens at the end of isometric contraction phase. So it begins clearly after the first heart sound. The murmur ceases when the left ventricle starts relaxing that is appreciably before the aortic valve closure (2nd sound). Therefore, the murmur is midsystolic and from the phonocardiographic appearance described as 'diamond' shaped murmur.

Blood pressure is usually normal at rest.

**ECG :** Shows left ventricular hypertrophy and strain pattern. Sinus rhythm is usual and presence of atrial fibrillation indicates co-existing mitral valve disease. A normal electrocardiogram, however, does not preclude aortic valve stenosis.

**Chest X-ray :** The heart is often of normal size, but has a rounded left contour indicating left ventricular hypertrophy. The ascending aorta is usually prominent owing to post-stenotic dilatation produced by the jet effect. When heart failure develops the heart size is enlarged and signs of pulmonary congestion appear in the lung fields. Left lateral view or left oblique view helps not only in assessing in left ventricular size but also in identification of aortic valve calcification.

**Special investigations**

**Exercise Test** — This helps in assessing the patient's functional capacity. If the patient's ECG and blood pressure can be monitored and supervised, he may be exercised to the limit of anginal pain, dyspnoea or exhaustion. Appearance of arrhythmia or a tendency to fall of blood pressure will necessitate termination of exercise test.

**Cardiac catheterisation** — It is performed for measurement of pressure gradient across aortic valve, cardiac output and for angiocardiographic studies. The left ventricle can be approached by brachial arteriotomy or by femoral puncture through Seldinger's technique or by transeptal puncture via right and left atria. The severity of the stenosis can be estimated from the systolic pressure gradient between left ventricle and aorta. Resting cardiac output is usually normal in absence of heart failure.

Left ventricular angiogram helps in visualising the anatomy of the stenosed valve and also in assessing the contractibility of the myocardium. It can be combined with selective coronary angiography, particularly if there is any angina.

**Echocardiography :** Helps in estimating the thickness of cusps and of the left ventricle cavity and wall dimension. It also gives an impression of the contractibility.

**Treatment :** Patients with physical signs of aortic stenosis without any subjective symptoms and who have a normal working capacity do not require any treatment nor any haemodynamic investigation. Prophylactic measures against infective endocarditis and secondary prevention of rheumatic recurrences are all that would be necessary. A clinical assessment including exercise test at one yearly intervals has been recommended. The patient should be advised to avoid sustained strenuous physical exercise. Appearance of symptoms and reduction of physical working capacity would necessitate haemodynamic evaluation in a cardiac laboratory. Heart failure should be treated with bed rest, digitalis and diuretic with potassium supplements. Angina pectoris usually responds to glyceryl trinitrate and prophylactic use of isosorbide-dinitrate, beta-receptor blocking agents and calcium antagonists. It is important to bear in mind that glyceryl trinitrate and vasodilators may occasionally produce syncope from a fall of blood pressure and beta receptor blocking agents should be avoided in presence of heart failure. Surgical treatment should comprise of commissurotomy provided the cusps are elastic and not calcified. Re-stenosis and post-operative incompetence may occur subsequently in many cases and eventually require valve replacement.

Valve replacement is carried out using either artificial valve prosthesis, homografts or frame supported porcine valves.

## AORTIC REGURGITATION
## AORTIC VALVE INCOMPETENCE

### Aetiology

(1) Rheumatic fever — is considered to be the most common cause of aortic incompetence.

(2) Subacute infective endocarditis — may affect the congenital bicuspid valve or a mildly incompetent aortic valve. The incompetence resulting from infective endocarditis is usually acute.

(3) Syphilis — accounts for only a small number of cases although it used to be major cause in the first half of this century.

(4) Degenerative — Some authorities believe that atheromatous changes can cause incompetence.

### Rare causes include

(1) Marfan's syndrome — Here the cusps are redundant and chordae are lax and result in incomplete apposition of cusps.

(2) Sero-negative arthritides — e.g. Ankylosing spondylitis and Reiter's syndrome.

(3) Rheumatoid arthritis and SLE rarely produce incompetence of aortic valve.

(4) Dissecting aneurysm of aorta with or without Marfan's syndrome.

(5) Coarctation of aorta.

(6) Congenital bicuspid valve — Usually produces trivial leak, but acute aortic incompetence may result following infective endocarditis.

(7) Ventricular septal defect associated with prolapse of aortic valve.

### Still rare causes are —

(1) Traumatic rupture of aortic cusp

(2) Pseudoxanthoma elasticum

(3) Methysergide poisoning

(4) Congenital aneurysm of the sinuses of Valsalva

(5) Mucopolysaccharoidosis — like Hurler's syndrome, Morquio's syndrome, etc.

### Haemodynamics

Since the aortic valve is incompetent only part of the ventricular output reaches the periphery and the remainder regurgitates back into the heart. This results in volume overload of the left ventricle which dilates and later undergoes hypertrophy. The myocardial compliance is reduced and end-diastolic pressure in the left ventricle increases causing a rise in left atrial pressure and development of pulmonary congestion. The stroke volume of the left ventricle is increased and the ejection phase is shortened. In early systole a large quantity of blood is quickly ejected into relaxed arteries because of low diastolic pressure. The low diastolic pressure is due to both aortic reflux and peripheral vasodilatation (Oram).

**Clinical features :**

**Symptoms**

Dizziness and palpitation are the common presenting symptoms. Throbbing sensation in the chest and/or head may result from rapid ejection of a large stroke volume. Palpitation is more intense in supine position. The throbbing sensation may induce anxiety and may produce other symptoms like fatigue, chest pain and difficulty in breathing.

*Dyspnoea* — Usually results from left ventricular failure and may be progressive.

*Angina pectoris* — Is less common than in aortic stenosis. The low aortic diastolic pressure may contribute to an insufficient diastolic filling of coronary arteries. A raised intracavitary pressure during diastole may also interfere with coronary diastolic flow. Compared to increased myocardial demands for oxygen of the dilated and hypertrophic left ventricle, the available supply is reduced due to poor coronary perfusion resulting in angina. Angina is more frequent in aortic incompetence of leutic origin and is usually more troublesome during the night.

**Signs :**

The pulse is of high amplitude and in the radial arteries produces a "water hammer" or collapsing pulse as a result of sharp pressure rise followed by an equally rapid fall in pressure resulting from regurgitation of blood back into left ventricle.

Capillary pulsation may be observed in the nail beds by applying light pressure on the tips. It can also be demonstrated in the inner aspect of the lower lips by pressing with a glass slide. It can also be detected in the retinal arteries by observing the variation of the small gap where the retinal arterioles and venules are running close to each other. It is important to remember that retinal veins pulsate but not the arterioles. Palpation of the precordium reveals displacement of the apical impulse downwards and to the left as an evidence of left ventricular enlargement. The apical impulse is forceful resulting from myocardial hypertrophy and a large stroke volume. Only in severe regurgitation a diastolic thrill is palpable along left sternal edge.

*Auscultation :*— The regurgitant flow of blood produces a high-pitched diastolic murmur starting after the second heart sound. There is no gap between the second sound and the onset of the murmur. Usually it is best heard along the left sternal edge in the third and fourth interspace. One can detect the murmur easily if the patient is asked to sit up, lean forward and to hold his breath after expiration. If the murmur is also heard over the right sternal border, it indicates that there is dilatation of aortic ring and of ascending aorta.

A concomitant systolic murmur is usually present in aortic incompetence and does not necessarily indicate the presence of co-existing aortic stenosis. The systolic murmur is explained by turbulence in the aorta caused by rapid ejection of a large amount of blood. If the aorta is dilated, a systolic thrill may also be felt. A low pitched diastolic murmur with or without pre-systolic accentuation may be heard over the apex suggesting a co-existing mitral stenosis. This murmur known as Austin-Flint murmur is produced by vibration of the anterior leaflet as the regurgitant stream impedes full opening of the mitral valve. Peripheral vascular signs apart from collapsing pulse and capillary pulsation are Traube's pistol shot sound audible over the femoral arteries and Duroziez double intermittent crural souffle which comprise of a systolic murmur over the femoral artery and diastolic murmur which is audible when pressure is applied distal to the point of auscultation.

The blood pressure is characterised by a wide pulse pressure caused by a low diastolic pressure. In younger patients the Korotkoff's 4th or 5th sound may be heard falsely down to zero. For accurate estimation of blood pressure, measurement of intraarterial pressure is required.

In patients with advanced disease arteriolar constriction compensatory to reduced cardiac output may cause rise in diastolic pressure.

### Investigations

**Phonocardiogram :** This reveals the presence of aortic diastolic murmurs which starts immediately after the aortic component of second sound. It is diminuendo in shape. A progressive decrease in the duration of the murmur indicates myocardial functional impairment. A diamond-shaped systolic murmur is also noticeable.

**Electrocardiogram :** It may remain normal for many years, but ultimately evidence of left ventricular hypertrophy with tall T waves (diastolic overload pattern) is seen.

**Chest Radiograph :**

Cardiac silhouette is enlarged, caused by left ventricular enlargement. Valvular calcification is less common in aortic stenosis. In presence of left ventricular failure, signs of pulmonary venous congestion will be evident in the lung fields.

**Echocardiography** — is useful non-invasive investigation. It also helps in assessing left ventricular function and in diagnosing Austin Flint murmur.

### Cardiac Catheterisation and Cineaortography

When the contrast medium is injected at about 4 cm. above the aortic valve, regurgitation of dye into the left ventricle can be demonstrated. The degree of reflux may also be estimated. In severe regurgitation there is almost complete opacification of the left ventricular cavity.

### Treatment

Patients with trivial aortic incompetence often remain asymptomatic but they are prone to infective endocarditis and should be protected by appropriate antibiotics before any dental procedure, invasive investigations etc. (see : chapter 19). Trinitrin tablets are helpful in relieving angina. Diuretics can be used as required but overdiuresis is dangerous. Valve replacement is the treatment of choice. Although one would usually like to wait until some symptoms appear, there is little advantage in waiting when the heart size is progressively increasing or the electrocardiogram is deteriorating. Patients presenting with effort syncope and intractable angina should be operated as early as possible. Coronary arteriography can be conveniently carried out during aortography.

### Valve replacement

Either a biological tissue valve or a prosthetic valve is usually used. Mortality from prosthetic valve replacement is less than 10 percent but occurrence of embolism should always be prevented by long-term anticoagulant therapy. The mortality of tissue valve replacement is little higher than replacement by prosthesis.

## INFECTIVE ENDOCARDITIS

*(Subacute Bacterial Endocarditis)*

*D.C. GHOSH*

### Introduction

Infective endocarditis remains, still one of the few dangerous conditions with a mortality rate of about 30 per cent in spite of the advent of so many antibiotics. The major cause for this high mortality is delay in diagnosis, because the clinical features in the early stage of the disease are unimpressive and more importantly inappropriate antibiotic therapy. The latter suppresses the fever but does not prevent the progression of the disease.

### Nomenclature

Since the infective agent is not always a bacteria, the term infective endocarditis is used in preference to bacterial endocarditis. With the advent of antibiotics, the clinical distinction between acute and subacute endocarditis has also become blurred. Acute infective endocarditis — also termed as malignant endocarditis occurs is a setting of depressed host resistance and forms a part of generalised overwhelming infection. The onset is rapid with high swinging fever with rigor and sweats. Healthy valves are often affected. The duration is short and outcome often fatal.

**Aetiology**

Subacute infective endocarditis occur in any patient with a cardiac lesion, and who has a bacteraemia.

**Predisposing causes**

The valves or other structures that are affected are nearly always abnormal either as a result of rheumatic or congenital defect (Oram). Of the acquired defects, old rheumatic valvulitis accounts for 80% of cases. The most vulnerable lesions being minimal mitral and aortic regurgitation. Severely damaged valves are less likely to be affected e.g. severe mitral stenosis, but in elderly subjects grossly sclerosed aortic valve can be affected. Of the congenital defects the important ones are persistent ductus arteriosus, bicuspid aortic valve, ventricular septal defects, coarctation of aorta, aneurysm of the sinuses of Valsalva, and arterio-venous fistula. It is important to remember that ostium secundum type of atrial septal defects are not affected and the occurrence of infective endocarditis in ASD suggests that the defect must have been of the primum type. Other conditions where infective endocarditis might occur include pulmonary stenosis and hypertrophic obstructive cardiomyopathy.

Infection is rare on the right side of the heart but right-sided endocarditis is being increasingly recognised amongst drug addicts who use unsterile syringes.

**Infective agents**

In acute bacterial endocarditis — which is rare, the infective agents are strepto pyogenes and staphylococcus albus. These organisms may affect a normal valve, particularly after cardiac surgery and in drug addicts.

In subacute infective endocarditis, most infections are caused by organisms of relatively low virulence i.e. by those which are regarded as common sets. Prior to the advent of antibiotics i.e. penicillin strepto viridans used to account for 80% per cent of cases. The majority of the infective agents were strepto viridans, strepto haemolyticus, strepto faecalis, staph pyogenes and albus. Other organisms include various aerobic and anaerobic streptococci, Neisseria gonorrhoeae, Haemophylus influenzae, Brucella abortus and Bacillus proteus.

These organisms gain entrance into the body from the following sources.

1. *Dental extraction* — This procedure is the commonest cause of endocarditis. Bacteraemia with strep. Viridans often occurs after tooth extractions. Scaling and filling are occasionally responsible. Even chewing with infected teeth may produce bacteraemia.

2. *Genito urinary and rectal procedure* —

Any stretching of tissue carrying commensal organisms can produce bacteraemia. Examples are urinary bladder catheterization, dilatation and curettage of the uterus and sigmoidoscopy. Strep. faecalis is the usual organism in these situations. But normal delivery is seldom a hazard.

3. *Bed sores* — may be source of infection in the elderly or debilitated patients. The organisms are often penicillin resistant staphylococci.

4. *Cardiac surgery* — including cardiac pacing and catheterisation may allow entrance of organism such as staph albus. In patients who has prior antibiotic cover there is also likelihood of fungus infection.

Rare infective agents include

Fungi — such as Candida, aspergillus,
histoplasmosis, torulosis —

Rickettsia burnetti (Q. fever)
Chlamydia type B.

**Pathology** : The hallmark of infective endocarditis are vegetations which are formed on the surface of damaged valves. The vegetations are comprised of irregular deposits of platelets white cells, red cells, and fibrin enclosing bacteria which are deeply embedded. "There is paucity of granulation tissues and cellular reaction and there is no walling off of the infection". Presumably the bacteria may be brought to the valve by blood vessels of the valve itself. This may explain why severely scarred valves are not affected (Oram).

The vegetations are larger than those found in rheumatic endocarditis. These are friable and get easily dislodged forming emboli. The vegetations may extend into the chordae and along the wall of atria and ventricles. In congenital heart disease the site of vegetation depends on the direction of blood flow for example in VSD with L-R shunt these are found on right side of the septum and the opposite wall of right ventricle.

Emboli from vegetations may cause infarction of kidney, spleen, brain and gut. An infected embolus may produce local arteritis of the occluded vessel, causing weakness of the arterial wall and thus forming mycotic aneurysm. Mycotic aneurysm may also be formed in the valve cusp, in the sinuses of valsalva, in the ventricular septum aorta and peripheral vessel. Rupture of the mycotic aneurysm may cause fatal haemorrhage. The septic emboli may cause abscesses.

Many of the manifestations of infective endocarditis which were formerly believed to be due to microembolism, are now thought to be due to deposition of complexes of antigen, antibody and compliment. Microscopical examination of skin lesions, such as petechia, splinter haemorrhages, and Osler's node have always shown evidences of vasculitis but not of embolism.

Both focal and diffuse glomerulitis occur in kidneys. The renal lesions is due to deposition of immune complex in the basement membrane of glomerulus. Neurological manifestations are due to vasculitis. Heart failure in infective endocarditis is due to rupture of valve or chordae.

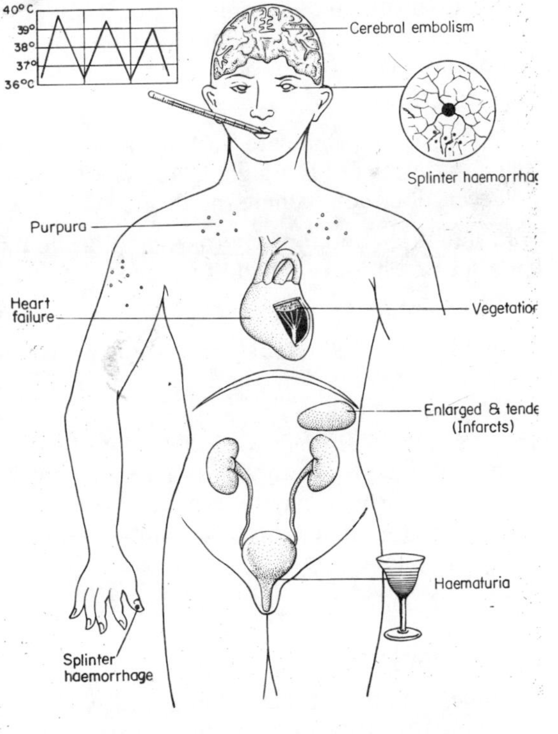


Fig.18.28 — Clinical picture of infective endocarditis

**Clinical Features**

The disease may occur in young adults of either sex. In recent years there has been an increased proportion of elderly patients with infective endocarditis.

A history of dental sepsis, tooth extraction or genito-urinary instrumentation may be obtained in about 50 per cent of cases.

The onset is gradual. The early symptoms comprise of malaise, anorexia and low grade pyrexia with intermittent sweats. Fever is sometimes difficult to detect. Subacute episodes of fever may alternate with afebrile periods (Fig. 18.28).

There is weight loss and progressive pallor. The classical description of cafe-au-lait complexion about the face and back of hand is a late sign and virtually non-existent now.

Finger clubbing and toe clubbing occur in about 50 per cent of cases and are diagnostic. It is important to remember that clubbing takes some 3-6 weeks to develop.

The spleen is usually palpable but rarely large. It is non-tender. Sudden enlargement of spleen with tenderness and appearance of splenic rub suggest infarction.

*Cardiac signs*

In a great majority of cases evidences of heart disease were already present. In absence of any cardiac involvement it is difficult to sustain the diagnosis. The alteration in the intensity and character of murmurs are strong confirmatory evidence in support of the diagnosis. The appearance of a new aortic diastolic or mitral systolic murmurs is highly suggestive. The features of acute valvular incompetence differ considerably from those of this usual established disease because there is no time for compensatory ventricular dilatation and hypertrophies. As a result, pulmonary oedema will occur with little cardiac enlargement.

*Embolic phenomenon*

Frank emboli from vegetation on the infected valve, may appear in any part of the circulation and may present as cardiac infarction, cerebrovascular accident, sudden loin pain and haematuria indicating renal infarction, and occlusion of the arteries of limbs. In right-sided endocarditis recurrent pulmonary emboli produce difficult diagnostic problems.

Minor emboli in the skin cause painful nodules in the pulp of the fingers. Osler's nodes are larger subcutaneous emboli (5 mm in diameters). These are pathognomonic. Emboli may occur in the retina and appear as exudate surrounded by haemorrhage.

Mycotic aneurysm involving cerebral vessels may produce subarachnoid haemorrhage.

Diffuse vascular change affecting small vessels may be part of an excessive immune process rather than of embolic origin and may manifest as petichiae splinter haemorrhages (Horder's line), haematuria due to glomerular lesion and generalised cerebral disturbances leading to a confusional state.

**Investigations**

Anaemia is normocytic and normochromic. White cell count is not of great value in the diagnosis but the ESR is high; a fall of more than 50 mm in the 1st hour is unusual. A normal ESR, however, does not exclude the diagnosis.

Proteinuria common. Microscopy of urine for red cells is a good confirmatory evidence. If a spun specimen is examined, it is almost invariably positive.

High plasma gamma globulin levels are seen and may produce a positive latex fixation test.

Blood culture is mandatory for diagnosis and management. Culture of bone marrow may sometimes prove positive in the presence of negative blood culture.

**Differential Diagnosis :** Any cause of pyrexia of uncertain origin must be considered. Sometimes it is difficult to differentiate between reactivations of rheumatic process and the features of infective endocarditis in a patient with pre-existing chronic rheumatic valvular disease. Left atrial myxoma may be confused with infective endocarditis because of identical clinical features. The former however is more common in female, (vide differential diagnosis of mitral stenosis). Systemic lupus erythematosus with verrucous endocarditis of mitral valve may simulate clinically because of arthralgia and heart murmur but embolic manifestation is very rare.

**Management**

Although most cases caused by strepto viridans infection respond to a standard treatment with Penicillin, the problem of antibiotic treatment is so great that in subacute infection it is usually wisest to delay antibiotic treatment until the causative organism has been identified. The best antibiotic regimen for the particular infection can then be outlined. Positive blood culture is needed to establish the diagnosis. It is a gross error to treat with inappropriate antibiotics an undiagnosed fever in a cardiac patient. Blood cultures should be taken with aseptic precaution. In subacute disease and with a good laboratory, no advantage is achieved by taking more than three cultures within 24 hours. In potentially complicated cases as in drug addicts or after cardiac surgery it is wise to collect six cultures within 12 to 24 hours. There is no advantage in timing the blood culture in relation to the body temperature or by taking samples of arterial blood.

Negative cultures usually result from ineffective antibiotic treatment or due to presence of fastidious organisms requiring special techniques for culture. Presistently, negative culture suggest, fungi, Q fever or psittacosis. Serological tests are necessary for their diagnosis.

If the clinical situation seems urgent and in any addicts, where rapid progression may be quickly fatal it is wise to start emperical treatment immediately after taking six sets of blood culture over one to one and half hour period before antibiotics are administered. The culture provides a valuable guide to the effectiveness of treatment.

**Choice of antibiotics**

The sensitivities of the organism to bactericidal antibiotics singly or in combination must be assessed by the bacteriologist in order to decide on appropriate treatment.

Bactericidal antibiotics such as Penicillin, Ampicillin, Cephalosporins and aminoglycosides must be used alone or in combination.

Bacteriostatic antibiotics such as sulphonamides, tetracycline, chloramphenicol suppress the infection but do not eradicate it. Erythromycin and novobiocin may be helpful in combination with other drugs. Cotrimoxazole has been found to be useful. Penicillin is safe because it can be given in high concentration without toxic effect. Probenecid although boosting the penicillin level carries the risk of drug reaction, e.g. skin rash.

More resistant infection responds well to penicillin and streptomycin. This regime of ampicillin and streptomycin are usually effective against strep. faecalis.

Staphylococcal infection may produce penicillinase and requires treatment with methicillin, cloxacillin or cephaloridine. Strepto viridans usually responds to penicillin but as it may take several days to establish sensitivities it is best to begin with four million units, six hourly I.V. and reduce the dose later and change to intramuscular regime if the organism is sensitive.

**Table — 18.8 : Antibiotic therapy in infective endocarditis**

| Organism | Drugs of choice | Dosage and route of administration |
|---|---|---|
| 1. Strep. Viridans | Benzyl Penicillin | 2-3 million units iv. 6 hrly. |
| 2. Strep. faecalis | (a) Benzyl Penicillin plus Streptomycin/Gentamycin | Benzyl Penicillin — as above.<br>Str. — 0.5 Gm 12 hrly.<br>Gentamycin — 3-5 mgm/kg in 3 divided doses. |
| | (b) Ampicillin plus Gentamycin<br>(Pts. sensitive to Penicillin-Erythromycin — 1 Gm. iv. every 6 hrs.) | Amp. 8-12 G/day in 3-4 divided by iv.<br>3-5 mgm/kg in 3 divided doses. |
| 3. Staph. aureus | (a) Benzyl Penicillin | 23 million units iv. 6 hrly. |
| | (b) Cloxacillin or Cephalothin<br>(Pts. sensitive to Penicillin-Vancomycin — 0.5 Gm. every 6 hrs. iv.) | 2 Gm. every 4 hrs. |
| 4. Staph. epidemidis | Vancomycin | 0.5 Gm every 6 hrs. iv. |
| 5. Yeast and Fungi | Amphotericin B | Amp. 1 mgm/1st day, 5 mgm 2nd day followed by daily increase 5-10 mgm/day until 1 mgm/kg/day is achieved (max 90 mgm/day) |
| | 5 fluorocytosine | 5 FC — 50 to 150 mgm/kg every 6 hrs. (Oral) |

**Effectiveness of therapy**

Clinical assessment is most important but wherever possible level of serum antibiotic level may be measured.

**Penicillin allergy**

If the patient is allergic to penicillin it may be possible to use an alternative antibiotic. Considering the fact that penicillin is often the best agent it is wise to give a test dose to confirm the patient's sensitivities. Desensitisation is a time-consuming process and steroids can conveniently be used before beginning treatment.

**Duration of treatment**

The protective effect of the immune response requires prolonged therapy. It is best to stick to the classical recommendation of treatment for six weeks. The shorter course although successful at times is associated with a high rate of relapse and relapses are difficult to manage. Careful observation for several weeks is needed after the course of treatment has been completed, as failure may occur when the damaged valves starts shrinking.

**Surgery in Infective endocarditis**

If severe valvular incompetence occurs urgent mitral or aortic valve replacement may be necessary.

**Prophylactic treatment**

In susceptible individuals, infective endocarditis must be prevented by effective bactericidal antibiotic before undertaking any procedure which might lead to a bacteraemia. All patients with known valvular lesions and congenital heart disease must be protected in this way.

## CARDIOMYOPATHY

**(Syn : Myocardiopathy : Myocardial disease)**

*G.C. MOOKERJEE*

**Introduction**

Heart muscle diseases of unknown aetiology are classed as cardiomyopathy (CMP). The disorder is usually a chronic myocardial disease usually ending in fatality once failure sets in. Acute or subacute myocarditis may also occur.

Aetiological classification varies but cardiac disorders due to coronary heart disease, hypertension, rheumatic heart disease, thyroid disorder, syphilis and congenital heart diseases are excluded from the list of aetiology of CMP. Previously CMP used to be classified into two types — primary and secondary but recently this classification is being revised.

The modern concept is to evaluate the cause whenever possible and call it a specific heart muscle disease. However, in most cases it becomes a guess-work as heart muscle biopsy is not routinely possible. Until more satisfactory classification and better methods of aetiological diagnosis are available, the following classification may be considered useful, at least to explain the ill-understood subject of CMP.

**Aetiology :**

Possible factors may be follows :

1) Idiopathic –– where no cause can be found, hence this was previously called primary CMP. Familial occurrence is well-known.
2) Viral — Coxsachie-B virus, influenza, infectious mononucleosis, diphtheria, toxoplasmosis, Chagas' disease, etc. may cause myocarditis, recognised during or weeks after the acute illness.

3) Alcohol, emetine, arsenic, cobalt, ethylene glycol etc. also may be responsible.
4) Infiltrative disorders : Sarcoidosis, amyloidosis, collagen diseases, gargoylism, glycogen storage disease, haemochromatosis can cause CMP.
5) Neuromuscular disorders e.g. Friedrich's ataxia, progressive muscular dystrophy and dystrophia myotonica may be associated with CMP.
6) Postpartum CMP occurs usually two to several weeks in post-partum period. Why it occurs is not clear.
7) Nutritional CMP (Beriberi) due to deficiency of vitamin $B_1$ (aneurin), is well known.

In this classification I have attempted to separate specific heart muscle diseases from the ill-understood idiopathic group.

However, from clinical angle three varieties are recognised based on haemodynamics and pathological data where available. Clinicopathological types based on haemodynamics are as follows :

## HYPERTROPHIC OBSTRUCTIVE CARDIOMYOPATHY (H O C M)
### [ Chronic obstructive cardiomyopathy – C O C M ]

In USA, this group is known as idiopathic hypertrophic sub-aortic stenosis (IHSS). Some of these cases may not have obstructive features, when they may be called as simple hypertrophic C M P.

**Pathology**

The diffuse hypertrophy with fibrosis specially involving outflow tract leads to narrowing of the left ventricle. The left ventricular cavity becomes small. Hypertrophy usually is not like generalised secondary hypertrophy as seen in systemic hypertension or aortic valve disease. It is asymmetric. often involving ventricular septum.

**Clinical features**

1) Usually familial but idiopathic and non-familial occurrence is also noted.
2) The lesion is sub-aortic valvular obstruction due to muscular hypertrophy in the outflow tract.
3) Clinical features are like aortic stenosis. L.V. heave, systolic ejection bruit, fourth heart sound and systolic thrill may be present.
4) There may be no symptoms in the early stage.
5) Later on anginal pain, effort intolerance dyspnoea develops.
6) Effort syncope and sudden death may occur. Family history of sudden death may be available.

**Investigations**

1) X-ray heart may or may not show gross cardiomegaly. LVH may be noted radiologically in some cases.
2) ECG – shows evidence of L.V.H.
3) Cardiac catheter studies and angiography reveals out flow tract obstruction and small L.V.

**Treatment**

There is no curative treatment. Beta-blockers are helpful by slowing heart rate and reduce contractile force of heart. Propranolol 40 to 80 mg daily is usually helpful. Surgical procedures to reduce outflow tract obstruction may be helpful in some cases.

Operative procedure consists of excision of hypertrophied areas, septal myotomy or myomectomy (Morrow's operation). Mortality may be around 10%.

## CONGESTIVE TYPE OF CMP

Grossly affected myocardium resulting in poor contractile power and dilatation of ventricles (pump failure). Clinical presentation is like CHF.

### Pathology

There are no specific histopathological findings excepting evidence of fibrosis especially in East African types. There may be intramural thrombus formation which may cause systemic embolism.

### Clinical features

Dyspnoea on exertion or nocturnal dyspnoea may be early manifestations and later signs of CCF will occur.

Heart is enlarged, JVP is raised and oedema appears. Third and fourth gallop sounds may be heard. Gross cardiac enlargement may result in reflux mitral and tricuspid incompetence. Diagnosis may be mistaken as rheumatic heart disease.

### Diagnosis

X-ray chest will reveal enlarged heart and pulmonary congestion.

ECG may show non-specific T-wave changes and sometimes low voltage complexes. Echocardiography helps in excluding valvular heart disease. If possible cardiac catheterization and angiography may be considered. Endocardial muscle biopsy may also be attempted but in any case prognosis is poor.

Alcoholism, pregnancy and presence of myopathy may be clues to the aetiology. General symptoms may be loss of weight, vague ill-health, fatigue, flatulence and joint pains. Usually they are chronic invalid patients and come to hospital with symptoms of dyspnoea on exertion, puffy face, ascitis and often with enlarged liver. Oedema legs is usually absent or not marked at all. Venous pressure is usually raised in advanced cases.

Tachycardia and auricular fibrillation may be present and heart is usually enlarged sometimes associated with pericardial effusion.

Prognosis is not considered satisfactory, especially in advanced cases. Early diagnosis however helps in planning proper medical care which may prolong life by a few years. Once failure is established patients usually die within two to three years.

If obvious cause is detectable e.g. alcohol, anaemia, thyroid disorder or syphilis appropriate action can be taken. In symptomless cases, avoidance of competitive sports and undue physical exertion should be avoided.

Congestive cardiac failure should be treated energetically with diuretics, digitalis and prolonged bed rest.

However, digitalis toxicity should be avoided. Vasodilators e.g. isosorbide dinitrates or hydralazine may be required in some cases to reduce after load and improve cardiac output. Side effects need careful watch. These can not be used if there is hypotension. $\beta$-adrenergic blockers may control tachycardia but must be cautiously used. Salbutamol, dopamine, captopril, dobutamine, steroids have been used with variable results.

Surgical treatment is not satisfactory due to underlying myocardial disease.

Anticoagulants may be considered if there is possibility of embolism (e.g. associated atrial fibrillation). Suitable cases may be put on beta-blockers to control tachycardia.

D.C. shock may restore sinus rhythm in some cases. Patients having syncope may be given pacemaker.

## RESTRICTIVE C M P

In this type,ventricular filling is affected during diastole due to development fibroelastic tissues in the endocardial lining of ventricles, left side more affected than right. This may extend in myocardium and pericardium in severe cases. Result is reduced diastolic filling and finally picture of constrictive pericarditis. The best example is African type of endomyocardial fibroelastosis (or endomyocardial fibrosis type of C M P).

This is quite rare and presents features of constrictive pericarditis. Echocardiography and left ventricular function studies may reveal constrictive features. Diagnosis can only be confirmed by biopsy if possible. Prognosis however is bad. Treatment is symptomatic, as surgery is not helpful.

However, many recent surgical procedures are being tried in endomyocardial fibroelastosis e.g. endocardial stripping, replacement of A-V valves, pericardio-peritoneal shunts in recurrent pericardial effusions.

Amyloid heart, also may present as restrictive CMP, these patients do not tolerate digoxin so well.

**General principles**

The practitioner should suspect C M P whenever there are features not atypical of valvular heart disease, I.H.D., systemic hypertension or pulmonary heart disease. There may be cardiac enlargement associated with gallop rhythm, tachycardia, abnormal rhythm due to conduction defects. Family history of C M P and sudden death may be present. If there is history of recurrent syncope a pacemaker may be given. Search for factors e.g. alcohol, toxic agents, nutritional deficiency etc., which can be avoided. Exertion should be avoided, protected living with sedentary jobs and supportive therapy prolongs life. Antiarrhythmic drugs and anticoagulation may be required where indication exists. DC shock with prior anticoagulation may be helpful in converting patients to sinus rhythm.

The ultimate prognosis however is bad in most cases.

## CONGENITAL HEART DISEASE

*SANJEEB K. MUKHERJEE*

Congenital heart disease is due to defective development of heart of the foetus in utero, resulting in structural or positional abnormality present at birth. Those with major defects may die soon after birth but others survive with some functional deficit. Most important developments take place during the third to eighth week of foetal life.

The primitive heart has four parts [(Fig : 18.29(a), (b) & (c)]

(1) Sinus venosus

(2) Auricle and auricular canal

(3) Ventricle

(4) Bulbus Cordis

The primitive heart resembles a tube. In the fourth week of foetal life, all these structures divide into two by a partition called septum. The interauricular septum divides the auricle into two chambers. A small valve-like opening (foramen ovale) closes after birth. The interventricular septum divides the ventricle into two parts. The septum of truncus arteriosus divides into two major vessels, the aorta and pulmonary artery.

During this time, the cardiac tube begins to get folded in such a way (S-shaped manner), that the left and right ventricles are juxtaposed with the division of truncus arteriosus viz. aorta and pulmonary artery respectively (Fig.18.29).

Sinus venosus joins right auricle at sino-auricular node (S.A. Node). The primitive auricular canal forms the A.V. node, bundle of His and its branches. The bulbus cordis gets incorporated in the right ventricle also to some extent in left ventricle. The spiral septum of truncus arteriosus divides it into aorta and pulmonary artery. [Fig.18.29(d)].

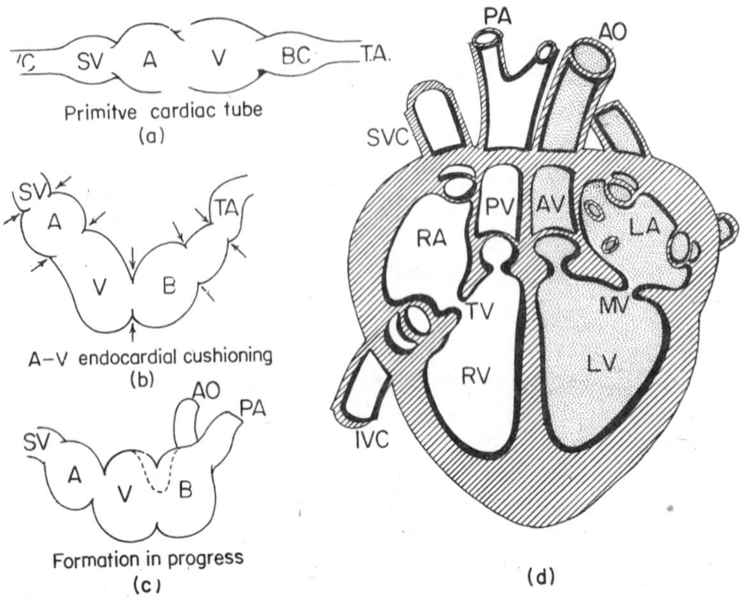


Fig.18.29 — Showing development of primitive heart (a), (b) and (c); (d) — shows completed development

Various processes during development occur simultaneously. So it is quite obvious that if some process or processes remain incomplete, single or multiple defects can result in heart of a newly born baby. It is easy to imagine, that many types of congenital heart disease may result, depending upon the site and stage of arrested growth. For instance if the septa dividing auricle, ventricle or truncusarteriosus remain completely developed, it will result in atrial septal defect (ASD), ventricular septal defect (VSD) and aorto-pulmonary window respectively.

In some congenital heart diseases (CHD) the arterial and venous blood may get mixed at the site of the defect. If venous blood is shunted to arterial side without passing through lungs, cyanosis will be evident. This happens in Fallot's tetralogy. If arterial blood is shunted to venous side from left ventricle to right ventricle (VSD) or left auricle to right (ASD), there will be no cyanosis. Fig. 18.30 shows foetal circulation in normals.

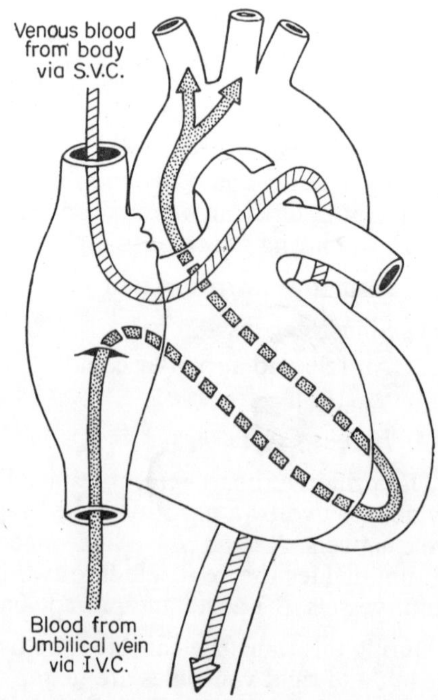


Fig.18.30 : Shows the foetal circulation.

**Hence congenital heart disease may be cyanotic or acyanotic. Acyanotic variety later on may become cyanotic if the reversal of blood flow occurs due to high pressure in pulmonary circuit.**

Congenital defect may occur without any shunt. For instance when truncus arteriosus does not develop normally, it may result in aortic valve stenosis, subvalvular stenosis or coarctation of aorta. Obviously there will be no cyanosis.

Clinicians have to remember that congenital heart lesions need radical cure but before patients are surrendered to knife, they have to be protected against infections, because they are liable to get infective endocarditis. In some of the lesions like PDA, VSD, ASD and even Fallot's tetralogy, surgical operation produce satisfying results.

It is difficult to pinpoint the aetiology of an established congenital heart disease. However, certain genetic factors such as chromosomal abnormalities, and hereditary diseases are important in the aetiology of congenital heart disease. The following factors are relevant :

(1) Trisomy 21 is associated with VSD, and ASD and trisomy 18 with VSD and PS.

(2) Some hereditary diseases associated with congenital diseases e.g. Ellis-Van-Crevel syndrome associated with single atrium. Holt-Oram associated with atrial septal defect, Garvell-Lange-Neilsen syndrome associated with prolonged QT interval and sudden death.

(3) Kartagener syndrome is associated with dextrocardia.

(4) Teratogens are well-known causes.

(5) Many other drugs include folic acid antagonists; anticonvulsive drugs-like dilantin, lithium chloride used in mental disorders and prolonged use of alcohol. Viruses like congenital rubella are associated with patent ductus arteriosus and stenosis of the pulmonary artery branches.

(6) Exposure to radiation and use of antimitotic drugs during pregnancy.

Congenital heart diseases can be broadly divided into three groups : cyanotic, acyanotic and miscellaneous types.

(A) **Congenital Cardiac Disease with Cyanosis**

(1) Tetralogy of Fallot
(2) Double outlet right ventricle with pulmonary stenosis
(3) Pulmonary atresia
(4) Tricuspid atresia
(5) Eisenmenger syndrome (ASD, VSD, PDA due to reversal of shunt)
(6) Transposition of the great vessels
(7) Ebstein's disease
(8) Truncus arteriosus
(9) Single ventricle

(B) **Without Cyanosis**

(1) Ventricular septal defect
(2) Atrial septal defect
(3) Osteum primum defect
(4) Endocardial cushion defect
(5) Patent ductus arteriosus
(6) Pulmonary stenosis in different forms
(7) Coarctation of the aorta
(8) Anomalous pulmonary venous return
(9) Congenital aortic stenosis
(10) Congenital mitral stenosis and mitral insufficiency.

**(C) Miscellaneous types**

(1) Anomalous origin of the coronary arteries.

(2) Marfan's syndrome primary pulmonary hypertension.

(3) Some abnormal metabolic diseases which are very rare.

It is customary to describe symptoms and signs of pure congenital lesions, but it should be realised that in many cases there is more than one congenital lesion present, hence signs are modified. Though various newer diagnostic tools are now available e.g. echocardiography (M--Mode and two-dimensional), Doppler echocardiographic studies, nuclear angiography, exercise testing, subtraction digital angiography and contrast angiocardiography, every physician should put great emphasis on clinical examination. History taking, symptomatology, routine radiology, screening of heart and ECG along with good physical examination should be the basis of routine cardiology. Provisional diagnosis must made before looking for advanced diagnostic aids. Certainly, congenital heart disease is a complex subject and needs wide area of discussion but in this concise textbook, only some important and common diseases will be presented (Fig.18.5 to 18.9 – *Echocardiography of Common Congenital heart diseases)*

## CYANOTIC HEART DISEASE

### Tetralogy of Fallot

**Definition**

Though tetralogy of fallot has been defined to be a combination of right ventricular hypertrophy, ventricular septal defect, obstruction of the right ventricular outflow tract and dextro-position of the aorta, the main determining relation producing these symptoms and signs are from obstruction of the right ventricular outflow tract either in the form of pulmonary stenosis or infundibular stenosis.

Ventricular septal defect is usually large and it is situated just below the aortic valve.

**Hemodynamics**

In this condition, venous blood is shunted from the right ventricle into the left ventricle because of the obstruction at the right ventricular outflow level resulting in cyanosis.

**Clinical features**

The physical signs are predominantly, cyanosis, which comes between the first month and the sixth month of life. Then at about two to four years of age, clubbing is noted and shortness of breath during exertion become the troublesome symptom. Later on characteristic squatting position occurs and finally in advanced cases, anoxic blue spells occurs. At this stage the child becomes suddenly dyspnoeic and restless. These attacks may last for a few minutes to a few hours and occasionally may be fatal.

Physical signs : There is central cyanosis and clubbing of fingers and B.P. is usually normal. Palpation of precordium reveals moderate right ventricular heave, as presence of VSD, ensures equalisation of pressure both ventricles, hence RVH is not too much. If VSD is unusually large, pansystolic murmur is not present.

Systolic thrill is present in 50% of the cases at the left sternal border in the third interspace. A grade II to IV ejection systolic murmur is heard. First sound is normal. There may be an ejection click heard at the second intercostal space. Second sound is usually single which is due to $A_2$.

Heart size is usually normal. The normal bulge due to pulmonary artery is absent. In the lateral view, right ventricular hypertrophy can be seen. Aortic arch may be right sided in 25% of cases.

Lung fields are too clear due to poor perfusion.

*The electrocardiogram* is very helpful. It shows right axis deviation and only moderate right ventricular hypertrophy, sometimes **rsR'** pattern can be seen.

*Echocardiography* is very helpful and sometimes it can differentiate conditions like double outlet right ventricle from truncus arteriosus.

*Cardiac catheterization* shows right ventricular pressure is elevated. There is a fall of pulmonary artery pressure, may be at the valvular level or at the subvalvular level. The level of arterial oxygen is approximately 75 to 85% at rest. This is due to the mixture of venous blood into the arterial system. The actual amount depends on the magnitude of right to left shunt. Selective right ventriculography is diagnostic.

The prognosis is usually not too good without surgery as most children die young due to cyanotic attack or brain abscess. Other complications include cerebral thrombosis due to polycythaemia, paradoxical emboli (from deep vein thrombus and bacterial endocarditis).

The treatment is surgical, which could be a total correction or initial palliative treatment, followed by total correction at a later date. Palliative treatment includes anastomatic procedures, anastomosis of subclavian to right pulmonary or pulmonary artery and descending aorta (Blalock's operation). Operation is usually rewarding, though there are some post-operative complications.

## DOUBLE OUTLET RIGHT VENTRICLE

In this condition, the aorta and pulmonary artery arise from the right ventricle. There is a ventricular septal defect through which the blood from the right ventricle goes into the left ventricle. Double outlet right ventricle (DORV) can be complicated by pulmonary stenosis. Subpulmonic ventricular septal defect with pulmonary stenosis. In addition, there may be transposition of the great arteries as well.

The history and the physical signs are more or less similar to those of tetralogy of Fallot. The echocardiography can differentiate these two conditions while angiocardiographic examination finally determines the nature of the congenital defects.

The prognosis, unless operated upon, is unfavourable.

The treatment is surgical correction, creating an intraventricular channel so that the left ventricle ejects blood through ventricular septal defect into the aorta. The pulmonary obstruction is relieved by either creating a valve conduit or just pulmonary valvotomy.

## PULMONARY ATRESIA

This condition is an extreme form of tetralogy of fallot. In this condition the cyanosis appears earlier than tetralogy of fallot. Symptoms are severe in early infancy. Cardiac failure occurs early. Cardiac enlargement is usual. Second sound is single. Right ventricular hypertrophy is noted.

Treatment is pulmonary valve operation, relief of the outflow tract obstruction by patch graft of various types are indicated.

## EISENMENGER SYNDROME

In this condition, the blood flow in patients suffering from atrial septal defect, ventricular septal defect, patent ductus arteriosus is reversed. Instead of the flow from left to right, it becomes from right to left. In patients with atrial septal defect, ventricular septal defect, or patent ductus arteriosus, there is increased blood flow into the pulmonary arterioles which causes pulmonary hypertension due to increased vascular resistance; therefore right ventricular pressure becomes higher than the left causing reversal of the shunt.

Symptoms are dyspnoea, fatigue and failure to thrive and recurrent pneumonia, cyanosis becomes obvious and is quite increasing in severity. Associated features are clubbing and polycythemia. In addition, the physical signs of the underlying disease, atrial septal defect, ventricular septal defect and patent ductus arteriosus are present.

Jugular venous pressure is increased when there is added congestive heart failure or tricuspid insufficiency. Heart size is variable. It could be normal in some cases in ventricular septal defect, but usually enlarged in atrial septal defect and patent ductus arteriosus.

*The X-ray* confirms previous findings in addition, the pulmonary arteries are seen to be significantly enlarged at the hilar areas and.they become diminished in their diameter in their peripheral branches.

*The electrocardiogram* shows definite right ventricular hypertrophy and strain pattern. The echocardiography shows right ventricular hypertrophy in addition to chamber dilatation and the presence of underlying lesion.

*Cardiac catheterization* shows redirectional shunt at the site of the defect.

Treatment in this condition is usually medical, once pulmonary hypertension and pulmonary vascular resistance has developed. Surgery is contraindicated.

## TRICUSPID ATRESIA

In this condition, the tricuspid valve is not developed. There may be a small dimple at the site of the anatomical tricuspid orifice. Sometimes only a small membrane is present, but there is no communication between the atrium and the right ventricle.

This condition could be associated with transposition or without transposition. Each again could be further sub-classified with having decreased pulmonary flow — (1) Pulmonary atresia and (2) Pulmonary stenosis, or with increased pulmonary flow.

The anatomical configuration of the right atrium is larger and sometimes hypertrophied and the right ventricle may be sometimes rudimentary. There is an atrial septal defect, as well as a small ventricular septal defect in most of the cases, the pulmonary valve may be stenosed or may be atresic.

There may be other associated cardiac abnormalities with tricuspid atresia usually, left superior vena cava entering the coronary sinus, abnormal bands in the left atrium, partial anomalous pulmonary venous drainage, subaortic stenosis or coarctation, etc.

*Clinical manifestations* — Shortness of breath develops early. After infancy, clubbing is a common finding in addition to fatiguability.

The heart may or may not be enlarged. Left ventricle is usually hypertrophied with apical heaving impulse present. There is a systolic ejection murmur audible best at the left sternal border. Second sound being single due to the absence of the pulmonary component.

*X-ray chest* shows heart is usually normal sized. Cardiac contour is variable, sometimes formed by the right ventricle, sometimes by the left ventricle. The right border of the heart is straight or rounded by the enlarged right atrium. Anterior border of the heart may be normal. The X-ray pictures are very much like that of Tetralogy of Fallot.

*Electrocardiogram* is highly diagnostic. There is left axis deviation, left ventricular hypertrophy and with an abnormal, tall, spiked P waves.

*Echocardiogram* is interesting, it shows increased echo refractability in an area which is usually occupied by the tricuspid valve. Certainly, there is no valve demonstrated. The right ventricle is small. Pulmonary artery may be atrophic or may have pulmonary stenosis. It may or may not have any transposition.

*Cardiac catheterization* may also document immediate visualization of the left atrium from the right atrium and followed by left ventricular filling into the aorta. There is complete absence of the dye into the right ventricle.

The prognosis is usually poor. Many infants die within the first few months of life.

Surgical treatment : Fontan operation is advised at the age between eighteen months to five years of age.

## TRANSPOSITION OF THE TWO GREAT ARTERIES

This condition accounts for the majority of deaths of infants under the age of one year with cyanotic congenital heart disease. Occurs predominantly in males and a significant number of patients have a family history of diabetes mellitus.

In this condition, the aorta arises from the right ventricle and pulmonary artery arises from the left ventricle. Hence the aorta carries the venous blood to the systemic circulation and the pulmonary artery carries blood back to the lungs, hence the life is impossible if there is no communication through atrial septal defect or ventricular septal defect or patent ductus arteriosus. In the majority, ventricular septal defect is the path of communications between the two chambers.

Transposition of great arteries may have the following associations :

(1) With A.S.D.

(2) With V.S.D.

(3) With large PDA

(4) With Pulmonary stenosis

(5) With tricuspid atresia

Clinical manifestations are predominantly cyanosis, congestive heart failure, and retardation of the growth. Cyanosis seems to appear within ten days of life and become progressively worse. Congestive heart failure is inevitable before six months.

In the way of physical signs, significant cardiomegaly with hyperactive precordium, right ventricular thrust is usual, and first heart sound is sharp. Second heart sound is single, or could be narrowly split. Radiology is very characteristic in transposition of the great arteries. Cardiomegaly, increased pulmonary vasculature and a narrow cardiac base due to super imposition of the two arteries in postero-anterior view, may be noted.

*The electrocardiogram* particularly shows right axis deviation, right ventricular hypertrophy, and frequently P pulmonale. There may also be biventricular hypertrophy or dominance of the left ventricle.

*The echocardiographic* pictures are also very characteristic. In the short axis view of two dimensional echocardiography, the normal anatomic configuration of the pulmonary artery and the aorta is changed, hence the typical circle and "sausage" is changed into double circles. The aorta may be situated on the right or posterior pulmonary artery vessels may not be side by side, the aorta may even be anterior to the left of the pulmonary artery. This depends upon whether it is levotransposition or dextrotransposition.

Through two dimensional view, the exit of the great vessels can be imaged through the long axis parasternal and apical four chamber views. Bifurcation of the pulmonary artery should be always be determined in order to identify properly the pulmonary artery distinct from the aorta. In the early neonates, when the great suspicion for transposition of the great arteries is there, an echocardiography is a must. It will also show the presence of VSD or ASD or PDA.

Prognosis of this condition is fatal unless treated by surgery. Urgent balloon atrial septostomy should be done in order to establish a mixture of venous and arterial blood.

## EBSTEIN'S DISEASE

In this condition, there is a downward displacement of the tricuspid valve into the right ventricle. The tricuspid valve, consists of three leaflets, has abnormal anterior leaflet which retains its attachment with the annulus, where as the septal leaflet and the posterior leaflet were inserted into the wall of the right ventricle. The anterior leaflet is very large and may be incompetent. *The right atrium is huge, while the right ventricle is relatively small* and hence inadequate in expelling the blood into the lungs.

**Symptomatology :** The majority of the patients are asymptomatic or the symptoms are very mild complaining of fatigue or some form of cardiac arrhythmias are the first presenting complaint. This may take paroxysmal tachycardia, usually supraventricular type.

Rarely, depending upon the presence of foramen ovale, there may be right to left shunt with consequent cyanosis.

On examination, usually the venous pressure is normal. Carotid pulsations are normally felt. Heart is quiet. Apex beat can be located outside the midclavicular line. There is systolic murmur present over the anterior chest. Diastolic murmur may also be heard. Sometimes there is a tricuspid opening snap or even a series of systolic ejection clicks are heard. Pansystolic murmur of tricuspid incompetence can also be recorded. Sometimes, in the presence of right bundle branch block, one may hear three distinct components of the first sound.

Second sound is usually single composed of $A_2$. Sometimes splitting of the second sound can be also present depending upon the conduction defect, such as right bundle branch block, which may cause wide splitting.

Third heart sound, right ventricular type is usually present following the $P_2$. It may be rather high in pitch resembling an opening snap. Fourth sound is occasionally present. Sometimes diastolic tricuspid murmur following the third heart sound may be heard indicating that it has right ventricular filling.

**Electrocardiogram** shows right bundle branch block, tall P waves, prolonged PR interval, sometimes the pattern of Wolff Parkinson White Syndrome is present.

**X-ray chest** shows cardiomegaly, may be from mild to massive and the pulmonary circulation is usually decreased or it could be normal. Aorta is small.

**Echocardiography** is very characteristic and almost diagnostic and particularly two dimensional echo shows the atrial portion of the right ventricle and unusual position of the tricuspid valve.

**Cardiac catheterization** is hardly necessary and treatment is usually symptomatic: Occasionally, surgical interference may be indicated, which means some form of tricuspid annularplasty and closure of the atrial septal defect.

## TRUNCUS ARTERIOSUS

**Definition :** In this condition, there is only one large anterior trunk, which leaves ventricular portion of the heart and then divides to supply the systemic circulation, pulmonary circulation and the coronary circulation. The large majority of the cases, there is ventricular septal defect. As expected, it is a large artery which has four semilunar valves. Though the semilunar valves may vary from two to six. Truncus arteriosus should be differentiated from pseudo-truncus and from truncus solitarious pulmonaries. In both these conditions, both the aortic and pulmonary trunk emerges from the heart, however, in the former there is pulmonary atresia while in the latter there is aortic atresia.

Associated cardiac abnormalities : truncus arteriosus communis could be associated with a fair number of other cardiac anomalies. They are persistant left superior vena cava, anomalous origin of left vertebral from aortic arch, origin of right subclavian from descending aorta, total anomalous pulmonary venous return, common atrio-ventricular orifice, dextrocardia, mesocardia tricuspid atresia, etc.

**Clinical manifestation —** Dyspnoea and fatigue are the most common symptoms. Cyanosis is however minimal. The patient may present with heart failure. On examination, the heart usually appears to be enlarged. Precordium is hyperdynamic and there is a systolic ejection murmur present at the left sternal border. The murmur is preceded with a *loud ejection click.* Second sound is loud and is always single and appears very superficial. A mild diastolic apical rumbling murmur may also be heard.

**Electrocardiogram** shows there may be right, left or combined hypertrophy.

**X-ray chest** shows cardiac enlargement, prominence of both ventricles and the truncus sometimes produce shadow, which follows the normal course of the ascending aorta and the aortic knob. Associated right aortic arch in 50% of the patients. Pulmonary vascularity is increased in Type I and Type II cases and decreased in the remaining two types.

**Echocardiography** shows the presence of ventricular septal defect, right ventricle independantly overriding of the large trunk, multiple cusps of the truncus could be seen in the short axis view. Mitral aortic continuity is maintained. No pulmonary valve could be seen, sometimes it is difficult to differentiate from pulmonary atresia with ventricular septal defect and severe tetralogy of fallot.

The prognosis is usually bad. The majority of the patients die during the first two years of life.

The treatment is surgical. Initially some surgeons prefer banding of the pulmonary arteries in order to reduce the pulmonary inflow in Type I and Type II cases and later on, radical corrective surgery could be done, which consists of the closure of the ventricular septal defect and the pulmonary arteries are amputated from the truncus and continuities are established between the right ventricle and pulmonary arteries with a valve conduit.

### Single Ventricle

In this condition, the right and left atrium, by means of separate interventricular valves or with common atrio-ventricular valves empty into a single chamber from which the two main arteries, aorta and pulmonary artery arise. This condition could be associated with transposition of great arteries, dextrocardia and pulmonary stenosis.

Presenting feature is usually shortness of breath and fatigue. Clinical examination shows polycythemia and cyanosis. There may be a left ventricular heave, may have a systolic thrill. A systolic ejection murmur is usually loud and the ejection click is heard. Second sound is single and loud.

**Echocardiography** is very characteristic. It shows the two separate atrio-ventricular valves, but there is no interventricular septum. This can be seen very clearly in the four chamber apical view, or in the subcostal four chamber view.

Treatment is essentially surgical and carries a high mortality.

## CONGENITAL MITRAL STENOSIS

This is relatively a rare condition. It may be an isolated condition or it may be associated with lesions such as PDA, aortic stenosis, and coarctation, of the aorta.

Anatomical defect here is the presence of a funnel-shaped mitral valve.

Symptoms usually appear earlier and is characterised by shortness of breath during exertion. There may be some lack of growth and frequent attacks of cough and cold and some children may have obvious episodes of pulmonary edema and congestive heart failure.

The heart is usually enlarged and there may be a diastolic thrill, loud first sound, rumbling diastolic murmur and an opening snap along with typical. Second sound is usually split with normal physiological variations.

**Electrocardiogram** shows right ventricle hypertrophy with bifid P waves characteristic of left atrial enlargement.

**X-ray** shows characteristic left atrial enlargement. Right ventricular enlargement and pulmonary congestion.

**Echocardiography** is very characteristic. It signifies reduction of the mitral valve surface area in the two dimensional echo and associated left atrial enlargement and small left ventricle, right ventricular enlargement.

Prognosis is usually poor. The majority of the children die in the first two years of life. Surgical treament is only advisable, but the mortality rate is higher than average.

**Congenital Mitral Insufficiency**

This condition could be isolated phenomenon or associated with PDA, coarctation of the aorta, ventricular septal defect, or corrected transposition of the great vessels, endocardial fibroelastosis. Mitral incompetence is the integral part of the endocardial cushion defects.

The essential feature is deformed mitral valve. The leaflets are thickened. The attached cords are also deformed, they may be short and may insert in improper places in the cordi. There may be endocardial fibrosis of varying degree present.

The left atrium enlarges significantly. Left ventricle is also hypertrophied and dilated. The pulmonary venous pressure is increased. Finally in late cases, right ventricle and right atrium are enlarged.

**Electrocardiogram** shows left axis deviation. Counterclock wise inscription of the QRS complex, biventricular hypertrophy and normal or spiky P waves.

## ACYANOTIC CONGENITAL HEART DISEASE

Dominant left to right shunt. 1) Ventricular Septal Defect 2) Atrial Septal Defect 3) Patent Ductus Arteriosus 4) Aortico-Pulmonary Septal Defect 5) Ruptured Sinus of Valsalva 6) Fistula of a Coronary Artery.

## VENTRICULAR SEPTAL DEFECT

Defect in the ventricular septa may present as an isolated phenomenon or isolated malformation or it may be associated with a variety of other congenital disorders, e.g. Tetralogy of Fallot, endomyocardial cushion defect, tricuspid atresia, etc.

According to the situation of ventricular septal defect, it can be classified into 1) Perimembranous, type when membranous portion of the septum is defective; 2) Supracristal type, when the defect is situated in the outflow tract of the right ventricle; 3) Muscular type, when central or muscular part of interventricular septum was involved; 4) Ventricular septal defect of the common atrio-ventricular canal type, when it is part of the complete endocardial cushion defect.

**Hemodynamics :** Blood from the left ventricle is shunted into the right ventricle and is then thrown into the pulmonary circulation, which is engorged and then returned to the left artium and left ventricle which is again shunted back to the right ventricle. Hence, there is significant enlargement of the left atrium, left ventricle and right ventricle. The pulmonary arteries are dilated in this condition. As time progresses, there is increasing resistance in the pulmonary circulation causing pulmonary hypertension and as a result of which, the shunt becomes less and less and finally there may be reversal of the shunt from right to left, the condition called Eisenmenger's Syndrome. Clinical manifestations are largely depending upon the size of the defect and the reaction of the pulmonary circulation. If the defect is very small, the majority of the children are asymptomatic. Where the defect is large, it may present with heart failure even at a very early stage of their life. Shortness of breath is a common symptom. Fatiguability and failure to thrive are the two symptoms for which the child presents to the pediatrician.

General condition is usually satisfactory except that they probably have increased respiration rate than average and there is a systolic thrill best heard at the second and third intercostal spaces. Pansystolic murmur heard loudest at the left lower sternal area. Second sound is normal. It is moderately split with increase in the pulmonary blood flow, there may be an ejection type systolic murmur at the left upper sternal area. There may be a rumbling mid-diastolic murmur heard best at the apex due to increase flow across the mitral valve.

**X-ray :** In the early stage heart size may be absolutely normal with moderate degree of shunt, there may be cardiomegaly, increased pulmonary vascular congestion and left atrial enlargement or combined ventricular hypertrophy.

Most cases can be diagnosed correctly with an echocardiography, particularly the two dimensional views which determine the site of the defect and the extent of the defect and with added Doppler tracings, the actual flow velocity and calculation therefore of the shunt is possible. The two-dimensional echocardiography, particularly the four chamber apical view, would detect the presence of any membranous type of ventricular septal defect, below aortic valve. The muscular defects are not very easy to diagnose, particularly if they are multiple, however, with some degree of reservations, it is possible to detect the large muscular type of ventricular septal defect.

**Angiogram** does show the actual shunting of the dye from the left ventricle to the right ventricle. Pressure studies would also indicate increase in the pressure and oxygen saturation in the right ventricle as well as pulmonary arteries.

The natural history of the ventricular septal defect indicates that a large majority of small defects are closed spontaneously. Unless the defect is large, all patients should have periodic check up through echocardiography examination. In addition, complications e.g. infected endocarditis, recurrent pneumonia, congestive heart failure and pulmonary hypertension need regular watch.

**Treatment** is usually surgical and includes if it is isolated phenomenon, closure of the ventricular septal defect. It is associated with other congenital malformations, the surgical treatment would be directed accordingly to the presence of those defects. Once the right to left shunt is established, surgical treatment is naturally contraindicated. Sometimes the repair of the ventricular septal defect is done in two stages, initially by pulmonary artery banding in the early infancy and later by proper closure of the ventricular septal defect. This again depends upon the different surgeons and different centres.

## ATRIAL SEPTAL DEFECT

In intrauterine life, the foramen ovale is the normal channel of communication as there is no pulmonary circulation for oxygenation of blood.

Foramen ovale normally closes after birth but some cases the communication persists, which is called atrial septal defect (A.S.D.). A.S.D. according to its site, can be classified into the following types :

(1) Fossa ovalis type, where the persistance of the defect at the fossa ovalis level.

(2) The atrial septal defect of the secondum in which the defect is near the region of fossa ovalis. Sometimes the defect could be multiple small openings, and sometimes usually there is one single large opening seen.

(3) The third type is sinus venosus defect, which is situated near the opening of the superior vena cava and is usually associated with partial anomalous pulmonary venous return.

(4) The fourth type is the septum primum defect, which is a part of the endocardial cushion defect in which the atrial septum defect is associated with a cleft mitral valve, with or without abnormal tricuspid valve. The defect in the atrial septum is at lower portion of the atrial septum adjacent to the atrio-ventricular valves.

**Hemodynamics :** Here the blood from the left atrium is shunted to the right atrium, which also accommodates the usual venous return. Hence larger volume of blood flows into the right ventricle and into the lungs. Lungs are congested and returned the blood to the left atrium and then again shunted quickly into the right atrium. As a result the pulmonary vascular resistance increases with increased pulmonary arterial pressure and subsequently right ventricular pressure, leading to pulmonary hypertension. Sometimes the shunt may be reversed causing central cyanosis (Eisenmenger Syndrome).

**Clinical manifestations** are alike in all these four types of the condition and the large majority of the children are asymptomatic, though some amount of exertional intolerance has been common.

Recurrent attacks of chest infection and pneumonitis is also common.

**Physical signs :** The pulse is usually normal. Venous pressure is normal. The heart is usually enlarged, with right ventricular preponderance. There is a systolic murmur which is of ejection type and is usually best heard at the pulmonary area and is produced by the torrential flow in the pulmonary artery. There may be an ejection sound following the loud first sound present due to the same reasons. The second sound however, is split widely and is fixed, that means it does not vary during inspiration and expiration. This auscultatory findings are really very characteristic of this condition. Sometimes a mid-diastolic murmur can be heard due to the torrential flow across the tricuspid valve and could be heard at the apex.

**Electrocardiogram** shows evidence of right ventricular diastolic volume overload, and they consist of right axis deviation, right ventricular hypertrophy with rsR' pattern in E.C.G. There may be tall P waves or sometimes normal P waves, PR interval may be prolonged. These may be associated other cardiac arrhythmias like atrial fibrillation and heart block and occasionally Wolff Parkinson White Syndrome.

The **echocardiographic** examination is very characteristic and in the large majority of the patients a diagnosis can be reached with echocardiography. Cardiac catheterization is usually not required, unless other associated congenital lesions are suspected.

The echocardiographic findings consisting of right ventricular volume overload, paradoxical interventricular septal motion, relatively smaller sized left ventricle and normal left atrial size. In two dimensional echocardiography examination the actual site of the defect can be established.

**Cardiac catheterization** will indicate increased oxygenation at the level of the right atrium. Right atrial, right ventricular, pulmonary arterial pressure elevation will be noted. Angiogram will also show the shunting of the dye at the level of the atrium.

**Complications** — Cardiac arrhythmias are not uncommon in this condition. Atrial fibrillation is the commonest cardiac arrhythmias seen, though Wolff Parkinson White Syndrome and heart block have been reported.

**Treatment** — In the Western World all patients with atrial septal defect, whether they are asymptomatic or symptomatic, undergo surgical repair operation because the mortality rate is almost nil.

## ENDOCARDIAL CUSHION DEFECT

(Common atrio-ventricular canal, and osteum primum defect)

In this condition, lack of fusion of embryonic endocardial cushion tissue leads to a variety of anatomic defects involving atrio-ventricular valves and the cardiac septum.

**Clinical manifestations :** Symptomatology are the same as in atrial septal defect. Physical findings are however diverse because of the associated presence of mitral incompetence from cleft mitral leaflet.

In this condition, as expected, the left ventricle is also enlarged along with left atrial enlargement, which is not present in atrial septal defect of the secundum type.

**Radiology** confirms cardiac enlargement of both the ventricles and right atrium. Pulmonary arteries are also large, and the pulmonary vascularity is increased.

**Electrocardiogram** is highly characteristic. This shows left axis deviation, counterclockwise inscription of the superiorly orientated QRS vector loop, biventricular hypertrophy, prolonged PR interval and tall P waves.

**Echocardiographic** examination shows the presence of atrial septal defect along with right ventricular volume overload, left ventricular enlargement, left atrial enlargement and defective anterior leaflet of mitral valve.

**Treatment** is corrective surgery with artificial heart lung machine and closure of the defect as well as the cleft of the mitral valve is repaired.

Endocardial cushion defect in its complete form, consists of a large central defect involving the lower portion of the atrial septum and upper portion of the ventricular septum. Instead of separate mitral and tricuspid valves, the large common anterior leaflet bridges the atrio-ventricular canal defect. The morphology and the attachment of this common anterior leaflet forms the basis of the Rastelli's classification.

**Hemodynamics :** There is a significant shunt from the left to the right both at atrial and as well as the ventricular level. Pulmonary congestion is increased resulting in earlier appearance of pulmonary hypertension.

This condition is usually symptomatic. The majority of the children show fatiguability, recurrent pulmonary congestion and infection, and shortness of breath. Some with obvious heart failure.

J.V.P. is increased, cardiac enlargement is moderate to massive. Systolic thrill is frequently palpable at the third intercostal space due to ventricular septal defect. First sound is normal. There is a harsh systolic murmur heard best at the third intercostal space. Second sound is widely split with increased pulmonary valve closure sound. Low frequency mid-diastolic murmur is also heard at the left parasternal edge.

**X-ray** shows significant cardiac enlargement with both ventricular enlargement, right atrial enlargement as well as severe pulmonary congestion. Selective right ventricular angiography is extremely helpful in diagnosis of endocardial cushion defects, deformity of the mitral or the common atrio-ventricular valve and the distortion of the outflow tract of the left ventricle, the so-called goose neck deformity can be well demonstrated in the large majority of the patients. They have cleft leaflet of the mitral valve and mitral incompetence also is demonstrated easily in the cin angiography.

Prognosis of this case depending upon the magnitude of the shunt and the degree of pulmonary vascular resistance and usually it involves surgery of an extensive nature and the mortality is higher than simple repair of the atrial septal defect. Pulmonary arterial banding can be done in the earlier stages and at later phase, complete correction of this defect is possible. According to Rastelli classification there are three types. Rastelli type A is the most common type, where there is a septal defect with cleft in the mitral or tricuspid valves but anchoring of either mitral or tricuspid or both to the crest of the ventricular septum on the ipsi-lateral side.

Rastelli type B where the chordal attachments from medial portions of the cleft mitral valve is related to the papillary muscle on the right side of the septum crossing the ventricular septal defect, requiring mitral valve replacement operation.

Rastelli type C in which it is a floater, free floater anterior leaflet without having any attachment to the chords. This condition is not amendable to surgery. The leaflets are anchored to the right or left ventricle respectively.

## PATENT DUCTUS ARTERIOSUS

During foetal life the ductus arteriosus conveys blood from pulmonary artery into the aorta and it closes soon after birth as soon as pulmonary circuit is opened up. If the ductus remains patent, the blood from the high pressure areas, aortic blood is shunted into the pulmonary artery. This is a common congenital cardiac defect, which may occur as an isolated anomaly or it could be associated with other congenital disorders.

**Hemodynamics :** Here the blood flows from the aorta into the pulmonary artery and hence the left ventricular output is reduced depending upon the magnitude of the shunt. Consequently the pulmonary blood flow is increased.

**Clinical manifestation :** Majority of the children having patent ductus arteriosus are symptomless. However if the ductus is large, the shunt is significant, so the patients develop signs and symptoms of left ventricular failure namely, shortness of breath during exertion, paroxysmal nocturnal dyspnoea, and finally left heart failure with pulmonary oedema. Retardation of the growth could occur as well.

**Physical signs :** Pulse is of the water hammer characteristic, the low diastolic pressure with increased pulse pressure is noted, jugular venous pressures is not increased, apical pulse is of the left ventricular type with some cardiac enlargement, a thrill may be present in the left second intercostal space. Classically the murmur has been described as machinery, humming top, rolling thunder in quality. It characteristically begins soon after the first sound reaches its maximum intensity at the end of the systole and wanes in late diastole. Second heart sound, when heard, may be normal splitting with A2 and P2 being equal.

**The electrocardiogram** may be normal or show left ventricular hypertrophy depending on the left ventricular volume overload.

**X-ray** chest shows significant pulmonary vascular markings with dominant pulmonary arteries. Cardiac size is usually enlarged with left ventricular preponderance. The left atrium is also enlarged. The aortic knob is usually normal, or sometimes prominent.

**Echocardiographic** examination is also characteristic and it shows the presence of left atrial enlargement, left ventricular enlargement and the ductus can be demonstrated in the large majority of the cases by means of two dimensional echo studies. Recent Doppler technique not only confirms the diagnosis but measures the flow calculating the amount of shunt.

**Cardiac catheterization** is usually unnecessary.

**Treatment** is surgical closure of the ductus.

## AORTICO-PULMONARY SEPTAL DEFECT

This defect consisting of a hole between the ascending aorta and the main pulmonary artery. Here there is no abnormality in the aortic valve, pulmonary valve, ventricular septum, or interatrial septum.

Symptoms resembles a large ventricular septal defect.

The *clinical manifestations* are similar as in patent ductus arteriosus. ECG and X-rays, are almost similar to patent ductus arteriosus. Cardiac catheterization and selective aortography with the injection of contrast medium into the ascending aorta would document the site of the lesion.

**Treatment** is surgical correction.

## FISTULA OF THE CORONARY ARTERY

Fistula of the coronary artery exists between the coronary artery and the vein or the coronary artery may directly empty into the right ventricle. The physical signs may closely simulate patent ductus arteriosus as the machinery murmur is also common. The anatomic abnormality can only be demonstrated by injection of the contrast material into the ascending aorta. The treatment consists of surgical repair of the fistula.

## RUPTURE OF THE SINUS VALSALVA

When one of the sinus of the valsalva of the aorta is weakened either due to congenital aneurysm or rupture and they open into the right atrium or the right ventricle. The clinical manifestations closely simulate that of the patent ductus arteriosus, except the machinery murmur which is heard so characteristically at the left upper intercostal space more on the right side. Cardiac catheterization may be indicated and aortography with injection of a contrast material into the ascending aorta determines the site of the aneurysm and rupture.

Surgical correction again is essential.

## PULMONARY STENOSIS

Pulmonary stenosis may present as an isolated anomaly or it may be associated with other congenital diseases. Hence the classification of the pulmonary stenosis is simple unless complicated with other diseases. Pulmonary stenosis can be valvular type when the stenosis of the valvular level or the infundibular type when the stenosis is at the infundibular level. But sometimes it can be valvular and infundibular.

Pulmonary stenosis could be associated with patent ductus arteriosus, ventricular septal defect, or atrial septal defect. Pulmonary stenosis could also be associated with other rare diseases like tricuspid atresia, transposition of the great arteries, etc.

**Hemodynamics :** Because the pulmonary valves are stenosed, either at the valvular level or at the infundibular level, the pressure in the right ventricle is increased. Subsequently, the right ventricle undergoes hypertrophy as a consequence of the increased pressure. Pulmonary artery pressure however is low. Arterial oxygen saturation remains normal.

**Clinical Features :** Usually with a mild form of the disease, there are no symptoms. According to the pressure in the right ventricle, the pulmonary stenosis is classified into three types; when the pressure is less than 50 mm, it is called mild, between 50 to 100 mm, it is called moderate; and above 100 mm, it is called severe.

The symptoms depend upon the severity of the lesion and usually manifestation is shortness of breath during exertion. Occasionally there is chest pain, which is substernal and sometimes the patient may have syncopal attacks.

General development is normal. With a mild degree of pulmonary stenosis, the blood pressure and pulse is normal and the only abnormal finding is a loud pulmonary systolic ejection murmur at the left second intercostal space. The heart size is normal.

**Electrocardiogram** may be normal or show very early right ventricular strain pattern. In moderate group the symptoms are slightly increased and there is definite electrocardiographic abnormalities present in the form of right ventricle hypertrophy. Here there is not only rough ejection systolic murmur heard at the pulmonary area, but it may be accompanied with a thrill and the second sound is split with reduced intensity of the pulmonary component. Radiology of chest shows some abnormality, right ventricular hypertrophy and post-stenotic dilatation of the pulmonary artery, if the lesion is of the valvular type.

**Echocardiography** will show characteristically the dome pulmonary valve which moves during systole and diastole. Similarly echocardiography can demonstrate the infundibular lesion as well. With the recent Doppler technique the severity of stenosis can be determined by analysing the doppler flow, and gradients can be measured.

In a severe grade of pulmonary stenosis the patient may have cyanosis due to the reduced cardiac output, the venous pressure may be elevated with increased A wave. The right ventricular lift may be palpable. Systolic murmur and thrill is well evident in the pulmonary area. The second sound is split with delay and diminished pulmonary component.

The *electrocardiogram* definitely reveals significant right ventricular hypertrophy associated with tall P waves.

Radiology shows decreased pulmonary vascularity, in addition to right ventricular hypertrophy. Cardiac size is moderately enlarged. Cardiac catheterization may be indicated and selective right ventriculography also clearly documents the nature of the obstruction and contrast may also be necessary in order exclude the possibility of any shunt.

### Course and Prognosis

The natural course of the disease is usually very slow and the majority of the patients with a mild or moderate disease can lead a normal life and the prognosis in these cases are usually good. In severe cases, symptoms come early. Progressive shortness of breath and fatiguability are the main symptoms. Treatment is surgical depending upon the nature of the lesion, either pulmonary valvotomy or pulmonary valvular plasty is indicated.

## PULMONARY VALVULAR INSUFFICIENCY

The patients are usually asymptomatic and the physical findings are similar to aortic insufficiency, only the carotid pulse and the aortic pulse do not show the characteristic water-hammer type of the aortic incompetence. The first sound and seconds are normal followed by low pitched early diastolic murmur, which increases intensity during inspiration.

**Radiology of** chest shows prominent main pulmonary artery. Electrocardiogram is normal. In severe cases E.C.G. may show right ventricular hypertrophy.

**Echocardiography** does shows abnormality of the pulmonary valve, but with the Doppler studies, pulmonary incompetence can be well demonstrated.

Absence of the pulmonary valve is usually associated with other defects like tetralogy of Fallot and ventricular septal defect.

The pulmonary arteries are widely dilated here. The condition is usually fatal in infancy.

Recently valve conduit is given in this type of patients and after correcting the ventricular septal defect and ventricular stenosis.

## COARCTATION OF THE AORTA

This condition is characterised by constriction of varying length in the aorta. The majority of them occur just below the origin of the left subclavian artery, though it can occur in any part from the arch down to the bifurcation of the aorta. Males are more affected than females. Turner Syndrome (XO) has frequent occurrence of coarctation of the aorta.

**Hemodynamics :** Because of obstruction in the passage of blood through the aorta at the level of origin of the subclavian artery, the extensive collateral circulation develops which does maintain blood flow from branches of the subclavian to the intercostal and internal mammary arteries by passing the constricted portion of the aorta.

**Clinical Feature :** The symptoms are that of either hypertension, which is accidently noted or the presence of a murmur or sometimes epistaxis. Throbbing headache, occasionally left ventricular failure, congestive heart failure or cerebral hemorrhage can occur. Intermittent claudication is not rare.

Classical sign of coarctation is the disparity of pulsations and the blood pressure between the arms and the legs. Pulsations of femoral, popliteal and dorsalis pedis arteries are all weak and delayed and the brachial and radial arterial pulsations are pounding and can be easily felt.

The blood pressure in the legs are lower than the blood pressure in the arms. There may be left ventricular heave with slight degre of left ventricular enlargement. Murmurs systolic ejection type best heard at the base of the heart radiates down to the sternum to the apex and interscapular area and frequently loudest at the back. Second sound is usually normal. There may be an early diastolic murmur due to the presence of congenital aortic insufficiency from bicuspid aortic valve.

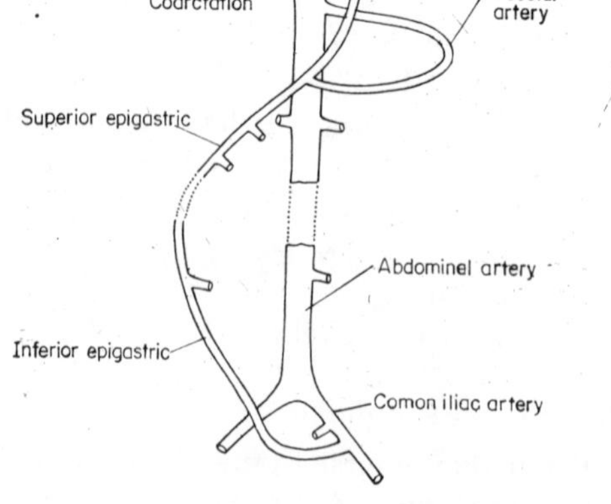


Fig.18.31 : Coarctation of the aorta showing collateral circulation.

**X-ray** chest shows left ventricular hypertrophy, notching of the inferior border of the ribs from pressure erosion by enlarged collateral vessels. There may be poststenotic dilatation of the descending aorta.

Associated anomalies of which most common is the presence of bicuspid aortic valve, which could be stenotic or incompetent. The next common association is Patent Ductus Arteriosus, Ventricular Septal and Atrial Septal Defect.

**Complications :** Usually subarachnoid hemorrhage and intracerebral haemorrhage result from rupture of congenital aneurysms, the circle of Willis. Abnormalities of the subclavian arteries may be present, such as stenosis of the orifice of the subclavian artery.

The natural history of the disease is that the majority of the patients die below the age of 40 because of complications.

**Treatment :** Is essentially surgical consisting of removal of the coarctated portions of the aorta with either primary anastomosis or if the length of the aortic constriction is large enough not to have a primary anastomosis possible, then Dacron grafts may be used instead. The operations are highly successful. Post operative complications are rare.

## ANOMALOUS PULMONARY VENOUS RETURN

In this condition, the pulmonary vein instead of opening into the left atrium, opens into the systemic veins completely or partially.

In partial anomalous venous return, usually the veins of one lung, most frequently the right, opens into the systemic venous system. Usually there is atrial septal defect of the sinus vensous type.

The history and physical signs and electrocardiogram, X-ray findings are distinguishable from those of atrial septal defect of the secondum thpe.

During cardiac catheterization, the catheter may enter one of the anomalous pulmonary vein which can be demonstrated by selective pulmonary arteriography.

Treatment is surgical, in which the pulmonary veins are joined with left atrium and closure of the atrial septal defect is done.

In total anomalous pulmonary venous return, all the pulmonary veins enter into the systemic circulation. Usually the pulmonary veins form a single trunk before entering into the systemic venous circulation at one of the following sites : (1) left superior vena cava, (2) coronary sinus, (3) right atrium. (4) right superior vena cava; in that order. The remaining part enters the portal vein or the ductus venosus.

**Clinical manifestations :** The majority of the infants develop symptoms before the end of two year with poor weight gain, cyanosis, congestive heart failure.

Signs are that of bulging of the left side of the chest. Heart is enlarged, there is gallop rhythm, and systolic murmur at the left sternal border, which may be followed by a diastolic murmur. Occasionally clinical signs of pulmonary edema can also be documented.

**Electrocardiogram** is that of right ventricular hypertrophy and P waves are usually tall and spiked.

Radiology of this chest is pathognomonic of this condition, if the pulmonary veins enter the innominate vein and persistent left superior vena cava. There is a large cardiac shadow, with a figure of eight or Snowman's sign. Supra cardiac shadow is produced by the dilated left superior vena cava, left pulmonic vein and right superior vena cava.

**Echocardiography** shows the right ventricular volume overload with paradoxical interventricular septal motion. Left ventricle is usually smaller than normal. Coronary sinus can be seen to be dilated when pulmonary veins open directly to the coronary sinuses. The common channel of the pulmonary veins can be seen sometimes and associated defects like atrial septal defect, ventricular septal defect can be documented.

**Angiography** is diagnostic and establishes the nature of abnormal venous connections.

**Treatment** is surgical correction whenever possible.

## CONGESTIVE CARDIAC FAILURE

*B.K. DAS*

### Introduction

"The very essence of cardiovascular practice is recognition of early heart failure and discrimination between different grades of failure". — *Sir Thomas Lewis* (1933) —

Heart failure is a pathophysiological state in which an abnormality of cardiac function results in failure of the heart to pump and maintain adequate blood supply for the metabolic requirements of the body.

Not all patients with congestive cardiac failure have myocardial failure. Heart failure may occur because the normal heart is faced with an excessive load that exceeds compensatory mechanisms or because ventricular filling is impaired. Conversely, myocardial failure (in the early stages) may be present without overt congestive heart failure, the latter only occurs once myocardial dysfunction is far advanced and compensatory mechanisms, including chamber dilatation, vasoconstriction, and fluid retention, come into play.

### Magnitude of the problem

Congestive cardiac failure is a common ailment with a variety of causes. An estimated 3.5 to 4 million Americans have chronic congestive cardiac failure. Data from the Framingham study suggest that the incidence (i.e. the number of new cases per year) averages 3.7 per 1000 for men and 2.5 per 1000 for women. The incidence of cardiac failure more than doubles for each decade of life from 45 to 75 years.

### Pathophysiology

It is convenient to consider separately the consequences of impaired function of the left and the right sides of the heart. Left sided failure is characterised by a reduction in effective left ventricular output for a given pulmonary venous or left atrial pressure, or conversely, an increase in the left atrial pressure needed to sustain a given cardiac output. An acute increase in left atrial pressure may cause pulmonary congestion or pulmonary oedema but with more gradual increase in left atrial pressure there tends to be, reflex pulmonary vaso-constriction which protects the patient from pulmonary oedema at the cost of increasing pulmonary hypertension.

In right-sided cardiac failure there is similarly a reduction of right ventricular output for a given right atrial pressure or a need for an increased right atrial pressure to maintain a given output. The increased right atrial pressure is manifested as an increase in Jugular venous pressure and as hepatic engorgement.

In both left and right sided cardiac failure the body attempts to compensate for the drop in cardiac output by activation of the sympathetic nervous system, causing tachycardia and vasoconstriction, and retention of salt and water by the kidneys. Fluid retention is accompanied by the development of oedema, in pure left sided failure this is principally pulmonary. In right sided failure or in a combination of right and left sided failure, most of the oedema is peripheral. It affects the ankles in ambulant patients and the thighs or sacrum in bed ridden patients. Considerable quantities of peripheral oedema may accumulate without causing distress. Massive accumulation of fluid may cause ascites or pleural effusion.

**Left heart failure**

**Causes**

(1) Primary disease of the left ventricle such as myocardial infarction, cardiomyopathy and myocarditis.

(2) Systolic overload of the left ventricle from systemic hypertension, aortic stenosis and hypertrophic obstructive cardiomyopathy.

(3) Diastolic overload of left ventricle from mitral and aortic incompetence, ventricular septal defect and persistent ductus arteriosus.

(4) Restriction of the left ventricle due to localised constrictive pericarditis externally and endomyocardial fibrosis internally.

(5) Left atrial failure from mitral stenosis.

**Symptoms**

The earliest symptom is dyspnoea on effort. Eventually dyspnoea occurs at rest and the patient is distressed if he lies flat i.e. orthopnoea. Finally paroxysmal cardiac dyspnoea appears, usually nocturnal, and is commonly associated with bronchospasm i.e. cardiac asthma. It is not clear why these attacks are more common at night. Acute pulmonary oedema results in severe dyspnoea, sweating, and cough associated with copious, frothy sputum, occasionally pink. Infection is apt to occur and frequently precipitates failure. Occasionally paroxysmal cough on effort is a symptom of left heart failure. Haemoptysis may be due to pulmonary infection or congestion, but if severe a pulmonary infarct should be suspected. Profuse sweating is an early characteristic of left sided failure. The reduction in forward flow may give rise to fatigue and reduction in renal flow may produce diurnal oliguria with nocturnal diuresis.

**Signs**

The signs of left heart failure are few and chronic left ventricular failure is the commonest missed cardiac diagnosis.

(1) Left ventricular hypertrophy.

(2) Triple rhythm — If it is presystolic it is less ominous, being usually associated with systolic overload of the left ventricle. Protodiastolic triple rhythm, due to exaggeration of the third heart sound, is common in the diastolic ventricular overload of advanced heart failure and is therefore more ominous. Tachycardia is always well marked.

(3) Basal rales are present with often expiratory wheezing. In acute pulmonary oedema medium to loud bubbling rales are heard all over the lungs.

(4) Pulsus alternans (alternate large and small pulse) which usually needs a sphygmomanometer for its detection implies that the heart is labouring.

(5) Cheyne-stokes respiration — A periodic form of breathing characterised by waxing and waning of the depth of respirations and regularly recurring periods of apnoea may occur.

(6) Signs of causative disease — e.g. hypertension.

**Right heart failure**

**Causes**

(1) Systolic overload of right ventricle due to pulmonary hypertension of whatever cause. Congestive heart failure is most commonly secondary to left heart failure. The next most common cause is chronic cor pulmonale.

(2) Systolic overload of the right ventricle due to obstruction of the right ventricular cavity

given rise to pure right ventricular failure e.g. pulmonary valvular and infundibular stenosis.

(3) Diastolic overload of the right ventricle. Atrial septal defect is relatively common. But tricuspid incompetence and pulmonary incompetence are rare as causes and almost invariably secondary to other lesions.

(4) Restriction of the right ventricle—localised constrictive pericarditis on the outside of the ventricle and endomyocardial fibrosis on the inside, can both lead to right ventricular failure.

(5) Right atrial failure rarely follows tricuspid stenosis and a right atrial tumour.

**Symptoms**

These are due mainly due to congestion. Pain may be experienced over right hypochondrium, commonly aggravated on exertion — so called hepatic angina. The patient may notice that his liver is tender and his abdomen has become distended. Jaundice may appear when cirrhosis develops. Congestion of the gut results in anorexia and sometimes vomiting. Oedema is not an early or reliable sign of heart failure. It may be minimal with a high venous pressure and may be massive when the venous pressure not very high. Dyspnoea is usually present even in the absence of pulmonary congestion. The low cardiac output gives rise to fatigue, sluggish mental state and oliguria.

**Signs**

(1) Raised venous pressure is invariable and is best seen in the neck. Pressure on the liver will produce elevation of the jugular venous pressure, the hepatojugular reflex.

(2) Hepatomegaly is present and in tricuspid incompetence systolic pulsation over liver may be appreciated.

(3) Oedema : the erect position favours collection of fluid in feet, ankles, lower parts of legs, whereas recumbent position favours accumulation of fluid in sacral region. If oedema is severe it may be associated with ascites, hydrothorax and hydropericardium.

(4) Peripheral cyanosis may be due to slow peripheral circulation.

(5) Signs of right ventricular or combined ventricular enlargement are present and triple rhythm is common. Tachycardia is always present.

A right ventricular protodiastolic triple rhythm carries a more serious prognosis than atrial gallop. A murmur of tricuspid incompetence, usually functional is common too.

**Investigation of heart failure**

(1) Skiagram Chest :—The silhouette of the heart will vary with the cause of the heart diseases, prominence of upper lobe veins and hilar congestion an early sign of left ventricular failure. Opacities feed to spread in a butterfly manner from the hila. In acute pulmonary oedema with more extensive oedema diffuse mottling of lungs will be seen.

(2) ECG :—will show changes hypertrophy, infarction, strain pattern.

(3) Non-invasive methods

(a) Measurement of the systolic time interval by using simultaneous records of the ECG, Phonocardiogram and carotid tracing for evaluation of left ventricular function.

(b) Apex cardiography will demonstrate various types of triple rhythm and other abnormal features.

(c) Echocardiography besides evaluation of left ventricular function (ejection fraction) helps in diagnosis of basic problem e.g. cardiomyopathy of various types, valvular heart disease and L.V. aneurysm.

(d) Radionuclide studies — multiple gated acquisition study (MUGA) using Technetium

99 helps in seeing the anatomy and function of the heart and in particular the assessment of left ventricular function and dyskinetic movement.

**Clinical approach to management**

Three general principles apply to the treatment of heart failure :—

1) Removal of the underlying cause.
2) Removal of the precipitating cause.
3) Control of the congestive heart failure state.
4) Be sure that bronchial asthma is excluded. L.V.F. may be diagnosed by mistake when patient has bronchial asthma.

**Removal of the underlying cause.**

Every patient who presents with congestive cardiac failure should be suspected of having a treatable underlying condition until proven otherwise. Practically, this entails search for a surgically correctable structural abnormality (eg, congenital cardiac malformation, acquired valvular lesion, localised large ventricular aneurysm) or a medically treatable condition (eg. infective endocarditis, rheumatic activity and hypertension).

**Removal of the precipitating cause**

The recognition, prompt treatment and, if possible, prevention of precipitating factors that produce or exacerbate heart failure are critical to successful management of congestive cardiac failure. Common precipitating factors include :-

1) Inappropriate reduction of therapy or dietary excesses of sodium.
2) Tachy or bradyarrythmias.
3) Systemic infection.
4) Pulmonary embolism.
5) High-output states (anaemia, pregnancy, thyrotoxicosis).
6) Administration of cardiac depressant drugs (Beta-adrenergic blocking agents, verapamil, disopyramide).
7) Development of an unrelated illness (eg, renal failure, hepatic failure, prostatic obstruction).
8) Injudicious fluid administration.

**Control of congestive failure state**

(1) Increase myocardial contractility and increase cardiac output.
(2) Decrease congestion by reducing preload.
(3) Decrease after load and increase cardiac output.
(4) Decrease workload by agents which alter preload and after load.

It is more convenient however to discuss the treatment of chronic cardiac failure under three principal classes of therapeutic agents, which may be employed : digoxin, diuretics, and vasodilator drugs.

**Digoxin**

For over 200 years, the place of cardiac glycosides in the treatment of congestive heart failure is secured. Digitalis has direct action on the myocardium. It improves the contractility of a failing heart. By its action on the AV node it slows the heart rate. The other effects, e.g., lowering of venous pressure, relief of hepatic congestion and increase of urinary output are indirect effects.

While it appears that some patients with heart failure do not require digitalis when they have normal sinus rhythm, the majority do benefit by chronic digitalis therapy. In fact the majority of patients with heart failure should receive digitalis. A good response often occurs in patients with hypertensive heart disease, valvular heart disease, heart failure due to ischaemic heart disease and congenital heart disease with left to right shunt. A less satisfactory response may be noted in patients whose heart failure is due to acute myocardial infarction, chronic cor pulmonale, myocarditis, chronic constrictive pericarditis.

Digoxin should be given orally unless the clinical situation demands more rapid action. The usual oral loading dose for adults and children over 10 years of age is 1.0 mg. The usual oral maintenance dose is 0.25 mg each day, six days in a week. Smaller doses may be effective for elderly patients. When the clinical situation does not demand speed, it may be preferable to start therapy with an average maintenance daily dose. This gradual method achieves an adequate steady-state : plateau in about 6 to 7 days. The maximum speed which may be obtained by oral dose is accomplished by giving 0.5 mg followed by 0.25 to 0.5 mg every 6 to 8 hours until the average total loading dose is given. If greater speed is demanded then digoxin may be given intravenously. If no digitalis preparation has been given in last 2 to 3 weeks, an initial dose of 0.25 to 0.5 mg may be given intravenously. The action starts within 15 to 30 mins and reaches its peak in one to 5 hours.

*Digitalis toxicity*

Anorexia, nausea, vomiting, slurring of vision and all types of cardiac arrhythmias are present, but multiple ventricular premature contraction, paroxysmal atrial tachycardia with A-V block, A-V dissociation, A-V block, paroxysmal ventricular tachycardia are common.

*Treatment :* Stop the drug, correction of hypokalemia and if required give phenytoin 100 mg intravenous which can be repeated if necessary.

**Other drugs which increase myocardial contractility**

Certain sympathomimetic amines (ephedrine, dopamine, dobutamine) increase contractility and may be helpful in certain acute situations but are not recommended for long term use.

Bipyridine agents are new drugs that increase cardiac contractility and cause arterial vasodilatation. Amrinone, the first bipyridine group of drug was not clinically useful for long time due to toxicity (thrombocytopenia).

Milrinone is a very potent bipyridine derivative and has got both inotrophic and afterload reducing properties. The drug appears promising and merits further study.

*Diuretics* : Diuretics form the corner stone of management of congestive heart failure and the main effects are :

(1) Reduction in oedema both pulmonary and peripheral.
(2) Reduction in blood and plasma volume. This reduces right and left ventricular preload, lower jugular and pulmonary venous pressure.
(3) There is also reduction in left ventricular afterload as a result of peripheral arteriolar dilatation.

Commonly used diuretics have been classified in three groups :

(1) High potency loop diuretics.
(2) Medium potency thiazide diuretics.
(3) Low potency potassium sparing diuretics.

1. *Loop diuretics* – Major action is on the ascending loop of Henle. (a) Furosemide average single dose is 40 mg oral or I.V. (b) Ethacrynic acid 50 mg oral once or twice a day, (c) Bumetanide 1 mg O.D. or BD.

2. *Benzothiazine compounds :* Site of action is on the cortical diluting segment of loop of Henle

and at the beginning of distal convoluted tubule where they interfere with active reabsorption of sodium ions.

(a) Thiazide—daily dose
  (i) Hydrochlorothiazide 50 mg.
  (ii) Polythiazide 2 mg.
  (iii) Hydroflumethiazide 100 mg.
  (iv) Chlorthalidone 50 mg twice weekly.

3. *Low efficacy diuretics* — (Potassium sparing diuretics).
  (i) Aldosterone antagonists — Spironolactone useful in patients resistant with thiazide groups. Its important clinical effect is the reduction of renal excretion of potassium which it shares with low potency diuretics. It should not be given with potassium supplement. Dose — 25 mg QDS.
  (ii) Triamterene best used in combination with thiazide because it not only potentiates the sodium loosing effect of thiazide but also reduces potassium loss.

It is logical to combine diuretics from different classes if an increased action is desired, but it demands for monitoring of fluid or electrolyte imbalance.

Complications of diuretic therapy.

(1) Hypokalemia — High potency and thiazide diuretics produce potassium depletion and is particularly serious since it may be responsible for increased sensitivity to digitalis. It can precipitate hepatic coma with patients having liver disease.

*Management* : Potassium chloride in solution 1.5 g. TDS or slow release preparation (600 mg per tablet) 4-6 tablets daily. Fruit juice, bananas and salads are rich in potassium and may be enough if mild diuretics are used.

(2) Hypovolaemia may occur high potent diuretics.

(3) Hyponatraemia seen in long standing congestive cardiac failure. Serum sodium may be less than 120 mEq/L.

**Management**

To restrict diuretic therapy, limit fluid intake to one litre daily and unrestricted diet.

(4) Hyperglycemia, hyperuricemia, urinary retention in presence of prostatic obstruction are seen.

*Vasodilators* : This is an important concept in the management of congestive cardiac failure. Venodilatation reduces central venous pressure and right ventricular output and slows the accumulation of pulmonary oedema, while arteriolar dilatation improves left ventricular function by reducing the afterload against which it has to work. Isosorbide dinitrate (sorbitrate) is predominantly venodilator, hydralazine, nifedepine and salbutamol are predominantly arteriolar dilators. Prazosine dilates both arteries and veins. Captopril is a powerful vasodilator and also reduces aldosterone production. Captopril, because of its ability to inhibit the effects of renin, is particularly valuable in the management of severe chronic cardiac failure, where plasma renin level tends to be high.

Vasodilator therapy can be adjusted to the patient's requirement, by using venodilator for relieving pulmonary congestion and arteriolar dilators to improve cardiac output. Choice of the therapy depends on patients tolerance. Side effects are headache, postural hypotension, some times increases peripheral oedema partly because fluid retention by the kidneys, higher doses of diuretics may be needed.

*Dose* : Hydralazine — upto 200 mg daily better not exceeded.
Salbutamol — 4-8 mg TDS

Prazosine — 0.5 mg and gradually increase 10 mg TDS.
Captopril — 25-100 mg TDS
Sorbitrate — 10 to 20 mg 6 hourly.

**Management of acute heart failure and acute pulmonary oedema**

(1) The majority of patients are more comfortable in the trunk up legs down position.

(2) 5 to 10 mg of morphine sulphate should be given intravenously, with close watch for respiratory depression.

(3) Oxygen should be given by mask or by intermittent positive pressure.

(4) Furosemide — 40 mg intravenously and may be repeated if necessary.

(5) It is important to reduce preload so as to decrease dyspnoea and pulmonary congestion. Sublingual nitroglycerine 0.4 to 1.2 mg may be given. Tourniquets have the advantage of being immediately reversible.

(6) If bronchospasm and wheezing are prominent, Aminophylline 250 mg diluted may be given intravenously slowly.

(7) When the patient is not receiving digitalis 0.5 to 0.75 mg digoxin may be given intravenously, followed by additional dose as indicated.

(8) Constant watch and monitor of vital parameters.

Do not make mistake in diagnosis between cardiac asthma and bronchial asthma.

*Restriction of physical activity*

Rest depends on the severity of failure

(a) Complete rest (confine to bed-chair) for 3-4 weeks. Should move lower limbs from the beginning.

(b) Confine to the house, another 3-4 weeks.

(c) Discontinue full time work, there must be rest period during the day.

*Restriction of Sodium intake*

(a) In severe failure there should be low sodium diet and eliminate salt from cooking and at table (Na 0.2 to 1.0 gm a day).

(b) With improvement, eliminate salt in cooking and at table (Na 1.2 to 1.8 gm a day).

(c) Eliminate salt taken on the dining table (Na 1.6 to 2.8 gm a day).

**Conclusion**

Medical therapy of congestive heart failure has improved markedly over the past few years. The wide variety of agents at our disposal have enabled us today to enuse better comfort although the effects on survival may be slight. The end-stage heart, however, like the end-stage kidney, liver disease is unlikely to respond dramatically to any therapy apart from organ replacement. Unfortunately, the resources available to support heart-transplantation, even in the wealthiest country in the world are limited.

It therefore seems appropriate that much greater attention should be directed towards the prevention and early detection of cardiac muscle dysfunction, before systemic decompensation ensues. This implies much greater attention to such antecedents as hypertension and coronary artery disease as well as other treatable causes of cardiac decompensation. It also implies a much more precise understanding of the derangements that occur at a subcellular level in a variety of conditions that culminate in "heart failure". Once the specific derangement is elucidated in a particular condition, it may be possible to direct more specific therapy to the problem that exists rather than to treat the consequences in an empirical manner. In this field, we are just beginning to scratch the surface.

# PULMONARY EMBOLISM

*SUKUMAR MUKHERJEE*

## Introduction

Recently the importance of pulmonary embolism as a relatively common cause of death has become more widely appreciated, despite gross underestimation of this problem by the prevalent statistics. Pulmonary embolism is quite common, but often unrecognised clinically which suddenly presents without much warning.

## Incidence

The true incidence of pulmonary embolism is unknown and estimates of its frequency vary, depending on the diagnosis i.e. clinical, following investigation or postmortem studies. A mortality survey estimated 21,000 deaths in U.K. each year from pulmonary embolism (DHSS, 1970). Recent survey shows that around 650,000 patients in U.S.A. are annually afflicted with symptomatic pulmonary embolism. No definite data is available in context to the incidence of pulmonary embolism in India.

## Aetiopathogenesis

Virchow in 1846 showed that pulmonary 'embolii' were due to impaction of dislodged venous thrombi formed elsewhere. Thus, when considering the etiology of pulmonary embolism, we primarily consider the causes of peripheral venous thrombosis. This involves the triad as postulated by Virchow, namely :

(1) Changes in blood flow (Stasis)
(2) Changes in vessel wall (Endothelial damage)
(3) Changes in blood (Hypercoagulability)

1) *Changes in blood flow* : Stasis may predispose to venous thrombosis, particularly in presence of other risk factors. Stasis can occur as a result of low cardiac output states (heart failure), prolonged bed rest or other causes of restriction of lower limb venous return e.g. in chronically hospitalised patients; it may also occur in passengers following long air flights.

(2) *Changes in vessel wall* : The current concept is that an injured vessel wall/platelet interaction is probably the starting point of a thrombus. Electron microscopy demonstrates, that under certain circumstances, platelets gain access to the subendothelial layers of blood vessels; ADP and other substances are released which helps platelets to stick together.

(3) *Changes in blood* : Attention has been focused on the interaction between blood platelets and coagulation mechanism in relation to vessel injury. Thrombosis begins by deposition on vascular endothelium of masses of platelets; platelets liberate thromboplastins which convert prothrombin to thrombin and thus result in clot formation. The coagulation mechanism is probably dominant in determining the ultimate size of thrombus.

## High risk patients :

Clinical, latest diagnostic aids and post-mortem studies have led to the identification of certain risk factors in the development of venous thrombosis and subsequent pulmonary embolism.

**Table : 18.9 – High risk factors for Venous thrombosis**

- Advanced age (above 50 years)
- Major operations (lower abdominal, pelvic, orthopaedic operations)
- Post operative immobility
- Heart failure
- Obesity
- Pregnancy
- Oral contraceptive pills
- Malignancy
- Previous H/O thrombosis

Although lower extremities are usually considered the source of emboli, they may also arise from other sites like axillary, hepatic, portal or renal veins. Embolus may also arise from the right heart in certain conditions, like acute right ventricular myocardial infarction, cardiomyopathy and most important in our country, rheumatic carditis, particularly in presence of atrial fibrillation where there is dislodgement of thrombus from right atrial appendage. Besides, amniotic fluid, fat, air and bone-marrow particles have been implicated on occasions in the production of pulmonary embolism.

**Consequences of impaction of embolus in pulmonary artery**

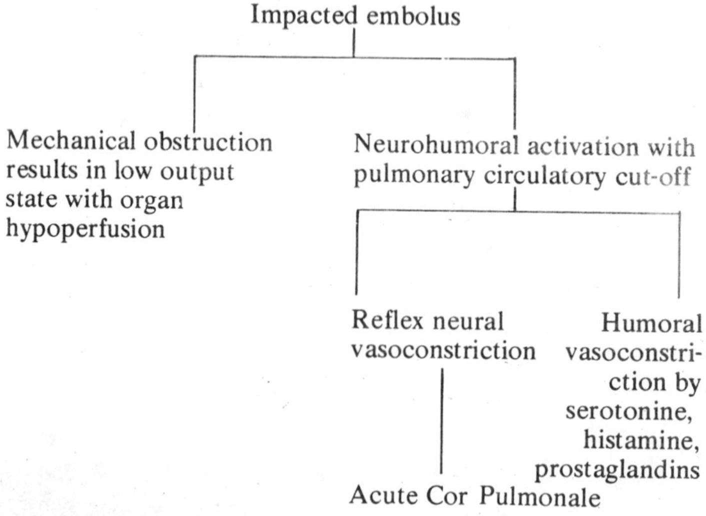


### Clinical spectrum of pulmonary thrombo embolism

Pulmonary embolism includes the following clinical syndromes

1) Acute minor embolism
2) Acute massive embolism
3) Subacute massive embolism
4) Recurrent thrombo-embolic pulmonary artery hypertension (vide infra)

*Acute minor embolism* : This occurs due to impaction of small blood clot in a distal pulmonary artery. Hence, there is preservation of collaterals and no haemodynamic consequences. Clinically it may be silent, or there may be features suggestive of pulmonary infarction like pleuritic pain, haemoptysis, pleural rub and occasionally fine crepitations.

*Acute massive embolism* : The volume of embolic material in this case must be sufficient to obstruct 50%, or more of the pulmonary arterial tree. In contrast to minor embolism, haemodynamic disturbances, rather than pleural involvement is the mode of presentation. Acute massive embolism is the commonest cause of acute cor pulmonale. The haemodynamic disturbances are categorized as follows a) Acute reduction in cardiac output

b) Acute disturbances of ventilation and perfusion.

c) Acute right ventricular failure

**Acute reduction in cardiac output**

The sudden reduction in cardiac output due to obstruction to right ventricular output is responsible for the common presenting symptom of massive embolism i.e. collapse in a patient who is severely dyspnoeic. The syncope and shock may be almost momentary or prolonged in severe cases.

**Acute disturbance of ventilation and perfusion :**

This results in acute dyspnoea, tachypnoea and hyperventilation. The resultant characteristic finding of low arterial $PO_2$ (average-50 mm Hg) and low arterial $Pco_2$ (average-35 mm Hg) may be found in proportion of cases due to right to left shunting across a patent foramen ovale. In some cases due to shunt like effect due to mismatched ventilation-perfusion of lung.

**Acute right ventricular failure**

This occurs as a result of sudden obstruction of right ventricular outflow tract leading to acute dilatation and poor contractibility of right ventricle. This resultant chest pain due to low cardiac output and coronary insufficiency erroneous diagnosis of myocardial infarction, however, while a patient of myocardial infarction is orthopnoeic a patient of pulmonary embolism prefers to lie flat. Clinically there is raised jugular venous pressure and appearance of summation gallop. Haemodynamically, there is moderate elevation of pulmonary arterial and right ventricular pressures.

**Subacute massive embolism :** In these cases, patients have a long history extending for days or weeks. Unlike in acute embolism, patients with subacute embolism frequently give history suggestive of deep vein thrombosis, along with episodic pleuritic pain, haemoptysis and gradually progressive dyspnoea. The longer duration results in higher pulmonary arterial pressure as compared to massive embolism.

**Aids to diagnosis :** Diagnosis of pulmonary embolism is aided by the index of clinical suspicion, particularly in presence of high risk factors e.g. sudden appearance of chest pain or syncope or shock in a patient with congestive cardiac failure. Confirmation of diagnosis requires a number of preliminary as well as sophisticated investigations like of following :-

**Diagnosis of deep vein thrombosis :—** Since it is deep venous thrombosis which leads to pulmonary embolism, hence a discussion on the diagnosis of pulmonary embolism must include recent advances in the diagnosis of deep venous thrombosis.

This involves :- 1) Clinical examination which must progress from foot end upwards. Homan's sign is often unrewarding.

2) Investigations likely to be valuable.
   a) Venography.
   b) Labelled fibrinogen technique :- This involves the incorporation of $^{131}I$ ($^{131}$ Iodine) labelled fibrinogen into the thrombus.
   c) Ultrasonic flow detector.

**Electrocardiogram :** Electrocardiographic abnormalities are seen in 85% of patients with proven acute pulmonary embolism. A normal E.C.G. does in no way exclude the diagnosis of pulmonary embolism since E.C.G. changes may be transient or delayed, serial E.C.G. recordings are particularly useful in the diagnosis of pulmonary embolism.

The electrocardiographic abnormalities are due to diminished coronary perfusion. The common abnormalities are as follows :

1) Sinus tachycardia is very common. $S_1$ $Q_3$ $T_3$ pattern which simulates acute inferior wall infarction. The absence of current of injury pattern in III, absence of Q in avF and presence of 'T' wave inversion in right precordial leads differentiates pulmonary embolism from acute inferior infarction.

2) Incomplete RBBB pattern is more common than complete RBBB pattern which may be transient.
3) Right ventricular strain pattern as characterised by T-inversion in right precordial leads.
4) Clockwise rotation due to acute dilatation of R.V.
5) On rare occasions left sided ECG abnormalities (e.g. ST-T wave changes over $V_4$-$V_6$) may be present due to coexistent coronary artery disease or due to development of coronary insufficiency.

Thus electrocardiography in a case of acute pulmonary embolism not only differentiates it from myocardial infarction, but also excludes coexistent ischaemic or valvular heart disease.

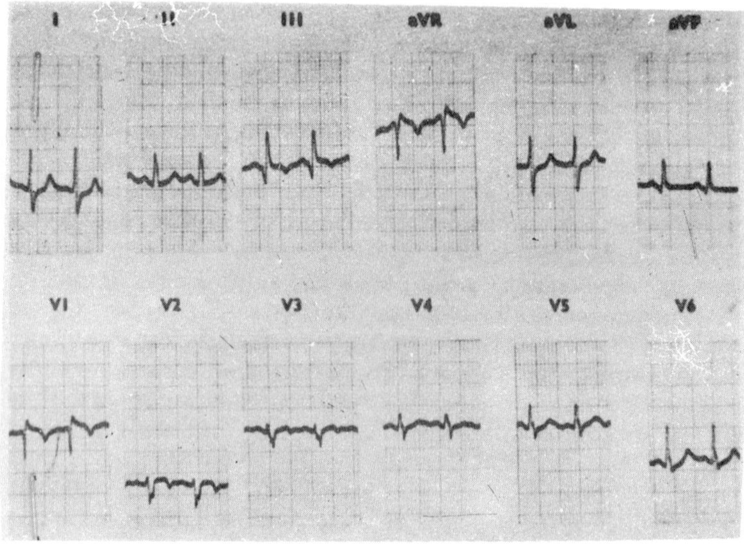


Fig.18.32 : E.C.G. in acute Pulmonary embolism.

**Plain Chest X-ray :** Radiography of chest is also useful in the differentiation of acute pulmonary embolism from other causes of collapse and shock. Besides, it helps in the identification of pre-existing heart or lung disease.

The common radiological abnormalities are :

1) Loss of lung volume as manifested by raised dome of diaphragm.
2) Patchy oligaemia.
3) Abnormalities of pulmonary artery perfusion : due to rapid cut off pulmonary artery there may be 'plump' or 'pear' shaped hilar shadows.
4) Infarct shadows which are initially wedge shaped but later on may leave linear scars.
5) Changes in the size and configuration of heart.

**Biochemical Investigations and other laboratory investigations**

The triad of high LDH, normal SGOT and elevated serum bilirubin though helpful for the diagnosis of massive pulmonary embolism is rarely obtainable.

Serum fibrinogen-fibrin degradation products are usually elevated following an attack of massive pulmonary embolism.

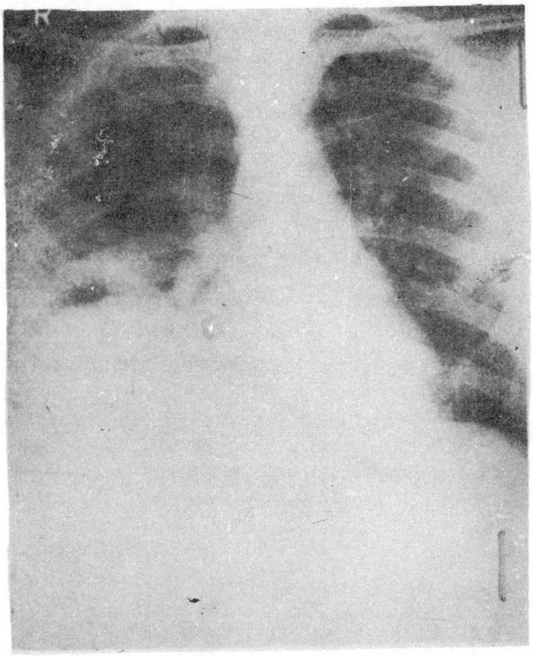

Fig.18.33 : Plain X-ray chest showing elevated right diaphragm, right basal shadows and oligaemic upper zones of pulmonary embolism

**Lung function studies :** Very few studies have been performed on the mechanical lung functions close in time to an embolic episode. Sasahara and his colleagues (1967) reported reduction in vital capacity and FEV in 80% or more of a large group of patients, 2/3rd of whom were studied within a week of suspected embolism.

Alveolar gas exchange studies in acute embolic period reveals :

(i) Mismatched VA/Q ratio.

(ii) Reduced diffusing capacity.

(iii) Widened arteriolar alveolar gradients for $CO_2$.

**Central Venous Pressure :** It is characteristically elevated due to acute right sided congestive cardiac failure.

**Haemodynamic responses :** Previously there were relatively few data on the hemodynamic studies in acute pulmonary embolism. It is only recently, that the National Co-operative study (Urokinase - Pulmonary Embolism Trial (1973) has recorded haemodynamic measurements in 143 patients with angiographically proved thromboembolism. The common abnormalities in decreasing order of frequency are :

1) Arterial hypoxaemia.
2) Right ventricular systolic pressure $>$25 mm Hg.
3) Elevation in total pulmonary resistance
4) Right ventricular end diastolic pressure$>$6 mm Hg
5) Mean pulmonary artery pressure$>$20 mm Hg
6) Mean right atrial pressure$>$6 mm Hg
7) Decrease in cardiac index ( 2.7L/min/$m^2$)

**Scinti-scan :** The use of perfusion scan utilising $I^{131}$ or Te-99m Labelled macroaggregated human albumin have been proved to be useful in the study of pulmonary embolsim.

This investigation was first described by Wagner in 1964 and allows the determination of pulmonary blood flow in vessels as small as 50 micro. m. It is a very sensitive investigation but lacks specificity.

However, combined ventilation-perfusion scan shows perfusion defects unaccompanied by defects of ventilation; a finding specific for pulmonary embolism.

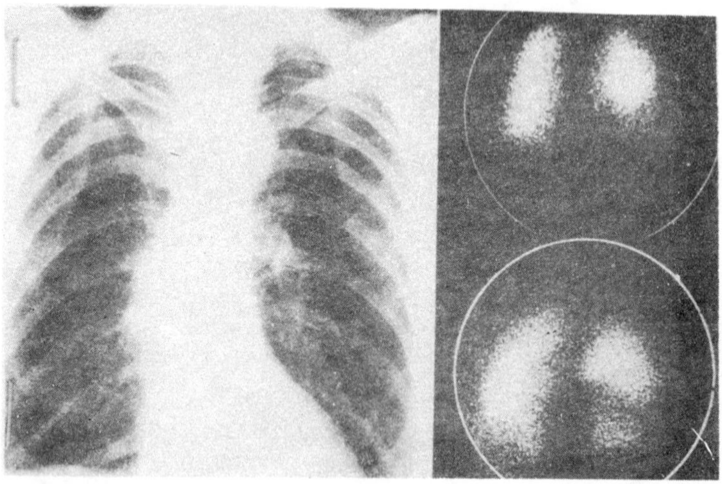

Fig.18.34 — Chest X-ray and Pulmonary Scinti-scan showing perfusion defect of right lower lobe.

**Pulmonary arteriography :** This established or excludes the diagnosis of pulmonary embolism beyond doubt and also accurately determines the severity and distribution of embolism. Besides,

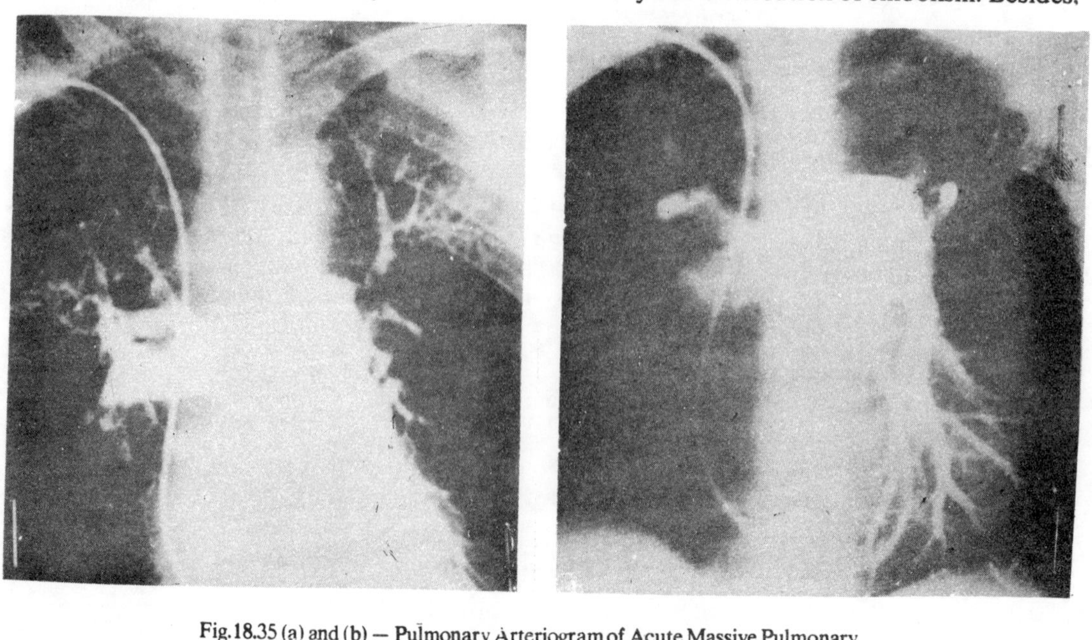

Fig.18.35 (a) and (b) — Pulmonary Arteriogram of Acute Massive Pulmonary Embolism.

to some extent it helps in determining the age of emboli; a recent emboli producing a convex filling defect while a lysed emboli produces a concave filling defect. (*Miller* – 1973).

The hazards of this investigation is perhaps overestimated.

There are two major angiographic signs of massive pulmonary embolism, namely, intra-luminal defects and cut-off an artery. Pulmonary angiography must be carried out via an arm vein in order to avoid dislodgement of thrombi from iliac veins or inferior vena cava that may happen when the femoral route is used.

**Differential Diagnosis**

Acute minor embolism must be differentiated from other causes of pleuritic pain and haemoptysis e.g. pneumonia.

Acute massive and subacute massive pulmonary embolism must be differentiated from other causes of collapse and shock.

The table 18.10 illustrates the different diagnosis of massive pulmonary embolism.

**Table – 18.10 : D.D. of massive pulmonary embolism**

| Distinguishing Features | Acute Massive Pulmonary Embolism | Acute Myocardial Infarction | Tension Pneumothorax | Septicaemic Shock |
|---|---|---|---|---|
| Chest pain | Present | Present | Present | Absent |
| Posture | Supine | Orthopnoea | Orthopnoea | OFTEN flat |
| Lung | No evidence of basal crepitations | Basal crepitations present | Hyperresonant percussion note Mediastinal shift Diminished breath sounds | Evidence of pulmonary oedema or ARDS |
| Heart | Features of Right ventricular failure $P_2$ not loud. $S_3$ & $S_4$ present | Features of Left ventricular failure | Apex beat shifted | Features of shock |
| Bleeding disorders | Nil | Nil | Nil | Features of D.I.C. present |
| Chest X-ray | Patchy oligaemia Raised hemidiaphragm | Features of pulmonary oedema | Hypertrans-luscency & mediastimal shift | Features of ARDS |
| E.C.G. | R.B.B.B. pattern Right ventricular strain pattern – $S_1\ Q_3\ T_3$ pattern or $S_1\ T_3$ pattern | Typical Q-wave and ST-T changes in appropriate leads | Nothing particular | Nothing particular |

**Recurrent thrombo-embolic pulmonary artery hypertension.**

The haemodynamic disturbance in this clinical syndrome gives rise to elevated pulmonary artery pressure and resultant right ventricular hypertrophy.

Investigations include preliminary X-ray demonstration of patchy oligaemia, with marked enlargement of main pulmonary artery and the electrocardiographic identification of right ventricular hypertrophy.

Catheterisation studies reveal high right ventricular and pulmonary arterial pressure. Diagnosis is confirmed by the angiographic demonstration of enlarged pulmonary arteries with asymmetric occlusions.

Pulmonary hypertension from recurrent thrombo-embolism must be distinguished from other causes of pulmonary hypertension like mitral valve disease or primary pulmonary hypertension.

*Pulmonary angiogram showing dilated pulmonary artery of recurrent thromboembolism* (Fig.18.35).

**Management of pulmonary embolism.**

In minor embolism where there is no haemodynamic disturbance, no treatment is required, except for the relief of symptoms. However, in cases of minor embolism associated with deep vein thrombosis anticoagulant therapy is perhaps a wise precaution against massive embolism.

In contrast, acute massive embolism always heralds therapy :-

This involves A. Immediate resuscitation

B. Definitive therapy.

*Immediate Resuscitation :* The following measures are adopted for the immediate resuscitation of a patient suffering from massive pulmonary embolism.

(i) Oxygen mask or endotracheal intubation.

(ii) External cardiac massage which may also help in the propagation of emboli.

(iii) Use of vasopressor drugs e.g. Metaraminol, Dopamine.

(iv) Correction of metabolic acidosis by I.V. bicarbonate.

(v) Use of plasma expanders like 500 ml of 70% Dextran.

(vi) High dose heparin intravenously (15,000 units) to combat serotonins—mediated vasoconstrictor effect.

If the above mentioned measures fail to resuscitate the patient then one may try :-

(i) Intrapulmonary urokinase infusion.

(ii) Emergency pulmonary embolectomy using inflow occlusion (modified Trendelenburg operation).

(iii) Immediate establishment of partial cardiopulmonary bypass (femoro-femoral bypass); pulmonary angiography may then be confirmed and patient transferred for emergency embolectomy.

*Definitive treatment* :—There exists much controversy about the correct treatment of massive pulmonary embolism. It must be remembered that the establishment of diagnosis is a must before performing definite treatment like pulmonary embolectomy, which will obviously be fatal in a case of shock due to any other cause.

The currently available forms of treatment are :

1. Anticoagulants.
2. Thrombolytics.
3. Embolectomy.

*Anticoagulants* :—This involves intravenous heparin therapy in the early stages, replaced later by oral anticoagulants as heparin is tapered off and patient begins ambulation. In the absence of contraindications, the current recommendation is 10,000 units of IV. heparin as a single dose, followed by 5,000-7,500 units of IV heparin every 4 hrs after confirmation of diagnosis or 1,000 units/hr by constant infusion.

During heparin therapy, tests for clotting time should be performed regularly and the value should be 2.3 times the normal.

*Thrombolytics :* Several studies have shown that thrombolytic therapy results in considerably accelerated resolution as compared to heparin therapy. Streptokinase 250,000 units in the first hour, followed by maintenance therapy of 100,000 units over 24 hrs by constant infusion, is the usual adopted regime under steroid cover.

Thrombolytic therapy is contraindicated in conditions like acute gastric bleeding, severe hypertension, H/O cerebrovascular accident. During thrombolytic therapy the thrombin clotting time must be checked regularly and kept at 2-3 time normal value.

*Pulmonary embolectomy* :— Pulmonary embolectomy is the treatment of choice in the patients in whom thrombolytics are contraindicated or in occasional patients in whom there is a rapid deterioration despite thrombolytic therapy. Lastly embolectomy is also indicated in these patients in whom thrombolytic therapy is unlikely to exert its effect soon enough to prevent imminent death.

Criteria of pulmonary embolectomy may be enumerated as follow :—

(i) Persistent shock unresponsive to treatment with fluids and vasopressors.

(ii) Massive pulmonary embolism with having 60% obstruction of pulmonary vasculature as revealed by angiography.

(iii) Right sided heart failure with an elevated and diastolic right ventricular pressure and C.V.P. above 15 cm.

**Follow-up**

All patients should be maintained on anticoagulants for atleast 3 to 6 months. Since patients having one episode of pulmonary embolism are at increased risk of subsequent embolism, hence they must receive anticoagulant coverage whenever they are exposed to risks of thrombosis (eg. surgery, bed rest).

There are a few patients in whom there is repeated pulmonary emboli despite anticoagulants control or in whom anticoagulants are contraindicated. These patients are at a risk of developing thrombotic pulmonary hypertension and in them there may be a place for inserting a filter in inferior vena cava. Lastly, an attempt to discover occult neoplasia is justified in many patients with unexplained pulmonary embolism.

**Prophylaxis :**

On the basis of several autopsy studies conducted, it seems, that an effective method of prophylaxis would prevent mortality and morbidity associated with the spectrum of pulmonary thrombo-embolic diseases. The chief methods employed are classified as follows :-

*Elimination of deep vein stasis in lower limbs :-*

This involves early ambulation, guided physical exercises and specific methods to increase venous return in lower limbs (eg. pneumatic compression or electrical stimulation).

*Counteracting blood coagulability.*

a. Drugs affecting platelet aggregation :- Evidence of antiplatelet agents in prophylaxis of deep vein thrombosis is unconvincing.

b. Drugs affecting coagulation :- This involves utilisation of low dose heparin therapy and long term therapy with oral anticoagulants.

**Prognosis :**

Acute massive pulmonary embolism is almost always fatal if left untreated. In those that are fatal, 75% of deaths occur within one hour of symptoms and remaining 25% within 48 hours.

In case of smaller embolism prognosis is much better and the patient can have one or more clinically unrecognised attacks.

A pulmonary embolus tends to resolve over a period of time. Complete resolution may occur as soon as two weeks but is usually delayed upto two months. The pulmonary artery pressure usually returns to normal by three weeks.

It is now clear that chronic thrombo-embolic pulmonary hypertension is seldom, if ever, a complication of acute massive embolism. It is probably due to numerous clinically unrecognised attacks of minor embolism.

**Special types of pulmonary embolism :**

*Fat embolism* :- Acute cor pulmonale due to fat embolism can occur when globules of liquid fat enter the systemic veins and are carried to the lungs.

Common causes of fat embolism includes severe fractures or crush injuries, amputations, osteomyelitis and burns.

Since fat globules are able to penetrate lung capillaries and enter general circulation they may become lodged in the vessels of brain. Therefore both pulmonary and cerebral symptoms and signs may develop usually within 72 hrs after an accident.

*Air embolism* :- Acute cor pulmonale can also be produced by air embolism. Unlike fat, air does not penetrate pulmonary capillaries. IV. infusion, angiography, vaginal insufflations,operations on neck veins, dural sinuses are the usual source of air embolism. The volume of air required to occlude the pulmonary circuit is atleast more than 10 cc/kg body wt.

*Amniotic fluid embolism* :- This is particularly seen in pregnant mothers in third trimester of pregnancy, in puerperium and as a hazard of amniocentesis. There are associated features of D.I.C.

## CHRONIC PULMONARY HEART DISEASE

(Chronic Cor Pulmonale)

*G. C. MOOKERJEE.*

### Introduction

The term Cor Pulmonale was introduced by Stuart Harris (1957), Chronic Pulmonary Heart Disease (CPHD) or chronic cor pulmonale is characterised by hypertrophy of the right ventricle, due to hypertension in the pulmonary circuit caused by chronic lung disease or pulmonary vascular pathology. But CPHD does not include cardiac damage due to pulmonary hypertension of mitral stenosis or congenital heart disease.

The expert committee of the W.H.O. (1961) defined C.P.H.D. as "hypertrophy of right ventricle resulting from disease affecting the function and/or the structure of the lungs, except where these pulmonary alterations are the result of the diseases that primarily affect the left side of the heart or congenital heart diseases".

### Causes of pulmonary heart diseases

A) *Diseases primarily affecting air passages of the lungs and the alveoli :*

1) Chronic bronchitis with generalised airway obstruction with or without emphysema
2) Bronchial asthma or chronic asthmatic bronchitis
3) Emphysema with or without bronchitis or asthma

4) Pulmonary fibrosis with or without emphysema due to :

(a) Tuberculosis
(b) Pneumoconiosis
(c) Bronchiectasis
(d) Other pulmonary infections
(e) Radiation therapy
(f) Mucoviscidosis etc.

B) *Pulmonary granulomata or infiltration*

1) Sarcoidosis
2) Chronic diffuse interstitial fibrosis
3) Berylliosis
4) Eosinophilic granulomata or histiocytosis.
5) Malignant infiltration
6) Dermatomyositis
7) Alveolar microlithiasis

C. *Pulmonary resection* may also be a significant factor when a major portion of lung is removed.

D. *Congenital cystic diseases of lungs* : a rare cause.

E. *Diseases primarily affecting the movement of the thoracic cage.*

(1) Kyphoscoliosis and other thoracic deformities
(2) Thoracoplasty
(3) Pleural fibrosis
(4) Chronic neuromuscular weakness e.g. poliomyelitis
(5) Obesity causing alveolar hypoventilation (Pickwickian syndrome)
(6) Idiopathic alveolar hypoventilation.

Recurrent subacute pulmonary thrombo-embolism or occlusive diseases of small pulmonary arteries may also lead to cor pulmonale but are rare.

**Clinical features**

Clinical features will depend on the background pathology and its effect on the heart though it can be acute, subacute or chronic. Chronic cor-pulmonale is most commonly due to chronic obstructive pulmonary disease, with emphysema. The ultimate effect is raised pulmonary artery pressure causing R.V.H. and high output failure.

Typical patient gives history of chronic cough over many years, due to some form of chronic obstructive airway diseases, (C.O.A.D.) e.g. chronic bronchitis, bronchial asthma and emphysema, the three major causes.

The patient is usually middle-aged, with history of recurrent winter bronchitis or bronchial asthma. He may be a heavy cigarette or 'Biri' smoker.

Careful history-taking in some patients may show past history of bronchiectasis, chronic pulmonary tuberculosis, pneumonectomy, thoracoplasty, spinal deformity, occupational lung diseases e.g. silicosis or asbestosis etc (vide supra).

Regardless of the type of onset, symptoms are almost similar in most patients. As the severity of pulmonary disease increases, gradual development of cardiac decompensation begins, finally leading to right heart failure.

There is history of recurrent cough and wheezing which gradually becomes continuous with gradually increasing dyspnoea. In advanced cases the subject is dyspnoeic at rest; chest expansion is poor; breath sounds are sometimes distant and rhonchi are present all over with scattered crepitations in both lungs. At this stage right heart failure usually occurs; J.V.P. is raised. Liver is enlarged and tender, cyanosis and peripheral oedema are late signs.

Physical signs will depend on the background diseases causing pulmonary hypertension, R.V.H. and finally right heart failure.

Due to emphysema, apex beat is impalpable. Right ventricular thrust is therefore is not easily palpable although it may be present over the epigastrium.

A systolic bruit due to tricuspid incompetence and right ventricular third heart sound may be heard on auscultation. Respiratory infection always makes the situation worse and may end in fatality, if not properly treated. Papilloedema may sometimes be present. In advanced cases,the patient may be drowsy or comatose.

**Laboratory findings :**

Polycythaemia may be present in established cases. In developing countries evidence of malnutrition often complicates the picture. The author has seen many cases of cor pulmonale associated with hepatic cirrhosis. In factory labourers "biri" smoking and cheap country made alcohol often are in the background. In addition there may be environmental pollution. Hence attention to hepatic function should be given, because malnutrition, alcoholic hepatocelluar injury and congestive failure are all agents in damaging the liver.

Radiography of chest may be normal in early stages but may show emphysematous changes with prominent bronchovascular markings, or features of primary pulmonary diseases. Heart shadow may show right ventricular hypertrophy; pulmonary artery enlargement may be seen in advanced cases. Low diaphragm and tubular heart is usually present.

**ECG :**

In early cases ECG may be normal. Evidence of right ventricular hypertrophy, right axis deviation, right bundle branch block, accompanied by S pattern across left chest leads may be present. P-pulmonale in ECG is a very typical finding.

**Lung function tests** will show diminished forced vital capacity from predicted normal, forced expiratory volume ($FEV_1$) is usually less than 75%, expiration is prolonged then normal. In restrictive lung disease there is hardly any obstruction and $FEV_1$ and EVC may be more than 75%. Blood gas analysis may show diminished $PO_2$ and increased $PCO_2$ of arterial blood depending upon degree of respiratory failure.

**Diagnosis :**

Disease is difficult to diagnose in early stage. Long history of respiratory disease, increasing exertional dyspnoea, appearance of mild oedema legs, with radiological and electrocardiographic evidence of right heart strain or enlargement, may help in early diagnosis. Blood gas analysis and lung function tests give supportive evidence. Finally fully developed picture of rightsided heart failure sets in. The most important point is to consider the possibility of pulmonary origin of heart failure.

**Prognosis**

Once congestive heart failure develops the prognosis is poor. Some patients may die within a year or two inspite of treatment. However emergency treatment of respiratory infection as well a heart failure must be done. Oxygen therapy and supportive treatment may prolong the life and comfort to a great extent. In elderly age group there may be associated I.H.D. and hypertensive heart disease to make the situation worse

**Treatment :**

By the time pulmonary hypertension and cardiac failure sets in, no curative treatment for the underlying lung disease is possible. But most patients are benefited by proper control of pulmonary infection and intensive therapy of congestive heart failure.

**Prevention of further pulmonary damage :**

Smokers should stop smoking for good. The patients should be prevented from exposure to hazardous dusts, fumes, or industrial pollutions. Change of occupation, though difficult, may be necessary. Economic problems often become the limiting factor. Environment and diet are very important.

**Control of respiratory infection :**

This is the most important part of treatment. Respiratory infection leads to myocardial hypoxia and usually precipitates heart failure. Proper antibiotics should always be given according to bacterial flora of the sputum. Hyposensitization against common respiratory allergens may sometimes help to prevent recurrent respiratory allergy.

**Bronchodilators :** Treatment with bronchodilators always necessary in patients with respiratory distress, as discussed in the chapters on bronchial asthma and chronic bronchitis.

**Diuretics**

Reduction of fluid overload improves peripheral circulation reduces C.V.P. and improves oedema. Right ventricular muscle function also improves due to decrease in intravascular volume.

Frusemide or ethacrynic acid are the two diuretics which should be used. Judicious use of diuretics prolongs left provide hypokalaemia is avoided and infection is combated with proper use of antibiotics. Oxygen therapy off and on several times a day also improves cardiac function by relieving hypoxia. Oxygen toxicity occurs due to pure or high oxygen concentration for too long a period.

To avoid hypokalaemia, potassium supplements or potassium-sparing diuretics e.g. spironolactone should be prescribed. Acetazolamide is not recommended.

**Corticosteroids :** are also used in cases associated with bronchial asthma. However, inhalational use of beclomethasone is preferable to systemic therapy. But when patients become refractory, bronchodilators and betamethasone inhalation also fails. Prednisolone should be used orally in doses of 20 to 30 mg per day in four divided doses and minimum dosage should be used. It may be possible to tail off the drug within two weeks or may be switched over to inhalation therapy. Parenteral steroids are used only as emergency measure (Refer to chapter on bronchial asthma).

**Oxygen therapy :** is of great help and often life saving. Regulated oxygen therapy should be given under close supervision. Best method is to hospitalise the patient but where it is not possible oxygen should be administered at home with usual precautions (risk of fire should be explained). The oxygenation should be adjusted to $PO_2$ level above 60 mmHg. At right, the flow rate of oxygen may have to be increased to prevent sleep-induced hypoxaemia and possible cardiac arrhythmias. While using nasal catheter, flow-rate of oxygen of 2 to 5 litres per minute ensures oxygen supply of 30 to 40% in inspired air.

In patient of COPD, respiratory centre (R.C.) may become tolerant to rising $PCO_2$ and the action of R.C. is principally influenced by the hypoxaemic stimulus, via carotid sinus and aortic bodies. Sudden removal of this hypoxaemic drive by rapid oxygenation may cause drowsiness, convulsion, coma or even death (carbon dioxide narcosis).

Hence careful oxygenation under close observation is necessary. However, where mechanical ventilatory support is available, this is not a problem.

Inhalation of oxygen above 60% and above, if continued over 36 hours may be damaging to respiratory epithelium and pulmonary surfuctant. This is also likely to occur during prolonged assisted ventilation with high percentage of oxygen.

Most dangerous complication is ventilatory failure (hypoxaemia and hypercapnic respiratory failure) which should be treated preferably in a respiratory care unit.

**Mucolytic therapy**

Thick tenacious sputum alone may cause severe dyspnoea cause small air way blockage. Bronchiolar drainage by suction-aspiration of mucus may even be life saving. Soft plastic catheters can be used but modern sophisticated instruments are also available (Askrad Lab. Cranford N.J. USA). Even fiberoptic bronchoscope can be used.

It should be realised that even simple suction by soft plastic catheter using local anaesthesia can be life saving.

Potassium-iodide mixtures and adequate hydration are helpful. Mucolytic agents e.g. bromhexine is commonly used. Bromhexine can be administered orally, parenterally and by inhalation. This is synthetic benzylamine compound obtained from an alskaloid vasicine from a plant *Adhatoda vascia.*

Oral dose — 8 to 16 mg three times daily.

**Acetyl cysteine** (Airbron; Mucomist) is also used in USA. It is a derivative of an aminoacid 1-cysteine. It is given by inhalation or through intratracheal catheter or via bronchoscope. Rubber or metal tubes should not be used.

**Pancreatic dornase** obtained from beef pancreas has been also used. These last two agents may also cause allergic reactions as well side effects.

**Right ventricular failure** — The picture resembles Congestive cardiac failure (CCF).

In cor pulmonale right ventricle ultimately fails and it should be treated with adequate rest, low salt diet, diuretics, digitalis and regulated oxygen therapy. Too much salt restriction may result in hypochloraemia. Water intake needs restriction in some cases. Effect of digitalis is not so good as in heart failure due to nonpulmonary cause, but myocardial function shows some improvement. (Refer to the chapter on Heart failure). However, it is probable that digitalis produces its good effects when there is associated left ventricular dysfunction. Occurrence of arrhythmias are likely due to existing hypokalaemia result of prolonged diuretic therapy.

**Vasodilators**

Vasodilators are being recently tried which may help, by decreasing right ventricular after-load. Though we are not yet certain about their efficacy in improving right ventricular function, drugs like isosorbide-dinitrate, nifedipine and hydralazine may be tried with caution.

**Phlebotomy**

Phlebotomy is an old procedure which may be helpful occasionally in preventing thrombo-embolic phenomenon and reducing viscosity of blood.

Exercise-conditioning, relaxation-training, use of home ventilators, occupational therapy and vocational rehabilitation may be rewarding. Yoga-therapy also helps to some extent. It increases relaxation and self-confidence due to controlled breathing. But these are of no use once right heart failure is established.

Finally it should be remembered that background disease also determines this prognosis and planning of treatment. Hence all effort should be made to investigate the nature of underlying pathological status.

## PERIPHERAL VASCULAR DISEASES

*N.K. MAJUMDAR*

They are of three types :

(1) Degenerative, (2) Inflammatory and (3) Vasospastic disorders.

**Degenerative vascular disorders**

Three types of disorders are known according to type of vessels involved.

Atherosclerosis principally affects large and medium-sized vessels i.e. aorta, cerebral and coronary arteries. Monckeberg's medial sclerosis consists of degenerative changes occuring in old age involving muscular coats of medium sized vessels i.e. radials.

Arterio-sclerotic involvement of small sized arteries or arterioles e.g. renal arterioles in malignant hypertension.

Atherosclerosis is related to aging and progresses as age advances. However, atherosclerosis can be accelerated by conditions like diabetes and hypertension. The basic lesion is the formation of plaque in arterial wall consisting of cholesterol and lipids. Plaque latter becomes sclerosed and calcified and thrombosis occur at that site. Thus thrombosis cerebral or coronary or peripheral arteries develop.

**Atherosclerosis obliterans**

Atherosclerosis occurs in large vessels of lower limbs usually affecting males over 50 years and less commonly females. Due to impairment of blood supply the following symptoms may develop :

(a) Pain on exercise (intermittent claudication)

(b) Cold extremities.

These symptoms may be initially unilateral but later bilateral.

Intermittent claudication appear on walking but disappears at rest. Commonly calf muscles are affected. In severe cases pain may occur even at rest. Ischaemia may lead to dryness, scaling and inelasticity of skin. Loss of hair, brittle nails, later ulceration and gangrene may develop. Loss of pulsation of arteries will indicate vascular disease.

X-ray may show arterial calcification. Arteriography will demonstrate arterial occlusion.

**Treatment**

Rather unsatisfactory. Associated factors like diabetes and hypertension need to be controlled. Tobacco habit should be forbidden as tobacco is known to aggravate ischaemia of arteries. Cold exposure should be avoided and suitable woollen clothing to be worn. Protection against trauma and treatment of sepsis are mandatory. Graduated exercise should be undertaken to improve blood flow. Role of vasodilators is doubtful. Surgical treatment i.e. sympathectomy may be helpful.

**Atherosclerosis and aneurysm**

Atherosclerosis in aorta may weaken the arterial wall and may lead to dilatation and aneurysm formation. This may occur in ascending aorta, arch of aorta or descending aorta. Aneurysm may lead to pressure symptoms. Sometimes atherosclerosis in aorta leads to dissection when blood stream makes its way into arterial wall through ulcerated intima. Dissection of aorta is found in young people in a connective tissue disorder named "Marfan's syndrome" characterised by long slim extremities high arched palate and subluxation of lens.

**Arterial embolism**

This may occur due to sudden lodgement of an emboli in a large vessel. The source of emboli may be rheumatic heart disease, myocardial infarction or an atrial myxoma. Emboli lodge commonly in aortic, iliac or popliteal artery at the bifurcation. Limb is painful, cold pale and numb. Pulses are absent distal to block. Treatment consists of rest, relief of pain, application of warmth, vasodilators or embolectomy.

**Inflammatory arterial diseases**

Peripheral diseases are as follows :-

(1) Polyarteritis nodosa

(2) Thromboangitis obliterans (Burger's disease)

(3) Cranial or giant cell arteritis

(4) Takayasu's syndrome (pulseless disease)

(5) Syphilitic aortitis.

**Polyarteritis nodosa :–** It is an immunological disorder affecting collagenous connective tissue in men commonly between 20-30 years. Characteristic lesions consist of multiple nodules on the small arteries. Clinically presents with fever, tachycardia, muscle wasting, sweating muscular pain. Due to multiple organ involvement, haematuria, abdominal pain, angina, myocardial infarction, pericarditis, neuropathy, subcutaneous nodules occur. Asthmatic symptoms, eosinophilia and hypersplenism may also occur (Refer to chapter on collagen diseases).

**Takayasu syndrome or pulseless diseases –** also known as aortic arch syndrome or reverse co-arctation. Common in Japan but also frequently encountered in India affecting young females. An arterial inflammation of unknown origin involves the aortic arch with narrowing of its branches. Tuberculous aetiology has been suspected in Indian patients. The arterial pulsations are diminished or absent in upper extremities, neck and head. Headaches, fits, visual disturbances and muscular wasting may occur. Prognosis is poor but corticosteroids may relieve the symptoms.

**Syphilitic aortitis**

It is now extremely rare, a manifestation of late syphilis affecting cardiovascular system. Disease begins above aortic valve cusps with loss of elastic tissue by fibrous tissue. Thus weakened aorta gradually dilates the ascending part of aorta. Initially there may be an aortic systolic murmur, later typical early diastolic murmur due to aortic regurgitation. The diastolic murmur is heard best on right of sternum. Diagnosis can be confirmed by serological tests for syphilis. Treatment is by penicillin and later surgical treatment for aneurysm, when possible.

**Vasospastic disorders**

(1) Raynaud's disease is peripheral vascular disturbance with spasmodic contraction of digital arteries of hand.

It may be primary when occuring commonly in young woman as a exaggerated response to cold. In secondary Raynaud's disease causes are as follows :

(a) Connective tissue disorder

(b) Obliterative arterial disease

(c) Occupation in which hands are exposed to vibrations e.g. pneumatic drills.

(d) Occasionally from cold agglutinins.

In all cases, obliterative changes with gangrene or thrombosis may occur.

Disorder is usually bilateral and fingers are more affected than toes. Numbness, tingling and burning sensations are more prominent than pain. Sensitivity to cold may be extreme and disabling. Colour change may vary from pallor, cyanosis and redness. Treatment consists of treatment of primary disease and avoidance of smoking. In severe cases sympathectomy may be done to remove vasomotor tone.

## HEART DISEASE IN PREGNANCY

*N.K. MAZUMDAR*

**Introduction**

Almost 2% of all pregnant woman suffer from some type of heart disease. Of these so affected, rheumatic heart disease accounts for 80-90%, which is the rather common in child bearing age. Most common rheumatic heart disease is mitral valve disease. Coronary artery disease and hypertensive heart disease are more common after 40 years but hypertension may occur in child bearing age.

Congenital heart disease may sometimes remain undiagnosed till pregnancy, most common lesions being A.S.D. and V.S.D., rarely P.D.A. and pulmonary stenosis. Thyrotoxicosis, myxoedema even syphilis should not be forgotten. Congestive heart failure (CCF) may occur due to chronic cardiac disorders but anaemia is an important common cause of CCF during pregnancy, specially in the tropics.

Heart disease produces an additional burden to mother due to the following reasons during pregnancy :

(1) $O_2$ consumption increases 20% above normal.

(2) Heart beat increased by more than 10 beats per minute.

(3) Total blood volume rises by 30-50% over normal during thirty fourth week (32nd-36th week) of pregnancy.

Additional stress on the heart during labour occurs due to :

(1) Exertion involved in the abdominal contractions during labour and more so when prolonged labour occurs.

(2) In immediate post-partum phase the heart is over burdened by volume of blood expelled by contracting Uterus.

Due to above reasons woman with heart disease are particularly prone to develop heart failure.

**Fallacies in the diagnosis**

(1) Oedema of feet occuring during pregnancy may not necessarily be due to heart disease. It may be due to retention of fluid due to pressure on abdominal veins by a gravid uterus.

(2) A functional systolic murmur may be heard over praecordium over the pulmonary area due to anaemia so common in India. A murmur over engorged mammary arteries also may simulate a heart disease.

(3) Heart may appear enlarged due to its horizontal position which in turn is caused by elevation of diaphragm.

(4) Minor E.C.G. changes of QRS-axis and ST segment or T wave may sometimes normally occur in pregnant woman.

**Clinical features :**

Increased load in the heart provokes or worsen symptoms in patients with heart disease. Symptoms usually occur before or after the 12th week and tend to be become maximal from 24th week onwards. Chief symptom of heart disease in pregnancy is breathlessness but oedema also may occur. Angina is very unusual. Some are asymptomatic, some may develop acute pulmonary oedema in late pregnancy or shortly after delivery. Commonest heart disease is mitral stenosis with or without incompetence.

**Hypertensive heart disease**

If toxaemia of pregnancy is excluded hypertension is uncommon in pregnant woman. If a pregnant woman is found to have high BP early in pregnancy, one can assume that the hypertension antedated the pregnancy and physician should look for some other cause e.g. kidney disease or aortic disease. If no cause is found it is probably essential hypertension.

If hypertension is found late in pregnancy it is difficult to say whether she has long standing hypertension with toxaemia of pregnancy or just toxaemia of pregnancy. Pregnant woman with severe hypertension is exposed to all obstetric hazards commonly associated with pregnancy toxaemia and in addition those due to severe hypertension itself e.g., left ventricular failure, C.V.A. and renal failure.

Hypertension is a difficult problem in pregnancy and teratogenicity of most modern hypotensive drugs are not established as yet. Therefore judicious treatment with salt restriction, dietary measures, careful use of diuretics and drugs like methyl-dopa should be carried out.

**Post-partum heart disease (Cardiomyopathy)**

This is a rare from of heart disease occuring during puerperium in women who had no apparent heart disease previously. The cause however is unknown. Heart at autopsy show changes typical of cardiomyopathy i.e. heart is large and flabby with generalised dilatation of all cardiac chambers. Microscopically the myocardial fibres show degenerative changes or fragmentation. It has been associated with malnutrition in Negroes in U.S.A. It has also been reported from Jamaica, South America, West Africa, Sudan and India.

Symptoms of heart failure begin one to four months after delivery and rapidly progresses. On examination heart is enlarged and gallop rhythm is found. E.C.G. shows non specific T wave changes. Murmurs are usually absent. Cardiac failure should be treated, with diuretics, digitalis and bed rest. Mortality may be about 30%.

**Rheumatic heart disease**

Common heart disease in pregnancy is mitral stenosis. Other heart diseases are uncommon. If the patient has severe mitral stenosis with functional class III or class IV changes, pregnancy should be deferred. If pregnancy occurs, termination of pregnancy or mitral valvotomy should be done early before 16th week of pregnancy.

With mild degrees of mitral stenosis or other forms of heart disease with class I and II functional changes, pregnancy may be allowed but careful follow up is necessary. If symptoms of failure develop in late pregnancy, careful management with rest, salt restriction, digitalis and diuretics should be carried out. Cardiac patients with pregnancy should be seen regularly at least once a fortnight during the antenatal period. The physician should always be alert to detect signs of failure i.e. oedema feet, engorged neck veins or basal rales in lungs.

The outcome of patients with heart disease in pregnancy may be as follows :—

(1) In rheumatic heart disease and acyanotic congenital abnormalities, patients with no cardiac symptoms or disability (functional Class I) may have uneventful delivery.

(2) Patients who complain of mild symptoms of dyspnoea and fatigue (Class II) require close observation throughout pregnancy. They should be advised to take rest as much as possible and do little housework. Such woman may develop more severe symptoms during pregnancy in which case digitalisation, diuretics and bed rest are indicated.

(3) Patients who are in functional class III with dyspnoea mild exertion have to be digitalis and diuretics throughout their pregnancy. At any time during antenatal or postnatal period they may develop failure. During the last trimester of pregnancy the patient may need hospitalisation for a few weeks.

(4) The most severe cases comprise functional Class IV. They are breathless even at rest. If they do not respond to digitalis or diuretics during first trimester, mitral valvotomy is indicated. If mitral regurgitation, aortic disease or congenital heart disease be present therapeutic abortion should be done in early stage.

## DRUG THERAPY IN CARDIOLOGY

*In early part of the present century very few drugs were available in the treatment of cardiac disorders. Of these drugs digitalis, quinidine, mercurial diuretics, opium derivatives, aminophylline and bromides are particularly mentionable.*

*Today we have numerous drugs for control of hypertension, I.H.D. and cardiac failure. Practitioners are often bewildered to choose proper drugs in a particular case. Pharmacology and drug interactions must be known and side-effects as well as adverse effects should be realised. Most new drugs are unsafe in pregnancy. Hence treatment of pregnancy hypertension is really a great problem. Methyl-dopa is only the sheet anchor with cautious use of diuretics. Though treatment of cardiac disorders has been discussed under various cardiac diseases, yet two special chapters on drugs used in the treatment of heart diseases have been included to assist the practitioners in choice of drugs — Editor.*

# DRUGS USED IN HEART DISEASE

*A.K. CHATTERJEE*

## Angina Pectoris

Nitrates — There are short acting and long acting nitrates. The short acting ones have been used for over 100 years.

The common side-effects are headache & fall of blood pressure (therefore not to be given where there is very low blood pressure). There is also a diminution of cardiac output.

Commonly used drugs are —

(1) Glyceryl trinitrate tab 0.3, 0.4 and 0.6 mg.

(2) Isosorbide dinitrate tab 5 & 10 mg.

(3) Pentrerythritol tetranitrate 10 & 20 mg.

(4) 2% Skin ointment for local application.

(5) I.V. nitroglycerine is also used in special situations.

*Combination of Nitrates and Sedatives*

Because anxiety plays a major role in ischaemic heart disease particularly in precipitating an anginal attack, there are some preparations available in which nitrites and sedatives or tranquilizers are widely used. Papavarine and aminophyllines are also combined along with nitrites and meprobamate.

*Beta Adenergic Blocking Drugs*

These drugs are very popular, especially in angina with hypertension, angina with cardiac arrhythmias and intractable angina. A few contraindications are bronchial asthma, presence of congestive cardiac failure and hypotension. It cannot be given in heart block. These have been discussed in the chapter on systemic hypertension.

*Other drugs used in Ischaemic heart disease*

Although the nitrates and beta blockers form the mainstay of drug regimen in I.H.D., these are the following useful drugs used in angina pectoris and I.H.D.

*Verapamil*

It reduces the myocardial oxygen demand and has very effective antiarrhythmic activity. It also slows the heart and lowers the B.P., so cannot be given in patients with low B.P. and bradycardia. Effective in coronary spasm. It is available as injection also (5 mg. in 2 ml).

*Oxyfedrine*

This drug increases coronary micro-circulation, reduces the oxygen demand of the heart, improves left ventricular function, normalises availability and utilisation of energy. It is contraindicated in aortic regurgitation, aortic stenosis and pregnancy. It can produce temporary loss of taste.

Dose — Available in tablet, oral drops and injection forms. Tablets 8 mg.-2 tab. thrice daily before food.

Drops — 10 mg. per ml. acts more quickly given sublingually (10 ml. vials.)

Injection — 4 mg. per 2 ml; 2 ml. amp should be given in a drip in post M.I. states.

Recently doubts have been expressed whether it is that effective.

*Phenylamine Lactate*

This drug dampens excessive sympathetic drive, has calcium transport inhibiting property, mild central sedative action and a mild coronary vasodilatation. Because of its first property (dampening excessive sympathetic drive) it is particularly useful in patients who face many stress situation in their everyday life and are hyper-reactors. This drug should always be used with another coronary dilator e.g. nitrates. It is contraindicated in the presence of conduction defects, in the presence of C.C.F., liver and kidney disease.

Dose — Dragees 60 mg. given two or three times a day. Rarely higher dose of 120 mg. tds may be necessary, to be reduced to two or three tablets daily.

*Lidoflazine*

This is a new addition to the group of antianginal drugs. It reduces the number of anginal attacks and improves exercise tolerance. It should be used for some weeks (minimum 6 weeks) to derive maximum benefit hence not so popular. It potentiates the action of adenosine which is a vasodilator contraindicated in pregnancy.

Dose — 60 mg. one tablet daily. Gradually increase the dose upto one tab. TDS after food.

*Nefidipine*

This is a dihydropyridine derivative which acts in angina pectoris by its calcium-entry-blocking effect to myocardial tissue.

Dose — 5 mg. x TDS upto 20 mg. TDS. To enhance effect it can be given sublingually by breaking the capsule in the mouth.

Adverse effects — Headache (usually passes off gradually after some time), dizziness, hypotension, tachycardia, fatigue, oedema, or allergic rash.

*Dilazep Hydrochloride*

This drug has a multifaceted action. It has anti-ischaemic property, protects sinus rhythm (antiarrhythmic) and prevents thrombogenesis.

It is contraindicated in first 10 days after, M.I. and should not be given in cerebral oedema. It is well tolerated but a few patients may complain of headache, giddiness, skin rash, diarrhoea and epigastric pain. In case of skin rash the drug should be stopped. It should be given for a minimum period of eight weeks.

Dose — Available in 50 mg. tablets. 50-100 mg. three times a day.

*Dipyridamole*

The drug increases coronary blood flow by reducing coronary vascular resistance. In recent years it has been found that increased adhesiveness of platelets and increase in the viscosity of blood play significant role in the pathogenesis of I.H.D. Dypyridamole reduces platelet adhesiveness and is very useful in the long-term treatment of angina pectoris, diabetes with I.H.D. and hypercholesteraemia. It is also given in combination with aspirin.

Dose — Available in 25 mg. and 100 mg. tablets. 30-300 mg. daily before food.

Side-effects — Bradycardia, hypotension, heart block, constipation and C.C.F.

*Aspirin*

Aspirin appears to be highly effective in long-term treatment of I.H.D. for prevention of myocardial infarction. The advantages are its easy availability and cheapness. It is contraindicated in peptic ulcer. Asthmatics sometimes do not tolerate aspirin.

Dose — one tab. 350 mg three times a day after food.

*Sulphin-pyrazone*

Attention to this drug was first drawn in 1965 when investigators observed that patients being treated for gout had fewer heart attacks than the general population.

The trials were started in 1975 in big hospitals in U.S.A. and Canada. In 1978 it was confirmed that sulphin-pyrazone indeed prevents further attacks and has a very significant role to play in prevention of sudden death in the first year after an attack of M.I. It is contraindicated in peptic ulcer, in patients who are on salicylate therapy and in aspirin-induced asthma.

Dose — One capsule (200 mg) four times a day.
Available in strips of 10 tablets and bottle containing 50 tablets.

**Treatment of variant angina or Prinzmetal's angina**

*(Coronary Spasm)*

In recent years considerable interest has been drawn on this subject. The condition was first described by *Prinzmetal* in 1957.

These patients have the following characteristics —

1) The pain occurs at rest — may disappear on exercise.
2) Nitrates may not relieve the pain as it always does in classic angina.
3) There is ST elevation in ECG during the attack instead of depression. The ECG may be normal.
4) Risk of sudden death is more if the spasm occurs in right coronary artery (sinus node artery).

**Drugs effective in variant angina**

1) *Verapamil* is the widely used drug for coronary spasm. It prevents the attacks and greatly diminishes their incidence. Dose 80 mg. to 240 mg. Injections of 40 mg. are also available.

   Contraindication — cannot be given in patients who have low blood pressure or conduction defects.

2) *Nifedipine* — is also very effective in coronary spasm. It has a direct cardiovascular effect without sympathetic inhibition. Dose : 5 to 10 mg. (capsule) three times a day taken with meals, it can be increased to 20 mg. three times a day. If immediate action is needed the capsule should be opened and liquid contents allowed to remain in mouth.

   Long acting preparations are now available.

   Side-effects : Well tolerated, minor side-effects like — headache, lethargy and flushing are transient. Skin rash may occur.
   Tachycardia, fall of B.P. and leg cramps may also occur.

3) *Diltiazem*

   This is the latest drug used in coronary spasm mainly in Japan and found to be useful. It is also a calcium blocker.

   Dose — Initially 30 mg QDS upto maximum — 60 mg QDS.

   Side-effects — Bradycardia, funny taste in the mouth can occur.

4) *Perhexiline Maleate*

   Effective in coronary spasm given in starting the dose of 200 to 400 mg. four times a day, and then reduced to 200 mg. daily. It decreases coronary vascular resistance and has some dilating effects on coronary vessels.

   Side-effects : Nausea, giddiness, polyneuropathy and proximal muscle (gluteus, quadriceps) myopathy, elevation of SGOT (when coronary spasm may be confused with myocardial infarction). Fortunately the side-effects disappear if the drug is discontinued. Hypoglycaemia, peripheral neuropathy, visual impairment, raised intracranial pressure and impotence may occur rarely.

**Treatment of Dysrhythmiass**

Treatment of dysrhythmia has been revolutionised during the last two decades as a large number of drugs are now available. In addition, introduction of modern pace makers and microsurgery of conducting tissues are also additional methods. Some drugs are more suitable for supraventricular dysrhythmias, which others are more useful in ventricular types. These ventricular dysrhythmias are also more dangerous.

Treatment of dysrhythmias should therefore be very cautiously prescribed. In view of this problem a separate chapter on anti-arrhythmic drugs follows this chapter. However, recognised therapy of common dysrhythmias is as follows.

*Dysrhythmias* arising in the sinus node.

1) *Sinus bradycardia* – The heart rate is below 60 per minute, regular in rhythm, ECG shows normal PQRS complexes. This rhythm disturbance occurs directly from a slow discharge rate from S.A. node. If tolerated well, it frequently needs no treatment. There are quite a few causes of sinus bradycardia. Bradycardia frequently occurs in patients having, digoxin, betablockers and verapamil. When it occurs in myocardial infarction (inferior wall type), it calls for prompt treatment.

   (a) *Atropine* – 0.6 to 1.0 mg. I.V. or subcutaneously.

   (b) *Isoprenaline* available in ampoules 4 mg. of 2 ml .

   Dose : 4 mg. to be given by drip in 500 ml of normal or dextrose saline.

   (c) Very rarely atrial pacing is required.

2) *Sick sinus syndrome – Sino Atrial Block : Sinus Arrest :*

   Considerable interest has been generated in Sick Sinus Syndrome in the last decade. This is a much more common condition than is generally believed. This is due to fibrotic changes in the S.A. node. The clinical features are dizziness and syncopal attacks. At times it can be fatal.

   Treatment is essentially the same as for sinus bradycardia. Atropine is useful in most cases but pacing may be required in a few. Ventricular pacing should be instituted as most patients of sick sinus syndrome has additional disease in A.V. junctional tissues and run the risk of complete heart block. In addition, suitable placing of the catheter in the atrium is difficult.

3) *Wandering pace maker in the sinus node*

   This is an E.C.G. diagnosis, very often seen in normal persons with sinus arrhythmia. It sometimes occurs in digoxin toxicity. No specific treatment is required except withdrawal of digitalis in case of digoxin toxicity.

*Sinus Tachycardia*

It is a very common condition. There are many causes : physiological, cardiac and extracardiac. It occurs in connection with heart disease in (a) Cardiac failure, (b) Rheumatic fever and rheumatic heart disease, (c) Subacute bacterial endocarditis and (d) Myocardial Infarction. Drugs used in sinus tachycardia are – (i) Digoxin : Initial dose is 0.25 mg. TDS or B.D. (ii) B - blockers; Propranolol : 80 to 240 mg daily orally, in divided doses. It is contraindicated in cardiac failure and dysrhythmias arising in the atrium.

*Atrial Premature Beats*

(Atrial Ectopic Beats)

It arises from the discharge of an ectopic focus anywhere in right or left atrium for no apparent reason. Occasionally they are produced in anoxia and low serum potassium.

The importance of atrial ectopics is that, they are very often a prelude to persistent dysrythmias e.g. atrial flutter and fibrillation.

Treatment – No specific treatment required except correction of electrolyte disturbance and anoxia.

*Atrial Tachycardia, Paroxysmal AV Junctional Tachycardia*
(Paroxysmal Supraventricular Tachycardia)

These two conditions are taken together because treatment is the same.

Impulses arise from an ectopic focus in the atrium with rates varying from 150 to 220 per minute. The condition is very distressing to the patient who complains of severe palpitation, giddiness, faintness, dyspnoea and angina. The patient may have a syncopal attack. It may occur in normal individuals, provoked by violent exercise, strong tea, coffee, alcohol or a sudden physical jolt. This type of dysrhythmia can occur in heart disease of any kind, particularly in ischaemic or rheumatic heart diseases and digitalis toxicity. It may complicate infection or surgical operation.

*Treatment*

The condition is not always serious as was previously thought. But if it is allowed to persist for days, it can precipitate an attack of pulmonary oedema, which may be fatal. For unknown reason some persons who are otherwise normal are more prone to attack of paroxysmal atrial tachycardia. Treatment can be divided into two groups.

*Physical Maneuvers*

The attack in many cases can be terminated by pressure on carotid sinus which lies at the level of upper border of thyroid cartilage or by soft pressure on eyeball, drinking ice cold water, putting the head between the knees and Valsalva maneuver (forcible expiration against a closed glottis). The author prefers massaging the carotid sinus as in his experience it has been almost always successful. Sometimes patients learns how to terminate the attack. If the above methods fail, drug treatment is required.

The following drugs are useful :

(1) *Digoxin* is still the drug of choice — 0.5 mg 8 hourly by mouth or 1 mg I.V. in 10 ml dextrose solution. For obvious reasons digoxin is contraindicated in digitalis toxicity.

(2) *ß-Blockers* — Propranolol can be given.

Dose of propranolol : 10 mg I.V. is most effective. It can also be given orally 80 mg initially, followed by 40 mg 8 hourly.

(3) *Verapamil* — is also useful, especially in tachycardias where there is preexcitation phenomenon, I.V. ampoules are available in 2 ml containing 5 mg of verapamil can be given as an I.V. drip - 5-10 mg hourly.

40 mg tablets are available, dose same as Propranolol.

Caution — Should not be given along with ß - blockers.

*All these three drugs mentioned above reduce the ventricular rate, but the atrial arrhythmia continues. The atrial arrhythmia can be converted to sinus rhythm by*

(a) Quinidine : 5-10 mg daily.
(b) Disopyramide : 200 - 300 mg daily
(c) ß - Blockers.

In refractory cases, D-C counter-shock should be given before which all the drugs must be withdrawn for at least twenty-four hours, otherwise there is danger of precipitating fatal ventricular fibrillation.

*Paroxysmal Atrial Tachycardia* with 2 : 1 AV Block (PATB). This condition most often is precipitated by digitalis intoxication and is aggravated by low potassium.

*Treatment* — The drug of choice is propranolol I.V. or orally, (dose mentioned before) and supplement of potassium. *D.C. counter—shock is absolutely contraindicated.*

*Atrial Flutter*

This dysrhythmia is due to atria discharging in a coordinated manner at rate of about 250-350 per minute. There is varying degree of A.V. block from 1 : 1 to 4 : 1. If the ventricular rate is rapid the patient gets symptoms. The danger of this condition is that, if ventricles beat 1 : 1 ratio there is severe haemodynamic impairment.

(i) Carotid sinus pressure may abruptly change 1 : 1 to 2 : 1, 3 : 1 or even 4 : 1 AV block and bring down the ventricular rate.

(ii) D.C. counter-shock is very effective, low energy 50W/second is required. No anaesthetic is required, 10 mg of I.V. diazepam will be sufficient.

(iii) Digoxin — I.V. route or oral route.

(iv) Propranolol — I.V. or oral route.

(v) Disopyramide : Available in 100 mg and 150 mg tablets
Dose — 200 to 300 mg daily.

*Long-term treatment of atrial flutters*

Atrial flutter is on exasperating dysrhythmia as it has a strong tendency to recur, particularly after closure of atrial septal defect. The following drugs are recommended for long-term treatment.

(a) Disopyramide — Loading dose 300 mg later 100 to 200 mg × six hourly.

(b) Quinidine sulphate available in 200 mg tablets, 200 mg three times a day. Quinidine phenyl ethyl barbiturate — 100 mg tab. three times a day can be given.

(c) Digoxin is also useful but quinidine is preferable. Digoxin in post-operation Atrial Flutter.

*Atrial Fibrillation*

This is one of the commonest forms of dysrhythmia which occurs mitral stenosis; thyrotoxicosis, myocardial infarction, after thoracotomy and in old people without any apparent cause.

Treatment — Same as Atrial Flutter.

(a) Digoxin is the drug of choice for slowing the ventricular rate by producing delay of conduction.

(b) D.C. counter-shock is helpful in A.F. of acute onset but it is not effective as a long-term measure in chronic A.F.

(c) Other drugs which can be used are quinidine and disopyramide.

Dysrhythmias arising in the A.V. node (A.V. Junction) should be called 'Junctional' in preference to 'Nodal' as it is often impossible to determine whether the focus is within the A.V. node. The conditions which will be mentioned below are all diagnosed by E.C.G., but these are often noted during constant monitoring in ICCU.

*Junctional ectopic beats and junctional rhythm* — This condition is recognised by configuration of P wave which is inverted occurring before QRS, with QRS or after QRS complex. If the P is buried with QRS, it is detected by an oesophageal lead or an intracardiac electrocardiogram.

Treatment — As these two conditions are benign and self-limiting, no treatment is necessary.

*Paroxysmal AV Junctional Tachycardia*

The treatment is the same as supra-ventricular tachycardia (atrial tachycardia). Verapamil and beta-blockers together must be avoided as shock-like states or cardiac asystole leading to sudden death has occurred in these circumstances.

**Non-Paroxysmal AV Junctional Tachycardia or Idionodal Tachycardia**

In this type of dysrhythmia, the ventricular rate is 70-140 per minute. The ventricular rate is regular and there may be retrograde conduction to atria or complete AV dissociation.

(a) *Procainamide* — Can be given orally 250-500 mg, 6 hourly or I.V. 100 mg every 5 minutes, not used widely nowadays :

(b) *Disopyramide* — ( Disopyramide phosphate).
Dose — 100 to 150 mg Q.I.D., Higher dose up to 1600 mg may be rarely required.

*Ventricular Tachycardia*

This is a serious arrhythmia as it may lead rapidly to serious haemodynamic consequence or may herald or fatal ventricular fibrillation. It occurs in ischaemic heart disease, myocardial infarction, myocarditis, cardiomyopathy and digitalis toxicity.

*Treatment* — All the measures must be prompt —

(i) *Lignocaine* (2%) — 100 mg I.V. as a bolus dose to be given slowly 5-10 minutes. Then the drug is followed by I.V. drip of lignocaine 1-4 mg per minute.

(ii) *Direct current counter-shock* (D.C. Shock) —
Should be given if there is no change after the bolus dose of lignocaine.

(iii) Other drugs mentioned in the treatment of premature ventricular contractions are also of value, but they have to be given I.V.

*Idioventricular Tachycardia* (Slow ventricular Tachycardia)

This is a benign form of dysrhythmia where the ventricles beat at the rate of 50 to 90 per minute. Diagnosis is made by E.C.G., the broad ventricular beats are not preceded or associated with usual 'P'-wave as pace maker is in the ventricle. Very often the ventricular QRS beat is wide with inverted T-wave.

*Treatment* : No treatment if infrequent. I.V. Atropine can be used to restore sinus rhythm.

*Ventricular Fibrillation*

This is the most serious form of dysrhythmia that occurs mostly in I.H.D., in the operation theatre, due to digitalis and quinidine toxicity. The patient loses consciousness and dies within a few minutes.

*Treatment*

(i) External cardiac massage.

(ii) D.C. Counter-shock — Defibrillator is necessary.

(iii) I.V. sodium bicarbonate is necessary to correct acidosis produced by circulatory arrest. 20% soln of sodium bicarbonate is available in 20 ml & 50 ml ampoules for I.V. use.

(iv) Propranolol 5-10 mg given I.V. is useful; one ml. ampoule is available containing 1 mg of Propranolol 1 mg - 2 mg is given I.V. per minute. Careful monitoring necessary.

*Parasystole* — This is a rare type of dysrhythmia. The normal sinus rhythm is not disturbed, only occasional extra beats (inter polated extra systoles) occurs in between two normal complexes.

This can occur in perfectly normal individuals but most commonly occurs in connection with myocardial infarction.

*Treatment* — Is not necessary in most cases. If the rate of parasystole is fast then suppression therapy with disopyramide, lignocaine,quinidine should be done. Rarely artificial pacing may be required to drive out the ectopic focus.

## CARDIAC ARREST

Epidemiological studies have shown that 60% of all deaths in ischaemic heart disease are sudden. This is also not infrequently seen in operation theatre, and post-operative patients and during postnatal period.

*Treatment — Stammer Technique*

S — Summon help, surface on which patient is lying should be hard.

T — Thumping which is done by a sharp blow on the midsternal region by closed fist from a distance of 12 inches above the anterior chest wall.

A — *Airway and artificial ventilation*

A clean and straight airway can be established by extending the neck with one hand under the neck and lifting it while the head is pushed backward. After doing this, mouth to mouth respiration is given directly or through a wide rubber tubing. *Air tight contact between the operator's mouth and the nose and mouth of patient is absolutely essential.* 12 to 16 inflations per minute is sufficient.

M — *External Cardiac Massage*

This acts by compressing the heart between the sternum in front and vertebra behind and sending the blood to the body. (Fig.18.36)

The correct site of compression is at the junction of upper 2/3rd of sternum and lower one-third. The compression should be of sufficient strength so as to depress the sternum by 4 to 5 cm. Rate of compression should be 60 to 80 per minute.

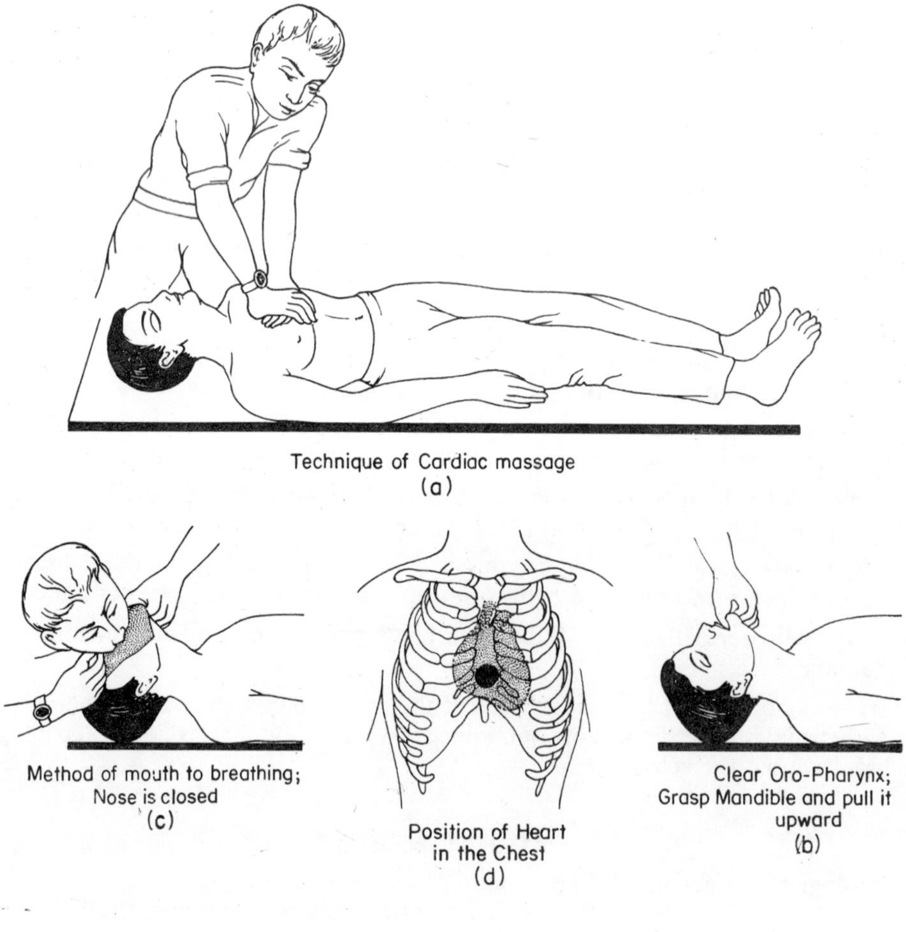


Fig.18.36 : Showing steps of external cardiac massage

M — *Medications and monitoring*

The immediately useful drugs are —

(i) Adrenaline solution (1 in 1000) — 0.5 ml given I.V. or intracardiac and can be repeated after five minutes if necessary.

(ii) Lignocaine (2%) — 50 to 100 mg I.V. followed by I.V. drip 1 to 4 mg per minute if there is any dysrhythmia.

(iii) Atropine sulphate 0.6 mg I.V. given every five minutes if there is bradycardia.

(iv) Sodium bicarbonate is essential to treat metabolic acidosis which is always present in cardiac arrest.

(v) Calcium chloride is given I.V. (can be given intracardiac) 5 ml of 10% solution.

(vi) Oxygen - 6 L/min.

Apart from the above the other useful drugs are —

Nor-adrenaline (one ml ampoule 4 mg) should be given in I.V. drip of normal saline or 5% glucose saline. Rate of drip 0.5-1 ml per minute (15 drops/minute).

**Wolff Parkinson White (W.P.W.) Syndrome**

W.P.W. syndrome occurs due to the establishment of an accessory A.V. pathway which is much shorter than the traditional A.V. pathway. It is classically found in right or left lateral atrio-ventricular groove and is known as bundle of kent.

*Treatment* — Drugs which block the accessory pathway are —

(i) Quinidine

(ii) Disopyramide

(iii) Procaine amide, 250 - 500 mg 6 hourly orally or I.V. 100 mg every 5 minutes.

(iv) Surgery — In recent years (since 1976) it has been possible to identify the site of accessory pathway using recording techniques to map the activation sequence of myocardium. Surgical interruption of accessory pathway has been carried out successfully in many cases. Surgery should be considered only in patients who have refractory drug resistant tachycardia.

**Dysrhythmia arising in the ventricles**

*Ventricular premature beat* (PVC — premature ventricular contractions) — This is the commonest type of dysrhythmia, it can occur in normal people or in any form of heart disease, more particularly so in ischaemic heart disease. Myocardial infarction, rheumatic heart disease, myocarditis, cardiomyopathy, hypokalemia and digitalis-toxicity occurring in M.I. They are very often harbingers of ventricular tachycardia which can be fatal.

*Treatment of PVC*

*Lignocaine* (Gesicard—SG Chemicals, Xylocard — Astia) 2% solution i.e. 20 mg in 1 ml available in 5 ml vials and 50 ml vials. Given as slow bolus dose — 100 mg I.V. or in a drip 1 mg per kg. body weight 100 mg in 500 ml of infusion solution (5% dextrose).

*Dopamine* — considered most useful and least dangerous drug given in shock (cardiogenic shock). Isoprenaline (Isoproterenol) — 4 mg per 2 ml ampoules (Isoprin – Unichem) given in drip method in 500 ml of normal saline or glucose saline solution. Rate 20 drops per minute.

*Corticosteroids* — It is now felt after a lot of controversy that its use in shock is definitely beneficial.

E. — Evaluation of the state of the patient.

R — *Rectification of complications* — A full record of cardiac arrest should be maintained properly. Complications arising should be carefully monitored, which include ECG monitoring, maintenance of respiration, correction of residual metabolic acidosis. All the above measures should be terminated and the patient declared dead if –

(i) The pupils remain dilated and fixed for more than 20 minutes.

(ii) If there is no signs of ventricular activity in ECG for more than 10 minutes.

**Congestive cardiac failure (C.C.F.) – Role of digitalis**

CCF has been fully discussed in a separate chapter. Though newer drugs including vasodilators are now being used in the treatment of CCF, the role of digitalis is still supreme hence it has been specially discussed here.

Digoxin – Since the discovery of William Harvey in Birmingham (England) that Foxglove leaves are useful in cardiac failure, this drug has established its permanent place in cardiac therapeutics. Foxglove is the source of digitalis alkaloids. It is better to be well acquainted with one of the preparations of digitalis.

Digoxin tablets are available as 0.25 mg white tablets and in Injection form as 0.5 mg. in 2 ml ampoule and also in syrup from (Lanoxin paediatric elixir) which contains 0.05 mg per ml of syrup.

*Actions* – 1) It lowers the venous pressure.
2) Raises the blood pressure in low output failure.
3) Slows the heart rate.
4) Relieves hepatic congestion (distension)
5) Increases capacity
6) Increases cardiac output.
7) Encourages diuresis.
8) Lowers pulmonary hypertension.
9) It has a direct action on myocardium and increases myocardial tone.

*Indications*

1) In all forms of congestive cardiac failure due to any cause.
2) Supraventricular tachycardia.
3) Atrial fibrillation.
4) Atrial flutter.

The dose schedules are of two types :–

Rapid digitalisation or slow (standard) digitalisation. Digoxin tablet is very quickly absorbed from stomach (the whole drug is absorbed within 15 minutes). So parenteral preparations are to be rarely used.

*Rapid Digitalisation* – 4 to 6 tablets stat then 4 tablets after 8 hours and 3 tablets after further 8 hours and fix-up them maintenance dose. By injection 1 mg. (2 ampoules) mixed in 25% glucose and injected slowly – useful in acute pulmonary oedema.

*Standard Digitalisation*

2 Tablets T.D.S. on 1st day.
1 Tablet Q.D.S. on 2nd day.
1 Tablet T.D.S. on 3rd day.
then 1 tablet daily or B.D.

It should be remembered that elderly patients above 60 years and children are very susceptible to digoxin so a lower dose have to be used for them.

*Side-effects and Toxic effects*

Unfortunately the gap between therapeutic dose and toxic dose of digitalis is very small. So constant watch has to be maintained for any toxic manifestation. Because of its toxic effects its use became less after 2nd world war. But in the last decade it has been seen that most toxic effects can be prevented with supplements of potassium. So the drug has again come back in the picture.

*Toxic effects :*

1) G.I. System — Anorexia, nausea, vomiting, diarrhoea, epigastric pain.
2) C.V. System — Ectopic beats, coupling nodal, rhythm, heart block, paroxysmal atrial tachycardia with block (PATB) sudden death due to ventricular fibrillation.
3) Others — Hypovolemia (very important), mental confusion, Headache, drowsiness, visual disturbance with yellow vision.

*Contraindications*

1) All types of heart block.
2) Marked bradycardia.

*Resistance to Digitalis*

This phenomenon, though rare, occurs sometimes in patients of mitral regurgitation, thyrotoxicosis, cor pulmonale and other hyperkinetic circulatory states. In this event other drugs or measures has to be resorted to.

*Low Sodium Diet*

After the discovery of powerful diuretics it is not mandatory for patients of C.C.F. to take a salt ree diet. However, taste is matter of habit and even with low salt diet patients gets used to salt restricted. However, physician has to look into the problem and convince the patient about it. If better result is obtained by salt restriction, side-effects of diuretics can be avoided.

## ANTI-ARRHYTHMIC DRUGS

*RAMANUJA DAS GUPTA*

In the past couple of decades numerous drugs with varied anti-arrhythmic properties and modes of action have become available. This in the background of more precise knowledge of the arrhythmias, has made detailed classification and knowledge of these drugs imperative, for the sake of correct usage.

On the basis of *in vitro* electrophysiological studies the anti-arrhythmic drugs are classified as follows :

**Classification (Vaughan, Williams and Singh)**

I. Inhibit fast $Na^+$ channel. Decrease phase O action potential. Membrane stabilizing agents :

A) Increase action potential duration and effective refractory period e.g. quinidine, procainamide and disopyramide.

B) Decreases action potential duration and increases outward $K^+$ current; decreases effective refractory period in ventricular tissue : e.g. lidocaine, phenytoin, mexiletine, tocainide and aprindine.

C) No effect on action potential duration or refractoriness, e.g. encainide, lorcainide, flecainide, cibenzoline and propafenone.

II. Beta antagonist : Block cardiac β receptors e.g. propranolol group of drugs.

III. Agents which widen action potential duration : e.g. amiodarone, bretylium, sotalol, β–n– acetyl procainamide, melperone.

IV. Inhibit slow $Ca^+$ channel (esp. AV node) : verapamil, diltiazem and bepridil.

**Anti-arrhythmic drugs**

**Quinidine (Class IA)**

**Action** – Quinidine slows phase O, resting membrane potential is unaltered. It depresses tendency for spontaneous diastolic depolarization and prolongs ERP in atria, ventricles. His Purkinje system and bypass tracts.

**Pharmacokinetics** – Quinidine is metabolised by hydroxylation in liver : small amount is excreted by kidneys. Therapeutic blood level 2.3-5 μg/mL.

**Administration** – Test dose – 0.2 gm Quinidine Sulphate by mouth. Dose – 0.2-0.3 gm orally every 3-4 hrs; total dose 1.2–1.6 gm/day (max. 2 g/day). Check with repeated ECG and plasma level (when possible). Long acting preparations – quinidine gluconate, quinidine polygalacuronate.

USE – Conversion of A.F. to sinus rhythm.

Maintenance of sinus rhythm after cardioversion.

**Side effects** –
1. Prolongation of QRS duration. May lead to Torsades de pointes.
2. Depression of sinus and AV node in sick sinus syndrome.
3. May worsen digitalis toxicity. Increases blood digoxin level.
4. Diarrhoea, nausea, headache, dizziness, cinchonism, visual disturbance, disturbed hearing, thrombocytopenic purpura, agranulocytosis and cardiovascular collapse.

**Drug interactions** – Quinidine increases blood digoxin level. There is interaction with β-blockers, coumarin anticoagulants and amiodarone. Low serum K decreases quinidine efficacy.

**Lidocaine (Xylocaine) (Class IB)**

**Action** – Lidocaine acts preferentially on ischaemic myocardium, it is more effective in absence of hypokalaemia.

**Pharmacokinetics** – Lidocaine is de-ethylated by liver microsomes.

Effective blood level 1.4–6.0 μg/mL (toxic over – 9 μg/mL).

Single bolus lasts only for few minutes.

**Administration** – Loading dose – 50-100 mg IV or 300 mg/IM.

This is followed by continuous infusion @ 1–4 mg/min.

The dosage should be reduced in case of poor liver blood flow, liver disease, cimetidine therapy and in elderly patients.

**Side effects** – Drowsiness, numbness, speech disturbance, and dizziness. Asystole has been reported.

**Procainamide (Class IA)**

**Action** – Procainamide resembles quinidine but QT prolongation is less. It may be used intravenously.

**Pharmacokinetics** — Rapid renal elimination occurs (half-life 3.5 hrs.). Effective blood level is 4-10 μg/ML. Plasma metabolism — acetylation converts it to N-acetyl procainamide (half life 6-8 hrs.).

**Use** — Effective is prevention of ventricular arrhythmias early after myocardial infarction. It is often effective when lidocaine fails.

**Contra-indication** — Shock, heart failure, myasthenia gravis, renal failure and heart block.

**Side effects** —
1. Fall of BP when used by IV route
2. Heart block
3. Vagolytic effect — may exaggerate post occlusion ventricular arrhythmias. It is can worsen myasthenia gravis.
4. Rash, fever, arthralgia, lupus like syndrome, and agranulocytosis.

**Newer Antiarrhythmic Agents**

**Disopyramide** (Class 1A) — It is a quinidine like drug.

**Action** — Like quinidine. Potent anticholinergic and negative inotropic action; increases peripheral resistance. Increases refractoriness of accessory AV Pathways.

**Indications** —
1. As quinidine. Controls ventricular tachyarrhythmias.
2. Reduces recurrence of arrhythmia after D.C. cardioversion.
3. Effective against atrial arrhythmias complicating WPW syndrome as it depresses conduction via bundle of Kent. It is less effective against other atrial arrhythmias.
4. Arrhythmias complicating mitral valve prolapse.

**Pharmacokinetics** — It is not metabolised in liver.

Half life 8 hrs but prolonged in renal failure, and acute myocardial infarction. Blood level 2—6 mg.ml (Toxic over mg/ml)

**Dosage** — Intravenously — 2 mg/kg/5 min (Max. 150 mg — upto 300 mg/1st hour). Then 0.4 mg/kg

Oral — 300 mg loading dose — then 100-200 mg 6 hourly.

**Side effects** — Hypotension, heart failure, tachycardia (Torsades de Pointes). Sinus node depression, coronary vaso-constriction, QRS widening and anti-cholinergic effects. Avoid loading dose if there is cardiomegaly.

**Contraindications** Uncompensated congestive heart failure, urinary retention, glaucoma, hypotension, This drug should not be used in presence of renal failure.

**Drug interactions** — Not effective in digitalis toxicity. Given intravenously, cardiac output falls when added to β-blockers and calcium channel antagonists. Combination with quinidine, digoxin, methyldopa is not advised.

**Phenytoin** (Class 1B)

**Uses** — Narrow spectrum of activity. Effective against :
1. Atrial and ventricular arrhythmias due to digitalis toxicity.
2. Torsades de pointes.

**Therapeutic plasma level** — 6 to 20 mg/L : Metabolism — eliminated by liver, after microsomal hydroxylation to parahydroxy-phenylhydantoin, which is devoid of antiarrhythmic properties.

**Dosage** — Intravenously 200 mg (@ 5 mg/min) (watch BP carefully). Oral maintenance dose 100 to 300 mg/day (single or divided doses).

**Toxicity** — Hypotension, sinus bradycardia, ventricular fibrillation, blurred vision, dizziness, vertigo, nausea, nystagmus, ataxia, drowsiness, megaloblastic anaemia, lymphoma-like syndrome, gingival hyperplasia, skin rash (rarely toxic epidermal necrolysis).

Prenatal exposure — Craniofacial and skeletal abnormalities (40%).

**Lidocaine-like agents** (Class 1B)

**Mexiletine (Class 1B)** This drug has been called oral lidocaine. It possesses additional quinidine-like (Class 1A) and anticonvulsant properties.

**Major therapeutic uses** — Chronic oral prophylaxis of ventricular arrhythmias after myocardial infarction). It may be combined with quinidine.

**Pharmacokinetics** — Half life — 10 hrs (longer after cardiac infarction).

**Blood level** — 0.5—2.0 µg/mL (toxic level = 1.5—3.0 µg/mL).

**Side effects** — Fine tremor, nystagmus, dizziness, diplopia, dysarthria, ataxia, indigestion, nausea, bradycardia, fall in BP, increased QRS duration. Not effective in supraventricular tachyarrhythmias. Skin rash can occur.

**Dose** — Intravenously 150-250 mg/5 min.
total 750 mg/3 hrs , followed by 0.5-1.0 mg/min.

**Oral** — 200-300 mg. every 8 hrs. Loading dose 400-600 mg.

**Tocainide (Class 1B)**

**Major use** — Serious ventricular arrhythmias resistant to quinidine, procainamide and propranolol. Used for prophylaxis. Effective in AV nodal re-entrant tachycardia and AV re-entrant tachycardia using by-pass tract.

**Pharmacokinetics** — Half life = 13.5 hours. Therapeutic level 5-15 µg/mL.

**Side effects** — Anorexia, nausea, vomiting, dizziness, cerebellar signs, visual disturbance. Increased systemic and pulmonary vascular resistances. Rash, blood dyscrasias pericarditis, pulmonary fibrosis, fibrosing alveolitis, interstitial pneumonitis. Occasional worsening of cardiac arrhythmia may occur.

**Dose** — Intravenously 0.5 — 0.75 mg/kg/min × 15 min. Oral loading dose 400-800 mg then 8 hourly.

**Aprindine (Class 1B)**

**Use** — Against VPC and VT (specially digitalis toxicity). Effective in SVT, WPW Syndrome, drug resistant ventricular arrhythmias associated with mitral valve prolapse. Prevents recurrence of AF.

**Pharmacokinetics** — Blood level 1 to 3 mg/L. Metabolised in liver.

**Toxicity** — Polymorphic VT can occur. It has negative inotropic properties. Other adverse affects include tremor, nervousness, dizziness, ataxia, seizure, psychosis, agranulocytosis, cholestatic jaundice.

**Dosage** — Intravenously 150-250 mg/5 min. total 750 mg/3 hrs. followed by 0.5—1.0 mg/min. or divided doses).

**Encainide (Class 1C)**

**Action** — Reduces conduction velocity in specialised tissue. Increases AV conduction time and QRS duration. No effect on action potential duration or refractoriness. Effective against experimental atrial arrhythmias, sometimes VPC and recurrent VT. Therapeutic plasma concentration 1-56 ng/ml. Toxic level — 135—570 ng/ml.

**Toxicity** — May cause or aggravate polymorphic VT (not necessarily with prolonged QT interval).

**Side effects** — Ataxia, diplopia, dizziness, tremor, headache.

**Flecainide acetate (Class 1C)**

**Action** — Slow and conduction increases refractoriness in slow and fast response tissues.

**Effects** — Suppresses VPC and non-sustained VT.

**Therapeutic plasma level** — 0.3 to 1.4 mg/L.

**Administration** — I.V. loading dose 1 mg/kg body wt./5 min. Additional boluses 0.5 mg/kg every 30 min. Total dose — 2.0 mg/kg.

Oral dose — 200-600 mg/day — given in two divided doses.

**Toxicity** — Blurred vision,abnormal taste, flushing, tinnitus, sleepiness, paraesthesias, increased serum alkaline phosphatase.

**Beta Adrenergic Receptor Antagonists (Class II)**

**Propranolol** — Competitively blocks effects of catecholamines on the heart. Indirectly reduces slow inward current that contributes to action potential. Exerts direct membrane stabilising effect in high dose.

**Anti-arrhythmic effects** —

Propranolol is effective against

1. Atrial tachyarrhythmias
2. AV nodal reentrant tachycardia
3. AV reentrant tachycardia using accessory AV pathway
4. Ventricular premature beats
5. Exercise provoked ventricular tachycardia
6. Torsades de Pointes (with prolonged QT)
7. Arrhythmias of digitalis toxicity
8. Reduces risk of sudden death in first year after acute myocardial infarction.

**Dosage** — Inravenously 0.1 to 0.2 mg/kg body wt. given @ 1-2 mg every 3-5 min. Oral administration — 40 mg to 1 gm — daily in 2 to 4 divided doses.

**Toxicity** — CVS — negative inotropy, sinus bradycardia, AV nodal block; circulatory collapse, peripheral vasospasm Extracardiac effects — nausea, vomiting, bronchospasm, diarrhoea, fatigue, insomnia, nightmares, impotence.

**Precaution** — Avoid its use in diabetes unless there is an overriding indication.

**Newer — Adrenergic receptor antagonists :-**

**Selective $\beta$ Blockers** — Metoprolol, Atenolol, Acebutol

**Less Lipophilic $\beta$ Blockers** — Atenolol, Nadolol, Timolol

**Intrinsic Sympathomimetic Activity** — Pindolol

(Refer also to the chapter on Hypertension and anti-anginal drags)

**Amiodarone (Class III)**

**Action** — 1. Increases ERP by prolonged action potential duration
2. Coronary and peripheral vasodilator
3. Calcium channel antagonist.

**Uses** — 1. Atrial flutter-fibrillation in WPW syndrome
2. Life threatening ventricular tachyarrhythmias. Recurrent cardiac arrest.
3. Paroxysmal atrial fibrillation or flutter.
Paroxysmal supraventricular tachycardia
4. Maintains sinus rhythm after cardioversion of atrial fibrillation
5. AV nodal reentrant tachycardia
6. AV reentrant tachycardia using accessory AV pathway.

**Pharmacokinetics** — Half life — 15 to 105 days.
A loading dose is required — peak effect may take weeks. Contains iodine; inhibits conversion of T4 to T3. Not excreted by kidneys.

**Dosage** — Intravenous 5 mg/Kg/5 min. then infusion @ 25 mg/hr. Oral — Loading dose 1200 — 1600 mg daily for 7—14 days. Maintenance dose 200-800 mg once daily.

**Contraindication** — SA block, AV block.

**Drug Interaction** — Digoxin, quinidine, procaine amide (increased blood level), coumarin (bleeding tendency).

**Side-effects** — Corneal microdeposits (whorl-like pigmentation, cornea verticillata), halovision, photo-sensitivity, slate-gray or bluish skin discolouration, proximal muscle, weakness, peripheral neuropathy tremor, impaired memory, insomnia, pulmonary infiltrates, hyper or hypothyroidism. Torsades de pointes, VF, hypotension, constipation, nausea, vomiting.

**Bretylium Tosylate (Class III)**

**Action and indication** —
1. VF refractory to lidocaine and multiple D.C. shocks
2. Resistant ventricular arrhythmias (may take 20-40 minutes)
3. Causes hypotension
4. Adrenergic neurone blocking properties.

**Pharmacokinetics** — No liver metabolism. Half life 7.5 hours

**Toxicity** — Nausea, vomiting, parotid pain, postural hypotension, worsening of arrhythmia.

**Contra-indication** — Digitalis toxicity.

**Dose** — Intravenous 5 to 10 mg/kg. D.C. shock may be applied if required.
Maintenance dose 5 - 10 mg/kg IV every 6 to 8 hours or infusion @ 1-2 mg/min.

**Calcium channel blocking drugs (Class IV)**

**Verapamil** — Actions :
1. Reduces slow inward current which contributes to action potential plateau of cardiac fast response tissue and AV node.

2. Depresses conduction of injured fast response tissues.
3. Slows ventricular response to atrial fibrillation or flutter but may speed up response in patients with WPW Syndrome.

**Use** — 1. Supra-ventricular tachycardia
2. Atrial fibrillation or flutter (beware of WPW syndrome)
3. Ventricular arrhythmias, e.g. ventricular tachycardia.

**Dose** — Intravenous 5-10 mg/given over 2-5 min. May repeat same dose after 10 min. It may be given as infusion @ 0.00 25 mg/kg/min. Oral dose 120 mg - 480 mg/day in divided doses.

**Toxicity** — CVS — hypotension, negative inotropy, bradycardia, asystole. AV block. Other adverse symptoms : headache, dizziness, vertigo, nausea, constipation, epigastric discomfort.

**Diltiazem**

**Action** — At low concentration it blocks slow inward $Ca^{++}$ current but at higher concentration it may also block fast inward $Ca^{++}$ current. It depresses both retrograde and antegrade AV nodal conduction. Diltiazem prolongs AV nodal refractoriness (less than verapamil). It is effective against AV nodal reentrant tachycardia and AV reentrant tachycardia using accessory AV pathway.

**Side effects** — CVS — Flushing, hypotension, bradycardia, palpitation, congestive heart failure and syncope.

Other adverse effects — oedema, headache, dizziness, paraesthesia, somnolence, tremor, constipation, dyspepsia, diarrhoea, vomiting, rash.

**Dosage** — Oral — 90-360 mg/day (in 3 or 4 divided doses). I.V. 0.15-0.25 mg/kg given over 2 mins.

**Antiarrhythmic drug therapy**

**Basic approach** — Assess the following :

1) What is the arrhythmia (i.e. recognition) ?
2) Is treatment necessary ?
3) If so, how urgently is treatment necessary ?
4) Are there any underlying or potentiating factors ? What measure are necessary to correct them ?

**Methods of Assessment**

1) Clinical assessment (including detailed history) and ECG (especially during dysrhythmia)
2) Holter monitoring — documentation of onset may be invaluable
3) Exercise testing — may be helpful.
4) Invasive electrophysiologic testing — in some cases.

GUIDELINES OF MANAGEMENT OF ARRHYTHMIAS

**Atrial Fibrillation (AF)**

1. Control ventricular response : Digitalis, β-blockers and verapamil
2. Cardioversion :
   (a) Drugs — Quinidine, procainamide, disopyramide and amiodarone;
   (b) Electrical D.C. Shock (Synchronised)

3. Drugs to prevent recurrences
   Quinidine, procainamide, disopyramide, aprindine and amiodarone
4. WPW Syndromes — Digoxin and verapamil may increase ventricular response. Quinidine, procainamide, disopyramide and amiodarone
5. Role of Surgery

**Atrial Flutter**

1. Drug therapy as for atrial fibrillation
2. Cardioversion — D.C. Shock (usually about 25-50 Joules is adequate)
3. Pacing techniques

**Atrial Tachycardias**

**Non-Paroxysmal atrial tachycardia with AV block**

Consider digitalis toxicity

Drugs — as for AF and flutter

Surgery — May help selected patients

**Paroxysmal Supra-Ventricular Tachycardia**

I. Maneuvers to augment vagal activity
II. Drugs-IV Verapamil, Propranolol, Digoxin.
III. Electrical cardioversion.
IV. Drugs to prevent recurrence —
   (a) Depress antegrade conduction through AV node — Verapamil, Digoxin, Beta blockers.
   (b) Depress retrograde conduction through AV node or accessory pathway — Quinidine, Procaine amide, Disopyramide.
V. Pacemaker therapy.
VI. Surgery

**Ventricular Tachycardia (VT) & Ventricular Fibrillation (VF)**

**ACUTE STAGE —**

TO RESTORE SINUS RHYTHM

VF — D.C. Shock.

VT — Lidocaine, Procaine amide, Bretylium ± D.C. Shock (Synchronised)

**CHRONIC STAGE — VT**

Nonsustained VT — Lidocaine like drugs including Aprindine, Mexiletine.

Psychologic stress — Provoked VT — Phenytoin, Propranolol, Digitalis.

Pacing provoked VT — Variable response to different drugs

Refractory VT — 1) Try Amiodarone
2) Antitachycardia pacing
3) Surgery

REFERENCES :-

(1) "Antiarrhythmic Agents" by B.N. Singh, L.H. Opie, F.I. Marcus in Drugs for the Heart (Ed. L.H. Opie 1984) Grune & Stratton Inc.

(2) "Clinical Pharmacology of Conventional and Newer Anti-arrhythmic Drugs" by T.E. Bump in Principles and Practice of Acute Cardiac Care (Ed. D.S. Dasgupta, 1984) York Book Medical Publishers, Inc.

# CHAPTER – 19
# MISCELLANEOUS

## MALARIA – UPDATE

*N.R. KRISHNAN*
*A.R. SUBRAMANIAN*

[ *Malaria has been discussed in the Chapter-7. In this chapter two senior and eminent specialists of the Armed Forces have presented the latest update on the subject, particularly contributing their experience from the Armed Forces with special reference to preventive measures. This, however, does not represent the official directive of the Army, Navy or Air Force. – Editor* ]

Malaria is a pyrexial disorder characterized by periodic fever, progressive anaemia and splenomegaly. It is caused by the sporozoa belonging to the genus plasmodium. The plasmodia which are infective to man are P. malariae, P. ovale, P. vivax and P. falciparum, the last two being responsible for almost all cases of malaria in India. The vector responsible for transmission of the infection from man or animal to man are the female mosquitoes of the genus Anopheles.

The parasite undergoes a life cycle of 8-20 days in 2 phases, the asexual cycle or schizogony in man followed by the sexual cycle in the female anopheles mosquito both of which are essential for survival of the species. The asexual cycle in case of P. vivax, P. ovale and P. malaria consists of a primary exoerythrocytic or tissue phase, an erythrocytic phase and a secondary tissue phase, the last one maintaining the infection in the host for a prolonged period resulting in relapses. In case of P. falciparum there is no secondary exoerythrocytic phase and hence relapses are absent.

**Pathology**

The main pathological process in malaria is the invasion and destruction of erythrocytes, by the parasites. When the falciparum merozoite enters the red blood cell (RBC) it produces inherent changes in the RBC itself, the external surface or membrane becoming sticky. This leads to aggregation of RBC especially in the deeper capillaries of brain and other organs causing obstruction. This results in peticheal haemorrhages and ischaemic changes in different organs like brain, kidney and liver. The reticuloendothelial cells of liver, spleen and bone marrow, react with intense phagocytic activity and proliferation causing enlargement of liver and spleen. The rupture of infected RBC leads to anaemia. Details have been discussed in chapter 9.

More severe and life threatening cases of falciparum malaria may present as – (a) hyperpyrexia, (b) cerebral malaria, (c) gastrointestinal type, (d) algid malaria, (e) black water fever or (f) renal failure

*In the hyperpyrexic form the temperature may be as high as 41 to 41.5° C* and may be mistaken for heat stroke and vice versa. It is often associated with cerebral manifestations.

Cerebral malaria is the most dangerous and often fatal manifestation of P. falciparum infection. There is often hyperparasitaemia and the parasite count exceeds 100,000 per cmm. More than 5% of the RBC may be infected and many RBC may show more than one parasite. In some cases this may not be seen due either to previous but inadequate treatment or to sequestration of parasites in deep capillaries. Cerebral oedema was supposed to be one of the causes of many of the neurological manifestations but the evidence for the same is very meagre. The autopsy finding of cerebral oedema is probably due to terminal phases of cerebral anoxia in the fatal cases.

Patient becomes drowsy and comatose. He may be disoriented and delirious and some cases may present as acute mania. Muscular twitchings, convulsions, aphasia, monoplegia or hemiplegia may occur. In some cases due to superadded infection septicaemia with shock may set in. Less than 5% of patients show overt signs of disseminated intravascular clotting (DIC). Acute renal failure is an important and fatal complication.

The gastrointestinal form of falciparum malaria may present as acute watery diarrhoea and vomiting, acute dysentry or increasing jaundice and acute liver cell failure. In the algid type there is acute peripheral circulatory failure and shock. Black water fever is due to acute haemolysis with haemoglobinaemia and haemoglobinuria.

**Treatment — update**

There is no single drug which is effective against all stages of the parasite i.e. sporozoite, schizont, tissue forms and the gametocytes. Table-19.1 shows the list of drugs available for the treatment of and prophylaxis against malaria.

The most important problem in modern malariology is the development of resistance of malaria parasites, especially P. falciparum to many anti-malarial drugs. Resistance to chloroquine is widespread including parts of India. Many of these strains are also resistant to pyrimethamine. In Thailand and the Philippines diminished sensitivity of P. falciparum to quinine has been reported. Resistance to long-acting sulfa-pyrimethamine combination is also spreading to many parts of the world. Although the newer drug mefloquine is at present used under the control and supervision of WHO, resistance to the drug has already been reported.

**Table-19.1 : Anti-Malarial Drugs**

| Group | Drug |
|---|---|
| A. Cinchona Alkaloid | Quinine<br>Quinidine |
| B. Acridine | Mepacrine |
| C. 5 Aminoquinolines | Chloroquine<br>Amodiaquine |
| D. 8 Aminoquinoline | Primaquine<br>Quinocide |
| E. Antifolates (Dihydrofolate reductase Inhibitors) | Proguanil<br>Pyrimethamine<br>Cycloguanil-Embonate<br>Trimethoprim |
| F. Para Aminobenzoic acid inhibitors | 1. *Sulfones* :<br>Dapsone<br>Acedapsone<br>2. *Sulfonamides* :<br>Sulfadoxine<br>Sulfalene<br>Sulfadimethoxine<br>Sulfamethoxypyrdiazine<br>Sulfadiazine |
| G. Antibiotics | Tetracycline<br>Doxycycline<br>Minocycline |

H. Newer drugs on trial — Mefloquine, Quinghaosu, Halofantrine

**Falciparum Malaria**

Chloroquine in a dosage of 25 mg/kg body weight over three days is the drug of choice in uncomplicated cases, in areas where resistance to the drug is not present. The schedule advised is 600 mg of the base initially given orally followed by 300 mg after 6 hours on the first day and then 300 mg daily for next 2 days. If the patient is having persistent vomiting or diarrhoea or is comatose or has parasite count over 100,000/cmm, parenteral therapy is advisable.Chloroquine 200 mg base given every 8 hours, if necessary. It should be given very slowly and well diluted. The dose of 800 mg of chloroquine base over 24 hours should not be exceeded. If the case is very serious and the sensitivity of the parasite in the area to chloroquine is not known, it is better to use quinine parenterally as mentioned under cerebral malaria. As soon as possible oral administration must be undertaken. In areas where resistance to 4 amino-quinolines is present but not to antifolate-sulfa combinations the schedule recommended in uncomplicated case is quinine 600 mg orally 8-hourly for 5 days and a single dose of sulfalene or sulfadoxine 1500 mg with pyrimethamine 75 mg on the 6th day. If there is resistance to antifolate and sulfas,also give quinine for 7 days together with tetracycline 500 mg twice daily for 7 days. When quinine is not available, quinidine in same doses may be used provided the patient has no cardiovascular complications.

In cerebral malaria i.v. quinine hydrochloride must be given and not chloroquine. If the patient has not had any quinine previously a loading dose of 20 mg/kg body weight diluted in 500 ml of glucose saline must be given as an intravenous drip over a period of 4 hours. If necessary, it can be repeated 8-hourly in a dosage of 10 mg/kg body weight till oral therapy is possible. Patient's blood glucose level has to be monitored to guard against hypoglycaemic attacks which is common in patients with severe malaria with hyperparasitaemia and pregnant women. The diagnosis of hypoglycaemia should be considered in all cases of falciparum malaria, but especially in those with severe disease, if there is a change in the level of consciousness, deepening coma, abnormal behaviour, fits or any other deterioration of the clinical condition of the patient. Recurring hypoglycaemic episodes depsite i.v. glucose administration presents a major problem in treatment. The pathogensis of hypoglycaemia is complex involving, (a) drug (quinine) induced hyperinsulinaemia, (b) glucose requirement of parasites and (c) possibly endotoxaemias. Corticosteroids though widely used in the past are better avoided as it has been found to significantly prolong unconsciousness and increase incidence of complications. As mentioned earlier there is little clinical evidence of cerebral oedema in cerebral malaria. If there is bleeding due to DIC, blood transfusion should be given and heparin avoided. Symptomatic treatment includes proper nursing care, good hydration, use of anti-convulsants and antimicrobials in case of superadded infection.

Prevention of further transmission of infection from patients to others can be ensured only by complementaryschizonticidal treatment with a gametocidal drug. A single dose of primaquine 30-45 mg is sufficient.

*P. Vivax Malaria*

Chloroquine is the drug of choice and is given for 3 days as for P. falciparum malaria. To eradicate the tissue form and provide a radical cure,primaquine 15 mg base daily in 2 divided doses, is started on the 4th day and continued up to 14th day. It should be avoided in patients with G-6 P.D. deficiency.

*Malaria and Pregnancy*

Malaria, especially P. falciparum infection during pregnancy poses a great danger to both the mother and foetus. The mortality is 10 times more. Fear that quinine in therapeutic doses may cause abortion is exaggerated. Chemoprophylaxis throughout pregnancy while the patient is in an endemic area is imperative. Chloroquine or sulfa-antifolate combination with supplements of folinic acid may be used.

**Chemoprophylaxis**

For a successful regimen of chemoprophylaxis several variable factors must be taken into consideration. These are drug resistance, the period of exposure, the degree of exposure, the season of exposure and the compliance of the drug regimen.

Range of drugs available is limited to 4 amino-quinoline and combinations of pyrimethamine, sulfadoxine and dapsone. Pyrimethamine alone is not adequate and status of proguanil is uncertain. If a drug is to be effective sufficient concentration must be obtained in blood by the time the parasite enters blood — 6 to 10 days after start of exposure to infection. Chloroquine 5 mg/kg body weight is given for 2 consecutive days and then repeated weekly. Start therapy one week prior to exposure and continue for 4 weeks after exposure is over. Alternatively, a weekly dose of one tablet containing 500 mg of sulfadoxine with 25 mg pyrimethamine started 1-2 weeks before exposure will be adequate. If total cumulative dose of chloroquine base exceeds 100g, risk of retinopathy is there. When the stay of an individual in an endemic area is going to be long, it is better to adopt other preventive measures and treat malaria as and when it occurs. The only semi-immune individuals in malarial area for whom suppression therapy is indicated are pregnant women.

Along with chemoprophylaxis other antimosquito measures and personal protection against mosquito bite must be undertaken for an effective malaria control programme.

**Immunoprophylaxis**

Recent immunological researches have opened up possibilities of a malaria vaccine though here one is faced with the problem of type specificity, strain specificity and phase-specificity of the antigens. Two stages stand out for use as potential antigen for immunoprophylaxis and both are asexual stages — sporozoites and the erythrocytic forms (trophozoites and merozoites). The different approaches to vaccination are complementary and the ideal should be to combine them, e.g. a merozoite/gamete antigen mixture that would alleviate clinical malaria and prevent spread of the infection. Malaria vaccine once produced should not be considered as a replacement for other control measures. Chemotherapy and vaccination could be combined effectively for a proper malaria control programme.

## DRUGS RESISTANCE AND CHEMOPROPHYLAXIS OF FALCIPARUM MALARIA

*N.R. KRISHNAN*
*A.R. SUBRAMANIAN*
*A.C. ANAND*

**Definition and assessment of drug resistance**

Drug resistance in malaria has been defined as "the ability of a parasite to survive and/or to multiply despite the administration and absorption of a drug given in dosage equal to or higher than those usually recommended but within the limits of tolerance of the subject". Recent data suggest that it may have to be qualified by a statement that 'the form of drug active against the parasite must gain access to the parasite or infected RBC for the duration of time necessary for its normal action'

Implicit in the definition is a wide spectrum of parasite response to an antimalarial drug, from mere survival at subclinical level with subsequent recrudescence to active multiplication during the course of therapy. It is assessed by *in vivo* and *in vitro* tests. Extended field test is the important *in vivo* test wherein the patient's blood smear is tested every day for first 7 days after chloroquine administration followed by twice a week for next three weeks. Results are expressed as S or sensitivity (clearance of a sexual parasitaemia within 7 days of initiation of treatment without subsequent recrudescence), $R_i$ or Resistance at level 1 (clearance of asexual parasitaemia but followed by recrudescence), $R_{ii}$ (marked reduction in parasitaemia but no clearance) or $R_{iii}$ (no or minimal reduction in parasitaemia).

One can also express the result as average parasite clearance time. Recent introduction of micro (*in vitro*) test, utilising 0.1 ml blood, has made the assessment of drug resistance convenient and quick.

**Distribution of drug resistance**

Chloroquine resistance in P. falciparum was first confirmed in Thailand in 1959 and almost simultaneously it appeared in a totally independent focus in Columbia. In the following years it showed a centrifugal spread to its present state extending from Vanuate to Central India in Asia, a wide area east of Panama Canal in South America and recently in some east African countries. In India the earliest reports appeared from Diphu and Nowgong (Assam) in 1973 and this was followed by several reports of drug resistance from other parts of North-Eastern states, from Delhi, U.P., Haryana and Maharashtra. Presently most of the drug resistance found in India is at the $R_i$ level with occasional sporadic reports of $R_{ii}$ and $R_{iii}$ resistance from various places, mainly from the North-Eastern region.

**Mechanism of drug resistance**

The knowledge of the exact mechanism of drug resistance is incomplete and the present views are summarised in Table-19.2(a) & 2(b). Hematin, a transient breakdown product of haemoglobin, readily disrupts plasmodia and host membranes. P. Falciparum synthesises a protein which combines with haematin to form a harmless pigment-haemozoin. Chloroquine probably binds to hematin to form even more haemolytic compound which disrupts plasmodial membranes.

How the resistant parasite avoids it at the molecular level is not clearly known but they have been shown to synthesise excessive amounts of segregating protein and have larger surface area permitting more efficient pinocytosis.

**Drug treatment of resistant malaria**

Several anti-malarials are available at present to treat drug resistant malaria. Present recommendations (Table-19.3) are based on experience in India and abroad. It is important that intravenous quinine be used wnen patient is having vomiting or severe diarrhoea, or patient is comatose or when parasite count is very high (100,000/cumm.).

Quinine remains the sheet-anchor of therapy for resistant malaria today and is given in the dosage of 600-650 mg 8 hourly for 7 to 14 days. Intravenous preparation is available and should be dissolved in 200 ml. of saline and infused over 20-30 minutes. In areas where higher grades of resistance are known to be present, quinine should be combined with tetracycline 250 - 500 mg six hourly for 7 to 10 days.

In India, single dose of sulfadiazine (or sulfaline) + Pyrimethamine combination continues to be effective alternative for the treatment of resistant P. falciparum infection, though reports of resistance to this combination have started appearing from Thailand. Another two drugs with good promise for such therapy are mefloquin and artimisinine (Qing - hao - su). Mefloquin is an aminoalcohol which is introduced in late 1970s. It is well-tolerated and has shown consistently good results (cure rate>95%) with the dose range of 12.5 to 20 mg base/kg (single dose). Malariologists all over the world are now thinking whether it would be wise to make widespread use of this drug or a rational combination can be used to delay the emergence of resistance. Presently fixed dose combinations of mefloquin, sulfadoxin and Pyrimethamine in the ratio of 10:20:1 are being evaluated by WHO for this purpose. Qing-hao-su is the active ingredient of the Chinese herb Qing Hao (Artemisia Annua L.). Although it was being used for over 1000 years in China, clinical trials with purified extract have been conducted only in the last decade and have shown good results in resistant cases with parenteral therapy. Presently the search for alternative drugs for treatment of resistant P. falciparum is still on and biological and biochemical aspects of Plasmodia are being scrutinised for rational developments of new drugs.

### Chemoprophylaxis

The range of drugs available for suppression of malaria is very limited and includes 4 aminoquinolines and fixed drug combinations of sulfadoxine/or sulfalene + Pyrimethamine, pyrimethamine or proguanil alone are not considered adequate due to widespred resistance among plasmodia to these drugs. It is important to remember that there is no drug that can guarantee complete malaria suppression and there is no significant difference between various drugs in terms of efficacy. The recommended regime is summarised in Table-19.3.

### Malaria vaccine

Development of a vaccine for malaria is difficult because falciparum strains show marked antigenic heterogeneity. Moreover, malaria infection *per se* may be able to induce some degree of immunosuppression leading to reduced ability to mount primary immune response to certain non-plasmodial antigens, leading to increased frequency and greater severity of intercurrent (viral and other) infections. The hypothesis that motivates present research efforts is that there are parasite antigens that may fail to elicit protective response by host during natural infection (e.g. sporozoites, merozoites and microgametes) but may impart protection if they were used in a vaccine.

The development of vaccine against P. falciparum sporozoites has been the work of Dr. Ruth Nussenzweig and is currently in most advanced stages. Vaccination against merozoites has been successful in simian malaria. Immunisation against sexual stages of parasite prevents transmission of plasmodia and has again been achieved in simian malaria. It is a possibility that malaria vaccination of future may be polyvalent one to include a variety of stage specific antigens.

Recommended for further reference :

1. Advances in Malaria Chemotherapy. Report of a WHO scientific group. Technical report series 711, WHO Geneva 1984.
2. Chemotherapy of Malaria. Ed. Bruce-Chwatt L.L, 2nd Ed, WHO Geneva 1981.

**Table-19.2(a)**

**Mechanism of drug resistance in blood schizonticides**

| Chemical class and Drug | Main site of Action | Mechanism of resistance |
|---|---|---|
| 1. Aminoqunoline<br>a. Chloroquin<br>b. Amodiaquin | Haemoglobin digestion products (Hematin) | Surface area of parasite and host membrane<br>Production of protolytic enzymes to lyse Hb |
| 2. Aminoalcohols<br>a. Quinine<br>b. Mefloquine<br>c. Halofantrine | Haemoglobin digestion Product | Same<br>Cross resistance develops more readily in chloroquine resistant strains |
| 3. Biguanides<br>a. Proguanil | DHFR inhibition | Modification of drug transport mechanism |
| 4. Pyrimidines<br>a. Pyrimethamine | DHFR inhibition | Gene amplification, Synthesis of blocked enzyme |

*Table continued to next page ....*

*Table contd.. from previous page*

| | | |
|---|---|---|
| 5. Sulfones (Dapsone) | PABA Blockers | Production of mutant enzyme with drug affinity |
| 6. Sulfonamides | PABA Blockers | Production of drug inactivating enzymes<br>Use of alternate pathway |
| 7. Sesquiterpene Lactone<br>a. Artemisinine (Qinghaosu) | Protein Metabolism | Change in drug transport mechanism into parasite |
| b. Artesuanate (ester) | Protein Metabolism | Production of drug inactivating enzyme |
| 8. Naphthacene derivatives (Tetracyclines) | Protein synthesis | Production of segregating protein to reduce hematin |

**Table-19.2(b)**

**Mechanism of drug resistance in tissue schizonticide**

| Drug Used | Stage effected | Site of Action | Mechanism of Resistance |
|---|---|---|---|
| 8 Aminoquinoline (Primaquin) | PE Schizont | Mitochondria | Synthesis of Mitochondria |
| Biguanides (Proguanil) | PE Schizont | DHFR inhibition | as noted in table 19.2(a) |
| Pyrimidine (Pyrimethamine) | PE Schizont | DHFR inhibition | |
| Sulfonamide (Sulfadoxine) | PE Schizont | PABA Blocker | |
| 8 Aminoquinoline (Primaquin) | Merozoite | | |

**Table-19.3**

**Recommendations for treatment of acute falciparum malaria — in areas where 4-Aminoquinolines are ineffective**

| Drug | Day-1 | Day-2 | Day-3 | Day 4-7 |
|---|---|---|---|---|
| a) Quinine | 1800 mg (600 × 8 hrly) | 1800 mg | 1800 mg | 1800 mg daily |
| or | | | | |
| b) Quinine plus | 1800 mg (600 × 8 hrly) | 1800 mg | 1800 mg | 1800 mg daily |
| Tetracycline | 1-2 gm (250-500 × 6 hrly) | 1-2 gm | 1-2 gm | 1-2 gm daily |
| or | | | | |
| c) Sulfadoxine | 1.3 gm | Given in a single dose | | |
| or | | | | |
| Sulfalene | 1.5 gm | | | |
| plus | | | | |
| Pyrimethamine | 75 mg | | | |

**Note :** I.V. Quinine for serious patients, comatose patients or patients with vomiting or severe diarrhoea or patients with high parasite count (over 100,000/cmm).

**Table-19.4**

**Recommendation for Chemoprophylaxis**

1. In areas of low grade chloroquin resistant P. Falciparum infection give Chloroquine or Amodiaquine 300 mg weekly (adult dose)
   - first dose should be repeated on second day of prophylaxis
   - To be continued for 4-6 weeks after leaving endemic area.
2. In areas of high grade chloroquine resistance where P. vivax infection coexists.

| | | | |
|---|---|---|---|
| Sulfadiazine (500 mg + Pyrimethamine (25 mg) plus (1 tablet) | Chloroquin or Amodiaquin 300 mg base (2 tablets) | or | Mefloquin 250 mg base (1 tablet) |

**Note :** To be given weekly along with folic acid supplements : breakthrough may occur — To be treated as any other resistant malaria.

## LEPROSY

*S.K. HAJRA*

### Introduction :

The estimated number of leprosy patients is progressively increasing and the world figure now stands between 12 and 15 million. The estimated number of leprosy cases in India was 2.5 million in 1961, 3.2 million in 1971 and 3.9 million in 1981. The probable factors for this increase are increase in population, life expectancy, increased activity in case-finding programme and greater emphasis on health education.

It is the general practitioners who have greater contact with the population at large in our country and enjoy their confidence regarding health matter. In the treatment of a disease like leprosy of which everybody is afraid, due to its social stigma, general practitioners have an important role. But it is however noted that general practitioners sometimes miss the diagnosis resulting in delay in starting specific treatment.

### Early diagnosis

The importance of early diagnosis in leprosy cannot be too strongly emphasised. Early treatment prevents complication and ensures cure and for this early diagnosis is essential. Early leprosy is often overlooked or not given due attention, as it usually does not cause any discomfort to the patient. Once the diagnosis is made in a house, all contacts should be thoroughly examined.

The commonest early manifestation of a patient of leprosy is a skin change which takes the form of either hypopigmentation or erythema. Any chronic dermatoses without any irritation and not responding to conventional treatment should make one suspicious of its being due to Hansen's infection. If there is some diminution of tactile or thermal sensitivity then leprosy is even more likely. Hence thorough examination of nude skin is necessary.

Leprosy presents spectrum of clinical manifestations which is dependent on cell-mediated immunological (CMI) status of the patient. For this reason classification of this disease is essential.

Indian Leprosy Association in its latest recommendation on classification of leprosy has recognised the following types : (1) Indeterminate, (2) Tuberculoid, (3) Borderline, (4) Lepromatous and (5) Pure neuritic.

Another widely used classification advocated by Ridley and Jopling, recognises the following spectrum : (1) Polar Tuberculoid (TT), (2) Borderline Tuberculoid (BT), (3) Mid Borderline (BB), (4) Borderline Lepromatous (BL) and (5) Polar Lepromatous (LL).

Subsequently further elaborations were made viz, recognition of an additional subpolar lepromatous (LLs) form and designating Polar Lepromatous as LLp. Since this classification is primarily based on histopathology, the former classification is more suitable for clinical purposes.

Since *Mycobacterium leprae,* the causative organism of leprosy primarily affects skin and peripheral nerves, the commonest clinical manifestations are skin lesions and sensory impairment.

## Skin manifestations of Leprosy

### Indeterminate Leprosy

The earliest change in the skin comprises of small areas of skin, single or multiple, with slight difference from normal skin — slightly hypopigmented and flat. Sensory impairment is slight. The margins are indistinct. Loss of hair or sweat function is usually not seen. These lesions usually appear in the back, forearms and thighs. Skin smears are negative for acid fast bacillus (AFB).

*Histopathology*

The histopathological picture comprises of non-specific granuloma consisting of collections of small round cells arranged partly diffusely and partly in perivascular and perineural foci with some occasional endoneural infiltration. A small proportion of epitheloid cells may be present. Staining for AFB may show an occasional organism inside Schwann cells or errectores pilli muscle cells.

This type of leprosy if left untreated may resolve spontaneously or gradually progress on to any of the determinate forms of the disease viz, tuberculoid, borderline or lepromatous depending on the immunological status of the patient.

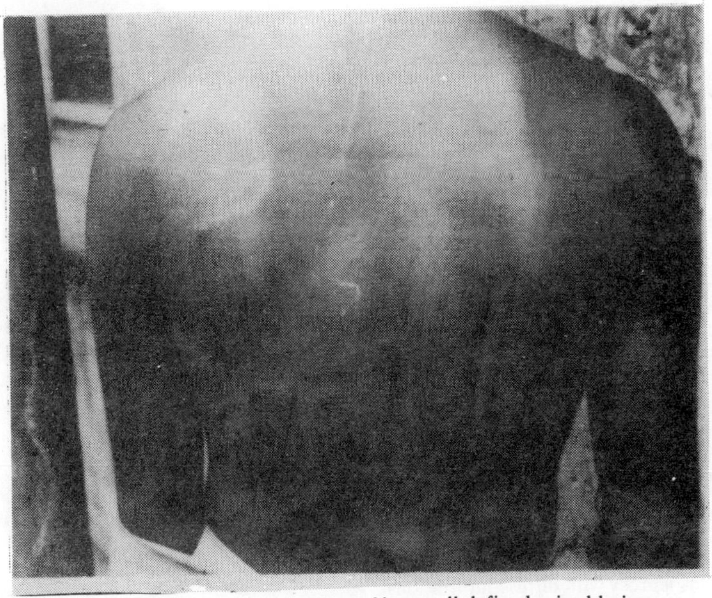

Fig.19.1 : Tuberculoid leprosy. Note well defined raised lesion

### Tuberculoid leprosy

The early lesions of tuberculoid leprosy are sharply defined, slightly erythematous or hypopigmented macules, in which sensation is definitely impaired. With progress of the lesions the borders become elevated and erythematous, sweating is diminished and loss of hair takes place.

The thickness may be confined to the margin or outer zone or the patch may be uniformly thickened. Cutaneous nerves or peripheral nerve trunks in association with the patches are frequently thickened. Skin scraping samples usually do not reveal AFB.

*Histopathology*

Typical tuberculoid granuloma comprising of epitheloid cells, Langhan's giant cells and surrounding zone of lymphocytes are found in the dermis, around skin adnexa and cutaneous nerve bundles which extends up to the subepidermal zone. The nerves show perineural and endoneural infiltration with the granuloma cells. Acid fast bacilli are very few and very difficult to detect.

**Lepromatous leprosy**

The macular lesions of early lepromatous leprosy appear as small multiple macules, either hypopigmented, erythematous or coppery red, with ill-defined margins, disposed bilaterally and symmetrically. Sensory disturbance may or may not be present. Gradually the macules will enlarge and coalesce to give rise to generalised infiltration of established lepromatous leprosy and nodules. Nerve involvement is symmetrical, giving rise to symmetrical sensory impairment in the extremities and bilateral nerve thickening. In some cases, particularly in light skinned persons, the disease may appear as diffuse ruddiness in face and forearms or trunks in the early stage. The nodules are usually manifestations of advanced stages but in some cases the earliest mainfestation of leprosy infection may be the presence of small discrete nodules in the ears.

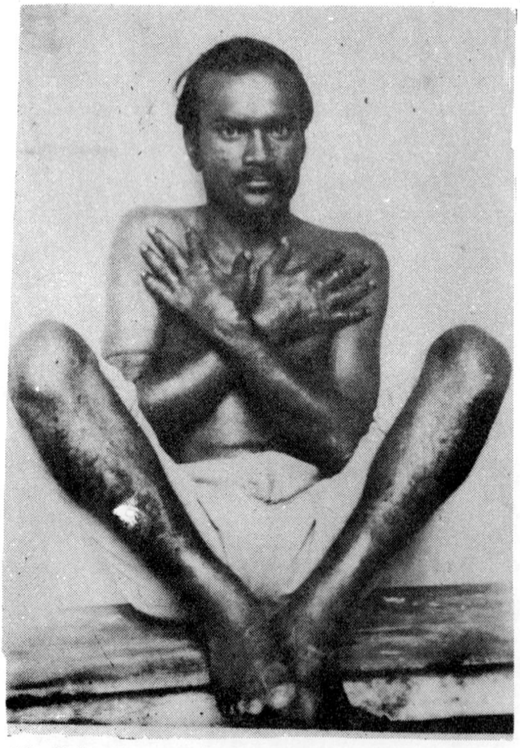

Fig.19.2 : Lepromatous leprosy with diffuse infiltrations and nodules.

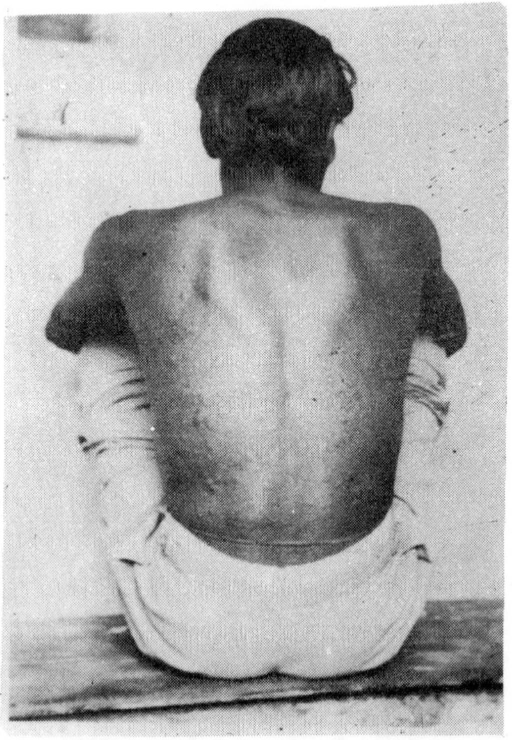

Fig.19.3 : Same patient-backside shows similar lesions.

Leonine facies with thickened skin and nodules in face, loss of eyebrows (madarosis), gynecomastia,sterility and impotency are the features of advanced lepromatous leprosy.

Microscopical examination of smears from skin and nasal mucosa shows large number of AFB.

*Histopathology*

Epidermis shows thinning and flattening of rete ridges with a clear subepidermal zone. The characteristic finding is diffuse granuloma consisting mainly of macrophages with foamy cytoplasm. Lymphocytes are absent or scanty with scattered plasma cells. Nerves show perineural and epineural infiltration but practically no endoneural infiltration. Acid fast staining of tissue section shows large number of bacilli in and outside macrophages and inside the nerves.

**Borderline leprosy**

This type of leprosy occurs in those persons whose degree of resistance to leprosy bacilli lies somewhere in the spectrum between tuberculoid and lepromatous. Clinical manifestation combines the features of both tuberculoid and lepromatous leprosy.

Skin manifestation consists of single or several patches of lesions, erythematous or copper - coloured, raised in the centre and sloping towards the periphery, presenting an inverted saucer shaped appearance. Depending on the patient's position in the borderline spectrum, the lesions vary greatly in number, size and shape. The nearer the disease is to the lepromatous end of the spectrum, the more numerous, more shiny, less well-defined and less anaesthetic they are. Annular lesions in leprosy are invariably borderline. Erythematous plaques with vague outer edges and punched out central portion are characteristic of borderline leprosy. Nerve damage is widespread. Routine skin smear examination usually shows lepra bacilli.

*Histopathology.*

There is feature of both tuberculoid and lepromatous histology in different areas of the body and in different depths below the epidermis. Clear subepidermal zone is visible. Langhan's giant cells and bacilli laden macrophages many co-exist in the same section. Acid fast staining shows presence of lepra bacilli.

**Pure Neuritic leprosy**

This is a form of leprosy in which there is no evidence or history of skin lesion. Larger nerve trunks or their branches are enlarged. There is sensory loss in the areas of distribution of the nerves. A single or multiple nerves may be involved. Skin smears are negative.

Histopathology of nerve section may present the picture of tuberculoid, borderline or non-specific reactions.

**Manifestations of nerve damage**

Early leprosy may usually present some typical manifestations in the skin but in some cases the features are due to damage to the dermal nerves or peripheral nerve trunks.

Persistent or recurrent paraesthesia in the area should arouse suspicion of leprosy. Shooting type of nerve pain or recurrent pain in the nerve trunks may be present.

In some cases there may be no skin manifestation, but there may be anaesthesia in the distribution of a particular nerve trunk which is thickened. These are pure neuritic leprosy. There may be associated weakness or wasting of the muscles, deformity or trophic ulcers.

In leprosy the peripheral nerve trunks commonly affected are :

(1) *The Ulnar nerve* — above the medial epicondyle or dorsal branch of the ulnar winding around the pisiform bone.

(2) *The Median Nerve* — in the antecubital fossa or just above the anterior annular ligament of the wrist.

(3) *The Radial Nerve* — in its groove in the arm.

(4) *The Lateral Popliteal nerve* — as it winds round the neck of the fibula.

(5) *The Posterior Tibial nerve* — midway between the medial malleolus and point of the hee

Certain superficial sensory nerves are commonly enlarged, which include :

(1) The great auricular branches traversing the sternomastoid muscle and is demonstrated by turning the head to the opposite side.

(2) The dermal fibres over the dorsum of the hand and forearm.

(3) Superficial radial nerve coursing over the lower end of the radius.

(4) Supra-orbital and supra-trochlear nerves.

(5) Sural cutaneous nerve.

Besides these, nerves may be thickened adjacent to any tuberculoid patch.

Skin patch, loss of sensation, thickened nerve and demonstration of acid-fast bacilli constitute the cardinal signs of leprosy of which any two must be present.

The sensations tested are for touch sensation, pain sensation and thermal sensation, and all these are mostly lost.

Touch sensation is tested with a wisp of cotton wool or a paper cone. The loss of this sensation is designated as superficial anaesthesia (Sa).

Similarly, pain sensation is tested with a pin. Loss of pain sensation is expressed as deep analgesia (Da).

The thickening of cutaneous nerves or peripheral nerve trunks must be sought for (Fig. 19.4).

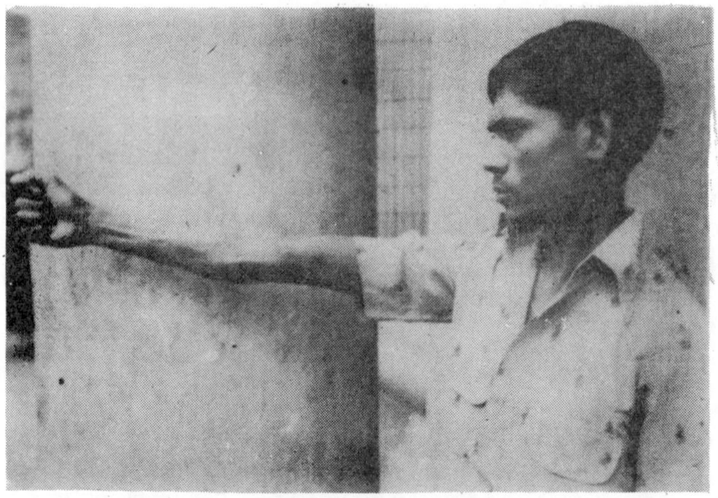

Fig. 19.4 : Showing much thickend cutaneous nerve of forearm

Examination of skin smears for demonstration of acid-fast bacilli is a very important sign and is routinely done to determine the infective status of the patient and to confirm the clinical diagnosis. If routine smear examination by 'slit' and 'scrape' method reveals acid-fast organism, the case is taken as 'infectious', and if no such bacilli are found the case is 'non-infectious'. The smears are routinely taken from the skin patch and the nasal mucous membrane on the antero-inferior part of the nasal septum. If the case is suspected to be an infectious on clinical ground, additional smears from the ear lobule should be examined.

Anhydrosis is a feature of a leprotic path and this is tested by giving pilocarpine injection over the suspected patch after painting it with tincture of iodine and dusting with starch powder. If the starch powder turns blue it indicates sweating which in turn signifies that the patch is non-leprotic.

Similarly, lack of triple response over the skin patch following local histamine introduction with the help of a needle prick is suggestive of a leprotic patch.

The above two skin tests may help in doubtful cases, but they are seldom required.

The lepromin test which is usually thought to be a diagnostic test of leprosy, is not really a diagnostic test. It indicates the immunological status of an individual against leprosy and helps in classification of leprosy cases.

Histological examination of skin biopsy specimens and or concentration method of bacterial examination may be undertaken to confirm the diagnosis in doubtful cases.

**Reactions in Leprosy**

All types of leprosy excepting indeterminate type may have periodic acute exacerbational phases known as "Reactions". Antileprotic treatment, treatment for any other disease, vaccination, child birth, associated infections, mental and physical strains, exposure to excessive heat or cold are well-known precipitating factors of reactions, but these exacerbations may also occur without any apparent cause.

Reactions in tuberculoid and borderline leprosy are characterised by sudden increase in thickness of some or all of the existing skin lesions which become more erythematous and in severe case may burst open. Similar new lesions appear in different parts of the body. They desquamate on subsidence. Most serious symptom is acute neuritis, particularly seen in borderline reaction, which may occur in single or multiple nerves and is characterised by acute pain, swelling and tenderness of the nerve trunks where abscess may form. There may be sudden muscle paralysis. Commonly affected nerves are ulnar, radial, facial and common peroneal nerves Other constitutional symptoms like fever, joint pain etc. are usually absent. But oedema of hands and feet may occur. Initial smear-negative lesions may show presence of bacilli during the reactional episodes.

Reactions in lepromatous leprosy are characterised by appearance of crops of erythematous, tender nodules in the skin which are evanescent (lasting for a few days). These lesions are known as *'Erythema Nodosum Leprosum'* (ENL). In severe cases they may become vesicular, pustular, bullous and finally break down. Commonly associated features are fever, joint pain, bone pain, nerve pain, muscle pain, iritis, iridocyclitis, lymphadenitis and epididymo-orchitis. There is often oedema of hands and feet. Smear examination from nodules reveal fragmented and granular bacilli. Blood examination shows polymorphonuclear leucocytosis and raised ESR.

**How to disclose and guide the patient**

Every leprosy patient is under severe mental stress. This mental agony in leprosy patients originates from three sources, viz. stress of inherited ideas, experience of suffering from leprosy and problems created due to stigma of leprosy in home and family life.

This fact should be kept in mind by doctors, nurses and all paramedical persons concerned with treatment and care of this disease. Before disclosing the nature of the disease to the patient his or her psychological make-up must be assessed.

Necessary courtesy, understanding and patience must be shown in dealing with these patients and they should not feel neglected.

**How to initiate treatment**

An average uncomplicated case may be treated in Leprosy-treatment centres, where treatment is supervised by trained medical officers who are assisted by paramedical workers, or treatment can be undertaken by the supervision of medical practitioners. In cases with complications such as deformity, trophic ulcer, lagophthalmos etc. where physiotherapy and surgical intervention is required, the patient should better be referred to an institution where facilities for specialist services are available. During the phases of reaction sudden nerve damage or eye damage may cripple or even blind the patient in a rather short span of time and management of those cases may require the expertise of a Leprologist.

**Treatment**

Leprosy and its complications present varied manifestations, in the management of which various disciplines of medicine have important roles to play. The whole management will be considered under the heading 'Treatment of uncomplicated leprosy' and 'Management of complications'.

*Treatment of uncomplicated leprosy*

General Treatment — It comprises maintenance of nutritional status of the patient and prevention and treatment of intercurrent infection. Diet should better be sufficiently rich in protein. In developing countries animal proteins are expensive , hence good vegetable proteins should be utilised from cereals and soya beans. Overstrain and exposures to sun and cold are to be avoided. A suitable vocation must be provided.

*Specific Treatment* — At present a number of effective drugs against leprosy are available. But prior to the introduction of sulphone in the treatment of leprosy in 1941, hydnocarpus oil was the main therapeutic agent available. This drug has become almost obsolete nowadays.

Hydnocarpus oil or its esters can be used by intradermal, subcutaneous or intramuscular routes. It can be administered on residual patches, along the thickened nerves, around the trophic ulcers and in the atrophied muscles, as a supplementary treatment with other antileprotic therapy.

*Dose* : Starting with a dose of 0.25 ml, gradually increased by 0.5 ml. every week up to a maximum of 10 ml. Injections are given on an average once a week or till the signs of irritation of previous injection subside.

Studies in mouse foot-pad have revealed that hydnocarpus oil has got bacteriostatic action against *Myco. leprae* and also that its mode of action differs from that of sulphones.

*Dapsone* — This is the most important drug in the treatment of leprosy and also the cheapest. It is 4:4 - diaminodiphenyl sulphone (DDS). It was first used in the treatment of leprosy (by intramuscular injection of oily suspension) by Cochrane in 1946 and John Lowe tried dapsone orally in 1947. The mechanism of action of dapsone is thought to be an interference in folic acid synthesis through competition with para-aminobenzoic acid. In the mouse, the minimum inhibitory concentration (MIC) of dapsone in the serum is 0.003 microgram/ml. Depending on the body weight adult patient should receive a daily dose of 50-100 mg (1-2 mg/kg body weight). With a dose of 100 mg the peak serum level exceeds the MIC of dapsone against *M. leprae* by a factor of about 500 and in this dosage the drug is weakly bactericidal.

In the recommended dose dapsone is well tolerated and side effects are rare. Some cases during the first few months may complain of weakness, tingling and burning sensation in the extremities, headache, nausea and vomiting. These symptoms usually pass off. Occasionally it may lead to haemolytic anaemia which is pronounced in glucose-6-phosphate dehydrogenase deficiency, leucopenia, methaemoglobinaemia, drug fever, peripheral neuritis, exfoliative dermatitis, fixed drug eruption and psychosis.

In borderline cases, dapsone, may precipitate acute neuritis and in some lepromatous and non-lepromatous patients may cause reactional episodes. Clinical improvement is usually observed within 3-6 months of initiating treatment. If clinical improvement is not observed within six months of regular intake of dapsone, drug resistance should be suspected.Dapsone resistance is more likely to emerge in patients taking the drug in small dose (100 mg or less per week) and irregularly (multiple breaks of one month or more in treatment). This type of dapsone resistance known as secondary resistance is noted in lepromatous cases and time taken for this development to occur may vary from 3 to 24 years. The pattern of resistance to dapsone is of multi-step type mutation. Infection with dapsone-resistant bacilli gives rise to primary dapsone resistance. Both these types of resistance are being reported with greater frequency from different parts of the world. If monotherapy with dapsone is continued there will be spread of primary dapsone resistance to such an extent as to make control by chemotherapy unattainable.

*Acedapsone*

This repository compound, 4.4 diacetyl-diaminodiphenyl sulphone (DADDS) very slowly releases dapsone and a dose of 225 mg. by injection may maintain effective blood concentration for over 2 months. However, it should not be used in preference to oral dapsone.

*Rifampicin*

It is the semisynthetic derivative of rifamycin S.V. which is derived from rifamycin B, the fermentation product of *Streptomyces mediterranei.* It is the most potent antileprotic drug available at present. A single dose of 600 mg kills majority of the bacilli within a few days. Although clinical improvement with this drug is good, decrease in bacterial count in smear examination is not better than dapsone. In spite of rifampicin being a strong bactericidal drug viable *M. leprae*, can be detected at certain sites in lepromatous patients. So it should not be used singly. Tolerance of the drug is good. It produces yellowish colouration of urine. It may cause skin rashes, gastrointestinal symptoms, joint pain, thrombocytopenia and/or hepatitis which may occur more frequently with intermittent dosage.

It has been found that daily administration of 600 mg rifampicin does not produce any better result than that of once monthly dose of 600 mg. As recommended by WHO, the drug is administered in dosage of 600 mg. once a month and to be given at least half an hour before food. The cost of treatment is therefore considerably reduced.

*Clofazimine*

It is a substituted iminophenazine bright red dye (Hansepran) available in 100 mg. capsules. This drug is an unique antileprotic drug, because it combines an antileprotic property which compares well with that of dapsone, with an anti-inflammatory action which is useful in reactional states.

When given as a component of triple drug regime recommended by WHO it is administered in dosage of 100 mg on alternate days or 50 mg daily plus an once-monthly dose of 300 mg. For treatment of reactive states it is given in a dosage of 300 mg daily and gradually diminished. It is a well tolerated drug. Its main drawback is pigmentation of skin which initially becomes red, then deepens to brown and eventually brownish black. This effect is reversible. This colouration also affects conjunctivae, urine and sputum. Dryness and ichthyosis of skin occur frequently which is also reversible. In some cases abdominal pain, nausea and diarrhoea may occur. Clofazimine resistance is also on record.

*Ethionamide and Prothionamide*

Both are bactericidal drugs. WHO has recommended either of these drugs as a substitute for clofazimine in those patients who are reluctant to take clofazimine for reasons of pigmentation. Recommended dose is 250-375 mg. daily. It may cause gastrointestinal disturbance and is hepatotoxic.

*Multidrug Therapy (MDT)*

Since introduction of dapsone in the treatment of leprosy it was being used as monotherapy. Prolonged treatment period spanning quite a large number of years, made the patient irregular in respect of drug intake. This factor along with low dosage of administration of dapsone contributed to the emergence of dapsone resistance leprosy, which was experimentally confirmed in 1964. Fortunately, rifampicin and clofazimine appeared in the arena of leprosy treatment around that period. Administration of rifampicin and clofazimine singly has also resulted in emergence of bacilli resistant to those drugs. To prevent drug resistance of *M. leprae*, to make the initially smear positive cases smear negative i.e. non-infectious in a shorter period, to shorten the period of treatment and for treatment of already drug-resistant leprosy patients WHO study group in 1982 recommended multi-drug treatment for all the leprosy cases whether untreated or already under treatment. For this purpose, the leprosy patients are divided into two groups according to their bacteriological status viz. paucibacillary (those with no bacillus or scanty bacilli in routine smear examination — Bacteriological Index (BI) less than 2 (Ridley's Scale) and multibacillary (those with large number of bacilli — BI more than 2). (Bacteriological Index is the average of degree of positivity of skin smears taken from multiple sites).

The proposed multidrug regimen is designed for the treatment of all categories of multibacillary patients, including :

1) Previously untreated patients
2) Patients who have responded satisfactorily to previous dapsone monotherapy
3) Patients who have not responded to previous dapsone monotherapy
4) Patients who have relapsed while on dapsone monotherapy or after its withdrawal.

The six-month chemotherapy course for patients with paucibacillary leprosy should be introduced with the following order of priority :

1) All newly diagnosed paucibacillary patients
2) All dapsone-treated paucibacillary cases with relapse, and
3) Paucibacillary patients who are currently on treatment with dapsone monotherapy and who have not yet completed two years of treatment.

**Table-19.5 : Multidrug chemotherapeutic regimes for adult patients recommended by the WHO study-group on Leprosy (1982).**

| Type of Leprosy | Paucibacillary (I,TT,BT) Leprosy | Multibacillary (BB, BL, LL) Leprosy |
|---|---|---|
| BI according to the Ridley Scale | Less than two at all sites | Two or more at any site |
| Regimen | Daily (taken at home)<br>Dapsone 100 mg. | Daily (taken at home)<br>Dapsone 100 mg.<br>Clofazimine (Hansepran) 50 mg or 100 mg on alternate days. |
| | Once a month (under supervision)<br>Rifampicin 600 mg. | Once a month (under supervision)<br>Rifampicin 600 mg.<br>Clofazimine (Hansepran) 300 mg. |
| Duration of treatment | Six months | At least two years or until negative skin smears are obtained whichever is later. |

**Table-19.6 : The dosage of anti-leprosy drugs for children with paucibacillary leprosy**

| Age groups | Dapsone : daily dose, Unsupervised (mg) | Rifampicin : monthly dose, Supervised (mg) |
|---|---|---|
| 3 - 5 years | 25 | 150-300 |
| 6 - 14 years | 50-100 | 300-450 |
| 15 years and above | 100 | 600 |

**Table-19.7 : The dosage of anti-leprosy drugs for children with multibacillary leprosy.**

| Age groups | Dapsone : daily dose unsupervised (mg) | Rifampicin : monthly dose, supervised (mg) | Clofazimine | |
|---|---|---|---|---|
| | | | Unsupervised dose (mg) | Monthly dose supervised (mg) |
| 3 - 5 years | 25 | 150 - 300 | 100 once weekly | 100 |
| 6 - 14 years | 50 - 100 | 300 - 450 | 150 once weekly | 150 - 200 |
| 15 years and above | 100 | 600 | 50 daily | 300 |

**Recommendation of Govt. of India**

(A) For multibacillary patients

**Adults**

(a) Daily supervised treatment should be given during the initial intensive phase for 14 days with the following drugs :

Rifampicin 600 mg
Clofazimine 100 mg
Dapsone 100 mg

(b) Continuation phase : Treatment is given for a period of 2 years or until smear negativity, whichever is later

Rifampicin 600 mg once monthly (supervised)
Dapsone 25 mg daily (Self-administered)
Clofazimine 300 mg once monthly (supervised) and 50 mg daily (self-administered) or 100 mg on alternate days.

**Table-19.8 : Recommended dose for Children**

| Phase | 6 to 9 years | 10 to 14 years |
|---|---|---|
| Intensive | Rifampicin 300 mg daily<br>Clofazimine 50 mg daily<br>Dapsone 25 mg daily | Rifampicin 450 mg daily<br>Clofazimine 50 mg daily<br>Dapsone 50 mg daily |
| Continuation for a minimum of 2 years or until smear negative whichever is later. | Rifampicin 300 mg once monthly<br>Clofazimine 100 mg once monthly and 50 mg twice weekly.<br>Dapsone 25 mg daily | Rifampicin 450 mg once monthly<br>Clofazimine 150 mg once monthly and 50 mg on alternate days<br>Dapsone 50 mg daily |

(B) For *Paucibacillary cases*

Rifampicin 600 mg once monthly (supervised)
Dapsone 100 mg daily (self-administered)
— To be continued for 6 months

In our experience six month regimen for paucibacillary cases does not render all the patients clinically inactive (signs of activity are erythema, increase or decrease in the size or number of lesions, thickness of skin lesion, nerve tenderness and presence of bacilli in smear examination). In those cases where the lesions become inactive, treatment is stopped but patients are kept under surveillance and those not becoming inactive should be continued with dapsone in full dosage till the stage of inactivity is achieved.

In case of multibacillary schedule the patients are to be followed for at least five years before final conclusion about the efficacy of the regimen can be drawn.

*Immunotherapy*

Persons suffering from lepromatous leprosy have a specific defect of cell mediated immunity (CMI) towards *M. leprae*. The main objective of immunotherapy is to induce effective CMI to *M. leprae* in patients with lepromatous leprosy. The following procedures have been tried to achieve this objective :

(1) Intravenous injection of peripheral blood lymphocytes obtained from patients with tuberculoid leprosy or from the donors who have strongly positive lepromin (Mitsuda) reaction.

(2) Intravenous injection of transfer factor (TF), an extract of lymphocytes from patients suffering from tuberculoid leprosy or from healthy donors who have strongly positive (Mitsuda) reaction.

(3) Intradermal injection of the vaccine, containing heat killed *M. leprae* from armadillos and living BCG. The injection is repeated three or more times at intervals of 2-3 months.

It would take several years before procedures of immunotherapy with long-lasting effect and suitable for wide-scale application are made available.

*Treatment of complications*

(1) Treatment of reactions

For successful management of lepra reactions early diagnosis and timely initiation of anti-inflammatory measures are to be made.

Management of reactional states should aim at —

1) Controlling acute neuritis and preventing paralysis and contracture;
2) Checking eye damage and preventing blindness;
3) Controlling disease state and
4) Controlling pains.

The possible precipitating factors are to be searched for and dealt with properly. Anti-leprosy treatment should be continued in full dosage without interruption as far as possible.

*For mild reaction :*

No nerve pain. Skin lesions are mildly inflammed with or without systemic disturbances.

Analgesics and anti-inflammatory drugs :

1) Aspirin — In daily dosage of 600-1200 mg after meals is helpful in controlling mild to moderate degree of pain. Avoid in small children.
2) Paracetamol — 650 mg twice daily is also helpful.
3) Ibuprofen or Oxyphenbutazone may be given if required in suitable dosage during acute phase of reaction.
4) Chloroquine : 150 mg (base) thrice or twice daily may be given and dose reduced with improvement. Prolonged chloroquine administration requires careful watch for skin rashes, photosensitization, pruritus, visual disturbances, tinitus. Chloroquine retinopathy is well known. Rarely it may also cause thrombocytopenia, agranulocytosis and pancytopenia.
6) Antimonials : The anti-inflammatory action of antimonials is particularly effective in mild ENL reactions.

Inj. Potassium antimony tartarate (PAT) — 0.02 gm I.V. on alternate days for three injections and later 0.04 gm I.V. alternate days for three more injections are given and freshly prepared 2% solution of the drug in 10 ml of normal saline or with 10% 10 ml calcium gluconate should be used.

Alternatively, Inj. Sodium Antimony Gluconate (Stibatine, Stibanate) 3-6 ml. by I.M. injection every day up to a total of 40-60 ml.

Antileprotic treatment is to be continued in full dosage.

In case of moderate reaction with rise of temperature above 100°F and mild nerve pain or joint pain, above mentioned treatment is to be given and specific treatment may have to be halved or temporarily suspended if reaction is not controlled.

*Severe reaction*

Reactions should be considered as severe, if any of the following is present —

1) Severe neuritis with impending paralysis
2) Skin ulceration
3) Iritis or orchitis

These conditions are medical emergencies in leprosy and immediate anti-inflammatory treatment with corticosteroids is to be instituted to prevent disability.

In cases of acute neuritis whether in tuberculoid, borderline or lepromatous reaction, systemic corticosteroid is to be started. The average initial dose is 20-40 mg prednisolone daily but in very severe cases higher dosage up to 60-80 mg daily may be required. The dose is to be gradually reduced according to response of the patient till at a maintenance dose of 5-10 mg daily it is to continued for several months. During severe acute phase of neuritis dapsone is better suspended temporarily and instituted as soon as acute phase is brought under control. Severe pain of acute neuritis may also be controlled by giving injections of steroid, lignocaine and hyalase intraneurally or preferably perineurally, repeated if required after two days. Inj. Vit $B_1$, $B_6$ and $B_{12}$ although empirically used, often gives relief. Proper splint should be applied with nerves in relaxed position along with passive and active exercises, which will stimulate muscle recovery and prevent joint stiffness.

Severe pustulating skin lesions with rise of temperature above 102°F will require suitable antibiotics.

Acute iridocyclitis will require application of 1% atropine drops, or ointment and steroid drops or ointment in the eyes, along with systemic steroids and non-steroid anti-inflammatory drugs. In severe cases sub-conjuctival injection of 0.2 ml of a solution containing 25 mg hydrocortisone per ml should be given.

Acute epididymo-orchitis will have to be controlled with prompt administration of prednisolone and scrotal suspensory bandage.

*Treatment of repeated steroid dependent lepra-reaction in lepromatous leprosy.*

Both thalidomide and clofazimine in a dosage of 300 mg daily are useful in dealing with ENL reaction. Some of the cases with recurrent reaction become steroid dependent and withdrawal of steroid becomes a problem. While clofazimine takes 6-12 weeks to control the reactive state, thalidomide does it in a much shorter time. Both the drugs help in controlling reactions as well as weaning the patients from steroid dependence and increase their sulphone-tolerance. Either thalidomide or clofazimine is started with 300 mg daily till reactive state is controlled and during this period dose of steroid is tapered off to be finally stopped. Afterwards, DDS is inducted and maximum dose is built up, the dose of thalidomide and clofazimine is gradually reduced till reaching maintenance dose of 50 mg thalidomide or 100 mg clofazimine on alternate days. Thalidomide is not helpful in tuberculoid and borderline reaction. It is not available in India and should not be given in patients of child bearing age.

2. *Treatment of eye in leprosy : treatment of exposure and anaesthesia*

Conservative treatment consists of massaging the facial muscles and eyelids along with active closure of eyelids. Dryness of conjunctiva is prevented by a tear-substitute, viz. 1.4% polyvinyl alcohol in water to be given one drop three times daily or 1% methyl-cellulose or 1% sodium bicarbonate drops may also be used. At night sterile liquid paraffin or vaseline is to be used. The eyes are to be protected with goggles.

In more severe degree of lagophthalmos and in presence of anaesthesia and pre-existing corneal damages tarsorrhaphy and temporalis tendon transplantation are done.

Acute iridocyclitis : Discussed under reaction.

3. *Plantar ulcers*

An ulcer which occurs on the weight-bearing part of the sole of the foot is called a plantar ulcer. Roughly 70% of the plantar ulcers occur on the forefoot and less that 30% on the heel and outer border of the foot.

It is to be noted that plantar ulcer is not a sign of activity of the disease because it may occur in the inactive and arrested stage of the disease; these ulcers are not caused by *M. leprae* and they are not a danger to the public, since the discharge does not contain leprosy bacilli.

*Causation of Plantar ulcers*

Predisposing causes

1. *Anaesthesia*

Any condition which causes anaesthesia of foot may predispose to plantar ulcer formation because with loss of sensation the most important protection for the body viz. pain and discomfort are lost, making the foot more liable to injury.

2. *Muscle paralysis*

Damage to posterior tibial nerve causes paralysis of the small muscles of the sole of foot leading to closing of the toes. The head of the metatarsals tends to project below and tips of the toes become liable to damage because of contact with ground.

3. *Blood supply*

Blood supply to sole of the foot is hampered because of the damage to the autonomic nerve fibres.

Direct causes :

1. *Shearing stress*

When the foot is pushed backwards in order to move forward, a shearing stress takes place in the region of the metatarsal heads. When this force acts together with the body weight, the tissues tend to get torn because there is a stress occurring between the layers of the skin, resulting in a blister formation. The blister may break down under local stress and infection takes place and finally an ulcer develops.

2. *Direct pressure*

When a patient stands on one foot pressure on the weight bearing area of foot is roughly ½ kg/sq. cm. equivalent to 380 mm of mercury. This squeezes out blood and no blood can enter the tissues between the skin and the bone. In leprosy, uncomfortable sensation felt by a normal person on prolonged standing is lost. So the patient stands in the same position for a prolonged time leading to progressive loss of softness of the tissues of sole of foot which become hard and fibrotic.

3. *Direct injury :*

It is caused by nails, thorns or sharp stones.

4. *Heat :*

Walking barefoot on a sun heated tar road may cause blisters on the sole of an anaesthetic foot.

*Prevention of ulcer in the first place*

Avoid injuries — by constant use of footwears with tough soles, resistant to thorns, sharp stones and short nails. Tyre side pieces are used as the outer sole in the footwear for leprosy patients. All fixation of straps and soles is done by stitching or with adhesives. No nail should be used in footware. Avoid infection through cracks. Skin of the sole of the foot should be kept hydrated and supple by daily soaking in water or saline, mopping excess of water and smearing the foot with a thin coat of oil or grease.

Prompt and proper treatment of an injury of foot is a must.

The patient must make it a habit to inspect his foot daily for injury.

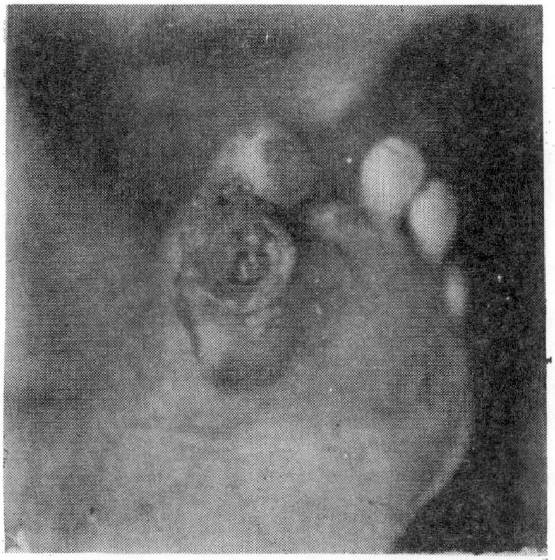

Fig.19.5 : Showing plantar ulcer of foot.

*Treatment of plantar ulcer*

Treatment of ulcer depends on the condition of the ulcer. From treatment point of view ulcers may be broadly classified as — acute, chronic, complicated and frequently recurrent.

Acute ulcers : Patient is put in bed. Stop walking.

Profusely discharging ulcer — dressed frequently with sterile dressing following aseptic technique. Sterile gauze soaked in freshly prepared EUSOL (12.5 gm of boric acid and 12.5 gm of bleaching powder dissolved in one litre of water) is best dressing.

If there is collection of pus, it must be drained out.

If toxaemia with fever is present use suitable antibiotics.

If infection of bone or joint is suspected, X'ray pictures should be taken for assessment and appropriate treatment. In a few days the ulcer is converted into a healing ulcer and treated as a chronic ulcer.

*Chronic ulcer*

The ulcer must be protected from excessive loading and other strains generated by walking. This is done by encasing the foot and leg in a plaster of Paris cast fitted with a walking iron. It is kept for about six weeks by which time the ulcer heals.

*Complicated ulcer*

The particular complication which is interfering with healing must be identified and treated by appropriate methods like exploration and removal of dead bones, dead tissue by surgical methods. Afterwards it is treated like a chronic ulcer.

*Prevention of recurrence of the ulcer*

Causes of recurrence

1) Original causes leading to the ulceration — anaesthesia of the sole of the foot, paralysis of small muscles and continued walking persisting.

2) Scar tissue is of inferior quality.

3) Associated deformities subjecting the scar tissue to increased stress.

Stress and strains generated by walking can be reduced by :

(a) Reducing walking

(b) Interposition of shock-absorbing material between ground and the foot. Reduce walking by using vehicles or taking rest periodically. Avoid running and jumping,etc.

Use of shock-absorbing insole

Sheets of microcellular rubber of 10° to 15° hardness is the best for the purpose. In some patients even these precautions are also not sufficient and the forces at the site of ulceration will need to be further reduced by other modification in the foot wear, like addition of metatarsal bar or moulding of the insole by Plastazote . These modifications increase the area of load bearing and thus reduce the intensity of load at any point. Thus by suitable footwear, one can relieve strain on the foot and the ulcer-bearing site to a great extent.

In certain cases, skin grafting of the ulcer or surgical revision of the scar will have to be done to improve the quality of the scar. A deformity throwing excessive strain on the scar should be corrected.

*Physiotherapy in the treatment of motor paralysis and deformity*

Physiotherapy has an important role in the medical and surgical management of leprosy.

Physiotherapy aims at preserving the physiological properties of affected muscles and preventing atrophy and also to strengthen them during recovery. One should try to maintain the activity as well as the bulk of the paralysed muscles because in spite of nerve conduction remaining impaired for a fairly prolonged period some function may return. The sooner physiotherapy is started the better.

The paralytic state has two phases :-

The expectant phase — when there is no sign of recovery being resumed. The active phase — when nerve conduction has returned to some extent.

The aims of physiotherapy in the expectant phase would be :-

(1) To retain joint mobility and to prevent contraction

(2) To prevent overstretching of paralysed muscles

(3) To prevent muscle atrophy.

These can be achieved by the following means :

Passive movements — The joints that are not inactivated due to paralysis of the muscles are moved passively through the full range of motion each day.

Massage — Light massage of the affected muscles may help maintain circulation and muscle tone.

Electrical stimulation — Faradic stimulation of paralysed muscles will help to maintain tone and prevent atrophy. It should be done twice daily.

Physiotherapeutic measures — in the treatment of deformity include daily massage, wax-therapy and exercise with corrective splintage in the intervening period.

Massage with any bland oil. The oil massage is done by the patient himself. The fingers should be rubbed downwards to the tips. The purpose is to straighten the fingers and to keep the joints mobile. When there is flexion-deformity without contracture, massage helps to maintain mobility of the fingers and prevents their contracture. With some degree of contracture due to skin tightness, regular massage helps to straighten the fingers gradually.

Wax therapy helps to loosen stiff joints and makes the skin smooth and supple. It may help to restore sweat function and give relief to nerve pain. This is given by dipping the hands a number of times in fairly quick succession into a bath of melted paraffin wax, the temperature of which varies from 50°C to 55°C, starting with lower temperature and increasing it with progress of treatment.

Exercises are the most important, and greatest stress should be placed on them. Exercises may be in the form of (1) passive movements, (2) assisted active movements, and (3) free active movements.

The passive movements of the fingers : In case of flexion deformity without contracture, the aim is to straighten the fingers passively and to retain their full mobility. Care must be taken not to hyper-extend the fingers. In case of contracture of the fingers effort should be made to decrease it by gradually loosening the stiff joints by passive stretching. Strong and forced passive movements should be avoided.

Assisted active exercises : The aim is to help the patient to perform certain movements which he is unable to do freely by himself.

Free active exercises : These are very important as they help the patient to practise some movements which are necessary in his day-to-day life, viz. opening and closing of the hand, meeting each finger-tip with that of the thumb in turn, making an "O" shape, picking up small objects with the thumb and one of the fingers in turn.

Splintage : The improvement gained in the deformity of the fingers with exercises and massage will not be effective if this is not maintained with the help of proper splints. In addition to their role of maintaining the improved condition the splints may actually help in improving the condition in between two successive sittings of physiotherapy.

## SEXUALLY TRANSMITTED DISEASES

*G.C. MOOKERJEE*
*B.U. KHAN*

### Introduction

The venereal diseases are group of disorders, which are spread by sexual intercourse. Syphilis, gonorrhoca, chancroid, lymphogranuloma venerum, and granuloma inguinale are legally defined venereal disease. Out of these syphilis and gonorrhoea are kept in major group among the veneral diseases. The other venereal diseases are caused by bacteria, virus and parasitic infections and they are described as nonspecific urethritis (non-gonococcal), chlamydia infection, viral infections e.g. herpes simplex and warts. Parasitic infections e.g. trichomonas, scabies and pediculosis can also be due to close sexual body contact but not truly sexually transmitted.

Incidence of venereal disease was at peak before the second World War. After that it was declining till 1950. Again its incidence is increasing during last three decades specially among younger generation, society being more permissive. However recently systemic diseases such as hepatitis B virus (HAB) causing hepatitis, are found to spread in sex partners by semen or saliva. Single or multiple infections may be present in same individual. Acquired immunodeficiency syndrome i.e. A.I.D.S. has been discussed in the following article.

## SYPHILIS

Syphilis is a chronic infection and its characteristic course involves every structure of the body. It is transmissible even to the offspring and its appearance may mimic many diseases causing difficulty in diagnosis.

*Mode of Infection*

The causative organism is a spirochaete, treponema pallidum and its incubation period as usually two to four weeks but it may be as short as nine days and as long as 90 days. Sexual contact is the main mode of infection. Organisms usually enter through minor abrasions in skin or mucous membrane of genital organ but it is also possible that they may enter through intact surfaces. They spread via lymphatics to surrounding lymph glands and to the other systems through blood stream.

**Pathology**

The primary lesion is a solitary macule which become papular and later ulcerates. Histologically there is infiltration of plasma cells, mononuclear cells and lymphocytes around perivascular lymphatics. Spirochaetes are also present around the perivascular lymphatics. If untreated this leads to obliterative of endarteritis with tissue destruction and fibrosis. Granulomatous inflammatory process is seen in syphilitic gumma due to delayed hypersensivity.

**Clinical course**

The disease is generally classified into acquired and congenital types as well as early and late syphilis. The sub-division between early and late syphilis is before and after two years from the onset of infection. In first two years it is highly infectious and it may even be transferable to the foetus from the infected parents.

*Stages of syphilis*

Syphilis may be acquired through sexual contact or be transmitted to offspring i.e. congenital.

(A) *Acquired syphilis*

(1) *Early stage*

(a) Primary

(b) Secondary

(2) *Late stage*

(a) Tertiary stage

(b) Quarternary stage

It also may remain latent over many years.

(B) *Congenital*

(a) Early stage at birth

(b) Late stage

(c) Stigmata may only be evident as healed scar.

*Primary stage*

Primary lesion is seen within three weeks after the exposure. The primary lesion is a chancre, which usually develops on the genitals or around the anus in homosexuals. Rarely lips, breasts, arm, fingers oropharyngeal cavity may also be involved. Chancre starts as a small pink macule which soon becomes papular and later on ulcerates. It has punched out margin and indurated border which is hard button-like on palpation. The regional lymph nodes are moderately enlarged, firm, discreet, rubbery, painless, nontender and seldom suppurate.

*Secondary stage*

The primary chancre tends to heal within six to eight weeks after primary infection and then secondary stage starts. Symptoms of generalised infection may then appear with malaise, fever, sorethroat, hoarseness, arthralgia and pain in bones and muscles. Secondary stage shows mainly involvement of muco-cutaneous surface. The four cardinal signs are (i) Cutaneous rashes (ii) Condyloma (iii) Mucous patches (iv) Lymphadenopathy.

Cutaneous rashes are present in about 75% of cases and it simulates generalised eruption without vesicles and bullae.

Condyloma are papules in warm, moist areas such as around the anus and they are heaped to form sessile warty moist lesions. This is highly infective and contain spirochetes.

The mucous patches are present in about 30% of the cases. It is a shallow ulcer with narrow red edge and its surface is covered by whitish membrane. It is seen on genitals, mouth and throat. The serpigenous type of this ulcer is called snail-track ulcer.

***Recurrent stage***

In first two years, after the early lesion, relapse is possible with inadequate treatment. The relapse is seen occurring at the site of primary chancre, known as *"Redux chancre"* or *"Mono-Recidibe"*. In some cases only positive serological test may be noted.

***Latent stage***

Early latent syphilis is infectious and it persists up to two years from the time of primary infection. In this stage without clinical evidence and negative cerebrospinal fluid report, the diagnosis is mainly based on specific blood test and routine STS. At this stage, the infection in women may result in congenital syphilis in the new-born.

Late latent syphilis appears within two years or more after the initial infection and it is not infectious. It may continue for many years or even through out the life. This stage is symptomless and usually detected in routine check-up during the blood donation or ante-natal clinics.

***Tertiary stage***

It takes about three to ten years to develop manifestations. Skin, mucous membrane, subcutaneous tissue or the covering structures of the body and the supporting structures of the body e.g. bones, joints and muscles are usually involved. The gumma is the typical lesion. It is a localised, necrotic painless swelling the usual lesion of tertiary stage. The lesions are non-infective but are chronic and destructive in nature.

***Quarternary stage***

In this stage, cardiovascular and neurological structures are mainly involved. This is usually 10 to 40 years after the original infection. The tissues are gradually destroyed, leading to serious complications.

The cardiovascular syphilis affects the aorta and leads various complications e.g. aortic insufficiency, constriction of the origin of the coronary artery and aortic aneurysm. Meninges are usually affected in neuro-syphilis and it causes meningitis with headache, convulsions, cranial nerve involvement and delirium. The meningo-vascular and parenchymatous changes in syphilis are very late features and it is manifested by hemiplegia, aphasia, transverse myelitis and progressive muscular atrophy. Cranial nerve palsies are also seen as well as Argyll Robertson pupil may be present.

The parenchymatous neurological manifestations may be present in two ways e.g. Tabes dorsalis and general paralysis of Insane (G.P.I.). Tabes dorsalis is a chronic and progressive degeneration of the ascending sensory neuron of the posterior column of spinal cord. While the G.P.I. involves the cerebral cortex and meninges and it results in varying degree of cerebral cortical atrophy.

*Congenital syphilis*

As the name suggests, it is acquired in the uterus from the infected mother, viz the placenta usually in second trimester of pregnancy. The foetus may die *in utero* or may have skin eruption at birth or child may be born normal but may develop signs of syphilitic diseases after a few months.

Rarely congenital syphilis present, *macules, papules and bullae as cutaneous eruptions. Snuffles, pot belly, saddle nose, (due to perforation of septum)* are usually seen. Bony lesions *e.g. epiphysitis, dactilytis, osteo-chondritis, osteomyelitis and osteoperiostitis* are commonly seen.

Late lesions in congenital syphilis are similar to features of acquired syphilis.

Syphilitic stigmata are features like *saddle shaped nose. Hutchinson's triad (malformation of upper central incisor tooth, corneal opacity and deafness) bulldog jaw, rhagades at the angle of* mouth. These are diagnostic aids in late life.

**Diagnosis**

Syphilitic lesions in all stages simulate other diseases so without careful history and definite signs, diagnosis becomes very difficult. Laboratory procedure helps in definite diagnosis.

Demonstration of treponema pallidum from chancre and mucous lesions with dark field microscopy is the best way to diagnose early syphilis.

Serological tests for syphilis (S.T.S.) are screening tests for specific tests.

Screening tests include (i) V.D.R.L. (Venereal diseases research laboratory test) (ii) W.R. (Wasserman's reaction) and (iii) Complement fixation test.

Screening tests are usually positive in secondary stage. They may show false positive results also. Specific tests are – (a) T.P.I. (Treponema pallidum immobilisation test) (b) F.T.A. – A.B.S. (Fluorescent treponema antibody) (c) R.P.C.F. (Reiter protein complement fixation) (d) T.P.H.A. (Treponema pallidum haemagglutination).

**Treatment**

In early stage or primary syphilis, penicillin is the drug of choice but it needs prolonged treatment. Procain penicillin-G, 600,000 units is given daily I.M. for 10 to 12 consecutive days. For secondary or tertiary stage and latent syphilis the course is increased for 15 days and in quarternary syphilis it is given for 21 days.

Benzathine penicillin 2.4 million units I.M. is also recommended for the treatment in early syphilis. However, 1.2 million units should be given in each buttock. This method is used in some clinics to avoid daily visits. Many patients may fail to come regularly specially in rural practice. In latent syphilis, three million units of benzathene penicillin in single dose repeated twice at weeks' interval is the ideal treatment. Half the dose is given in each buttock.

In case of allergy to penicillin, tetracycline (500 mgm) six hourly or erythromycin (500 mg) 6 hourly is given orally for 2-3 weeks.

Erythromycin is preferred in pregnancy.

## GONORRHOEA

Gonorrhoea is caused by Gram negative diplococcus niesseria gonorrhoea. It is highly infectious and usually effects the genito-urinary mucous membrane, anal canal, rectum, cervix and eyes in newborn. It may spread to synovial and serous membrane.

**Mode of transmission**

Gonorrhoea commonly results from, sexual intercourse, with an infected person. In the infants and babies, eyes may be involved from mother. Anal and buccal cavity infections come through perverted coitus. The incubation period is 2-10 days but it may be even longer in some cases. Asymptomatic infection in women especially prostitutes, provides common source of infection.

**Clinical features**

*In the male :* Anterior urethera is the most commonly infected site. It causes acute purulent uretheritis with dysuria. Gradually it spreads to posterior urethera and increases the frequency of micturation with serous discharge which turns soon to profuse and yellowish purulent discharge, with dysuria and pain. The external meatus becomes swollen and red. This infection spreads to the prostate and occasionally to epididymis and urinary bladder. In untreated cases, phimosis, paraphymosis and uretheral stricture may occur.

*In the female* : Urethra, the cervix, the Bartholin's glands, labial folds and occasionally rectum are sites, where infection first starts. Among infected women 50% may remain symptomless. But some case may show evidence of gonococcal vaginitis and urethritis during or after next menstrual period.

Oral intercourse may produce gonococcal pharyngitis, a diagnosis which can be missed.

Classical symptoms are dysuria, frequency of micturition, vaginal discharge and swelling of vulva. These symptoms may escape attention of the patient and extension of infection may lead to cervicitis and acute salphingitis. In young women, gonorrhoea may cause sterility due to stricture of fallopian tubes, chronic dysparunia and chronic relapsing pelvic inflammatory disease.

In female children, gonococcal infection causes inflammation and oedema of vulva with profuse purulent, vaginal discharge.

In newborn babies, infection may occur in the eyes during birth and may cause profuse purulent ocular discharge and may lead to blindness. Gonococcal conjunctivitis in newborn is also known as ophthalmia neonatorum.

Systemic infection occurs usually with skin lesion and it spreads with septicaemia, gonorrhoeal arthritis is the most common systemic infection. Iritis, iridocyclitis and keratoderma blennorrhagia may be associated with arthritis. Gonococcal myositis, tenosynovitis, pleuritis, meningitis, endocarditis and perihepatitis are some of the rare systemic complications. Reiter's syndrome is urethritis, conjunctivitis and aseptic arthritis.

**Diagnosis**

Diagnosis is confirmed rapidly even in outdoor by demonstration of Gram negative, kidney shaped, intracellular diplo-cocci, from the stained, pus smear from urethra. In smear negative case, culture of exudate on selective media such as Mcleod's chocolate agor or Thayer's Mortins selective media, shows more reliable and positive diagnosis. Specific serological test in gonorrhoea is not helpful.

**Treatment**

A single dose treatment with 2.4 million units of procain penicillin with 1 gm. of probenacid orally is sufficient to cure the male patient but female patient should get the same dose on two consecutive days. Ampicillin 2.0 g with probenacid 1.0g orally is also sufficient to treat mostly uncomplicated cases.

In patients allergic to penicillin, co-trimoxazole, eight tablets (480 mgm) single dose or three doses of five tab. at 12-hour interval is usually adequate to treat infection.

Oral tetracycline or oxytetracyclins (500 mgm) six hourly for three days or kanamycin 2 g or spectinomycin hydrochloride 2 g. by intramuscular injections are the alternative treatment.

Resistant cases require four to eight million units of procain penicillin or 3.5 g. of Ampicillin orally each preceded by 1.0 g. orally probenacid, Cefuroxime, cifoxitin and spectinomycin are also now used in resistant gonorrhoea. Recently a quinoline derivative rosoxacin (Eradacil) has been introduced for single dose treatment of gonorrhoeal urethritis in males and gonorrhoeal cervicitis in females and oral or rectal gonorrhoea of both sexes. Each capsule is of 300 mg and one dose is claimed to be effective. It is however still quite expensive.

To ensure complete cure, repeated clinical examination, smear test and culture of urethral as well as prostate massage or cervical swab are done 3 months after the treatment.

**Non-specific uretheritis**

Non-gonococcal urethritis is more prevalent nowadays than gonococcal urethritis. Cervix, prostate, urinary bladder, fallopian tubes are involved other than ureters. The causative organisms are unknown in majority of cases. In known cases they may be protozoa (e.g. trichomonas), fungus (e.g. candida albicans), bacteria (e.g. staphylococcus, diphtheroids, corneybacterium vaginale or may be due to mechanical or chemical trauma.

Chlamydia, trichomona and mycoplasma T.strains are principal organisms causing non-specific urethritis. They are obligatory intracellular organisms containing RNA and DNA and they multiply by binary fission. They are neither bacteria nor virus. Their growth is inhibited by sulphonamides or tetracyclines. Sexual intercourse is mode of transmission.

### Clinical features

Pain in urethera, glans penis, testis, perineum and inguinal region are the common symptoms. Dysurea is uncommon whereas pruritis around the urethera is the most common symptoms in non specific urethritis. Purulent, mucopurulent or serous urethral discharge may be present. Only examination of smear and culture may exclude from gonorrhoea. Uretheral exudate may be cultured for chlamydia. In females, it is even more difficult to diagnose on clinical evidence. However, presence of urethritis, vaginal discharge and cervicitis helps to settle the diagnosis.

Non-specific urethritis with associated systemic manifestation e.g. non-suppurative arthritis, conjuctivitis and distinct lesion of skin and mucous membrane (Keratoderma blennorrhagica) constitutes Reiter's syndrome.

### Treatment

Tetracycline (250-500 mg) orally given six hourly for 5 to 21 days is the usual treatment. Long acting sulphonamides (e.g. sulpha-methoxy-pyridazine) in dosage of 1.5 g. on the first day and 0.5 g daily for four consecutive days are also helpful. Refractory cases are treated by erythromycin (250 mg) six hourly orally for two weeks.

## CHANCROID

Soft chancre or chancroid is an acute venereal disease. It is localised and caused by Haemophilis ducreyi. The site of inoculation is tender and causes necrosis as well as ulceration.

### Clinical features

The initial lesion is a vesicle or papule and seen one to eight days after intercourse. It breaks down to form shallow irregular tender ulcer. The inguinal lymph nodes are enlarged, matted and may suppurate. Malaise and fever may be associated with local lesion. Prepuce, glans, frenulum and anus in males and vulva, urethra, clitoris, cervix or fourchette in females are usually involved but by auto-inoculation ulcers on the other part of the body may be present.

The ulcer is soft and bleeds on gentle touch and it may erode deeply on shaft of penis even to penetrate the urethera resulting in the sinus formation. The enlarged inguinal lymph nodes may form a suppurative fluctuant tender mass.

### Diagnosis

The multiple tender irregular genital ulcers with enlarged or suppurating inguinal lymph node, usually suggest the diagnosis but chancroid should be carefully differentiated from primary and secondary syphilis, lymphogranuloma venereum, granuloma inguinale and genital herpes.

Haemophilis ducreyi may be identified by gram staining, from exudate of genital ulcer. Special media (Brochardt and Hoke's inactivated serum medium) is used for the culture. Biopsy of the genital ulcer and its histopathology are the most efficient methods of diagnosis. Syphilis should always be excluded but it may be present in association of chancroid.

### Treatment

Sulphonamides are the antibodies of choice. Sulphadimidine is given 2.0g orally, followed by 1g. six hourly for 7-14 days. Co-trimoxazole in full dose is given for 7 to 10 days. Tetracyclines (500 mg) six hourly, streptomycin 1 gm intramuscular daily for 10-20 days are also effective.

Saline bath of local ulcer is also very helpful in inguinal abscess. Incision is not given but repeated aspiration of pus along with usual antibiotics is the ideal treatment.

## LYMPHOGRANULOMA VENEREUM

Lymphogranuloma Venereum is sexually transmitted and caused by chlamydia trachomatis. It is highly contagious, widely distributed in tropics and characterised by constitutional symptoms, suppurative adenitis, inguinal bubo and secondary ulceration.

### Clinical features

Small genital ulcer appears within one to five weeks after sexual exposure. In males,papular erosion or ulcer is seen on glans, prepuce or penis or external meatus. Vulva, vagina or cervix is involved in females.The regional lymph nodes are enlarged, tender, matted and adherent to skin and deeper structures, giving a characteristics dusky pink colour. They are usually unilaterally affected and forms a fused tender mass known as bubo which finally ulcerates and forms multiple sinuses. "Grooving sign" of L.G.V. is a groove between the enlarged inguinal and femoral group of lymph nodes corresponding to inguinal ligaments. Fever, chill, malaise, anorexia, weight loss, conjuctivitis and hepatomegaly are the possible constitutional symptoms.

In untreated cases, pelvic lymph nodes are also enlarged and lead to abscess and sinus formation resulting in peri-rectal or ischio-rectal abscess or fistulae. Rectal structure may develop due to chronic proctitis.

Elephantiasis of the vulva or penis may result due to involvement of genital lymphatics. This may even lead to ulceration of skin, pendunculated tumours on vulva in females and lobulated polypoid growth around anus in both sexes may occur.

### Diagnosis

It is made by clinical feature, isolation of chlamydia trachomatis as well as confirmed by Fries intradermal test and serum complement fixation test. Syphilis must be excluded by serological and dark background microscopic examination test.

### Treatment

Tetracyclines (500 mg) six hourly for two weeks are recommended dose but acute severe cases may require even higher doses in early stages. Chronic cases need more prolonged treatment. Co-trimoxazole in full doses e.g. two times daily for two weeks is very effective treatment. Aspiration of abscess is done but incision is avoided.

## GRANULOMA INGUINALE

It is sexually transmitted chronic progressive disease of the genitals, anus and surrounding area. It is contagious, auto inoculable disease affecting the skin and lymph node around genitals.

Donovania granulomatis is a causative organism demonstrated in scraping from genital lesions. Organism is characterised by presence of bipolar Donovon's bodies. Disease occurs in coloured persons of tropics and subtropics.

### Clinical features.

The incubation period is 8 days to 3 months. The disease starts with a small papule or nodule on the genitalia which enlarges and breaks down to form an ulcer with buffy red granular base. By autoinoculation or extension, the ulcer enlarges and spreads to thigh, perineum and natal cleft. The lesion is neither tender nor it spreads to surrounding lymph nodes. Due to cicatrisation, the lymph channels are blocked and pseudo-elephantiasis of genitals usually occurs. Untreated lesions may continue for years and leave an unhealthy scar which always tends to break down. Fibrosis may leads to stenosis of urethera, vagina or anus.

Liver, other visceras, eyes, face, larynx, chest may be involved by haematogenous or lymphatic spreads. This may be precursor of epidermoid carcinoma.

### Diagnosis

Syphilis must be excluded. Diagnosis is performed by histological appearance of Donovan's bodies in mono-nuclear cells from the scraping or biopsy of lesion. Giemsa's or Wright's stain is used to see the Donovan bodies.

### Treatment

This is treated with streptomycin 1.0g. I.M. twice a day for 10 to 20 days or oxytetracyclines 500 mg 6 hourly for two to three weeks. Tetracyclines are avoided till syphilis is excluded, and S.T.S. repeated three months after the treatment to exclude syphilis.

## SEXUALLY TRANSMITTED VIRAL DISEASES

Virus also spreads by sexual contact. Anogenital herpes simplex, hepatitis B-virus, warts, molluscum contagiosum, cytomegalovirus disease are usually commoner among sexually transmitted viral diseases. Most of them have usually subclinical course.

## ANOGENITAL HERPES SIMPLEX

It is to herpes simplex type II virus and resembles herpes or cold sores. Virus spreads by sexual intercourse.

### Clinical feature

Lesion is noticed with local discomfort around genitalia followed by a crop of vesicles as seen in herpes zoster lesions. These vesicles rupture and usually fresh crops of vesicles reappear. Vesicles are widespread on genitalia with fever, malaise and regional lymphadenopathy. Retention of urine and severe pain in sacral 2-3 dermatomes may be present due to root involvement. The illness lasts 2-4 weeks and about 50% cases have recurrent attacks which last 2-4 days. It gradually heals. Females may infect their babies during delivery.

### Treatment

It is self-healing disease, local saline bath, antiseptic lotions help in healing of lesion. Acyclovir (antiviral drugs) may shorten the course of disease. Co-trimoxazole in full dose twice a day for a week is given to prevent secondary infection.

## HEPATITIS B-VIRUS

It is more common in homosexual men and it is usually transient and sub-clinical. Few cases may develop chronic active hepatitis or cirrhosis of liver.

Vaccine is developed and used for prevention of this disease in homosexuals.

## SKIN CONDITIONS

Scabies is also transmitted in young adults by body contact during sexual intercourse. The modified lesions on genitals are seen along with burrows on other parts of body. The burrows are coiled on genitalia and looked like dull red papule. Local application of benzyl benzoate treat the condition.

*Crab-louse* or phthiris pubis is transmitted by infestated person to the pubic hairs as well as other hairy parts of the body. Treatment is the local application of benzyl benzoate or gamma benzene.

# ACQUIRED IMMUNODEFICIENCY SYNDROME (AIDS)

*G.C. MOOKERJEE*
*K.A. KABIR*

Acquired Immunodeficiency Syndrome (AIDS) is a recently discovered viral disease which has produced a tremendous and dreadful impact in our society. The disease destroys the T-Cells of the patient and thus makes him helplessly vulnerable to infective disorders. The disease was first reported from USA in 1981 (in the "Mortality and Morbidity" weekly report No.30, 305--1981). Since then many cases are being detected in many cities and towns of the Western World, chiefly USA. By 1986 more than 30,000 cases were reported out of which approximately 80% were from USA and the remaining from Europe, UK and Africa. It is uncommon in Russia and the eastern parts of the world, though some recent reports suspect its occurrence in India.

The disease specially occurs among homosexuals, bisexuals, promiscuous heterosexuals, drug abusers (taking I.V. drugs) and also young and old people receiving blood transfusions.

It is now established that AIDS is a viral disease due to a retrovirus now called "Human Immunodeficiency Disease (HIV)", previously known as LAV/HTLV-III.

## Types of AIDS

Depending on the availability of antibody tests, HIV infection has been classified as follows :—

1) Acute infection with seroconversion
2) Asymptomatic infection
3) Persistent generalised lymphadenopathy
4) Typical clinical complexes
   (a) Constitutional disease (AIDS related complex)
   (b) Neurological disease
   (c) Immunodeficiency infection
   (d) Secondary tumours in HIV infection

The last two types were previously considered as full blown AIDS.

It should be noted that in this immunodeficient state the subject becomes susceptible to other viral, bacterial, fungal or even protozoal infection.

## Clinical features

1) *Acute HIV infection* : It may present as acute infectious disease. Presenting features are : recurrent transient fever, diarrhoea, truncal rush, acute peripheral/or cranial neuropathy, thrombocytopenia, mild encephalopathy and lymphadenopathy. HIV antibody can be demonstrated at this stage.

2) *Asymptomatic HIV infection* : In this group the person does not have any evidence of the disease, but they belong to high risk groups e.g. persons with promiscuous sexual habits, homosexuals, persistent drug addicts, newborn from affected mothers, medical and laboratory workers handling infected materials, persons receiving large and/or frequent blood transfusions especially in countries where AIDS is widely prevalent. They have strong antibody levels in blood.

Only about 12% develop full-blown AIDS. Others will develop minor illness or lymphadenopathy and this latter group may be designed as carriers.

3) *Persistent generalised lymphadenopathy (PGL)*

   Extrainguinal lymph glands are enlarged and persist for more than three months in a person of high risk group in absence of a concurrent illness. About 10% of the patients develop constitutional disease.

4) *Constitutional disease*

Any person of high risk group having temperature for more than one month, weight loss of greater than 10% with diarrhoea and in absence of concurrent illness, should be strongly suspected.

5) *Clinical AIDS*

This is characterised by evidence of an immunodeficiency state. It may be associated with opportunistic infection and/or malignancy (Kaposi's sarcoma). There is absolute decrease in OK-T4 lymphocytes. Dementia and other neurological signs are present in this group.

AIDS virus have been demonstrated in both white and grey matter of human brain while elsewhere it is in T4 lymphocytes.

Lymphadenopathy may or may not be present.

**Diagnosis**

Presence of persistent fever, continuous loss of weight, oral candidiasis, diarrhoea, cough with thick expectoration, lymphadenopathy, leucopenia, anaemia, thrombocytopenia are very suggestive features. Such cases should be selected for *ELISA test* for HIV-III virus. Positive *ELISA Test* should be confirmed by other tests e.g. Western blot (W B) & immunofluorescence test. Virus can also be confirmed by electron microscopy.

**Treatment**

No curative treatment of AIDS is available up to date. Main theory today depends on :

(1) Immunodulation.

(2) Direct effect on the virus or its enzymes.

Immunodulation means boosting up of immune response of the patient by which the virus may be eliminated. It may be done by the following methods :

(a) Interleukin-2 therapy

(b) Alpha and gamma interferon therapy.

Several antiviral agents have also been tried without convincing results.

In some cases autologous bone marrow transplant has been tried. Palliative radiotherapy, chemotherapy, even vaccines have been tried but with no success.

No effective drug therapy is available for prevention, progression or spread of the disease. However, counselling is most valuable.

Will it be possible to make AIDS vaccine ? What to do tell them ?

"Avoid pregnancy, use barrier contraception, avoid needle sharing, avoid immunosuppressive drugs. Prevent recurrent infections. Suspected person should not donate blood, tissue or semen".

*"Healthy persons who do not have any promiscuous sexual habits and who do not indulge in intravenous drug addiction should have no fear from AIDS."*

## MEDICAL MANAGEMENT OF MALIGNANT DISEASES

*M. BHATTACHARYA*
*S.H. ADVANI*

There are various types of malignant diseases which can affect any system of the body. Prevention of cancer by altering the mechanism by which a normal cell changes into an invasive malignant cell is not yet known. However, some cancers can be prevented or minimised by protecting people from exposure to known carcinogens, viz. cigarette smoking, industrial pollutants etc. Medical management of cancer known as medical oncology, constitutes the application of drugs including hormones (chemotherapy) and alteration in cell mediated immunity (immunotherapy) for the cure, control and palliation of malignant diseases. Drugs can be used alone or adjuncts to surgery and radiotherapy. It is no use to refer cases for treatment in state of malignant cachexia (Fig.19.6).

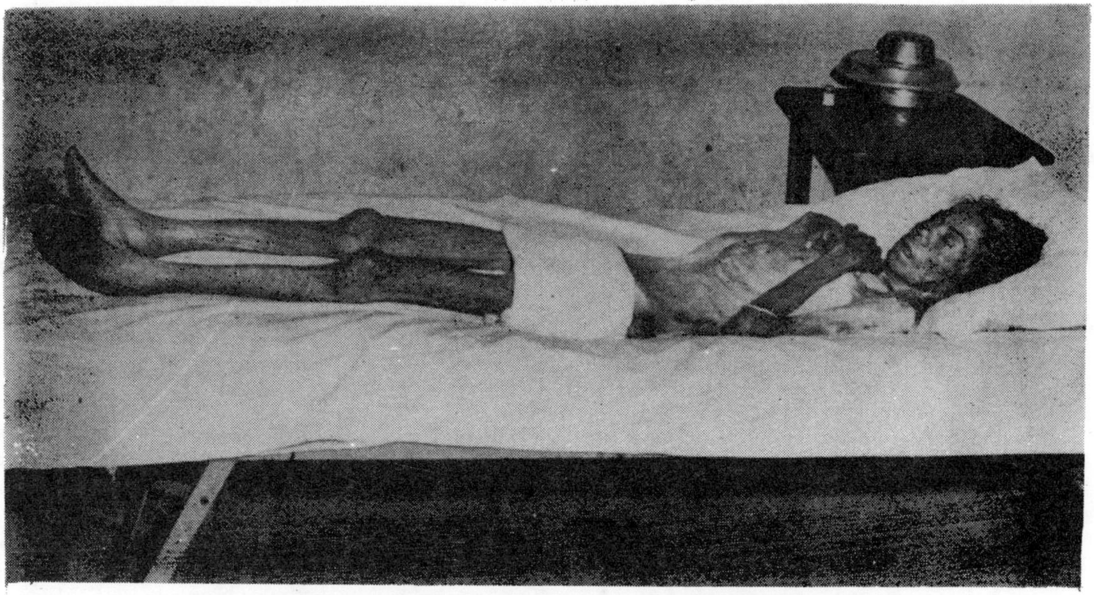

Fig.19.6 : Photo of a patient on admission. A case of Carcinoma stomach. What anti-cancer drug can be prescribed ? *(From Editor's record)*

## Chemotherapy

Chemotherapy is a major form of treatment for a variety of cancers and long-term complete control of disease amounting to cure has been achieved in several malignant diseases like childhood acute lymphoblastic leukaemias, Hodgkin's and non-Hodgkin's lymphomas, choriocarcinoma, embryonal rhabdomyo-sarcoma and certain testicular cancers.

*Mode of action of anticancer drugs*

The essence of any living cell is embedded in the three complex chemicals, viz. deoxyribonucleic acid (DNA), ribonucleic acid (RNA) and proteins. DNA is the basic blue print of life and RNA translates this blue print into the structural and functional unit of life i.e. proteins. Any drug that interferes substantially with normal synthesis of DNA, RNA or proteins can retard cell growth and may cause cellular death.

Some chemotherapeutic agents act to inhibit the synthesis of DNA, others destroy already formed DNA, some block production of RNA while still others destroy specific proteins (Fig.19.7).

*Cell division :*

One of the major factors influencing the response of a neoplasm to drug therapy is the fraction of the tumour cells that are in the replicative phase, the so-called growth fraction. The life cycle of cells starts with mitosis (M). This is followed by either differentiation or a series of biochemically distinct phases known in sequence as $G_1$ (the first 'gap' phase), S phase (DNA synthesis), $G_2$ (the second 'gap' phase) and again to mitosis (Fig.19.8). After 'M' phase, cell can enter into dormant phase $G_0$ (extended $G_1$) and such cells are relatively resistant to chemotherapy. The anticancer drugs may act on specific phase of a cell cycle (phase specific) or they may kill cells during all or most of the cell cycle (phase non-specific). (Fig.19.8).

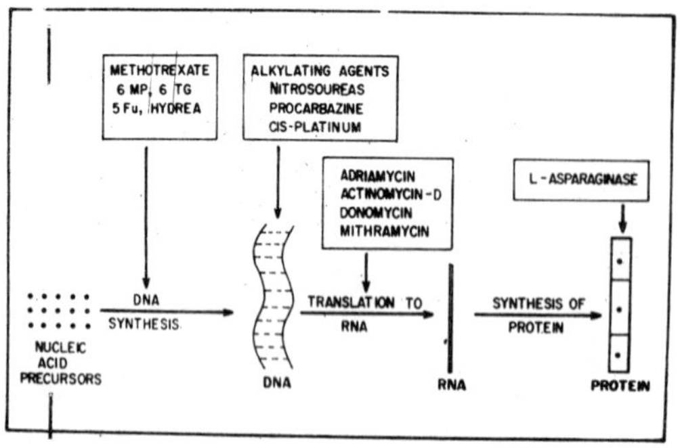


Fig.19.7 : DNA & RNA factors in oncological therapy

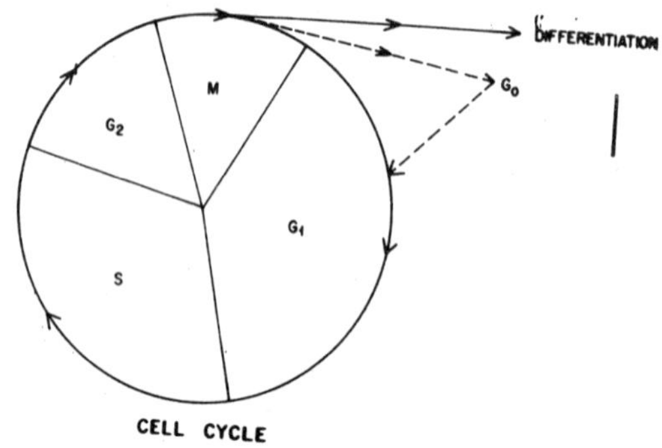


Fig.19.8 : Life cycle of malignant cells.

**Table-19.9 : Anti-cancer drugs.**

| *Predominantly phase specific drugs* | *Predominantly non-phase specific drugs* |
|---|---|
| 1. Vinca allkaloids | 1. Alkylating agents |
| 2. Hydroxyurea | 2. Nitrosourea |
| 3. Cytosine Arabinoside | 3. Antimitotic antibiotic |
| 4. Methotrexate | 4. Imidazole Carboxamide (DTIC) |
| 5. 6-Mercaptopurine | |
| 6. 6-Thioguanine | |
| 7. Procarbazine | |
| 8. Podophylotoxins | |

**Adverse effects and toxicity :**

All the anticancer agents affect mostly the rapidly dividing cells and, therefore, apart from the cancer cells, the brunt of toxicity is borne by the normal rapidly proliferating tissues of the body viz. bone marrow (neutropenia, thrombocytopenia, anaemia, infection), gastrointestinal tract (mucositis, diarrhoea), gonads (sterility) and skin (alopecia). Neurotoxicity occurs with vinca alkaloids and pulmonary toxicity (interstitial fibrosis) is a limiting factor to bleomycin and busulfan. Cardiac toxicity is a dose limiting problem with adriamycin. Immunosuppression and teratogenic effects are common to all. Table-19.10 shows the commonly used anti-cancer agents with their mode of action and major indications and toxicity.

**Table-19.10 : Commonly used anti-cancer drugs.**

| Compounds | Major Indication | Presentation and route of administration | Toxicity |
|---|---|---|---|
| I. *Alkylating Agents* (attack formed DNA chains) | | | |
| 1. Nitrogen Mustard (Mustargen, $HN_2$) | Hodgkin's & Non-Hodgkin's Lymphomas | 1 mg/vial I.V. intracavitary | Marrow, Gastrointestinal, local vesicant effect. effect. |
| 2. Cyclophosphamide (Cytoxan, Endoxan) Endoxan) | Lymphomas, Multiple Myeloma, Carcinoma Breast | 50 mg/tab Oral 100, 500, 1000 mg/ vial I.V. | Alopecia Haemorrhagic cystitis. Bone marrow (↓) |
| 3. Chlorambucil (Leukeran) | CLL | 2 mg, tab Oral | Marrow (↓) |
| 4. Melphalan (Alkeran) | Multiple myeloma, Ca-Breast | 2 mg, 5 tab Oral | Marrow (↓) |
| 5. Busulfan (Myleran) | CML, Polycythaemia vera | 2 mg/tab Oral | Marrow; Pulmonary |
| 6. Triethylenethio phosphosamide (thio-tepa) | Hodgkin's, Ca-Bladder, Ca-Breast | 15 mg/vial I.V. Intravesical | Marrow (↓) |
| 7. Decarbazine (DTIC) | Hodgkin's Melanomas, Sarcomas | 100, 200 mg/ampoule I.V. | Marrow (↓) Gastrointestinal |
| 8. Carmustin (BCNU) | Brain Tumours, Hodgkin's | 100 mg/vial I.V. | Marrow, Local Pain, Nausea |
| 9. Lomustin (CCNU) | Brain Tumours, Hodgkin's | 10,40,100 mg/ capsule Oral | Nausea, Marrow (↓) |
| II. *Antimetabolites* (Block DNA synthesis) | | | |
| 1. Methotrexate | ALL, Ca-Breast, Ca-Lung, Choriocarcinoma, Carcinoma of Head & Neck | 5 mg, 50 ml/vial 2.5 mg/tab Intrathecal Oral | Marrow, (↓) GT Tract, Mucositis (Antidote-Folinic acid) |
| 2. 6 Mercaptopurine (Purinethol-6 MP) | ALL, AML, CML | 50 mg/tab Oral | Marrow, (↓) Hepatic |
| 3. 6 Thioguanine (6 TG) | AML, ALL | 40 mg/tab | Marrow, (↓) Hepatic |
| 4. 5 Fluoro-racil (5 FU) | Gastrointestinal cancers, Ca-Breast | 250 mg, 500 mg/ vial I.V. | Nausea, Diarrhoea, Marrow (↓) |

*Table Continued to next page.....*

*Table Continued from previous page....*

| Compounds | Major Indication | Presentation and route of administration | Toxicity |
|---|---|---|---|
| 5. Cytosine Arabinoside (Cytosar, Alexan) | AML, ALL | 100 mg/vial I.V. SC. Intrathecal | Marrow (↓) |
| III. *Anticancer Antibiotics* (interfere with RNA synthesis) | | | |
| 1. Doxorubicin (Adriamycin) | Ca-Breast, ALL Lymphomas | 10 mg/vial I.V. | Marrow (↓) Cardiac (dose related) Alopecia, Local Irritation. |
| 2. Daunorubicin (Daunomycin) | AML, ALL Neuroblastoma | 20 mg/vial I.V. | —do— |
| 3. Actinomycin D (Cosmegen) | Chorio-Carcinoma, AML Sarcomas | 0.5 ml/vial I.V. | Marrow, (↓) Gastro-intestinal, Local Irritation |
| 4. Bleomycin (Blenoxane) | Lymphomas, Squamous cell Carcinomas, Testicular Carcinoma | 5 Units, 15 units/vials I.V. I.M. | Lung, skin hyper-pigmentation, Mucositis |
| 5. Mithramycin (Mithracin) | Testicular Carcinoma | 2.5 mg/vial I.V. | Haemorrhagic Diathesis, Marrow, (↓) G.I |
| 6. Mitomycin C (Mutamycin) | Gastrointestinal Adenocarcinoma | 2 mg, 5 mg/vial I.V. | Delayed severe marrow toxicity, Local vesicant effect |
| IV. *Vinca Alkaloids* (Interfere spindle formation in mitotic cell division) | | | |
| 1. Vincristine (Oncovin) | ALL | 1 mg/vial | Neurotoxicity, Ilius, Alopecia |
| 2. Vinblastine (Velban) | Lymphomas, Ca-Testes | 10 mg/vial I.V. | Marrow (↓) Neurotoxicity. |
| V. *Miscellaneous Agents* | | | |
| 1. Procarbazine (Natulan) | Lymphomas | 50 mg/capsule Oral | Marrow (↓) Nausea (Monoamine Oxidase inhibitor) |
| 2. Hydroxyurea (Hydrea) | CML, AML | 500 mg/capsule 2 mg/vial Oral I.V. | Marrow (↓) |

*Table Continued to next page*

*Table Continued from previous page*

| Compounds | Major Indication | Presentation and route of administration | Toxicity |
|---|---|---|---|
| 3. Mitotane (Lysodren, O'p-DDD) | Adrenocortical Carcinoma | 500 mg/tab Oral | G.I. upset, CNS toxicity, skin rash. |
| 4. L-asparginase (Leunase) | ALL | 10,000 I.U/vial I.V. | Anaphylaxis |
| 5. Cisplatinum (Platinol) | Ca-Testis, Ca-Ovary, Ca-Bladder | 10 mg/vial I.V. | Nausea, vomiting Marrow toxicity, Renal toxicity, Auditary toxicity |
| 6. Hexamethylemelamine (HMM) | Ca-Ovary, Ca-Lung. | 50 mg/cap Oral | Marrow (↓) Nausea Vomiting |
| 7. Podophyllotoxin (VM 26) | Lymphoma, Brain Tumours | 50 mg/vial I.V. | Marrow (↓) Nausea Vomiting, Alopecia |
| 8. Streptozotocin | Islet cell CArcinoma Carcinoid tumours | 1 mg/vial I.V. | Nausea, vomiting Marrow (↓) Hepatic Renal toxicity. |

**Principles of chemotherapy**

Chemotherapeutic agents are usually used in combination based on pharmacologic, kinetic and toxicologic considerations. Such combination chemotherapy allows the use of multiple agents without increasing toxicity and prevents the development of resistant cancer cells. Intermittent use of combination chemotherapy helps to maximize tumour cell killing along with regeneration of normal cells.

**Antitumour Hormones**

Antitumour hormones act on hormonally responsive cancers. Probably they influence synthetic process related to RNA or protein synthesis and influence production of anterior pituitary hormones. Their main indications are in cancers of breast, prostate, ovary and endometrium. Clinically, useful hormones belong to androgens (testosterone etc.), oestrogens, antioestrogens (tamoxifen), Progestrins (hydroxyprogesterone) and glucocorticoids (prednisolone, dexamethasone).

**Immunotherapy**

Immunotherapy is in experimental stage, though seems to be the ideal answer to cancer problem. No specific anticancer vaccine has so far been isolated. The principle is based on the concept that immune deficiency disorders are associated with increased risks of cancer and so enhancement of immune system may play a vital role in the control of cancer. Active non-specific immune stimulation by use of levemisole, BCG and corynebacterium parvum vaccines in lymphomas, leukaemias and solid tumours have been tried whereas passive immunisation with transfer factor, lymphocyte transfusion and interferon have found favour with some workers on cancer therapy.

Cancer chemotherapy should be carried out under expert supervision. Adequate laboratory facilities are important prerequisites. Supportive therapy like blood and blood components and intensive care are frequently needed in cancer management. Renal and hepatic function are to be assessed routinely prior to therapy and periodically during the course of treatment. Often the treatment is prolonged for months or years and frequent doctor-patient dialogue and good inter-relationship are essential.

Uric acid nephropathy is frequently encountered, particularly during treatment of haematological malignancies due to rapid breakdown of cancer cells with drugs. Adequate hydration and institution of allopurinol (Zyloric 100-200 mg three times a day) can prevent complication like gout or nephropathy.

The following discussion gives the outline of management of common haematological and other malignancies. Schedule of treatment widely varies on the type of the case at presentation, previous therapy received and experience of the physician.

**Management of Acute Leukaemia**

During the past two decades, the progress in acute lymphocytic leukaemia (ALL) of childhood has been impressive. Before the discovery of methotrexate, these children survived upto three months. The recent advances in chemotherapeutic drugs, chemical prophylaxis, and use of intensive supportive treatment have resulted in a 50% five year survival and perhaps a cure.

The treatment of ALL is divided into :-

1. Induction therapy — using vincristine and prednisolone achieving complete remission in 80 to 90% of children. Adriamycin and L-asparaginase are added in resistant cases.
2. Consolidation therapy is a continuation of intensive therapy after complete remission.
3. Central nervous system (CNS) prophylaxis.

Systemic treatment can not kill the leukaemic cells in certain anatomic sanctuary like CNS and thymus, CNS leukaemic involvement increases with the length of remission. Hence, CNS therapy (cranial irradiation 2400 rads and intrathecal methotrexate) given prophylactically does prevent the meningeal relapse.

4. Maintenance therapy : The continuation of therapy with 6-mercaptopurine and methotrexate can prolong the period of remission. Intensification therapy (periodic reinduction) is the intermittent use of the induction regimen during the maintenance phase.

The patient in remission has no symptoms or signs of disease and peripheral blood and bone marrow does not show abnormal blast cells.

Acute myelogenous leukaemia (AML) occurring frequently in adults in relatively resistant to therapy. Induction regimen including cytosine arabinoside, 6-thioguanine with or without Dauomycin can achieve complete remission in 50% of patients. Maintenance therapy usually uses same induction therapy given at less frequent interval. Immunotherapy and bone marrow transplantations are now being used in AML.

In chronic myeloid leukaemia (CML), the objective is to reduce the granulocyte mass. Busulfan 0.1 mgm/kg by mouth is the treatment of choice till total white cell count comes down to 5-1000/cmm. Hydroxyurea, and di-bromomanitol can be used in resistant cases. Splenic irradiation has also been used. Once blastic phase sets in the disease takes an acute course and does not respond to induction therapy.

In chronic lymphatic leukaemia (CLL), chlorambucil (0.1 to 0.2 mgm/kg body weight) is the drug of choice when treatment is necessary to reduce lymphocyte mass. In the presence of autoimmune haemolytic process, treatment with oral prednisolone is rapidly effective.

**Multiple Myeloma**

The protean manifestations of this condition are determined by proliferation of plasma cells and the production of abnormal gamma globulin.

Phenylalanine (Melphalan) in dosage of 0.05 to 0.25 mgm/kg daily by mouth produces relief in a few weeks. It has been shown that continuous treatment is not as effective as using the drug intermittently in courses of 4-6 weeks. A better and more sustained response is produced by using prednisolone in addition to melphalan.

Cyclophosphamide given orally is equally effective. Procarbazine, BCNU and vincristine alone or in combination have also shown their effectiveness especially in resistant patients.

**Malignant Lymphoma**

Treatment of Hodgkin's and non-Hodgkin's lymphomas depends on the pathological classification and stage of the disease.

*Classification of Hodgkin's disease (HD)*

1. Lymphocytic predominance (LP)
2. Nodular sclerosis (NS)
3. Mixed cellularity (MC)
4. Lymphocytic depletion (LD)

*Classification of non-Hodgkin's Lymphomas (NHL)*

**Nodular or Diffuse**

1. Lymphocytic well differentiated
2. Lymphocytic poorly differentiated
3. Mixed (Lymphocytic and Histiocytic)
4. Histiocytic
5. Undifferentiated

*Stage :*

I. Involvement of a single lymph node region.
II. Two or more lymph node regions on the same side of diaphragm.
III. Lymph nodes on both sides of diaphragm.
IV. Diffuse or disseminated disease involving marrow, liver & lungs.

Suffix E is used for extranodal disease.

Even stage is subdivided into A or B depending on absence (A) or presence (B) of systemic symptoms like loss of body weight fever and night sweats.

**Treatment :**

By and large radiotherapy is used for stage I and II disease. Extranodal disease may need surgical extirpation. Chemotherapy has been effective in all stages but preferably used in advanced stages (III and IV). Common chemotherapeutic regimes used are 'COP' (Cyclophosphamide, Oncovin, Prednisolone), 'MOPP' (Nitrogen mustard, Oncovin, Procarbazin, Prednisolone), 'COPP' (Cyclophosphamide, Oncovin, Procarbazin, Prednisolone) given in sequential order every 3—4 weeks for 6 cycles. Other combination regimen including vinblastin, leukeran, Bleomycin, Adriamycin, DTIC, CCNU are also used in resistant or poor risky patients.

Lymphocytic depletion in Hodgkin's disease and diffuse and histiocytic varieties of NHL constitute poor risk categories. They need more aggressive treatment. Non-Hodgkin's lymphoma can undergo leukaemic transformation during the natural course of the disease.

Prognosis of all types and stages of HD and NHL have improved remarkably with modern combination chemotherapy and significant percentage of patients will be in long term remission or even cured.

**Chemotherapy of Solid Tumours**

Unlike haematological malignancies including lymphomas wherein chemotherapy has definitive curative role; solid tumours are by and large treated with surgery and radiotherapy. Drugs are used with the aim of (a) eradicating micrometastatic tumours following or preceded by chemotherapy with the idea of long-term remission and cure viz. choriocarcinoma, carcinoma breast, Wilm's tumour, neuroblastomas, Ewing's sarcoma, (b) for reducing the tumour mass to make it amenable to surgery or radiotherapy viz. carcinoma of the head and neck region, pelvic tumours etc., (c) Palliative chemotherapy to provide symptomatic relief from pain and give a sense of well-being in metastatic and advanced inoperable cancers.

Benefit accrued to the patient from chemotherapy should be weighed against the inherent risk involved in the institution of anticancer agents. Principal drugs used in the management of common tumours are enumerated below :—

1. *Choriocarcinoma :* In good risk patients, Methotrexate alone gives high rate of cure (over 95%). In low risk or resistant cases Actinomycin D alone or in combination with methotrexate is used.

2. *Carcinoma Breast* : 'CMA' (Cyclophosphamide, Methotrexate, 5-Fluouracil) is a popular combination regime. In resistant or extensive or relapse cases, Adriamycin, Vincristin and hormonal manipulations are done.

3. *Carcinoma of Head and Neck Region :* Methotrexate and Bleomycin are very useful drugs. In resistant cases, Mitomycin and Cisplatinum are used. Single agents and various combination regimes have been used.

4. *Gastrointestinal Adenocarcinoma* : Mitomycin and 5-FU combination, are drugs of choice. Adriamycin, cyclophosphamide, cisplatium are used in resistant cases.

5. *Testicular Carcinoma :* Combination therapy of Endoxan, methothrexate, Actinomycin D or Vinablastin with Bleomycin are found to be effective in large percentage of cases. Cisplatinum has converted many hopeless cases into potentially curable problem.

6. *Paediatric Solid Tumours* : Paediatric solid tumours are more responsive to chemotherapy amounting to cure. The combination regime of 'VAC' (Vincristin, Actinomycin D. Cyclophosphamide) given at a monthly interval for 6-12 cycles. This combination has been used in Wilm's tumour, neuroblastomas, teratocarcinomas and Ewing's sarcomas. In Ewing's sarcoma and other resistant tumours,Adriamycin is used in place of Actinomycin D.

7. *Soft Tissue Sarcomas :* These tumours are usually resistant to chemotherapy. However, Adriamycin, DTIC, Methotrexate, Actimomycin,Endoxan and Vincristin either singly or in combination have been used with variable results.

# SNAKE BITE

*P. K. SETHI*

## Introduction

The snakes are among the most widely distributed reptiles. They inhabit all tropical, subtropical and most temperate zones of the earth. As a result of this broad distribution and their relatively great numbers, there are more accidents involving snakes than any other kind of venomous animals. Among the 2,000 species of snakes about 400 species are venomous. They are classified into four families :-

1. Elapidae (Cobras, krait, coral snakes, membas)
2. Hydrophlidae (Sea snake)
3. Crotalidae (rattle snakes, pit vipers)

Venomous snakes possess a complete venom apparatus, containing highly specialized glands and venom ducts draining into the fangs. Snakes are indeed more timid than aggressive towards humans. They only bite if they are threatened, frightened or stepped upon when hidden under grass or leaves.

**Estimate of the problem**

According to statistics based on hospitalized cases only (but not taking into account the USSR, Cuba and Europe), there are 40,000 fatalities per year, nearly 50% of this occur in the Indian subcontinent. In reality the number of cases may be higher as many cases go unreported. These are unofficial estimates, for the Asian subcontinent (comprising India, Bangladesh, Pakistan and adjoining areas) of approximately 1,00,000 fatalities per year. Hence it is imperative to be thoroughly conversant with the clinical presentation and management of these cases.

**Pathogenesis**

**Snake Venoms :** The venoms of most species which have been analysed have been found to be a mixture of several toxic proteins, and enzymes with diversified and complicated pharmacological effects. Venomous properties come from specific toxins, peptides with 60-70 amino acids. Most of these are cardiotoxins or neurotoxin. In addition to the toxins, the crude venoms contain many enzymes, e.g. phospholipases, endopeptidase, exopeptidases, proteinases. These are also toxic causing rapid decrease of blood pressure, change in the clotting properties of blood or damage to blood vessels and tissues.

**Clinical Symptoms/features** (Table — 19.11)

The clinical symptoms of snake bite depend upon three factors :

1. On the amount of venom injected : In defensive bite relatively little venom is ejected, but just the opposite is true in predation.
2. Relative toxicity of venom in different species.
3. Symptoms depend on the site of the bite : Venom injected into a muscle produces less dangerous symptoms than if a blood vessel has been punctured.
4. The general physical condition of the victim is very important, since cardiac and/or circulatory distress are frequent. Primary shock and collapse are not rare occurrences.

Venomous snakes leave characteristically two or occasionally one fang mark at the site of bite whereas bites from non-poisonous snakes produce a semi-circular set of teeth mark.

(a) *Local Effects* : Pain and swelling around the bite is a prominent symptom of cobra bite but not of other elapid bite. Tissue necrosis is particularly likely in bites from viperadal and crotalidae.

(b) *Systemic effects* : Venom may cause the following effects :-

(i) Gastrointestinal : Vague pain abdomen, necrosis vomiting, excessive salivation;;

(ii) Cardiovascular system : Hypertension and circulatory collapse due to vasodilatation and hypovolaemia;

(iii) Haematological system : Increased blood coagulability may occur in rattle snake bite. In others these may be increased tendency for bleeding, extensive echymoses and disseminated intravascular clotting.

(iv) Renal : Acute renal failure may occur following shock or due to disseminated intravascular clotting.

**Central Nervous System :** In elapid bite especially due to Krait, ptosis is very quick to occur followed by total external ophthalmoplegia and bulbar palsy and difficulty in handling the secretions. This in turn is followed quickly by respiratory difficulties and flaccid paralysis affecting neck in 2 to 5 days. Recovery occurs in reverse order with power in limbs improving first and ptosis last.

**Sea Snake Bites :** Are characterized by little pain and swelling at local site. There is massive necrosis of voluntary muscles with myoglobinuria and hyperkalemia. The renal failure may occur.

Some of the clinical features have been summarised in Table 19.10.

**Management**

1) Careful cleansing of the wound with sterile saline or water.
2) Most of the authorities now feel that there is no evidence that there is any value in the use of tourniquets or incision and suction of the injection site, in fact these may be harmful in unskilled hands.
3) Tetanus toxoid boester injection should also be given.
4) Reassurance is very important.
5) Antivenin : Polyvalent anti-snake venom serum (Haffkine Institute, Bombay or similar product should be given I.V. in dosage of 20 ml initially, after proper test dose, and repeated six hourly. A total dosage of 100 to 200 ml may be required.
6) In cases of neuromuscular paralysis neostigmine has been advocated by some, but majority of workers have not found it of much use.
7) As in other poisonings, maximum stress should be given to intensive supportive care of respiratory and circulatory parameters.

**Table-19.11 : Clinical picture of snake bites**

| Family | Local Effects | Systemic effects |
|---|---|---|
| **Elapidae** | | |
| 1. Cobra | Swelling, necrosis pain | Neurotoxics cardiotoxic |
| 2. Kraits | None | Neurotoxic |
| 3. Micrurus | Pain | Neurotoxic |
| **Viperidate** | Swelling, strong pains : necrosis very rare | Tissue destruction (Haemorrhages, breakdown of coagulation cardiovascular shock) |
| **Hydrophidae** | None | Myotoxic |
| **Crotalidae** | | |
| 1. Crotalus | Strong pains changing to apathy | Neurotoxic |
| 2. Bothrops | Strong pains | Proteolytic |
| 3. Lechesis | Necrosis | Breakdown of coagulation |

## POISONING

*G.C. MOOKERJEE*
*AROTI MOITRA*

### Introduction

In a study carried out by the authors in NRS Medical College Hospital, Calcutta (1975) it was observed that 469 cases of poisoning cases were admitted in a year, total admission from all causes being 30,287. These 469 cases were due to self-inflicted or accidental poisonings but snake bites were not included.

Although ICU's are now available in many city hospitals, it is unfortunate that 'Respiratory care' units are not available in many hospitals. For proper treatment of poisoned individuals 'Respiratory support' is most valuable.

Poisoning may occur due to the following causes : (1) Accidental (2) Suicidal (3) Homicidal

The substances that are commonly involved are drugs like phenobarbitone, diazepam, anti-depressants, aspirin, salicylates and even iron-salts as well as household substances like paraquet, carbolic acid, detergents, weed killers, rat poisons and sometimes poisonous fruits like berries etc. In Indian villages datura seeds are sometimes used. Children are often victims.

**Accidental poisoning**

It appears that deaths due to suicidal poisoning have increased considerably in last 30 years and women are more often involved. Except in children, many cases which are recorded as accidental may be actually intentional. Such incorrect reporting is often made to save family prestige.

Another type of accidental poisoning may be due to industrial hazards. In the recent Bhopal tragedy in India, thousands of people were affected due to methyl isocyanate gas leak from an Union Carbide Plant (1985).

**Intentional poisoning**

Patients in pathological stae of mind of often indulge in self-destruction by committing suicide. Some of these patients do not really want to die but demand sympathy. Therefore they indulge in "self poisoning" not always to really kill themselves but to threaten their relatives. This is called "para-suicide". In self-poisoning, the patients may often take positive precautions to ensure that help will be available, although misjudgements may also occur.

**Substances and methods used in intentional poisoning**

The easy availability of a number of drugs and chemicals has made this method one of the commonest modes of self-poisoning. Pesticides (e.g. TIC 20 (Sumithien) and corrosive materials (e.g. phenol and carbolic acid) are used very often.

Kerosene is often taken usually by poorer and illiterate class of people. Small children have often consumed kerosene accidently while playing in the kitchen.

Some of the drugs used are : Morphine, opium, pethidine, methaqualone (Mandrax), tricyclic antidepressants, barbiturates, benzodiazepenes, salicylates, dextropropoxyphene in combination with paracetamol.

Corresives especially acids are also swallowed by emotionally agitated patients especially women.

The methods used for suicide often vary with sex. Females prefer drugs while males seem to indulge in self-injury such as hanging and shooting. Previously when coal-gas lines were available for domestic purposes, this method constituted an important cause in both accidental and intentional poisoning but nowadays also gas cylinders are available. Accidental coal gas poisoning is also possible.

**Diagnosis**

Careful history taking environmental clues and clinical findings are the basis of diagnosis. No time should be lost in starting emergency care, whenever possible in an I.C.U. In most cases diagnosis is not difficult if the history and environmental circumstances are carefully taken into account. The poisoned patient may have left a note of his intention to die by taking poison. Be sure to verify his signature.

Poison-consultancy centres are not yet available as in the West. Therefore, the clinical has to work with lots of practical difficulties. However, much good work can be done in most cases without the accurate knowledge of the poison. A general practitioner should always refer cases of poisoning or suspected poisoning, to hospitals but unfortunately in our world even hospitals are not available within miles in many villages. So the local practitioner has to give the possible treatment, hence he should be aware of his medico-legal responsibilities.

Treatment consists of the following principles :

1) *Prevention of further absorption of poison :*

If the poison has been ingested :
Try to empty the stomach by — (a) Induction of vomiting. (b) Gastric lavage.
This should not be done in corrosive poisoning if patient comes several hours after ingestion of poison.

2) *Minimising gastrointestinal absorption :*

Neutralisation and precipitation for acids or alkalies with water, milk or a neutralizer (use of aluminium hydroxide, milk of magnesia or dilute vinegar depending on the case).

Absorption by powered activated charcoal may be helpful. Give 20 to 30 g. of charcoal or 15 to 20 ml of sorbitol it helps elimination of digoxin, pheno barbitone and theophylline.

3) *Catharsis*

Sodium sulphate in 10 to 30 g dosage is cathartic. But cathartics are contraindicated after ingestion of corrosives.

*Poisoning by other routes*

If the poison has been inhaled — remove the patient to fresh air and assist ventilation. Skin contact-wash with water and soap.

**Details of Management**

No time should be lost in starting immediate emergency care, if possible in an I.C.U. In many cases diagnosis can be made if the history and environmental evidences are taken into account. Some poisons have definite diagnostic clues as follows :

*Morphine or opium* — pinpoint pupil, slow and deep respiration.

*Coal gas* — Circumstances and its smell give clue at once.

*Methaqualone (Mandrax)* — Exaggerated reflexes, myoclonus and hypertonic limbs.

*Tricyclic compounds* (used in Psychiatry) — may cause coma presenting with dilated pupils, pyramidal signs, even cardiac arrhythmias.

*Corrosive poisons* — (Corrosive burnmarks can be seen in skin tongue and oral mucosa. *(Refer also to Table 19.12)*

**Clinical picture**

*Respiration depression* — Note if the patient is maintaining his own airway and ventilation. Respiratory depression from sleeping pills is less hazardous and resuscitation is more effective, as the B.M.R. is lowered in barbiturate poisoning and so permanent brain damage is less likely.

*Cyanosis* — If cyanosis is present administer oxygen and note its effect.

*Gag-reflex* — Good gag-response is invariably coupled with the functioning pharyngeal reflexes.

Minute volume (MV) — A Wright's respirometer is used to measure minute volume (MV). If MV is satisfactory and the rate of respiration is around 16 to 18 per minute, ventilatory exchange is considered adequate. If in doubt measure arterial carbon dioxide ($PCO_2$) and oxygen tensions ($PO_2$) wherever possible. Normal values are $PCO_2 = 40$ mm Hg. $PO_2 = 100$ mm Hg.

**Shock**

Clinical appearance : A warm pink patient with full veins indicates adequate tissue perfusion. Urine flow should be at least 30 ml per hour.

Monitoring of pulse rate — rate and depth of respiration, relationship of skin (surface) to rectal (core) temperature and acid base balance are to be noted.

Blood pressure : Should the systolic fall below 90 mm Hg, it is worth administering a plasma expander.

Hypothermia – Rectal temperature below 36°C indicates a significant degree of hypothermia.

**Identification of poison**

Samples of gastric lavage, blood, urine and vomitus should be sent to the nearby Forensic Laboratory or the Regional Poisons Centre for analysis which is a must for medico-legal purposes. However, in developing countries even in large cities poison consultancy centres are not available.

**Removal of absorbed poisons from the body**

*Detoxification* – Enzyme induction – Certain enzymes act as cholinesterase reactivators e.g. Pralidoxime in insecticide poisoning.

*Biliary excretion* – Interruption of enterohepatic circulation.

*Urinary excretion* – Forced diuresis by administering osmotic diuretics such as mannitol or urea.

Mannitol 10 to 20 g/hr. Urea 25 to 50 gm. loading dose may increase the urinary output by one litre/hr.

Frusemide 40 mg I-V administration further increases the flow. Osmotic diuretics should not be used in presence of congestive heart failure, shock or renal failure. Forced diuresis has a beneficial effect in salicylate, barbiturate, meprobamate and glutethimide poisoning.

This method is potentially applicable to all unfiltered poisons which are passively reabsorbed.

*Alteration of pH* – increases renal clearance of some poisons.

**Dialysis**

Peritoneal dialysis, hemodialysis, charcoal or resin haemoperfusion, exchange transfusion, as well as chelation or chemical binding are all practised. However, both peritoneal and haemodialysis are very useful in suitable cases.

**Administration of systemic antidotes**

*Chemical Agents*

Chemicals combine with toxic substance and thus reduce the concentration of the toxic substance e.g. ethylene diamine tetra-acetate with lead and dimercaprol with mercury.

*Pharmacologic antagonists*

Other systemic antidotes complete with the poison for the receptor site.

e.g. Atropine with muscarine
Nallorphine and Naloxone with morphine
Vitamin K with coumarine.

**Supportive therapy**

Most chemical poisonings are reversible, self-limited diseased state. Skilful supportive therapy can keep seriously ill patients alive, detoxifying & keeping excretory functions active till the concentration of toxic agent has fallen to a safe level.

As mentioned already very few poisons have specific antidotes and it is the supportive therapy which brings them back to life.

**Central nervous system depression**

This may result in coma but if the patient is given meticulous nursing care and is kept under close observation he will emerge from the state of unconsciousness as if from prolonged anaesthesia. Depression of medullary centre may result in respiratory and circulatory failure and this has got to be supported by chemical and mechanical means.

The use of analeptics in the treatment of poison induced central nervous system depression has been largely abandoned for the following **reasons** :–

(1) Their effect is unpredictable and their use in intoxicated patient produces an abnormal pattern of nervous activity in which paroxysmal excitation and convulsions may be superimposed on depression.

(2) The availability of artificial ventilation and of effective measures to support the circulation has lessened the need of rapid restoration of normal medullary function.

(3) Picrotoxin and bemegride are analeptics which were commonly used in the past.

It is doubtful that analeptics shorten the duration of coma sufficiently to justify their risks, and they have not been shown to improve prognosis.

If central venous pressure is low, fluid replacement is the first therapeutic approach.

In shock resulting from central depressions vasoactive drugs are helpful. Intravenous hydrocortisone or dopamine drips may be helpful. In spite of certain disadvantages (e.g. vasoconstriction) I.V. mephentermine drip 300 mg in 5% glucose may tide over hypotensive crises, especially if dopamine is not available.

Most of the complications of poisonings are due to :—

(1) Hypoxia
(2) Hypoglycaemia
(3) Metabolic disturbances.

Hypoxia may be due to lack of proper pulmonary ventilation and inadequate ventilation causes of the following :—

1) Central respiratory depression
2) Muscular paralysis
3) Airway obstruction
4) Retained secretions
5) Laryngeal oedema and
6) Bronchospasm.

Alveolar-capillary diffusion may be impaired by e.g. pulmonary oedema.

Interference with oxygen transport may be due to :

1) Anaemia
2) Methemoglobinemia
3) Carboxyhaemoglobinemia
4) Shock.

Inhibition of cellular oxidation occurs in continued hypoxia.

1) Cyanide poisoning
2) Fluroacetate poisoning
3) General protoplasmic poisons

Maintenance of an adequate airway is a must which may require frequent use of suction apparatus and insertion of an oropharyngeal airway or endotracheal tube or tracheostomy. The following emergency equipment should be always available :—

1) Laryngoscope
2) Cuffed endotracheal tubes
3) Ambu bag or positive pressure breathing machine
4) A portable mechanically or electrically operated suction machine to remove pulmonary secretions, foreign body, etc. from the upper respiratory tract.

If the patient does not breathe after the airway has been established, a positive pressure breathing (PPB) is to be utilised. A cuffed tube is desirable so that positive pressure breathing (PPB) may be accomplished if needed. The cuffed tube prevents aspiration of fluids into the lungs of an unconscious patient.

When insertion of endotracheal tube is difficult, tracheostomy may be done. In desperate emergency the trans-tracheal intubation is essential.

**Transtracheal Resuscitation**

Insertion of an oxygen carrying needle into the tracheal lumen may prevent respiratory death. Hypoxaemia of arterial blood may be normalised or alleviated within minutes by this technique. However, oxygen by this route will be effective only when there is some respiratory effort by the patient. Oxygen used should be humidified.

Needle is inserted through cricothyroid membrane or by cutting a point in the trachea 2 to 3 cm. below the larynx.

Patients on artificial ventilation require careful attention to endotracheal tube. Dilute (8.4%) sodium bicarbonate is instilled into the tube to wash out the secretions if required.

Administration of high concentration of oxygen is indicated whenever tissue hypoxia occurs. When central nervous system is severely depressed oxygen administration often results in apnoea and must be combined with artificial ventilation. Hyperbaric oxygen may be helpful in some situation. The treatment of methemoglobinemia, carboxyhemoglobinemia and inhibition of cellular oxidation is discussed under the specific poisons.

**Cardiac Arrhythmias**

Disturbances of cardiac impulse generation or conduction in the poisoned patient arise from the effects of certain poisons on the conductivity or due to myocardial hypoxia or metabolic disturbances. Both hypoxia and metabolic disturbances should be connected and antiarrhythmic agents administered as indicated by the nature of arrhythmia.

**Pulmonary oedema**-may be caused due to :—

(1) Depressed myocardial contractility
(2) Alveolar injury from irritant gases or aspirated fluids.

This may be associated with laryngeal oedema Action

(1) Suction : Clear airway
(2) $O_2$-4L to 5L/min may raise the $O_2$ saturation of blood. Positive pressure ventilation may be essential if the clinical state and blood gas indicates so.
(3) Aerosols of surface active agents.
(4) Bronchodilators
(5) Adrenocortical steroids
(6) Heavy doses of frusemide IM/IV

**Acute renal insufficiency**

Oliguria and anuria as a result of renal failure may occur in poisoned patient because of :

(1) Shock
(2) Dehydration or electrolyte disturbances
(3) Nephrotoxic poisons e.g. mercury, phosphorus, carbon tetrachloride and bromate.

**Treatment**

(1) Correction of electrolyte disturbances
(2) Fluid administration to treat shock and combat the dehydration.

electrolyte and water disturbances.

Imbalances of fluid and electrolytes are common features of chemical poisoning.

They are the result of :—

(1) Vomiting
(2) Diarrhoea
(3) Renal insufficiency
(4) Therapeutic manoeuvres such as catharsis, forced diuresis or dialysis.

Refer to the chapter on water and electrolyte balance.

**Table-19.12 : Common poisons and treatment guide**

| Name | Diagnostic features | Specific management |
|---|---|---|
| *Organophosphorous compounds* | Salivation, nausea, vomiting, diarrhoea, twitching convulsions, bronchospasm & bronchorrhoea, constricted pupils, pulmonary oedema, cold perspiration and bradycardia. | General measures : Wash contaminated skin; wearing gloves for safety.<br>Gastric lavage (if ingested). Give $O_2$ rapidly 5 L/min; Atropine-2 mg/I.V. repeat every 10-15 minutes till full atropinisation. This may be required for 2-3 days;<br>*Pralidoxime chloride (Protopasm). 25 mg/kg I.V slowly in about 4-5 min. If cyanosed, use $O_2$ first, before atropine.<br>Morphine, aminophylline and phenothiazine should not be given<br>[* Obidoxume recently reported better than Protoplasm.] |
| *Opium alkaloids and morphine* | Respiration very slow even less than 8 p.m.; Nausea, vomiting, pallor, pinpoint pupils, coma; respiratory depression causes death. Alcohol potentiates effects. | Nalorphine hydrobromide (Lethidrone Naloxone) to be given 15 mg (.4 mg - .8 mg) I.V. and repeat one or two more doses I.V., till respiration improves and till patient is conscious. Repeat only if relapse of coma. Effect is usually dramatic.<br>Gastric lavage with potassium permanganate solution 1:10,000 (if ingested). |
| *Dextropropoxyphene and pethidine* | SAME AS OPIUM ALKALOIDS | |
| *Petroleum and paraffin distillates* | Vomiting, diarrhoea, pallor, cough and dyspnoea. | DO NOT WASH STOMACH. If aspiration into lungs occurs respiratory support is essential. Antibiotics given with general measures to combat secondary infection.<br>Fluid and electrolyte balance essential. |
| *Salicylates* | Blurring of vision, tinitus, deafness, sweating, restlessness, hyperventilation, respiratory alkalosis-vomiting & dehydration; hypokalemia metabolic acidosis and coma in children; patient seems well despite gross abnormalities in laboratory reports. alkalosis is followed by acidosis. | General measures :<br>Gastric lavage. Forced Alkaline diuresis. Fluid-electrolyte balance is very important. Give one bottle of 5% glucose saline adding 50 ml 7.5% $NaHCO_3$ or 10 ml KCl (5%) in alternate bottles. Sometimes 20% mannitol 200 ml may be useful, encourage better diuresis. Inj. frusemide and antibiotics may be necessary.<br>Occasionally peritoneal or haemodialysis may be required. Patients may not look very ill but there may be severe acidosis leading to sudden cardiac arrest. |
| *Paracetamol* (Acetaminophan) | Large doses e.g. 8.0 g or more taken in single dose causes liver damage.<br>If mild nausea, vomiting, sweating and pallor proclaims onset of poisoning.<br>Moderate to severe hypotension, metabolic acidosis, hypothermia, hypoglycaemia, delirium and bleeding-diathesis may follow. | General measures :<br>If within 12 hours N-Acetyl cysteine to be given orally 150 mg/kg diluted in fruit juice or barley water with lemon flavour.<br>Repeat half the above dose four to six hourly for three days. Do not use charcoal.<br>(Arch. Int. Med. 141 : 138, 1981)<br>Plasma paracetamol level helpful. I.V. glucose to correct hypoglycaemia. Prothrombin time ratio to detect impending liver failure (if above 3.0) |

| | | |
|---|---|---|
| *Tricyclic compounds* | Dry mouth, urinary retention, dilated pupils, absent bowel sounds, hallucinations, slurring of speech, cardiac arrhythmias, hypotension, spasmodic torticollis, ataxia, tonic-clonic spasm, and loss of consciousness due to ventilatory depression. | Gastric lavage within twelve hours. Physostigmine 1-2 mg I/V slow or I.M. repeat after 30 to 60 min as necessary. For refractory arrhythmias 40 mEq $NaHCO_3$ I/V plus propranolol or phenytoin. Avoid digitalis or quinidine. Diazepam 10 mg I.M. or I.V. for convulsion. |
| *Amphetamine* | Excitement, tremor, insomnia, alertness, confusion, hallucinations aggressive homicidal tendencies, lethargy, depression, tachycardia, hypertension, nausea, vomiting, diarrhoea, abdominal colic, reflexes, convulsions, deep unconsciousness. | Chlorpromazine 100 mg I.M. or Droperidol/ Haloperidol (5-15 mg) may be used. A forced diuresis if severe; $NH_4Cl$ orally to acidify urine. General supportive measures. |
| *Barbiturates* | Restlessness, drowsiness, coma, delirium convulsions. Hypothermia hypoventilation, hypotension, renal failure, pupillary changes, variable reflex changes, bullous lesions in short/ medium acting barbiturates. | General measures : Treatment of cases with respiratory depression should be done in ICU as assisted ventilation is necessary. Treat hypotension and shock with pressor agents. Alkaline forced diuresis is life saving. In severe cases charcoal haemoperfusion. Haemodialysis given for phenobarbitone & barbitone. Charcoal haemoperfusion for short/medium acting barbiturates. |
| *Benzodiazepines* | Ataxia, drowsiness, hypotension, ventilation,dizziness. | General supportive measures : |
| *Cyanides and Hydrocyanic acid* | Cyanides are used in metal polishing. It is also used as pesticide, gold extraction, electroplating, rubber industry and photography. Calcium cyanide is used as fertilizer. HCN gas polluting air may cause death in seconds. Toxic symptoms are shallow respiration, smell of bitter almonds, dilated pupils, pink colouration of skin and mucosa, shock and rapid death, Many fruit seeds contain amygdalin e.g. apple, bitter almond, cassava beans, cherries, jet beans etc. | General measures. Ingestion of 50 mg of HCN or 200-500 mg of its salt, may lead to fatal issue if not urgently treated. Suicidal cases rarely are available for treatment. Amyl nitrite is easily available and can be given by given by inhalation; 2 or 3 capsules are inhaled. Then slowly give 3% soln, 10 ml I.V. in 3-5 min followed by 25% sod. thiosulphate. As cobalt compounds from an inert stable compound with cyanide, its given now-a-days as treatment of choice. dicobalt edetable (keyocycenor). Read instructions carefully. Do not give if diagnosis doubtful supportive measures include oxygen & vitamin $B_{12}$ parentrally. (Vogel S.N. etal — cyanide poisoning. Clin. Toxicology 18,367, 1981) Gastric lavage with 25% sodium thiosulphate may be given. |
| *Dhatura* | These plants grow wild all over India. Poisoning occur due to eating datura seeds, fruits and dried leaves. Symptoms are dry mouth, vomiting, dizziness, ataxia, dilated pupils, delirium and high fever. | General measures : Inj. Neostigmine 0.5 to 1 mg I.M. is a specific antidote to be repeated cautiously, if required. Antipyretics and sponging required for hyperpyrexia. Barbiturates, diazepam or paraldehyde may be used to control delirium and restlessness. Treat hyperpyrexia with cold sponging and paracetamol. |

| | | |
|---|---|---|
| *Arsenic* | Used as weed killers, insecticides, anti-fungal agents and glass industry, presenting symptoms are severe epigastric pain, vomiting, diarrhoea, resembling cholera. In cholera evacuations are painless. Circulatory collapse, coma and death may occur. | Gastric lavage; Treat hypotension energetically with I.V. fluids and dopamine. Fluid electrolyte balance needs careful attention. BAL is specific antidote. |
| *Iron salts* | Usual victims are children, Epigastric pains, nausea, vomiting, haematemesis and shock, rapid pulse and respiration, lucid interval-black stools, circulatory failure, later renal and hepatic failure, encephalopathy may occur. | Gastric lavage may be done as soon as possible with solution of desferioximine 2 g/litre of warm water and keep 5 g in stomach after washing out stomach.<br>Desferioxamine B-mesylate is used in doses of 2 g in 6 ml of distilled water by I.M. route. Slow I.V. dose is also recommended. Calcium EDTA 30 to 40 mg/kg 24 hours orally or sometimes I.V. route. |
| *Dinitro-orthocresol* | Burns of lips and mouth, yellow skin, restlessness, anxiety, fatigue, convulsions, coma, dyspnoea, pulmonary oedema, hyperpyrexia, sweating, liver/renal failure. | Wash exposed areas thoroughly with water chlorpromazine is given 100 mg I/M. Hydrotherapy to reduce temperature and supportive therapy. |
| *Corrosives — Acids or alkalies and phenol* | Burns of mouth and lips, fauces, stains, abdominal pain-shock-hepatic or renal damage. | Wash mouth, lips and immediately with plain water. Give gastric lavage to be done very carefully. Neutralise acid or alkaline poison with magnesia or dilute vinegar. Morphine or pethidine for pain. Combat shock. Give egg yolk or milk to drink. Supportive treatment most important. |
| *Carbon Monoxide (CO)* | CO-poisoning may become rapidly fatal. The most important diagnostic sign is cherry-red discolouration of skin and mucous membrane, Convulsions may occur.<br>Respiratory failure causes death. | Treatment is to ensure oxygenation. Pure oxygen should be given. Hyperbaric oxygen is most useful Delay in oxygenation leads to irreversible brain-damage. |
| *Methyl alcohol (methanol)* | Incidence of increased alcohol consumption among industrial labour often leads to consumptions of methazol as a substitute of more expensive alcohol. It is also an agent of adulteration with country liquor. | Gastric lavage as urgently as possible as it will be of very little use after 2-3 hours.<br>Sod. bic (7.5%) sol 100 ml given I.V. stat. I.V. ethanol 1 g/kg in 5% dextrose given to combat methanol poisoning in severe cases. (Blood methanol level above 20 mg%). Dialysis is best and life saving method. |

## MEDICAL PROBLEMS AT HIGH ALTITUDE

*N.R. KRISHNAN*
*A.R. SUBRAMANIAN*

Effects of high altitude (HA) have been encountered in aviation and mountaineering, but here the aviator or mountaineer goes fully prepared for a short stay. With introduction of pressurised planes many of the high altitude problems in commercial aviation have been solved. But in case of men who have to go to the mountains at short notice and stay there for a long time, the problems are many.

## ENVIRONMENTAL FACTORS AT HIGH ALTITUDE

The environmental factors at high altitude which influence the physiological processes are : the low atmospheric pressure and low partial pressure of oxygen, extreme cold, high velocity winds, low humidity, solar radiation, especially ultraviolet rays and isolation from society. The major factors responsible for the ill-effects are the low atmospheric pressure, low oxygen pressure and cold.

### Atmospheric Pressure and $PO_2$

The atmospheric pressure at sea level is 760 mm of Hg and that of Oxygen 159 mm of Hg. At about 11,000 ft, it is reduced by one-third (502 & 105 mm Hg) and at 18,000 ft to half the atmospheric pressure (379 & 79 mm of Hg).

Though $PO_2$ in atmospheric air is 159 mm Hg, on entering respiratory tract the inspired air becomes rapidly saturated with water vapour which exerts a constant pressure of about 47 mm Hg. So the partial pressure of oxygen and nitrogen in respiratory tract is reduced. At sea level, the pressure is 760-47 = 713 mm Hg and $PO_2$ is 20% of this viz. 149 mm Hg. At 18,000 feet $PO_2$ is only 69 mm Hg. At 63,000 feet where atmospheric pressure is 47 mm only, there is no room for other gases in respiratory tract.

Although the tracheal oxygen pressure can be safely predicted for any given altitude the pressure in the alveoli involves many complicated physiological conditions including partial pressure of carbon dioxide which is 40 mm Hg. At sea level the alveolar concentration and partial pressure of the gases are fairly constant, that of Oxygen being 96-110 mm Hg (103 mm Hg) and carbondioxide 36-44 mm Hg (40 mm Hg). At 18,000 feet though the atmospheric pressure is just less than half that at sea level (379 mm Hg), the alveolar $O_2$ pressure is only about one-third (39 mm Hg).

### Oxygen diffusion and its transport in blood

The transfer of oxygen from the lungs into the blood stream depends upon the pressure gradient between the alveolar oxygen and oxygen tension in mixed venous blood entering the lungs.

When the alveolar oxygen pressure found at various altitudes is projected on to the oxygen dissociation curve, it is seen that at about 10,000 ft. the oxygen pressure is already reduced by 40 mm Hg. But the oxygen saturation is still at 90%. Though there is an additional drop of 30 mm of Hg only in $PO_2$ at 22,000 feet, the oxygen saturation has dropped to 58%. The characteristic shape of oxygen dissociation curve explains the relatively mild effects of hypoxia up to 10,100—12,000 feet and the more severe effects at higher altitude.

Another important factor to be considered at high altitude is what is called the oxygen cascades. The total oxygen pressure can be broken down into 4 separate steps. The first step is the result of water vapour saturation, a fall of about 9-10 mm Hg. The second is between the tracheal and alveolar air — a fall of about 46 mm Hg and then a small gradient of 3 to 4 mm Hg between alveolar air and arterial blood due to physiologic arteriovenous shunts in the pulmonary circuit. The final step is between the systemic arterial and venous mixed blood which is about 60 mm Hg. With increasing altitudes the tracheal-alveolar gradient becomes smaller, but more significant is the artery to mixed venous blood gradient. At 22,000 feet this is only 7 mm Hg as against 60 mm Hg at sea level.

## EFFECTS OF HYPOXIA

As mentioned earlier,up to 10,000 to 12,000 feet there are no adverse effects. There is increased ventilation up to not more than double that at sea level. As altitude increases it is irregular and periodic, and may even stop while the heart is still beating. Heart rate increases (up to maximum of 30-40 beats per min) due to rise in systolic pressure. The stroke volume and cardiac output are decreased. There is redistribution of blood to vital organs with reduction of flow to unimportant organs. In some, hypoxia causes rise in pressure in pulmonary trunks causing exudation into alveoli and right ventricle may dilate. A certain degree of pulmonary hypertension is inevitable but the cause is not exactly clear. With brief exposure there are no appreciable changes. During acclimatization and on prolonged stay Hb and RBC increase.

The most objective neuropsychiatric manifestations are behavioural changes and neuromuscular incoordination. At 12,000 feet there is slight decrease in memory and onset of psychological complaints. At 14,000 feet, there is impairment of handwriting, mental fatigue and deterioration of voluntary muscular control. There is incoordination of fine muscular movements. There may be change in moods. At about 18,000 feet there is a decrease in sensory perception, loss of memory, development of fixed or irrational ideas and loss of judgement. There is a profound deterioration of neuromuscular control. Above 20,000 feet, as the altitude increases there are explosive emotional outbursts and sense of time is lost. There are tremors and finally paralysis. Ultimately consciousness is lost, visual acuity, accommodation, field of vision and depth of perception, all get affected. In addition, there is snow blindness. Hearing is impaired. In the initial stages sense, touch and pain tend to be exaggerated but later on become dulled.

Tone and mobility of gastrointestinal tract is reduced and the secretions are reduced. Liver metabolism may be affected. The intestinal gases expand with increasing altitude. At 26,000 feet the volume is double that at sea level. There is increased adrenaline secretion. Adrenal cortical insufficiency has been postulated as a cause for some of the effects of high altitude hypoxia. Thyroid function also is reduced.

## MEDICAL SYNDROMES AT HIGH ALTITUDE

1. Acute mountain sickness (AMS)
2. High altitude pulmonary oedema. (HAPO)
3. Chronic mountain sickness (Serocha-Monge's Disease)
4. Pulmonary hyertension of high altitude
5. Others — Snow blindness
   Ill Effects of cold
   High altitude retinopathy

The predisposing factors for development of AMS and HAPO are —

1. The altitude : The critical altitude is 10,000 to 11,000 fect.
2. Age : Teenagers and young children are at high risk. Young healthy people are affected.
3. The rate of ascent; especially ascent above 10,000 feet without acclimatisation.
4. Non-acclimatization.
5. Severe physical activity immediately after reaching high altitude.
6. Individual predisposition.
7. Re-entry to hypoxia is very important. It occurs at re-entry to high altitude in those already living at such elevations after going down to low altitude for a period of even as little as a week or less.
8. Pre-existing organic disease, especially of cardiovascular and respiratory systems.

**Pathogenesis of AMS and HAPO**

These two conditions seem to be clinical variants of the same condition. There is definite time lag between arrival at HA and onset of illness. The pathogenesis is not fully understood. Hypoxia causes reduction of peripheral blood flow leading to increased pulmonary blood volume and pulmonary congestion. This results in low arterial saturation and reduced splanchnic blood flow resulting in oliguria. At the same time hypothalamic-pituitary-adrenal axis is stimulated causing disturbed equilibrium of vasopressin and adrenal steroids again leading to oliguria. There is increased cerebral blood flow which causes cerebral oedema. There is also constriction of venous reservoirs which leads to dumping of an excess volume of blood in the pulmonary bed.

HAPO is apparently associated with marked pulmonary hypertension and pulmonary arteriolar constriction but normal pulmonary capillary pressure. It is possible that development of HAPO is related to an unusually marked non-uniform vasoconstriction of terminal pulmonary arterioles leading to excessive blood flow in other areas where capillary bed may be relatively unprotected from high pulmonary artery pressure. An additional factor is the presence of preterminal arterioles which are short non-muscular vessels that arise at right angle from small medium-sized pulmonary arteries, bypass the pulmonary arterioles and empty directly into the venous side of the capillary bed. Some believe HAPO to be a form of neurogenic pulmonary oedema. Widespread platelet and fibrin thrombi have been detected in the pulmonary capillaries. It is postulated that at HA a primary coagulopathy develops causing a temporary thrombotic occlusion of large number of pulmonary capillaries and those areas where capillaries are normal will be flooded with entire cardiac output leading to an 'Overperfusion oedema' of patchy distribution.

**Pathology**

In HAPO lungs are congested with serosanguinous oedema fluid. Bronchiolar and alveolar oedema with hyaline membrane over the internal walls of alveoli, alveolar sacs and ducts are characteristic findings. Preterminal arterioles are dilated; septal capillaries and small and medium sized pulmonary arteries show thrombi. Right ventricle may be dilated but left ventricle is normal. Small muscular pulmonary arteries show medial hypertrophy and crenation of elastic laminae consistent with vasoconstriction. Pulmonary arterioles are muscularized.

## ACUTE MOUNTAIN SICKNESS

Very few symptoms occur below 11,000 feet in majority of people, especially if the ascent has been gradual. In the Rockies of America, symptoms have been noted at heights of 7,000 to 8,000 feet. Above 12,000 feet majority have some symptoms and still more above 14,000 feet. Majority of persons suffer for a short time only and most of them recover without any treatment. All the symptoms disappear within 7-10 days. Between 11,000 and 14,000 feet headache, insomnia or disturbed sleep, occasional palpitation, nausea and rarely vomiting are common symptoms. Above 14,000 feet severe headache, giddiness, disinclination to work, depression and persistent insomnia are common. There is anorexia. Patients may develop breathlessness and cheynestokes respiration. Muscular weakness and fatigue may occur. Depression, apathy and drowsiness may be marked. In some there may be excitement, loss of control and abnormal and dangerous behaviour. Hallucinations and mental irritability may be seen. Above 15,000 feet symptoms are more common and severe.

Gradual ascent with periodic halts of several days to allow acclimatization will prevent or reduce symptoms. In some symptoms are severe and unrelieved except by oxygen or descent to a lower altitude. A high carbohydrate and low fat diet is said to be beneficial. Diuretics especially acetazolamide 250 mg 8-hourly prior to and during exposure to high altitude is said to reduce frequency and severity of symptoms. Increased ventilation and alveolar oxygen, decreased carbon-dioxide tension and bicarbonate and absence of alkalosis have been noted in treated subjects. Frusemide 80 mg, 12-hourly produces relief of symptoms in 48 hours, but its role appears to be controversial. In addition to being a diuretic it is said to act as a fibrinolytic also. In many cases simple aspirin will help and that is all what may be required.

## CHRONIC MOUNTAIN SICKNESS

(Monge's disease. Seroche — Monge's disease)

This is a disease due to progressive loss of acclimatization to high altitudes, first described by Monge in 1928 in the Peruvian Andes. It is usually seen in altitudes above 14,000 ft. It is rare in women and their exemption may be ascribed to menstrual loss. It is also not seen in children.

The signs and symptoms are due to hypoxaemia of high altitude and are relieved by descent to lower altitudes. In these patients the hyperventilation which usually maintains the alveolar $PO_2$ around 50 mm Hg at high altitude stops because of failure of respiratory centre to respond to carbon dioxide. This leads to hypoventilation. These persons are devoid of ventilatory response to hypoxia also.

The symptoms are headache, dizziness, cough, palpitations, easy fatiguability, paraesthesiae, sleeplessness and decreasing mental activity. Right heart failure may develop. Cyanosis and clubbing of fingers are marked.

Haemoglobin and haematocrit values are increased with haemoglobin value as much as 25 gms/100 dl. Oxygen saturation may be 70% or less. $PCO_2$ is increased. Total blood volume is elevated. Roentgenogram of chest shows cardiomegaly due to increase in size of right cardiac chambers and clear lung fields. ECG shows right ventricular strain.

The pulmonary arterial pressure is twice as high as that of a healthy person at that altitude. This returns to normal or reduces considerably after stay at sea level. Living at lower altitudes ameliorates the symptoms. Trials with acetazolamide are promising.

## HIGH ALTITUDE PULMONARY OEDEMA

It is a serious and fatal complication of rapid exposure to HA. This syndrome was first described by Hurtado in 1973 and was first reported in English literature by Houston in 1960. Since then many cases have been reported from the Himalayas, Peruvian Andes and the Rocky mountains.

The incidence of HAPO appears to be 1 in 200 ascents. Symptoms appear 3-48 hours after exposure to HA in the Andes and within 72 hours in the Himalayas. It may be delayed up to 10 days. Symptoms of AMS may precede an attack of HAPO.

Dry cough, dyspnoea on exertion, palpitation, weakness, malaise and precordial discomfort are the initial symptoms. Headache, nausea and vomiting may be present. These are followed by noisy respiration, rales, cyanosis, orthopnoea, pink frothy sputum and even haemoptysis. Cerebral symptoms may be present. In some patients there is apprehension, fear of death, incoherence and irrational behaviour, hallucinations and coma. On examination there is pallor of skin with cold and clammy skin. There is tachycardia and low grade fever may be present. Tachypnoea and cyanosis are common. Blood pressure is low. $P_2$ is loud and may be palpable. Chest reveals crepitations and even bubbling rales.

Urine is acidic with a high specific gravity. Roentgenograms of chest reveals pulmonary vascular congestion and patchy pulmonary opacities often most marked in the middle and upper zones and more on the right than on the left side. Pulmonary conus and artery may be prominent. With clinical improvement shadows disappear in 6-48 hours. ECG shows sinus tachycardia, peaked P waves, tall R in VR, prominent R in $V_3R$ and deep S in $U_6$. T waves are tall and peaked in right precordial leads. Sometimes T wave may be inverted in chest leads. There may be even positive displacement of RS-T segment.

In the management of HAPO prophylaxis in the form of proper acclimatization is the best. Oral administration of frusemide as a prophylactic measure is hazardous and has been given up. Cases of HAPO must be put to bed and promptly evacuated to altitude below 8,000 feet. 100% oxygen should be given continuously at rate of 4-8 litres per minute. Frusemide 20-40 mg every 12-24 hours has been used extensively in the armed forces on troops at high altitude but its use appears to be controversial. The dehydrating effect of frusemide under mountain conditions, themselves predisposing to dehydration, may be dangerous. Digoxin has no place in the treatment of HAPO and morphine may produce depression of respiration, especially if cerebral oedema is present. Intravenous aminophylline has been used by some and parenteral corticosteroid administration has been found to be useful by others but the value of these drugs in HAPO is doubtful.

## HIGH ALTITUDE PULMONARY HYPERTENSION

A certain degree of pulmonary hypertension is inevitable at high altitude. It manifests itself after about 5-6 months' stay above 12,000 feet. Individuals who have had HAPO and have returned to high altitude, after living in the plains for some time, are particularly predisposed.

The exact cause is not known. Hypoxia does not appear to be a direct cause though it is well-known that hypoxia leads to pulmonary vasoconstriction. There is fibrin deposits in alveolar capillaries and branches of pulmonary arteries which leads to obstruction to the blood flow and hypertension. There is also intra-alveolar deposition of fibrin to form typical hyaline membranes. Polycythaemia is another factor to be considered in the causation of pulmonary hypertension. The increased pulmonary vascular resistance leads to right ventricular hypertrophy and later failure.

Majority of individuals get only mild pulmonary hypertension and their physical fitness is not adversely affected. The predominant symptoms are dyspnoea and anginal pain. Less common symptoms are cough, puffiness of face, muscular weakness particularly in lower limbs, intermittent claudication, anorexia, syncopal attacks, haemoptysis and profuse perspiration on exertion.

Jugular venous pulse shows a prominent "a" wave. Right ventricular hypertrophy is evidenced by a right ventricular heave and a loud palpable split pulmonary second sound. A grade I or II midsystolic murmur with or without an ejection click may be present. In severe cases there is right ventricular failure. Electrocardiogram shows right axis deviation, inversion of T-waves in chest leads especially V1-V4, right ventricular hypertrophy and peaked 'P' waves. There may be an RBBB pattern. Chest X-ray shows dilatation of main pulmonary artery and its branches and peripheral oligaemia.

All symptomatic individuals must be evacuated to sea level. Congestive cardiac failure is treated on usual lines. Drugs like Tolazoline, guanethidine and reserpine have been tried. Nitroglycerine and nifedipine may be used for the angina.

## OTHER DISABILITIES

There are other disabilities like snow blindness, upper respiratory disorders due to cold, dry air and psychological disturbance due to isolation from society, boredom and hypoxia itself. Many changes in the retina in those exposed to HA have been reported. Hypothermia, frostbite and other ill-effects due to the extreme cold associated with high wind velocity are not uncommon.

# LIFE IN EXTREME COLD

*J.S. BHALLA*

Deleterious effects of extreme cold are inherent in the atmospheric environments at high altitude. At high altitudes humidity is low (as in the high altitudes of Ladakh, western Himalayas and Andes) whereas high atmospheric humidity is seen in areas like Sikkim and Arunachal.

Man's reaction differs if there is acute exposure with short-term adjustment as may appear in mountain climbing or in case of emergency parachute jumping at high altitude, from long-term acclimatisation to the low temperature,natural in permanent mountain dwellers.

### Acute exposure to cold

Human body loses heat to its surrounding by convection, conduction, evaporation of sweat and radiation in which electromagnetic energy passes to the surroundings.

Thus the loss of heat can be restricted by diminishing the area of skin directly exposed to the surrounding air and avoiding direct contact of body to snow. The type of clothing and footwear will be described in the later part of this chapter.

### Long-term acclimatisation to cold

Man can meet his climatic problems at high altitudes by evading them and by use of clothes. Acclimatisation to cold is, therefore, of lesser importance except among troops manning the borders at high altitudes or explorers.

Adaptive responses consist of circulatory adjustments protecting the temperatures of exposed portions of the body; metabolic adaptation results in greater heat production to compensate for increased heat loss.

Primary tissue which brings about increase in metabolic rate is identified as 'Brown Fat'. It is deposited in the abdomen, cervical, inter-scapular and axillary regions. The role of non-shivering thermogenesis in high altitude areas is modified due to hypoxia since the process consumes lot of oxygen. It has been observed experimentally as well as in certain animals that after acclimatisation to hypoxia heat production under cold exposure returns to normal. This is accompanied by hyperplasia of brown fat. Non-shivering thermogenesis also appears to operate in the infants naturally exposed to hypoxia and cold. Sudden exposure to severe cold causes shivering but non-shivering thermogenesis is a long-term metabolic process to combat cold due to acclimatization.

Thus the reactions to cold among the native mountain dwellers and plain dwellers differ in that the highlanders do not shiver much, non-shivering thermogenesis is maintained even in hypoxia and the blood-flow in face and extremities is high.

**Factors determining cold injuries**

1) *Environmental (Extrinsic) Factors* :

(a) Severity of cold and abruptness increases the liability of incidence of cold injuries.

(b) Wind movements hasten tissue cooling. It is the wind-chill factor (combination of low temperature and wind movement) rather than the temperature alone which determines the severity of cold injury.

(c) Duration of exposure matters in determining the final injury.

(d) Presence of moisture enhances cooling.

(e) Hypoxia at high altitude decreases the cardiac muscle oxygen and thus tissue oxygen saturation is decreased. Also capillary endothelium is, devitalised and exudation of fluid appears in tissue spaces.

2) *Subjective (Intrinsic) Factors* :

(a) Local circulatory stagnation allows lowering of temperature, exudation of fluids into tissue spaces through devitalised vascular endothelium. Shoes and tight-fitting clothes become tighter still. Physical inactivity and forced immobility cause circulatory stagnation.

(b) Malnutrition predisposes a person to cold injuries. Individual's subcutaneous fat increases tissue protection in a well-fed individual.

(c) Chronic disease, convalescence from acute illness, intercurrent infection, physical exhaustion — all diminish the power of acclimatisation.

(d) Local trauma and skin injuries predispose to cold injuries.

(e) Mental apathy, fatigue, fear, and anxiety present in cold and high altitude lead to neglect of essential precautions and enhanced liability to cold injuries.

(f) Nicotine increases vasospasm and thus risk of frostbite is increased among smokers.

(g) Alcohol consumption in large quantities increases the chances of adverse effects to cold.

(h) Adaptation to cold is an important factor determining individual vulnerability to cold injuries.

**Cold injuries in high altitude**

The various clinical conditions can be grouped as under :

(a) Hypothermia
(b) Local effects — viz, frostbites, trench foot, chilblain.

## Hypothermia

Normally the temperature of the inner trunk and brain remains constant at 37°C even though the surface temperature of extremities may be considerably low in the extreme cold climate. The rectal temperature below 34°C is recorded in what is called 'Pathological Hypothermia'. This condition occurs if low temperature and high wind velocity are present.

Early recognition of the condition is very essential. The clinical features depend upon the severity of the hypothermia and the speed with which it appears. The rectal temperature is usually 0.2° to 0.5°C higher than the others (sublingual, aural etc.).

*Clinical manifestations of hypothermia*

(a) Pallor, coldness, tiredness, light-headedness, muscle cramps, unreasonable and violent behaviour. This is followed by bouts of shivering, outbursts of energy with tendency to stubbornness, staggering gait and fainting. Listlessness and confusion are often followed by amnesia of events at the time of low body temperature.

(1) When rectal temperature is still above 30°C, clouding of consciousness with slow mentation, depressed power of comprehension appears. Speech is inarticulate and incoherent. Drowsiness supervenes, shivering bouts are more frequent, respiratory rate, pulse rate and blood pressure all are raised.

(2) Unconsciousness, stupor and light coma occur at rectal temperature of 30°C to 26°C. Incontinence of bladder and bowel occur followed by lowering of blood pressure and cardiac output. Shivering appears less frequently, pupillary and other reflexes become weak. There is generalized stiffness heralding further deterioration. Pulse and respiration slow down.

(3) When rectal temperature falls below 25°C to 26°C, deep coma sets in. Progressive respiratory and circulatory failure is followed by either rigidity or relaxation of muscles. The cardiac output becomes insufficient and death ensues.

(4) Atrial fibrillation is common between 28° and 35°C (rectal temperature) and ventricular fibrillation may occur at temperature below 28°C. Cardiac activity is known even at 11°C. Gastric haemorrhage and pancreatitis occasionally follow severe hypothermia.

## Metabolism in hypothermia

(1) Hypothermia depresses respiratory rate in proportion to the metabolic needs, thus there is slight respiratory acidosis; gradual cooling producing frequent shivering in early stages leads to lactic acid accumulation and certain degree of metabolic acidosis.

(2) Severe degree of hypothermia produces anoxic liver damage.

(3) Glucose metabolism is depressed and blood glucose and serum potassium rise as body temperature falls.

(4) In the beginning cold diuresis leads to salt and water depletion. It aggravates if hypothermia persists. Also there is extravasation of fluid into injured tissues, thus there is hypovolaemia. There is fall of blood pressure on rewarming a victim of prolonged hypothermia.

## Management of Hypothermia

Remove the patient to sheltered place immediately. Do not allow physical exertion. All measures which cause vasodilatation and further heat loss like massage and alcohol consumption are contraindicated. Aim is to raise the temperature of brain and trunk fast, at the same time avoid undue vasodilatation. Frequent recording of deep body temperature by rectal thermometer must be carried out. Warming though fast, should be carried out by stages; immediately wrap the individual in blankets and insulate it all around especially from the ground.

Subsequent management consists in immersing the individual in a warm bath at 35°C and gradually raise the temperature to 42°C in 10-12 minutes. If rectal temperature is 31°C or below at the time of rescue, immerse in bath at 42° - 44°C or not hotter than the temperature tolerable to the hand of the observer. If heart beat and respiration are absent then give artificial respiration and external cardiac massage at a slower rate than usual. Do not give artificial respiration if spontaneous breathing is present. Cardiorespiratory stimulants have no role. Intravenous fluids warmed to 35° - 38°C are helpful. Once the patient is able to swallow hot and sweetened drinks should be provided but do not give alcohol. In the absence of water bath, warming up of thorax and abdomen with hot-water bags must be achieved.

**Local effects of severe cold climate**

They are frostbite, (trench), immersion foot and chilblain. Frostbite is due to freezing of protoplasm. Trench foot is mainly due to stagnation of circulation. Chilblain is due to local ischaemia and circulatory stagnation in susceptible individuals.

**Pathogenesis**

Local cooling for many minutes below 12°C without freezing causes sensory and motor paralysis. After several hours of exposure, nerve and muscles undergo local damage and subsequently degenerate when normal temperature and blood flow are restored. Cooling below 0.54°C can freeze tissues, however biological process of super cooling, well before actual freezing which occurs at 5°C-7°C, helps.

*Frostbite* occurs in extremities and exposed areas like nose-tip and ear lobes. When the tissue temperature drops below the critical level the cellular protoplasm gets frozen and cellular framework gets disrupted causing irreversible changes in the affected tissue. Clinically the violent reaction in surrounding tissue may completely mask the tissue destruction due to actual frostbite. Two clinical types are recognised : acute and insidious.

*Acute frostbite* develops with high wind-chill factor, especially with palms and touching cold metal. The skin becomes white and crystalline. During thawing a red area appears around the frozen patch. The effects vary with the degree and duration of the exposure. There may be recovery or it may progress to a state of itching, swelling with blister formation or it may end in frank gangrene of skin. Insidious frostbite develops on rather prolonged exposure of parts to sub-critical temperature. The skin may appear normal, white or grey. If freezing continues there is extensive exudation causing oedema and haemorrhage. **Generally a frost bitten area looks worse than it really is.** *Recovery* may often be near complete, however susceptibility to discomfort on re-exposure to cold is increased. Very rarely, carcinomatous changes occur in the frostbite scar at a later period.

*Immersion (Trench) foot* develops where temperature is above the critical level and dampness is also present. Catabolites accumulate owing to circulatory stagnation, cooling and thawing producing fluctuation of temperature and capillary damage produced by cold as well as tissue hypoxia. There is pain followed by numbness due to nerves becoming insensitive. On thawing there is swelling with dusky blue discolouration; there may be desquamation of the superficial skin which may actually be gangrenous in severe cases. In more severe cases the swelling and other pathological changes described above may extend to the leg and some toes may become gangrenous. Healing is very slow and recovery may be incomplete. Restriction of joints movements and paraesthesias may remain permanent.

**Chilblain** : There is redness, intense irritation especially when in bed or on sitting near fire. Gradually cyanosis of the affected parts replaces the initial redness and pain replaces the irritation. Desquamation may supervene and bullae or ulceration may develop. The predisposing factors are assumed to be defective circulation, increased vascular permeability and deficiency of Vit.B complex and Vit.K. Chilblains may precede trench foot.

**Treatment** (of local effects of cold)

Immediate treatment consists mainly in rewarming as in case of hypothermia. Apply firm pressure with warm hands (without rubbing). Remove moist socks and clothes, apply warmth and replace by dry socks and clothes.

Avoid trauma, e.g. pressure or friction. Give bed rest and do not apply bandages or dressings. Anti-infective measures must be strictly followed after the rewarming. Skin blebs should be protected from physical contact. Treat with mild soapy water soaks, a hexachlorophene compound, cetavlon or betadine etc. Clean the skin of superficial blebs and shreds of skin by warm whirlpool therapy for 15 minutes twice a day for 3 weeks or more.

Drugs are of marginal help. Aspirin 60-120 mg three times a day reduces thrombus formation (anti-coagulants like rapid-acting Heparin should be given for one week starting within first 24 hours, if any active anti-coagulation is desired). Use of low molecular weight dextran (Dextran-40: Lomodex etc.) one unit twice a day IV helps prevention of sludging in capillaries. Vasodilators usually are of doubtful value. Tetanus toxoid should be given and antibiotics are required to deal with infection.

Surgical treatment of any kind in the early stages is contraindicated. It is impossible to judge how much of a toe or finger will finally be lost. A natural falling of dead tissues followed by plastic procedure gives the best results.

Regional sympathectomy 24-48 hours after thawing is followed by rapid resolution of oedema, earlier demarcation of destroyed tissue and faster healing.

**Life in Cold and Snow :**

**Preventive measures**

Attention of the reader is drawn to the paras dealing with factors determining the cold injuries. The factors enumerated should be guarded against. Basic dictum should be "keep warm, keep moving the limbs and toes, and keep the parts dry". **(Fig. 19.9 & 19.10)**.

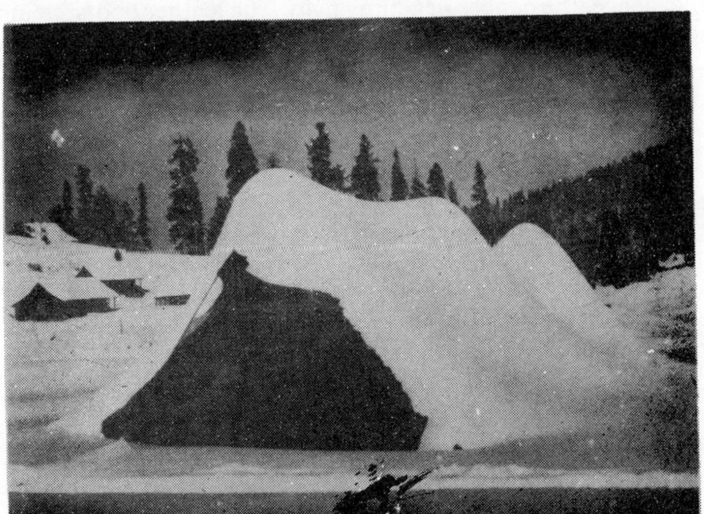

Fig. 19.9 : Problems of high altitude. Cold and snow : Wonderful to enjoy if limitations are known *(photo : Editor)*.

**Clothing :** Clothes should be loose and in many layers. The outer layer should be impervious and wind-proof. Earlier mountain-dwellers used hide of the animals like Yak, Reindeer, Mithun etc. treated with the animal fat. Now lighter and synthetic materials are available fastened with strong non-metallic zip-fasteners to keep the outer covering impervious and wind-proof. Wool, fur or cotton padding still forms the main layers of clothing. Special care should be taken for head and face which lose 30% of the body heat through poor vasomotor control. This can be prevented by use of woolen scarf in loose padded layers around the neck and Balaclava caps of wool. Damp clothing should be immediately changed (avoiding drought of wind). Gloves should be padded and loose fitting for slipping over hands in mittens.

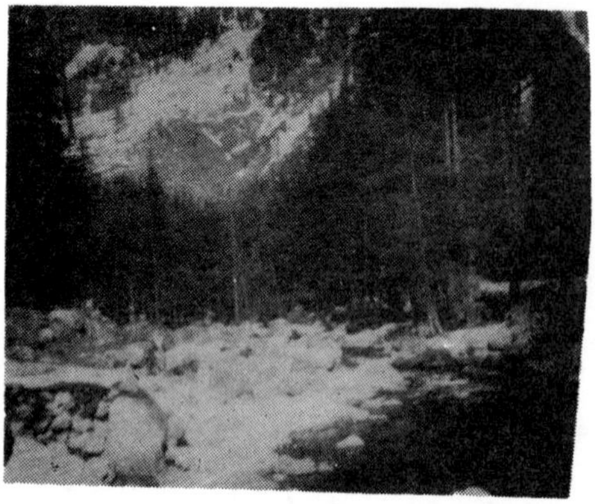

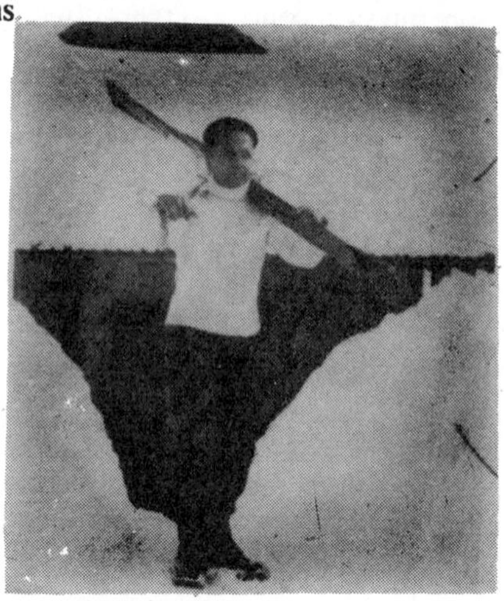

Fig. 19.10 . Living in cold and snow — Dr.Bani Ghosh ready to go on skating *(Photo : Editor)*

**Boots :** A special care should be taken in selecting boots which do not get tight on wearing double pad of socks. In cold, the felt get swollen due to exudation and prolonged dependence on standing or walking, hence, the danger of getting tight. The leather boots should be kept soft and water-proof as far as practicable by use of dubbin. For those who have to work or walk in snow and slush, gum boots are of advantage.

**Socks :** Socks should be new or not badly-darned, and they should not be tight nor any garters be worn. Spare pairs of dry socks must be readily available. Badly darned socks become dangerous by adding an element of trauma. Damp socks should be changed immediately.

**Care of the feet :** Foot should be inspected carefully before retiring to bed. Wash them with warm water and dry thoroughly. Apply animal fat or vaseline on cleaned, dried, feet every evening before sleeping. This prevents forstbite.

**Shelter :** Shelter from strong wind is essential especially when resting or sleeping. Inside the pucca-built permanent or semi-permanent structures, an arrangement for warming is made by *Bukharies* which are made of wrought iron like *Hamams* with the provisions of smoke-outlets and burning of kerosene where fire-wood is not locally available (due to trees being absent above 3000 meters) or using coke to keep the room temperature warm through convection. Kangries (a small earthenware with cane-casing and handle) with lighted coal are kept in contact with abdominal wall by Kashmiris, wrapping them inside the loose garment in cold area of Jammu and Kashmir (Incidence of skin cancer is higher among these people as a result of thermal trauma).

**Exercise :** Regular moderate exercise to keep the circulation, yet without causing any exhaustion or sweating, should be undertaken regularly. When there is reason to stay indoors for long, there should be frequent vigorous movements of limbs and wriggling of toes, fingers and wrinkling of face should be carried out from time to time.

**Nutrition :** Caloric requirement in cold is higher. Ensure well-cooked, tasty nourishing, hot food and drinks. This increases resistance to cold, promotes mental and physical well-being. Added supplement of Vit. C is desirable.

**General principles :** Personal cleanliness, dry clothing, ventilated shelter without drought, warm bed and adequate recreational activities are helpful. Bathing places should be sheltered from wind and snowfall. Avoid excess use of soap as it washes away useful sebaceous secretions.

Contact with cold metal should be avoided. Torches and metal binoculars and weapons should have velvet/flannel covers. Alcohol should not be consumed when likely to be exposed to cold wind or undertake excessive exertion, while climbing or when proper shelters to sleep are not there.

Smoking should be avoided, if possible. In case cold injury has appeared it is contraindicated.

Persons who once suffered from cold injuries should not be exposed to a similar risk.

**Adaptation to cold**

Adaptation to cold is slower and less efficient than acclimatisation to heat. However, it slowly occurs when subjects are inducted to cold areas in summer and are gradually taken on to the mountains in stages. When sudden induction to cold areas is necessary in winter, systematic acclimatisation to cold is carried out by exposing the individuals to atmospheric temp. of 0°C to 5°C for three to four hours a day for three weeks consecutively. This is called 'Hardening', 'Conditioning' or 'Seasoning'. During this period the individual should be under-cover and not in direct drought of wind and should not be carrying out exercise which may warm him and delay adaptation.

**Snow blindness**

Snow blindness is not due to effect of cold. It may occur at high altitude areas where sunglare is reflected from heavily covered snow peaks. It is best prevented by using snow goggles which completely cover the eyes and protect from the ultra-violet light. The sides of the goggles in touch with the skin are of velvet or felt materials. If an individual develops snow blindness he is kept in a dark room and bland ophthalmic creams are applied locally in the event of redness and conjuctival oedema. Generally, recovery occurs in a few days to a week.

## DISORDERS DUE TO THERMAL STRESS

*N.R. KRISHNAN*
*A.R. SUBRAMANIAN*

Climatic extremes impose their stress on man by altering the heat balance, leading to loss of vital functions, endangering life itself. Man responds to repeated exposures to a thermal stimulus in many ways, most importantly by behavioural changes like wearing special clothes or building of shelters that prevents or minimises exposure to extremes of climate. Acclimatization to climate may be defined as an enhanced ability to maintain functions at an optimal level in the face of climatic stress. The changes brought about by acclimatization to heat may be classified into primary adaptive and secondary changes. The primary changes are increased capacity to sweat, a higher blood flow through the skin and fall in resting body temperature. Less is known about cold acclimatization though it does occur in man. The temperature threshold for shivering (Ts) to augment thermogenesis is affected by the deep body temperature, insulation of subcutaneous fat and other indiviudual characteristics. The non-shivering form of thermogenesis is a complex metabolic response to cold thought to be mediated by neurotransmitters.

### EFFECTS OF HEAT

Ability to lose heat depends upon : (a) The power of body to sweat, fluid reserve in body, efficiency of thermoregulatory homeostatic mechanism and (b) evaporating power of atmosphere which in turn depends upon atmospheric humidity and air movement. When adequate sweating is associated with good evaporation and replenishment of water and salt, there is effective thermoregulation and acclimatization with a suitable level of sweating and economical loss of salt. (Fig.19.11).

**Table-19.13 – Heat disorders**

**Major** –

1. Heat stroke
2. Heat Exhaustion
   a) Pure water depletion type
   b) Pure salt depletion type
   c) Mixed type
3. Heat cramps.

**Minor** –

1. Prickly heat
2. Anhidrotic heat exhaustion
3. Heat syncope
4. Heat fatigue
5. Heat oedema
6. Sunburn

Factors which predispose to ill-effects of heat may be primary which are extrinsic environmental factors or secondary intrinsic factors. The former include high atmospheric temperature and wind velocity of more than 32 km per/hour, direct exposure to sun and high atmospheric humidity. The secondary factors are excess fluid loss, severe exhaustion, non-acclimatization, dirty skin, overcrowding, unsuitable clothing, ill-health, alcohol consumption etc. (Fig.19.11).

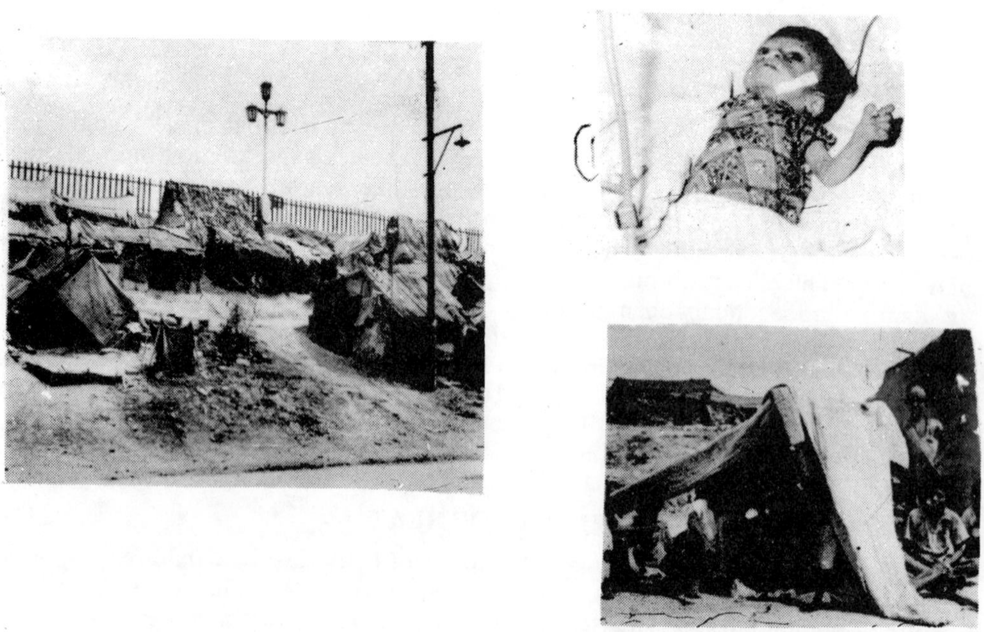

Fig.19.11 : Living condition in improvised huts leads to dehydration and Heat stroke. Inset shows a dehydrated child under fluid therapy *(Photo : Editor)*

## HEAT STROKE

Heat stroke is a medical emergency and is easily diagnosed when expected, as in young adults working hard in a hot atmosphere. But it is more common and more serious in the old and children in whom history of exposure may be lacking and hence easily missed. Use of drugs like atropine and phenothiazines may induce an attack even when temperature is not very high.

There is a central failure of sweating leading to breakdown of heat regulating mechanism and hyperpyrexia. The clinical features are due to extensive cellular damage of the central nervous system, kidney, liver and intravascular coagulation. Cerebral and cortical neurons show degeneration and haemorrhage; liver shows centrilobular necrosis. Haemorrhages may occur in serous linings, intestines, adrenals and myocardium. There is also renal tubular degeneration.

Prodromal symptoms which may be present are diminished sweating, intense thirst, polyuria, faintness, dizziness, staggering, headache and nausea. Clinical manifestations include impairment of consciousness, from lethargy to deep coma, restlessness, delirium and even convulsions. Muscular twitching may be seen. The muscles may be flaccid with absent reflexes. Skin is dry and flushed but rarely, in individuals who have been doing severe exercise, some sweating may be there. There may be tachypnoea and Chyne Stokes respiration. The temperature is 40°C or more, pulse is fast and bounding and jugular venous pressure may be raised. There may be transient cardiac arrhythmias and occasionally, pulmonary oedema. Pupils are fixed and do not react to light. The prognosis is worse when the temperature is very high and it has been present for a long time. Usual complications are shock, pulmonary oedema, myocardial infarction, acute renal and hepatic failure, cerebellar damage and consumption coagulopathy.

The laboratory findings are : low urine volume with a high specific gravity, albuminuria and renal casts, haemoconcentration, leucocytosis, raised blood urea and bicarbonate levels, low serum potassium with normal or high chloride levels, elevation of serum enzymes and reduced blood coagulation with low prothrombin and low platelet counts.

Heat stroke has to be differentiated from malignant tertian malaria, cerebrospinal fever and pontine haemorrhage.

Treatment should begin at once. The airway must be kept open and the patient moved to a shady area. The clothes should be removed and he should be covered with a wet sheet, and an air movement around the patient must be produced. In the hospital first aim of treatment must be to bring down the temperature as quickly and as aggressively as possible and maintain circulation. The most effective and quickest way to bring down the temperature is to put the patient in a tub of ice cold water. The other less effective methods are applying water cooled sheets, massaging the body with ice bags and wet sheets with a strong fan in a cold and dry room. During cooling, rigorous massage of limbs is advised to prevent vasoconstriction. Cooling is continued till the temperature comes down to 38.5°C but not to normal or sub-normal levels. Monitoring of temperature should be continued to prevent an after-drop of temperature and recurrence of hyperpyrexia. Sedation may be required to control patients who are restless and struggling or having convulsions. Tranquilizing cocktails containing chlorpromazine, pethidine and promethazine hydrochloride may be used to control shivering and convulsion.

Hypovolaemia and electrolyte imbalance, if present, must be corrected but overloading must be avoided. To correct adrenal insufficiency, shock and cerebral oedema, betamethasone 4 mg or hydrocortisone hemisuccinate 100 mg may be given intravenously slowly. Isoproterenol has been advocated by some to treat shock. Further management depends upon the nature of complications. If the treatment is delayed by more than 4 hours, mortality is very high and permanent neurological sequelae may result in those who survive. These are some changes in temperament, motor dysphasia and signs of cerebellar dysfunction like dysarthria and alexia, tremors, incoordination and nystagmus.

**Heat Exhaustion**

The clinical syndrome of heat exhaustion which is more common than heat stroke, is the result of water and salt depletion due to excessive sweating. There may be pure water depletion, pure salt depletion or more commonly depletion of both water and salt.

In pure water depletion the extracellular fluid (ECF) becomes hypertonic leading to outflow of water from the cellular compartment to restore ECF volume, resulting in cellular dehydration. Finally the ECF volume also shrinks and fails to maintain an effective circulation. Plasma sodium, chloride and urea levels rise. The clinical features are increasing thirst with a dry mouth and tongue with difficulty in swallowing. Mental capacity and judgement are impaired. Patients develop paraesthesia, giddiness, restlessness, incoordination and in severe cases even, delirium and coma, temperature is normal. Signs of dehydration are present. Respiration is rapid and may even lead to tetany. There is oliguria with high specific gravity of urine. Sodium chloride is present in urine. Treatment consists mainly of rest in bed in a cool room, and fluid intake of 6-8 litres of 5% dextrose in first 24 hours and until urine excretion is satisfactory.

Pure salt depletion results in hypotonicity of ECF. Kidney excretes more water causing fall in ECF and extracellular dehydration. Some fluid passes into the cells also. Water loss is more in the tissue compartment than in the vascular compartment. Acid base equilibrium may be upset. Patient complains of extreme fatigue, apathy and lassitude and may even go into a stupor. Anorexia, diarrhoea and vomiting reduces the intake of salt further. There is often painful muscular cramps and weakness. Due to fall in systolic blood pressure, patient may feel giddy and faint on assuming an upright posture. Here thirst is often absent. Body temperature is normal. Sodium and chloride are reduced in plasma and absent in urine. Fanta's test for chloride in urine is a useful test in diagnosing pure salt depletion heat exhaustion. Plasma volume is decreased and blood urea is raised. Patient should be put in a cool room and given plenty of salt in the form of salted fruit juices, soups and drinks. In severe cases intravenous infusion of isotonic solution, 2-4 litres in 12-24 hours should be given.

Combined salt and water depletion is more common. Dehydration is more universal and clinical picture is mixed.

**Disorders due to cold**

Harmful effects of cold, though inherent in the atmospheric environments of high altitude and the arctic and subarctic zones, can also occur in the low altitudes of plains of the northern parts of our country as in the elderly people living in unheated homes, drunks falling asleep out of doors, slum-dwellers and people accidentally immersed in very cold water. At altitudes above 3000 metres the temperature is similar to arctic climate and at altitudes between 2000 and 3000 metres it is like a subarctic zone. Effects of cold are as follows :

**Table 19.14 : Ill effects of cold**

A Generalised effect :
  1 Hypothermia

B Localised effects :
  1 Frostbite
  2 Trench foot
  3 Children

**Hypothermia**

Pathological hypothermia is due to universal lowering of body temperature as a result of acute exposure to cold. The rectal temperature falls below 34°-35°C. Injury, blood loss, shock and excessive alcohol consumption especially by a fatigued person predispose to hypothermia. If the condition is not recognised early, it rapidly progresses to a fatal end. Since the lowest reading in the clinical thermometer is 35°C, and the patient's shivering reaction ceases at about 32.5°C the condition is often missed. It is also likely that a patient with severe hypothermia may be presumed to be dead since the vital signs are so depressed and hence no resuscitative measures are undertaken.

The early manifestation of hypothermia are pallor, coldness, light headedness and muscle cramps. Unreasonable and even violent behaviour may precede the syndrome. The early symptoms are visual disturbances, slurred speech, staggering, falling and fainting. All cerebral activity ceases when the rectal temperature falls below 30°C and coma results. Bowel and bladder incontinence is common. Blood pressure falls and there is bradycardia. There is progressive failure of respiration and circulation. Cardiac pace makers fail and ectopics and ventricular fibrillation may supervene. There is generalised rigidity. Death is due to cardiac arrest or cerebral failure. In a typical case patient is absolutely cold to touch. Skin is pale and greyish. Rigidity simulating rigor mortis may be present. Vital signs appear to be absent.

Patient must be first removed to a sheltered place and all efforts made to raise his body temperature by the fastest means without overwarming the body. Till he is taken to the hospital, he can be put in a sleeping bag or wrapped in a blanket providing insulation all around. One or two healthy persons can even lie alongside him to give bodily warmth. Resuscitative measures may be required to revive the patient.

The most effective method of increasing the body temperature is by immersing the patient in a warm bath at 35°C which is gradually brought up to 40°C in 10-15 minutes. To restore the vascular tone gradual and gentle massaging can be done. When this is not possible, regional warming can be carried out by placing hot water bottles on head and abdomen. Intravenous glucose at 35°C has been advocated by some. If the patient is conscious and able to swallow, hot drinks can be given. More sophisticated but often impractical methods are inhalation of heated $O_2$ at 40°C by special equipment, warm peritoneal dialysis or extra corporeal blood circulation with a heater. (Details of life in extreme cold discussed in the previous article).

## MANAGEMENT OF AGED PATIENTS

*G.C. MOOKERJEE*
*P.N. BISWAS*

### Introduction

Treatment of elderly patients is not always away. It is important to realise that age is not always the true indication of the ageing process. Many people look aged even at fifty-five when they usually retire from services, while others look healthy and relatively younger even at sixty or seventy years. The study of the ageing process is known as "Gerontology". In medical practice it is now a speciality, known as "Geriatrics".

Modern research suggests that the ageing process may be related to immune mechanism. The involution of the thymus gland is a universal accompaniment of ageing process. Involution of cellular mass of the thymus begins at a sexual maturity and completes by 45 to 50 years. Several poly-peptide hormones are synthesized in the thymus and released into the blood, which influence life cycle of lymphocyte. These thymic hormones can no longer be detected in normal humans over 60 years of age. (The Medical Clinics of North America, March 1983). A physician must assess the patient from that angle to decide how much ageing has taken place.

### Clinical profile

An active, extrovert patient at seventy-five with diabetes mellitus, high blood pressure or coronary ischaemia may be less difficult to treat than an introvert, sedentary, senile looking patient with constipation and flatulence at sixty or even at fifty years. A careful inspection of the patient is very rewarding if the doctor is conversant with the art of clinical methods. Old people may have grey hair, arcus senilis, loss of subcutaneous fat, wrinkled skin, but his attitude and mobility, his gait and posture will indicate a lot about his ageing process. Note specially his muscle strength, spinal curvature, evidence of osteoporosis, his coordination and balance. Hearing is often impaired, specially in high frequency range. Vision may be impaired, especially if there is cataract.

Sense of smell is often impaired considerably. Sideroblastic anaemia may sometimes be encountered, which responds to pyridoxin therapy.

**Psychological aspect**

This is a very important aspect in the assessment of an aged patient. A few simple questions will suffice to assess the patient roughly. It is essential to assess his memory, orientation, thinking power and personality. Some old people ignore symptoms, so that they may attribute anginal pain to gas and gastrointestinal symptoms of carcinoma, to wind in the tummy or dyspepsia. Self-treatment is common with the assistance of lay magazines, till the disease is far advanced. On the other hand, some old hypochondriacs may develop a mountain of symptoms. Psychological attitude is to be considered carefully. At times sound advice offered by the relatives is often ignored by the old folk until the same guidance comes from the doctor. Thus a general practitioner can do a great deal to maintain health of the old people. The old has to be advised to learn the art of enjoying their old age through hobbies or some kind of pleasant occupation.

**Investigation**

The most important thing is to take a good history from the patient as well as from his close relatives or friends, who have known him for quite some time and intimately. Direct questioning is very necessary. How much activity ? How much food ? How much sleep ? Drug habit, alcohol and smoking habits ? All these must be noted. Besides a thorough physical examination, special examination, including ophthalmoscopy and rectal or vaginal examination may be necessary. Look for varicocoeles, hernia, enlarged prostate, operation scars, lumps in breast, testes and epididymis.

Routine urine test and blood sugar test two hours after full meal must be done, while lipid profile, X-ray chest and ECG may be ordered if indicated. In case of sedentary people who indulge in rich food, alcohol and smoking etc., six-monthly check-up must be recommended by the family doctor. Many symptoms, e.g. non-articular rheumatism, constipation, insomnia, fatigue, acidity and gas etc. can be cured without many drugs but by adjustment of posture, regular exercise, walking in fresh air and adjustment of diet and eating habits. A patient aged 55 years was referred to me for suspected coronary disease because of nocturnal discomfort off and on. History revealed that he used to leave his house after breakfast (consisting of two fried eggs, vegetables, "parathas" and coffee) and did not eat anything but tea or coffee during the whole day. On return at 8 p.m. to his house, he used to consume three large pegs of whisky followed by one full chicken curry and a few "chapaties" before going to bed. No wonder, his eating and drinking habits needed change. No coronary dilators were necessary.

An aged patient came for consultation with symptoms of dyspnoea on slight exertion. He smoked about 40-50 cigarettes a day and his alcohol consumption was little over half a bottle of whisky per day. He wanted to be treated, if possible without any change in his habits.

**Management**

Management of old patients depends not only on the age and degree of senility, but also upon the background disease, if any. Common causes of severe disablement are :—

(a) Hemiplegia or paraplegia
(b) Parkinsonism which is often missed in early cases
(c) Cardiac diseases, such as I.H.D. or hypertension with or without failure.
(d) Chronic bronchitis leading to emphysema which can be a leading factor of disability in the elderly. These patients are usually heavy smokers.

(e) Obesity alone can be a cause of great handicap. It can lead to hypoventilation and even cardiac failure.
(f) Result of fractures or effects of accidents
(g) Chronic bowel diseases including severe constipation or chronic diarrhoea. Colonic carcinoma can remain silent for a long time.
(h) Osteoarthritis, non-articular rheumatism, cervical spondylosis and gout.
(i) Intellectual failure — may be due to cerebral arteriosclerosis or confusional states due to infection, electrolyte imbalance, drugs, alcohol and narcotic habits.
(j) Progressive visual and auditory failure.

Management therefore should include review of family background, economic and housing condition, feeding problems, toilet and hygienic facilities as well as diagnosis of underlying diseases.

The following principles should be remembered in the management of very old patients :—

(a) Proper nursing care by nurse or domestic attendant. The nurse may train a domestic assistant in such a way that the patient can be taken care of ultimately without a regular nurse.
(b) The family doctor is the person who should supervise by periodical visits or calling the patient, if possible.
(c) Drugs should be used very carefully and encouragement should be made to "Do it yourself" way, as much as possible.
(d) Advice should be given regarding bath, toilet, care of mouth, denture, as well as how to combat pressure-sore. Pressure-sore is one of the most horrible complications in very old patients and bed-ridden people.

Some of the common symptoms in old people should be treated as follows, while investigation may be carried out :

(a) **Anorexia**

Light physical exercise, especially yogic exercise or walking, may be helpful, Acid-bitter-mixtures or alkaline-bitter mixtures may be prescribed :—

Acid-bitter-mixture —

| | | |
|---|---|---|
| Acid Hydrochlor dil | 2.0 ml | Dose : 5 ml half an hour before meals; wash mouth after taking the medicine. Better sip it with a straw. |
| Tinc. Gentian Co | 5.0 ml | |
| Aqua Chloroformi | 100.0 ml | |

Occasionally small dose of steroids, e.g. prednisolone 2.5 mg. twice a day for a week or so, may be very useful, provided there are no contraindications.

(b) **Halitosis**

This can be a very unpleasant symptom and is often due to neglect of oral hygiene.

(c) **Hiccough**

May be due to too much chillies, betel chewing, tobacco chewing, alcohol or even serious organic disorders. If persistent, it needs investigation to exclude local causes but may be relieved with antacid, non-spicy diet, regular meals and drugs like metclorpropamide or chlorpromazine.

**Skin rash and pruritus**

Unhygienic condition of the skin, nail, hair, genitalia, perineum and body folds may lead to skin infection and ulcer. Pruritus may be due to allergic dermatosis, drug rash, fungal infection, diabetes mellitus, chronic renal failure, also lack of skin care.

(e) **Chest pain**

Should always be taken seriously and properly investigated. Investigation of chest pain includes ECG as well as proper clinical evaluation.

**Dyspnoea**

Chronic bronchitis, emphysema, pulmonary fibrosis, gross obesity, cardiac failure, anaemia, skeletal fixation, are the most common causes of dyspnoea in old people. Rarely, myasthenia gravis may be responsible. Chronic renal failure or spondylitis may also cause dyspnoea when the disease is advanced.

(f) **Cough**

Treatment depends on the underlying pathology. Do not neglect a persistent cough which may be due to chronic bronchitis, cardiac failure or pulmonary carcinoma.

(g) **Joint pains and Rheumatism**

Inactivity is often responsible for so-called rheumatism in the old. Stiffness and slowness of movements are common especially during early hours in the morning. This is due to replacement of elastic tissue by fibrous tissue in the structure around the joints, gentle exercise, local heat and massage are helpful. Osteoarthritis is not uncommon, but encouragement to active life as much as possible, is the real answer. Osteoporosis should be looked for and properly treated with calcium, Vitamin D, Vitamin C and short course of anabolic steroids. Active physiotherapy is more valuable than drugs in old age.

However, drugs when necessary should be cautiously used. Avoid corticosteroids. Ibuprofen, Diclofenoc sodium, Flurbiprofen etc. may be prescribed in exceptional cases under careful supervision. Some old people tolerate aspirin quite well while others may not. In any case, investigate the underlying cause and treat cautiously.

(i) **Insomnia**

Old people may keep good health with five to six hours of sleep. Proper assessment is necessary before sleeping drugs are prescribed. Sometimes small dose of tranquilisers or even placebo may help. A night cap of warm milk or artificial milk-preparation may be useful. A table-spoon of brandy well diluted with soda or warm water may be useful and more effective as well as harmless than continuous use of sleeping tablets in old people. Psychological problem is the most important and single cause of insomnia. This factor can be carefully investigated by psychoanalysis and treated by psychoanalysis and psychotherapy. Lastly, be careful about the use of sleeping drugs, tranquilisers and narcotics in the old. Sometimes combination of drugs may be fatal.

(j) **Constipation**

May occur when the patient is dehydrated, hyperpyrexic or is acutely ill. Insufficient food intake, lack of roughage in food, drugs, e.g. opium and ganglion-blocking agents, aluminium hydroxide etc., may lead to constipation. But organic causes should be kept in view, e.g. rectal or pelvic and colonic diseases, diabetes mellitus and myxoedema. Psychological disorder may sometimes cause severe constipation. For treatment of constipation diet adjustment and regular exercises are methods of choice. Avoid regular use of paraffin-containing drugs or proprietary laxatives as far as possible. Many Ayurvedic drugs like "Trifala", 'Isabgool', 'Senna pod', Bael-fruit etc., if properly used, are far more effective and safe. Adequate water should be ingested.

(k) **Bleeding P.R.**

Do not diagnose it as bleeding piles and dismiss the case. Rectal examination and proctoscopy must not be forgotten. There may be underlying rectal or colonic malignancy in old age group.

(l) **Bleeding P.V.**

Any unusual bleeding per vagina should be taken seriously. Opinion of gynaecologist is a must. If a gynaecologist is not available in rural practice, the doctor himself must do a P.V. examination and if in doubt refer the patient to the nearest hospital.

(m) **Miscellaneous symptoms**

Painful feet often result from callosities and other minor abnormalities, relieved by local treatment. Peripheral vascular disease may lead to burning sensation or paraesthesia in the feet, mostly felt at night. Foot bath with warm water is helpful. Some drugs are useful such as nicotinic acid 50 to 100 mg twice or thrice a day or other vasodilators are of some use. Muscular cramps especially of calf muscles usually precipitated by sudden stretching movement. Relief may be obtained by standing up and thrusting the feet downwards. If not relieved, drugs such as tolazoline may be needed.

*Dizziness* — It is a distressing symptom in advanced old age. It is mostly subjective symptom to describe the effects of different clinical syndromes. Commonly light headedness, postural hypotension, instability and cerebral ischaemia. A proper history and symptomatic treatment is of value.

(Revised and updated from an article from Management of Common Diseases Vol.II by Dr. G.C. Mookerjee published by Allied Book Agency, Calcutta).

## ANTIBIOTICS

*G.C. MOOKERJEE*
*JAYANTA CHAKRABORTY*

**Introduction**

The success of antimicrobial therapy depends upon the host and parasite factors. As different drugs are handled differently by the tissues and micro-organisms, knowledge of basic biochemical and pharmacological factors is necessary for planning successful antimicrobial therapy. These factors may be briefly summarised :—

*Susceptibility of the organisms*

A simple laboratory method to determine the bacterial susceptibility to antibiotics is a disc diffusion method. It is a quick method but the results are qualitative. Quantitative data can be achieved from broth dilution (MIC) of the drug, which is the lowest concentration of the antimicrobial agent that inhibits visible growth after 18 to 24 hours incubation period. An organism is susceptible when its MIC is one-fourth of the peak serum concentration of particular antimicrobial agent. Another quantitative index of susceptibility is minimal bactericidal concentration (MBC). It is the concentration of the drug which is necessary to reduce the original growth by 99.9% as evidenced by subculture on antibiotic-free medium.

**Antimicrobial resistance**

Knowledge of resistance of micro-organisms to antimicrobial agents is mandatory for effective therapy. The organism causing infection should not be susceptible to the killing action of the antibiotic but the toxic or side-effects, if any, should be within safe level.

The development of resistance to antibiotic involves a change in the genetic material of micro-organisms. This may occur through mutation of the gene of micro-organism exposed to antimicrobials in sub-lethal concentrations for prolonged period or it may occur through transfer of genetic material from one group of organism which has already gained resistance to a particular antimicrobial to another group by process of transduction, transformation or conjugation.

*Host factors*

Metabolism of an antimicrobial agent by the body is dependent on age of the host, as some hepatic and renal bio-mechanisms are related. Premature or new-born infants are in dearth of enzyme glucuronyl transferase and are liable to develop the "gray baby syndrome" when treated with chloramphenicol. Kernicterus may develop when new-borns are treated with sulfonamides as these drugs compete with bilirubin for binding sites on serum albumin. Tetracyclines should never be used for infants and small children as it is deposited in growing bones and teeth.

*Pregnancy and lactation*

When planning an antimicrobial therapy in pregnancy one has to consider three questions. (a) Is it toxic to pregnant mother ? (b) Will it it pass through the placenta ? (c) Is it possibly harmful to the foetus ? Penicillin is quite safe drug except if allergy exists, while the cephalosporins and erythromycin are considered non-toxic to pregnant mother and possibly safe to foetus, provided there are no hepato-renal insufficiency. Following drugs should not be given to pregnant and lactating mothers.

1) Streptomycin is toxic to accoustico-vestibular system of foetus.
2) Tetracycline is toxic to pregnant mother and several cases of acute necrosis of liver and renal failure have been described when used in pregnant females. It also crosses the placenta and reach the foetal skeletal system.
3) Sulphonamides are excreted in breast milk and may cause haemolysis and kernicterus in infants.
4) Chloramphenicol should be avoided as far as possible.

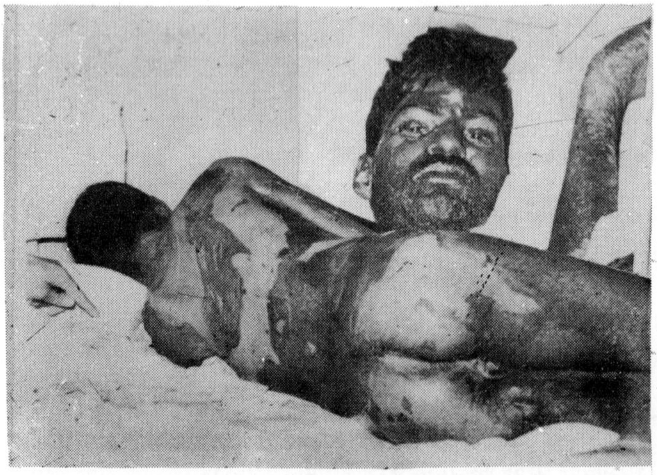

Fig.19.12 : TOXIC epidermal necrolysis in a case of Jaundice who had Inj. Penicillin (originally reported by the Editor in Naval Medical Bulletin published by Naval H.Q. New Delhi Vol.13 No.2 P.13, 1971).

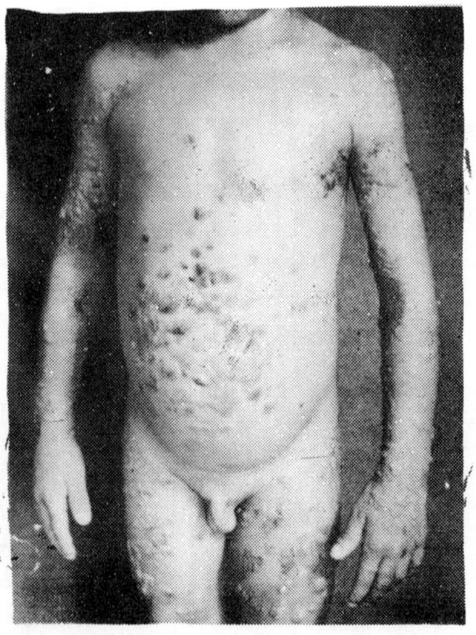

Fig.19.13 : Bullous Dermatosis due to Penicillin allergy.

*Drug allergy*

A detailed history of allergy to antimicrobial agents should always be taken and skin tests (though controversy exists) is necessary before administering an antibiotic. Penicillins, sulfonamides, and aminoglycosides are responsible for highest percentage of hypersensitivity reactions. *Keep an anti-anaphylaxis tray ready for emergency. Drug allergy may occur without warning, sometimes with dramatic suddenness.* Therefore, do not prescribe antibiotics (or even any drug) without real necessity.

1) A healthy patient has some skin disorder and was prescribed oral penicillin. As she was not improving she was given penicillin injection I.M. She collapsed and died within a few minutes.
2) An elderly executive went to his company doctor for common cold and was given a penicillin injection by the medical officer. Within a few minutes he felt unwell and was sent to a hospital by ambulance. The patient was found dead on arrival at the hospital.
3) The picture in Fig.19.12 and 19.13 are examples of drug allergy due to penicillin.

The lesions are :

1) Be cautious in indiscriminate use of drugs.
2) Penicillin is a very effective and cheap antibiotic but produces fatalities on rare occasions.
3) Keep emergency tray ready before any drug is given by injection.
4) Enquire past history of allergy.
5) Never allow patient to leave the clinic after an injection. Let him wait for half an hour.

Many common febrile illnesses are viral and do not respond to antibiotics. A patient having fever for one or two days is often given an antibiotic along with an antimalarial. Even steroids are used indiscriminately to reduce fever.

Chloramphenicol is often prescribed if the temperature does not come down within three or four days. This is not correct.

***Liver disorders***

Some antibiotics e.g. erythromycin, chloramphenicol, linconoids, macrolides, rifamycin and imidazoles are metabolised by hepato-biliary system. So in hepatic disorders the use of these antimicrobial agents should be avoided.

7) *Renal disorders* — Though most of the antimicrobial agents are excreted by kidney some of them e.g. aminoglycosides, vancomycin, flucytosine and polymixins are solely dependent or renal excretion. In renal diseases or in old age when renal function is partly impaired the usc of these agents should be properly monitored or better avoided.
8) *CNS disorders* — Some antibiotics e.g. penicillin G reduces the seizure threshold of CNS. So these drugs should be avoided in high doses to epilepsy patients. Aminoglycosides should be avoided in myasthenic patients as they have some inherent neuro-muscular effect.
9) *Genetic factors* — Fatal haemolysis or methemoglobinaemia may develop when patients with glucose 6-phosphate dehydrogenase deficiency or some haemoglobinopathy are prescribed, sulfonamides, chloramphenicol and nitrofurantoins.
10) *Immunological status* — It is an important modifying factor of the host-defence mechanisms, both humoral and cellular. Antimicrobial therapy in this immunocompromised patients (e.g. AIDS) should consist of administration of most rapidly bactericidal drugs in combination with antifungal agents, where necessary.
11) *Local factors* — Presence of pus, blood, foreign body, devitalised tissue at the site of infection interfere with penetration and efficacy of antibiotics. Particularly presence of prosthetic material may produce a protected environment where host-defence mechanism cannot assist the antimicrobial agent in eliminating the pathogen.

**Penicillins**

Since the discovery of penicillin in 1929 by Fleming, many newer penicillins have become available.

Penicillins can be classified according to their antimicrobial activity into following classes :

(1) Penicillin G. and Penicillin V
(2) Amino-Penicillins
(3) Penicillinase-resistant penicillins
(4) Carboxy-penicillins
(5) Ureido-penicillins
(6) Miscellaneous penicillins.

**Penicillins G and Penicillin V**

Penicillin G is active through oral, intramuscular and intravenous routes. We do not generally recommend oral penicillin. It may cause allergic reactions when penicillins are parenterally used later on. It also becomes expensive as long-term therapy while absorption may not be guaranted.

Penicillins are highly active against many species of Gram-positive and Gram-negative cocci e.g.

(a) Streptococci — β-hemolytic streptococci, st. pneumonae, st. viridans, micro-aerophilic and anaerobic streptococci.

(b) Staphylococci — S. aureus and S. epidermidis were sensitiye to penicillin-G but now-a-days about 90% of them are resistant to penicillin G.

(c) Neisseria — N. meningitidis and N. gonorrhoeae are β lactamase producing, hence resistant.

(d) Clostridia — Most of the strains of clostridia are highly sensitive to penicillin G.

(e) Other infrequently encountered organisms e.g. corynebacterium, treponema, listeria monocytogenes, erisipelothrix, pasturella, strepto-bacillus monilliformis, spirillium, fusospirochaetes, actinomyces israelii and leptospira are susceptible to penicillin G. Generally Gram-negative bacilli are resistant to penicillin G but in high concentrations of the drug some organisms e.g. proteus mirabillis and some strains of E.Coli are susceptible.

**Aminopenicillins**

The aminopenicillins have the spectrum similar to penicillin-G but in addition they are active against many Gram-negative bacteria. They are all destroyed by β-lactamase hence inactive against staphylococci. Aminopenicillins may cause allergic reactions like penicillin-G. So they should not be given to patients with known penicillin hypersensitivity.

There are many aminopenicillins available at present but among these ampicillins, amoxycillin and bacampicillins are presently available in our country. Amoxycillin and bacampicillin are absorbed twice as fast as ampicillin in similar doses. So oral amoxycillin and bacampicillin give effective concentration in serum comparable to ampicillin administered parenterally. On the other hand, due to rapid absorption of amoxycillin and bacampicillin from gut they are less effective against shigella and salmonella organisms.

The aminopenicillins are very much effective against streptococi, pneumococci, meningococci, gonococci, haemophilus influenzae and streptococcus viridans. They are also used in the treatment of infections caused by E. Coli, B. mirabilis, salmonella, shigella though increasing number of resistant strains are now being discovered.

**Penicillinase resistant penicillins :-**

In this group are included those penicillins which are resistant to the enzyme β-lactamase (penicillinase) elaborated by S. aureus and other micro-organisms e.g. S. epidermides, S. pyogenes etc. There are now several compounds used for this purpose e.g. methicillin, nafcillin, oxacillin, cloxacillin, dicloxacillin and floxacillins are also effective.

Methicillin cannot be administered orally as it is destroyed by acid gastric juice. It has a short half life, so 4 hourly intramuscular injections are needed. It may cause interstitial nephritis, so its use is restricted nowadays.

Nafcillin should not be used orally as its absorption is irregular after oral dose. However, when administered parenterally its concentration in CSF is sufficient for treating staphylococcal meningitis.

The penicillinase-resistant penicillins are not effective against Gram-negative organisms. It should be remembered that though Gram-positive organisms are susceptible to them, they are not subsititute for penicillin-G in the treatment of organisms susceptible to it.

*Carboxy-penicillins*

These are penicillinase-susceptible penicillins derived from 6-aminopenicillanic acid. They are unique in that they are active against pseudomonas aeruginosa and certain indole positive proteus species. These carboxypenicillins act synergistically with aminoglycosides to inhibit the Gram-negative organisms. But they cannot be given in same solutions with aminoglycosides, since they combine with aminoglycosides rendering the latter inactive. Two of them are now used – carbenicillin and its indanyl-ester, indanyl-carbenicillin and tricarcillin Carbenicillin is not absorbed from the G.I. tract and hence is given parenterally. The pseudomonas are inhibited by a concentration of the drug about 100 μg/ml in plasma, which can only be achieved by giving about 4 to 5 gm daily in four hourly divided doses by I.V. injections.

It should be remembered that suboptimal doses of carbenicillin may result in emergence of resistant strains of pseudomonas in vivo. Carbenicillin is excreted primarily by the kidneys. So dose adjustment is necessary in renal failure. Carbenicillin preparations available in the market, have high sodium content, therefore this aspect needs due consideration while administering it to cases of C.C.F. It may also cause hypokalaemia due to obligatory excretion ,of cation when large amounts of non-absorbable anion (carbenicillin) is presented to distal renal tubules. Carbenicillin may also cause prolonged bleeding time or actual bleeding diathesis as it binds itself to ADP receptor sites on platelets and hence prevents platelet aggregation. Carbenicillin indanyl can be given orally as it is acid stable. But when given orally it does not reach optimal plasma concentration for treatment of systemic pseudomonas infection. However it is very effective for urinary tract infections caused by proteus species, other than proteus mirabilis and pseudomonas aeruginosa as massive portion of the drug is excreted rapidly in urine.

Tricarcillin is four times more potent than carbenicillin. The antibacterial spectrum and excretion are similar to carbenicillin but the doses required are a little less.

**Ureido-penicillins**

The ureido-penicillins are derivatives of ampicillin, they are mezlocillin, azlocillin and pipercillin. They are unstable when given orally and should be administered intravenously as large doses are required (15-20 gm/day). They are rapidly excreted by kidneys. Dosage modification is necessary in advanced renal insufficiency.

Azlocillin is more potent than tricarcillin against pseudomonas. It has the same activity as ampicillin against streptococci.

Mezlocillin is also similarly active against streptococci especially S. faecalis. It is also active against klebsiella, H. influenzae and B. fragilis in contrast to carbenicillin or tricarcillin.

Pipercillin in many respects has the combined properties of azlocillin and mezlocillin. It is of greatest value in treatment of abdominal and female genital tract infections where anaerobic or mixed aerobic-anaerobic organisms are likely pathogens. It is active against streptococci., neisseria, hemophilus, klebsiella and bacteroides in addition to pseudomonas species.

**Miscellaneous Penicillins & Enzyme Inhibitors**

There are some newer penicillins e.g. amongst which temocillin is a derivative of tricarcillin. It is a β-lactamase resistant penicillin but it has less activity against Gram-positive bacteria. It is effective against E. Coli, klebsiella, enterobactor, proteus and serratia.

Table-19.15 : presents commonly used penicillins and semisynthetic penicillins.

**Table-19.15 : Commonly used penicillins and semisynthetic penicillins**

1) *Penicillins* : Benzyl-penicillin (crystalline penicillin-G), Procaine benzyl-penicillin (procaine penicillin), Procaine penicillin fortified (procaine penicillin G containing procaine penicillin 300,000 units + crystalline penicillin 100,000units), Benzathine penicillin (long acting penicillin, available as $LA_6$ and $LA_{12}$ with antibiotic action remaining for two to four weeks.

   Procaine penicillin in oil (suspension in oil with 2% aluminium monostearate) action maintained for 48-72 hours.

2) *Semisynthetic penicillins* :
   (a) Penicillinase resistant and acid resistant : Oxacillin, cloxacillin, nafcillin, etc.
   (b) Penicillinase resistant but acid sensitive : Methicillin.
   (c) Broad spectrum effects : Ampicillin, amoxycillin, bacampicillin are also acid resistant while carbenicillin, ticarcillin and piperacillin are acid resistant.

In addition oral penicillins are also available e.g. potassium phenoxymethyl penicillin and potassium phenoxyethyl penicillin.

We do not recommend the use of oral penicillins in general as they are not always therapeutically reliable. Allergic reactions are more likely to occur when parenteral penicillin is used at a later date. It is also expensive (Editor's view).

**Cephalosporins**

The original discovery of cephalosporin by Prof. G. Brotzu of Sardinia is no less dramatic than the discovery of penicillin by Dr. Alexander Fleming. Prof. Brotzn collected sewage water from the drainage out-fall of the town to the sea and discovered a fungus cephalosporium acremonium. This material was sent to Dr. Florey in 1948 and after seven years of research he found in 1955 that this fungus produced seven antibiotics.

Cephalosporins are chemically 7-amino cephalosporinic acid nucleus.

The cephalosporins can be conveniently classified into three generations according to the antimicrobial activity, metabolic stability and resistance to cephalosporinases.

**Table-19.16 : Important Oral & Parenteral Cephalosporins**

| Oral use | Parenteral use only | |
|---|---|---|
| | β-lactamase sensitive | Beta lactamase resistant |
| Cephalexine | Cephaloridine | Cefuroxime |
| Cephadrine | Cephalothin | Cephamandole |
| Cefactor | Cephazolin | Cefoxitin |
| Cefaclor | | Cefotaxime |
| Cephadroxil | Cephradine | Cefoperone |
| | | Moxalactum |

**First generation cephalosporins**

Included in this group are cephalexin, cephalothin, cephaloridine, cephazolin, cephradine, cefaclor and cefadroxil. They are active against most streptococci, some strains of streptococcus viridans, S. aureus and epidermidis. Among the Gram-negative bacteria, E. Coli, klebsiella, Pr. mirabilis, hemophilus influenzae are susceptible. They have little or no effect against serratia, enterobactor, indole-positive proteus, pseudomonas aerugenosa and B. fragilis species.

*Cephalothin, Cephaloridine and Cephazoline :*

They are the earliest cephalosporins, Cephalothin has very short half life and requires frequent I.V. administration. So it is not very popular.

Cephalosporins destroy cell wall of bacteria and are bactericidal. Cephalosporins have wide range of anti-bacterial action against many Gram-positive and Gram-negative organisms and are quite effective against pneumococci, $\beta$-haemolytic streptococci, C-diphtheriae and staphylococci. Many Gram-negative organisms e.g. E.Coli, K. pneumonae, N. gonorrhoea, Pr. mirabilis, Ps. aeruginosa, B. proteus, S. typhae and paratyphae. Sensitivity varies depending on the type of cephalosporins used.

**Cephaloridine :** This drug is nephrotoxic, hence its use should be restricted, better be avoided as far as possible where any possible damage to kidneys is suspected. It is administered in doses of 0.5 to 1 gm six hourly by intramuscular or intravenous route. It is useful in therapy of osteomyelitis due to staph. aureus or endocarditis due to strep. viridans in patients allergic to penicillin.

*Cephalexin and Cephradine :* These are well absorbed after oral administration. They are useful in staph aureus and entero-bactor infections but not effective in H. influenzae infections. These two are also useful in patients allergic to penicillin. High concentration in urine is achieved after oral administration so they are also helpful to treat urinary infections.

*Cefaclor :* It is similar to cephalexin but it is more effective in treating infections with H. influenzae and also effective in staph. aureus and entero-bacterial infections.

*Cefadroxil :* It has similar spectrum of activity as the other oral cephalosporins but its longer half life makes a twice daily doses schedule possible.

*Second generation Cephalosporins :* Included in this group are Cefuroxime, Cephamandole and Cefoxitin, Cefonicid, Ceforanide and Cefolism. All the second generation cephalosporins are administered by parenteral route and they are more resistant to $\beta$-lactamases.

Cefuroxime is active against staphylococci and H. influenzae. It also enters the C S F in adequate concentration, so it is useful for treatment of meningitis due to H. influenzae, S. pneumonae and N. meningitidis. It is not active against S. faecalis, ps. aeruginosa and B. fragilis.

*Cefamandole* — has comparable antibacterial spectrum but it is not useful to treat meningitis as its concentration in CSF is not adequate.

*Cefoxitin* — It is very much effective in treating infections with mixed aerobic and anaerobic organisms e.g. pelvic inflammatory disease. It is also very resistant to $\beta$-lactamases. Its concentration in C S F is not adequate for treatment of meningitis. It is excreted through kidney. *Cefonicid* has similar spectrum as cefamandole but its long half life makes it convenient to be used in single daily dose, but dose adjustment is necessary in renal failure.

Ceforanide is similar to cefamandole but it is less active against H. influenzae. Cefoliam — $\beta$-lactamase labile cephalosporin whose spectrum is wider than cefamandole.

**Third generation cephalosporins**

Four compounds of this group are used presently. They are : cefotaxime, latamoxeff, cefsulodine and ceftazidine. These third generation drugs are more active against Gram-negative organisms and are also much more resistant to $\beta$-lactamases.

**Cefotaxime** — It is effective against S. pneumonae, N. meningitidis, H. influenzae but it is not very active against ps. aerurginosa and anaerobic organisms.

**Latamoxef** also called moxalactum has a wide spectrum of activity against gram-negative and anaerobic organism. e.g. H. influenzae, E. Coli, klebsiella, ps. aeruginosa and B. fragilis. However, it has decreased antistreptococcal and anti-staphylococcal activity. Latamoxeff enters the CSF in sufficient concentrations. It may cause hypoprothombinaemia and decreased platelet adhesiveness, so bleeding and clotting time should be monitored when it is used in high doses.

**Ceftazidine**:— It is effective in treating pseudomonas infections though it is less effective against streptococcal, staphylococcal and infections with anaerobes. It enters the CSF in concentration adequate to inhibit the majority of organisms producing meningitis. It is excreted through kidneys, so dose adjustment is necessary in renal failure.

Finally it is stressed that cephalosporins are not only expensive but also potentially nephrotoxic, though degree of nephrotoxicity varies, indiscriminate use of these drugs has resulted in renal failure especially in old age. *It's use for common infections, for which safer and cheaper drugs are available is not at all justified.* Cephalosporins are also well-known to produce sensitisation causing fever, skin rash, anaphylaxis, nephritis, haemolytic anaemia and granulocytopenia. Patients allergic to penicillin may also be allergic to cephalosporins. Very few of these preparations are available in India.

I.M. injections are painful, I.V. injections may produce thrombophlebitis. Some newer cephalosporins are reported to cause hypoprothrombinaemia requiring Inj. Vitamin K.

**Vancomycin :—** Vancomycin a glycopeptide produced by the actinomycete streptomyces orientalis. Vancomycin is active only against Gram-positive bacteria. It is widely used for the treatment of methicillin resistant staphylococcal infections and for S. faecalis endocarditis in penicillin allergic patients.

**Vancomycin** is poorly absorbed from G.I. tract and should be given I.V. However, for treatment of C. difficile enterocolitis it should be given orally to get local action. The usual dose of vancomycin is 0.5 to 1 gm every 12 hours by I.V. injections. About 20% of the agent is excreted through kidney. The drug is nephrotoxic. So it should not be combined with other nephrotoxic antibiotics. It is also ototoxic in higher doses. A macular skin rash may develop during I.V. infusion which is usually controlled by anti-histaminic drugs.

(D) **Aminoglycosides**

They are divided into several families as follows :

(1) *Neomycin family* — neomycin-B, paromomycin, ribostamycin and lividomycin.
(2) *Kanamycin family* — Kanamycins A & B, amikacin and tobramycin.
(3) *Gentamycin family* — Gentamycins $C_1$ & $C_2$, sisomycin and netilimycin
(4) *Streptomycin*

The aminoglycoside antibiotics are generally active against aerobic gram negative organisms. They are bactericidal, act directly on bacterial ribosome. They have little or no action against most gram-positive bacteria. However they are active against S. aureus and S. epidermidis. They are poorly absorbed from the G.I. tract. But repeated oral administration in patients with renal impairment may result in accumulation of the drug and toxicity. Similarly instillation of these drugs to serosal cavities or topically in large wounds may result in toxicity particularly in renal insufficiency. They are not recommended for treatment of meningitis as they poorly cross the blood brain barrier (BBB) except in neonates where BBB is immature. The aminoglycosides are excreted almost entirely by glomerular infiltration. Since the incidence of nephrotoxicity and ototoxicity is directly related to the accumulation of the drug in plasma, it is necessary to reduce the maintenance dosage of the drugs in renal impairment. Either the dose of the drug can be reduced or the interval between the two successive doses can be prolonged. Usually the dose of the drug is reduced in direct proportion to the reduction of creatinine clearance.

The aminoglycosides cause acute tubular necrosis. Concurrent use of other nephrotoxic drugs increases the incidence of renal damage. Ototoxicity results in progressive destruction of vestibular and cochlear sensory cells. Diuretics potentiate the ototoxic effect of aminoglycosides. Streptomycin and gentamycin predominantly produce vestibular effects whereas neomycin, kanamycin and amikacin has a predilection for auditory sensory cells. Tobramycin affects both equally. Neuromuscular blockade produced by aminoglycosides is mostly manifested when they are administered in patients of myasthenia or during anaesthesia with neuromuscular blocking agents.

**Neomycin** — It is poorly absorbed from the G.I. tract. It is administered orally for preparation of bowel for surgery in association with erythromycin and or metronidazole. It is also used by many physicians used orally for treatment of hepatic coma — in doses of 4 to 8 gm daily *but it may be absorbed to some degree causing hepatotoxicity hence not recommended (Editor).* It is used more commonly in a variety infections of skin and mucous membranes as a topical antibiotic.

**Kanamycin** — It is not widely used nowadays except in children with gram-negative septicaemia. It is nephrotoxic. Dose is 5-15 mg/Kg of body wt. daily given in two to three intramuscular injections in divided doses.

**Amikacin** — Amikacin has the widest spectrum of antibacterial activity. It is specially used in situations of aminoglycoside resistant organisms as it is not inactivated by aminoglycoside inactivating enzyme. It is administered in dosage of 15 mg/kg of body weight daily in divided doses intramuscularly or intravenously. It is used to treat hospital-borne gentamycin resistant Gram-negative infections. It is also active against M. tuberculosis and atypical mycobacteria.

**Tobramycin** — The antibacterial spectrum of tobramycin is similar to gentamycin except that it is more active against P. aeruginosa. It is also less nephrotoxic than gentamycin. Dosages are identical to that of gentamycin (3-5 mg/kg/day). Tobramycin in combination with Tricarcillin is widely used nowadays for control of pseudomonas infections.

## NUTRITIONAL FACTORS IN DISEASES

*J.R. BARUA*

*Proper nutrition is essential for good health. It is easy to prescribe an ideal diet but proper food supply to total population is becoming a serious global problem. Population explosion, floods, droughts as well as poverty are the chief reasons for undernutrition especially of the people living in underdeveloped and developing countries. Control of population explosion by family planning, improved agricultural methods and finding additional resources of food e.g. sea-food, must be effectively implemented.*

*Waste of food in rituals and festivals also should be abandoned. Milk-producing animals should be cared for and their health to be well maintained. Ancient Hindus worshipped cows like demi-gods and cared for them as mothers.*

*We are recommending 'breast-feed' for all the babies. How many mothers in poor countries are fit to produce adequate amount of breast milk for their babies ?*

*Over 400 million people in the world are suffering from malnutrition. The number will be increasing unless global food policy can be effectively and successfully implemented. We are talking about health for all by 2000 A.D. We have to work sincerely and be honest in implementing food policy and food production as well as ensure very strict family planning if we want to survive beyond 2000 A.D.*

*In his article Dr. Barua has presented the problems of under-nutrition and disease. Editor —*

## Aetiology of Nutritional Disorders

Nutrition relates to the constituents of food, which are known as nutrients. They are protein, fat carbohydrate, minerals, vitamins and water.

Proteins are the chief substances in the cells of muscles and other tissues, of blood, of enzymes and antibodies (immunoglobulins) and hormones. They are necessary for growth and for replacement of wear and tear of the tissues. Hence they are called "Body building foods" though they can also supply energy, in times of necessity proteins are broken when down to yield energy. Ingested proteins are broken down in the digestive tract to aminoacids, before being absorbed and metabolized. Out of 20 aminoacids in the body, the following aminoacids are not formed by the human tissues.

1) Isoleucine
2) Leucine
3) Lysine
4) Methionine
5) Phenyl-alanine
6) Threonine
7) Tryptophan
8) Valine
9) Histidine (for infants and children).

Hence, they are called essential aminoacids which are found in animal proteins (first class proteins) like milk, egg, meat and fish. Vegetable proteins (second class proteins) are present in cereals, pulses, and vegetables and individually they do not contain all essential aminoacids. Rice and wheat are deficient in lysine and pulses lack in methionine but contain enough lysine. If the cereals and pulses are taken at the same time these deficiencies can be met.

According to the Indian Council of Medical Research (I.C.M.R.), one gramme of protein per kg. per day is sufficient for an adult Indian. Additional protein allowance must be made during pregnancy and lactation.

For infants and children milk should supply most of the proteins. Average protein content of mother's milk in India is 1.2 gm/dl. Protein requirements for infants and young children are as follows :—

0 - 3 months ...... 2.3 g/kg.
3 - 6 months ...... 1.8 g/kg.
6 - 9 months ...... 1.8 g/kg.
9 - 12 months ...... 1.5 g/kg.
1 - 3 years ...... 1.83 kg.

## Energy Producing Nutrient

The body needs energy for metabolic processes to maintain body temperature to support growth and physical activity. Fats and carbohydrates are the best sources of energy. Food energies are expressed in calories (kilocalories). Recently, WHO/FAO, International Union of Sciences have adopted "Joule" in place of "Calorie".

1 Calorie = 4.184 joules (approx. 4.2 joules)

Adequate energy should be provided to promote growth in infants and children and to maintain body weights in adults, consistent with good health. Factors influencing energy needs are age body weight, sex, physical activity, climate, pregnancy and lactation.

**Influence of basal metabolism :** In computing total energy need, basal metabolism and amount of physical activity should be taken into account.

Allowance for infants (I.C.M.R.) during 1st year of life is 112 calories or 470 joules/per/kg/per day.

1-3 years .... 1220 C .... 5100 Joules
4-6 years .... 1720 C .... 7200 Joules
7-9 years .... 2050 C .... 8600 Joules

**Energy Allowance for Adults (K/Calories)**

Level of physical activity in adequate quantities

| | Body Weight | Light | Moderate | Heavy |
|---|---|---|---|---|
| MALE | 55 kg | 2400 | 2800 | 3900 |
| FEMALE | 45 kg | 1900 | 2200 | 3000 |

* Very heavy activity e.g. wood cutters or soldiers on operational duty etc. may require higher calories.

**Fats**

Dietary fats are concentrated source of energy (1 g = 9 C). They serve as vehicles for fat soluble vitamins; lipids form structural cell-membranes and are also sources of essential fatty acids (EFA).

*Two Poly-unsaturated fatty acids linolinic acid and arachidonic acid are essential for nutrition.* Linolinic acid cannot be synthesized in the body. EFAs are precursors of prostaglandins, which are required in various metabolic functions. Deficiency of EFA in infants or young children results in phrynoderma (toad skin).

In developed countries fats provide 30-40% of total energy. But in developing countries like India, low income group people cannot afford expensive fats like ghee, butter, vanaspati, and oils in adequate quantities. They subsist usually on available fats, present in almost all foods e.g. cereals, pulses, tubers, vegetables, a little milk, oil seeds and/or occasionally meat, fish, eggs etc. They provide about 10% of energy in poor people.

For Indian male and female adults, 20% of energy should come from fat and half of it should be animal fats. Children's requirements are usually available from saturated fats like ghee, butter, vanaspati, coconut oil which may enhance cholesterol in the body, and is considered as one of the factors for causing ischaemic heart disease. So poly-unsaturated fats contained in sunflower oil, groundnut oil, mustard oil should also be taken.

**Carbohydrates**

All starchy food and sugar are carbohydrates. These are important sources of energy. Pure carbohydrates like glucose, maltose, lactose or sucrose are not required for good health, as lots of starch are present in cereals. Starch being cheap it is the main source of energy in poorer countries. Cereals are the staple diets in India. Cellulose and hemicellulose carbohydrates are present in leafy vegetables, fruits, condiments and spices. They are important as they form "fibres" or "roughages" which stimulate peristalsis and help in elimination of waste products. They prevent constipation.

In ideal diet schedules, requirement of proteins and fats should be calculated first and then sufficient carbohydrates are to be added to meet total energy needs. But ideal diet is an impossibility in developing countries for most people.

## DEFICIENCY OF PROTEINS AND ENERGY

Protein Energy Malnutrition

*(Protein Calorie Malnutrition : P.C.M.)*

*Undernutrition* — Starvation undernutrition is a form of malnutrition with which 66% of world's population are affected and most of them are in India and developing countries.

In developed countries undernutrition is not due to lack of food but due to causes, e.g. difficulty in intake of foods, their digestion, absorption or metabolism. Examples in adults are anorexia nervosa, obstruction of oesophagus, idiopathic steatorrhoea, chronic pancreatitis, liver diseases, malabsorption syndrome, chronic infections, etc. Examples in infant and children are hypertrophic pyloric stenosis, severe habitual vomiting, difficulty in sucking due to cleft lip, congenital heart diseases, chronic infections like congenital syphilis, tuberculosis, empyema, osteomyelitis, persistent vomiting, mental diseases, following gastroenteritis, coeliac disease and fibrocystic disease of the pancreas.

But in developing countries as in India, the main cause is lack of foods, both qualitative and quantitative, due to poverty. Use of foods of low nutritive value, non-availability of foods like milk, lack of knowledge about relation of food to health, religious beliefs, taboos and rituals which deny proper nutrition. Chronic infections like malaria, tuberculosis, worm infestations and diarrhoeal disease, urbanisation with low sanitary conditions, poor housing conditions, lack of cooking facilities are important factors. Pure starvations occur during famine due to floods, droughts, earthquakes or political upheavals. In acute starvation, ketosis is present and hunger usually disappears in couple of days. But in chronic undernutrition ketosis is not present while hunger and desire to eat are dominant features. There is apathy and depression, muscle wasting is evident associated with lethargy and lack of endurance. Bradycardia, hypotension, and anaemia are present, sometimes oedema is noted (famine oedema). In India along with undernutrition vitamin deficiencies are also present. Vitamin A deficiency causes xerophthalmia, vitamin $B_1$ deficiency causes beri beri, nicotinic acid deficiency causes pellagra,riboflavine deficiency leads to glossitis, folic acid and iron deficiency cause megaloblastic/iron deficiency anaemia, and iodine deficiency causes goitre in millions in sub-Himalayan people.

### Treatment

For management of chronic malnutrition, it is always necessary to exclude underlying pathological conditions e.g. cancer, tuberculosis or malabsorption syndrome. For improving nutrition careful controlled feeding is done in the beginning and then increased gradually, otherwise semi-starved individuals may suddenly develop congestive heart failure, if large amount of food is ingested. Vitamins and mineral deficiencies should also be treated. Infections and infestations need appropriate treatment but treatment of helminths may be delayed till some improvement has occurred.

## PROTEIN CALORIE MALNUTRITION (P.C.M.)

P.C.M. covers a wide range of diseases prevalent among children of economically underdeveloped countries of the world. In India it is largely responsible for high rate of mortality and morbidity among poor children. P.C.M. includes :

1) Kwashiorkor
2) Nutritional marasmus
3) Marasmic Kwashiorkor

## KWASHIORKOR

Though this condition was known long ago, it was first described by Cicily Williams, a paediatrician, while working in West Africa in 1933. She found this condition in children between six months and four years. After weaning these children were fed chiefly on starchy foods, like

Cassava, without milk or any protein. Kwashiorkor is a world-wide condition, in which there is deficiency of protein and some deficiency of calories as well.

Aetiology –

1) Early weaning of the child without adequate supplementary food, or prolonged breast-feeding without supplementary food or inappropriate supplementary food e.g. barley or arrowroot without any milk of any kind.
2) Unhygienic feeding habits which predispose to diarrhoea.
3) Drastic medication and withholding of food in treating diarrhoea.

Kwashiorkor is common between one and four years though no age is exempt.

In a classical case the symptoms are :–

Growth retardation of children; muscle wasting with retention of some subcutaneous fat; oedema of legs and feet, peevish mental apathy, hair and skin changes. Hairs may become light coloured, sparse or coarse. Alternate light and dark colour of the hair (flag sign) may be present. Skin changes are variable. Skin may become light-coloured or develop dermatoses with hyperpigmentation intervened with raw-red skin (crazy pavement) or dermatosis mosaic dermatoses or pellagra-like lesions. Some anorexia is present. Diarrhoeal diseases are superadded and infections like malaria, tuberculosis or pneumonitis may be present. The appearance of pot-belly with hepatomegaly is quite characteristic. Clubbing of fingers has been reported. Deficiencies of vitamins A, B-complex, vitamin C, D and E are usually associated with mineral deficiencies of iron, potassium and magnesium. Anaemia may be mild to moderate. Low serum enzymes, serum cholesterol, glucose and urea are present. Liver biopsy shows fatty infiltration and degenerative changes in pancreas. Kwashiorkor may be mild, moderate and severe.

## NUTRITIONAL MARASMUS

Marasmus arises from subsistence diet markedly deficient in all nutritional principles in which there is no excess of carbohydrate. The victims are usually under one year of age. The condition develops when breast feeding is withheld or fails for some reasons or erratic and insufficient artificial feeding is given to the child or when the child suffers from some disease which prevents utilisation of the foods e.g. diarrhoea or malabsorption. Marasmic child is always under-weight. The muscles are grossly wasted. The skin is thin to the touch, as there is no subcutaneous fat and is tightly stretched over the bony prominences with protuberant belly.

Oedema is not present and changes do not occur in hairs. Skin, liver and pancreas are usually normal. Apathy and refusal of foods are not seen. Anorexia, intercurrent infections and infestations and vitamin deficiencies may be present.

## MARASMIC KWASHIORKOR

This condition shows features of both kwashiorkor and marasmus. Presence of oedema is essential for diagnosis. When a marasmic child is treated with enough calories without sufficient protein, hypoproteinaemia and oedema may develop. Other features of kwashiorkor may or may not develop.

### Treatment

Severe P.C.M. should be hospitalised for about two to three weeks. Dehydration and electrolyte imbalance should be corrected by I.V. drip. Blood transfusion should be given only if necessary. Potassium by mouth and parenteral magnesium should be given. Antibiotics may be required for infections and vitamin supplements should be prescribed for appropriate deficiencies. Vitamin A one to three lac units should be given at the onset. No diuretics should be used. Treatment for helminthiasis may be delayed till the child is fairly recouped.

**Feeding :** In kwashiorkor where there is marked anorexia, tube-feeding may be necessary. But usually there is no difficulty in feeding the marasmic child, when small and frequent feeds are given. Skimmed milk with cane-sugar, honey or jaggery is quite acceptable.

Lactose is expensive and may cause lactose intolerance. Soyabean milk is a very good food. Starting with 50/C/kg/Bw/day one to 1.5 gm. protein/Kg food should be increased to 100-120 C per kg/Bw/day with 3-4 gm protein/kg. As the condition improves,solid food may be added. Several mixtures have been tried. A good mixture is skimmed milk, Bengal-gram powder, ashed leafy vegetables, jaggery and oil. The aim is to supply enough food to offer sufficient calories. It may take for the child to reach the weight according to its height in two or three months. Diarrhoea disappears and skin and hair become normal. After nutritional rehabilitation in some cases, nutritional recovery syndromes appear which consist of abdominal distension, enlarged liver, ascitis, hypertrichosis, parotid swelling,gynaecomastia, transient rise of intracranial tension and encephalitis-like syndrome. The aetiopathogenesis of this syndrome is not properly understood. Infants and small children suffering from P.C.M. over prolonged period may develop permanent irreversible shunting of growths.

There is also mental impairment which may not be completely cured and such children will have low I.Q. Cirrhosis of liver is very rare after P.C.M.

**Parenteral nutrition**

In many situations oral or even routine I.V. fluid therapy with glucose and electrolytes are not adequate. In these cases central venous catheterisation should be done to supply total parenteral nutrition (TPN) without risk of thrombophlebitis.

Lipid emulsions are now available, which contain glycerol, triglycerides and phospholipids.

Daily supply of lipids along with additional glucose and aminoacid solutions will be adequate.

**Prognosis**

In severe P.C.M. cases mortality is very high. But with good hospital treatment, mortality can be lowered. Diarrhoea, dehydration, vitamin deficiencies, congestive cardiac failure, hypoglycaemia and hypothermia are the main causes of deaths. Observation of the child has to be continued for a long period, otherwise relapses are common. Of course, the earlier the treatment is started, the better is the prognosis.

**Prevention** : P.C.M. is a global problem. Individually mothers should be educated about breast feeding, weaning, food hygiene and, of course, birth control.

## BERIBERI

*G.C. MOOKERJEE*

**Introduction**

Beriberi is a nutritional disease due to deficiency of thiamine. In acute form it presents with features of congestive cardiac failure (wet beriberi). It may also present as syndrome with symmetrical peripheral neuropathy (dry beriberi).

Beriberi used to occur in rice-eating areas (south-eastern India) and was formerly widespread in South-East Asia. Incidence has now declined due to awareness of the dietary requirements. Beriberi may also occur due to malabsorption, chronic colitis and in chronic alcoholics.

**Aetiology**

Beriberi may occur due to prolonged subsistence on a diet grossly deficient in thiamine. The daily requirement of thiamine is 1 mg. It is specially common in people eating polished (milled) rice. Rice-husk which is a rich source of thiamine, is removed during milling. Parboiling before milling of rice however can prevent loss of thiamine. Rich sources of thiamine in our diet are :

whole cereals, peas, beans, yeast, eggs and liver. Green vegetables, fruits and dairy products also contain significant amounts but are not so rich in thiamine.

**Pathology**

The main changes are seen in the heart and the nervous system :

*Heart* – The heart is usually dilated. Microscopically there is separation of muscle cells and oedema of muscle bundles. There is no cellular infiltration or muscle necrosis. Lungs are oedematous and serous effusion may occur in the pleura. Liver, spleen and kidneys reveal passive oedema but sometimes there may be petechial haemorrhage.

*Nervous system* – The brain substance may show bilateral haemorrhagic and sometimes necrotic foci. Peripheral nerves show degeneration and demyelination. Spinal cord and optic nerves may also show these changes.

**Clinical features**

Three clinical types are usually described e.g. wet beriberi, dry beriberi and infantile beriberi.

The presenting features are anorexia, malaise, heaviness and weakness of the limbs which cause difficulty in walking. There may be palpitation, tachycardia with high volume pulse. The tendon jerks are depressed and calf muscles may be tender on palpation.

*Wet Beriberi*

It is also called cardiac beriberi. Onset is usually insidious with shortness of breath on mild exertion, with or without precordial pain. Tachycardia, collapsing pulse, cardiac enlargement, cardiomegaly and signs of congestive heart failure may be present. Oedema of the legs is, however, very well-marked. The skin is warm to touch due to vasodilatation. Urinary output gradually falls but urinary findings are usually normal. Sudden death may occur in untreated cases.

*Dry Beriberi*

Onset is usually insidious with weakness, anorexia, loss of weight, pain and tenderness of leg muscles. Patient may find difficulty in getting up from squatting position. Deep reflexes in lower limbs are depressed or absent. Wrist drop and foot drop with high stepping gait may finally occur in untreated cases.

*Infantile Beriberi*

The baby shows signs of failure to thrive. There may be weight loss, restlessness, abdominal cramps, crying, refusal to take feeds and vomiting. Deep reflexes are sluggish. Therapeutic trial with thiamine is the best method.

**Treatment**

Thiamine hydrochloride should be administered orally or by IM or IV route for about two weeks.

Dose – 20 to 50 mg daily, depending on the urgency, Brewer's Yeast is also a good source but dose is 30 g three times daily. Liver, pork, kidney and whole grain cereals are the dietary sources.

## PATANJALI ASTANGA YOGA

*P.S. DAS*

*'Yoga' is an ancient art which has been practised in India since ancient times. Indian sages lived healthy lives by practising Yoga and survived over centuries in those days when medical science was in infancy. It is a system of mental discipline as well as physical culture which simultaneously ensure excellent musculo-skeletal health, improves function of deep organs, including improved oxygenation of brain and skin surface as well.*

*'Psyche' and 'Soma' are joined in the technique, hence called 'Yoga'. It is a health promoting system but does not cure diseases like I.H.D., diabetes mellitus, hypertension, asthma, gout, rheumatism or sinusitis etc. But no doubt many chronic diseases may be considerably benefited provided doctors and Yoga-therapists work together in planning of Yoga-therapy of modern times. Psychosomatic diseases are particularly benefited but supportive drug therapy may also be necessary. Indiscrete Yoga therapy especially by half-baked Yoga-instructors without medical supervision may be dangerous. Diseases e.g. hypertension, I.H.D., asthma, diabetes, gout, rheumatism etc. will require supervision and periodic medical check-up. Many so-called experts claim to cure diabetes, heart disease and even cancers, these "Yogis" should be avoided.*

*In this article Prof. P.S. Das who is attached as Yoga-expert to the famous Ghose's College of Physical Education, explains the basic principles of the art of Yoga for benefit of our readers.* — Editor — |

## PATANJALI ASTANGA YOGA

*P.S. DAS*

In the process of salvation through meditation there are eight stages to be practised and the comprehensive name is ASTANGA YOGA which means eight limbs of communion. The yogic limbs,Asana (postures of yoga) and Pranayama (controlled breathing) are only parts of these eight stages of activities.

However, the seven stages of yoga i.e. self realisation have correlation with PATANJALI's ASTANGA YOGA. Patanjali, the great yogic authority emphasised the importance of ASTANGA YOGA (eight limbs of yoga) for self-realisation. Some modern interpreters say that Astanga Yoga refers only to Hatha Yoga (which is a part and parcel of Karma Yoga). Actually, whatever be the type of field of Yoga, it ought to undergo the eight limbs of Yoga viz. :-

(1) Yama
(2) Niyama
(3) Asana
(4) Pranayama
(5) Pratyahara
(6) Dharana
(7) Dhyana
(8) Samadhi.

Yama — The first step of Yoga is to free ourselves from all kinds of malicious thoughts, hatred, jealousy, ill-will, greediness, unlawful desire for things (both animate and inanimate), thievish tendency and over-indulgence in sex. All kinds of evil thoughts have to be curbed by the Yogic aspirant and only then he can rise to the next rung of the Yogic ladder. 'Ahimsa' is most important i.e. "do not envy others" is the principal idea.

Niyama — After having mastered YAMA, the Yogic aspirant should begin to practise NIYAMA. Niyama here refers to disciple with regard to food, sleep, pleasure, profit and pain.

To achieve success 'Yoga' is impossible for the man who overeats, the man who starves, or for the man who sleeps too much or for the man who does not sleep enough. The Yoga which dispels sorrow or misery is for the man who is temperate in his food, recreation, activity and sleep. NIYAMA implies limit in all respects. Yoga does not prescribe one's pleasure, nor does it prescribe any kind of pain. Tamasik (or pleasure-seeking) attitude should have certain limits. It is a wrong notion that God is accessible to a man who renounces the world and has gone to the forests as an ascetic. It is only by realising the joys of creation, man can unravel the mysteries of the nature's Riddle-Me-Ree. The aspirant of Yoga should avoid bad company. He should indulge in Satsang (good companionship). SVADYAY (study), EESWARA PRANIDHANA (devotion to the Almighty), he must be pious, chaste and he must consume SATVIK food (balanced and normal diet which is not too spicy or stimulating).

*"Ashara Shuddo Satva Shuddihi*
*Satva Shuddo Druva Smrutihi".*

Consumption of good Satvik food leads to Satva Shuddhi (purification of mental outlook) and Satva Shuddhi leads to enlightenment.

All kinds of inebriating intoxicants should be avoided. His dictum is 'Chastity is life and sensuality is death'. Of course, what is life without natural piety and religious sanctity ?

*Asana* — The Asanas or Yogic postures have been given so much of importance in Yogic texts only beoause they help in reaching the ultimate limits of Yogic realisation and also in maintaining the body in a state of good health, free from all kinds of psychosomatic diseases. According to Yogic texts, it is not possible to be rid of diseases or to improve health without performing Asanas. Primarily, the Yogic postures, which have a remarkable therapeutic value, are practised to improve the physical and mental health. Our great poet Kalidas has remarked :

*Shareeramadyam Khalu Dharma Sadhanam'.*

A good healthy 'Shareera' (body) acts as a vehicle for 'Dharma Sadhanam' (righteousness). Life is like a journey in a vehicle between birth and death. The body is the vehicle in which we are motoring to death. The less luggage we carry the better it is. (Here the word luggage has an ironical meaning, for it represents 'Karma' (your own actions in life). Even the great Greek scholar Aristotle too has rightly remarked;

*'A sound body with a sound mind'.*

Sickly person cannot aspire for any kind of salvation, neither materials nor spiritual relief, since his illness acts as an obstacle. The physical body acts like a rampart or wall for the sacred inner temple of our soul and if the rampart is sound enough, then the inner temple of soul could be kept clean. If the house is not covered with a wall or any kind of good protection then it will have all kinds of intruders and the treasures in the house will be carried away by unknown elements.

Even the attainment of 'Samadhi' is a matter of greatest importance. Yoga, is not possible without Asanas. Patanjali has described the 'Asana' as a poised and relaxed manner of body postures :-

*'Sthira Sukamasanam'*
*(Patanjali Yoga sutra)*

Therefore, this means that the student should try to get fully disciplined in the various Yogic postures, so that he can sit motionless and relaxed for considerable periods. Only then will he be prepared for the various advanced disciplines and practices in Yoga.

When perfection is attained in any 'Asana', the external movements of the 'Yogic' gradually and progressively diminish till they cease altogether. This aphorism, thus not only corroborates the idea contained in the preceding one but also indicates that the attainment of perfection in the Yogic postures and leads to the attainment of 'Samadhi'.

On attainment of perfection in the Yogic postures, the individual becomes immune to dualities.

The body of the Yogic remains unaffected by environmental heat or cold and other dualities on the attainment of perfection in Asanas.

It means that the body acquires enough strength and tolerance to withstand stresses and strains of all types which disturb the 'Chitta' (mind) and by making the mind unsteady, disturb the practice of 'Yoga'. These aphorisms taken together very distinctly indicate that the stage of 'Samadhi' is attained by a Yogic only by mastering the 'Asanas'.

The Yogic postures have in fact assumed new significance in modern times. The occidental system of gymnasium exercises, aimed at developing the bulk and the power of the muscle masses, is the most commonly used system all over the world. This system is primarily, if not entirely, based on processes generating great tension in the muscles.

There is no corresponding relaxation of any group of muscles. There is exertion in performing these exercises which lead to depletion of energy and it is harmful to the osteo-articular surfaces which are utilised in these movements. Consequently a pent-up tension in the motor organs of the body is sometimes accompanied by varying degrees of organic injury. Chronic arthritis and arthomyalgic incapacity, which cripple the able-bodied, can to some extent be traced to this single cause. The performance of Yogic postures, on the other hand, results in renewal of energy and they aim at a homogenously integrated system of neuro-muscular movements in which contraction of the muscles is always consciously followed by their relaxation or the relaxation of some other muscle masses.

At every step, a mental association is established with the physical action, so that the unfathomable reserves and powers of the mind are harnessed for the essential interest of achieving a perfect physical culture of the body. Accordingly a few yogic postures have 'Pranayama' or breath control as an internal part of the procedure, but even it ceases generating great tension in the muscles. Others are preceded or followed by exercises in breath control as part of the general plan of the 'Eight-limbed Yoga' (Astanga Yoga).

*It is now being recognised that the mind and the body, the 'psycho' and the 'soma' interact and influence each other. Yoga maintains that far-reaching effects can be produced by the effect of the mind. These effects not only affect the physical health of the body but may even overflow into the states which are beyond the average.*

Yoga affords an opportunity ,for a bold departure from this limitation. However, it must be realised that deal as they do with matters of far-reaching and vital importance. The Yogic practices require the utmost precision and care due to them. It is, therefore, not advisable to completely rely on books to learn the yogic postures. It is essential that a good 'Guru' should introduce the student to the exciting mysteries of Yoga to obtain maximum physical, mental and spiritual benefits from it.

*Yoga acts as a rejuvenating tonic which revives vigour and vitality, for it not only keeps the practitioner slim, trim and happy but also enables him to transcend to higher spiritual plains. We have instances of great men and women who have excelled in their professional career and they have attributed their success in their respective fields to Yoga.*

Dr. Thorpe has said that he seldom has cold and no disease of any kind. He got rid of the fear-ridden world and his mental and emotional control improved and yoga had given him a reserve of mental and physical energy and inner harmony and poise.

Some people do ask whether yoga is a religion or science. Religion is a way of life and yoga, of course, is a healthy way of life and should be considered as science.

*Pranayama (Breath control)* — 'Prana Vayu' is the life force, and the movement of Prana in the human body is always upwards whilst the movement of 'Apana Vayu' (bad air etc.) is always downwards. Therefore, the art of controlling the upward movement of 'Prana Vayu' and making it flow downwards and expelling the 'Apana Vayu' is called pranayama. 'Yama' in Yoga means to suppress.

Deep breathing is integral to the discipline and 'Pranayam' or breath control is the key not only the bodily stamina but also for supersensory development. The 'Pranayam' prescribed by the yogic system is one by which the respiratory system is kept in efficient working order, thereby enabling one to throw out waste matter (Apana) and take in the most essential requirement of life viz., oxygen.

Yogi Charan Das has said that one must attain control on the routes of Pavana through Asanas and Pranayam and through transcending the six chakras (six nerve plexuses) one must concentrate one mind on the void. The term Pavan implies a double meaning, i.e., of the various Vayus (airs), viz., Prana, Apana, Samana, Udana and Vyan in the body, as also the Prana Sakti. The latter faculty of Prana be clearly defined by any single term. As in the Yogic texts this term has been made to mean the life force as well as that of cosmic fund of energy of which vitality is only one of the many manifestations.

There are, however, eight different types of Pranayam which starts from the practice of Suryavedhana and ends with the perfection of Plavini. To sum up Pranayam, it can be said that it is the secret of the phenomenal energy and mental powers of comprehension and retention.

*Pratyahara* — We are all too much involved in the activities of this material world and unless we develop a sense of detachment in the midst of attachment, we cannot escape from this snare net of material complications and commitments. Therefore, Pratyahara means developing a sense of detachment in the midst of attachment or a kind of dissociation in the midst of association or it could even be defined as :

*'Relationless relationship'*

However, Pratyahara does not mean that we would renounce this material world for we need this material world to know the subtle aspects of spiritualism. To know the reality, we have to survive and for survival we need 'Annam' (food). Only then comes the knowledge of Brahma.

A friend of Sri Ramakrishna asked him whether he could realise the self by living in this material world or should he go to the forest to know the truth. Sri Paramhansa cited an example :

"Take out a fish swimming in a stinky pond of water and you will see that nothing of the stinkyness of the pond is attached to its body and it remains to be slippery. But the fish cannot survive without the stinky water. Similarly this material world could be compared to a stinky pond. But we should remain like a fish attached and yet detached as a drop of water on a lotus leaf. This is the very meaning of Pratyahara".

*Dharana :* It is a state of concentration of the infinite or on some particular object. The human body and mind keep on undergoing stresses and strains of different kinds every day. The stresses and strains of the body get relieved at the time of sleep. The stresses and strains experienced by the mind get relieved in the form of appearance of dreams.

There are about two billion cells in the human brain and each brain cell acts like a tape-recorder cassette, for the brain cells record various kinds of things which results in the accumulation of different kinds of impressions. Such impressions get discharged in the form of dreams during our sub-conscious dreamy state (which is the first state of consciousness among the seven different types of conciousness) and relieves the strain caused upon the human mind. The human mind is like a white screen and the very mundane stresses and strains experienced by the serene mind from the black dots on the screen of the mind. The black dots get released during the course of sleep. The working of mind during sleeping hours is called 'Dreaming' and the working of the mind during working hours is called 'Thinking'. The dreams of different kinds are experienced during the state of sleep. However, the dreams after playing these roles before the screen of mind in our sleepy state will vanish and at that moment we shall be in a deep sound sleep state (Second type of consciousness) where we shall be literally dead like a wooden log. So this is the subconsciousness pleasurable experience of sound sleep state of nothingness. According to Yogic analysis it is said that *human mind is like a monkey which keeps on jumping from place to place, might be from somewhere to nowwhere or nowhere to somewhere. This activity of the mind is the very cause of our experiencing the dreams of different kinds. The human mind has no rest* and in Yoga it is said that the mind will have a moment's respite in the *Brahma Nadi and this stage of mind's respite in the Brahma Nadi represents the state of sound sleep, in which state a person neither experiences dreams nor his state of being alive.* However, only after getting up from the bed, he could recollect the pleasurable experience of sound sleep, and he would of course long to have it for ever. Now the person is awake and he is conscious of what he is (Third Type of Consciousness) i.e., state of being alert or alive. The person will be seeing so many things, and the mind will be experiencing different kinds of stresses and strains.

Let us now come to the analytical approach to Dharana or Concentration :

You will now begin to concentrate on some particular object (say, burning candle fire) by keeping your eyes closed.

The reason why you are asked to keep your eyes closed is to make the eyes free from external distractions. The thought of fire appears before your mind's eye, once in a way, for the mind will be wavering and different kinds of thoughts will glide before your mind's eye.

*Dhyana :* Dhyana is a state of meditation. Meditation could be defined as a gentle process of disciplining the naturally diffused rays of mind. In meditation, the distracted rays of mind will be gently disciplined and the different kinds of thoughts will vanish and you will only have the thought of the very object of your concentration. Therefore, meditation means no stress and no strain on the mind. Meditation is the fourth state of the spiritual consciousness, for it transcends the height of the individuals to a higher state of consciousness which is known as the "Transcendental Consciousness". The stream of consciousness is an unimpeded one and therefore the object on which you are meditating is constantly appearing before your mind's eye, although the perspective of the fire perceived in your mind's eye might often wobble and shake forward and sideward. Therefore, the distractred rays of mind or thought have now vanished and only a ray or thought is constantly directed towards the very thought of the object of meditation. And now the burning fire is ever before the inner vision.

*Samadhi :* (Contemplation) — Samadhi is a state of pure consciousness. It is a crystal-clear state of being alert and union with the infinite. The Buddhists call it Nirvana. Nirvana/Samadhi is not like the black dead peace of the grave but the living peace and living happiness of a soul which is conscious of itself.

It is a state of utter extinction of all that is based in us, all that is vicious in us, all that is corrupt and corruptible in us. In the state of contemplation the line we had drawn on the graph sheet becomes the axiomatic straight line, for the fire has now merged with the vision, the body and soul have all merged together. This is the very meaning of yoga — the union of the body and soul with the supreme consciousness, namely Universal or Cosmic Conciousness — God consciousness and now merged with the Brahmic consciousness — the state of Supreme Delight.

Let apart the subconscious pleasurable experience of sound sleep, the highest material fleshy pleasure that man can derive on earth is the transient or momentary pleasure of sex.

The ancient students of yoga asked their Masters as to how the Moksha (Salvation) would be. Their Masters could only give one small example, which is as follows :—

*'Priyaya Samparshvaktaha Bahya Nakinchanaveda'*

The pleasure derived at the climax of conjugal process of sexual love is after all momentary, and evanescent; whereas Moksha/Salvation is a delight in itself and is eternal.

The present-day concept about yoga is that it is a method of religious discipline aimed to achieve transcendent state of Brahmic conciousness or God realisation. In fact, yoga philosophy teaches us how to control the mind and how to bring about developments pertaining to the physical, intellectual and spiritual well-being. Yoga is a science of introspectional psychology. Hence, the school of philosophy has not only a spiritual or psychological significance; it has also something very important to do with regard to the body which is to be properly built up for higher intellectual acquisition. The principles of the Yoga system of Hindu philosophy can be traced even to the days of the Rig Veda as has been pointed out by eminent scholars in this field. Even in the Upanishads there are several references to the basic principles of yoga. The Yoga Sastra or the Yoga Darshana of Patanjali is taken to be the most important work, nó doubt. As a matter of fact, the establishment of God's Kingdom is a co-operative enterprise between God and man. And man is after all a co-sharer in the work of creation with God.

No doubt, ancient sages had a profound understanding of the subtle interdependence of the physical and the mental.

Kingland in his *Rational Mysticism* says :—

> 'Modern scientific cries are largely a reversion to the ancient teaching with the added force of experimental evidence and greater knowledge of detail'.

Woodroffe in his *The World as Power Reality* says :—

> 'An examination of the Indian Vedantic doctrine shows that it is an important aspect in conformity with the most advanced scientific and philosophical thought of the West, and where it is not so, it is the science which will go to Vedanta and not the reverse'.

In this connection it might not be wrong to say that much of the credit of discovering the wisdom of the Oriental likes rightly with the Western scholars.

To conclude :—

> *Asatoma Sadgamaya, Tamasoma Jyotirgamaya, Murtyrma Amritahgamaya Om Shanti, Shanti.....*

**Some of the important 'Asanas' are illustrated as follows :**

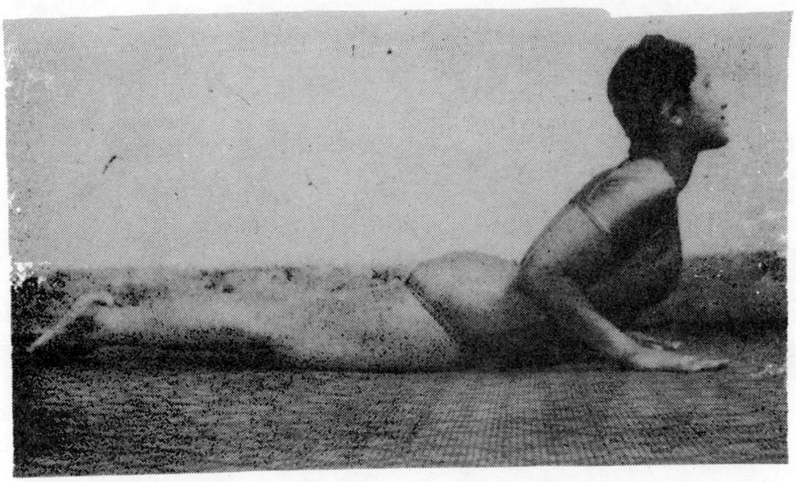

*BHUJANGASANA (Cobra Posture) :* (Fig.19.14) — Maya Kundu —

Benefits : It helps pain in the lower back, indigestion, gastritis, spondylosis, defect of the spine, menstruation trouble, pigeon chest, respiratory troubles etc.

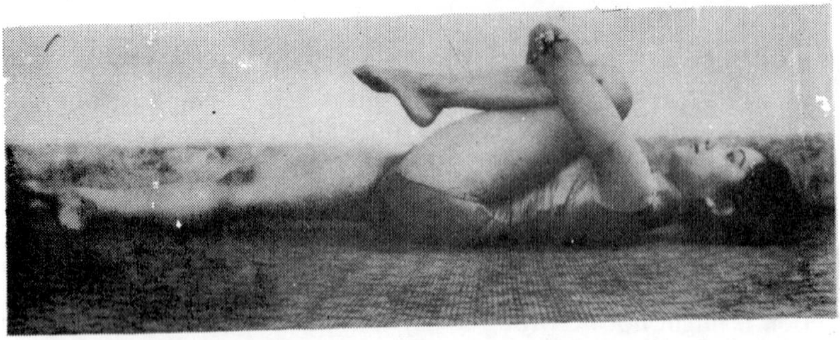

*PABANMUKTASANA (Anti-flatus posture)* : (Fig.19.15) — **Maya Kundu** — Benefits : It helps wind trouble, acidity, dyspepsis, colitis, constipation, loss of appetite and rheumatism.

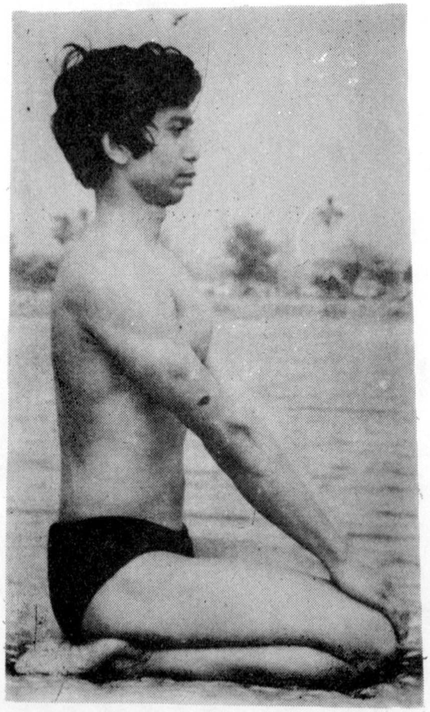

*VAJRASANA (Thunder Posture)* : (Fig.19.16) — Dibya Sundar Das — Benefits : It relieves pain in the hip, knees and ankle joints and improves the appetite and cures functional digestive troubles. It also helps sciatica, varicose veins etc.

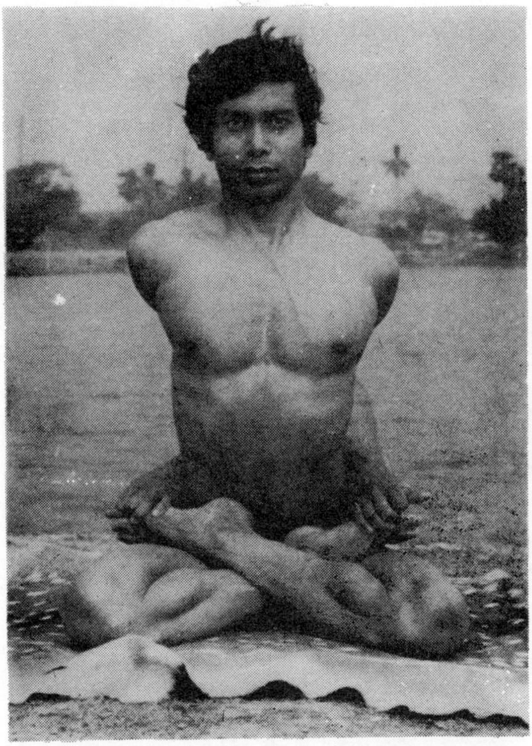

*PADMASANA (Lotus Posture)* : (Fig.19.17) – Dibya Sundar Das –

Benefits : It helps to cure pain in the lower limbs (the knees and the ankle joints).

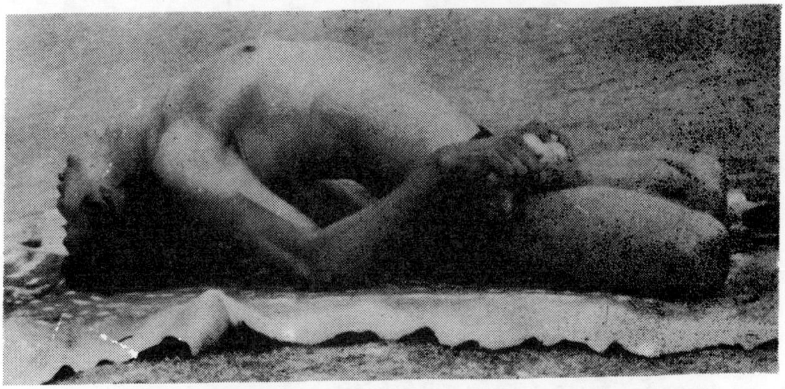

*MATSYASANA (Fish Posture)* : (Fig.19.18) – Dibya Sundar Das –

Benefits : It is very helpful for chronic bronchitis, pharyngitis, asthma, tonsillitis, susceptibility to cough and cold, lumbago, fatigue, headache and insomnia.

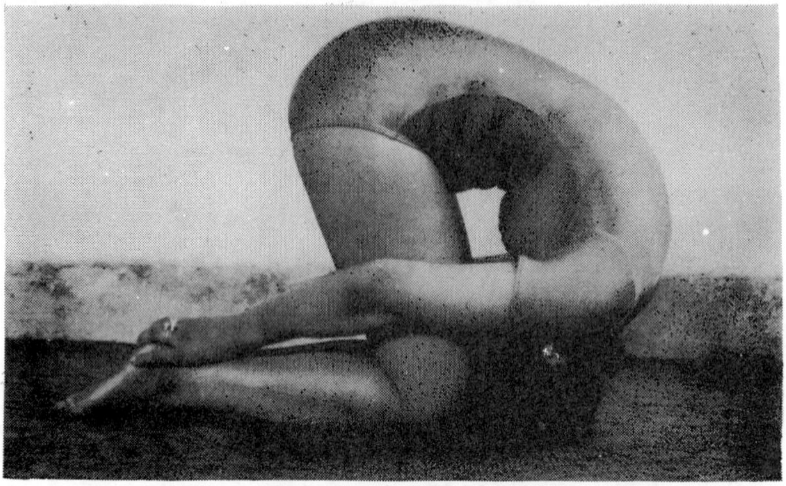

*SHASHANGASANA (Rabbit Posture)* : (Fig.19.19) — **Maya Kundu** —

Benefits : Susceptibility to cough and cold, tonsillitis, weak memory, brain fatigue, and insomnia. It helps to increase height.

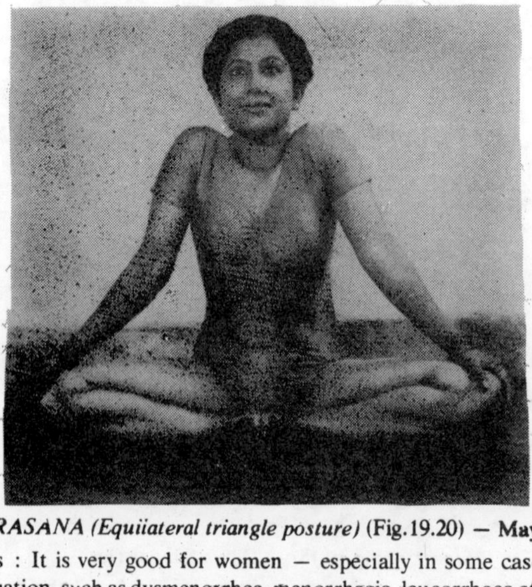

*BHADRASANA (Equiiateral triangle posture)* (Fig.19.20) — **Maya Kundu** —

Benefits : It is very good for women — especially in some cases of irregularities of menstruation such as dysmenorrhea, menorrhagia leucorrhoea etc. For men — it helps to cure excessive nocturnal emission. This Asana improves the flexibility of the lower limbs and hip-joints, and is effective in some cases of lowback pain.

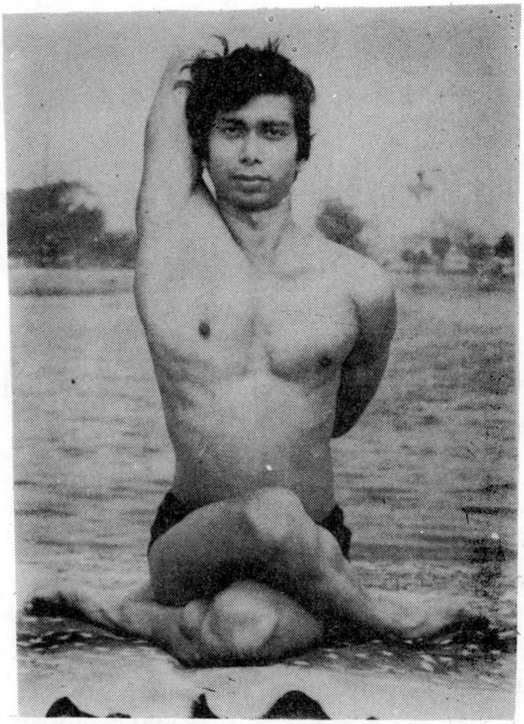

*GOMUKHASANA (Cow face posture)* : **(Fig.19.21) – Dibya Sundar Das –**

Benefits : Neuralgia of the limbs, insomnia, inability to control urine, spermatorrhoea and frozen shoulder (in the arly stage) may improve by this Asana.

# CHAPTER – 20
# APPENDIX

## SELECTION OF LABORATORY TESTS

*S.K. DUTTA*

With advancement of biochemistry and bioscientific technology large number of new diagnostic tests are now available for purposes of diagnosis. Many of these tests are expensive and facilities of getting these done are available in large city hospitals and special laboratories only.

Good clinical assessment of the patient is essential before ordering these tests. These tests do not relieve the physician of his responsibilities to go through proper history taking and relevant clinical examination.

In this article important laboratory tests which are often required for diagnostic purposes are discussed with comments on their interpretation.

**Febrile illness :**

(1) *Total and differential count of WBC, haemoglobin level, E.S.R. and malaria parasite* should be checked on or after third day of a febrile illness if diagnosis is not made. Peripheral blood film must be checked for abnormal cells and platelet population. Very high E.S.R. is strongly suggestive of tuberculosis, active rheumatic process, malignancy and myelomatosis.

(2) *Blood culture* : Best results are obtained if it is done before starting antibiotics and chemotherapeutic agents. In bacterial endocarditis repeated blood cultures are helpful. Results available after 3 to 10 days.

(3) *Urine analysis* : Chemical and microscopic examination is usually done routinely on 3rd or 4th day of fever and if abnormal, culture and drug sensitivity test should be done especially where urinary tract infection is suspected.

It is always better to examine midstream samples, particularly in female patients, for routine and culture examination. Cultures may be false positive due to improper collection and undue delay in despatch. False negative results are common if therapy is started beforehand. A positive culture report has to be evaluated by colony count and associated pyuria (number of pus cells per h.p.f.). Colony count less than 100.000/ml of unspun urine in absence of any therapy is not considered suggestive of infection. *Unfortunately some laboratories do not bother to report the colony count.* The number of pus cells in high power microscopic field of less than five per field is not abnormal.

*N.B.* *Throat swab culture and smear examination* should be done before antibiotics are started and drug sensitivity tests should be done if pathogens are isolated. The sample should be collected in fasting state and before washing mouth.

(4) **Serological tests**

(a) *Widal test* is performed after 7 to 10 days of fever, when enteric group of fever is suspected. A rising titre or 'O' agglutination over 1/100 and 'H' agglutination over 1/200 are considered significant. In persons who have received TAB Vaccine, only definite rise of titre at an interval of 3 to 5 days will be considered significant.

(b) *Paul Bunnell test* is done when glandular fever or infectious mononucleosis is suspected. Rapid slide test are presently done.

(c) *Brucella agglutination or* Weil-Felix reaction : when Brucellosis or Typhus fever is suspected.

(d) *Antistreptolysin* 'O titre : high titre above 200 units strongly suggests acute rheumatic infection.

(e) *Aldehyde and complement fixation tests* are done when kalaazar is suspected.

(5) *Bone marow study* is important particularly for diagnosis of chronic Kalaazar.

(6) *Antinuclear factor and L.E. cell tests* are recommended particularly in protracted illness not responding to common therapy with a clinical suspicion of collagen disease.

(7) *Antigen detection* is most simple and rapid method for detection of bacterial antigens from blood, C.S. fluid, sputum and throat swab. Results not affected by previous drug therapy. Tests are performed by counter immunoelectrophoresis (CIEP) or latex agglutination tests. Rapid diagnosis of bacterial meningitis, bacterial and viral infections of upper and lower respiratory tracts are possible.

(8) *Diabetes mellitus* has to be excluded in protracted and complicated case. Rare infections should be excluded in immunocompromised patients (particularly after cancer chemotherapy).

(9) *Cerebrospinal fluid* examination is essential in suspected cases of meningitis. Physical examination, cytology (cell count and type), Sugar and protein levels are determined. Staining may be done with Gram's stain, acid fast stain and Indian ink for staining ordinary bacteria, acid fast bacilli and fungi respectively.

**Anaemic conditions**

(1) *Complete Haemogram* — Hb, TC, DC, PCV, MCV, MCH, MCHC and study of peripheral blood film usually gives idea to the type of anaemia — normocytic, microcytic or macrocytic and whether it is normochromic or hypochromic in type. Peripheral blood film study also helps in the diagnosis of hypoplastic or aplastic anaemias and leukaemias.

(2) *Reticulocyte count* is done by staining a blood film with 3% cresyl blue. High count indicates haemolytic anaemia or response to specific therapy. a low count indicates hypoplastic/aplastic marrow.

(3) *Bone marrow study* — most useful in the diagnosis of chronic Kalaazar, megaloblastic anaemia, acute leukaemias, multiple myeloma and idiopathic thrombocytopenic purpura. This is not routinely necessary in all anaemia cases.

(4) *Haemoglobin electrophoresis* — is essential for the diagnosis of thalassaemia and haemoglbinopathies.

(5) *Serum Iron, iron binding capacity* and ferritin level is helpful in the diagnosis of iron-deficiency anaemia or iron overload.

(6) *Serum $B_{12}$/folic acid* levels confirm the diagnosis of megaloblastic anaemia.

(7) *Renal function tests* sometimes diagnostic of chronic renal failure, undiagnosed but producing anaemia. Hookworm disease, malabsorption syndrome, protein calorie malnutrition, menorrhagia and bleeding piles are often overlooked by the inexperienced.

**Hepatitis (particularly with jaundice)**

(1) In many cases clinical history physical inspection of stool and urine colour will help. Basic information is obtained by urine examination for bile pigment, salt and levels of serum bilirubin and SGPT (ALT). In diagnosis of complicated cases and when there is doubt other tests should be ordered.

(2) However, if there are no limitations of finance and facilities, performance of the following tests are valuable :

(a) *Serum bilirubin-serial* levels of conjugated and unconjugated fractions.

(b) *SGPT (ALT) and/or SGOT (AST)* — in liver disease both the enzymes are raised, but SGPT is more elevated and lasts longer.

(c) *Alkaline phosphatase* — particularly important in cholestatic jaundice. Intra or extrahepatic cholestasis cannot be differentiated biochemically hence ultrasound, C.T. scan or cholangiography, may have to be done.

(d) *Total protein,* albumin and globulin levels are determined in hepatic diseases. Albumin is solely synthesised in liver and reflects functional synthetic capacity of liver cells.

(e) *Detection of hepatitis-B surface antigen (HBS Ag)* or Australia antigen : It is a very useful and important test for diagnosis of HAB virus infection and is best done by Elisa technique. Reversed passive haemagglutination may also be used in the diagnosis of hepatitis-B virus.

There is no test for the diagnosis of non — A non — B hepatitis. Presence of $HB_SAg$ indicates infective state and antibody to hepatitis-B surface antigen indicates clinlca recovery and immunity.

(f) *Frequent blood tests* are not necessary in uncomplicated cases. Initial and one or two final tests after 4 to 6 weeks may be sufficient. Routine urine test for bile pigment may be used to monitor the progress of the recovery.

(g) *When jaundice does not improve* i.e. serum bilirubin level remains at high level, some special tests should be done :

(i) *Prothrombin time :* It is the most sensitive test to detect synthetic function of liver which is prolonged in impending hepato-cellular failure.

(ii) *Ammonia level* (serum/plasma) is also increased in impending hepatocellular failure.

(h) *Chronic hepatitis and other liver diseases :* In chronic hepatopathies the patient may be anicteric but transaminase levels remain elevated for over 6 months. BSP excretion test may be helpful. Needle biopsy of liver confirms diagnosis. $HB_SAg$ also persists in serum in many cases.

(i) *Chronic active hepatitis :* Immunoglobulin-G is increased.

(ii) *Cirrhosis of liver* — IgG and IgA levels are increased with beta-gamma fusion noted in electrophoresis of serum proteins.

(iii) *Lupoid hepatitis*

Antinuclear, smooth muscle, and mitochondrial antibodies are present.

(iv) *Alcoholic hepatitis*

Elevated level of GGTP occurs and it is out of proportion to the rise of SGOT/PT and bilirubin values.

(v) *Primary biliary cirrhosis* — elevated IgM is diagnostic.

(iv) *Hepatic malignancy* — There is raised alpha-fetoprotein level in primary hepatocellular carcinoma.

Most of the other hepatic function tests are usually normal.

(viii) *Inherited hyperbilirubinaemia :* Both conjugated and unconjugated forms may be slightly raised. Some of them are harmless.

**Diabetes mellitus**

(1) If symptoms of diabetes are present, fasting value above 140 mgm % or value over 200 mg % after two hours of 75 gms glucose intake are considered abnormal.

(2) In absence of clinical symptoms, high values should be checked by repeat examination or by oral glucose tolerance test (G.T.T).

(3) *W.H.O. recommends* glucose estimation by enzymatic method (true glucose) using serum or plasma.

(4) *Serum or plasma glucose* levels are about 15% higher than whole blood.

(5) *Folin Wu method* glucose values are 10-15% higher than true glucose values.

(6) *Whole blood Folin Wu method* values (practised widely so long) are close to plasma/serum true glucose values.

(7) Astoor and King, Nelson-Somogyi and O-toluidine methods produce results, which are considered true glucose values.

(8) *Post-prandial blood glucose* should be estimated two hours after ingestion of 75 g. of glucose dissolved in 250 ml water at the time of initial investigation for diagnosis. Once diagnosis is established, G.T.T. is not necessary.

(9) Confirmed diabetics should have their post — prandial glucose level checked two hours after the recommended diet and with usual antidiabetic drugs.

(10) *Fasting blood glucose* level increases approximately two mg% and post prandial approximately ten mg% per decade of life above the age of 50 years.

(11) *Frequency of testing* should be more in uncontrolled cases and fewer in stable cases.

(12) *Lipid profile and renal function tests* including chemical, microscopical and bacteriological examination of urine along with clinical examination and ECG should be done at least twice a year.

Even if there is no suspicion of respiratory problem, an X-ray chest should be ordered. Diabetics are susceptible to tuberculosis.

(13) *Glycosylated haemoglobin indicates* the level of blood glucose in the preceding two to three months period. Commonly, total $HbA_1$ is estimated and this correlates well with specific $HbA_1C$.

(14) *W.H.O.* has recommended the following values with reference to diagnosis of diabetes :

| *Diabetes mellitus* | Venous whole blood | Capillary whole blood | Venous plasma/serum |
|---|---|---|---|
| Fasting-over and/or | 120 | 120 | 140 |
| Post prandial-over (2 hrs after 75 gm glucose) | 180 | 200 | 200 |
| *Impaired glucose tolerance* | | | |
| Fasting-Less than and | 120 | 120 | 140 |
| Post prandial (as above) between | 120-180 | 140-200 | 140-200 |

(These values refer to enzymatic true glucose in mg/dl)

(15) *Impaired glucose tolerance* patients are often controlled without drugs. However, some of them may require drug therapy.

(16) *Pregnant patients* with impaired glucose tolerance must be treated with insulin. Similarly juvenile diabetics with so called IGT also will require insulin therapy.

(17) *Testing urine for glucose* with Benedict's qualitative reagent or clinitest tablet is not specific. Dip sticks (Diastix and others) are convenient and specific.

(18) *Home monitoring instruments* measure capillary true glucose level of whole blood. If the patient can afford this is the best way to *"live well with diabetes"*. These self-monitoring instruments are now available in India.

**Hypertension**

Routine studies

(1) Haemoglobin and Haematocrit value

(2) Blood urea/urea-nitrogen and creatinine

(3) *Electrolytes* — Serum Na, K and chloride level should be estimated whereever possible as initial baseline tests prior to diuretic therapy and also to screen primary aldosteronism. This is however not routinely possible hence clinical judgement is of supreme importance.

(4) *Blood glucose level* to exclude associated diabetes mellitus.

(5) *Lipids-serum* cholesterol and triglycerides to assess lipid profile, an important aspect of atherosclerotic complication.

(6) *Serum Calcium, Phosphates* and uric acid particularly in patients with renal impairment.

(7) *Urine-chemical examination* for protein and glucose, microscopic examination for RBC, pus cells and casts and cultural examination with drug sensitivity when required. This must be done in all cases and at least once in two or three months.

*Special studies*

(1) *V.M.A. and catecholamines* in 24 hrs urine when pheochromocytoma is suspected.

(2) *$T_3$, $T_4$ and TSH* when thyrotoxicosis is suspected.

(3) *Plasma cortisol level* with dexamethasone suppression test when Cushing's syndrome is suspected.

**Cardiac risk evaluation (Lipid profile)**

(1) Blood to be collected after strict overnight fasting.

(2) Total cholesterol and triglyceride levels are basic minimum tests.

(3) *HDL, LDL and VLDL fractions* of cholesterol are very helpful.

(i) *HDL (corresponds to alpha lipoprotein).* Normal range 30-95 mg/dl. Risk factor if less than 35 (men) and if less than 45 (women).

(4) *LDL (corresponds to beta-lipoprotein).* Normal range 65-175 mgms/dl. Suspicious if above 150 mg/dl. Abnormal if elevated above 190 mg/dl.

(5) *VLDL fraction (corresponds to pre-beta lipoprotein).* Normal range 14.5 - 28 mg/dl.

(6) *Ester (60-75%) and free (25-40%) fractions* of cholesterol important in liver diseases (esterification is a function of liver).

(7) Coronary Heart Disease (CHD) risk or atherosclerotic risk may be predicted as follows :

CHD risk (HDL/total cholesterol %). Atherosclerotic Risk (Total/HDL ratio)

| | Male | Female | Risk | Male | Female |
|---|---|---|---|---|---|
| Dangerous | 7 | 12 | ½× average | 3.4 | 3.2 |
| High | 7-15 | 12-18 | 1× average | 4.9 | 4.4 |
| Average | 15-25 | 18-27 | 2× average | 9.5 | 7.0 |
| | | | 3× average | 23.3 | 11.0 |

(8) *Cholesterol triglyceride levels* varies with age, sex and diet habit.

(9) *Lipoprotein electrophoresis* clearly indicates the levels of different lipoprotein fractions and chylomicrons.

(10) *Inspection of serum-clear or opalescent or lipaemic* is also very important. Presence of chylomicron and high triglyceride level produces lipaemic serum.

**Myocardial infarction**

(1) Blood tests are very useful for the diagnosis and monitoring of the course of the disease.

(2) Serum enzymes are routinely studied :

| Serum Enzymes | Starts to rise (Hours) | Peak elevation (Hours) | Duration of rise (days) |
|---|---|---|---|
| 1. CPK/CK with MB fraction | 3 - 6 | 24 - 36 | 3 |
| 2. AST/SGOT | 6 - 8 | 24 - 48 | 4 - 6 |
| 3. LDH | 10 - 12 | 48 - 72 | 11 - 13 |
| In myocardial infarction, MB fraction is over 6% of total CPK activity. | | | |

$LDH_1$ (fast moving fraction) this isoenzyme is specific for cardiac damage. Serum alpha-hydroxy-butyrate dehydrogenase (SHBD) level indicates $LDH_1$ activity.

(3) Estimation of myoglobin in serum and urine by latex agglutination test is a very simple and rapid method for diagnosis. Results are almost similar to CPK study.

(4) Flipped LDH means $LDH_1 > LDH_2$, highly significant in infarction.

(5) Rise of total CPK may sometimes be found after multiple intramuscular injection (not CPK-MB). In cardiac surgery or cardioversion both total CPK and MB fractions will rise. Increase of LDH (total) is nonspecific, but $LDH_1$ is specific.

However, when the clinical diagnosis and E.C.G. findings are characteristic, many of these sophisticated tests need not be done as a routine matter. These are also quite expensive tests but can however be done with modern laboratory-kits available.

(6) *Differentiation from other causes of chest pain.*

| | SGOT | SGPT | LDH | SHBD | CPK |
|---|---|---|---|---|---|
| AMI | ↑↑ | ± | ↑↑ | ↑↑ | ↑↑ |
| Angina pectoris | N | N | N | N | N |
| Pulm. infarction | ± | ± | ↑↑ | ± | ± |
| Pneumonia or Atelectasis | N | N | N | N | N |
| CCF | ± | ± or ↑ | ± | N | N |

(7) *Non-specific findings*

(a) Neutrophilic leucocytosis — from 2nd day

(b) Raised ESR from 2nd or 3rd day

(c) Glycosuria and hyperglycaemia (in 50% cases)

(d) Glucose tolerance decreased

**Renal function tests**

(1) Blood examination - urea/urea-nitrogen (BUN), creatinine and uric acid levels rise in renal failure. Urea and creatinine should be the basic tests.

(2) Urine - routine chemical, physical and microscopical examinations required. Increased protein excretion with presence of RBC, pus cells and casts in urine are highly suggestive.

(3) If necessary 24 hours urine to be collected — total volume and amount of protein excreted are to be measured, important in nephrotic syndrome.

(4) If infection is suspected-culture, colony count and drug sensitivity tests to be performed. In cases of persistent pyuria with negative bacterial culture report, tuberculosis should be excluded.

(5) Other blood tests required.

(a) Haemoglobin level and haematocrit values

(b) Na, K, chloride, calcium, phosphate and bicarbonate levels.

(c) Total protein, albumin and globulin level.

(d) Glucose level.

(6) Glomerular filtration function assessed by creatinine clearance test.

(7) Selective protein excretion in urine is helpful in glomerulonephritis.

**Collagen diseases**

(1) Blood count (Hb, TC, DC, ESR) — normochromic normocytic anaemia, high ESR and leucopenia are typical features of SLE in most cases.

(2) C-reactive protein — increased (nonspecific).

(3) LE cell test positive in 60 to 70% of SLE cases. Also positive in some cases of rheumatoid arthritis.

(4) Antinuclear antibody (ANA or ANF) are of different types. Antibody against double stranded DNA is highly specific for SLE.

(5) Lupus band test (direct immunofluorescence on biopsy of normal skin in SLE patients) positive in 50-80% of SLE.

(6) Blood urea, creatinine and urine analysis necessary to assess renal involvement.

(7) Thrombocytopenia, Coombs positive haemolytic anaemia and biologically false positive serological tests for syphilis are sometimes found.

(8) Decreased levels of complement $C_3/C_4$ and presence of circulating immune complexes.

(9) Analysis of body fluids e.g. pleural, ascitic or joint fluids.

(10) Tissue biopsy.

**Acute abdominal pain**

(1) Clinical impression to be supplemented by routine blood count — leucocytosis with neutrophilia in acute pyogenic infection.

(2) Examination of stool to exclude worms/presence of frank or occult blood. To exclude protozoa, exudate and specific bacteria in cases of diarrhoea/dysentery.

(3) Examination of urine for presence of haematuria/pyuria/renal stone/urinary infection and porphyria.

(4) Serum amylase and lipase in suspected acute pancreatitis.

(5) Bilirubin and alkaline phosphatase when gallstone suspected.

(6) Urea, and creatinine levels when renal disease suspected and for IVP urea level is necessary.

(7) Blood glucose level to exclude diabetes mellitus.

(8) Serum electrolyte level — Na, K, chloride and bicarbonate to assess the condition of patient, particularly in intestinal obstruction.

**Patient in comatose/semicomatose state :**

(1) *Diabetic coma and hypoglycaemic* coma-blood glucose, urinary glucose and ketones. Serum Na may be low. Blood pH and bicarbonates should be checked for diagnosis of metabolic acidosis. Hypokalemia may occur after therapy.

(2) *Chronic end-stage renal failure (Uraemia)* —

(i) High urea/creatinine

(ii) Na — low, K — high, chlorides and bicarbonates — low, calcium — low, phosphates high.

(3) *Hepatic coma* — (Acute hepatic failure)

Bilirubin — may or may not be high, SGOT/SGPT very high prothrombin time increased; blood ammonia is high.

(4) *Septicaemic conditions* — Blood count and blood culture will be helpful.

(5) *Lactic acidosis* — increased serum lactate

(6) *Hyperosmolar coma* — serum osmolality and blood glucose increased.

(7) *Reye's syndrome* — ferbile illness in childhood treated with aspirin group — normal CSF with findings of hepatic coma.

(8) Alcohol, sedative drugs, narcotic and poisons may cause coma. These should be carefully considered and excluded.

**Thyroid diseases**

(1) Clinical — hypo or hyper-thyroid states. ($T_3$, $T_4$, and T.S.H. levels.

(Elevated TSH is essential to prove hypothyroid state)

Cholesterol — is raised in myxoedema.

(2) In enlarged thyroid — these tests not always helpful. Uptake studies with $I^{131}$ or $I^{123}$ or technetium are necessary. Clinical presentation and family history are inportant points.

**Bleeding disorders**

(1) Bleeding and coagulation time
(2) Platelet count and study of peripheral blood film
(3) Prothrombin time
(4) Activated partial thromboplastin time
(5) Fibrinogen level and fibrin degradation product = in disseminated intravascular coagulation (DIC)
(6) Bone marrow study in I.T.P.
(7) Haemoglobin/haematocrit values.

**Bone, joint and muscle disease**

(1) Calcium, phosphate and alkaline phosphatase in some bone diseases.
(2) Uric acid (gout), rheumatoid factor, (rheumatoid arthritis) LE cell test and ANF (SLE) & ASO titre (rheumatic) are helpful investigations.
(3) Assessment of kidney function and anaemia.
(4) *CPK and aldolase* are increased in muscle diseases.

**Malignant conditions**

Biological markers —

(1) *Alpha-fetoprotein (AFP)* in hepatoma, in gonadal tumours
(2) *Carcino embryonic antigen* (CEA) — particularly in colonic carcinoma
(3) *Beta HCG* — in choriocarcinoma.
(4) *Acid phosphatase* — carcinoma prostate (prostatic fraction)
(5) *Alkaline phosphatase* level rises with metastatic malignancy in bone, in space occupying lesions in liver and a placental like isoenzyme found in some bronchial tumours.
(6) *Immunoglobulin level* high in multiple myeloma (G or A or M)
(7) *LDH leves* rises non-specifically in all disseminated malignancy. Also uric acid and calcium levels may increase.

**Sexually transmitted diseases**

(1) *Urethral discharge* — Gram stained smear and culture in suspected gonococcal infection. In females endocervical smear is necessary. G.C.F.T. sometimes helpful in gonorrhoea, particularly chronic form.
(2) *Dark ground examination* of serous discharge from genital ulcers in suspected syphilitic infection. VDRL and TPHA tests are confirmatory.
(3) *Chancroids* caused by H. ducreyi confirmed by smear and culture.
(4) *Non-specific or non gonococcal urethritis* (NSU/NGU) are caused by chlamydia (confirmed by ELISA test or cell culture) and mycoplasma (confirmed by culture).

**Infertility**

(1) Both male and female partners to be investigated to exclude diabetes mellitus and STD
(2) Male partner — semen analysis
(3) Female partner — vaginal cytohormonal pattern and blood hormone analysis depending on the clinical presentation.

**Determination of immune status**

(1) Electrophoretic fractionation of serum proteins and immunoglobulin level for humoral immunity status.
(2) Cutaneous delayed type of hypersensitivity test with tuberculin, candida or mumps antigen and DNCB test for assessment of cell mediated immunity status.

**Tuberculin Test (Mantoux Test) :**

Tuberculin PPD. has been recommended by WHO for Mantoux test. Source material is Batch RT23 and it is commercially available as a ready-to-use solution in a special buffer stabilised with Tween 80. It is well known that old tuberculin (OT) contains nonspecific substances which may give false positive reaction.

*Principle* – Infection with M. tuberculosis results in hypersensitivity to tuberculoprotein. Intradermally injected PPD produces "induration" and erythema of the skin around the site of injection. The diameter of the induration is directly proportional to the degree of sensitisation. The test becomes positive 4 to 6 weeks after infection. A positive reaction does not necessarily signify the presence of active disease. A negative reaction in a well-nourished child below the age of 3 years excludes tuberculosis.

*Dilution used*

In adults = 1 TU ( = 1/10,000 OT)

In children = 10 TU (=1/1,000 OT) Mass screening 5 TU.

In ophthalmology = 0.1 TU ( = 1/100,000 OT).

(Of course it is not advisable to equate the two products OT & PPD).

*Test procedure*

0.1 ml of PPD of desired strength is injected "intradermally" of the ventral surface of the forearm. Readings are taken 72 hours after injection. The diameter of induration is measured transversely to the long axis of the forearm.

*Interpretation*

Area of induration of diameter of 10 mm or more is considered significant. Diameter of 5 to 9 mm is considered "doubtful" reaction. In a strongly positive case the diameter is over 20 mm with blisters or even ulcer.

*False negative reaction found*

(1) In incubation period (2) in advanced disease (3) after measles, pertussis, Hodgkin's disease, sarcoidosis (4) after steroid or immunosuppressant therapy (5) due to technical errors like loss of potency of PPD, subcutaneous injection.

**'Tine' test** = PPD is injected by multiple puncture method with a disposable set.

**B.C.G. test** (accelerated BCG reaction) use of BCG has been found to be more sensitive than tuberculin, particularly in malnourished children.

## GENERAL LABORATORY PRINCIPLES AND PATHOLOGICAL DATA

*S.K. DUTTA*

**Collection of blood and urine**

1. Identification of patient and labelling of vials are very important.
2. Fasting samples are necessary for fasting blood sugar and lipid profile. In most other cases strict fasting not necessary.
3. Sterile disposable or autoclaved or boiled syringe and needle after drying should be used.
4. The puncture site should be cleaned with spirit.
5. Tourniquet must not be applied for a prolonged time.
6. Great care should be taken to avoid haemolysis – by use of dry containers and syringes, gentle manipulation and putting the blood in the container after removing the needle. Gentle shaking has to be done for mixing blood and anticoagulants and clotted blood should be left at room temperature for about 30 minutes. Plasma is obtained from anticoagulated and serum from clotted blood.

7. Blood collection vial and tubes –
   (a) Routine blood count and ESR = Vial containing EDTA salt.
   (b) Blood sugar = vial containing mixture of oxalate and fluoride.
   (c) Biochemical tests are better done from serum (clotted blood).
8. Urine (Routine examination) = morning samples.
   Stool – fresh specimen is better.
9. Urine culture – fresh midstream sample.
10. Urine (24 hrs. collection) – Urine to be kept from the 2nd sample of 1st day to 1st sample of 2nd day. Preservatives to be added when required.
11. In the interpretation of results of the laboratory values more importance should be given to the normal values given by the laboratory. Values differ widely according to many methods followed and many kits used.

## CONVERSION FACTORS FOR S.I. UNITS

| | From S.I. Units | To S.I. Units |
|---|---|---|
| 1. Bilirubin | mc mol/1 × 0.058 = mg/dl | mg/dl ÷ 0.058 = mc mol/1 |
| 2. Calcium | m mol/1 × 4 = mg/dl | mg/dl ÷ 4 = m mol/1 |
| 3. Cholesterol | m mol/1 × 39 = mg/dl | mg/dl ÷ 39 = m mol/1 |
| 4. Creatinine | mc mol/1 × 0.011 = mg/dl | mg/dl ÷ 0.011 = mc mol/1 |
| 5. Glucose | m mol/1 × 18 = mg/dl | mg/dl ÷ 18 = m mol/1 |
| 6. Phosphorus | m mol/1 × 3 = mg/dl | mg/dl ÷ 3 = m mol/1 |
| 7. Proteins | g/1 ÷ 10 = g/dl | g/dl × 10 = g/1 |
| 8. Urate | m mol/1 × 17 = mg/dl | mg/dl ÷ 17 = m mol/1 |
| 9. Urea | m mol/1 × 6 = mg/dl | mg/dl ÷ 6 = m mol/1 |

## USEFUL EQUIVALENTS

| | | | |
|---|---|---|---|
| 1 cc | = 17 minims | 1 mgm | = 1/65 gr |
| 0.1 cc | = 1½ minims | 1 gr. | = 65 mgm |
| 1 fl dr | = 4 cc | 1 oz. | = 28 gms |
| 1 fl oz | = 30 cc | 1 lb | = 454 gms |
| 35 fl oz | = 1 litre | 1kg. | = 2.2 lbs |

## HAEMATOLOGICAL VALUES

1. Haemoglobin – Male 15.5 ± 2.5 g/dl Female 14.0 ± 2.5 g/dl (Colorimetric Cyanmethaemoglobin method)
2. Haematocrit value (PCV) Male 40-54 %, Female 37-47 %
3. M.C.V. = 76 - 96 fl.
4. M.C.H. = 27 - 32 pg.
5. M.C.H.C. = 30 - 35 g/dl.
6. Reticulocytes = 0.2 - 2.0 %
7. Total count -
   (a) RBC Male 4.5 - 6.5 mill/cmm Female 3.9 - 5.6 mill/cmm.
   (b) WBC 4000 - 10,000/cmm
   (c) platelets 150,000 – 400,000/cms

8. Differential count of WBC
   - Neutrophils = 40 - 75%
   - Lymphocytes = 20 - 45%
   - Monocytes = 2 - 8%
   - Eosinophils = 2 - 6%
   - Basophils = 1%

9. E.S.R. Westergern method

| | < 50 years | > 50 years |
|---|---|---|
| Male | 0 - 15 mm/hr | 0 - 20 mm/hr |
| Female | 0 - 20 mm/hr | 0 - 30 mm/hr |

10. Hb F < 2% $HbA_2$ < 3.5%

## ENDOCRINE PROFILE (BLOOD)

1. Pituitary hormones —
   (a) Gonadotrophins
   Women mature, premenopausal, except at ovulation
   FSH = 5 - 20 mu/ml
   L.H. = 5 - 25 mu/ml
   Ovulatory surge
   FSH = 12 - 30 mu/ml
   LH = 25 - 100 mu/ml
   Post menopausal women
   FSH > 50 mu/ml
   LH > 50 mu/ml
   Men (mature)
   FSH 5 - 20 mu/ml
   LH 5 - 20 mu/ml
   Children, both sexes, prepubertal
   FSH > 5 mu/ml
   LH > 5 mu/ml
   (b) T.S.H. 1 - 4 u/ml (1 - 4 mu/1)
   (c) Prolactin Female < 25 ng/ml
   Male < 16 ng/ml
   (d) Growth hormone < 5 ng/dl
   (after 100 g glucose orally)
   (d) A.C.T.H. (8 AM) < 80 pg/ml
2. Thyroid hormones —
   (a) $T_3$ (Triiodothyronine) 0.7 - 2 ng/ml (70 - 200 ng/dl)
   (b) $T_4$ (Thyroxine) 45 - 125 ng/ml (4.5 - 12.5 mcg/dl)
   (c) PBI 4 - 8 mcgms/dl
3. Adrenal steroids —
   (a) Cortisol AM = 5-25 mcg/dl
   PM = approximately half of AM value
4. Gonadal steroids
   (a) Oestradiol
   Women = 20 - 60 pg/ml
   Men < 50 pg/ml
   (b) Progesterone

Women (Preovulation, prepubertal, post-menopausal) and Men < 2 ng/ml
Women (luteal peak) < 5 ng/ml

(c) Testosterone
Women < 100 ng/dl
Men 300 - 1000 ng/dl
Prepubertal boys and girls 5 - 20 ng/dl

5. Human chorionic gonadotrophin (Beta HCG)
Men and non-pregnant women <3 IU/1
Normal pregnancy up to 150 IU/1
6. Insulin (fasting) 6 - 26 mu/ml
7. Glucagon 50 - 100 pg/ml
9. Gastrin < 120 pg/ml

**URINE** (TIMED OR 24 hrs. COLLECTION)

1. Amylase 35 - 260 somogyi units/hr.
2. Calcium (200 mgms calcium diet)
<150 mgms in 24 hrs.
3. Copper up to 25 mcg/24 hrs.
4. Creatine (as creatinine)
Adult male <50 mgms Adult female < 100 mgms/24 hrs.
5. Creatinine 1 - 1.6 g/24 hrs.
6. Glucose (true) 50 - 300 mgms/24 hours.
7. Potassium 25 - 100 mEq/24 hrs.
8. Protein < 150 mgms/24 hrs.
9. Sodium 100 - 260 m Eq/24 hrs.
10. Hormone metabolites
(i) Catecholamine < 100 mcg/24 hrs.
(ii) V.M.A. < 8 mg/24 hrs.
(iii) 5 HIAA 2 - 8 mgms/24 hrs.
(iv) Oestriol Menstrual cycle 0 - 72 mcgms/24 hrs. with midcycle peak.
Pregnancy 10 - 40 mgms/24 hrs. (30-36th week).
(v) Pregnanediol Menstrual cycle 2-10 mgm/24 hrs.
Pregnancy 5 - 47 mgms/24 hrs.
(vi) 17 Oxosteroid Adult female 5 - 15 mgms/24 hrs.
(17 Ketosteroid) Adult male 8 - 20 mgms/24 hrs.
(vii) 17 Oxogenic steroid Adult female 5-15 mgms/24 hrs.
(17 Ketogenic steroid) Adult male 0-20 mgms/24 hrs.
(viii) 17 hydroxy — Adult female 4-8 mgms/24 hrs.
Corticosteroids Adult male 4-12 mgms/24 hrs.

**Stool**

Stool fat excretion — less than 5 gms/24 hrs.
(3 days collection).

**Cerebrospinal fluid —**

1. Clear colourless.

| | | |
|---|---|---|
| 2. Protein | 20 - 40 mgms/dl | |
| 3. Glucose | 40 - 70 mgms/dl | |
| 4. Cell count | Less than 5/cmm all lymphocytes | |
| 5. L.D.H. | 10% of serum value | |
| 6. IgG | Less than 4 mgms/dl. | |
| 7. Electrophoresis | Prealbumin | 0.4 - 4.5% |
| | Albumin | 47 - 66% |
| | $Alpha_1$ glob | 4.6 - 8.0% |
| | $Alpha_2$ glob | 5.0 - 9.0% |
| | Beta glob | 9.0 - 14.0% |
| | Thau glob | 4.6 - 8.0% |
| | Gamma glob | 8.0 - 13.0% |

**Serology**

1. ANF/ANA (Antinuclear antibody) Negative (Double stranded DNA antibody specific for SLE)
2. ASO (Antistreptolysin O) Normal upto 160 Todd units or 200 I.U.
3. Rheumatoid factor —
   Latex fixation test Normal upto 1/20
   Rose waaler test (Sheep cell) upto 1/16.
4. Widal test (typhoid agglutinin)
   'H' and 'O' titres above 1/80 or a rising titre significant.
5. Paul Bunnell test — heterophile antibody titre
   above 1/56 (latex agglutination spot test — positive).
6. Brucella agglutinin titre above 1/80
7. Weil Felix reaction Four fold rise of titre with paired sera.

## BLOOD - BIOCHEMICAL VALUES - NORMAL RANGE

*S.K. DUTTA*

| | | |
|---|---|---|
| Albumin | 3.5 - 5.6 Gms/dl. | |
| Aldolase | Less than 8 u/l | Values twice high in children |
| Alpha Fetoprotein | At birth 0-30 ng/ml<br>Adult less than 10 ng/ml<br>Normal pregnancy = maximum up to 520 ng/ml (in 3rd trimester). | |
| Aminotransferases | See SGOT/SGPT | |
| Ammonia (enzymatic) | 25 - 94 mc/dl | Immediate analysis |
| Ammonia - nitrogen (diffusion method) | 26 - 52 mcg/dl | —do— |
| Amylase | 60 - 180 Somogyi units/dl<br>110 - 330 u/l | |
| Bicarbonate | 20 - 31 mEq/1 | Oxalated blood under liq. paraffin. |
| Bilirubin | Total 0.2 - 1.0 mgms/dl<br>conjugated 0 to 0.3 mgms/dl<br>unconjugated 0.2 to 1.0 mgms/dl. | Higher values in new born. |

| | | |
|---|---|---|
| B.S.P. excretion test (Bromsulphthalein) (5 mgms/Kg body wt.) | Less than 5% retention after 45 minutes. | |
| Calcium | 9 - 11 mgms/dl (4.5 - 5.5 mEq/1) | |
| Ceruloplasmin | 25 - 40 mgms/dl | |
| $CO_2$ combining power | 40 - 60 vols/dl | as bicarbonate |
| Copper | 75 - 160 mcg/dl | |
| Chloride | 98 - 108 mEq/1 | |
| Cholesterol (total) | 150 - 250 mgms/dl | |
| Creatinine | Less than 1.8 mgms/dl | |
| Creatinine clearance test | 95 - 140 ml/min. (av 120 ml) (male)<br>85 - 125 ml/min. (av 110 ml) (female) | |
| C.P.K/ | 24 - 195 u/1 (male) 24 - 170 U/1 (female) | |
| C-reactive protein | 0-8 mgms/1 | |
| C.E.A. | $<$ 2.5 ng/ml (healthy nonsmokers) | |
| Electrophoresis (Haemoglobin) | Chiefly Hb A, and 1.8 - 3.5% Hb $A_2$ | |
| Electrophoresis of serum proteins | Albumin 50-70% 3.2 - 5.6 g/dl<br>$Alpha_1$ glob. 2 - 6% 0.1 - 0.4 g/dl<br>$Alpha_2$ glob. 5 - 11% 0.4 - 0.8 g/dl<br>Beta glob. 7 - 16% 0.5 - 1.0 g/dl<br>Gamma glob. 11 - 22% 0.7 - 1.5 g/dl | |
| Fatty acid (free) | 8 - 25 mgms/dl | |
| Ferritin | Male 15 - 200 mcg/1 Female 12-150 mcg/1 (adult) | |
| Fibrinogen | 200 - 400 mgms/dl | Plasma |
| F.D.P. | $<$10 mcgm per ml | |
| Folate (serum) | 3 - 20 ng/1 | |
| (RBC) | 160 - 640 ng/1 | |
| Globulin | 1.2 - 3.5 Gms/dl | |
| Glucose (fasting) | 70 - 110 mgms/dl<br>60 - 100 mgms/dl | Serum/plasma<br>Whole blood. |
| Glucose (Post prandial) (2 hrs. after 75 Gms glucose) (Plasma/serum values) | Less than 140 mgms/dl<br>Between 140 & 200 mgms/dl<br>Over 200 mgms/dl | (normal)<br>(I.G.T.)<br>(D-mellitus) |
| G 6 P D | 120 - 240 u/$10^{12}$ RBC<br>Screening method — Decolourisation time 30-60 min. | |
| Glutamyl transpeptidase (G.G.T) | Male 11 - 50 u/1<br>Female 7 - 32 u/1 | at 37°C. |
| Glycosylated Hb ($HbA_1$) | Normal 5-8% Diabetes mellitus>10% | |
| Glutamic oxaloacetic transaminase (SGOT/AST) | up to 40 u/1 at 37°C | Varies with method and reaction temperature. |
| Glutamic pyruvic transaminase (SGPT/ALT) | upto 35 u/l at 37°C | Do |

| Test | Normal value | Remarks |
|---|---|---|
| Haptoglobin | 83 - 267 mgms/dl (RID)<br>(Mean = 175 (Varies with method) | |
| Hydroxybutyrate dehydrogenase ( HBDH or LDHl) | Adults 72 - 182 u/l at 37°C | |
| Immunoglobulins | IgG 550 - 1600 mgms/dl<br>IgA 60 - 330 mgms/dl<br>IgM 45 - 170 mgms/dl<br>IgD 1-5 mgms/dl<br>IgE Less than 0.025 mgms/dl. | |
| Iron (total) | Male 80 - 175 mcgms/dl<br>Female 60 - 160 mcgms/dl | |
| Iron binding capacity (total) | Male 280 - 400 mcgms/dl<br>Female 200 - 430 mcgms/dl | |
| Lactate dehydrogenase (LDH, total) | 70 - 300 u/l | Varies with method and reaction temperature. |
| Lipase | Upto 190 u/l | |
| Lipids (total) | 400 - 800 mgms/dl | |
| Lipoproteins | Beta : Alpha upto 2.5 | |
| Lithium | Negative normally<br>Therapeutic level = 0.5 - 1.5 mEq/1<br>Toxic level over 2.0 mEq/1 | |
| Magnesium | 1.4 - 2.3 mEq/l (1.7 - 2.8 mgms/dl) | |
| Non-esterified fatty acid | See Fatty acid (free) | |
| Non-protein nitrogen | 15 - 35 mgms/dl | |
| 5 - Nucleotidase | 4 - 14 u/l | |
| Phosphatase | | |
| acid | 1 - 4 K.A. units/dl<br>0.5 - 1.2 Bodansky units/dl<br>1.8 - 8.2 U/l | |
| alkaline | 3 - 13 K.A. Units/dl<br>1.5 - 4.5 Bodansky units/dl<br>22 - 92 U/l | Higher values found in children and during pregnancy. |
| Phospholipids | 150 - 380 mgms/dl | |
| pH (blood) | arterial 7.38 - 7.44<br>Venous 7.36 - 7.41 | |
| Phosphorus (inorganic) | 2.0 - 5.0 mgms/dl adults<br>1.2 - 3.0 m Eq/l<br>4.0 - 7.0 mgms/dl children<br>2.3 - 4.1 m Eq/1 | |
| Potassium | 3.5 - 5.0 mEq/l | |
| Proteins Total | 6 - 8 Gms/dl | |
| Albumin | 3.5 - 5.6 Gms/dl | |
| Globulin | 1.2 - 3.5 Gms/dl. | |
| Protein bound Iodine (PBI) | 4 - 8 mcgms/dl | |

| | | |
|---|---|---|
| Sodium | 137 - 148 mEq/1 | |
| Thymol turbidity | 1 - 4 units | |
| Transaminases | See GOT/GPT | |
| Triglyceride | Usually upto 150 mgms/dl elevated if above 200 mgms/dl (enzymatic). | |
| Urea | 15 - 40 mgms/dl. | |
| Urea nitrogen | 8 - 20 mgms/dl | |
| Uric acid | Usually up to 5 mgms/dl Upper limit of normal = 6.5 to 7 mgms/dl. (enzymatic) | Values differ with method used, diet habit and age. |
| Vitamin $B_{12}$ | 200 - 600 pg/ml | |
| D-xylose absorption test (5 Gms dose, urine collected for next 5 hrs). | Normally excrete more than 1.2 Gms. Lower value in malabsorption. | |
| Zinc sulphate turbidity test | Less than 12 units. | |

## DIET-THERAPY

*G.C. MOOKERJEE*
*RAM UDAYAN RAY*
*GOWRI KRISHNA*

Good health depends on properly balanced diet. In diseased state also, appropriate diet is, extremely essential. Wrong diet, wrongly cooked and unhygienically served may cause numerous medical problems. Cardiovascular disorders, obesity, chronic diarrhoea, malnutrition, malabsorption state, renal disorders etc. require special diet as well as calorific adjustments. Diabetics need restriction of sugar and calories while juvenile diabetics and pregnant diabetics will require special allowances particularly in respect of protein and fats.

This chapter presents some important data and information in construction of diets in various common disorders. However it should be remembered that it is neither possible nor necessary to calculate calories and nutritional values to any mathematical accuracy. Because food values are also variable depending on the source and types of item. For instance, calorific value of broiler Chicken is 151 per 100 g while fried chicken is 109 calories for same weight. Meat sausage is about 310 per 100 g while mutton is 194 calories. Calorific value of fish varies considerably. Lobster is 90 calories per 100 g while pomfret is about 90, medium Rohu 90 but Hilsa is 273 calories per 100 g.

However butter, oil or ghee gives 900 calories per 100 g (9 cal/g.). A small egg is 50 calorie. Calories of milk also will vary considerably depending on the source. One glass of butter milk is about 25 calories while 100 g. ice cream is about 200 calories and milk cake (100g) is 330 calories.

Vegetables have very little calorific value. 100 g of bottle gourd (Lauki) gives 12 calories while same amount of potato provides about 100 calories. So selection of items is most important. Some basic data for planning of diet are presented :

Calorific content of some common food for ready calculation

| Food | 2000 Cal | 1800 Cal | 1600 Cal |
|---|---|---|---|
| Rice/Atta | 200 g | 200 g | 175 g |
| Dal | 60 g | 60 g | 50 g |
| Egg 50 g. | One | One | One |
| Meat | 150 g | 150 g | 100 g |
| Oil for cooking | 30 g | 30 g | 30 g |
| Butter | 15 | | |
| Milk | 500 ml | 500 ml | 500 ml |

EXCHANGE LISTS FOR MEAL PLANNING

| No Food | Quantity = 1 exchange (g.) | Calories | Carbohydrate (g) | Protein (g) | Fat (g) |
|---|---|---|---|---|---|
| 1. Cereals | (Raw Wt. 20) | 70 | 15 | 2 | 0 |
| 2. Pulses | (Raw Wt 20) | 70 | 13 | 4 | 0 |
| 3. Meat Lean | 30 | 55 | 0 | 7 | 3 |
| High fat-meat | 30 | 100 | 0 | 7 | 8 |
| 4. Fat - ghee, oil (one tsp) | 5 | 45 | 0 | 0 | 5 |
| 5. Fruits (average) | 30 | 40 | 10 | 0 | 0 |
| 6. Vegetable — Group: A* | 150 | Negligible | Negligible | Negligible | Negligible |
| Group - B | 150 | 40 | 7 | 2 | 0 |
| 7. Milk-standard | 250 ml | 170 | 12 | 8 | 10 |
| Skimmed | 250 ml | 80 | 12 | 8 | 0 |

**House hold measures**

One tea cup = 150 ml
One large breakfast cup = 200 to 250 ml
One tumbler glass = 200-300 ml
One teaspoon = 5 ml, one table spoon = 15 ml. one dessert spoon = 10 ml.
One cup full of rice (uncooked) = 180 g.
One cup full of atta (uncooked) = 130 g.

**Diet for Diabetics**

Diet will depend on age body weight and nature of activity. It is better to have six meals than three standard meals — breakfast, lunch and dinner. Timings have to be adjusted depending on your duty. The doctor will advice calorie-intake as well as various items of good you need.

(1) Sugar and sweets should be avoided.
(2) Meat, fish or chicken should be taken in normal quantities — 120 to 150 g. daily. Avoid red meat and fatty meat.

(3) Milk for non-vegeterians may vary from 150 to 250 ml per day.
(4) Egg may be allowed for children and pregnant ladies, Adults may be allowed an egg, depending on blood cholesterol level and lipid profile.
(5) Vegetarians may take 500 to 750 ml of milk per day and children up to one litre. This can be taken as plain milk or curd or 'Chhana' (clotted milk).
(6) Pulses allowed 30 to 60 g day.
(7) Starchy food i.e. Rice/atta depends on weight and physical activity. For sedentary persons it varies between 120 to 200 g daily.
Vegetables — (total about 500 g daily). Leafy vegetables allowed 120-180 g; others 100 — 200 g; (except potato, Yam, beet) etc. Raddish, onion and green carrot allowed.
(8) Ghee and oil — depends on age, pregnancy and lactation. Usually obese adults will take only 30 g of cooking oil. Others may be allowed up to 60 g an average. Children and pregnant women and lactating mother will be allowed butter, 5 to 10 g daily, depending on sugar level.
(9) Do not take any sugary food e.g. candy, honey, jam jelly, marmalade and ice creams.
(10) Sausages and pork not allowed. Fried food have high calories so better be avoided.
(11) Most proprietory tinned food contain a lot of sugar; special products may be allowed by your doctor.
(12) Alcoholic and cola drinks are not allowed.
(13) If diabetes is well controlled and patient is not obese and he is used to take alcohol, small amounts of whisky or brandy may be allowed.

**Diabetic Menu**
(2000 calories)

**Daily Ration**

*(Values in g or ml)*

| | | | |
|---|---|---|---|
| Cereals | 200 | Carbohydrate | 52% (260 g.) |
| Dal | 60 | Protein | 17% ( 85 g.) |
| Egg | One | Fat | 31% ( 69 g.) |
| Meat (low fat) | 150 | | |
| Vegetables | Group A and B | | |
| Fruits | 100 | | |
| Oil | 30 | | |
| Butter | 15 | | |
| Milk (skimmed) | 500 | | |

**Food distribution :**

| *Breakfast* | | *Lunch* | |
|---|---|---|---|
| Cereal or bread | 60/80 | Rice or atta | 60 |
| Egg | one medium | Dal | 30 |
| Milk from allowance | | Lean Meat/fish | 75 |
| Tea or coffee without sugar | | Vegetables | 2 servings |
| Fruit | one | | |
| Butter | 15 | | |

| *Afternoon Tea* | | *Dinner* | |
|---|---|---|---|
| Tea | | Cereal | 60 |
| Puffed rice (Muri) | 25 g. | Dal | 30 |
| or Biscuits | 2 pcs. | Meat/fish | 75 |
| | | Vegetables | 2 servings |

*Bed time*
*Left over milk from allowance*

---

**Daily Ration**

| *(In g. or ml.)* | |
|---|---|
| Cereals | 200 |
| Dal | 60 |
| Egg | one |
| Meat (low fat) | 150 |
| Vegetables A group | 2 servings |
| Vegetables B group | 2 servings |
| Fruits | 100 g. or 1 apple |
| Oil | 30 |
| Milk (skimmed) | 500 |

| 1800 calories | |
|---|---|
| Carbohydrate | 242 g. (53%) |
| Protein | 83 g. (18%) |
| Fat | 58 g. (29%) |

**Food distribution**

*Breakfast*

| | |
|---|---|
| Cereal : 60/Bread : 80 | |
| Egg | one |
| Milk from allowance | |
| Tea or coffee without sugar | |
| Fruit | one |

*Lunch*

| | |
|---|---|
| Cereals | 60 |
| Dal | 30 |
| Lean meat/fish | 75 |
| Vegetables A and B one serving each | |

*Tea*

| | |
|---|---|
| Tea or coffee (without sugar) | |
| Cereal | 30 |
| Or | |
| Bread | 40 |

*Dinner*

| | |
|---|---|
| Cereals | 50 |
| Dal | 30 |
| Meat/fish | 75 |
| Vegetables | |
| Group A and B | one serving each |

*Bed-time*
Left over milk from allowance

---

**Daily ration**

| *(Value in g. or ml)* | |
|---|---|
| Cereals | 175 |
| Dal | 50 |
| Egg (one) | 50 |
| Meat (lean) | 100 |
| Vegetables Both groups | |
| Fruit | one |
| Oil | 30 |
| Milk (skimmed) | 500 |

| 1600 calories | |
|---|---|
| Carbohydrate | 212 g. (53%) |
| Protein | 67.7 g. (18%) |
| Fat | 51 g. (29%) |

**Food distribution**

*Breakfast*

| | |
|---|---|
| Cereal or | 50 |
| Bread | 70 |

*Lunch*

| | |
|---|---|
| Cereal | 50 |
| Dal | 25 |

| | | | |
|---|---|---|---|
| Egg | one | Lean meat/fish | 50 |
| Milk from allowance | | Vegetables | |
| Tea or coffee without sugar | | Group A & B | one serving each |
| *Tea* | | *Dinner* | |
| Tea or coffee without sugar | | Cereal | 50 |
| Fruit | one | Dal | 25 |
| Biscuits | 3 pcs | Lean meat/fish | 50 |
| or cereal | 25 g. | Vegetables | |
| | | Group A and B | one serving each |
| *Bed time* | | | |
| Left over milk from allowance | | | |

## List of Fruits and Vegetables

**Group A vegetables**

*very little calories (around or less than 20 cal/100 g.*

Sag, Brinjal, Lady's finger, cabbage, drumstick, onion stalks, cucumber, raddish, pumpkin, lauki, ash-ground, bottle gourd, bittergourd, snakegourd, fresh beans, plantain flower (mocha) lettuce, green tomato, turnip,knol-khol.

**Group B Vegetables**

*(around 50 calories/100 g portion)*

Cluster beans (guarphali), peas, double beans, green mango, carrot, onion, barbati, green papaya, cauli-flower.

**Fruits**

*(containing 10 g CHO = 40 cal)*

| | | |
|---|---|---|
| Apple | one small | 80 |
| Banana | one small | 40 |
| Grapes | Ten small | 60 |
| Guava | one small | 80 |
| Mango | one portion | 80 |
| Melon | | 150 |
| Pineapple | 1/3 cup. | 80 |
| Papaya | | 120 |
| Safeda (Chikoo) | | 40 |
| Pears | | 80 |
| Musambi (sweet lime) | one medium size | |
| Orange | one (medium size) | |

**Foods allowed without restriction**

(useful for diabetics and obese people)

1. Tea or coffee without sugar
2. Thin butter milk
3. Clear soups
4. Lime juice without sugar
5. Cucumber
6. Tomato juice without sugar

**Avoid**

1. Fried foods
2. Sweets and sweetened foods, cakes, pastries, puddings.
3. Thick sauces
4. Sugar, glucose, jams, honey, syrup, glucose drinks, fruits tinned and preserved in sugar syrup.
5. Red meat and oily fish.
6. Alcoholic drinks

**Use in moderation**

1. Starchy vegetables and dried fruits
2. Oils, butter, cheese, cream etc. (Restricted amount with doctor's approval)

**Diet for Obesity (In g. or ml) :**

(1000 calories approx.)

**Daily Ration**

| | |
|---|---|
| Cereals | 120 |
| Dal | 50 |
| Lean meat or fish | 75 |
| Skimmed milk | 300 |
| Vegetables | only low calorie |
| Vegetables of Group A | |
| Oil in cooking | 15 |
| Fruit | one |

**Diet plan**

*Breakfast*

| | |
|---|---|
| Bread or | 40 |
| Rice flakes | 30 |
| Tea or coffee without sugar | |
| Milk ½ cup from allowance | |
| Fruit | one |

*Tea*

| | |
|---|---|
| Tea/coffee without sugar | |
| Biscuit — two pieces | (10) |

*Mid-morning*

Lime juice one glass (without sugar)

*Lunch*

| | |
|---|---|
| Rice/Atta | 50 |
| Dal | 25 |
| Lean meat/fish | 75 |
| Vegetables — Group A as desired | |

*Dinner*

| | |
|---|---|
| Rice/Atta | 30 |
| Dal | 25 |
| Vegetables — group A as desired | |

LOW FAT DIET

*(Fat — 30 g)*

| Restricted foods. | In g | Fat. (g). |
|---|---|---|
| Lean meat e.g. chicken, low fat/fish | 120 | 17 |
| Egg — one small | 30 | 3.5 |
| Cereals as desired up to | 180 | 1 |
| Dal | 90 | 0.6 |
| Oil in cooking (2 teaspoons) | | 10 |
| use only skimmed milk | — | — |

*Morning*

| | |
|---|---|
| Bread with jam | 60 |
| Egg | (one) |
| Fruit (one) (Fruit juice or as fruit) | |
| Skimmed milk (one cup) | 150 ml. |

*Tea*

| | |
|---|---|
| Tea or coffee with sugar | |
| Fruit — one apple or other fruit about | 100 |
| Low fat biscuits | (2 pieces) |

*Mid-morning*

Juice with sugar

*Lunch*

| | |
|---|---|
| Cereal | 60 |
| Dal | 30 |
| Lean meat or fish | 40 |
| Vegetables — as desired | |

*Dinner*

| | |
|---|---|
| Cereal | 40 |
| Dal | 30 |
| Lean meat/fish | 30 |
| Fruits : Apple, pear, guava or banana (small size) | one |

---

LOW PROTEIN DIET : (In g. or ml.)

*(Protein 40 g. approx.)*

| Restricted food items : | | Protein (g.) |
|---|---|---|
| Cereals | 130 | 9 |
| Low protein vegetables as desired | | 3 |
| Low protein fruit (up to 300 g. orange or 600 g. of most other fruits of low protein value) | | 3 |
| Meat/fish | 50 | 21 |
| Dal | 50 | 4 |
| Milk | 120 | |

*Breakfast*

| | |
|---|---|
| Cereal or | 30 |
| Bread | 40 |
| Milk from allowance. | |
| Tea or coffee with sugar | |
| Fruit : one apple or any fruit | 100 |

*Tea*

| | |
|---|---|
| Tea or coffee with sugar and milk from allowance. | |
| Biscuits — 2 pcs. | 20 |
| Fruit | 100 |

*Midmorning*

Fruit or juice

*Lunch*

| | |
|---|---|
| Cereal | 50 |
| Meat/fish/egg | 50 |
| Dal | 20 |
| Vegetables | |
| Jelly with cream | |

*Dinner*

| | |
|---|---|
| Cereals | 30 |
| Dal | 30 |
| Vegetables | |
| Fruit with sugar and cream | |

**Vegetables and fruits with low protein content**

Carrot, raddish, green papaya, beat root, ashgourd, cabbage, cauliflower, bottle gourd,cucumber, ridge ground (Jhinga) snakegourd, brinjal, tomato.

Most fruits except guava, banana, jackfruit, chiku (safeda) contain less than or about 5 g protein for each 100 g portion.

**Low cholesterol foods**

Vegetables
Fruits
Cereals
Flour
Spaghetti
Juice
Biscuits (arrowroot)
Skimmed milk
Curds using skimmed milk
Cottage cheese
Vegetable seed oils
Black tea and coffee
Soft drinks, spirits, wines, beer

**High cholesterol foods**

Whole milk, butter, cheese, margarine, cream, ice cream, egg, shell fish, duck, goose, mutton, pastry, lard, suet and clarified butter (ghee).

Chicken and white fish contain moderate amounts hence permitted in average helpings.

**Potassium rich food**

*Fresh vegetables*
Asparaus
Bean
Brussels sprout
Cabbage
Potato
Corn
Peas
Raddish

*Fresh fruits*
Apple
Apricot
Avoçado
Banana
Date
Grape-fruit
Orange
Peach
Raisin

**Low sodium diet for cardiac failure**

*General principles :*

1. Avoid foods cooked or tinned with salt, mono-sodium glutamate, baking powder and baking soda and other preservatives containing sodium.
2. Restrict high sodium foods and include fruits, vegetables, cereals, all prepared without salt.
3. Restrict milk intake to 250 ml/day.
4. Where possible,avoid salted foods like bread, salted butter and sausages and food with large amounts of milk and egg.
5. Wherever necessary, yeast/and sodium free baking powder can be used. Sodium free baking powder can be made by mixing 40g potassium carbonate, 30g. corn flour and 8g. tartaric acid. One and a half teaspoon of this mixture can be used instead of one teaspoon of baking powder.
6. Give smaller meals at frequent intervals rather that large meals for apart.
7. Reduce weight wherever necessary.
8. Use of spices can enhance the monotony of a salt free diet. Avoiding external salt can bring down the sodium intake to less than 1 gm/day.

**Protein, fat, carbohydrate and caloric values of cooked food**

*Cereals and cereal food*

| No. | Name | wt. (g) | Pro (g) | Fat (g) | CHO (g) | Calori K. Cal. |
|---|---|---|---|---|---|---|
| 1. | Arrowroot (one tbsp) | 8 | — | — | 7.0 | 29 |
| 2. | Bajra 30 g. flour (one chappati) | 45 | 3.5 | 1.5 | 20.1 | 108 |

| No. | Name | wt. (g) | Pro (g) | Fat (g) | CHO (g) | Calori K.Cal. |
|---|---|---|---|---|---|---|
| 3. | Barley (pearled) 2 tbsp | 30 | 2.3 | .3 | 22.3 | 99 |
| 4. | Corn flakes (one cup) | 25 | 2.1 | 0.1 | 21.0 | 95 |
| 5. | Corn flour (¼ cup) | 25 | 2.1 | 0.1 | 21.0 | 95 |
| 6. | Farex 2 tbsp | 30 | 3.7 | 0.7 | 20.7 | 97 |
| 7. | Jowar flour (30g) (one chappati) | 45 | 3.1 | 0.6 | 22.2 | 106 |
| 8. | Macaroni cooked (2/3 cup) | — | 3.6 | 0.1 | 21.7 | 107 |
| 9. | Maize flour (30g) (one chappati) | 45 | 3.3 | 1.1 | 19.8 | 102 |
| 10. | Oat meal porridge (one cup) | 236 | 5.4 | 2.8 | 26.0 | 148 |
| 11. | Ragi flour (30g) (one chappati) | 45 | 2.1 | 0.4 | 21.6 | 98 |
| 12. | Rice milled, boiled one cup (cooked) (= 3 tbsp dry rice) | — | 2.9 | 0.1 | 30.2 | 134 |
| 13. | Rice, puffed (one cup) | 13 | .8 | 0.1 | 11.5 | 51 |
| 14. | Spaghetti plain, cooked (one cup) | 146 | 7.4 | 0.9 | 44.1 | 216 |
| 15. | Wheat bread (one slice) | 30 | 2.3 | 0.5 | 15.0 | 75 |
| 16. | Wheat bread (one slice) with one tsp. butter and one tsp. jam | 40 | 2.6 | 4.6 | 19.7 | 130 |
| 17. | Wheat bun (one average) | 35 | 2.6 | 3.2 | 20.0 | 120 |
| 18. | Wheat chappati/khakhra (15 g flour) one small | — | 1.2 | .1 | 8.0 | 40 |
| 19. | Wheat paratha using atta-60 g, fat 2 tbsp one paratha | | | | | 256 |
| | Allo paratha (one) | | | | | 260 |
| | Fried potato (60 g) | | | | | 200 |
| | Doughnuts (60 g) | | | | | 225 |
| | Puri (one) 3½″ diameter | | | | | 115 |
| | Dumplings (60g) | | | | | 120 |
| | Clear soup (250 ml) | | | | | 35 |
| | Thick soup (250 ml) | | | | | 100 |

**Table of food values**

Approx. calorific values of alcoholic beverages

| | | (cal.) |
|---|---|---|
| Beer | 200 ml | 98 |
| Benedictine | 20 ml | 69 |
| Brandy | 30 ml | 73 |
| Cider | 180 ml | 71 |
| Gin | 43 ml | 105 |
| Rum | 43 ml | 105 |
| Sherry | 100 ml | 120 |

| | | |
|---|---|---|
| Toddy (fermented) | 240 ml | 24 |
| Toddy (sweet) | 240 ml | 144 |
| Whisky | 30 ml | 90 |
| Wine<br>one glass | 100 ml | 160 |

Alcohol content varies in different alcoholic drinks depending on the brand of manufacture.

Approx. calorific value of beverages with protein, fat and carbohydrate

| Name | Wt. (g). | Pro. g | Fat. g | CHO g | Calories |
|---|---|---|---|---|---|
| Bournvita 2 tbsp in one cup cow's milk | 230 | 10.2 | 11.1 | 28.8 | 265 |
| Cola drinks one bottle | 170 | — | — | 20.4 | 78 |
| Cocoa powder 2 tbsp | 30 | 5.8 | 6.6 | 9.9 | 128 |
| Cocoa one tbsp in one cup of cow's milk | 215 | 9.9 | 12.3 | 14.5 | 224 |
| Coffee 2 tbsp cow's milk 2 tsp sugar | 200 | .9 | 1.1 | 11.4 | 60 |
| Horlicks 2 tbsp | 30 | 4.1 | 2.3 | 20.1 | 113 |
| Lemonade / Fresh lemon } juice 2 tbsp, sugar 3 tsp | 240 | — | — | 17.4 | 73 |
| Tea 2 tbsp cow's milk 2 tsp. sugar | 200 | .9 | 1.1 | 11.4 | 60 |
| Limca one bottle | — | — | — | — | 50 |
| Coconut water * one glass | 240 ml | 0.2 | 0.2 | 10.8 | 46 |
| Tomato juice one glass (using 200g. fruit) | 200 ml. | 1.8 | 0.4 | 7.3 | 40 |

* varies a lot depending on Kernel content

Milk and milk Products

| No. | Name | wt. (g.) | Pro. (g.) | Fat. (g.) | CHO (g.) | Calories K.(cal.) |
|---|---|---|---|---|---|---|
| 1. | Butter one tbsp | 5 | — | 4 | — | 36 |
| 2. | Butter milk (one tbsp of water curd making 3 cups) one cup | 200 | 2.7 | 4.6 | 2.1 | 62 |
| 3. | Butter milk using cow's milk (one cup) | 200 | 2.3 | 3.0 | 2.1 | 45 |

*Table contd...*

*Table of food values contd. from previous page*

| No. | Name | wt. (g.) | Pro. (g.) | Fat. (g.) | CHO (g.) | Calories K. cal. |
|---|---|---|---|---|---|---|
| 4. | Cream, light 2 tbsp | 30 | .8 | 5.4 | 1.2 | 56 |
| 5. | Milk, Buffalo milk, (one cup) | 200 | 8.0 | 14.0 | 10.4 | 206 |
| | Buffalo, skimmed (one cup) | 200 | 8.4 | 0.2 | 10.8 | 78 |
| | Cow's milk (one cup) | 200 | 7.0 | 9.0 | 9.6 | 160 |
| | Cow's milk skimmed (one cup) | 200 | 7.2 | .2 | 10 | 70 |
| | Milk, condensed, sweetened (one tbsp) | 20 | 1.5 | 1.7 | 10 | 62 |
| 6. | Milk, goats (½ cup) | 100 | 3.3 | 4.1 | 4.7 | 75 |
| 7. | Milk, whole, powdered (one tbsp) | 7 | 1.9 | 1.9 | 2.7 | 35 |
| 8. | Milk, skimmed, powdered (one tbsp) | 7 | 2.6 | trace | 3.7 | 26 |

| Biscuits and cakes | | Calories |
|---|---|---|
| 1. | Biscuit, salted (one pc.) | 15 |
| 2. | Biscuit, sweet (one pc) Cream cracker, Nice, Marie | 24 |
| 3. | Arrowroot | 20 |
| 4. | Cake, chocolate (one pc) 45 g. | 165 |
| 5. | Cake, fruit, (one slice) 30g. | 117 |
| 6. | Cake, plain (one slice) 40 g | 146 |

| Snacks and savouries : | | |
|---|---|---|
| 1. | Chat | 474 |
| 2. | Chewra (fried) | 420 |
| 3. | Dal Vadha (one pc.) 30 | 200 |
| 4. | Dhokla | 122 |
| 5. | Pakora | 200 |
| 6. | Potato chips (10 pcs) 20 2″ diameter | 110 |
| 7. | Potato kachori | 166 |
| 8. | Samosa | 256 |
| 9. | Tapioca chips | 570 |
| 10. | Balushahi | 469 |
| 11. | Burfi (25 g.) | 100 |
| 12. | Gulab Jamun (25 g.) | 100 |
| 13. | Jalebi (100g) | 412 |
| 14. | Rasgulla (30 g.) | 100 |

| No. | Name | Wt. (g.) | Pro. (g.) | Fat. (g.) | CHO (g.) | Calories K. Cal. |
|---|---|---|---|---|---|---|
| *Nuts* | | | | | | |
| 1. | Almond (12 - 15) | 15 | 2.8 | 8.1 | 2.9 | 90 |
| 2. | Cashewnut (6 - 8) | 15 | 2.8 | 7.2 | 4.1 | 88 |
| 3. | Coconut fresh (1 pc.) | 15 | 0.5 | 5.2 | 2.1 | 54 |
| 4. | Groundnut (roasted, one tbsp) | 15 | 4.0 | 7.0 | 3.3 | 86 |
| 5. | Peanut butter (one tbsp.) | 15 | 3.9 | 7.2 | 3.2 | 86 |
| 6. | Pistachi nut | 15 | 2.9 | 8.0 | 2.8 | 88 |
| 7. | Walnut | 20 | 3.2 | 12.8 | 3.2 | 128 |
| 8. | Peas, roasted | 100 | 22.9 | 11.4 | 58.1 | 340 |
| *Pulses, dried peas and Beans* | | | | | | |
| 9. | Dals Mung, Masur and others (one cup cooked thin dal) | 200 | 7.0 | 2.3 | 14.0 | 105 |
| *Sugar, Jams, honey, etc :* | | | | | | |
| 1. | Chocolate,nut (1 pc) | 28 | 2.4 | 7.9 | 16.9 | 142 |
| | Chocolate, milk (1 pc) | 28 | 2.4 | 9.5 | 15.9 | 152 |
| | Honey (1 tbsp) | 21 | 0.1 | — | 16.4 | 64 |
| | Jams (1 tbsp) | 20 | 0.1 | 0.1 | 14.2 | 55 |
| | Jaggery (1 tbsp) | 15 | 0.2 | 0.1 | 14.0 | 56 |
| | Glucose (1 tbsp) | 12 | — | — | 11.0 | 45 |
| | Sugar granular (1 tbsp) | 5 | — | — | 5.0 | 20 |
| | Cube (one cube) | 6 | — | — | 6.0 | 24 |
| | Syrup, golden (one tbsp) | 20 | — | — | 14.8 | 59 |

## ITEMS OF FOOD TO BE AVOIDED BY PATIENTS WITH RENAL CALCULI

(1) *Calcium rich food :* Egg, milk, spinach, cauliflower, beans, figs, potatoes and molasses.

(2) *Oxalate rich food :* Beef, cashewnuts, chikoo, chocolates, custard apple, spinach, strawberries, tomatoes.

(3) *Uric acid rich food :* Fish roe, liver, kidneys, sweet-bread.

## DIET IN COELIAC DISEASE

In coeliac disease, gluten containing food must be avoided. High protein diet e.g. chicken, meat, fish, eggs as well as all types of fat may be taken. Sugar, honey, jam, marmalada, jaggery and starchy food prepared from rice is allowed.

*Avoid the following :*

Wheat products, oats, semolina, spaghetti, macroni, including cakes, chocolates, icecreams and Horlicks and milk-products which contain wheat and rye.

In Western countries gluten free products are available over the country according to the recommendation of the Coeliac Society.

**Diet for Galactosaemia :**

Avoid milk and lactose (disacharides ⇌ glucose + galactose). Milk, cream, milk powder cheese, sour-milk (Yoghurt) or baby food e.g. Yard etc. cannot be used.

## PARENTERAL FEEDING

*G.C. MOOKERJEE*
*RAM UDAYAN RAY*

**Introduction**

Intravenous administration of the preparations of fats and aminoacids may be advised in patients with non-functioning alimentary canal. In such patients, the basic requirement of energy, water, electrolytes and nitrogen to be supplied by parenteral feeding through I.V. route.

A number of preparations are now available for intravenous nutrition.

**Techniques**

It is very important to follow the proper technique of infusion. Occurence of thrombophlebitis is a common problem, usually found in the patients receiving intravenous administrations for some days. Large veins should be selected for infusion where prolonged administration may be necessary But this technique may produce the problem of septicaemia during passage of aminoacids and fats for a longer period through the venous catheter. The following precautions may be adopted :

(1) The electrolyte supplements should not be added by opening the bottle containing infusion fluid.

(2) Regular changing of infusion sets can help to prevent sepsis.

(3) Another technique can be followed in which millipore filters are introduced in the infusion line. This technique prevents chances of septicaemia, but may create a problem on the other side because lipid emulsions may not pass through properly.

(4) Addition of drugs in the aminoacid preparation may cause interreactions and as a result, allergic reactions may be observed.

(5) In case of fat preparations, drugs may break the emulsions, and therefore, addition of drugs in these solutions should not be done.

**Dosage**

The infusion dosage depends on the necessity of the patient, but generally it is advised to infuse lipid preparation at the rate of 3 g of lipid per Kg body wt, daily in an adult. Similarly, 200 ml of amminoacid preparation is given by I.V. infusion for 2-3 hours daily.

**Side-effects**

The above mentioned dosage can be continued for a patient for up to 20 or even 30 days with a rare chance of any acute transfusion reaction, provided the necessary sterilization and other protective techniques during infusion are ensured. But possibilities of liver function impairment, rise of alkaline phosphatase level etc., are there following long term infusions. Fat infusion is contraindicated in cases of liver damage, acute shock and hyperlipidimea etc.

Plasma proteins level, serum bilirubin and hemoglobin content of blood may change after infusion of fats and aminoacids, and therefore if any such estimation is proposed, infusion should be witheld for at least four hours before taking blood sample.

**Uses**

In poorly nourished postoperative patients, loss of nitrogen from the tissues can be compensated by supplying amino-nitrogen and calories through infusion, but in well-nourished patients this is not necessary.

A combination of oral and intravenous feeding is found to be helpful in patients with poor assimilation of nutrients from the gut but requiring large amount of energy. Similarly, burnt patients are benefited in this process as their energy and anabolic demands are high, which can be supplemented in this way.

Intestinal fistula or paralytic ileus lead to acute alimentary insufficiency and if this condition lasts for few days, intravenous nutrition is required to prevent death due to starvation. Chronic diarrhoea in Crohn's disease and ulcerative colitis also may lead to protein loss. Protein loss is also observed in chronic malnutrition. Parenteral feeding may also be necessary in these cases as a preoperative measure, and it is also useful in neonates with congenital anomalies of the gut. After massive intestinal resection, long term intravenous feeding provides necessary supplements.

## AVAILABLE PREPARATIONS OF FATS & AMINOACIDS

### Intralipid (10% & 20%)

It is a sterile fat emulsion containing fractionated soyabean oil 100 or 200 g. fractionated egg, phospholipid 12 g. Glycerol 22.5 g. water for injection to 100 ml. It's pH is approx 8. It is available in 100 ml & 500 ml. pack, costing about Rs. 100 and Rs. 300 respectively for 10% preparations and Rs. 160 and Rs. 450 respectively for 20% preparations.

**Wintrolipids (10%)** — This is also another fat emulsion contains purified soyabean oi! 50 g, purified yolk phospholipids 6 g; purified glycerine 11.05 g per 500 ml. Available in 250 ml. and 500 ml. pack costs Rs. 200 = 00 and Rs. 300 = 00 respectively.

**Hermin :-** This is a parenteral protein suppliment, contains L-Lysine HCI (23 mg); L-Threonine (7 mg); L-methionine (6.8), L-tryptophan (3 mg); L-Leucine (10 mg); L-isoleucine (6.6 mg); L-phenylalanine (9.6 mg); L-Valine (6.4 mg); L-arginine HCI (10.9 mg.) L-histidine HCI (monohydrate, 4.7 mg); glycine (6 mg), sorbitol 50 mg per ml. Available in 200 ml pack costs Rs. 110 = 00.

**Astymin** — 3 : Amino acids preparation containing essential aminoacids 81.2 mg; glycine 10 mg; sorbitol 50 mg per ml. Available in 200 ml. bottle costs Rs. 60.71.

All of the above productions are rich in calories, because simultaneous supply of calories along with the supplement of aminoacids helps in the incorporation of the aminoacids into the body protein.

## VITAMINS

*G C MOOKERJEE*
*RAM UDAYAN RAY*

### Introduction

The word "Vitamine" has come from the conjugation of two different words "Vital" and "amine", as this organic compound was found to be essential (vital) factor in life and previously it was thought to be an amine in nature. This term was used at the suggestion of Dr. Max Nierenstein. In 1920, Prof. J.C. Drummond introduced the term "Vitamin" after dropping the Word "e".

### Definition

The vitamins are organic compounds, present in variable amounts in different foodstuffs. responsible for maintaining normal physiological functions, vital to life. They have no calorie value like fat, protein and carbohydrate.

### Distribution

Vitamins are widely distributed in all natural foodstuffs. Usually plants can manufacture all vitamins. The animals can manufacture a few only, but can store them all to some extent.

### Requirement

The daily requirement of vitamins varies with age, physical activity, during disease, growth period as well as in pregnancy and lactation etc.

### Classification

The vitamins are classified according to their solubility, namely, fat soluble vitamins and water soluble vitamins. Fat soluble vitamins include vitamin A (Retinol), vitamin D (Calciferol), vitamin E (alpha-Tocopherol) and vitamin K.

Water soluble vitamins are vitamin of B complex groups, vitamin C (Ascorbic acid) and vitamin P (Citrin, Rutin, Hesperidin).

(Vitamin P is called as permeability factor, closely related to vitamin C and helps its action. It prevents capillary fragility).

**Synthesis in body**

Vitamin A and D are synthesized in human body from their pro-vitamin precursors. Some intestinal bacteria are capable of synthesizing some of the members of vitamin B-complex family. Rats and some other lower animals can synthesize vitamin C.Beyond that, all vitamins should be supplied with diet to maintain normal physiological activities of all organs and systems.

**Storage and fate**

As per requirement, body can store some vitamins to some extent and after completion of their action, vitamins are partly destroyed and partly excreted as such.

The following table summarizes the sources, daily requirements, role and deficiency symptoms of the vitamins.

| No. | Vitamin (Daily requirement) | Major sources | Effect of deficiency |
|---|---|---|---|
| 1. | Vitamin A 750 ug (retinol), retinol equivalent | Dairy fats; fish oil; egg yolk; liver | Night blindness, keratinization of mucosal membrane. |
| | Carotene | Carrot; pumpkin, spinach, broccoli, apricots, yellow peach papaya, mango, red palm oil. | As vitamin A. |
| 2. | Thiamine (Vitamin $B_1$ 1.3 mg | Milk, meat, particularly organ meats, whole grain products green leafy vegetables. | Beri-beri in severe cases. In moderate deficiency cases loss of appetite and weight, emotional and psychological symptoms. |
| 3. | Riboflavine 1.6 mg | Milk, meat, particularly organ meat, whole grain products, green leafy vegetables. | Cheilosis (cracks at the corners of the mouth), burning eyes and affected vision. |
| 4. | Niacin 18 mg | Whole grain cereals; lean meat, poultry fish and organ meats; green vegetables. | Pellagra, Early symptoms; loss of appetite and weight weakness. |
| 5. | Vitamin $B_{12}$ 3 μg | Liver and kidneys; meat; milk; | Pernicious anaemia; Long-term deficiency results in sub-acute degeneration of the spinal cord. |
| 6. | Folic acid 28 μg | Dark green vegetables; liver and kidneys, yeast | Megaloblastic anaemia. |

| No. | Vitamin | Requirement | Major sources | Effect of deficiency |
|---|---|---|---|---|
| 7. | Ascorbic Acid (Vitamin C) | 30 mg | Citrus fruits, tomatoes, potatoes, strawberries | Scurvy evidenced by bleeding gums, subcutaneous bleeding cork screw hair follicles. |
| 8. | Vitamin D | 0-10 $\mu$g | Sunlight, fish liver oil fortified milk, margarine | Rickets; soft, fragile bones, skeletal deformities, retarded growth. Osteomalacia in adults, dental caries, tetany. |
| 9. | Vitamin E. (tocopherols) | 15 I.V. | Oils of vegetable origin, (e.g. sunflower seed oil, nut oils) peas, beans, leafy vegetables. | Not seen in humans under normal conditions. |
| 10. | Vitamin K | Dietary deficiency unlikely | Green leafy vegetables. | Haemorrhagic disease of the new born increased tendency to bleed. |

## PRACTITIONER'S EQUIPMENT FOR EMERGENCY BAG

## USEFUL DATA

*P.N. BISWAS*

Besides a stethoscope, blood pressure apparatus and thermometer, a portable ECG machine may be of great value. In vast rural areas of our country the G.P. should know how to interpret an ECG in emergency.

Unlike practice in towns and cities, in rural practice a doctor has to be properly equipped, as many life-saving Kits are not readily available locally. The following list is for guidance :

1. DIAGNOSTIC SET
2. DISPOSABLE STERILE SYRINGES & NEEDLES (VARIOUS SIZES)
3. RYLE'S TUBE, STOMACH TUBE
4. RUBBER TOURNIQUET
5. RUBBER CATHETER/FOLEY'S CATHETER
6. CATGUT, SCALPEL, SCISSORS & INSTRUMENT FOR SUTURING
7. LUMBAR PUNCTURE NEEDLE
8. MOUTH, TONGUE FORCEPS & PHARYNGEAL AIRWAY TUBE
9. ENDOTRACHEAL TUBES
10. VENESECTION NEEDLE
11. SURGICAL SCALPELS
12. COTTON WOOL & GAUZE (AUTOCLAVED)
13. BANDAGES OF DIFFERENT SIZES
14. A PAIR OF GLOVES & FINGER STALLS

15. STERILISING FLUIDS
16. BLOOD SLIDES
17. A BOTTLE OF MULTISTIX (BOEHRINGER & KNOWLES FOR SIMPLE BEDSIDE TESTING OF URINARY CONSTITUENTS
18. BLOOD SUGAR TESTING STRIPS (IF NOT A GLUCOMETER)
19. AMBU BAG
20. TINC. BENZOIN CO
21. RECTIFIED SPIRIT

NOW AVAILABLE IN INDIA.

Blood sugar testing strips (Boehringer & Knowles) can be used to roughly check blood sugar in rural practice. Glucometers are also available now for electronic measurement of blood sugar directly and immediately. Cost is approximately six to seven thousand rupees. Each test costs about five rupees.

INJECTABLE DRUGS FOR EMERGENCY BAG

| TRADE NAME | PHARMACOLOGICAL NAME | M F G CO. | STRENGTH | ML-AMP |
|---|---|---|---|---|
| AMINOPHYLLINE | THEOPHYLLINE-ETHYLENE-DIAMINE | B & W<br>B D H | 25 mgm/ml | 10 ml |
| ALUPENT | ORCIPRENALINE | GERMAN REMEDIES | 0.5 mg/ml | 1 ml. |
| ATROPINE | MYUCYAMINE | C I P L A | 0.6 mg/ml | 1 ml. |
| ADRENALINE | EPINEPHRINE | B & W | 1 : 1000 | 1 ml |
| ANTISTINE | ANTAZOLINE METHANE SULPHONATE | C I B A | 0.5 gm/ml | 2 ml |
| AVAFORTAN | AVAPYRAZONE<br>METAMIZOLE | AST<br>KHANDELWAL | 24 mg/ml<br>0.24 gm/ml | 3 ml/amp |
| BARALGAN | ANALGIN<br>PHENPIVERINIUM<br>PITOFENONEHAE | HOECHST<br>HOECHST<br>HOECHST | 500 mg<br>0.02 mg/ml<br>5 mg/ml | 2 ml & 5 ml |
| BUSCOPAN | MYOSCIN-N-BUTYL BROMIDE<br>ANALGIN | GERMAN REMEDIES | 20 mg<br>2.5 g/ml | 2 ml & 5 ml AMP. |
| BUSCOPAN 1 ml | DOES NOT CONTAIN ANALGIN | | | |
| CIPLAR | PROPRANOLOL HCL | CIPLA | 1 mg/ml | 1.0 ml |
| CEDILANID | DESLANOCIDE | SANDOZ | 0.2 mg/ml | 2 ml |
| CORAMINE | NIKETHAMIDE | C I B A | 0.25 g/ml | 2 ml & 5 ml |
| CARBACMOL | CARBAMOYL CHOLINE CHLORIDE | B D H | 0.25 mg/ml | 1 ml. |
| CALCIUM | CALCIUM LACTO GLUCONATE | CIPLA | 10% | 10 ml |
| CALMPOSE | DIAZEPAM | RANBAXY | 10 mg/2 ml | 2 ml/AMP |
| DECADRON | DEXAMETHASONE SODIUM PHOSPHATE | MERIND | 4 mg/ml | 2 ml bulb |

* BETAMETHASONE AVAILABLE AS BETACORTRYL (PFIZER); INJ. WYCORT FROM WYETH: BETNESOL, (GLINDIA) 4 mg/ml. DEXONA-20 mg/5ml FROM CADILA (CONTAINING DEXAMETHASONE).

| TRADE NAME | PHARMACOLOGICAL NAME | M F G CO. | STRENGTH | ML-AMP |
|---|---|---|---|---|
| DOPAMINE | DOPAMINE HCL | T K K | 200 mg/5 ml | 5 ml AMP. |
| DEXTROSE | d. GLUCOSE | CIPLA | 25%<br>50% | 25 ml<br>25 ml |
| DILANTIN | SODIUM DIPHENYL HYDANTOIN | P & D | 100 mg/bulb | Powered form |
| EFCORLIN | HYDROCORTISONE SODIUM SUCCINATE | GLAXO | 100 mg | Powered Bulb |
| FORTWIN | | BOEHR-KNOLL | 30mg | amp |
| GARDENAL | PHENOBARBITONE SODIUM | MAY & BAKER | 200 mg/ml | 1 ml. |
| INSULIN (Regular) or INSULIN (Sol.) | INSULIN SOLUBLE | BOOTS CO. INDIA LTD.<br>NOVO INDUSTRIES | 40 Units/ml<br>40 Units or 80 UNits/ml | 10 ml. |
| ISOPTIN | VERAPAMIL HCL | BOEHR-KNOLL | 5 mg/2 ml | 2 ml AMP. |
| ISOPRIN | ISOPRENALINE | UNICHEM | 2 mg/amp | 2 ml AMP. |
| LANOXIN | DIGOXIN | BURROUGHS WELLCOME | 0.25 mg/ml | 2 ml |
| LASIX | FRUSEMIDE | HOECHST | 10 mg/ml | 2 ml |
| LARGACTIL | CHLORPROMAZINE | MAY & BAKER | 25 mg/ml | 2 ml |
| LEVOPHED | L - NORADRENALINE | BITRATE | 1 in 1000 solin | 4 ml AMP. |
| MICOREN | ETHYLBUTAMIDE AND PROPYLBUTAMIDE | GEIGY | 75 mg & 75 ml | 1.5 ml |
| MEPHENTINE | MEPHENTAMINE SULPHATE | GEOFFREY MANNERS | 30 mg/ml<br>15 mg/ml | 10 ml bulb<br>1 ml AMP |
| MORPHINE | MORPHINE SULPHATE | BURROUGHS & WELLCOME | 20 mg/ml | 1 ml |
| NOVALGIN | A N A L G I N | HOECHST | 0.5 Gm/ml | 5 ml |
| PETHIDINE | PHENYL PEPEPADINE | BURROUGHS WELLCOME | 50 mg/ml | 2 ml |
| PARALDEHYDE | PARACETALDEHYDE | PHARMAX INDIA PVT. LTD. | | 5 ml |
| PRONESTYL HCL (Squibb) | PROCAINEAMIDE HYDROCHLORIDE | SARABHAI CHEMICALS | 100 mg/ml | 10 ml bulb |
| PHENERGAN | PROMETHAZINE HYDROCHLORIDE | MAY & BAKER | 25 mg/ml. | 2 ml |
| SIQUIL | TRIFLUPROMAZINE HYDROCHLORIDE | SQUIB | 10 mg/ml | 1 ml AMP<br>10 ml bulb |
| SYNKAVIT | VIT. K | ROCHE | 10 mg/ml | 1 ml |
| SERPASIL | RESERPINE | CIBA | 1 ml/ml | 1 ml |
| SODIBICARB | SODIUM BICARBONATE | BENGAL IMMUNITY | 7.5 % | 10 ml bulb |
| STYPTOCID | ADRENO-CHROME MONOSEMICARBAZONE | | 5.0 mg/ml | 1.0 ml<br>2.0 ml<br>10 ml AMP |
| SPASMINDON | ATROPINE<br>PARAVERINE HYDROCHLORIDE<br>CODEINE | INDOPHARMA | 0.4 ml<br>32 mg<br>per<br>16 mg' ml | 2 ml/AMP<br>10 ml bulb |

| TRADE NAME | PHARMACOLOGICAL NAME | M F G CO. | STRENGTH | ML-AMP |
|---|---|---|---|---|
| TAGAMED | (CEMETIDINE) | | 200 mg | 12 ml/AMP |
| TERRAMYCIN | OXYTETRACYLINE | PFIZER | 250 mg in 3 ml | 3 ml |
| XYLOCARD | LIGNOCAINE | SUHRID GEIGY LTD. | 2 %<br>20 mg/ml | 50 ml bulb<br>5ml/AMP |

Equivalent dosage of different glucocorticoids

| Glucocorticoid | Relative anti-inflammatory dose in mg. |
|---|---|
| Cortisone | 25 |
| Hydrocortisone | 20 |
| Prednisone | 5 |
| Prednisolone | 5 |
| Methylprednisolone | 4 |
| Triamcinolone | 4 |
| Dexamethasone | 0.75 |
| Betamethasone | 0.6 |

[Adopted from Grollman and Grollman, Pharmacology and Therapeutics, Sixth edition, Published by Lea & Fibger, Philadelphia, 1965. P. 889]

Height — Weight Tables of Average Values for Indian Females and Males *

H = Height F = Females M = Males

| H | 20 Yrs. | | 25 Yrs. | | 30 Yrs. | | 35 Yrs. | | 40 Yrs. | | 45 Yrs. | | 50 Yrs. | |
|---|---|---|---|---|---|---|---|---|---|---|---|---|---|---|
| Cm. | F | M | F | M | F | M | F | M | F | M | F | M | F | M |
| 148 | 38.6 | 42.7 | 41.0 | 44.2 | 42.6 | 46.2 | 44.0 | 47.6 | 45.1 | 48.8 | 46.3 | 50.0 | 47.1 | 50.9 |
| 150 | 40.3 | 43.6 | 41.6 | 44.9 | 43.5 | 46.9 | 44.8 | 48.5 | 46.9 | 49.7 | 47.0 | 50.8 | 47.7 | 51.5 |
| 153 | 41.9 | 45.4 | 43.5 | 47.0 | 45.3 | 49.0 | 46.6 | 50.4 | 47.9 | 51.7 | 48.4 | 52.3 | 49.5 | 53.5 |
| 155 | 42.8 | 46.3 | 44.3 | 48.1 | 46.2 | 49.9 | 47.7 | 51.5 | 48.8 | 52.7 | 49.5 | 53.5 | 50.1 | 54.2 |
| 158 | 44.9 | 48.6 | 46.3 | 50.0 | 48.1 | 52.0 | 49.5 | 53.5 | 50.4 | 54.5 | 51.6 | 55.7 | 52.1 | 56.3 |
| 160 | 46.0 | 49.7 | 47.3 | 51.1 | 49.1 | 53.1 | 50.6 | 54.7 | 51.5 | 55.6 | 52.4 | 56.7 | 53.0 | 57.4 |
| 163 | 47.3 | 51.1 | 48.8 | 52.7 | 50.8 | 54.9 | 52.1 | 56.3 | 52.2 | 57.6 | 54.1 | 58.5 | 54.9 | 59.4 |
| 165 | 49.1 | 53.1 | 50.6 | 54.7 | 52.16 | 56.9 | 54.1 | 58.5 | 55.3 | 59.7 | 56.0 | 60.8 | 57.9 | 62.0 |
| 168 | 50.0 | 54.0 | 52.1 | 56.3 | 53.8 | 58.1 | 55.6 | 60.1 | 56.8 | 61.5 | 57.7 | 62.4 | 59.0 | 63.7 |
| 170 | | 56.5 | | 57.9 | | 60.3 | | 62.2 | | 63.7 | | 64.7 | | 65.8 |
| 173 | | 58.1 | | 60.1 | | 62.2 | | 64.0 | | 65.8 | | 67.0 | | 68.3 |
| 175 | | 60.1 | | 62.2 | | 64.2 | | 66.0 | | 68.1 | | 69.7 | | 71.0 |
| 178 | | 61.9 | | 64.0 | | 66.3 | | 68.5 | | 70.6 | | 71.9 | | 72.4 |
| 180 | | 64.0 | | 66.2 | | 68.5 | | 71.0 | | 73.3 | | 74.4 | | 75.1 |
| 183 | | 66.0 | | 68.5 | | 71.0 | | 73.3 | | 75.6 | | 77.1 | | 75.8 |

* Adopted from Data : Medical Council of India & Life Insurance Corporation of India Standards

HEIGHT AND WEIGHT CHART FOR
INFANTS AND CHILDREN

| AGE (Years) | HEIGHT (Cms) | WEIGHT (Kg.) |
|---|---|---|
| 2 | 76 to 94 | 10 to 14 |
| 3 | 81 to 102 | 11 to 16 |
| 4 | 89 to 109 | 13 to 18 |
| 5 | 91 to 114 | 14 to 20 |
| 6 | 102 to 114 | 16 to 25 |
| 7 | 114 to 135 | 21 to 30 |
| 8 | 114 to 142 | 21 to 34 |
| 9 | 114 to 147 | 21 to 37 |
| 10 | 119 to 152 | 23 to 41 |
| 11 | 119 to 160 | 23 to 47 |
| 12 | 127 to 160 | 26 to 53 |

## DENTITION TABLE

Dentition begins at the sixth or seventh month and should be completed within two or sometimes three years.

**MILK TEETH :** (Total = 20 teeth; ten in each jaw)

| | |
|---|---|
| Central incisors .. .. .. | (1) lower, 6th month<br>(2) upper, 7th month |
| Lateral incisors .. .. .. | (1) upper, 9th month<br>(2) lower, 10th month |
| First molars .. .. .. | 12th month |
| Canines .. .. .. | 18th month |
| Second molars .. .. .. | 2nd or 3rd year |

**PERMANENT TEETH :** (Total = 32 teeth; 16 in each jaw)

| | |
|---|---|
| First molars .. .. .. | 6½ years |
| Lower central incisors .. .. .. | 7 years |
| Upper central incisors .. .. .. | 8 years |
| Lateral incisors .. .. .. | 9 years |
| First bicuspid .. .. .. | 10 years |
| Second bicuspid .. .. .. | 11 years |
| Canines .. .. .. | 12 years |
| Second molars .. .. .. | 13 years |
| Third molars (Wisdom) .. .. .. | 17 to 25 years or sometime many years later |

**Pulse and Respiration rates in different ages**

| | *Pulse per min.* | *Respiration per min.* |
|---|---|---|
| In utero | 150 to 140 | |
| In newborn | 140 to 130 | |

| | *Pulse per min.* | *Respiration per min.* |
|---|---|---|
| During 1st year | 130 to 115 | 1st year = 35 |
| During 2nd year | 115 to 110 | 2nd year = 25 |
| During 3rd year | 100 to 95 | Puberty = 20 |
| 8th to 14th year | average 84 | Adult = 18 |
| Adult | average 72 | |
| Old age | average 76 | |

## INCUBATION PERIOD

Symptoms of any disease do not appear immediately after invasion of infectious agent. Some time is required to manifest the characteristic symptoms of the disease. The latent period, after an invasion by a pathogenic organism and appearance of the first sign or symptom of the disease is known as *incubation period.* During the *incubation period,* the organisms multiply in the host. When sufficient concentration of the infecting agent is built up in the host tissues, the balanced state of health is disturbed and the disease becomes apparent. The duration of this period varies from disease to disease. The factors which determine the incubation period include growth time of the organisms, dose of infection, portal of entry and individual susceptibility.

All infectious diseases are not communicable during the incubation period, but there are exceptions such as measles, chickenpox, whooping cough etc. During the incubaton period the patient may feel a little malaise or remain perfectly healthy. During this incubation period the affected individual should be segregated or placed under quarantine. The quarantine system is important to control some communicable diseases.

The table below shows the incubation period of the different diseases and period of isolation recommended when necessary.

| **Diseases** | **Incubation period** | **Period of Isolation recommended** |
|---|---|---|
| Chicken pox | 14 to 15 days | Until all lesions crusted, usually about 6 days after onset of rash. |
| Measles | 8 to 15 days | From the onset of catarrhal stage through 3rd day of rash. |
| Cholera | A few hours to 5 days | 3 days after tetracyline started. |
| Diphtheria | 2 to 6 days | 2 to 4 weeks or until virulent bacilli disappeared from the secretions and lesions. |
| Enteric fever | 12 to 14 days | 6 weeks or as long as organisms are found in excreta. |
| Influenza | 1 to 4 days | 3 days after onset |
| Mumps | 12 to 26 days | Until swelling subsides. |
| Whooping cough | 7 to 10 days not exceeding 21 days | 4 weeks or until paroxysms cease |
| Meningococcal meningitis | 3 to 4 days | Until first 6 hours of effective antibiotic therapy. |
| Poliomyelitis | 7 to 14 days | 2 weeks adults and 6 weeks children |
| Viral hepatitis | 15 to 50 days (usually 28 days) | 3 weeks |

| | | |
|---|---|---|
| Ascariasis | 2 months | |
| Ancylostomiasis | 6 to 8 weeks | |
| Tetanus | 6 to 10 days | |
| Leishmaniasis | between 1 and 4 months | |
| Shigellosis | | Until 3 consecutive negative stool culture. |
| Malaria | Falciparum 12 days;<br>Vivax and ovalae 13 to 17 days<br>Quartern 28 to 30 days | |
| Rabies | 1 to 3 months | |
| Leprosy | 2 to 5 years | |
| Syphilis | 10 to 90 days | |
| Gonorrhoea | 2 to 10 days | |
| AIDS | 6 months to 5 years. | |

## ANTI-RABIC VACCINE FOR HUMAN

### Purified Chick Embryo Cell Rabies Vaccine

Vaccines prepared in earlier years since Pasteur's method, are all associated with possible neurological reactions. Suckling mouse-Irain vaccine (Fuenzalida type) are less dangerous but still reactions may occur.

Duck embryo vaccines (DEV) produce much less complications (1/10,000) but are of lower antigenicity.

The WHO expert committee on Rabies recommended the following in September 1983 :

"The committee supports the trend to limit or abandon completely — where economically and technically possible the production of such encephalitogenic brain tissue vaccines, and strongly advocates the production and use of inactivated cell culture rabies vaccines in both developed and developing countries.

Virus grown in duck embryos and inactivated by $\beta$-propiolactone is also used as a vaccine. This vaccine was developed to avoid the neuroparalytic factors contained in brain-tissue vaccines, but the indications are that although neuroparalytic hazards have been reduced, allergenic risks still exist".

Recently, however, a rabies vaccine has been produced from human diploid cells (HDC), which is very good with reference to potency, safety and tolerability. (Vide infra) Rabipur (Behring) which is purified chick-embryo cell Rabies Vaccine (PCEC Rabies Vaccine), is now quite expensive at present, and Human Diploid cell vaccine is still costly but available from Serum Institute of India. It is hoped that in the near future, it will be more freely available in cheaper cost.

### Contraindications :

These may be many routine contraindications but considering gravity of the disease and possible outcome, vaccination should not be postponed, when Rabies is suspected. It is felt that most routine contraindications are secondary when life is at serious risk. Therefore, expert advice should be taken and patients should be referred to special treatment centres for expert opinion.

Of the vaccines available today. Human diploid cell inactivated vaccine is the safest but most expensive. Its cost for six doses is little over Rs.2000/-

## IMMUNIZATION

*P.N. BISWAS*

Infant mortality rate is very high in any developing country. To protect the children from common infectious disease various measures are adopted. The aim is to prevent as many of infectious disease as possible, through immunization. Various trials are going on all over the world. Each country forms its own immunization programme keeping in view the epidemiological pattern of the disease. In our country immunization programme has been taken at the national level. Following schedule is recommended in India by the Ministry of Health, Government of India.

| Beneficiaries | Age | Vaccine | No. of doses |
|---|---|---|---|
| Infants | 3–9 months | DPT | 3 |
| | | Polio | 3 |
| | | BCG | 1 |
| | 9–12 months | Measles | 1 |
| | 18–24 months | DPT | 1 (booster) |
| | | Polio | 1 (booster) |
| Children | 5–6 years | DT | 1 |
| | | Typhoid | 2 |
| | 10 Yeats | T T | 1 |
| | | Typhoid | 1 |
| | 16 years | T T | 1 |
| | | Typhoid | 1 |
| Pregnant women | 16 to 36 weeks | T T | 1 |

Measles vaccine is available only at special centres.

Booster given in two doses,if not vaccinated previously.

Immunization should be done in a healthy child, usually three months after birth; by this time immune system is well developed to respond to vaccine. Interval between the doses should not be less than one month. The recommended course of each vaccine should be completed as early as possible. If for some reason or other the child misses the schedule the particular dose may be given within 4 to 8 weeks, without starting the course again. While starting D.P.T. and polio vaccine which are given together, BCG vaccine can be given with any one of the three doses. One should take care that the injection site should be different.

**Reaction**

Vaccines used to immunize the child are safe. Rarely, complication may develop. Natural reaction following use of vaccine is generally of short duration. Reaction of the first dose is little more than subsequent injections. Usually reactions are mild e.g. fever, local pain, swelling at the site of injection, transient rash may develop following a measles vaccine.

In case of BCG vaccine sometime a lump or papule may appear in the third of fourth week after vaccination. It is usually not painful but tender to touch. It increases in 6 to 10 mm in diameter, softened with formation of pus. No treatment is necessary. Occasionally after 10 to 12 years of age, DPT vaccine may cause convulsion or collapse. In such cases further DPT should be stopped. In these cases two doses of DT vaccine can be given, DPT vaccine should be limited to the children under two years of age and D.T. vaccine under six years. These reactions increase in the older age group.

Vaccines are most effective tool to protect the child from many infectious diseases. The children are exposed to risk of complications if the schedule is delayed. It is dangerous to withhold the immunization from any child. Vaccines are available in most of the chemist's shop, most of the health centres and special immunization areas where health service provides it free of charge. Mild illness such as low grade fever, mild respiratory infection, diarrhoea, malnutrition and other minor illnesses are not contraindication to vaccination. In oral polio-vaccine to ensure full doses given to the child with diarrhoea should not be counted as part of the series. At the first available opportunity the child should be given another dose. In case of actually ill patients immunization should be deferred. Whenever a child is admitted in a hospital the immunization status should be checked and should be given appropriate immunization before discharge where indicated. Mother should be informed about its future need for subsequent doses. Child having severe reaction with first DPT vaccine injection second and third DPT vaccine injection should not be given. A single dose of DT vaccine to be given.

**Universal immunization programme**

In May 1974, WHO officially launched a global immunization programme known as Expanded Programme of Immunization (EPI) to protect all children of the world against six preventible diseases e.g. diphtheria, whooping cough, tetanus, polio, tuberculosis and measles by 2000 A.D. EPI was launched in India in January, 1978.

The programme is now called universal child immunization (1990). The name given to a declaration sponsored by UNICEF as a part of the United Nation's 40th Anniversary in October, 1985. It is aimed at adding to the global programme of EPI.

Indian Version — The Universal Immunization Programme was launched in November, 1985, in the memory of Smt. Indira Gandhi. The national health policy is aimed at achieving universal immunization coverage of the legible population by 1990.

# BIBLIOGRAPHY


1. Emery AEH : *Elements of medical genetics.* 4th Ed., Churchill Livingstone, London, 1975.
2. Hamerton J : *Human cytogenetics,* Academic Press, New York, Vols. I & II, 1971.
3. Harris, H. *The Principles of human biochemical genetics.* 2nd Ed., North Holland, London, 1975.
4. NuKusick, VA. *Mendelian inheritance in man.* Johns Hopkins Press, Baltimore, 1975.
5. Nora JJ and Fraser F : *Medical genetics principles and practices.* Lea and Febiger, 1974.
6. Sharma A and Talukder G : *Laboratory Procedures in human genetics.* Vols. I & II, Nucleus, 1974, 1976.
7. Stanbury, JB, Wyngaarden JB and Fredericksen DS : *Metabolic basis of inherited disease.* McGraw Hill, NY, 4th Ed., 1978.
8. Sorsby A. *Clinical genetics,* 3rd Ed., Butterworths, 1978.
9. Talukder G and Sharma A. : *A handbook of clinical genetics.* Oxford & IBH, Calcutta, 1979.
10. Fudenberg, H.H., Stiles, D.P., Caldwell, J.L., and Wells, J.V. (1976) *Basic and Clinical Immunology,* Lange Medical Publications.
11. *The HLA System* — British Medical Bulletin (1978), 34, No.3.
12. *Immunological Tolerance* — British Medical Bulletin (1976), 32, No.2.
13. Miescher, P.A. and Muller-Eberhard, H.J. (Eds.) (1976), *Text Book of Immunopathology,* 2nd. Ed. (2 volts), Grune and Stratton.
14. Movat, H.Z. (1979). *Inflammation, Immunity and Hypersensitivity Cellular & Molecular Mechanism of Hypersensitivity,* Harper & Row, New York.
15. Taussig, N.J. (1979) — *Processes in Pathology,* Blackwell Scientific Publications.
16. Turk, J.L. (1978) *Immunology in Clinical Medicine,* 3rd Ed., William Heinnemann Medical Books Ltd.
17. Weir, D.M. (1977) — *Immunology, An outline for students of Medicine and Biology,* 5th Ed. Churchill Livingstone.
18. *Recent advances in Gastroenterology* No.3 — Jan A Bouchier; Pub : Churchill Livingston (1976).
19. *Renal Biopsy,* D.B. Breeocr; Pub : Edward Arnold (1973), 2nd Ed.
20. *Diseases of nervous system* — WB Mathews & Henry Miller. Pub : Black well Sci 3rd Ed. (1979).
21. *Drug. Ther.* Bull. 3,38, 1965.
22. FAO/WHO Expert Group. *Nutrition meetings,* 1965, report No.37.
23. *Prognosis for Juvenile diabetics with nephropathy and failing renal functions* — Anderson, A.R. (1978) Act Med. Scand. 203 : 131.
24. *Treatment of diabetic patients with End Stage Renal failure : Some clinical Aspects* — Eberhard Ritz, J Eomer, K Andrassy (1981), In Proc. 8th Int. Congr. Nephrol. Athens 1981.
25. *Proceedings of the European Dialysis and Transplant Association,* Robinson BHB, Hawbins, JB and Davison, A.M., 1981, Ritman, London.
26. *Early functional and Morphological changes in diabetic nephropathy,* Viberti, G.C., Clin. Nephrol 12, 47-53, 1979.
27. *The Medical Clinics of North America,* W.B. Saunders Company, Philadelphia, Philip Raspen (1982).

28. *Proc. of the International symphosium,* Ed : Nandy A, Chaudhury A.B., Sengupta A.B., Sen N.N., Jan 17—19, 1980, Calcutta, India.

29. *An introduction to Electrocardiography,* Leo Schamroth, 6th Ed; Blackwell Scientific Pub : Oxford (1982).

30. *Congenital heart disease,* Ed : Maccartney F.J., MTP, Press Ltd., Lancaster, England (1986).

31. *Dermatology for the Physician,* Rhodes, E.L., Bailliere Findall London 1st Ed; (1979).

32. *Inflammatory Bowel disease,* Ed : Allan, R.N. Keighley J. Alexander — Williams and Clifford.

33. Hawkens, Churchill Livingstone, Edenburgh 1st Ed (1983).

34. Keynes, W. Milo and Fowler; P.B.S. (ed.)

35. *Clinical Endocrinology :* William Heineman; Med. Books, London.

36. *Stroke* — a critical approach to diagnosis, treatment and management.

37. *Chapter on Respiratory Diseases;* Vishwanathan R. Editors : Datey K.K. and Shah S.J., Bombay 1978, A.P.I. Text Book of Medicine 3rd Edition.

38. *Chest Medicine,* 2nd Edition; Shankar P.S., Oxford & IBH Publishing Co., New Delhi — 1979.

39. *Respiratory Diseases,* Crofton, J and Douglas, A.C., 2nd Edition, Oxford Blackwell 1975.

40. *Principles and Practice of Respiratory Therapy;* Young J.A., and Crochier D., 2nd Edition; year Book Medical Publishers, Chicago, 1976.

41. *Classification of hyperlipidaemias and hyperlipoproteinemias,* Beaumont, JL, Carlson, LA, copper GR, FeyFar, Z, Fredrickson, D.S. and Stasser, T (1970); Bulletin of W.H.O. 43.891.

42. *A Physician guide to hyperlipidaemia, Modern concepts Cardiovasc diseases* 41 : 31, 1972, Fredrickson, D.S.

43. *Metabolic control & Laboratory practice;* Bondy P.K. & Resenbery LE (1980); Oxford Black well Scientific Publications.

44. *The Medical clinice of North America on approach to the patient with hyperlipidaemia,* Vol.66, Number 2, Richard J Haval, (1982); W B Saunders Company.

45. Co-operative trial on primary prevention of Ischaemic heart diseases using clofibrate to lower serum cholesterol, Lancet 2 : 379, 1980 : World Health Organisation (WHO).

46. *Text Book of Endocrinology;* Wiliams D H (1981), Philadelphia W.B. Saunders.

47. *Clinical aspects of the arachidonic acid-thromboxane pathway :* Mitchell, JRA; British Medical Bulletin (1983); 39, 3, 289—295.

48. *Chronic Beta Blockade therapy in patients after myocardial Infarction :* Pratt, CM and Roberts, R; American Journal of Cardiology, (1983); 52, 7, 661.

49. Heart Disease, 2nd, 1984; Braunwald.

50. *Treatment of cardiac emergencies,* (1977); Gold Berger.

51. *Recent Advances in Cardiology,* 1973; Hammer.

52. *Clinical Heart Disease;* Oram Samuel; 2nd, 1981.

53. *Man at High Altitude & Cold* — Heath D, and Williams R, (1982); 2nd Ed; Churchill Livingstone; Edinburgh and London.

54. *Effect of Altitude Exposure on Thermoregulatory response of man to Cold;* Blatteis, CM & Lutherer, LO (1976); Jounral of Applied Physiology 41, 848.

55. Brown Fat and Thermogenesis Physiological Review; Smith R. & Horowitz, BA (1969); 49, 330; Effect of altitude and cold acclimatisation on the basal metabolism in man.

56. Aerospace Medicine 42, 1056; In Mountain medicine; A clinical study of Cold and High Altitude; Ward, M (1975); London.

57. Crospy Lockwood Staples : The role of sympathectomy in frost bite with a review of 68 cases; Golding M.R. et al (1965); Surgery 57 : 774.

58. Current Medical Diagnosis and treatment; Disorder due to cold; Milton J. Chatton (1978); Lange Medical publications, Muruzen Asian Edition.

59. Field Surgery Pocket Book (1982) : Issued under the authority of the Director General Armed Forces Medical Services, New Delhi.

60. Mannual of Health for the Armed Forces (1968) : Issued under the authority of The Director General Armed Forces Medical Services, New Delhi.

61. Neurological aspects of ophitoxemia (Indian Krail); P.K. Sethi and J.K. Rastogi; Ind. Jour. Med. Res. 73 (1981), 269.

52. *Immunological Diseases* (Vol.I & II); Samter M (1971), Little Brown N.Y.

63. *Mixed Connective Tissue Disease;* Sharp GC et. al (1975), Amer. Jour of Med. 52, 148.

64. *Sjogren's syndrome;* Huges GRV; and Whaby K (1972) Brit. Med. Jour. 4, 523.

65. *Scleroderma or Sclerodermas :* Leading article; Brit. Med. Jour 4, 249.

66. Symposium on Scleroderma; Moyo Clin. Roe. (1971) 46 83.

67. *Essential Immunology;* Roitt, I (1974) 2nd ed. Oxford.

68. Antiarrhythmic Agents by B.N. Singh; L.H. Opie, F.I. Marcus in drugs for the Heart (ed. L.H. opic 1984) — Grmc & Stratton Inc.

69. *Clinical Pharmacology of commentional & Newer Antiarrhythmic drugs* by T.E.B......... in principles & Practice of Acute Cardiac care (ed. D.S. Das Gupta 1984), York Book Medical Publishers, Inc.

70. The clinical Pharmacology of Antiarrhythmic Drugs by P.C. Adans, RWF Campbell, D.G. Julian in Cardiac drug therapy (Ed. C.R. conti 1984), F.A. Dairs' Co.

71. Management of serious cardiac arrhythmias with drugs by D.S. Echt, J.W. Mawon in cardiac drug therapy (ed. C.R. Conti 1984), F.A. Dairs Co.

72. In Man at High Altitude : Health D. and Williams R. (1982), Cold 2nd ed. Churchill Livingstone, Edinburgh and London.

73. Effect of Altitude Exposure on Thermoregulatory response of man to Cold. Blatteis, CM & Lutherer, LO (1976), Journal of Applied Physiology 41, 848.

74. Brown Fat and Thermogenesis Physiological Review 49, 330 Smith R. Em & Horowitz, BA (1969);

75. *Effect of altitude and cold acclimatisation on the basal metabolism in man;* Nair, C.S.; Malhotra, M.S.; Gopinath, P.M.; (1971 a). Aerospace Medicine 42, 1056.

76. *In Mountain medicine; A clinical study of cold and High Altitude;* Ward, M (1975) London; Crospy Lockwood Staples.

77. *The role of sympathostomy in frost bite with a review of 68 cases :* Golding M.R. et. al (1965); Surgery **57 : 774.**

78. *In Current Medical Diagnosis and treatment; disorder due to cold.* Milton J. Chatton (1978); Lange Medical publications. Maruzen Company Limited. Maruzen Asian Edition.

79. In Oxford Text Book of Medicine — 1st Edition; ELBS edition 1985; W.R. Keatinge (1982); *Environmental Extremes effects of Cold on the body.*

80. Issued under the authority of the Director General Armed Forces Medical Services; Field Surgery Pocket Book (1982), New Delhi.

81. Issue under the authority of the Director General Armed Forces Medical Services; Mannual of Health for the Armed Forces (1968); New Delhi.

82. *The Nutritive Value of Indian Foods and Planning of Satisfactory diets;* Aykroyd, W.R., Gopalan, C., Balasubramaniam, S.C., I C M R Speiral Report Series No.42, 6th Revised Edition, 1966.

83. *Nutrition and dietetics in health and disease;* Joan M. Huskisson, Cassel Ltd., 1981.

84. *Clinical Nutrition and Dieteties,* Antia, F.P., Second Edition; Oxford University Press, 1973.

85. *Human Nutrition and Dietetics,* Sir Stanley Davidson, Passmore, R., Broik, J.F., Truswell, A.S., Churchill Livingstone, 6th Edition, 1975.

---

*H. Contd...*



*H. Contd...*

V Contd...



V. Contd...



**W**



**X**



**Z**